PRINCIPLES OF ADVANCED
TRAUMA CARE

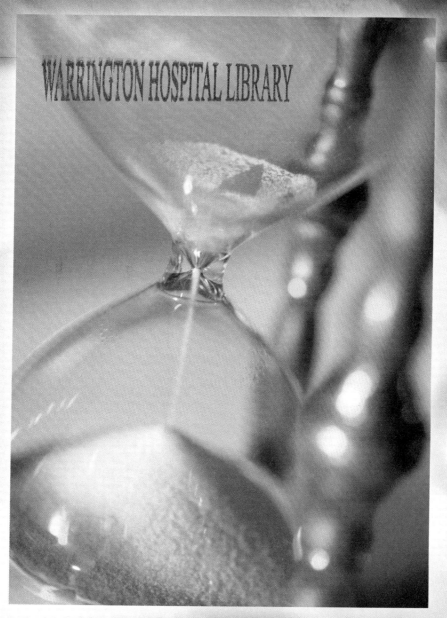

DELMAR

THOMSON LEARNING ™

Africa • Australia • ~~Canada~~ • ~~Spain~~ • ~~United Kingdom~~ • New Zealand • Philippines
Puerto Rico • ~~Singapore~~ • ~~Spain~~ • ~~United Kingdom~~ • United States

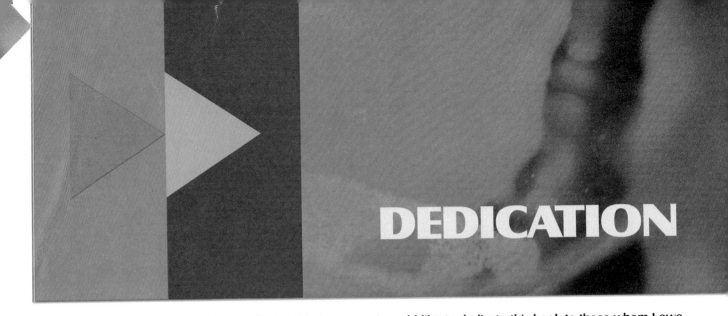

DEDICATION

Although I have lived sufficiently long to be indebted to many, I would like to dedicate this book to those whom I owe the most—my parents, Walter and Lucille Hubble. Among many other things, they taught me that hard work was the key to success, no matter how humble my beginnings. I would also like to dedicate this book to the EMS professionals who have devoted their lives to helping others.

M.W.H.

I dedicate this book to my mother, the late Mary Spring Page, whose never ending zest for life and courage in death continually awe and inspire me. Mom, your constant correction of my English has finally been appreciated. Also, to my father, Robert N. Page, III, for giving me love, a love of education, and an education—and who still answers all my legal questions. I love you Dad.

J.P.H

PRINCIPLES OF ADVANCED TRAUMA CARE

Principles of Advanced Trauma Care
Michael W. Hubble, PhD, NREMT-P
Director of Emergency Medical Care
Western Carolina University

Johnsie Page Hubble, BSN, CEN, MPH
Emergency Department Nurse
Medical Intensive Care Nurse

DELMAR

™

THOMSON LEARNING

Africa • Australia • Canada • Denmark • Japan • Mexico • New Zealand • Philippines
Puerto Rico • Singapore • Spain • United Kingdom • United States

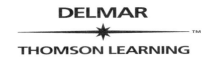

DELMAR
THOMSON LEARNING

Principles of Advanced Trauma Care
by Michael W. Hubble and Johnsie Page Hubble

Health Care Publishing Director:
William Brottmiller

Executive Editor:
Cathy L. Esperti

Acquisitions Editor:
Marie M. Linvill

Developmental Editor:
Darcy M. Scelsi

Editorial Assistant:
Jill Korznat

Executive Marketing Manager:
Dawn F. Gerrain

Channel Manager:
Tara Carter

Project Editor:
Mary Ellen Cox

Production Editor:
James Zayicek

Art and Design Coordinator:
Robert Plante

For permission to use material from this text or product, contact us by
Tel (800) 730-2214
Fax (800) 730-2215
www.thomsonrights.com

Library of Congress Cataloging-in-Publication Data
Hubble, Michael W.
   Principles of advanced trauma care / Michael W. Hubble, Johnsie P. Hubble.
      p. cm.
   Includes bibliographical references.
   ISBN 0-7668-1987-6 (alk. paper)
   1. Wounds and injuries. 2. Emergency medical technicians. I. Hubble, Johnsie P. II. Title.

   RC86.7 .H83 2001
   617.1—dc21

                              2001028448

NOTICE TO THE READER

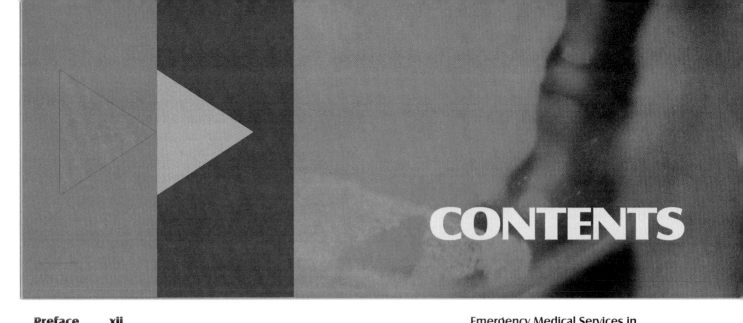

CONTENTS

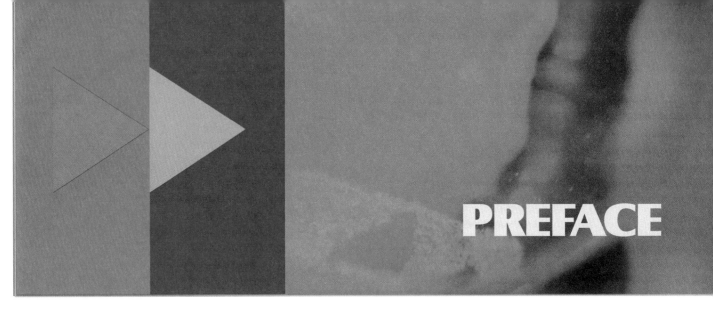

PREFACE

Amid the myriad of challenges to EMS professionals, none is more demanding in complexity of knowledge, physical stress, or emotional fortitude than caring for trauma patients. The paramedic has a keen awareness and intimate familiarity with the reality of the events surrounding the millions injured and thousands killed each year from trauma. The paramedic's firsthand knowledge and eyewitness perspective of traumatic injury solidifies for this profession a critical, special, and unique place in the world of trauma care. Injury is the leading cause of death and disability for persons aged 1–34 in the United States, and persists as a leading cause of death for all Americans. To these thousands of victims of trauma—individuals with names, loved ones, and friends—nothing could be more crucial than being cared for by EMS professionals educated with a sound clinical science knowledge base. Equally important is the need for paramedics to remain abreast of the latest changes in the science of their profession, avoiding the "pitfalls" of simply following hallowed traditions.

This book was written to meet the need for a specialized, evidence-based text in EMS trauma management. It is designed to provide a trauma textbook for students in baccalaureate and associate degree paramedic programs that expands upon the 1998 United States Department of Transportation's National Standard Curriculum for the EMT-Paramedic. It has been successfully piloted with students in community college and university settings. This textbook reflects current trends in education of paramedics of broader and more intense instruction, and encourages the extension of evidence-based medicine into prehospital care.

Though designed to meet the needs of EMS degree program students, others including nurses, allied health professionals, EMS physicians, critical care transport and air medical transport personnel, as well as graduate paramedics, should find this book a valuable reference.

The textbook is intended to serve as a complete source of paramedic education on trauma. Paramedic students utilizing this book should have completed a college level course in anatomy and physiology and possess a general familiarity with EMS, including EMT certification. Chapters 1 through 8 provide the underlying principles of trauma care and trauma care systems, beginning with epidemiology and prevention, and continuing through field assessment and triage of the traumatized patient. The intent of these chapters is to describe trauma as a public health problem and to provide the student with insight into the magnitude of injury in America. These chapters also place trauma care into perspective, additionally outlining rapid patient assessment procedures which are expanded upon in later chapters.

Chapters 9 through 17 address specific injuries to the human systems. Each chapter opens with a brief overview of the epidemiology and etiology of trauma pertaining to that human system. These chapters form the core of paramedic trauma care.

Chapters 18 through 21 are devoted to developing competency in specific advanced life support skills and procedures. Each chapter presents the skills presently available to paramedics and also introduces new procedures, techniques, and equipment. Controversies surrounding the use of certain techniques are also explored.

Chapters 22 through 31 address specialized situations and patient populations. Hazardous materials, environmental emergencies, extrication, air medical transport, and forensics are covered, as well as the special care needs of the elderly, children, pregnant women, and organ donors. Unique to this book, Chapter 27 also addresses the complications of trauma, as well as rarely discussed issues surrounding traumatic arrest.

The student and instructor should note the consistency in chapter structure. Each begins with the objectives and key terms, then discusses epidemiology, anatomy and physiology, pathophysiology, current management and treatment, hospital treatment, and promising research. Brief summaries are provided at the end of each chapter. Dispersed throughout the chapter are Internet activities designed to enhance and supplement the student's learning. These activities are current and create an interactive learning environment for the student. Internet activities also encompass the latest trends in trauma care and knowledge. Each chapter is followed by review questions and critical thinking questions with scenarios.

In addition to Internet activities, unique facets of this textbook include an increase in the depth of field and hospital treatment and the incorporation of evidence-based writing. Topics of special interest include injury epidemiology and injury prevention, organ and tissue donation, complications of trauma, traumatic arrest, air medical transport, advanced airway techniques, and forensics in trauma management.

A supplemental guide for the instructor is available from the publisher. The instructor's guide contains a list of the Department of Transportation National Standard Curriculum objectives covered in each chapter and answers to the chapter review questions.

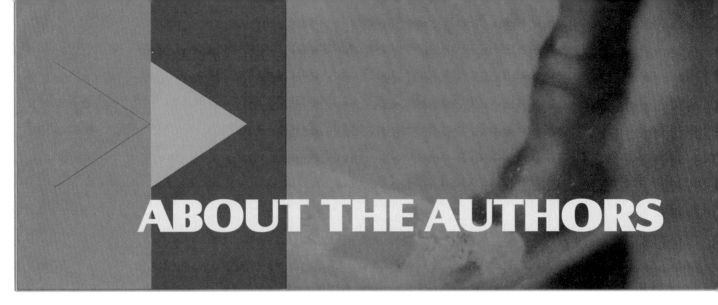

ABOUT THE AUTHORS

Michael W. Hubble, PhD, NREMT-P

Dr. Hubble is the director of the Emergency Medical Care Program at Western Carolina University. He received a B.S. degree from High Point College in Business Administration and Economics, followed by a Master of Business Administration Degree from the University of North Carolina at Chapel Hill in 1990. He received a Ph.D. from the University of Maryland-Baltimore County in 1997 with a concentration in Emergency Health Services Policy and Administration. Dr. Hubble's research focus is EMS system design. He has published several articles in EMS and scientific journals. Dr. Hubble has been a paramedic since 1982 and continues to work in that capacity in addition to his administrative, teaching, and research responsibilities at WCU.

Johnsie Page Hubble, BSN, CEN, MPH

Ms. Hubble, a North Carolina native, is an emergency department nurse and MICN with a special interest in prehospital care. She received a Master of Public Health degree from the University of North Carolina at Chapel Hill in 1991 and in the pursuit of that degree concentrated on the field of injury prevention and control. Ms. Hubble also completed baccalaureate degrees in nursing and Spanish. Ms. Hubble has worked in rural and tertiary care hospitals in both emergency departments and intensive care units. She has taught in paramedic classes and served as a preceptor of paramedic students.

ACKNOWLEDGMENTS

The authors wish to acknowledge the contribution of invaluable support of several talented people. We thank all of our authors and contributors; their effort and participation in this book have been invaluable—we couldn't have done this without each of you! We wish to pay special tribute to the Department of Health Sciences at Western Carolina University, and particularly to Dr. Barbara Lovin and Dr. David Trigg.

As many chapters as we read and re-read, we could not have produced this textbook without the critique of the many professional reviewers; though anonymous to us, we thank you. We are indebted to Crystal Spraggins and Lynn Caldwell at F.A. Davis Publishing who assisted us in developing the original concept of this book.

Special thanks are extended to our close friend and colleague, Elizabeth Zeringue who gave us much needed support and friendship, talented writing and editing, and who went above and beyond the call of duty in helping us finish this textbook. We are also grateful to the contributions of several photographs from her husband, Mark J. Zeringue, M.D. Thanks are also in order for several others who assisted with photography: John Ayling, Greg Bauer, Sherry Beal, Rick Brady, Ernest Grant, Elaine Frye, MGF Gilliland, Sarah Hicks, David Reeves, Jose Salazar, Barry Saunders, Tom Walsh, Denise Wilfong, and Regina Woodard. Thanks also to Paul Chelminski, M.D. for his expert review of the pediatric chapter and the improvements that were the result.

Finally, we extend profound gratitude to the staff at Delmar Thomson Learning and Argosy Publishing, particularly Darcy Scelsci, Mary Ellen Cox, Robert Plante, Daniel Rausch, and Beatrice Ruberto, who worked diligently to ensure the success of this text.

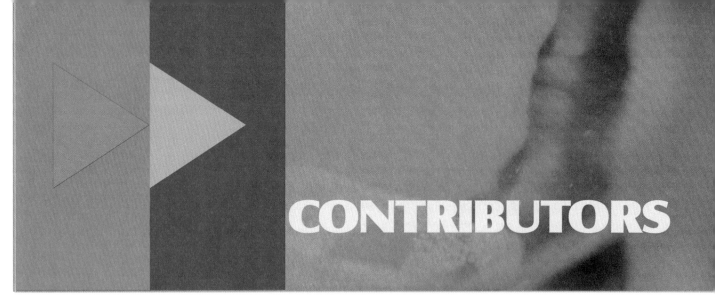

CONTRIBUTORS

Jeffery L. Beinke, BS, REMT-P, CCEMT-P
Division Chair
Allied Health Sciences Technology
Montgomery Community College
Troy, North Carolina
Chapter 10: Spinal Injuries

Lynda K. Black, PhD
Wilkes Community College
Wilkesboro, North Carolina
Chapter 4: Psychosocial Aspects of Trauma

Jane H. Brice, MD, MPH
Assistant Professor
Department of Emergency Medicine
University of North Carolina-Chapel Hill
Orange County Emergency Medical Services Medical
Director
Chapel Hill, North Carolina
Chapter 14: Abdominal and Genitourinary Trauma

John R. Clark, BS, NREMT-P
President - National Flight Paramedic Association
Salt Lake City, Utah
Chapter 26: Pediatric Trauma

Kerry Collins, MD
Department of Emergency Medicine
East Carolina University
Greenville, North Carolina
Chapter 27: Complications of Trauma

Craig DeAtley, PA-C, CCT
EMS Degree Program
George Washington University
Fairfax, Virginia
Chapter 22: Hazardous Materials Incidents

Elaine Frye, MT (ASCP), CLS (NCA)
Blood Bank Supervisor
Chatham Hospital
Siler City, North Carolina
Chapter 20: Fluid Resuscitation

Bill Garcia, MICP
EMS Department
Asheville-Buncombe Technical Community College
Asheville, North Carolina
Chapter 15: Extremity Trauma

Ernest J. Grant, RN, MSN
NC Jaycee Burn Center
UNC Hospitals
Chapel Hill, North Carolina
Chapter 17: Burns

Todd Hatley, EMT-P, MBA, MHA
Performance Improvement Coordinator
New Hanover Regional Medical Center
Wilmington, North Carolina
Chapter 24: Geriatric Trauma
Chapter 29: Air Medical Transport of the Traumatized
Patient

Johnsie Page Hubble, RN, CEN, MPH
Chatham Hospital
Asheville, North Carolina
Chapter 1: Epidemiology of Injuries
Chapter 2: Role of EMS in Injury Prevention and
Surveillance
Chapter 26: Pediatric Trauma
Chapter 31: Forensics in Trauma

Michael W. Hubble, PhD, NREMT-P
Assistant Professor
Director - Emergency Medical Care Program
Department of Health Sciences
Western Carolina University
Cullowhee, North Carolina
    Chapter 5: Biomechanics of Trauma
    Chapter 13: Chest Trauma
    Chapter 15: Extremity Trauma
    Chapter 18: Airway and Ventilatory Management

L. Lee Isley, PhD (c), MBA, NREMT-P
Vice President of Strategic Services
Westcare Health System
Sylva, North Carolina
    Chapter 7: Trauma Scoring Systems
    Chapter 8: Principles of Triage
    Trauma Management During Major Incident
        Response, *see* www.ems.delmar.com

David Kruse, MD
Department of Emergency Medicine
University of North Carolina-Chapel Hill
Chapel Hill, North Carolina
    Chapter 13: Chest Trauma

Virginia G. Lickel, MEd, LPC
Health Choices (Counselor)
Petra Leadership (Consultant)
Greensboro, North Carolina
    Chapter 4: Psychosocial Aspects of Trauma

Barbara Keelor Lovin, EdD
Head - Department of Health Sciences
Western Carolina University
Cullowhee, North Carolina
    Chapter 21: Pneumatic Anti-Shock Garment

Scott Morgan, NREMT-P
Flight Paramedic
UNC Air Care
Chapel Hill, North Carolina
    Chapter 13: Chest Trauma

Paul Murphy, BS, EMT-P
Director of Marketing
PMX Medical
Murray, Utah
    Chapter 3: Overview of Trauma Care

David Reeves, BS, NREMT-P
Department Chair
Emergency Medical Science
Guilford Technical Community College
Jamestown, North Carolina
    Scene Assessment and Personal Safety,
        see www.ems.delmar.com

Michael E. Richards, MD, MPA
Assistant Professor
Department of Emergency Medicine
University of New Mexico
New Mexico State EMS Medical Director
Injury Prevention and EMS Bureau
New Mexico Department of Health
Albuquerque, New Mexico
    Chapter 11: Head and Neck Trauma
    Chapter 12: Facial and Ocular Trauma
    Chapter 16: Compartment Syndrome and Crush
        Injuries

Jose V. Salazar, MPH, NREMT-P
Jose Salazar and Associates
Sterling, Virginia
    Chapter 19: Principles of Spinal Immobilization

Jeffery P. Salomone, MD, FACS, NREMT-P
Assistant Professor
Department of Surgery
Emory University
Atlanta, Georgia
Assistant Medical Director - National Prehospital Trauma
   Life Support
    Chapter 9: Pathophysiology of Shock

David C. Trigg, MD
Assistant Professor
Department of Health Sciences
Western Carolina University
Cullowhee, North Carolina
    Chapter 25: Trauma in Pregnancy

Denise E. Uhlin, RN, TNS, NREMT-P
Carolina Organ Procurement Agency
Chapel Hill, North Carolina
    Chapter 30: Tissue and Organ Donation

Regina Woodard, RN, BSN, EMT-P
North Carolina State Prehospital Trauma Life Support
  Coordinator
Westcare Emergency Medical Services
Sylva, North Carolina
  Chapter 6: Assessment of the Trauma Patient

S. Austin Yeargan, III, MD
Department of Emergency Medicine
East Carolina University
Greenville, North Carolina
  Chapter 12: Facial and Ocular Trauma

Elizabeth Zeringue, RN, BSN, MICN
North Carolina Nurse Consultant
NC TB Control Program
Siler City, North Carolina
  Chapter 20: Fluid Resuscitation
  Chapter 23: Environmental Emergencies
  Chapter 27: Complications of Trauma

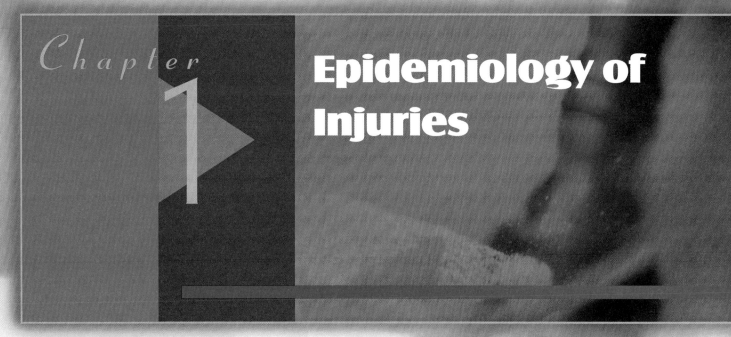

Chapter 1

Epidemiology of Injuries

OBJECTIVES

Upon completion of this chapter, the reader should be able to:

● Recognize the magnitude of traumatic injury as a public health problem.

● Compare and contrast incidence and prevalence.

● Describe the mathematical concept of rate and define mortality and morbidity rates.

● Explain the importance of surveillance of injuries, surveillance methods, and E codes and N codes.

● Discuss the financial and human cost of trauma.

● Calculate life years lost and years of potential (or productive) life lost.

● Describe the major causes of injury mortality and morbidity in the United States.

● List the basic facts of motor vehicle crashes, including motorcycles, bicycles, and pedestrians, as well as the impact of alcohol on motor vehicle injuries and deaths.

● Describe the epidemiology of drowning and water-related activities, fires, burns, fireworks, falls, poisonings, occupational injuries, firearm deaths, homicide, and suicide.

KEY TERMS

Category-specific rate	Morbidity rate
Crude rate	Mortality rate
Epidemiology	Prevalence
Incidence	Surveillance
Intentional injury	Unintentional injury
Life years lost	Years of productive life lost (YPLL)

Emergency medical service (EMS) professionals participate every day in the collection of epidemiologic information on injuries. Equally important to this data collection is their awareness and understanding of the extent of traumatic injury and death in the United States, its states, and its locales.

This chapter is written to impart an overview of the epidemiology of traumatic injury and as such is replete with statistical information, particularly mortality data. Though tedious to some, these statistics are vital to a basic understanding of the depth and severity of trauma in America and should be read to gain an appreciation of the profile of injuries. Data are also necessary so that comparisons between different causes of injuries and the specific populations at risk can be made. Keep in mind that these statistics represent the lives of real people—someone's mother, baby, father, brother, sister, or grandparent—individuals with names, families, and friends whose hopes and dreams for the future were permanently altered by traumatic death or serious injury.

No textbook can keep pace with the latest statistics available; therefore the reader is encouraged to find more current information through publications and Internet sources. Currently, injury mortality statistics are published about 20 months after the end of a given year. The National Center for Injury Prevention and Control of the Centers for Disease Control and Prevention is an excellent source of information and maintains a computer Web site at www.cdc.gov.

INJURY IS A PUBLIC HEALTH PROBLEM

Injury is the leading cause of death and disability among children and young adults in the United States. In 1998, unintentional injuries were the leading cause of death for Americans 1–34 years of age and the second most frequent cause of death for ages 35–44. Approximately 150,000 people die each year from a traumatic injury (see Figure 1-1). In 1997, this included 43,647 from motor vehicle crashes (MVCs), over 30,500 from suicide, nearly 20,000 from homicide, 13,301 from falls, more than 10,000 from unintentional poisonings, 5,096 from drowning, and 3,146 from residential fires.[1]

Major causes of injury mortality
By total number of deaths —1995

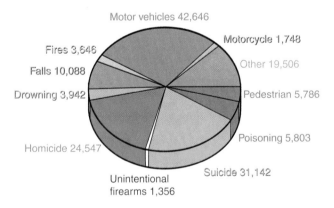

FIGURE 1-1 Major causes of injury mortality in the United States by total number of deaths for the year 1995. Note the major contribution of motor vehicles, suicide, homicide, and falls. It is important to note that although actual numbers of deaths have changed since 1995, the "portions of the pie" each consumes relative to the others has not substantially changed.

In those aged 15–34 years, unintentional injuries, homicide, and suicide are the top three leading causes of death. Homicide is the leading cause of death for African-American males aged 15–34. Overall, deaths from homicide increased almost 30% from 1985 to 1992, and if that trend had continued, homicide death rates would have surpassed that of motor vehicle crashes in the United States around the year 2003.[1] However, homicide death rates began declining in the late 1990s. Groups at particular risk for injury and traumatic death include males, the elderly, children, and minorities.[1]

Nearly 40% of all nonfatal emergency department (ED) visits are trauma related. Falls, MVCs, injuries caused by falling or thrown objects, lacerations or punctures, and violence are the major reasons for ED visits. More males than females are treated for injuries in EDs, and those under 15 and over 65 years have higher rates of injury-related visits. In 1992, $9.2 billion were spent for ED care of injured patients.[2]

WHAT IS EPIDEMIOLOGY?

The fundamental principles embedded in epidemiology can be illustrated by work done in the 1800s by British physicians William Farr and John Snow. In 1839, Farr organized a system to collect the numbers and causes of all deaths and for the next 40 years carefully examined the link between these statistics and the public's health. Farr observed a link between elevation above sea level and cholera deaths.[3] In the 1850s, Snow hypothesized that cholera deaths were a result of drinking contaminated water from the Thames River, although the exact causal agent in the water supply was unknown at the time.

In 1854, Snow noted that a severe outbreak of cholera took place in Broad Street, Golden Square, in London: "Within two hundred and fifty yards of the spot where Cambridge Street joins Broad Street, there were upwards of five hundred fatal attacks of cholera in ten days."[4] Going door to door, Snow investigated each cholera death by location, discovering which of two water companies supplied water to each home where a cholera death had occurred. The two companies both drew their water supply from the Thames River; however, the Lambeth Company changed its source of water to a sewage-free area of the Thames in 1852. Snow showed that the rate of cholera deaths from 1853 to 1854 varied dramatically with which company supplied water to a household. The death rate for persons receiving water from the Southwark and Vauxhall Company was 114 deaths per 100,000 living persons; the rate for the Lambeth Company was zero deaths per 100,000 living persons. Documenting the frequency and distribution of cholera deaths, Snow determined the cause of the cholera outbreak. Snow's approach to examining the cholera outbreak is still used by epidemiologists today; he used all three components of the definition of epidemiology: (1) measurement of disease or injury frequency; (2) distribution of the disease or injury, which includes the "who, where, and when" of the injury or disease; and (3) the causes or determinants of the outbreak, disease, or injury, based on 1 and 2 above.[3]

Epidemiology is the study of the distribution and causal factors of injury (and disease) in human populations and is based on two assumptions: (1) injury does not occur at random and (2) injury has causal and preventive factors that can be identified through systematic investigation using scientific principles and methods.[3]

INCIDENCE AND PREVALENCE

The two most common measures of injury frequency are prevalence and incidence. **Prevalence** is a measure of the proportion of individuals in a population with an injury (or disease) at a given point in time. Prevalence (P) equals the number of cases of an injury divided by the total population at a given point in time:

$$P = \frac{\text{number of cases of an injury}}{\text{total population at a specific time}}$$

For example, the number of persons with quadriplegia caused by an injury per 100,000 persons in 2001 includes all living persons with quadriplegia from injuries regardless of when the injury occurred and quantifies an estimate of the probability that an individual will have quadriplegia at the given point in time.[3]

Incidence is a measure of the number of new cases of an injury (or disease) in a population of people at risk during a specific time period. Incidence (I) is equal to the number of new cases of an injury during a given time period or point in time, divided by the total population at risk for that injury or disease:[3]

$$I = \frac{\text{new cases of injury}}{\text{total population at risk for a specific time period}}$$

Using the same example of quadriplegia, the number of new cases of quadriplegia from traumatic injury per 100,000 population in 2001 is an incidence measurement. Incidence, therefore, provides an estimate of the probability, or risk, that an individual will develop an injury during a specific time period. Incidence measures can be compared from one time period to the next; comparisons are important in studying trends as well as the impact of interventions and laws.[3]

Prevalence is a function of both the incidence and duration of a disease or injury. The prevalence of quadriplegia in 2001 is a function of the incidence of the injury and the duration of the condition. Duration, in turn, is affected by three factors: the recovery period of the injury, deaths in the affected group, and migration in and out of the geographical area under investigation. Changes in prevalence from one time period to another, therefore, can result from fluctuations in incidence rates, changes in the duration of disease or injury, or changes in both incidence and duration.[3]

Pay particular attention to the mathematical concept of rate; it is often misused. The numerator is the number of cases, such as the number of persons killed in MVCs. The denominator is the group at risk, such as all persons in the United States in the year 2001. Remember that the denominator must include a measure of time; for example, the number of persons injured in MVCs per 100,000 persons during the year 2001. Be aware of how reported measurements are obtained and calculated and exactly what they include.[3]

Mortality and Morbidity Rates

Commonly used incidence rates include the mortality rate and the morbidity rate. The **mortality rate** is a measure of the incidence of death (all deaths or deaths from a specific cause) in a specific population during a given period of time; it is calculated by dividing the number of fatalities (numerator) during that time period by the total population (denominator) of that same time period. In the United States during 1982, there were 1,973,000 deaths in a total population of 231,534,000, yielding a mortality rate from all causes of death of 852.1 per 100,000 persons per year. Because death statistics are widely and uniformly collected by legal mandates, mortality rates are readily available and thus commonly utilized when studying trauma.[3]

The **morbidity rate** is an incidence rate measuring the number of new cases of a nonfatal injury or disease (numerator) divided by the total population at risk (denominator) during a specific time period. For instance, the morbidity rate of tuberculosis for 1982 in the United States was 11.0 per 100,000 persons, the number of nonfatal, newly reported cases of tuberculosis in 1982 divided by the total population of 231,535,000. There exists a general lack of morbidity information for injuries. With the exception of certain infectious diseases, there are few instances in which the compilation of morbidity data is legally required.[3]

A rate is sometimes presented for an entire population, called a **crude rate**. Rates are also presented for specific groups by such criteria as race, age, and sex, and are called **category-specific rates**. Category-specific rates are calculated by dividing the number of deaths or injuries among individuals in each specific category, age for instance, by the total number of persons in that age category for the specified time period.[3]

Remember that statistical measures can be misleading. For instance, in 1996 several Honda automobile models were in the top five most frequently stolen vehicles. Honda maintained, however, that the statistics were misleading. They simply listed the total number of vehicles stolen, not the number of vehicles stolen per 100,000 owned vehicles of a particular model; Honda, being one of the most widely owned vehicle types in the United States, argued that a rate (the number of stolen vehicles per 100,000 owned vehicles of a particular model per year) would more accurately reflect the truth about stolen vehicles.

MORBIDITY AND MORTALITY: THE TIP OF THE ICEBERG

Fundamental to scientific investigation of injuries is access to adequate data concerning both morbidity and mortality. However, these fundamentals of injury epidemiology are often missing, fragmented, or limited. The majority of scientific information on injuries is mortality data. By law, deaths must be recorded in all 50 states. Morbidity data, on the other hand, are, at best, sketchy or localized and, at worst, nonexistent. Nonfatal injuries are less accurately recorded, and data are not available to ascertain trends in injury morbidity.[5] Furthermore, with both mortality and morbidity statistics, there are often central pieces of the puzzle missing, including many of the characteristics of persons injured, the factors that influence injury causation, and the events leading up to the trauma. The only exception to this lack of data is motor vehicle injuries. The incidence, prevalence, injury effects, and injury prevention measures of motor vehicle injuries have been studied in depth since the 1960s, their epidemiology well understood in comparison to other injuries. Federal funding for epidemiologic research through the National Highway Traffic Safety Administration and the Insurance Institute for Highway Safety has facilitated this advance in motor vehicle epidemiology. Lower rates of motor vehicle deaths and injuries have resulted, illustrating the potential for reducing rates of other injuries, given sufficient knowledge into their epidemiology. Continuous, systematic data collection is of paramount importance in planning and evaluating prevention programs. The lack of appropriate data systems has resulted in ineffective and expensive preventive programs.[6]

Although some very recent advances in the study of morbidity data have been made, there still exists a substantial gap between mortality and morbidity injury data. The disparity between mortality and morbidity data is what is referred to as "the tip of the iceberg" (see Figure 1-2). What is known about injuries chiefly involves mortality statistics, or the part of the iceberg we can readily see. Beneath that floating tip is a much larger chunk of ice, and the deeper it gets, the less about that part of the iceberg is known. Morbidity data lie below the visible part of the iceberg, including admissions to hospitals, patients treated in EDs, patients seen in clinics, urgent care environments, physician's offices, and those cared for at home. Unfortunately, this "submerged" information is vital to a complete understanding of the epidemiology of injuries.

SURVEILLANCE

One of the factors necessary to gaining adequate data is the establishment of effective, widespread injury surveillance systems, particularly for nonfatal injuries.[7] **Surveillance** is the systematic collection of population-based information on the occurrence, outcome, and cost of injury and disease.[8] John Snow went house to house to collect information, which is not practical or cost-effective for most data today. However, the advent of microcomputer technology makes widespread surveillance of injuries a realistic and attainable goal. Difficulties arise in establishing uniform, standardized computer data sets and facilitating the rapid collection, compilation, and retrieval of information.

Nationally, the National Highway Traffic Safety Administration and the National Transportation Safety Board collect data on highway and aircraft fatalities, respectively. The National Center for Health Statistics (NCHS) compiles incidence and demographic information from death certificates.[9] Recently, the NCHS began tabulating some nonfatal injury data from ED visits, releasing the first such information for the year 1992 in February 1995.[2]

The only long-term national data on nonfatal injuries come from the National Electronic Injury Surveillance System (NEISS).[8] Operated by the U.S.

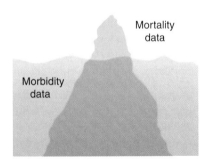

FIGURE 1-2 Mortality data for injuries are readily available. However, morbidity data are rare and more difficult to find, and are frequently compared to an iceberg, where what lies below the water's surface is much harder to determine.

Consumer Product Safety Commission in Washington, D.C., NEISS is composed of a sample of hospital EDs and collects information on a broad range of injury issues associated with consumer products. NEISS collects data on hundreds of different product categories, but not all products; for example, firearms are excluded. NEISS uses the data to project nationwide estimates of the number and severity of product-related injuries.[10] The discovery and subsequent investigation of injuries associated with all-terrain vehicle (ATV) use is an example of the work of the NEISS surveillance system, providing a good example of the benefit surveillance systems possess.[8] Further information on ATV injury prevention issues is provided in Chapter 2.

Trauma registries are also sometimes used to monitor injuries, but their use and content vary from location to location and are generally only maintained by "trauma centers." Police and state highway patrol agencies often identify locations of frequent trauma, helping to facilitate the improvement of highway measures, such as intersection traffic signals, to lessen the number of crashes in an area. However, they are less likely to be used to identify areas of severe trauma to persons than to identify clusters of property damage.[9]

E Codes and N Codes

Risk factors for fatal and nonfatal injuries differ for various causes of injury. Therefore, data about the causes of all injuries are needed to complete the epidemiologic information necessary to reduce trauma. One way of obtaining more complete information about injuries and their causes is through the International Classification of Disease (ICD) schema, primarily used in hospitals for insurance purposes.[11] Two codes exist within the ICD code system regarding trauma: the nature of injury code, called an N code (e.g., laceration), and the external cause of injury code, called an E code (e.g., passenger in a single motor vehicle crash, the vehicle leaving the road and striking a guardrail). There also exist E codes to identify where an injury occurred, such as "on a farm," and are called "place of occurrence" E codes. By assigning both N codes and E codes, researchers can compile much more information about injuries.[11] One problem with hospital and ED records is that E codes are frequently not included.[5] Setting national guidelines for use of E codes for all hospital records, ED, and in-patient would be one method to obtain more injury information. Additionally, national standards for trauma registries and other trauma care data systems would greatly improve trauma surveillance.[9]

Prehospital care providers are an essential link in collecting injury data for epidemiologic use. Frequently, they are the only members of the health care team to witness the scene and the environment of an injury event. Thorough documentation of the events leading up to the injury, the environment, and the statements of the patients and other witnesses should be included in the prehospital record. This information is vital, not only to the receiving health care team, but also to medical records personnel who document N codes and E codes.

INTERNET ACTIVITIES

Visit the Centers for Disease Control and Prevention (CDCP) Web site, http://www.cdc.gov/publications.htm. Scroll down to the Software area and click to download the *Doepi* program. Follow the instructions for downloading and installing the software. This program is a computer-assisted instruction (CAI) program that teaches the student the basics of epidemiology. While the examples are not trauma related, the exercises highlight some of the principles of epidemiology and surveillance that are common to all illnesses and injuries regardless of etiology.

THE COST OF INJURY

The total cost of injuries is impossible to estimate. Human physical suffering and emotional torment are the greatest cost. The tragedy of trauma cannot be quantified. However, the financial cost of injury, estimated by experts and ever changing, is certain to be outdated in this textbook. In 1989, an in-depth publication was produced for the U.S. Congress entitled *Cost of Injury in the United States: A Report to Congress, 1989.*[12] Though outdated, the book still serves as a resource manual and has been instrumental in increasing the national recognition and support for injury research and federal projects.

In 1994, the financial cost of injury was estimated to be more than $224 billion, an increase of over 42% in one decade.[1,13] These costs include medical care, rehabilitation, and lost wages and productivity of the injured and killed. In 1994, public money from federal, state, and local governments paid around a third of the cost of all injuries. Private funds, chiefly insurance, covered about two-thirds of injury costs. The federal government alone paid $12.6 billion in medical costs and $18.4 billion in disability and death benefits.[1]

Once injured, there is little difference in the medical cost of injury treatment for males and females. However, males have much higher national injury costs because of their higher injury incidence.[7,14] Medical care costs are highest for those 15–24 years old, and injury accounts for the largest source of medical care expenditure for young persons. Overall, MVC injuries are the most costly, followed by injury from falls, firearms, poisonings, fires and burns, and drowning.[15]

One of the major costs of injury is the loss of young, healthy persons to society. For the community, the future productivity of a 20-year-old is much greater than for a 75-year-old. The years of life lost due to premature death or morbidity from traumatic injury can be estimated. The number of productive years lost from work and care of the home and children can be estimated for both morbidity and mortality by two major types of calculations: (1) life years lost and (2) years of productive or potential life lost. **Life years lost** can be calculated by subtracting the age at premature death from the current life expectancy for someone of the deceased's age. Life expectancy is the age to which a person is predicted to live, based on current death data of the U.S. population. In a hypothetical example, life years lost for a black male killed in a homicide at age 20 in 2002, who has a life expectancy of 70 in 2002, is 50. Fifty life years are lost because of that homicide. Life years lost are much higher for injuries than for heart disease or cancer, because those two diseases chiefly affect older persons.[6,12]

The CDCP uses its own measure of productivity costs, called **years of productive (or potential) life lost**, or **YPLL**. Instead of using life expectancy as an endpoint, the YPLL uses age 65, because that is an average retirement age. The YPLL provides an estimate of the loss of the productive or working years of the injured person's life. In 1994, there were over 3.5 million YPLL resulting from injuries, far surpassing the second and third leading causes of YPLL, cancer and heart disease[16] (see Figure 1-3). The YPLL does not take into account persons who are injured after age 65 or the loss of life beyond age 65. It is strictly a measure of the loss of economic productivity.[12] In the United States, trauma is the leading cause of YPLL, far surpassing the other leading causes of death in the United States.[6]

UNINTENTIONAL INJURY

Unintentional injuries are injuries resulting from events that are inadvertent, unlike **intentional injuries**, which result from acts designed to injure or kill. Unintentional injuries are responsible for the deaths of over 90,000 persons each year. Unintentional injuries are the leading cause of death for Americans aged 1–34 years, the second leading cause for those aged 35–44, and the third leading cause of death for those aged 45–54 years.[1] For each injury death, there are an estimated 18 hospitalizations, 233 emergency department visits, and 450 physician office visits.[1,9]

Motor vehicle crash injuries are the leading cause of injury death for those aged 1–25 years. Among Americans aged 1–24, drowning is the second leading cause of unintentional injury deaths. Alcohol plays a major role in injuries, accounting for almost half of all MVC and residential fire deaths.[1] Other major sources of injury mortality and morbidity include pedestrian incidents, bicycles, motorcycles, poisoning, falls, occupational injuries, and recreational activities.

MOTOR VEHICLE CRASHES

Worldwide, more than half a million people die each year in MVCs. This is the equivalent of a jet crash killing over 1,350 people every day. In the United

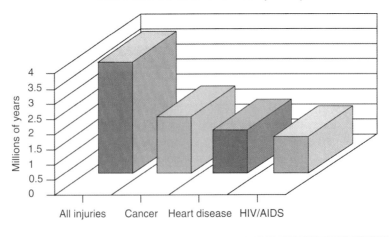

Years of Potential Life Lost (YPLL)

FIGURE 1-3 Years of potential life lost from injury far surpasses that of the nation's leading killers, heart disease and cancer. This is because injuries often take the lives of young, productive citizens as well as children.

States, MVCs have killed over 2.8 million people since 1900. This figure is more than two times the number of Americans killed in all wars involving the United States since 1775. Approximately one baby in 70 born in the United States will eventually die from a fatal injury sustained in an MVC. [9] Motor vehicle crashes hospitalize more than half a million people a year. They are also the major cause (between 30% and 60%) of head and spinal cord injuries, often resulting in permanent disabilities.[9]

In the United States, MVCs are the leading cause of death from age 1 to 34.[1] The largest number of years of life lost before age 65 is the result of MVC injuries.[17] In 1998, more than 43,000 individuals died as a result of injuries sustained in MVCs; the MVC death rate for all Americans was 16 per 100,000 population (28 for those 15–19 years old and 28.5 for 20–24-year-olds). Rates then decline until age 70 and above, when rates rise again; however, the total number of deaths is a much lower number than for young Americans. The death rate for males is over two times that for females but is roughly equal for whites and blacks. Although the overall death rates and numbers of deaths are down since the early 1980s (23.42 per 100,000 in 1980 with over 53,000 total deaths), death rates (and number of deaths) increased until 1995, then began to slowly decline. Motor vehicle crashes remain a significant public health problem, resulting in premature deaths of many young people, with significant economic costs to society.[1]

The statistics for MVCs are sometimes calculated based on the number of miles traveled. In 1966, the traffic fatality rate was 5.5 deaths per 100 million vehicle miles traveled. In 1993, the rate had dropped to 1.8 deaths per 100 million vehicle miles traveled, the lowest on record.[18] The number of vehicle miles traveled per person, however, continues to grow. From 1965 to 1990 the vehicle miles traveled for the U.S. population increased from under 900 billion to over 2.1 trillion miles per year. Therefore, reducing death rates from MVCs may be dependent on strategies other than reducing exposure, given current trends and lifestyles.[9]

Adolescents

For adolescents, MVCs are the leading cause of injury death.[5] Fatality rates for those 15–19 years of age are 10 times higher than for children under age 10. Males in the 15–19 age group have death rates twice that of females of the same age, and alcohol is involved in about half of all adolescent motor vehicle crash deaths. [17]

The overall profile of deaths for teenagers is different than that of adults. Although driving only 20% of the time at night, more than half of teenage crash fatalities occur between the hours of 9 PM and 6 AM, and males are twice as likely as females to become a night-

time crash fatality. Adolescents are disproportionately responsible for the deaths of other vehicle occupants, as well as pedestrians, and are much less likely to use seat belts than other age groups, even when mandated by law. However, nighttime curfews and raising the drinking age to 21 have resulted in significant declines in fatal adolescent MVCs. Studies have shown that driver education programs increase the number of teenage crashes, most likely by increasing the number of adolescent drivers.[5] Thirty-six states now have some form of graduated driver's licensing, although the exact terms of the graduated license varies from state to state. Graduated licenses involve night curfews for teens and license suspension or revocation for traffic violations or crashes. Data should be available soon on the effect of graduated licensing.

Impaired Driving

Alcohol and drug use are major factors in highway crashes and fatalities. Drivers with blood alcohol levels of 0.10% or higher are 12 times more likely to be involved in a fatal crash than drivers with lower levels or no detectable blood alcohol content. Studies show that other drugs are detectable in 10%–22% of injured drivers, although alcohol is also frequently present.[9] Although there have been significant declines in alcohol-related fatalities per motor vehicle miles traveled and per population since the 1980s, 39% of deaths from MVCs in 1997 were alcohol related.[1] (By comparison, in 1982, approximately 57% of all fatal crashes involved alcohol.[9]) The impact of eliminating alcohol-related deaths can be illustrated by noting that over 16,000 deaths would have been prevented in 1997 alone.[1]

Nearly a quarter of all children killed in MVCs are involved in an alcohol-related crash, and over a half of those killed are riding in the car with the impaired driver. Some states have enacted child endangerment laws that charge a driver with the additional violation of driving while impaired with a child in the car.[1]

Efforts to reduce impaired driving-related fatalities include raising minimum drinking age laws to 21 years (a measure which saved 1,100 lives in 1988[9]). Other interventions include strengthening impaired driving laws and raising community awareness through campaigns such as Mothers Against Drunk Driving (MADD), designated drivers, and alcohol-free social events.

Speed, Aggressive Driving, Fatigue, and Literacy

It is a well-known fact that as speeds increase, so do MVC fatalities. Speed is considered to be the second most significant problem in driver behavior, behind alcohol, and is a factor in about one-third of all fatal crashes.[9]

The effect of speed on highway fatalities is vividly outlined in American history. In 1973, foreign oil embargoes prompted Congress to pass the Emergency Highway Conservation Act. Effective in January of 1974, this law set a national speed limit of 55 miles per hour in an effort to reduce the country's oil consumption. A side benefit from that action was a significant reduction in the nation's motor vehicle death rate. In 1974 there were 9,000 fewer MVC deaths than in 1973, the largest single-year drop in U.S. history. Recent Congressional amendments to the National Maximum Speed Limit Law in the 1990s, which increased maximum speed limits on many highways, are predicted by highway safety advocates to result in upward trends in the number of MVC deaths compared to highways with lower speed limits.[18]

Aggressive, reckless driving is receiving more attention as a cause of crashes and fatalities. Aggressive driving may be the result of the increasing congestion on American roadways. Some experts have termed severely aggressive driving behavior as "road rage." Presently, there are few statistics on crashes involving aggressive driving. Vehicle and roadway design can help responsible drivers who have momentary lapses in judgment but may be of no help or be outweighed by aggressive, reckless driving behavior.[9]

Driver fatigue is increasingly being recognized as a cause of MVCs. The National Highway Traffic Safety Administration attributes 100,000 crashes each year to drivers who fall asleep at the wheel. In those crashes, an estimated 1,500 are killed and 71,000 are injured. Fatigued and sleepy drivers suffer from physical problems similar to impaired drivers: slowed reaction time, impaired judgment, and decreased awareness and attention to traffic conditions.[19]

There also appears to be a link between literacy and driving performance. Those not literate in the English language have more crashes than the average driver. Literacy is also related to socioeconomic status.[9]

Occupant Protection

Safety belts save thousands of lives every year—more than 4,800 lives of front-seat occupants over age 4 in one year alone. It is estimated that most (3,000) of those saved lives were related to safety belt laws. If every front seat occupant had been secured in a lap-shoulder belt in 1990, over 15,000 deaths and several hundred thousand injuries could have been prevented.[18] In 1997 the majority (over 60%) of children killed in MVCs were unrestrained.

It is clear that safety belt laws dramatically increase usage. New York passed the first state safety belt law in 1984.[18] Now, only New Hampshire does not have a safety belt law (as of May 1999).[1] Before laws were enacted in the United States, the usage rate was about 15%. Laws increased rates to around 50%; public enforcement campaigns have raised usage to over 70% in some states. Laws combined with educational and enforcement campaigns are attributed with producing the 87% national safety belt usage rate in Canada.[18]

Child and infant safety seats and belts are believed to have saved thousands of lives. Most MVC deaths of children under age 5 could be prevented if all children were secured in an appropriate safety seat.[18] Child-restraint laws (now in effect in all 50 states) and child seat loan programs are credited with increasing the usage of child-restraint seats and safety belt usage. Experts note, however, that better seat and safety belt designs are needed to reduce failure and misuse of these safety devices; in response, many law enforcement agencies now hold free educational programs on child safety seats.[9]

Motor Vehicle Safety Standards

Biomechanics research has led to the design of vehicle safety improvements, such as side impact protection, windshield safety glass, collapsible steering mechanisms, brake improvements, head restraints, door retention, and instrument panel padding. Vehicle safety experts estimate that improvements in vehicle design prevent thousands of deaths and injuries (over 5,000 deaths and 155,000 injuries between 1975 and 1985).[9]

Roadway Safety Improvements

The impact of roadway improvements on MVCs can be illustrated by the U.S. Interstate Highway System. Interstate highways physically separate opposing traffic, limit access, eliminate crossing traffic, and are designed to meet higher safety standards than are other roads. As a result, the Interstate Highway System has a crash fatality rate about one-half of the national average. Roadways with low safety design standards, such as local roadways, have crash fatality rates 25% higher than the national average. Since 1974, Federal Aid Highway Safety Improvement projects have saved more than 55,000 lives. These projects include guardrail improvements, crash cushions, traffic signs, improved lighting, and obstacle removals.[9]

MOTORCYCLES

Over 16,000 people died in motorcycle crashes in the first 7 years of the 1990s, and more than 50,000 died in the prior 11 years. Over half of these died from head injuries. However, deaths represent only a small part of the head injury problem resulting from motorcycle crashes; many survive but with significant disability.[9] A motorcyclist death is most often a young, white male. (In 1997 there were over 1,600 deaths from motorcycle crashes; all but 164 of those were males.) The death rate for white males is nearly twice that of black males. The largest number of deaths in recent years has occurred in the 20–24-year-old category, and most deaths occur between the ages of 15 and 40.[1]

One factor in motorcycle deaths is the experience and licensure of the driver. In 1989, it was estimated that over 40% of motorcycle deaths occurred among unlicensed or improperly licensed operators.[9,20]

States enacting mandatory helmet laws have many fewer motorcycle fatalities than states without laws.[20] As noted, most motorcycle-related deaths involve head injury; helmets are designed to reduce the risk of such injury. A study of crashes in Washington state found that although unhelmeted motorcyclists were hospitalized at just slightly higher rates than helmeted riders, they were three times more likely to suffer a head injury, four times more likely to sustain a severe head injury, and more likely to die from their injuries.[21]

PEDESTRIANS

Pedestrian deaths rank second behind motor vehicle crash occupant deaths in all motor vehicle–related fatalities and represent approximately 13.5% of all traffic-related fatalities.[1,22] "Hit-and-run" events are responsible for one in five fatalities. In 1998, over 5,000 persons were killed in pedestrian traffic events. Pedestrian traffic-related death rates have declined 42% from 1975 to 1997. In 1997, rates were highest in the over-age-80 group (5.79 per 100,000 population); though declining, this group continues to have the highest pedestrian death rates. This stems from decreased hearing, vision, and agility. The elderly are most likely to be hit at an intersection.[1] Although older persons have higher rates of pedestrian fatalities, the largest number of deaths has fluctuated—20- to 29-year-olds from 1979 to 1987, 30- to 34-year-olds from 1988 to 1993 (603 to 551), and 35- to 39-year-olds (510 to 481) from 1994 to 1997—perhaps reflecting total population trends more than any other factor.[1] Most deaths (70%) occur in urban areas, but rural highways are witness to a higher ratio of deaths to pedestrians struck due to higher driving speeds.

The rate for males is higher in every age category, including those 4 years and under; and, with the exception of the 4-and-under group, male pedestrian traffic-related death rates are nearly double that for females in every age category. Death rates for nonwhites are significantly higher than for whites in nearly every age category.[1]

Pedestrian deaths and injuries are a significant problem for the pediatric population. One-third of all children killed between ages 5 and 9 are pedestrian deaths.[1] Somewhere between 50% and 70% of pedestrian injuries among children under age 9 are "dart-out" incidents, occurring when a child "darts out" into the street in the middle of a block.[17]

Male children's pedestrian fatality rates are double that of female children. Nonwhite children have fatality rates one and a half times those of white children.[1] In addition, poor children are two or three times more likely to sustain a pedestrian-related injury than other children.[17]

Pedestrian deaths are often divided into traffic related and nontraffic related, with the latter encompassing deaths occurring in driveways or on private property. Pedestrian nontraffic deaths account for about 15% of all motor vehicle–related deaths in children from 1 to 4 years old.[23] It is often toddlers who are crushed underneath a slow, reverse-traveling automobile in a driveway. There is a threefold increase in the risk of a nontraffic-related fatality if a residential driveway is not physically separated from a child's play area.[24]

Children aged 5 and over are more likely to be involved in a traffic-related incident at higher speeds and often suffer leg, spinal, and pelvic trauma.[25] The elderly are more prone to chest and pelvic injuries, are more likely to require intensive care, have higher injury severity scores (see Chapter 7), and have significantly higher fatality rates than children.[26]

Overall, a substantial number of fatal pedestrian collisions involve head injuries in addition to lower extremity injuries. Furthermore, pedestrian deaths are more likely to occur at night, and night collisions most often involve adults. More fatalities occur on weekends, especially on Saturdays.[27] Fatalities are more common when the pedestrian is struck by the vehicle's front end, propelling the victim forward or onto the hood or windshield, called a wrap trajectory. Wrap trajectories are more common with passenger cars and forward projection more common with light trucks and vans (see Chapter 5). Vehicle damage is an ominous sign for the pedestrian.[26]

Trends in pediatric pedestrian injury mortality have been on the decline, not only in the United States but in several other countries as well, including England, Denmark, Sweden, and New Zealand. In a comparison between these countries for children under age 14, Denmark has achieved the greatest reduction in deaths, the smallest occurring in New Zealand. It has been found that the countries that show the largest strides in decreasing childhood pedestrian deaths are those that have emphasized environmentally based prevention strategies rather than pedestrian education[28] (see Chapter 2).

The decrease in childhood pedestrian deaths over the last 20 years is in direct contrast to what is known about risk factors for pedestrian deaths. Historically, as traffic volume increased, so did the pedestrian deaths for children.[29] Through the 1970s and 1980s traffic volume in the United States increased exponentially while child pedestrian injury rates declined. This unexpected finding is called the "safety paradox." This paradox is attributed to a decline in children's mobility. As roadways become more heavily traveled and dangerous for pedestrians, fewer children are afoot.[30]

Alcohol

Consumption of alcoholic beverages by drivers or pedestrians is a risk factor for motor vehicle collisions with a pedestrian. From 1982 to 1992 the percentage of persons over age 14 killed in a pedestrian traffic-related incident decreased 22%, but throughout the decline, the number of pedestrians who had consumed alcohol was higher than the number of drivers (hitting the pedestrian) who had drunk alcohol.[31] While the number of drivers with detectable blood alcohol levels involved in fatal pedestrian crashes has declined substantially, the number of pedestrians with detectable alcohol levels has decreased only slightly. Over half (55%) the pedestrians over age 14 who are killed have consumed alcohol.[1,31] In contrast to risk factors for impaired drivers, the risk factors for alcohol-impaired pedestrians are not yet well understood.[31]

BICYCLES

Bicycle–motor vehicle crashes occur less frequently than pedestrian–motor vehicle crashes. However, motor vehicles are a factor in 90% of bicyclist deaths.[32] Between 700 and 800 persons die from pedal cyclist traffic-related events and over 550,000 persons are treated in emergency departments for bicycle-related injuries in the United States every year.[1] Approximately another 100 bicyclists are killed in nontraffic-related pedal crashes, bringing the annual total from all causes to between 800 and 900 per year.[2] Overall, the rates of bicycle-related deaths have declined since the early 1980s, though not substantially.[1] The vast majority fatally injured are male (of the 757 traffic-related deaths in 1997, 656 were male).[1] Compared to females, males take 2.5 times the number of bicycle trips, are 2.4 times more likely to be killed per trip taken, and have a death rate six times higher.[32] Male pedal cyclist

deaths peak in the 10- to 14-year-old age category but are also high throughout the range from 5 to 19 years old and rise again from age 35 to 39.[1] For females, ages 5–14 are at highest risk. In contrast to male rates, female rates drop off significantly by ages 15–19. Overall, black males have higher death rates than white males, particularly between ages 10 and 14, and ages 35 and 54.[1]

Both speed and alcohol are factors in bicycle deaths. About a third of pedal cyclist deaths occur on roadways where the speed limit is 55 miles per hour or faster. Not all of the bicyclists who are killed are tested for alcohol consumption. However, research has shown that of the two-thirds who are tested, one-third have positive blood alcohol levels.[32]

An estimated 80% of fatally injured bicyclists suffer significant head injury. Bicyclists hospitalized with head injuries are 20 times more likely to die than those with no head trauma.[32] Bicycle helmets have been found to reduce the incidence and severity of craniocerebral trauma, the leading cause of death from pedal cyclist collisions.[33] Almost all deaths under age 16 occur to riders who are not wearing helmets.[1] Universal use of bike helmets could save one death per day and one head injury every 4 hours in the United States.[34] Bicyclists who don helmets have an 85% reduction in their risk of head injury.[35] Studies have also shown that bike safety education, and legislation combined with education, can substantially increase helmet use among children, whose national helmet use is a dismal 25%.[1,36] As of early 1999, 15 states have adopted laws requiring helmets for various specified ages of minors, ranging from 18 years and under in California to age 12 and under in Connecticut and Tennessee. There are additional locales across the United States where bicycle helmet laws exist.[37]

Although less life threatening than head injury, bike crashes are also a common source of facial, oral, and ocular trauma.[38,39] The zygomatic and orbital regions are the most frequently fractured, followed by the mandible and nose. Helmets, as they are currently designed and worn, do not prevent facial injuries but may reduce them.[1,40] The majority of eye injuries and some oral injuries can be prevented with sports oral guards and safety glasses.[41]

Death rates for male cyclists between 20 and 54 years of age have increased since the 1980s. The number of deaths has increased from around 200 per year in the early 1980s to about 350 per year in 1997.[1,32] In part, this increase may be due to a surge in the number of bicyclists, rising with the popularity of recreational biking.

It is known that the increasing popularity of mountain biking has increased the number of young adult riders who are injured. However, in mountain biking there is often less contact with motor vehicles owing to the use of off-road trails. The mountain biker is more likely to use protective head gear, which may help explain the lower number of head injuries in that group. A California study found that 51% of mountain bicyclists experienced some injury while cycling in a 1-year period. Extremity injuries were the most common type of trauma; serious head and neck trauma was relatively rare, and 88% regularly wore bicycle helmets, a figure much higher than overall helmet usage.[42]

DROWNING AND WATER-RELATED ACTIVITIES

Unintentional drowning deaths have decreased substantially over the period between 1980 and 1997. In 1980 there were over 7,000 unintentional drowning deaths (rate of 3.2 per 100,000 population).[1] In 1997 there were 4,051 fatal submersions (rate of 1.51 per 100,000 population) and in 1998 there were 4,406 drowning deaths.[1] The steady decline in drowning death rates spans all age groups, racial groups, and both sexes, with one exception: there has been a slight increase in the rates for infants (babies under age 1).[1,43] Drowning is the second leading cause of injury-related death in children aged 1–14.[1]

Drowning deaths remain a significant problem for children under 5 years (rate of 2.69 per 100,000 population in 1997) and for adolescents from age 15 to 19 (rate of 1.83 per 100,000 in 1997).[1] Between 1995 and 1997 1,600 children under age 5 died in submersion incidents; of these, roughly 1,000 (64%) were male.[1] In those same years, over 2,000 persons between ages 15 and 24 died in drowning events; over 1,900 were male (or 90%).[1] The disparity in male-female rates is present in every age category.[1] Studies suggest that the higher rates for males over females result from behavioral differences rather than differences in exposure to water or aquatic activities, although some studies do suggest that men may have greater exposure to water activities.[44] Men are more likely than women to engage in aquatic risk-taking behaviors and are more likely to consume alcohol while on or near the water.[45,46]

Most children under age 5 who drown unintentionally fall into a body of water, most often a pool, bucket, or a bathtub (85%).[9,47,48] Within the United States, Florida has the highest rates of drowning for this young age group (7.67 per 100,000 population in 1997) due to the large number of swimming pools.[1] For those under 5 years, up to 90% of drownings and near drownings in swimming pools are attributable to the lack of an isolated pool fence or a four-sided pool fence, failure to properly latch the gate entrance, or

lapses in adult supervision.[49] Pool isolated fencing, or four-sided pool fencing, physically separates the pool from both the house and the yard and should be at least 5 feet high.[9,49,50] New Zealand and Australia have nearly eliminated childhood drowning through mandatory pool isolated fencing. A study in Phoenix, Arizona, found that 35% of drownings and near drownings could be prevented with isolated fencing.[9]

In at least one area in Texas more drownings occur in apartment pools than in private home pools.[51] The role of fencing, gates, supervision, and children's exposure to apartment pools needs further investigation.

Teenagers are more likely to drown in a natural body of water: a lake, pond, or river, rather than a swimming pool. Alcohol is a factor in up to 50% of teenage drownings, particularly among teenage boys. Other factors, such as how and why this age group engages in risk-taking behaviors, are not well understood.[5]

As expected, May to August are the peak months for near-drowning and drowning deaths. Peak days are Saturday and Sunday.[47,49]

Locations of drownings vary by region, state, or geographical features. In North Carolina, for example, a large number of drownings occur in rural lakes and ponds.[52] In Florida and Arizona most occur in residential pools. Despite the large amount of ocean coastline, most drowning deaths in Maryland occur in rivers and creeks where currents are treacherous, footing is unsure, and supervision is minimal.[46] Imperial County, California, which adjoins the Mexican border, has the highest drowning rate in that state (around 21 deaths per 100,000 population). Eighty-five percent occur in irrigation canals, particularly the "All-American Canal," when water velocity and water levels increase. The vast majority are Mexican citizens attempting to illegally cross into the United States.[53] In Oklahoma, some drowning deaths have been attributed to electrocution that occurred during swimming or work activities in or near lakes.[54]

The state of Alaska has the highest drowning rates in the United States.[1,9] Rates have been declining, dropping from 13.45 in 1989 to 5.17 in 1997 (rates are per 100,000 persons).[1] Reasons for Alaska's number 1 position include cold water temperatures, the large number of water bodies, the swiftness of its rivers, the frequency of travel over water, and the large number of persons employed in fishing, logging, or other occupations that increase water exposure.[9] Commercial fishermen in Alaska are at particularly high risk. Between 1990 and 1994, fishermen in Alaska had fatality rates between 145 and 195 per 100,000 workers; almost all of those fatalities (over 90%) resulted from drowning.[55,56] This is especially alarming given the overall occupational fatality rates for all U.S. commercial fishermen: about 47 per 100,000 workers; Alaskan commercial fisherman have an occupational fatality rate 30 times higher than the U.S. rate for all workers. Many Alaskan fishing-related drownings result from overboard falls. Wearing personal flotation devices (PFDs) and training in prevention and recovering overboard falls has been shown to reduce drowning deaths of Alaskan commercial fishermen.[55,56]

Behind Alaska, Hawaii, Idaho, Louisiana, and Montana have the next highest drowning rates per state, respectively.[1]

Racially, Native Americans suffer the unfortunate distinction of having the highest drowning rates in America. This is postulated to be, at least in part, due to the large number of Native Americans who reside in Alaska.[9] Drowning rates for black Americans are approximately one and a half times higher than white Americans. Children between 1 and 4 years of age are an exception, with whites having twice the rate of blacks in this age group, believed to be related to residential swimming pool access. However, this gap is narrowing. Additionally, fewer blacks than whites drown in boating-related events.[9]

About 16% of all drownings are associated with boating activities; but 90% of all recreational boating deaths are due to drowning.[9,44] The Coast Guard estimates recreational boating deaths to be about 800 per year.[1] The ratio of male to female drownings associated with boating is 14 to 1, compared to 5 to 1 for other drownings.[57] Boating-related drownings are highest for those over age 15; motor boats are involved in about half, and the majority are boats under 16 feet in length. In other words, fast boats and small boats (including jet skis) are associated with drowning deaths. Capsizing or overboard falls are implicated in a large number of boat-related drowning fatalities. Personal flotation devices are in inadequate supply on the victim's boat 20% of the time.[47] Coast Guard data show that over 80% of boat-related drownings are the result of improper or nonuse of PFDs.[58] An Ohio study showed that the majority of boating fatalities occurred on the weekend, Friday through Sunday, and between June 1 and September 30; the peak hours were late afternoon and early evening.[59]

Alcohol is often a factor in drowning deaths. In addition to impairing judgment, alcohol increases the possibility of laryngospasm and aspiration, and suppression of the gag reflex.[47] Between 25% and 50% of adults who drown have consumed alcohol near the time of death.[57] In a North Carolina study of drowning deaths between 1980 and 1984, more than half of those tested (752 drownings) over age 15 had positive blood alcohol levels, one-third over the 100-mg/dL level.[52] Also, men are known to be more likely than women to consume alcohol when on or near the water. In addition, about a third of boat owners drink alcohol during water activities. Up to two-thirds of boating's drowning victims have consumed an alcoholic beverage close to the time of death.[9] It should be noted that obtaining data on alcohol and drowning is often difficult because alcohol tests can be inaccurate if the victim has been submerged for more than 6 hours.[47]

Surprising many, there are a number of children who drown in bathtubs and buckets of water. Once a toddler's head is submerged, his or her may not possess the strength or agility to raise he or she head from the water. An estimated 88% of children who perish in the bathtub are under 2 years old.[60] Lapses in adult supervision of children under 5 years, often 5 minutes or less, are implicated in a large number of these drownings.[9] In addition to being left unattended, children are often left with only an older sibling in the tub.[48,60] It is possible that some childhood drownings are misclassified as unintentional drownings. There should exist a high index of suspicion for child abuse and neglect when a child under 5 years of age drowns or suffers a near-drowning incident in a bathtub. Percentages of pediatric patients in bathtub drownings who have a history of child abuse are estimated to be as high as 67%.[61] For older children and adults who perish in bathtubs, the most common risk factor is a seizure history.[47,60,62]

Drowning in a bucket of water most commonly occurs to a toddler in the home environment. In the latter 5 years of the 1980s there were 160 bucket-related drownings in the United States; nearly all (88%) were infants and toddlers between the ages of 7 and 15 months. African-American babies are six times more likely to drown in a bucket than white babies, and males are at a much greater risk than females. Bucket drownings are more likely to occur in the summer. In the past, states with the highest bucket drowning rates were (1) Vermont, (2) Arizona, and (3) Illinois.[63]

The ability to swim and its relationship to near drowning and drowning has not been well established. The few studies examining swimming ability have not shown that the ability to swim reduces the chance of drowning. These studies have focused on comparisons between males and females, noting that with the numbers of males and females who are able to swim being relatively equal, the rates of drowning are, nevertheless, much higher for males.[45,64] Male risk-taking behaviors and overestimation of aquatic abilities, particularly when coupled with the use of alcohol, are thought to be more important factors in drowning deaths than the ability to swim.[45]

More research is also needed on the possible benefit of the presence of lifeguards, bystanders performing lifesaving functions, and early emergency medical services intervention. Lifeguards on Australian beaches have proved to play an important role in drowning prevention, successfully resuscitating 40% of initially apneic near-drowning victims.[65]

The best predictors of the outcomes for pediatric near-drowning victims are those obtained by field personnel. Good outcome predictors are neurologic responsiveness, reactive pupils, and sinus rhythm. Predictors of poor outcome are submersion duration of more than 10 minutes and resuscitation durations of over 25 minutes.[66]

As many as 1,000 persons suffer spinal cord injuries each year in the United States while diving into natural bodies of water and swimming pools. Males from age 15 to 24 are predominantly affected.[67] Fifty percent to 80% of spinal cord diving injuries occur in cervical vertebrae numbers 4–6, and between 50% and 65% are a complete transection of the spinal cord.[68] Dry summer conditions often lower the water levels of lakes, ponds, and rivers, increasing the chance that a diver will suffer a spinal cord injury due to miscalculation of water depth. Swimming pools often designate "no diving" and post water depth markings; however, those warnings are usually not available at natural water body sites.[67]

FIRES AND BURNS

Over 20,000 persons died unintentionally from fires from 1992 to 1997. Over 80% of those deaths occurred in residential fires; a residential fire happens every 78 seconds.[1] Deaths from fires and flames declined in the 1980s and 1990s, attributed to the widespread use of home smoke detectors. In 1980, over 6,000 died; this declined to under 4,000 by 1998.[1,9] Home property loss from fires was nearly $4.6 billion in 1997.[1]

House fires are the number 1 cause of fire-related mortality, and two-thirds of those deaths are caused by smoke inhalation resulting in carbon monoxide poisoning.[9] In the 1980s over 15,500 Americans died from fire-related carbon monoxide poisoning.[69] Those living in mobile homes have much higher mortality from fires; studies show that they have from two to three times the mortality rates of those living in non-movable houses or apartments.[70–72] Although house fires are the leading cause of fire mortality, scalds are the leading cause of burn hospitalizations. Scalds account for only 3% of all fire deaths, however.[70] Although less common than scalds, flame burns are the most severe type of burn.

Close to 1.5 million people seek medical treatment for burns every year, and another 50,000–60,000 are hospitalized with burn injuries.[1,73] Significant declines have occurred in burn deaths and injuries in the last two decades. Declines in deaths and burn hospitalizations approximate 50%, given the 25% increase in population over those 20 years.[73] Those at highest

risk are children under age 5 and the elderly (65 and older), particularly those over age 80.[1] Both those age groups are at high risk during a house fire; the elderly are also at risk for unintentional ignition of their clothing, particularly while cooking. The elderly are also more likely to be burned from faulty or misused electrical equipment, often electric blankets.[74]

Nationwide, it is estimated that 27,000 children are hospitalized due to a burn injury every year, and over 400,000 are treated by medical personnel in outpatient environments. About 80% of fire and burn deaths in children under age 19 are the result of house fires. Electricity-related fires and burns claim the lives of close to 10%.[75] Chemical burns are rare and are usually occupational injuries.[76] For children 10–15 years old, gasoline-ignited burns are a major source of hospitalizations, as are children playing with matches and cigarette lighters.[1,9,77] A study of all injury deaths to children under age 15 in Milwaukee, Wisconsin, from 1989 to 1990 found residential fires to be the number 1 cause of injury deaths, accounting for 34% of the total number of deaths.[78] Young children, chiefly those under age 4, are at high risk for nonfatal burns, with around two-thirds being scald injuries.[9,79] Hot food, grease, water, and drinks spilled on the skin of this age group is a leading cause of hospitalizations.[9,70] Many scald burns to children as well as elderly people are caused by contact with hot tap water, chiefly because their skin is thinner, burns at a lower temperature, and burns faster than adults' skin. Many experts recommend water temperatures not exceed 120°F, a temperature sufficient to sanitize eating and cooking utensils. In response to pressure from physicians, hot water manufacturers agreed to voluntarily preset hot water heaters at the time of installation to 120°F in 1990, an action designed to reduce the number of unintentional scaldings. It is important to note that scald injuries to infants and toddlers are often the result of child abuse.[70] It is estimated that up to 8% of all children's burn injuries are inflicted abuse.[79]

As with most other injuries, males are at higher risk than females, although the disparity is less for fire-related deaths than many other injury fatalities.[9] Male fatality rates are 1.5 times that of female rates.[1] The highest mortality rates for residential fire deaths are in the elderly black male population; 1997 black males from age 80 to 84 experienced a mortality rate of 37.38 per 100,000 population. Compare this to the overall fire death rate for all races and both sexes of 6.72 per 100,000 population. Black females, though their rates are much less than black males, still have death rates higher than either white males or females.[1,9] Black children comprise around 15% of the nation's childhood population, but account for 34% of all pediatric fire and burn fatalities; they are three times more likely to die in a fire than white children.[1,75] These rate dispariti-ties are considered a result of socioeconomic status rather than race differences. Higher income is associ-ated with lower risk.[70]

States with the highest fire-related mortality rates are concentrated in the southeastern United States: Mississippi, Arkansas, Alabama, South Carolina, Missouri, and Kentucky (in order of rates for 1997).[1,9,70] As expected, the winter months witness the highest number of fire deaths, particularly from December to March.[9,70,77] This is due to the seasonal use of portable heaters, fireplaces, and Christmas trees.[77] Nighttime is the high-risk period. In New Jersey more than half of all fatal house fires between 1985 and 1991 began between the hours of 11 PM and 7 AM.[80]

Cigarettes are commonly thought of as a cause of cardiorespiratory morbidity. However, they are also a common cause of house fires. Cigarettes are responsi-ble for about a quarter of all fire fatalities and are a leading source of ignition for fatal house fires.[70,80,81] Careless smoking is the leading cause of residential fire-related deaths for those over 70 years of age.[77] Typically, a cigarette is inadvertently dropped on furni-ture or bedding. Children playing with cigarette lighters are also a major cause of deadly house fires.[9,77] The capability exits to make cigarettes that are less likely to ignite furniture; however, such a cigarette has not yet been manufactured for widespread use.[9]

In addition to smoking materials, a large number of residential fires are ignited by heating devices, such as woodstoves and kerosene heaters. A North Carolina study found heating-related fires to account for one-third of all fires in which someone perished.[70]

Alcohol is implicated in more than 40% of fatal fires.[9] In one study, over half of the examined fire vic-tims had blood alcohol levels over 50%.[70] The combi-nation of alcohol consumption and smoking materials often sets the stage for a deadly house fire.[72]

Persons living in houses without smoke detectors are two times more likely to die in a house fire than those living in homes with smoke detectors.[9] In a study of 10 cities, the U.S. Fire Administration found that in five cities, Birmingham, Chicago, Cleveland, Dallas, and Detroit, smoke detectors were absent in most fatal residential fires.[82] Smoke detectors are present in over 80% of American homes; however, many contain a dead battery or no battery.[9] In addition, there are geo-graphical pockets within the United States where smoke detectors are present in a much smaller per-centage of residences. In 1993, for instance, in Appa-lachian Kentucky up to 30% of homes lacked smoke detectors, and in the Fond du-Lac Reservation in Minnesota 80% of the homes lacked smoke detectors until a community installation project was begun.[83,84]

Community smoke alarm giveaway projects have shown to decrease the incidence of residential fire injuries.[85] The CDCP recommends smoke detectors with 10-year lithium batteries and hush buttons to tem-porarily silence alarms from cooking smoke and steam.[1] Residential sprinkler systems are also available and, though not widely installed, are estimated to cost less than 1% of the total cost of a new home. Clothing burns are reduced with flame-resistant clothing and by wearing garments that are not bloused or loose. Children's sleepwear is manufactured with fire resist-ance; robes and gowns with fire-resistant features would also benefit the elderly.[9]

FIREWORKS

While house fires are usually associated with fire deaths, fireworks are often the cause of severe or disabling injuries. Internationally, fireworks injuries are most fre-quent during New Year and holiday celebrations. In the United States the majority of fireworks injuries occur around the week of July 4th—Independence Day.[86,87] Between 8,500 and 12,000 persons per year are treated for fireworks injuries in U.S. emergency departments, and although deaths are rare, they do occur.[1,86,88] Fireworks are also responsible for thousands of fires and their subsequent property damage.[89] Three times as many males as females are injured, and the highest injury rates occur in the 10- to 14-year-old age group (up to 22.3 per 100,000 persons per year).[87] Overall, bystanders are injured as often as 25% of the time; however, active participants are most often the victims and tend to have more severe injuries than do bystanders.[86,87] Class C fireworks, such as firecrackers, bottle rockets, Roman candles, fountains, and sparklers, are associated with the preponderance of injuries (two-thirds), particularly in adolescents and adults.[1,87,89] But, federally banned class B fireworks — rockets, cherry bombs, and M-80s—cause the most severe injuries.[1] It is no surprise, then, that the major-ity of fireworks-related injuries requiring hospitaliza-tion are connected to the use of federally illegal fireworks.[89]

The hands and the eyes are the most frequently injured body parts, comprising over half of all injuries, usually burns, but amputations do occur.[1,86,87] The U.S. Eye Injury Registry (USEIR) compiling data from 32 states from 1990 to 1994 cataloged 255 unintentional fireworks-related eye injuries, with injured bystanders comprising a significant portion of those injured, 123 (45%). Most eye injuries are caused by bottle rockets, a fact that has led to the banning of bottle rockets in at least 10 states, the bans being strongly supported by the American Academy of Ophthalmology, American Academy of Pediatrics, and American Public Health

Association.[88] In one study of children, 10% had permanent damage from their fireworks' injuries, including partial and complete blindness.[86] Though seemingly benign, sparklers burn at 1000°F, can ignite clothing, and are the leading cause of fireworks injury for children under 5 years old.[1,89]

The inconsistency of laws governing fireworks at the local, state, and federal levels and the ease with which fireworks can be transported across state lines are credited with increasing the availability of fireworks. Increased availability is associated with more injuries.[89]

FALLS

Falls are the leading cause of nonfatal injuries and are the leading cause of injury death for Americans 65 and older, though most deaths occur to those over age 74.[1,9] In 1998, over 12,000 Americans perished from unintentional falls, and over 43,000 died from 1994–1997. Mortality rates from unintentional falls is extremely high in the elderly, reaching over 104 deaths per 100,000 population in those 85 and older. Rates for fall deaths are increasing, as are the number of persons dying as a result of a fall.[1] Medical costs for falls exceed $20 billion a year. Males surpass females in the number of deaths and mortality rates for falls in every age group, with the lone exception being the number of deaths (not mortality rates) in females aged 80 and above. Fall mortality rates for whites are significantly higher than for blacks. Death rates for falls are highest in white males, followed by white females, black males, and black females.[1]

One-third of all hospitalized injured persons have sustained injuries during a fall.[9] Fall morbidity occurs across the life span, but the elderly, infants, and toddlers are most often injured. Fractures are common injuries for the elderly, and head injuries are common for infants and toddlers, owing to this age groups' relatively large head mass.[9] Older persons also experience a disproportionate number of deaths from falls.[90]

Among the elderly, falls are responsible for almost all (around 87%) fractures and are the second leading cause of spinal cord and brain injury. Hip fractures in this group generate the greatest morbidity and mortality. The death rate for hip fracture patients in the year after injury is between 12% and 20%. Just as important is that half of these older citizens do not return home and/or are unable to function independently. Risk factors for falls include dementia, visual impairments, neurological and musculoskeletal problems, weakness, medications, as well as gait and balance difficulties.[91] The vast majority of falls occur at home, about a third in public places, and the remainder in health care settings.[1] Complicating factors in the home environment include uneven floors, slippery surfaces, poor lighting, loose rugs, unstable furniture, and tripping hazards, such as objects lying on the floor or pets.[91] In health care facilities additional hazards include wet floors, poor lighting, improper bed height, and wheelchairs.[1] Osteoporosis, a demineralization of bone, is associated with an increased risk of fracture, particularly vertebral compression fractures and hip fractures. Osteoporosis is particularly a major health problem for older women but is also a problem for men over the age of 80.[92,93] Exponential increases are seen in hip fractures among women over age 70, such that by age 90 one of every three women has experienced a hip fracture.[92]

Falls account for over 100,000 hospitalizations for children (under age 19) and over 3 million emergency department visits. Trends in children's falls are directly related to development. Infants' falls usually involve furniture, such as changing tables and baby walkers. Toddlers' falls are often from stairs, windows, or toys; in urban areas, falls from high-rise buildings are rarely survivable. Window guard installation in high-risk tenements in New York City in the "Children Can't Fly Program" significantly reduced fall deaths in young children. School-age children often fall from bicycles, playground equipment, roofs, trees, and horses.[9]

Playground-related injuries send 200,000 children to emergency departments each year; most (60%) of those visits are due to falls to the ground surface.[94,95] Falls are the leading factor in playground injuries. Playground swings, monkey bars, climbing equipment, and slides are where the fall usually begins.[95] A one-foot fall onto concrete or asphalt or a four-foot fall onto packed ground can result in a fatal head injury if the head strikes the ground first.[94] One-third of playground injuries are severe: fractures, internal bleeding, amputations, and concussions. Of the 20 playground deaths per year, the majority are from strangulation, followed by falls.[1]

Although not in large numbers, young and middle-aged adults do succumb to fatal injuries from falls, and men perish much more often than women.[1] Men are at higher occupational risk than women. Falls account for about 10% of occupational fatalities and are the leading cause of occupational death for roofers, construction laborers, and structural metal workers.[96,97]

Pleasurable pursuits also lead to injury. For example, tree stands, which are elevated platforms used for hunting deer and other large game, are often sites of fall injuries in men, predominantly those aged 17–35. Victims fall from the stands, fall while ascending and descending, and fall with the collapse of the stands.[98] In Georgia, a 10-year study found that over 20% of all deer hunting–related injuries were the result of falls involving tree stands, causing fractures in 73% of the patients, often the cervical and lumbar spines.[98] In Louisiana, 28 deer stand falls resulted in permanent paralysis from 1985 through 1994, costing more than $4.2 dollars in first-year medical costs.[99] Treatment of the injured is often delayed because these falls occur in locations not readily accessible to EMSs.

Although hunting-related injuries are rare in women, horseback riding injuries are not. NEISS estimated that there were over 92,000 emergency department visits (48,000 females and 44,500 males) in the United States during 1987 and 1988 for horseback riding–related events, and falls account for most horseback riding-associated trauma.[100,101] Almost 10% of those injured (roughly 9,000 persons) required hospitalization. Falls from horses most often result in soft tissue injury followed by extremity fractures, but serious head and neck, pelvic, and thoracic trauma do occur. The majority of deaths are associated with head trauma. Studies also show that, at the time of the fall, fewer than 20% of injured riders were wearing helmets.[100]

POISONINGS

There are over 5 million unintentional poisonings each year. Deaths include the unintentional ingestion, unintentional overdose, or adverse reactions to legal and illegal drugs, either solids, liquids, or gases. Deaths are increasing. In 1984, 4,911 people in the United States died of unintentional poisoning. In 1997, that figure had risen to 10,163 persons.[1] Young men, aged 20–44 are responsible for the vast majority of the increase. Mortality rates for males are three times that for females. Black males have the highest mortality rates, followed by white males.[1,102] Misuse of drugs, primarily opiates, other narcotics, and cocaine, is the foremost factor in unintentional poisonings of young men. Cocaine is involved in the majority of ED visits; heroin, morphine, other narcotics, and cocaine are culprits in more than one-third of deaths.[102]

Because small children are much more likely to be poisoned by prescription medications, unintentional poisoning deaths for children under 5 have decreased more than 70% since the 1970 Poisoning Prevention Packaging Act. This act required screw-type closures or other child-resistant caps for over-the-counter and prescription drugs.[103] Poisoning fatalities among children under 5 declined from 226 in 1970 to 36 in 1998 (fluctuating in the late 1990s from 36 to 57).[1,9] Among children, those between the ages of 18 months and 3 1/2 years are at highest risk. Most ingestions occur in the child's home, usually in the kitchen or bedroom. The most frequently taken medications are antibiotics, birth control pills, analgesics, and cardiovascular drugs. Problems occur when the child-resistant cap is improperly reapplied, when medicines are secured in a weekly

dose container, or when medicine is not stored in the original container.[103] Children are also injured when ingesting household materials, most frequently petroleum products or cleaning products. Keeping these items in child-proof or out-of-reach cabinets can prevent these incidents.

The geriatric population is also subject to unintentional poisoning, particularly those over age 85.[1] Poison Control Centers report numerous calls for older adults who ingest extra doses of medicines due to forgetfulness.[104] Other problems include mistaking the identity of a medication, using an incorrect route of administration, or storing medications improperly.[105] In addition, older persons are more likely to require hospitalization than younger persons.[104,106]

Carbon monoxide (CO) is another significant source of poisoning in the United States; around 10,000 people seek treatment for this toxicity each year. Unintentional CO poisoning results most frequently from motor vehicle gasoline combustion or the use of coal, kerosene, and wood for heating or cooking. Deaths are most common in the winter months; those living in homes with old heating systems, gas-powered space heaters, or wood stoves are at higher risk.[107–109]

OCCUPATIONAL INJURY

Around 7 of 100 workers are injured, and roughly 2 million workers receive disabling injuries while at work each year.[9] In the United States approximately 6,000 persons die every year from injuries sustained while at work.[96,97] Occupational injury costs are conservatively estimated in triple digits of billions of dollars.[9]

Occupational fatalities are often difficult to accurately count due to inconsistences in death certificate reporting, so there may exist a bias toward underreporting.[9] Current statistics are also difficult to obtain. An average of 17 workers die from workplace injuries per day.[96] The CDCP's National Institute for Occupational Safety and Health estimates that the number of worker fatalities are decreasing (from 7,400 in 1980 to 5,800 in 1989—decreasing overall fatality rates in that period from 8.9 deaths to 5.6 deaths per 100,000 workers). Mortality rates for males are 10 times higher than for females and slightly higher for blacks than whites.[110]

The six leading causes of occupational death are (in order) motor vehicle incidents, machine-related injuries, homicides, falls, electrocutions, and being struck by falling objects.[96] Motor vehicle–related deaths are highest for those employed in transportation and public utilities. Around 30% of all machine deaths occur in agriculture, forestry, and fishing. Homicides are most often seen in retail trade, public administration (including law enforcement), and services. In contrast to homicides outside the workplace, where only a small percentage (13% in 1992) are in conjunction with a robbery or other crime, the vast majority (82% in 1992) of workplace homicides involve such activity. Seldom are occupational homicides perpetrated by family, coworkers, or acquaintances in personal disputes, whereas in the general population over half are.[110] Workers at highest risk are those who work alone, work late-night hours, and handle money. Specific high-risk groups are taxicab drivers, gas station cashiers, grocery store employees, workers in eating and drinking facilities, hotel and motel workers, and law enforcement officers.[97,111] Between 1980 and 1992, over 2,000 women and 7,000 men died in work-related homicides, and although many more men perish than women, homicide is the leading cause of occupational death for women.[111,112]

Almost half of all work-related fall deaths and about 40% of electrocutions take place in the construction industry. Those struck by falling objects are most often hit by trees, limbs, or logs during construction, agriculture, forestry, fishing, logging, and sawmill operations.[96]

Industries with the highest injury death rates are (in descending order) mining, construction, transportation/public utilities, and agriculture/forestry/fishing. Although rates are declining, they are still much higher than for the average worker. The largest number of deaths occur in the construction industry, followed in descending order by transportation/communication/public utilities, manufacturing, and agriculture/forestry/fishing. Table 1-1 lists the industry with the largest number of deaths in each state. Occupational mortality profiles vary from state to state, so it is important to obtain local data. For example, in Hawaii and Nevada air transport crashes are the leading cause of worker death.[96] In Alaska, the leading causes are water and aircraft transport incidents, which often result in drowning.[96,113] For West Virginia, Kentucky, and Oklahoma the largest number of deaths occur in mining.[96]

Youth workers, including both adolescents and children, should not be overlooked. Although occupational death rates are not as high as for other age groups, deaths do occur, and permanent disabilities are a problem as well.[114] An estimated 186 youths perish each year and another 4,000 are injured in farm-related incidents, most often with machinery, particularly tractors.[5,112] In addition to agriculture, injuries are also frequent for youths who are employed in manufacturing, at gas stations, convenience stores, and restaurants.[5,114] Males are more predominant than females among occupationally injured teens. Adolescents are more frequently injured during the summer months, when their work time increases.[5,112]

In the U.S. government, there exist two large agencies involved in occupational safety. Both were created by the Occupational Health and Safety Act of

Table 1-1
Industries Contributing the Largest Number of Occupational Deaths by Total Numbers of Deaths per State

Mining	Agriculture/Forest/Fishing
Oklahoma	Alaska
West Virginia	Idaho
Kentucky	North Dakota
Construction	South Dakota
Arizona	Nebraska
District of Columbia	Wisconsin
Rhode Island	Iowa
Texas	Missouri
Florida	Minnesota
Tennessee	Hawaii
North Carolina	**Transportation/Communication/ Public Utilities**
Connecticut	Wyoming
Massachusetts	Delaware
Virginia	Ohio
Maryland	Illinois
Pennsylvania	Indiana
New Jersey	Arkansas
New York	Louisiana
New Hampshire	Kansas
Manufacturing	Colorado
Maine	Nevada
Michigan	New Mexico
Washington	California
South Carolina	Utah
Georgia	Montana
Alabama Oregon	**Construction and Manufacturing (an equal number)**
Mississippi	Vermont

Source: Based on data from the Centers for Disease Control, 1980–1989.[96]

1970, the National Institute of Occupational Safety and Health (NIOSH), under the CDCP, and the Occupational Safety and Health Administration (OSHA), under the Department of Labor. Each agency has distinctly different responsibilities. NIOSH is responsible for conducting research and making recommendations for the prevention of work-related injuries and illnesses. OSHA is charged with creating and enforcing workplace safety and health regulations.[115]

INTERNET ACTIVITIES

Visit the National Center for Injury Prevention and Control Web site at http://www. cdc.gov/nc.pc/ovip/dvip.htm and www.cdc.gov/ ncipc/cmprfact.htm.

- Get the latest statistics on motor vehicle, fire, fall, and poisoning deaths.
- Select some of the injuries that interest you from the list of fact sheets. What are the latest statistics on incidence, prevalence, prevention activities, risk factors, and treatment costs for this injury?

INTENTIONAL INJURY AND UNINTENTIONAL FIREARM DEATHS AND INJURIES

Intentional injuries include homicide, suicide, and non-fatal injuries as a result of the violent behavior inflicted by one person on another or self-inflicted. Some ambiguity arises when there is not an intent to injure another person, but a violent action results in injury. In most of those cases, legal intervention ensues and these incidences are usually included in discussions of intentional injuries. In shaken-baby syndrome, for example, there may be no intent to injure the baby, but rather to quiet the infant; however, the aggressive, violent behavior of the adult shaking the baby often results in death or injury.[9]

Intentional injuries occur at an alarming rate in the United States. Every year, more persons die from suicide and homicide combined than from motor vehicle crashes. In 1997, there were 50,026 suicide and homicide deaths compared to 42,473 motor vehicle deaths.[1]

FIREARMS

Firearms are of particular public health concern in suicides, homicides, and unintentional shooting deaths, especially in adolescents and children. Firearm violence is the second leading cause of injury-related death behind motor vehicle crashes. If current trends continue, the national death rate from firearms will surpass motor vehicle death rates by the year 2003.[1,116,117] In 1991, both Texas and Louisiana wit-

nessed the number of firearm deaths surpass the number of motor vehicle–related deaths. Eight states and the District of Columbia now report more deaths from firearms than motor vehicle crashes.[1] Firearm mortality rates are increasing at a faster pace than any other cause of death in the United States, with the exception of AIDS-related fatalities.[116]

Firearms were the cause of traumatic death for 31,799 people in 1997 (suicide: 17,566; homicide: 13,252; unintentional shootings: 981). Between 1985 and 1991, firearm fatalities rose 25.4% but more recently have begun to decline.[1,2] (In 1997, the overall firearm fatality rate was around 12 per 100,000 persons compared to 14 in 1990.) Male firearm death rates are six times higher than females rates, and blacks rates are three times higher than whites. Black males 20–24 years old have very high firearm death rates (over 154 per 100,000 black males).[1,2] Firearm injuries cost over $20 billion a year, 80% of which is paid for with taxpayer dollars.[1] Figure 1-4 illustrates the impact firearms have on both homicide and suicide in the United States by comparing the number of deaths by firearm means to the number of deaths by all other means.

Internationally, the United States leads the industrialized nations in firearm mortality rates. The U.S. firearm fatality rates are over eight times higher than the next country, Italy.[118]

Unintentional shootings are likely to occur at home and are more prone to happen when a gun is kept loaded in an unsecured location.[119,120] Over one-third of unintentional firearm deaths occur in children aged 19 and under. Between 1995 and 1997, 144 children aged 9 and younger and 461 aged 14 or younger were unintentionally killed by firearms, or one child every day.[1] Studies show that a quarter of all gun owners store their firearms loaded in an unlocked area, and over half

**Homicides, suicides, and firearms:
The number of deaths in the United States, 1997**

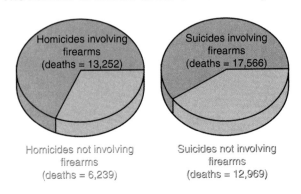

FIGURE 1-4 The number of deaths from firearms in both homicides and suicides is significant.

of parents who have guns in the home do not lock the gun away from the children.[121]

Although many people keep guns in the home for self-defense, the presence of a gun in the home increases by five times the likelihood of a suicide occurring and three times the likelihood of a homicide occurring when compared to homes without firearms.[122,123] The gun kept in a home is 43 more times likely to kill a household member than an intruder.[124]

Not all firearm injuries result in death. There are an estimated 4–12 firearm injuries for each gun-related death, or somewhere between 190,000 and 515,000 per year.[125]

HOMICIDE

Nationally, there are over 19,000 homicides each year, down from over 24,000 in 1994.[1] Homicide is the second leading cause of death for persons 15–24 years (17 victims per day); the leading cause of death in this same age group in African-American males, and the second leading cause of death in Hispanic youths. Mortality rates for ages 15–24 are more than double the overall rates. For African-American males aged 15–34, homicide is the leading cause of death.

Males have much higher homicide death rates than females. Eight of 10 homicide victims are male. Compared with 21 other industrialized countries, the homicide rates for U.S. males from 15 to 24 years old is

4.4 times higher than the next highest country, Scotland.[126]

Although females have lower homicide rates, they are at much higher risk of injury due to rape, child sexual abuse, and violent assaults by intimate partners. Researchers note that partner violence affects one in every six American homes each year, with over two-thirds of those encompassing multiple incidents. Black couples have 8.4 times higher spouse homicide rates than white couples.[9]

Racially, homicide rates for blacks are much higher than for whites. Hispanics have an estimated three times higher homicide rate than whites. Poverty is believed to be a factor in the increased rates of homicide for nonwhites.[9] Figure 1-5 illustrates the disparity in the homicide death rates of black males compared to white males and black and white females.

Firearms are the cause of injury in at least 70% of all homicide deaths in the United States. Firearms are the cause of injury for almost 80% teens and young adults.[1] For black males from 15 to 19, 95% of all homicides involve firearms. Deaths from firearm homicides in the United States increased close to 45% from 1985 to 1995, mostly due to handgun-related deaths. Handgun firearm deaths increased over 65% in that time period. Representing approximately one-third of all guns owned in the United States, handguns are responsible for 58% of all homicides and over 80% of all firearm homicides.[127]

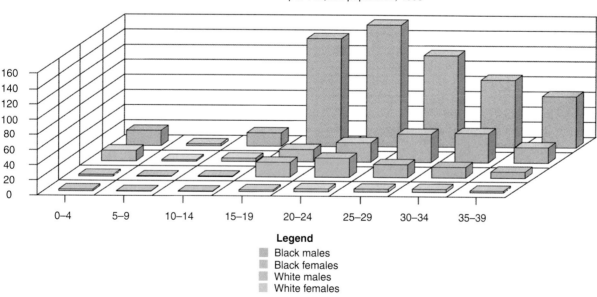

Homicide death rates by race and sex

per 100,000 population, 1995

Legend
Black males
Black females
White males
White females

FIGURE 1-5 Note that the homicide death rates for black males from ages 15 to 39 far surpass all other groups. Also note that black females have homicide death rates higher than white males and white females.

The majority of gun-related violence occurs in the home. Despite being in the media forefront, less than 1% of homicides of school-aged children occur on or around school grounds, though most events do involve firearms.[1] Drug crimes and gang killings together comprise only 7% of all firearm homicides.[128,129] The most common reason cited for a homicide is an argument.[128]

SUICIDE

In 1981 the number of suicide deaths in the United States overtook the number of homicide deaths, a statistic that has remained true since that time. Suicide ranks second in all causes of death for those from ages 25–34, and for those aged 10–24 suicide is the third leading cause of death. Suicide is the fifth leading cause of Years of Potential Life Lost in the United States.[130] From 1994 through 1997, 123,864 suicide deaths were reported in the United States. Since the mid-1940s, however, the U.S. age-adjusted suicide rates have remained nearly constant, at around 11 suicides per 100,000 population. Regardless of this stability, suicide risk and methods of suicide differ across age, race, gender, and geographical location.[130]

While those aged 10 to 34 have a larger number of suicide deaths, suicide death rates are highest among elderly Americans. Those over age 80 have the highest rates. Older persons' suicide rates began rising in the 1980s but remained relatively stable in the early 1990s.[1,130]

Suicide rates for adolescents have also increased substantially since the 1950s (from a rate of 2.7 per 100,000 population in 1950 to 11.0 per 100,000 population in 1994).[1,5] This trend can be primarily attributed to a fourfold increase in the teenage suicide rates for white males.[5] Particularly alarming is the 121% increase in the number of suicides in children aged 10–14, irrespective of the low total number of suicides in that age group. In contrast, rates among adults have generally declined since the 1950s.[130]

Around 90% of all suicides are among whites, and over 70% are white males. Among blacks, the rate for males is nearly six times higher than for females. Among both Native Americans and Hispanics male suicide rates are around five times higher than for their female counterparts. All races of males have sharp increases in suicide rates between ages 15 and 24, with Native American young men experiencing particularly sharp increases. Overall, Native American suicide rates are 1.5 times the national rates. For women by race, white female suicide rates peak in their fifties whereas black female rates peak in their thirties.[1,130]

By marital status, widowed and divorced persons have the highest suicide rates (around 30 per 100,000 population). Married persons have the lowest rates, with single persons' rates between married and widowed or divorced persons.[130]

Firearms are the method of suicide in 60% of the cases, followed, respectively, by poisonings (18%), strangulation (15%), other or unspecified means, and cutting. Strangulation by hanging is often the method chosen by children, adolescents, and young adults. Middle-aged adults account for the largest proportion of poisoning suicides. The largest percentage of male suicides for whites, blacks, Hispanics, and Native Americans are accomplished using firearms (about 65%). Firearms are also responsible for the largest percentage of female suicides for the same racial groups, but the percentages are much lower for females (around 45%). Poisonings rank second behind firearms for females, but a reduction in the number of poisoning suicides has fueled a decreasing trend in suicides by females. Strangulation ranks second in method by percentage for males. Strangulation is a prominent method among Asian men and women.[130]

By location, suicide rates are highest in the western states, highest in Nevada followed by Utah, Arizona, New Mexico, Oklahoma, Colorado, Wyoming, Idaho, Montana, Oregon, Alaska, and Florida. The higher rates in western states correspond with higher rates of firearm suicides. The lowest rate is in the District of Columbia. In recent years the greatest increases in suicide rates have occurred in Nebraska, Montana, Idaho, and South Carolina, increasing 20% or more. Poisonings and firearm wounds account for the majority of the increase in Nebraska. Firearm deaths accounted for most of the increases in South Carolina and Idaho.[130]

Firearm suicides are increasing, up 18% between 1980 and 1995. Firearms accounted for 77% of the increased number of suicides during that time period. Firearm suicides increased the most in 10- to 19-year-olds and those over the age of 80. Suicide rates by firearm trauma increased most rapidly in young and elderly males and black males.[130]

It is not known exactly how many nonfatal suicide attempts there are each year, but thousands more are attempted than are completed. In every age group males are more likely to complete suicide, although females attempt it three to four times as often as males. Survivors of suicide attempts are likely to attempt suicide again, with the chance of suicide completion at a later time as high as 10%. Suicide attempters and victims often have a history of depression, substance abuse, feelings of helplessness, and a family history of suicide.[5]

INTERNET ACTIVITIES

Visit the e-medicine Web site at www. emedicine.com. Click on the Emergency Medicine on-line book and select Epidemiology. Then click on Introductory Biostatistics. Review the chapter on the presentation of data in scientific studies.

SUMMARY

In the United States, over 400 people die every day from potentially preventable injuries. Thousands more suffer life-altering injuries and permanent disabilities. Motor vehicle deaths, suicides, homicides, and firearm deaths are leading causes of injury death. Males, particularly those from ages 15 to 34, are overrepresented in traumatic deaths, as are African Americans, Native Americans, the very young, and the very old for many causes of injury. Alcohol plays a significant role in all causes of trauma.

REVIEW QUESTIONS

1. What is the leading cause of death and disability among ages 1–34 in the United States?
2. What is the leading cause of death of African-American males aged 15–34?
3. What are the three components of epidemiology?
4. What is a measure of the proportion of individuals in a population with a disease at a given point in time?
5. What is a measure of the number of new cases of an injury in a population during a specific period of time?
6. What kind of rate is the morbidity rate?
7. Which rates are presented based on such characteristics as age, sex, and race?
8. Which cause of injury codes are part of the ICD classification system?
9. What are the life years lost and the YPPL for a 30-year-old suicide victim, using 75 as the life expectancy figure?
10. At least what three factors discussed in this chapter are causes of motor vehicle crashes?
11. What is the leading cause of injury-related death in children aged 5–9?

CRITICAL THINKING

● What are some common traits or characteristics of the people who are most at risk for injury or traumatic death?

● What etiologies of injury are most common in the United States? How does this compare with other industrialized nations? Why do you think the United States is different?

● Choose a specific injury common in your response area. Devise a plan for how your EMS system could prospectively monitor the frequency and outcomes of these injuries. How could this information be used to improve patient care in your system?

REFERENCES

1. Centers for Disease Control and Prevention. National Center for Injury Prevention and Control. Available at: http://www.cdc.gov/ncipc; 2000.
2. National Center for Health Statistics. Injury-related visits to hospital emergency departments: United States, 1992. Advance data no. 261. Available at: http://www.cdc.gov/nchswww/releases/fs_ad261.htm; February 1, 1995.
3. Hennekens CH, Buring, JE.: Mayrent, SL, ed. *Epidemiology in Medicine*. Boston: Little, Brown and Company; 1987.
4. Snow, J. On the mode of communication of cholera. In: Hennekens CH, Buring JE: Mayrent SL, ed. *Epidemiology in Medicine*. Boston: Little, Brown and Company; 1987; 6.
5. Runyan CW, Gerken EA. Epidemiology and prevention of adolescent injury. *JAMA*. 1989; 262 (16):2273.
6. Committee on Trauma Research, Commission on Life Sciences, and the Institute of Medicine. *Injury in America: A Continuing Public Health Problem*. Washington, DC: National Academy Press; 1985.
7. Malek M, Chang BH, Gallagher SS, Guyer B. The cost of medical care for injuries to children. *Ann Emerg Med*. 1991; 20(9):997.
8. Garrison HG, Runyan CW, Tintinalli JE, et al. Emergency department surveillance: an examination of issues and a proposal for a national strategy. *Ann Emerg Med*. 1994; 24(5):849.
9. Department of Health and Human Services: Public Health Service, Centers for Disease Control, National Center for Environmental Health and Injury Control, Division of Injury Control in conjunction with National Institute for Occupational Safety and Health, and National Highway Traffic Safety Administration. *Injury Control: Position Papers*

from the Third National Injury Control Conference. U.S. Department of Health and Human Services, Denver, April 1991; 22–25.

10. Consumer Product Safety Commission. National Injury Information Clearinghouse: The National Electronic Injury Surveillance System (NEISS). Washington, DC; 1996. Available at: http://www.cpsc.gov/about/clrnghse.html; 1997.

11. Page, JG. *Views about E-Coding Among Staff at a Small, Rural Hospital.* Chapel Hill, NC: University of North Carolina; 1991. Thesis.

12. Rice DP, MacKenzie EJ, Associates. *Cost of Injury in the United States: A Report to Congress.* San Francisco, Calif: Institute for Health and Aging, University of California and Injury Prevention Center, The Johns Hopkins University, San Francisco; 1989.

13. Stephens JA, Branche-Dorsey, CM. *Home and Leisure Injuries in the United States.* Atlanta, Ga: National Center for Injury Prevention and Control; 1996.

14. Runyan C. Injury prevention lecture. January 18, 1989.

15. Runge JW. The cost of injury. *Emerg Med Clin North Am.* 1993; 11(1):241.

16. Centers for Disease Control (CDC): National Center for Injury Prevention and Control. Years of potential life lost (YPLL) before age 65, by cause of death—United States, 1994. Available at: http://www.cdc.gov/ncipc/osp/ypll94.jpg; 1997.

17. Rodriguez JG, Brown, ST. Childhood injuries in the United States. *Am J Dis Child.* 1990; 44:627. Available at: http://www.saferoads.org

18. Advocates for Highway and Auto Safety; 1995.

19. Zepatos T. Silent cause of traffic deaths: falling asleep. *USA Weekend.* May 16, 1997; 12.

20. McSwain NE, Belles A. Motorcycle helmets: medical costs and the law. *J Trauma.* 1990; 22:587.

21. Rowland J, Rivara F, Salzberg P, Soderberg R, Maier R, Koepsell T. Motorcycle helmet use and injury outcome and hospitalization costs from crashes in Washington state. *Am J Public Health.* 1996; 86(1):41.

22. Centers for Disease Control. Alcohol involvement in pedestrian fatalities—United States, 1982–1992. *MMWR.* 1993; 42(37):716.

23. Waller AE, Baker SP, Szocka A. Childhood injury deaths: national analysis and geographic variations. *Am J Public Health.* 1989; 79(3):310.

24. Roberts I, Norton R, Jackson R. Driveway-related child pedestrian injuries: a case-control study. *Pediatrics.* 1995; 95(3):405.

25. Olson LM, Sklar DP, Cobb L, Sapien R, Zumwalt R. Analysis of childhood pedestrian deaths in New Mexico, 1986–1990. *Ann Emerg Med.* 1993; 22(3):512.

26. Lane PL, McClafferty KJ, Nowak E. Pedestrians in real world collisions. *J Trauma.* 1994; 36(2):231.

27. Kong LB, Lekawa M, Navarro RA, et al. Pedestrian-motor vehicle trauma: an analysis of injury profiles by age. *J Am Coll Surg.* 1996; 182(1):17.

28. Roberts IG. International trends in pedestrian injury mortality. *Arch Dis Child.* 1993; 68(2):190.

29. Roberts I, Crombie I. Child pedestrian deaths: sensitivity to traffic volume—evidence from the USA. *J Epidemiol Commun Health.* 1995; 49(2):186.

30. Roberts I. What does a decline in child pedestrian injury rates mean? *Am J Public Health.* 1995; 85(2):268.

31. Curtin D. Alcohol involvement in pedestrian fatalities—United States, 1982–1992. *MMWR.* 1993; 42(37):716.

32. Johns Hopkins Injury Prevention Center, Bicycle Helmet Safety Institute (BHSI). A compendium of statistics from various sources. Available at: http://www.bhsi.org; 1997.

33. Kelsch G, Helber MU, Ulrich C. Craniocerebral trauma in fall from bicycles: what is the effect of a protective helmet? *Unfallchirurg.* 1996; 99(3):202.

34. Sacks JJ, Holmgreen P, Smith SM, Sosin DM. Bicycle associated head injuries and deaths in the United States from 1984 through 1988. *JAMA.* 1991; 266:3016.

35. Thompson RS, Rivara FP, Thompson DC. A case-control study of the effectiveness of bicycle safety helmets. *N Engl J Med.* 1989; 320:1361.

36. Macknin ML, Medendorp SV. Association between bicycle helmet legislation, bicycle safety education, and use of bicycle helmets in children. *Arch Pediatr Adolesc Med.* 1994; 148(3):255.

37. Johns Hopkins Injury Prevention Center, BSHI. Mandatory helmet laws: a summary. Document no. 513; July 22, 1996.

38. Zeng Y, Sheller B, Milgrom P. Epidemiology of dental emergency visits to an urban children's hospital. *Pediatr Dent.* 1994; 16(6).

39. Kutschke PJ. Ocular trauma in children. *J Opthalm Nurs Technol.* 1994; 13(3):117.

40. Delank KW, Meldare P, Stoll W. Traumatology of the facial skull in bicycle accidents. *Laryngorhinootologie.* 1995; 74(7):428.

41. Kutschke PW, Lokshin MF. Preventive oral health care: a review for family physicians. *Am Fam Physician.* 1994; 50(8):1677.

42. Chow TK, Bracker MD, Patrick K. Acute injuries from mountain biking. *West J Med.* 1993; 159(2):145.

43. Brenner RA, Smith GS, Overpeck MD. Divergent trends in childhood drowning rates, 1971 through 1988. *JAMA.* 1994; 271(20):1606.

44. Centers for Disease Control. Alcohol use and aquatic activities—Massachusetts. *JAMA.* 1990; 264:3320.

45. Howland J, Hingson R, Mangione TW, Bell N, Bak S. Why are most drowning victims men? Sex differences in aquatic skills and behaviors. *Am J Public Health*. 1996; 86(1):93.

46. Baker SP, Guohua L. The risk of drowning: males in Maryland rivers. *JAMA*. 1991; 265(3):356.

47. Runyan CW. Drowning lecture. UNC School of Public Health; February 22, 1989.

48. Jensen LR, Williams SD, Thurman DJ, Keller PA. Submersion injuries in children younger than 5 years in urban Utah. *West J Med*. 1992; 157(6):641.

49. Centers for Disease Control. Drownings and near drownings in Maricopa County, Arizona, 1988 and 1989. *MMWR*. 1990; 39(26):441.

50. Brenner RA, Smith GS, Overpeck MD. Divergent trends in childhood drowning rates, 1971 through 1988. *JAMA*. 1994; 271(20):1606.

51. Warneke CL, Cooper SP. Child and adolescent drowning in Harris County, Texas, 1983 through 1990. *Am J Public Health*. 1994; 84(4):593.

52. Patetta MJ, Biddinger PW. Characteristics of drowning deaths in North Carolina. *Public Health Rep*. 1988; 103(4):406.

53. Agocs MM, Trent RB, Russell DM. Activities associated with drowning in Imperial County, California, 1980–1990: implications for prevention. *Public Health Rep*. 1994; 109(2):290.

54. Centers for Disease Control. Electricity-related deaths on lakes—Oklahoma, 1989–1993. *MMWR*. 1996; 45(21):440.

55. Perkins R. Evaluation of an Alaskan marine training program. *Public Health Rep*. 1995; 110(6):701.

56. Centers for Disease Control. NIOSH alert: request for assistance in prevention of drowning of commercial fishermen. *MMWR*. 1994; 43(24):449.

57. Centers for Disease Control. Alcohol use and aquatic activities—United States, 1991. *MMWR*. 1993; 42(35):675.

58. Centers for Disease Control. Drowning in the United States, 1978–1984. *MMWR*. 1988; 37(SS-1):27.

59. Centers for Disease Control. Recreational boating fatalities—Ohio, 1983–1986. *MMWR*. 1987; 36(21):321.

60. Budnick LD, Ross DA. Bathtub-related drownings in the United States, 1979–1981. *Am J Public Health*. 1985; 75:630.

61. Lavelle JM, et al. Ten-year review of pediatric bathtub near-drowning: evaluation for child abuse and neglect. *Ann Emerg Med*. 1995; 25(3):344.

62. Diekema DS, Quan L, Holt VL. Epilepsy as a risk factor for submersion injury in children. *Pediatrics*. 1993; 91(3):612.

63. Mann NC, Weller SC, Rauchschwalbe R. Bucket-related drowning in the United States, 1984 through 1990. *Pediatrics*. 1992; 89(6):1068.

64. Langley J, Silva PA. Swimming experiences and abilities of nine-year-olds. *Brit J Sports Med*. 1986; 20(1):39.

65. Maniolios N, Mackie I. Drowning and near-drowning on Australian beaches patrolled by life-savers: a 10-year study. *Med J Aust*. 1988; 148:165.

66. Quan L, Kinder D. Pediatric submersions: prehospital predictors of outcome. *Pediatrics*. 1992; 90(6):909.

67. Centers for Disease Control. Diving-associated spinal cord injuries during drought conditions—Wisconsin, 1988. *MMWR*. 1988; 37(30):453.

68. Kraus J. Spinal cord injuries lecture. UNC School of Public Health; April 5, 1989.

69. Cobb N, Etzel RA. Unintentional carbon-monoxide-related deaths in the United States, 1979 through 1988. *JAMA*. 1991; 266(5):659.

70. Runyan CW. Fire lecture. UNC School of Public Health; March 20, 1989.

71. Parker DJ, et al. Fire fatalities among New Mexico children. *Ann Emerg Med*. 1993; 22(3):517.

72. Chernichko L, Saunders LD, Tough S. Unintentional house fire deaths in Alberta 1985–1990: a population study. *Can J Public Health*. 1993; 84(5):317.

73. Brigham PA, Mcloughlin E. Burn incidence and medical care use in the United States: estimate, trends, and data sources. *J Burn Care Rehabil*. 1996; 17(2):95.

74. Elder AT, Squires T, Busuttil A. Fire fatalities in elderly people. *Age-Ageing*. 1996; 25(3):214.

75. Rodriguez JG, Brown ST. Childhood injuries in the United States. *Am J Dis Children*. 1990; 44:627.

76. Carlotto RC, et al. Chemical burns. *Can J Surg*. 1996; 39(3):205.

77. Centers for Disease Control. Deaths resulting from residential fires—United States, 1991. *MMWR*. 1994; 43(49):901.

78. Weesner CL, Hargarten SW, Aprahamian C, Nelson DR. Fatal childhood injury patterns in an urban setting. *Ann Emerg Med*. 1994; 23(2):231.

79. Herndon CN, Rutan RL, Rutan TC. Management of the pediatric patient with burns. *J Burn Care Rehabil*. 1993; 14(1):3.

80. Barillo DJ, Goode R. Fire fatality study: demographics of fire victims. *Burns*. 1996; 22(2):85.

81. Brunnemann KD, Hoffmann D, Gairola CG, Lee BC. Low ignition propensity cigarettes: smoke analysis for carcinogens and testing for mutagenic activity of the smoke particulate matter. *Food Chem Tox*. 1994; 32(10):917.

82. Federal Emergency Management Agency (FEMA). Arson in America fact sheet; Arson in America's cities fact sheet. Available at: eipa@fema.gov; May 2, 1996.

83. McKnight RH, Struttmann TW, Mays JR. Finding homes without smoke detectors: one step in planning burn prevention programs. *J Burn Care Rehabil*. 1995; 16(5): 548.

84. Shults R, Harvey P. *Efforts to Increase Smoke Detector Use in U.S. Households*. Atlanta, Ga: National Center for Injury Prevention and Control; 1996.

85. Mallonee S, Istre GR, Rosenberg M, Reddish-Douglas M, Jordan F, Silverstein P, Tunell W. Surveillance and prevention of residential-fire injuries. *N Engl J Med*. 1996; 335(1):27.

86. Smith GA, Knapp JF, Barnett TM, Shields BJ. The rockets' red glare, the bombs bursting in air: fireworks-related injuries to children. *Pediatrics*. 1996; 98(1):1.

87. See LC, Lo SK. Epidemiology of fireworks injuries: the National Electronic Injury Surveillance System, 1980–1989. *Ann Emerg Med*. 1994; 24(1):46.

88. Centers for Disease Control. Serious eye injuries associated with fireworks injuries—United States, 1990–1994. *MMWR*. 1995; 44(24):449.

89. Centers for Disease Control. Fireworks-related injuries—Marion County, Indiana, 1986–1991. *MMWR*. 1992; 41(25):451.

90. Mosenthal AC, Livingston DH, Elcavage J, Merritt S, Stucker S. Falls: epidemiology and strategies for prevention. *J Trauma*. 1995; 38(5):753.

91. Stevens JA, Thomas TA. *Major Causes of Unintentional Injuries Among Older Persons: An Annotated Bibliography*. Atlanta, Ga: Centers for Disease Control and Prevention, National Center for Injury Prevention and Control; 1996.

92. Birge SJ. Osteoporosis and hip fracture. *Clin Geriatr Med*. 1993; 9(1):69.

93. Runyan CW. Falls lecture. UNC School of Public Health; March 27, 1989.

94. Centers for Disease Control. Playground-related injuries in pre-school-aged children—United States, 1983–1987. *MMWR*. 1988; 37(41):629.

95. University of Northern Iowa: National Program for Playground Safety. U.S. Consumer Product Safety Commission, National Electronic Injury Surveillance System, 1990–1994, Cedar Falls, Iowa.

96. Centers for Disease Control and NIOSH Division of Safety Research. Occupational injury deaths—United States, 1980–1989. *MMWR*. 1994; 43(14):262.

97. Toscano G, Jack T. Occupational injury fatalities—1994. *Stat Bull Metrop Insur Co*. 1996; 77(2):12.

98. Centers for Disease Control. Tree stand-related injuries among deer hunters—Georgia, 1979–1989. *MMWR*. 1989; 38(41):697.

99. Lawrence DW, Gibbs LI, Kohn MA. Spinal cord injuries in Louisiana due to falls from deer stands, 1985–1994. *J La State Med Soc*. 1996; 148(2):77.

100. Centers for Disease Control. Injuries associated with horseback riding—United States, 1987 and 1988. *MMWR*. 1990; 39(20):329.

101. Bixby-Hammett D, Brooks WH. Common injuries in horseback riding. *Sports Med*. 1990; 9:36.

102. Centers for Disease Control. Unintentional poisoning mortality—United States, 1980–1986. *MMWR*. 1989; 38(10):153.

103. Centers for Disease Control. Unintentional poisonings of prescription drugs in children under five years old. *MMWR*. 1987; 36(9):124.

104. Kroner BA, Scott RB, Waring ER, Zanga JR. Poisoning in the elderly: characterization of exposures reported to a Poison Control Center. *J Am Geriatr Soc*. 1993; 41(8):842.

105. Haselberger MB, Kroner BA. Drug poisoning in older patients: preventive and management strategies. *Drugs and Aging*. 1995; 7(4):292.

106. Klein-Schwartz W, Oderda GM, Booze L. Poisoning in the elderly. *J Am Geriatr Soc*. 1983; 31(4):195.

107. Centers for Disease Control. Carbon monoxide poisoning associated with a propane-powered floor burnisher—Vermont, 1992. *MMWR*. 1993; 42(37):726.

108. Centers for Disease Control. Unintentional carbon monoxide poisoning following a winter storm—Washington, January 1993. *MMWR*. 1993; 42:109.

109. Baron RC, Backer RC, Sopher IM. Fatal unintended carbon monoxide poisoning in West Virginia from non-vehicular sources. *Am J Public Health*. 1989; 79:1656.

110. Stout NA, Jenkins EL, Pizatella MS. Occupational injury mortality rates in the United States: changes from 1980 to 1989. *Am J Public Health*. 1996; 86(1):73.

111. Jenkins EL. Homicide against women in the workplace. *J Am Med Womens Assoc*. 1996; 51(3):118.

112. Dunn KA, Runyan CW. Deaths at work among children and adolescents. *Am J Dis Child*. 1993; 147(10):1044.

113. Schnitzer PG, Bender TR. Surveillance of traumatic occupational fatalities in Alaska—implications for prevention. *Public Health Rep*. 1992; 107(1):70.

114. Belville R, Pollack SH, Godbold JH, Landrigan PJ. Occupational injuries among working adolescents in New York State. *JAMA*. 1993; 269(21):2754.

115. Centers for Disease Control. Home page. Available at: http://www.cdc.gov.

116. Centers for Disease Control. Deaths resulting from firearm and motor-vehicle-related injuries: United States, 1968–1991. *MMWR*. 1994; 14:37.

117. Fingerhut LA, Jones C, Makuo D. *Firearm and Motor Vehicle Injury Mortality—Variation by State and Race Ethnicity: United States, 1990–1991*. National Center for Health Statistics No. 242; 1994; Hyattsville, Md.

118. Gunfree: The extent of gun violence. Available at: http://www.gunfree.inter.net/csgv/bsc_int.htm; July 1996.

119. Weil DS, Hemenway D. Loaded guns in the home: analysis of a national random survey of gun owners. *JAMA*. 1992; 267:3033.

120. Hemenway D, Solnick SJ, Azrael DR. Firearm training and storage. *JAMA*. 1995; 273(1):47.

121. Talmey Drake Research & Strategy, Inc. *The Family Safety Survey: A National Survey of Parents Compliances with the Family Safety Check*. Washington, DC: National SAFE KIDS Campaign; May 8, 1995.

122. Kellermann AL, Rivara FP, Somes G, et al. Suicide in the home in relation to gun ownership. *N Engl J Med*. 1993; 327(7):467.

123. Kellermann AL, Rivara FP, Rushforth NB, Banton JG, Reay DT, Francisco JT, Locci AB, Prodzinski J, Hackman BB, Somes G. Gun ownership as a risk factor for homicide in the home. *N Engl J Med*. 1993; 329(15):1084.

124. Kellerman AL, Reay D. Protection or peril? An analysis of firearm-related deaths in the home. *N Engl J Med*. 1986; 314(24):1557.

125. Ryan GW. National estimates of nonfatal firearm-related injuries. *JAMA*. 1995; 273(2):1749.

126. Fingerhut LA, Kleinman JC. International and interstate comparisons of homicides among young males. *JAMA*. 1990; 263:3292.

127. Wintemute G. Firearms as a cause of death in the United States, 1920–1982. *J Trauma*. 1987; 27:532.

128. Federal Bureau of Investigation. *Uniform Crime Reports*; 1994.

129. Federal Bureau of Investigation. *Uniform Crime Reports*; 1995.

130. Kachur S, Potter L, James S, Powell K. *Suicide in the United States, 1980–1992: Violence Surveillance Summary Series, No. 1*. Atlanta, Ga: National Center for Injury Prevention and Control; 1995

Chapter 2

Role of EMS in Injury Prevention and Surveillance

OBJECTIVES

Upon completion of this chapter, the reader should be able to:

- Define injury prevention, injury control, and trauma.
- Explain why the term *accident* is not used by injury prevention specialists.
- Briefly summarize the history of injury prevention.
- Describe the Haddon matrix and its purpose.
- Describe the Public Health Model.
- Describe the Pat Barry Four Square and the meaning of the terms mandatory, voluntary, active, and passive.
- Describe six criteria for evaluation of injury control strategies.
- Define and provide examples of the five E's of injury prevention: education, enforcement, engineering, economic incentives, and evaluation.
- Design an effective "fear message" as part of an educational program.
- Discuss the role of legislation, litigation, and regulation in injury control.
- Explain the importance of evaluation in injury control programs.
- Describe the role of the individual paramedic in injury prevention.
- Describe the role of EMS in injury prevention.

KEY TERMS

Accident
Active intervention
Equity
Event phase
Horizontal equity
Injury prevention
Mandatory intervention
Outcome evaluation

Passive intervention
Post-event phase
Pre-event phase
Process evaluation
Vertical equity
Victim blaming
Voluntary intervention

Chapter 1 describes the human and financial cost of injury morbidity and mortality in the United States. Historically, the principal weapon against injuries has been medical care. However, as vital as treatment is, it can never substitute for prevention. Treatment is costly, and despite advances in trauma care, medical teams are unable to save many victims. Fifty percent of trauma deaths occur immediately or within an hour of injury.[1] Suffering from major trauma to vital organs, these victims will die regardless of the level and availability of medical care.[1] For these trauma victims, prevention is the only means of reducing traumatic mortality and morbidity.

THE IMPORTANCE OF INJURY PREVENTION

Paramedics are firsthand witnesses to unnecessary injuries and deaths and are observers of injury scenes; thus they play a vital role in injury prevention. EMS's close contact with trauma and high credibility with the general public mean EMS injury prevention efforts can have a substantial impact on the community. In Washington State, for example, EMS providers are major participants in a regional drowning prevention program. They are represented in coalitions, participate in statewide training, present health fair displays, testify in support of children's life vest legislation, and evaluate life vest use.[2] EMS providers are using the manual *Safety Advice from EMS (SAFE): A Guide to Injury Prevention* in community service work in various places across the United States. This manual contains predesigned formats and information for traffic safety, impaired driving, yielding to emergency vehicles, and bicycle and pedestrian safety.[3] These are but a few instances of the pivotal role EMS plays in injury prevention.

WHAT IS INJURY PREVENTION?

The term *trauma* is predominantly a medical word and is defined as "a wound, especially one produced by sudden physical injury";[3] major trauma refers to especially severe or critical injury;[4] injury is also defined as "a wound" or physical damage to a person.[5] **Injury prevention**, therefore, encompasses everything that serves to eliminate or reduce trauma. Injury control is sometimes used interchangeably with injury prevention, but the meaning of injury control can be broader, encompassing prevention, treatment, and rehabilitation.[6] However, injury prevention is more than these simple definitions. It is a scientific approach to identi-

fying groups or populations of persons at high risk for specific injuries or events that lead to injury.[7] Utilizing a multidisciplinary approach, which includes EMS, strategies are developed to prevent or minimize injury. Through evaluation of these strategies, scientific knowledge for today and for the future is obtained.

Nowhere in the definition of trauma or injury is the use of the word *accident*. This is not coincidental. The word **accident** means that the event is unexpected and random and happens by chance.[5,8] Scientists assert that injuries are not the result of random, chance, or unexpected events. Injury-producing events are predictable and, therefore, preventable. Thus, using the word accident is misleading. Holding to the tenet that injuries are not accidents, it can be determined how, when, where, and to whom they occur, and by using this information, interventions can be targeted to prevent specific types of injuries.[8]

HISTORY OF INJURY PREVENTION

Trauma has been a problem for humans throughout history. Homer's *Iliad* and Edwin Smith's *Papyrus* are early documents describing a variety of injuries and their treatments.[4] Hippocrates believed war to be the best school for surgeons. The first "trauma centers" were developed by the Romans during wartime and were strategically located to care for army soldiers.[4]

In 1942, Hugh De Haven published work on the importance of injury thresholds. De Haven analyzed the survival of falls from heights of 50–100 feet. Concluding that the normal body can withstand substantial but brief energy exchanges, DeHaven facilitated the design of "crash injury absorbing" automobiles.[9] In 1961, J. J. Gibson noted that all injury events were the result of the exchange of the five forms of energy: kinetic (mechanical), chemical, electrical, thermal, and radiation.[10,11] Using Gibson's energy form data, William Haddon, Jr. pioneered work in injury prevention in the 1960s, laying the foundation for today's injury prevention.[9]

An important historical figure, Bela Barenyi, specialized in automobile design safety. Barenyi, an inventor, designed automobile crumple zones in 1951. He also designed side-impact bars, rollover bars, and padded interiors. During Barenyi's lifetime he held over 2,500 patents related to safety design. He is referred to by some as the "father of passive safety."

In 1966, *Unsafe at Any Speed* was published by Ralph Nader, highlighting automobile crash injuries and deaths. This book was instrumental in drawing national attention to the high rate of automobile crash deaths in the United States.

THE HADDON MATRIX

In 1963, Haddon divided the injury process into three phases: pre-event, event, and post-event.[8,10] The **pre-event phase** refers to the time before energy exchange. During the **event phase**, one of the five forms of energy is transferred to body tissues. The **post-event phase** includes everything that treats, minimizes, or rehabilitates an injury. This important breakthrough work conceptualized that each of these injury phases provides a unique opportunity for preventing or minimizing the severity of injury.[10] Using the 1963 model, he developed the Haddon matrix.[9,12] This matrix is a combination of his event phase model and the traditional Public Health Model.

The Public Health Model asserts that there are three major factors involved in a health problem: the host, the agent, and the environment. Historically used in describing infectious diseases, it can be used with injuries as well. The Public Health Model is pictured as a triangle (see Figure 2-1). Using malaria as an example, the host is the patient, the agent (or vector) is the mosquito, and the environment is a wet or swampy area.[8] Interventions are developed to "break" the triangle, such as vaccines for the host, pesticides for mosquitos, and eliminating stagnant water in the environment. In a house fire, for example, the host is the family members living in the home, the agent is the fire (thermal energy), and the environment is the dwelling. In many cases the agent injures by interfering with normal body energy exchange.[9] For instance, in a drowning the agent, water, prevents adequate air exchange.

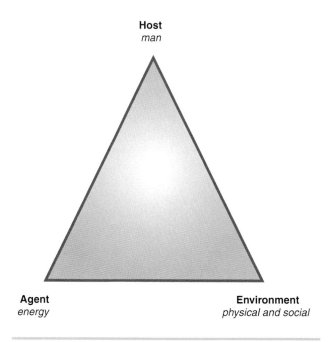

Host
man

Agent
energy

Environment
physical and social

FIGURE 2-1 Public Health Model.

Haddon combined the phases of injury with the host, agent, environment model to form the Haddon matrix[8,11,12,13] (see Table 2-1). Each block of the nine-cell matrix represents a point of intervention. The blocks of the matrix are filled with prevention strategies using a "brainstorming" approach; what seems like an outrageous idea may later evolve into a usable strategy. Airbags, for example, were originally invented for airplanes but were never used. When they became technologically available in the 1950s for automobiles, they were rejected by manufacturers who believed the public would not be willing to pay the extra cost of airbags. They are now accepted as an important "event" strategy for motor vehicles.

In the Haddon matrix, the "environment" section can be divided into the social and physical environment. The social environment includes human social interventions, such as education and laws. The physical environment pertains to the structure and physical properties of the agent or the event's vicinity.

The Haddon matrix provides for intervention at every point and every level in the injury process. This is important; it prevents dwelling solely on one area, such as medical treatment. The model also helps to avoid a phenomenon called **victim blaming**. In victim blaming the injured party is viewed as being responsible for the injury, confining the problem to the host. American society emphasizes individual responsibility, which, though often of value, can divert attention from other causes and contributing factors to an injury event. For example, thousands of people are injured every year falling down stairs, often attributed to clumsiness, lack of agility, or failure to pay close attention to the task. This fails to consider that stair design is often responsible. In fact, the depth and height of stairs in many buildings and homes today are based on dimension standards from hundreds of years ago, when people had much smaller feet.

Victim blaming also facilitates avoiding the feeling of vulnerability, in other words, saying to ourselves "that could never happen to me." While victim blaming may succeed in reducing immediate fear and anxiety, it also leads to a false sense of security. Victim blaming substantially narrows the possibility of finding strategies to prevent injury. The host's role in injury events is an important one but should not be the sole focus when developing injury prevention strategies.[9]

MOTOR VEHICLES AND BEYOND

Haddon, the first director of the National Highway Traffic Safety Administration (NHTSA), spent a substantial part of his career addressing the problem of motor vehicle crashes. A great deal of progress in this

Table 2-1
Haddon Matrix for Near Drowning

	Host Person	Agent Water	Physical Environment Pool, Lake, or Beach	Social Environment Community or Home
Pre-event: before submersion	Pool safety education; swimming lessons; feet-first programs	Water depth	Pool cover; four-sided pool fence; swimming warning signs at beaches	Boating and swimming regulations; adult supervision; lifeguard actions
Event: submersion	Host's physical condition; wearing a life jacket; alcohol consumption	Water temperature; water currents	Dual pool drains; pool depth; pool alarm	Buddy swimming; lifeguard present
Post-event: near drowning	Physical condition of the host; alcohol intoxication	Temperature, depth, and clarity of the water	Location of life preservers, boats, ropes, resuscitation equipment, cellular phone	Emergency medical services; community cardiopulmonary resuscitation (CPR); 911 services; cellular services

area has occurred since the 1950s. The National Motor Vehicle and Traffic Safety Act of 1966 charges the U.S. Department of Transportation (DOT) with establishing motor vehicle safety standards, research, and overseeing recall of defective automobiles. The 1966 Highway Safety Act requires the DOT to collaborate with local governments in the development of comprehensive highway safety programs. The DOT includes both the NHTSA and the Federal Highway Administration (FHWA); both are involved in motor vehicle safety.[4]

Also in 1966, the National Research Council published a report entitled[11] Accidental Death and Disability: The Neglected Disease of Modern Society.[11] This report, often referred to as the White Paper, noted that little progress had been made in applying the science of injury control to trauma and that quality EMS could realize improvements in the care of injured patients.

In 1973, with the Consumer Product Safety Act, Congress established the U.S. Consumer Product Safety Commission (CPSC) to collect injury data on consumer products. The CPSC is also responsible for advising the public about various hazardous consumer products. However, the agency is not responsible for motor vehicles, drugs, cosmetics, alcohol, tobacco, firearms, or work-related equipment not used in the home.[6]

In 1983, Congress instructed the secretary of the DOT to procure a study on trauma from the National Academy of Sciences. To accomplish this, the Committee on Trauma Research was formed. In 1985, this group published the report[11] "Injury in America: A Continuing Public Health Problem."[11] This work identified the extent of the injury problem and the recent progress in injury control, and recommended action for the future. Focusing attention on injuries, this report stated that "injury is a public health problem whose toll is unacceptable. The time has come for the nation to address this problem."[6]

Based on the impact of "Injury in America," Congress authorized funding ($10 million) for a 3-year pilot program in the Division of Injury Control of the Centers for Disease Control (CDC).[14-16] Giving special attention to five areas (epidemiology, prevention, acute care, rehabilitation, and biomechanics), the CDC began establishing regional injury research centers.[15] Now 10 in number, the locations of the regional injury control centers are listed in Table 2-2.

In 1987, Congress directed the CDC and NHTSA to evaluate the economic impact of injury. The culmination of this project was a report to Congress in 1989 entitled "Cost of Injury in the United States."[16] The two reports, "Injury in America" and "Cost of Injury in the United States," impressed upon Congress the depth of the traumatic injury problem in the United States. In 1992, the Division of Injury Control became the National Center for Injury Prevention and Control (NCIPC). The NCIPC was funded for $45 million in 1994; this supported eight regional injury control centers, numerous research projects, surveillance, and intervention programs. However, despite budget increases, there exists a lack of adequate funding for injury control projects.[14]

Table 2-2
Injury Prevention Research Centers in the United States, 1997

University of Alabama, Injury Control Research Center, University of Alabama at Birmingham, 403 Community Heath Services Building, Birmingham, AL 35294; Phone: 205-934-7845, Web address: http://www.uab.edu/icrc

University of California, Los Angeles, School of Public Health, Southern California Injury Prevention Research Center (SCIPRC), 10833 Le Conte Avenue, Room 76-078CHS, Box 951772, Los Angeles, CA 90095-1772; Phone: 310-206-4115, Web address: http://www.ph.ucla.edu/sciprcl.htm

University of California, San Francisco General Hospital, the San Francisco Injury Center for Research and Prevention (SFIC), Department of Surgery, 1001 Potrero Avenue, Ward 3A, Box 0807, San Francisco, CA 94110; Phone: 415-206-4623, Web address: http://itsa.ucsf.edu/·sfic/INDEX.html

Harvard School of Public Health, Harvard Injury Control Center (HICC), Department of Health Policy & Management, 677 Huntington Avenue, Room 445, Boston, MA 02115-6096; Phone: 617-432-2123, Web address: http://www.hsph.harvard.edu/hicrc

University of Iowa, Department of Preventive Medicine and Environmental Health, Injury Prevention Research Center, 158 IREH, Oakdale Research Campus, Iowa City, IA 52242-5000; Phone: 319-335-4458, Web address: http://www.pmeh.viowa.edu/iprc

Johns Hopkins University School of Hygiene and Public Health, Center for Injury Research and Policy, Hampton House, 5th Floor, 624 N. Broadway, Baltimore, MD 21205-1996; Phone: 410-614-4026, Web address: http://www.jhsph.edu/Research/Centers/CIRP

University of North Carolina, Injury Prevention Research Center (UNC IPRC), 233 Chase Hall-CB 7505, Chapel Hill, NC 27599-7505; Phone: 919-966-2251, Web address: http://www.sph.unc.edu/iprc

University of Washington, Harborview Medical Center, Harborview Injury Prevention and Research Center, Box 359960, Public Affairs, 325 9th Avenue, Seattle, WA 98104-2499; Phone: 206-521-1520, Web address: http://depts.washington.edu/hiprc

University of Pittsburgh, Center for Injury Research and Control (CIRCL), 200 Lothrop Street, Suite B400-PUH, Pittsburgh, PA 15213; Phone: 412-648-2600, Web address: http://www.circl.com

Colorado State University, Department of Environmental Health, Colorado Injury Control Research Center (CICRC), Environmental Health Building, Fort Collins, CO 80523-1676; Phone: 970-491-0670, Web address: http://www.colostate.edu/Orgs/CICRC

CONCEPTUAL MODELS AND INTERVENTIONS

The Haddon matrix promotes the conceptualization of injury control interventions in an easily understandable format. Once potential strategies have been placed into the matrix, a decision must be made about which strategy to plan, implement, and evaluate. Decision making is facilitated by the use of six criteria: efficiency, freedom of choice, equity, social stigma, consumer preference, and feasibility.[17]

Efficiency involves both the effectiveness of the intervention and its cost. Effectiveness and cost are weighed against the severity and probability of a particular injury. For example, are automatic sprinkler systems efficient? How do the probability of a fire and the severity of its consequences weigh against the effectiveness and cost of the sprinkler system?

Freedom of choice, fundamentally important and highly revered in American society, must also be considered. To what degree does the strategy restrict freedom of individual choice? Although important, individual choice affects, sometimes detrimentally, the community. For example, if an individual chooses not to wear a seat belt and is disabled during a car crash, there is a cost to society over and beyond the cost to the individual. Society loses the individual and the individual's future productivity while gaining the financial burden of medical care costs. Whose freedom is being restricted is also an important issue. For example, in the past, Americans have shown more willingness to restrict a child's freedom than an adult's freedom.

Equity refers to fairness or justness of an intervention. There are two types of equity: horizontal and vertical. In **horizontal equity** all groups are treated in the same fashion, for instance, requiring all children under 5 years to ride in child safety seats. **Vertical equity** treats unequal groups unequally in an attempt to make them more equal, for example, providing free child safety seats to low-income families—child safety seats are not provided for all children, only those with incomes below a certain level.[17] This is an attempt to make all children "more equal."

Social stigma is often involved in programs and interventions, for example, those targeted at alcoholics, drunk drivers, or the poor. Ethical questions are raised in response to programs that label or negatively stigmatize people into specific groups.

Preferences of consumers and manufacturers are vital to an intervention's success. When a device or program is not liked by the public, they are not likely to use it. This was the case with automobile seat belts for years.

Lastly, feasibility refers to the ability to carry out the project technologically, financially, and politically.

Often, difficult decisions must be made about where to place human and financial resources.[17]

Using these six criteria helps EMS, individuals, communities, policymakers, and manufacturers with critical decision making. Note, however, that there are no guidelines on how much weight to assign to each of the six criteria.[17,18]

HADDON'S TEN COUNTERMEASURES

In 1970, Haddon published a landmark paper entitled "On the Escape of Tigers: An Ecological Note,"[19] in which he outlined 10 countermeasures for injury control. These countermeasures with examples, are outlined in Table 2-3.[19] The countermeasures, are intended to prevent damage to both persons and property. They focus on the energy damage or hazard (the agent). Using the 10 countermeasures as a framework, interventions are generated. For example, when it became apparent that flammable vapor from liquids, such as gasoline for lawnmowers, posed a fire danger when stored in the same room with gas-fired water heaters, two ideas were suggested using countermeasure 5: Separate the hazard from the person or property. Removing the gasoline from the room containing the gas-fired hot water heater separates the flammable liquid from the source of ignition. Raising the hot water heater 18 inches off the floor safely separates the ignition source from the flammable liquid.

PAT BARRY FOUR SQUARE

Another method of classifying interventions is through the Pat Barry Four Square.[20] This method divides interventions into categories: active versus passive and mandatory versus voluntary. **Passive interventions** protect an individual without active participation on the part of the individual (e.g., circuit breakers). **Active interventions**, of course, are the reverse (e.g., motorcycle helmets). **Mandatory interventions** are those required by law (e.g., child passenger restraint laws), and **voluntary interventions** are just that, voluntary (e.g., protective gear for rollerblading). The interventions fall into one of four groups: active-voluntary, active-mandatory, passive-voluntary, or passive-mandatory. For examples see Table 2-4.

Research has shown that passive-mandatory (e.g., safety bars in car doors) interventions are the most effective, while active-voluntary (e.g., not driving during snow or ice) are the least effective; the other two categories fall in between.[9,20] Use of this square helps us predict the likelihood of an intervention's success. Although passive interventions produce the best results, they may require both education and some

Table 2-3
Haddon's Ten Countermeasure Strategies

Countermeasure	Examples
1. Prevent the creation of the hazard (energy).	Prevent the accumulation of snow where avalanches are possible. Do not manufacture nuclear weapons.
2. Reduce the amount of the hazard being made.	Reduce the number of aspirins in a bottle. Lower the temperature setting on hot water heaters.
3. Prevent the release of the hazard.	Chain wild and dangerous animals. Place prescription medicines in a locked cabinet.
4. Slow the rate of hazard release or the spatial distribution of the hazard.	Limit the muzzle velocity of firearms. Reduce the slope of skateboard ramps. Breakaway bases for softball.
5. Separate, in time and space, the hazard from the person or property.	Evacuate the community before a hurricane makes landfall. Construct bicycle lanes separate from roadways.
6. Impose a material barrier.	Fence dangerous animals. Knee pads for rollerblading. Firefighters' protective clothing. Bullet-proof vests.
7. Modify the contact surface of the hazard or basic quality of the hazard.	Pad and round vehicle interiors. Use Velcro darts in place of sharp, pointed darts.
8. Strengthen the person or property.	Maintain optimal physical condition. Construct buildings to current earthquake-proof standards.
9. Rapidly detect and evaluate damage to minimize the extent of damage.	Emergency medical services. 911 systems. Automatic fire alarms.
10. Stabilize and rehabilitate.	Emergency departments. Occupational and physical therapy.

Source: Prepared from "Energy Damage and the Ten Countermeasure Strategies," by W. Haddon, 1973. *Journal of Trauma,* 13, p. 321.

active participation for effectiveness. Parents must know the correct way to use a child-restraint seat; instruction is required for the proper placement and maintenance of smoke detectors; and so on.

Table 2-4
Pat Barry Four Square for Motor Vehicle Crashes

	Active	Passive
Voluntary	Educational driving programs Mothers Against Drunk Driving Keeping one's vehicle in good mechanical condition Avoiding driving in hazardous weather Emergency medical services	Side-impact air bags Voluntary production of vehicles with lower maximum speed capabilities Antilock brakes Automatic collision avoidance warning system
Mandatory	Driver education programs for specific ages Eye exams for driver's license renewal Motor vehicle inspections Obeying driving laws, such as speed limits Traffic citations	Automobile front-seat passive restraint systems: lap-shoulder restraints, airbags Motor vehicle lights, windshield wipers, turn signals, brake lights Infant restraint seats

THE FIVE E'S

EMS professionals can plan injury prevention efforts based on the five E's: education, enforcement, engineering,[6] economic incentives,[7] and evaluation. Using these greatly increases the chances of program success. Note, however, that rarely is any one E sufficiently effective.[21] To enhance the possibility of success, combine education with other E's. For example, teach bicycle safety practices (education) in conjunction with bicycle helmet distribution (environment), bicycle lane construction (environment), and/or laws requiring bicycle helmets (enforcement).

Education

Education is frequently the first strategy selected. Although an important strategy, it is often the only one chosen and, when used alone, rarely has a significant impact. Often educational programs, when evaluated, result in no measurable change in attitudes or behavior. Most motorists are aware of the dangers of speeding;

however, speed-related injuries remain a problem. Many injuries occur from the failure to apply knowledge we already possess. This is because behavior concerning health is extremely complex and is changed very gradually.[8] It is precisely because safety education is designed to change behavior, which often takes months or years, that limits its effectiveness as a lone intervention. Sometimes, however, education is the only option available for a prevention program.[22] In these cases, do not hesitate to use it. In the early 1980s, when the hazards of widely owned all-terrain vehicles (ATVs) were first realized, education was the only immediate intervention available. At that time, educational messages to the public were chiefly provided by the media.[23] Later, ATV design changes, helmets, and legal action joined educational efforts to reduce ATV-related injuries. For optimal results, one should neither exclude educational efforts, nor rely exclusively on them.[22]

EMS personnel can increase the effectiveness of educational programs by following certain principles. First, tailor the educational program to a specific population, for example, preschoolers or parents.[8] Second, explain both the danger of the hazard (e.g., a child falling from a high-rise building) and the effectiveness of the intervention (e.g., installation of window guards). Any appropriate opportunity to teach patients and families should be utilized. If, for example, smoke detectors are not present in a patient's home, an opportunity exists for counseling and action, but exercise care in the appropriate timing and setting of any educational message.

Fear is often believed to motivate behavior change; therefore, educational programs often contain elements designed to invoke fear. To gain the desired impact, however, fear messages must be carefully constructed. "Fear-only" messages, with no long-term plan for individual action to reduce injury risk, fail to produce changes in either attitudes or behavior (e.g., the old prom-night car crash movies shown in high school driver's education). Educational messages containing a high level of fear often result in short-term changes in behavior. Low-level fear messages are less likely to alter short-term behavior. However, the goal of most educational programs is to change behavior on a long-term basis. If, for instance, a high-level fear message is delivered to adolescents on the hazards of driving drunk, the message is most likely to decrease the behavior of drinking and driving on a short-term basis. The high risk of trauma occurring while driving after alcohol consumption necessitates long-term behavior change to significantly impact injuries resulting from this behavior. Note that "low-fear" and "high-fear" messages are equally effective in changing long-term behavior when they are coupled with a specific "action plan" to avoid injury. Because fear can "paralyze" some people, it is important to instill confidence in the individuals receiving the education program; they must believe they are capable of taking the actions required to reduce or avoid injury.[24] Properly designed fear messages can produce desired behavioral changes. When devising fear strategies, the following information must be included as part of the educational program:

1. Fear information: Target the information at the risky behavior, not the individual (e.g., the behavior of driving while intoxicated).

2. Cognitive information: Include the causes and consequences of the behavior.

3. Action plan: Include steps to take to reduce risk (e.g., designated driver).

4. Self-efficacy information or instilling confidence: Offer encouragement that the individual can take the action necessary to reduce the risk of injury.[24]

Enforcement

"Law is one of the most effective tools of injury prevention."[23] Laws are made to modify or change behavior, with the goal of increased safety.[11] Examples of effective injury control laws include speed limits, driving age laws, child poisoning prevention caps for medicines, motorcycle helmet laws, and prohibition of "Saturday Night Special" firearms.

Enforcement takes one of three forms: legislation, regulation, or litigation.[8] Legislation is a law, statute, act, or ordinance passed by a legislative body, such as Congress. Regulatory agencies, such as the Occupational Safety and Health Administration (OSHA), enact rules and standards and are given this authority by legislative bodies. Courts, through litigation, also create common law, which is the body of decisions stemming from litigation. Tort law is the litigation of civil wrongs, such as injuries obtained through careless actions or defective products. Product liability law is a form of tort law and is decided on the basis of precedent, or the actions of prior courts in similar cases.[23]

Compliance is basic to the success of laws (e.g., motorcycle helmets are not protective if not worn, regardless of a law requiring their use). Compliance increases with high rates of violation detection and when penalties are assigned. It increases when the law is not perceived as unpleasant, inconvenient, or uncomfortable and if there are few exceptions in the law. Compliance is greatest when violation of the law is swiftly and severely punished.[15]

Laws are very effective tools in injury control, but laws are often controversial. Arguments against injury prevention–related laws include the concern for individual rights and individual freedom.[15] Many Americans value the freedom to take risks with their individual safety while in pursuit of individual enjoyment, for example, driving a motorcycle without a helmet.[25] A major dilemma for American society is balancing the protection of individual rights and risk-taking behavior against the loss to society when injuries result.

The legal concept of "fault" is also intertwined in individual concerns. The concept of fault attempts to settle disputes in legal courts by placing blame or fault for an injury on an individual or a company. When an injury occurs, the legal system is often called upon to decide who was "at fault" and therefore liable for damages and suffering.[25]

Economic concerns can also be barriers to legislation. The National Transportation Safety Board (NTSB), the agency responsible for making airline safety recommendations, reported that a 9-month-old infant died because he was not secured in a child safety seat in a 1994 airline crash. Before this crash, the NTSB had recommended to the Federal Aviation Administration (FAA), which is the agency responsible for generating airline safety regulations, that child safety seats be required for children under age 2. Continuing to refuse to require them, the FAA has reasoned that the airlines would suffer large economic losses if parents had to purchase tickets for their infants. Whether this point of view is true or not true, the FAA is the agency responsible for weighing economic costs against potential safety gains.[26]

Regardless of controversy, regulation, legislation, and litigation are central to American culture and will continue to be used as injury prevention strategies. The legal history of all-terrain vehicles provides an example of all three types of enforcement and is detailed in Table 2-5.[23]

Engineering

Engineering builds safety into a product or the environment. Engineering uses inherent designs to protect people, often passively, without any individual conscious thought or action. In the injury control arena, technological advancements are highly successful.[8] Success is dependent on the inventiveness and creativity of individuals and corporations. Examples of engineering in injury prevention are numerous, so much so that they are often taken for granted. This ability to "take it for granted" ("it" meaning protection) is the ultimate goal of safety engineering.

Not all technological changes are completely "passive." Seat belts require that the motorist buckle the lap belt or lap-shoulder belt.[8] Babies must be placed properly into infant safety seats. Boaters must don life jackets. Therefore, inventions are often integrated with educational campaigns and regulatory efforts to increase overall success. For instance, at one

Table 2-5

Enforcement: Legislation, Regulation, and Litigation of All-Terrain Vehicles (ATVs)

1967	American Honda Motor Company seeks to market a product for winter use to offset seasonal declines in motorcycle sales.
1980s	Widespread ATV sales, including sales of vehicles for operation by children. Two factors make ATVs hazardous: weight (up to a quarter ton) and speed (up to 65 mph). Also, lack of rear-wheel differentiation requires using body weight to balance the ATV during turns, often resulting in riders being thrown.
1983	There are 85 reported deaths from ATVs in the United States.
1984	There are an estimated 67,000 ATV-related injuries treated in U.S. emergency departments. Half the deaths (161) are in children under 16 years of age.
1985	There are 295 reported deaths from ATVs in the United States.
	May 31: The Consumer Product Safety Commission (CPSC) publishes its "Advance Notice for Proposed Regulation," in which it plans analyses of ATV hazards; public meetings to discuss safety risks; monitoring the manufacturer's education efforts; and development of a voluntary standard. The plan does not include the available options of a CPSC standard, product banning, or court action.
1986	July: Congress begins hearings on whether the 1985 CPSC action sufficiently safeguards the public.
	Congressional committee report finds ATVs an unreasonable risk of injury and that CPSC has failed to adequately protect the public.
	December: CPSC asks the Justice Department to begin litigation against manufacturers, including a mandatory refund plan for ATV owners.
1987	Congress finds unconscionable delay at the Justice Department.
	Against CPSC request, Suzuki refuses to end marketing of ATVs to children under age 12.
	Justice Department files lawsuit against ATV manufacturers.
1988	From 1983 to 1988 there are 403,300 injuries and 1,465 deaths related to ATVs in the United States.
	Justice Department litigation is settled. In the settlement the ATV manufacturers must stop three-wheeled ATV sales and offer to repurchase stock from retailers; recommend that four-wheeled ATVs with engine sizes of 70–90 cm^3 be operated only by persons over 12 and over 90 cm^3 by those over 16; provide warning labels on all new four-wheel vehicles; conduct training; not oppose state legislation for licensing and age limits. The settlement does not provide consumer refunds or place fault on the manufacturers. The consent decree is heavily criticized by Congress. Individual lawsuit against Honda is won by manufacturer on the basis of comparative risk with minibike or snowmobile. The risk of injury on an ATV is viewed as no different from that of a minibike or snowmobile.
1989	Individual, K. Oberg, wins $920,000 in compensatory damages and $5 million in punitive damages against Honda for ATV crash-related injuries.
1990	Congressional report notes that 41 states have laws of varying comprehensiveness to regulate ATVs. Deaths from ATVs are down significantly.

Source: "All-Terrain Vehicles: A Case Study in Law and the Prevention of Injuries of Head Trauma," by S. P. Teret and J. Jagger, *Journal of Head Trauma, Rehabilitation,* 6, p. 60. 1991.

time the rate of U.S. motorists wearing seat belts was a dismal 15%.[27] Laws were enacted to increase seat belt usage in all but two states by 1994. In December of 1994, the national seat belt use rate rose to 67%.[28] Modeled after a Canadian plan, which combined seat belt technology with public education and law enforcement, North Carolina's "Click It or Ticket" program reached seat belt use rates over 80% in the early 1990s.[27] After a 1985 North Carolina law requiring that front seat passengers use seat belts, the state experi-

enced a drastic 42% decline in serious injury and death in children.[29] Combining engineering with other legal strategies can have a great impact on reducing injuries.

Engineering is frequently planned into the environment, an important part of injury control. Often accomplished by the use of space and cushioning, environmental modifications save lives. Imagine a ski slope littered with trees versus one with wide trails and soft snowbanks. Railings on steps, bridges, and highways and the development of sidewalks and bicycle lanes are part of the plethora of environmental modifications with one goal in mind: injury prevention. Table 2-6 provides examples of some of the many strategies designed to prevent injuries.

Economic Incentives

Injuries drain the economy. The financial and social impact of trauma is staggering. Significant economic pressures exist to reduce the amount of resources spent on the total cost of injury. The business community has become especially savvy in this area. Many corporations value the savings incurred through programs and engineering designed to prevent injuries in the workplace, beyond the regulations of OSHA.

Litigation, or the threat of litigation, is a powerful economic force. Product manufacturers and employers alike are motivated by the possible negative economic impact litigation may have. Many toys, for instance, have been redesigned or removed from the market due to safety problems, as have been specific models of motor vehicles.[22] The financial impact of litigation is intensely magnified by media intervention. Publicly trumpeting the dangers of a product affects consumer buying and confidence in a product or corporation; the

threat of financial damage is an incentive to produce safe products, albeit an insufficient one by itself.

As a nation, just as individuals, our pocketbooks are not limitless. Controlling expenditures on traumatic injuries is imperative and is most effectively done by injury prevention measures.[30]

Evaluation

Often overlooked, evaluation needs to be planned concurrently with any program or intervention. Evaluation is essential to success; it is the only way to know if a program, countermeasure, safety design, or regulation has accomplished the intended objectives. Unfortunately, evaluation is a missing element in some injury prevention efforts. Past problems with program evaluation have included no evaluation; evaluation with inappropriate methods; or appropriately evaluated, found not to be effective, but continued anyway.[10] Scientifically, evaluation is critical to establishing a knowledge base, and the same holds true in the injury control field. The paramedic is encouraged to review the basics of research methods, with particular attention to evaluation.

Evaluation of a program, law, product, or intervention serves multiple purposes, seven of which are (1) determining if the program objectives have been met; (2) examining the reasons for program success and failure; (3) describing why the program was a success for a particular group; (4) determining whether or not the program should be repeated, and, if so, under what circumstances; (5) evaluating what impact the program had on reducing injuries; (6) preparing the foundation for further research; and (7) substantiating the rationale for funding the program or future programs.[8,31]

Scrutiny of these seven items and determining if the goals of the program have been met are known as **outcome evaluation**—or seeing the "bigger picture." Evaluation of the details of a program is known as **process evaluation**—describing such things as how many people participated in the program, how many bicycle helmets were distributed, who staffed the project, did the program proceed on schedule, and what media groups participated. Process evaluation details how and where funds for the project were spent and is sometimes called "bean counting."[8]

It is imperative that evaluation is planned along with objectives and is continually in progress. Consider, for example, the goal of adding passenger side airbags to vehicles. Ongoing evaluation has shown that these bags are dangerous to rear-facing infant car seats and are also causing injuries to small children and small adults. Continuous evaluation of a product is critical to determining what, if any, changes are needed.

Table 2-6 Examples of Injury Prevention Through Engineering	
Mesh fan covers	Skid-resistant tires
Electrical wire coating	Automatic machine shut-off systems in manufacturing plants
Pedestrian bridges and crossings	Automatic sprinkler systems
Circuit breakers	Smoke alarms
Automobile airbags	Four-sided pool fencing
Child-resistant medication caps	Breakaway ski boots
Windshield safety glass	Shoes
Lawn mower automatic shut-off mechanisms	Nonremovable pop-top soda cans
Electrical outlet and switchplate covers	Electrical outlet caps
Crushable automobile zone	Padded automobile interiors
Airplane radar warning systems	

INTERNET ACTIVITIES

Visit the National Center for Injury Prevention and Control Web site at http://www.cdc.gov/ncipc/. Scroll down to the announcements section and click on the RealPlayer satellite broadcast of the Healthy People 2000 Progress Review on Intimate Partner Violence, Youth Violence, and Suicide. This 60-minute video will play on your computer screen. You must have the RealPlayer media application installed on your computer. If you do not have this program, it is available free of charge from http://www.real.com.

INJURY PREVENTION PROJECT DEVELOPMENT

Conceptual frameworks help EMS professionals to organize thoughts, ideas, and actions for injury prevention projects. Like a road map, these models assist in choosing which highway to take. However, success depends on many factors. If possible, consult injury prevention professionals to assist with program development. Regardless of whether or not experts are available, there are some key elements that can enhance the success of an injury prevention program. First, the injury problem should be carefully and completely identified. Second, a problem that is important to the community should be chosen. Third, before beginning any intervention, the injury problem should be thoroughly researched. For example, an emergency department in a Florida hospital examined all pediatric trauma records retrospectively for 1 year. Results showed that pedestrian and bicycle collisions with automobiles were among the most common causes of severe injury. Failure to don bicycle helmets was a common finding; in response to this investigation, an extensive bicycle helmet campaign was developed.[32]

A program from a Florida county illustrates the effort often involved just in problem identification. A group of interested public health professionals in Hillsborough County, Florida, conducted an observational study in child bicycle helmet usage over a 6-month period in 1993. Observation sites were selected from schools, parks, playgrounds, bike paths, and intersections and were observed three times a week. Results showed that local use was on par with the national average of 3.6%. Interventions aimed at increasing helmet use were planned based on the data.[33] In another example, EMS professionals in Cleveland, Ohio, examined the percentage of Clevelanders over 60 years of age and the percentage (27.5%) of EMS transports in this group due to fall

injuries. Based on these local statistics, EMS developed a fall prevention program for senior citizens that included an EMS in-home safety assessment.[34]

It is helpful to find out what has been done in the past and who has done it; then those persons can be consulted, as well as other organizations that can support the project or have overlapping interests. In the Hillsborough County, Florida, study, the organizers designed their protocol from guidelines prepared by the Harborview Injury Prevention and Research Center and obtained their evaluation guidelines from the Washington Bicycle Helmet Study published in 1989.[33] Measurable objectives and goals should be outlined and how those goals are to be met precisely defined. The target population of the program should be defined and localized and how they can be reached most effectively determined. For example, a coalition of EMS professionals in Pinellas County, Florida, developed a drowning registry to prospectively collect data in response to the alarming number of EMS calls for submersions in the summer of 1991. Those under age 3 were found to experience submersion events most frequently in residential swimming pools, while those over 19 were more likely to experience submersion events at public beaches or lakes. Clearly, interventions targeted at one group would not be effective or appropriate for the other.[35] Program designers must remember that a combination of strategies is needed to tackle most injury problems. Also, one should not shy away from recommending regulations, such as bicycle helmet laws, for the community. Sources of antagonism and opposition should be anticipated. A source of adequate funding needs to be secured and a budget finalized. It is important not to underestimate the "manpower" needed to complete the project, at the same time anticipating where additional resources can be obtained, if necessary. Establishing a timeline is vital to the project. If media will be involved, they should be met with early and media experts consulted if available. It is imperative to evaluate every aspect of the project. If the project fails, finding out why is very valuable in future endeavors.[8,36] Finally, information about the project should be shared and discussed in professional organizations, journals, conferences, and meetings. Cooperation and collaboration are vital to controlling and preventing injury.

INTERNET ACTIVITIES

Visit the National Center for Injury Prevention and Control Web site at http:// www.cdc.gov/ncipc/pub-res/pubs.htm. Scroll down the list of publications. Select a publication that interests you, such as motor vehicle injury prevention or statistics on firearm-related deaths, and order the publication. These publications are free of charge and can be ordered on line.

EMERGENCY MEDICAL SERVICES IN INJURY PREVENTION

You know, sometimes it feels like this. There I am standing by the shore of a swiftly flowing river, and I hear the cry of a drowning man. So I jump into the river, put my arms around him, pull him to shore, and apply artificial respiration. Just when he begins to breathe, there is another cry for help. So I jump into the river, reach him, pull him to shore, apply artificial respiration, and just as he begins to breathe, another cry for help. So back in the river again, reaching, pulling, applying, breathing, and then another yell. Again and again, without end, goes the sequence. You know, I am so busy jumping in, pulling them to shore, and applying artificial respiration that I have no time to see who the hell is upstream pushing them all in.

Irving Zola[11]

Most EMS professionals have no trouble identifying with Irving Zola's story. Continually running from one call to the next, they seem to have little time to dwell on what happens before the next call comes to 911. Responding to the scene of an injury and providing the best care possible are a critical part of injury control. EMS has the primary responsibility to provide life-saving treatment at the scene and in transport to a medical facility; in addition, EMS provides interventions that prevent further injury, reduce morbidity, and begin the rehabilitation process. Despite these important contributions, escalating the involvement of EMS professionals and EMS organizations is vital to the control of the injury problem in America: "The injury problem is too large and too complex, and resources are too limited for any one group to solve" alone.[37]

EMS providers are the first line of response to any traumatic event, are ubiquitous in most communities, and possess high community credibility. In addition, economic incentives to provide more comprehensive services, or role expansion, encourage paramedics to expand in the injury prevention arena.[38,39] How can the paramedic or EMS organization intensify participation in injury prevention efforts? EMS providers can utilize the fundamentals of injury prevention: the Haddon matrix, Pat Barry Four Square, the five E's, and Haddon's 10 countermeasures. Injury prevention roles for the paramedic and EMS include individual, family, community, professional, organizational, and coalition of organizations.

INDIVIDUAL

Individually, the paramedic can become well educated about injury prevention. Also, the paramedic can properly use safety devices, such as motorcycle helmets and seat belts. It is important to engage in safe behavior in all aspects of life. This decreases the chance of becoming injured and makes the paramedic a positive role model in the community. Perhaps the paramedic can also become involved in designing his or her own safety device, such as a stretcher to decrease back stress. Or, the paramedic may design and collaborate on a broad-based invention, such as a device to prevent railroad crossing crashes. Individually, the paramedic can become a community advocate, lobby for legislation, and participate in litigation as necessary.

FAMILY

Many of the most serious and most frequent injuries occur in the home, particularly to children. Ensuring that one's family engages in safe behavior and properly uses safety equipment is injury control in the home. Home safety checks can be performed. Examples include providing functioning smoke detectors, safe storage of poisons and hazardous materials, wearing bicycle helmets, using mouth guards for sporting activities, and setting the hot water heater at a safe temperature. Results are best when the entire family is involved in the effort to prevent injuries.

COMMUNITY

Local communities are one of the best places to begin intensifying participation in injury prevention. Community agencies, such as schools and businesses, are frequently planning and conducting injury control projects. Many volunteer organizations, such as Safe Kids and the American Red Cross, participate in injury prevention strategies. The National Safe Kids Campaign is a national organization with nearly 200 local coalitions with the goal of reducing unintentional childhood injuries.[40] Find out who is doing what and become involved, or start a project that has meaning to you and your community. Collect and analyze local statistics on injuries. Has there been a cluster of pedestrian injuries at one corner in your neighborhood? Use the Haddon matrix or five E's to define strategies to attack the problem.

PROFESSIONAL

Professionally, be well informed on current topics in trauma. Subscribe to professional journals and participate in professional organizations and conferences. Share your injury control knowledge with other EMS professionals at work, at conferences, and in professional publications. Become an advocate for organizational involvement in injury prevention, not only in the workplace, but in professional organizations as well.

Data collection, or the lack thereof, is one of the foremost problems in injury prevention today. The paramedic is at the scene of injury events; the documentation provided by on-scene personnel is invaluable in discovering information on the circumstances preceding these events. Documentation ideally includes an "injury score." These scores also provide critical information to researchers.

How many highway crashes involve emergency vehicles? Safe emergency vehicle operation and participation in other strategies designed to reduce these crashes are other valuable ways to participate in injury control.[38]

ORGANIZATIONAL

Organizations can have a powerful effect on injury prevention. Their access to resources and their position in the community enable them to accomplish what an individual often cannot. EMS organizations participate internally and externally in injury prevention. Internally, the EMS organization is charged with providing a safe environment for the practicing paramedic. Programs to decrease back injuries through education, exercise, and optimal equipment are an example. Externally, EMS organizations have multiple roles. An organization can participate at any level and with any strategy, including lobbying for legislation, education, program development and evaluation, data collection, and surveillance. In Wisconsin, the State EMT Association conducted a Statewide Injury Prevention Program using EMS providers to increase community awareness of the effects of impaired driving and the benefits of correct safety belt and child safety seat use. Funded by a grant from the NHTSA, the program trained 360 EMS volunteers to disseminate information into local communities.[41]

COALITIONS OF ORGANIZATIONS

Organizations often work together to accomplish injury prevention goals. Coalitions of organizations have even more resources and affect a greater number of people than do single organizations. Government organizations, both legislative bodies and functioning agencies, are actively involved in injury control, often working together to accomplish national goals. For example, a coalition of organizations participate in the formation of health objectives for the nation through the CDC. These objectives outline measurable health goals for the nation to reach in a specified time period. These objectives guide governmental organizations' decision making on which programs are funded and provide a standard for evaluation of how well the goals are met. A copy of these objectives can be obtained from the CDC.

An excellent example of EMS organizational efforts and cooperative participation is the Drowning Prevention Program in Pinellas County, Florida.[35] During the summer of 1991, local paramedics noticed an alarming number of drownings and near drownings. Using epidemiology and quality assurance, they collected data to define the drowning problem in their county and to identify causes of the problem and strategies to reduce it. They continued data collection to evaluate the effectiveness of the selected strategies over subsequent years. Pinellas County EMS, along with the Pinellas County Fire Chief's Association, city and county governments, the American Red Cross, and the Florida Suncoast Safe Kids organization, coalesced efforts to form the Pinellas County Fire and EMS for Safe Kids Coalition. By joining forces and combining resources, they were able to conduct an extensive community injury prevention project. The coalition initially designed a drowning registry for paramedics to collect data in the field. Subsequent to defining the problem and events leading up to submersions (defined by the program as respiratory difficulty from immersion in water resulting in a call to 911), the coalition planned a prevention program. One intervention was a pool safety survey, offered free of charge to families with pools, and conducted by local fire departments. In addition to evaluating individual residential pools for safety hazards, the fire department representatives provided written information for both children and adults on pool safety. The coalition also conducted an extensive media campaign in May of 1992 to raise awareness of the local drowning problem and to educate the public on water safety. This campaign included articles in local newspapers, 30- to 60-second public service television messages, radio interviews, and county utility bills that included a phone number to request a free pool survey. The coalition found a 43% decrease in the number of submersions from 1991 to 1993. Continuing to analyze and collect data, the coalition has determined that many submersions of children occur under parental supervision and that different strategies must be developed for different age groups. The coalition has begun more intensive investigation into the location of submersions and is planning to conduct future interventions in the areas with the highest incidences of submersions.[35]

Lastly, EMS organizations should not underestimate the importance of voting, letter writing, and lobbying activities. Both individuals and organizations influence political decisions. Legislative activities have a great impact on injury control. Injury control activities are underfunded, given the extent of this public health problem. Be aware that funding for governmental organizations, such as the NHTSA, is sometimes given from Congress with stipulations. For example, in 1996 Congress approved funding for the CDC's National Center for Injury Prevention and Control at similar levels to the 1995 budget; however, Congress also prohibited research on gunshot injuries, reducing funding to the CDC by the $2.6 million that would have been spent on a gunshot project. In response, the American Academy of Pediatrics requested other national health care organizations concerned with the gunshot injury problem in the United States to sign a letter requesting restoration of funding for this project.[42] EMS organizations have an invaluable role in lobbying activities for injury prevention, both at national and local levels.

INTERNET ACTIVITIES

Visit the Center for Emergency Medicine Web site at http://www.hsc.wvu.edu/crem/. Scroll down and click on Educational Programs. Click on Review the ENPP Curriculum. Watch the RealMedia presentation of Injury Prevention and the Emergency Department Patient. This 22-minute video will play on your computer screen. You must have the RealPlayer media application installed on your computer. If you do not have this program, it is available free of charge from http://www.real.com.

SUMMARY

EMS professionals participate in injury prevention through a multitude of roles and a variety of strategies. EMS involvement is critical. No one individual, organization, strategy, or safety device is sufficient to reduce the staggering financial, emotional, and human cost of

trauma. It takes a team of individuals, communities, and organizations working toward the goal of preventing injuries to realize a significant impact on this public health problem. EMS members and professional groups are challenged to become involved at every level.

REVIEW QUESTIONS

1. Why is the use of the word *accident* discouraged by injury prevention specialists?
2. Pick an injury problem important to you and fill in the cells of your own Haddon matrix.
3. Select 10 interventions in the Haddon matrix in question 2 and evaluate each based on the following six criteria: efficiency, freedom of choice, equity, social stigma, consumer preference, and feasibility.
4. Differentiate between vertical and horizontal equity and give an example of both.
5. Abstaining from alcohol while swimming or boating is an example of a:
   a. Mandatory-passive intervention
   b. Voluntary-passive intervention
   c. Mandatory-active intervention
   d. Voluntary-active intervention
6. Using the same choices as in question 5, home smoke detectors are: a, b, c, or d.
7. List the five E's for planning injury prevention interventions.
8. Selecting an injury problem of importance to you, follow the five E's and outline a plan for intervention for the selected problem.
9. Educational efforts alone are sufficient to prevent injuries:
   a. True
   b. False
10. Educational efforts are not sufficient but are necessary to reduce injuries:
    a. True
    b. False
11. What is outcome evaluation?
12. What is process evaluation?
13. Describe three ways the individual paramedic can participate in injury control.
14. List three ways you actively participate in injury control in your own life or home.
15. The Drowning Prevention Program in Pinellas County, Florida, included a pool safety survey conducted by the fire department, written information on pool safety, and a media campaign to

increase awareness and educate the public on water safety. Determine where in the Haddon matrix and the Pat Barry Four Square each of these interventions belongs.

16. Using the intervention examples in question 15, plus a law requiring four-sided fencing around each residential swimming pool, a law prohibiting the consumption of alcohol at swimming locations, and voluntary installation of residential pool alarms, evaluate each on the criteria of efficiency, freedom of choice, equity, social stigma, consumer preference, and feasibility.

▶ CRITICAL THINKING

● Choose a specific injury or etiology of injury common in your response area. Develop an injury prevention program to reduce these injuries using the Haddon matrix.

● Evaluate your injury prevention program from above based on the following six criteria: efficiency, freedom of choice, equity, social stigma, consumer preference, and feasibility. Also assess your program's vertical and horizontal equity.

● Why do you think morbidity data are so difficult to obtain? Develop a plan for how your EMS system could prospectively collect morbidity data for a specific injury. How could this information be used to develop and evaluate the effectiveness of a prevention program for this injury?

▶ REFERENCES

1. Sampalis JS, et al. Impact of on-site care, prehospital time, and level of in-hospital care on survival in severely injured patients. *J Trauma*. 1993; 34:252.
2. Washington State Drowning Prevention Project. Washington State EMSC grant develops a regional approach to drowning prevention. *EMSC News: EMSC Newsletter*. 1997; 10(1):2.
3. North Carolina Office of Emergency Medical Services. Safety advice from EMS (SAFE) traffic safety lesson plans for EMS, fire & rescue personnel. *North Carolina EMS Rep*. 1997; 23(5):4.
4. U.S. Department of Health and Human Services. Injury control: Position papers from the Third International Injury Control Conference; April 22–25, 1991.
5. *American Heritage Dictionary*. 2nd ed. Boston, Mass: Houghton Mifflin Company; 1985.
6. Committee on Trauma Research, Commission on Life Sciences, National Research Council, and the Institute of Medicine. *Injury in America: A Continuing Public Health Problem*. Washington, DC: National Academy Press; 1985.
7. Martinez R. Injury prevention: a new perspective. *JAMA*. 1994; 272:1541.
8. New Mexico EMS for Children Project. *EMTs and Injury Prevention: Advocates for Children*. Albuquerque, NM: University of New Mexico Department of Emergency Medicine, 1995.
9. Haddon W. Advances in the epidemiology of injuries as a basis for public policy. *Public Health Rep*. 1980; 95:411.
10. Waller, JA. The epidemiologic basis for injury prevention. *Public Health Rep*. 1985; 100:575.
11. Hargarten SW, Karlson T. Injury control: a crucial aspect of emergency medicine. *Emerg Med Clin North Am*. 1993; 11:255.
12. Liller K. Using the Haddon matrix in injury prevention education. *J Health Educ*. 1994; 25:112.
13. Holden JA, Lumpkin, JR. Injury prevention and control. In: Rosen P, Barkin M, eds. *Emergency Medicine: Concepts and Clinical Practice*. St. Louis, Mo: Mosby Year-Book; 1992.
14. Runyan C. Letter from the Director. *IPRC News: Univ North Carolina Injury Prevention Res Ctr*. 1995; 7:2.
15. Jacobs BB. Epidemiology of injury. In Sheehy SB, ed. *Emergency Nursing: Principles and Practice*. 3rd ed. St. Louis, Mo: Mosby Year-Book; 1992.
16. Rice DP, MacKenzie EJ, Associates. *Cost of Injury in the United States: A Report to Congress 1989*. San Francisco, Calif: Institute for Health and Aging, University of California and Injury Prevention Center, Johns Hopkins University; 1989.
17. Margolis LH, Runyan CW. Accidental policy: an analysis of the problem of unintentional injuries of childhood. *Am J Orthopsychiatry*. 1983; 53:629.
18. Runyan CW. Personal communication; January 1990.
19. Haddon W. Energy damage and the ten countermeasure strategies. *J Trauma*. 1973; 13:321.
20. Runyan CW. Personal communication; February 1989.
21. Sheridan DJ. Letter to the editor. *J Emerg Nurs*. 1994; 20:5.
22. Runyan CW, Runyan DK. How can physicians get kids to wear bicycle helmets? A prototypic challenge in injury prevention. *Am J Public Health*. 1991; 81:972.
23. Teret SP, Jagger J. All-terrain vehicles: a case study in law and the prevention of injuries. *J Head Trauma Rehab*. 1991; 6:60.
24. Moore J. Personal communication; February 1989.
25. Barry PZ. Individual versus community orientation in the prevention of injuries. *Prev Med*. 1975; 4:47.

26. Beck M, et al. How safe is this flight? *Newsweek.* April 24, 1995: 18.

27. Advocates for Highway and Auto Safety. The scope of the problem: deaths and injuries on our nation's highways; 1995.

28. National Highway Traffic Safety Administration, 1994 Performance Report; 1994.

29. Steele J, ed. Death and serious injuries decline after seatbelt laws go into effect. *IPRC News. Univ North Carolina Injury Prevention Res Ctr.* 1996; 8:2.

30. Runge JW. The cost of injury. *Emerg Med Clin North Am.* 1993; 11:241.

31. Schuman EA. *Evaluation Research: Principles and Practice in Public Service and Social Action Programs.* New York: Russell Sage Foundation; 1967.

32. Martin V, Langley B, Coffman S. Patterns of injury in pediatric patients in one Florida community and implications for prevention programs. *J Emerg Nurs.* 1995; 21:12.

33. Liller KD, Knowles A, McDermott RJ. Bicycle helmet use among children in Hillsborough County, Florida. *J Health Education.* 1995; 26:292.

34. Sanadi NE. Geriatric injury prevention. *Emerg Med Services.* January 1996: 51.

35. Harrawood D, et al. Drowning prevention: a case study in EMS epidemiology. *JEMS.* June 1994: 34.

36. Kirkwood HA. Before the call comes in: EMS and injury prevention. *JEMS.* June 1995: 21.

37. Martinez R. Putting it together: a model for integrating injury control system elements. *Prehospital and Disaster Medicine.* 1995; 10:72.

38. Garrison HG. The role of EMS in injury prevention. Presented at the Emergency Medicine Today 1995 Conference; October 4, 1995; Greensboro, NC.

39. Brown B. Are paramedics an endangered species? *JEMS.* March 1996: 56.

40. National Safe Kids Campaign. *Family Guide*; 1996.

41. Edwards R, Evans D. Wisconsin EMT Association: a statewide injury prevention program. United States Department of Transportation: DOT HS 807 804; September 1990.

42. *Etcetera: Official Newsletter of the Emergency Nurses Association.* 1996; 20:8.

Chapter 3

Overview of Trauma Care

OBJECTIVES

Upon completion of this chapter, the reader should be able to:

- List and describe the major etiologies of traumatic death.
- Discuss the trimodal distribution of trauma deaths and provide examples of the types of interventions necessary to decrease the number of deaths in each category.
- Briefly trace the history of trauma systems development in this country.
- Compare and contrast the various levels of trauma centers.
- Define the role of EMS in trauma care.
- Discuss the problems encountered in rural trauma situations.
- Discuss the White Paper and its effect on EMS system development.

KEY TERMS

Early death
Golden hour
Immediate death
Late death
Level I trauma center

Level II trauma center
Level III trauma center
Level IV trauma center
Level V trauma center

Trauma can affect any person at any time in any location. When a shooting or other "major" traumatic incident occurs, it becomes headline news. While the occurrence of trauma is by no means a "new phenomenon," approach and attitude toward the topic have changed. In the last 30 years considerable improvements have been made toward the management of trauma. Remember that trauma is the most common cause of death for persons under the age of 34. Each year 2 million people are hospitalized following traumatic events.[1–3]

Despite these numbers, only a relatively small percentage of all trauma patients will require specialized care. In fact, less than 10% of all trauma victims will require prehospital advanced life support or a level I trauma center. Fifteen percent of all trauma patients will benefit from receiving prehospital advanced life support; however, they do not necessarily need a level I trauma center. The majority of trauma patients (75%) can be managed by basic life support in the field and local hospital emergency care. However, the "critical 10%" of the trauma patient population will require more services than the remaining trauma patient population.[3,4]

WHY TRAUMA PATIENTS DIE

Why, despite the advances in medicine, do trauma patients die? The answer requires some background information. First, when the time of death is plotted against the number of deaths on a graph, death from trauma occurs in a "trimodal fashion" (Figure 3-1).[5] There are three types of trauma deaths: immediate deaths, deaths occurring shortly after injury, and later death. **Immediate-death** victims often have suffered an acute injury to the brain, spinal cord, heart, or major blood vessels. These deaths account for more than 50% of all trauma fatalities. The injuries are so severe that death would probably occur regardless of what services were available.[5]

The second group of patients, categorized as **early death**, are those who die within a few hours after injury.[5] These deaths account for about 30% of the trauma patient population. Their injuries, such as intracranial hemorrhage and airway compromise, are considered to be treatable. The key to saving these patients is early and aggressive EMS intervention and treatment and transport to a definitive care facility, such as a trauma center. This group must "beat the clock" in order to survive.[5]

The third group of patients, categorized as **late death**, are those dying several days or weeks after the initial injury. A majority of these deaths are related to infection or systemic failure (e.g., multisystem organ failure, sepsis, respiratory distress syndrome).[5] These patients require intensive care and extensive follow-up. The goal is to avoid infection and organ failure.[5]

Injury prevention is the only intervention for the immediate-death population.[5] In fact, because the injuries in this group are so severe, preventing the injury from ever occurring is the only means of salvaging these patients. Unless the immediate death population is reduced to zero, there will be a need for injury prevention (see Chapter 2).

The early-death group benefits from a systems approach to trauma care.[5] This includes prehospital care providers, EMS, and trauma centers. Prehospital care providers have the knowledge and skill level necessary for providing initial field resuscitation.[6,7,8] Aggressive airway control and proper fluid resuscitation reduce the trauma patient's morbidity and mortality from hypoxia and circulatory collapse. Prehospital care providers treat patients on-scene and continue care while transporting to the closest trauma center. Providers strive to keep on-scene times to a minimum, thus helping the patient to arrive in a surgical suite in sufficient time.[6,7]

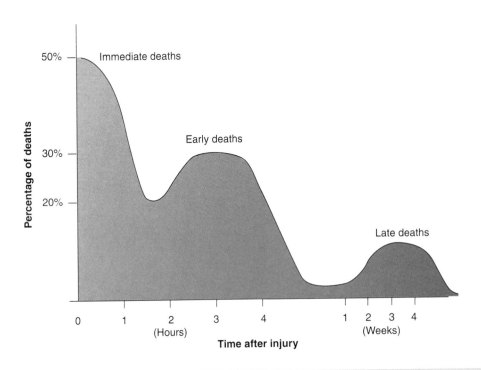

FIGURE 3-1 Trimodal distribution of trauma deaths. The first peak, "immediate deaths," corresponds with patients who die very soon after an injury, usually as a result of severe brain, heart, spinal, or major vessel injuries. The second peak, "early deaths," corresponds with patients who die within the first few hours following injury. These patients typically die from airway complications or hemorrhage. The third peak, "late deaths," corresponds with patients who die days or weeks following the initial injury, usually as a result of sepsis, organ failure, or adult respiratory distress syndrome.

The early-death patient population also benefits from transport to a trauma center. In fact, studies have shown that trauma patients taken to a trauma center have better outcomes than those taken to the local hospital.[5] EMS may need to bypass the local hospital. If distance or traffic is a concern, air transportation is an alternative, if available. In comparison to small, local hospitals, there will be minimal (or no) waiting for specialized staff to arrive at a trauma center. Surgeons and operating suites are available within minutes of notification. Depending on the health care system in the area, bypassing the local hospital may not be allowed or possible. Establishing statewide or regional trauma systems facilitates transport of the injured patient to the most appropriate facility.

The late-death patient population benefits from comprehensive care following the initial resuscitation. These patients need extensive rehabilitation and life support measures. Research continues on ways to reduce the incidence of infection and organ failure in the trauma patient.[5]

INTERNET ACTIVITIES

Visit the National Center for Injury Prevention and Control Web site at http://www.cdc.gov/ncipc/dacrrdp/dacrrdp.htm. How many visits to the emergency department each year are trauma related? What proportion of the population lives in an area served by a trauma system? How many trauma deaths could be prevented each year if appropriate acute care were accessible?

HISTORY OF TRAUMA CARE

The history of the U.S. trauma system and EMS are similar. Both have been influenced by major military events, government, and motor vehicle crash (MVC) deaths and injuries. In fact, the number and the severity of MVCs, in combination with the lack of prehospital care, led to the development of EMS and trauma care as it is known today (Table 3-1).[4]

The first government involvement in health care occurred in 1946 with the passage of the Hill Burton Act.[9] This act was designed to determine the number of existing hospitals versus the number of hospitals that were actually needed.[4] There was little or no mention of the need for special facilities, such as "trauma centers," let alone the establishment of statewide trauma systems. Nor was there any mention of the morbidity and mortality associated with MVCs.

Over the next few years, however, the number of MVC injuries and fatalities soared. The level of on-

Table 3-1
Medical Events, Trauma Care, and EMS

1913	American College of Surgeons formed.
1933	American Red Cross prints the first *First Aid Manual*
1941	World War II creates a need to educate and train persons quickly in first-aid skills.
1946	Hill Burton Act—determines the number of hospitals necessary to provide care.
	Hospital Survey and Construction Act
1950	Mouth-to-mouth resuscitation is introduced
1953	Korea and MASH units—helicopters used with success for transport
1960	Cardiopulmonary resuscitiation (CPR) developed at Johns Hopkins Hospital
1961	Civilian trauma care starts in Baltimore
1966	Comprehensive health planning—plan and regulate funds
	The White Paper
1969	EMS Council is established; emergency medical technician (EMT) certification, 81 hours
	First civilian air medical unit
1971	First statewide trauma system, Illinois
	EMT certification offered on a national basis.
1973	EMSS Act
1974	American Red Cross revises their first aid manual.
1975	National Health Planning and Resources Development Act of 1974
1976	EMS amendments
1977	MIEMSS established
1979	EMS extension
1981	Block Grant Program
1990	Trauma Care Systems Planning and Developing Act

scene care was usually less than adequate; there was no standard of care for "field providers."[4] In this early phase of "field response" it was not uncommon for a hearse with a mortician to respond to the scene of a collision. An early event supporting the improvement of civilian trauma care occurred in 1960, when John F. Kennedy publicized that car crashes were a national problem.[2] At the same time, the Division of Emergency Health Services, of what was then the Department of Health, Education, and Welfare, the Division of Medical Sciences, the National Academy of

Sciences, and the National Research Council began to review the level and quality of initial care that was available to injured persons "in the field."[2,4]

In 1965 the President's Commission on Highway Safety published a document titled "Health, Medical Care and Transportation of the Injured." This report offered recommendations to improve the initial response to MVCs. It suggested measures to improve the level of on-scene care. The suggestions included medical training for police officers and firefighters, creation of a national certification process, and utilization of both ground ambulances and aircraft to transport patients. It was proposed that ambulances, not hearses, staffed with trained medical personnel, not morticians, respond to crash scenes. Prior to the passage of the Emergency Medical Services Systems Act of 1973, most ambulances were operated by mortuary personnel with minimal training in first aid.[2,4] In 1966, the National Academy of Sciences and the National Research Council (NAS/NRC) released a report that set the criteria for the implementation and development of the modern-day EMS system. This document, titled "Accidental Death and Disability, the Neglected Disease of Modern Society" (also referred to as the White Paper), publicly revealed that the level of morbidity and mortality from MVCs was an epidemic problem.[2,10] The White Paper outlined plans for trauma systems development across the nation. It included topics such as injury prevention, trauma registries, mass casualty plans, ambulance services, rehabilitation, disaster management, autopsy, and trauma research.[2,3,4]

In 1966, Congress passed the Highway Safety Act, which called for additional changes to the current EMS systems. It was suggested that (1) all states include EMS in their highway safety program, (2) funding be provided to upgrade prehospital care, (3) highway safety standards be developed, and (4) funding for the purchase of rescue vehicles and equipment be made available to EMS systems. This act required that each state develop a highway safety program in accordance to the standards suggested by the Secretary of Transportation. As a result of these legislative proposals and the increased awareness of the need for EMS and trauma care, trauma systems began to emerge across the country.[3,4]

Throughout the 1970s the federal government remained involved in the development of EMS and trauma systems. One of the most important EMS legislative proposals during this time was the Emergency Medical Services Systems (EMSS) Act of 1973, which was modified in 1976 and 1979.[4] This act mandated that emergency care programs (those supported by federal funds) utilize a systems approach toward providing care. With this act the "15 components" of an EMS system were introduced. In addition, seven ill-

nesses and injuries were selected to be the basis for EMS systems development. These conditions included trauma, burns, spinal cord injuries, poisonings, cardiac conditions, psychiatric emergencies, and high-risk infants and mothers. This act also required the creation of a lead agency within the Department of Health and Welfare and for trauma education. In essence, the EMSS act of 1973 offered an outline to assist any state in developing a statewide EMS system[2,3,4] (see Tables 3-2 and 3-3).

In 1981 the federal government stepped down as the lead agency for EMS development following the passage of the Reconciliation Act.[4,9] This act placed EMS under the Health Prevention Block Grants, which in turn placed the responsibility of EMS development with each individual state. As a result, funding for system development became limited. Due to these reductions, several states were unable to continue EMS system development. Unfortunately, and simultaneously, the level of uncompensated trauma care took a

Table 3-2 **EMSS Act of 1973**
Finances provided to organize
National EMS care
Establish trauma courses
Department of Transportation (DOT) specifics
EMT, 911
Advanced life support in prehospital setting
Medical control
Research for EMS systems*

*From ref. 4.

Table 3-3 **Fifteen Components of EMSS Act**	
Manpower	Access to care
Training	Client transfer
Communications	Standardized medical records
Transportation	Consumer information and education
Facilities	Independent review/evaluation
Critical care units	Disaster plans
Public safety agencies	Mutual aid policies
Consumer consultation/participation	

financial toll on "trauma centers," and several were forced to reduce their status or close.[2,4]

Trauma received federal attention and funding, once again, in 1990. The Trauma Care Systems Planning and Development Act was implemented to provide funding for the development of trauma systems in states that lacked them.[11] This act also recognized injury as a public health problem and offered a model trauma system plan that was considered to be "inclusive." The inclusive system implies that all available resources within the trauma system are included in providing trauma care. The act recommended that support for research, training, and education for trauma be maintained and that an advisory council for trauma care systems exist.[2,3,12]

Despite these positive trends, multiple barriers have affected the survival of EMS and trauma systems. These barriers include (but are not limited to) political, economic, professional, and educational issues. The benefits and necessity of trauma systems have been scrutinized. Financial issues are cornerstone, as the cost of trauma care is often excessive, especially when the patient is uninsured. Fortunately, there are donations, such as those from the Robert Wood Johnson Foundation, made available for EMS and trauma systems development. For trauma systems to survive, they must be evaluated and modified as health care and trauma needs change.[1,3,4,11,13,14]

MILITARY CONTRIBUTIONS

EMS and trauma systems have been influenced by the military. Medical lessons learned from World War I, World War II, Korea, and Vietnam (e.g., field treatment, use of helicopters, use of traction splints, and triage) are often cited as being the foundation for current civilian trauma care, but field medicine dates back much further. "Field hospitals" were available during the Roman Empire, Napoleonic Era, Crimean War, and U.S. Civil War. The concepts of triage, horse-drawn ambulances, and surgeons have been recorded as early as the 1800s.[2] During the Civil War a "systems approach" was implemented and there was an increase in field survival rates.[2,3,4]

In each military conflict since World War I there has been a decline in mortality: The World War I death rate was 8%, World War II less than 5%, Korea just over 2%, and 2% in Vietnam.[4,15] The military's approach to trauma care helped to reduce wartime mortality rates. The same concepts and approaches that the military uses to provide "field medicine" have been successfully adapted and applied to civilian trauma care. Examples include field triage, patient packaging, radio communications, and rapid patient transport. By adapting these skills, there has been a decrease in civilian morbidity and mortality rates.[4,15]

EMERGENCY MEDICAL SERVICES

Emergency medical services have a significant role in trauma care. Despite the fact that the current EMS approach to trauma has only been in existence for a few decades, ambulance services have been in existence for more than 100 years. The first "ambulance service" in this country was established in 1865 in Cincinnati, while the first "city" ambulance service was established in New York City in 1866.[8] Over 100 years later, in 1969, the first national EMS conference was convened. At this conference the topics of discussion included establishing the curriculum for emergency medical technician (EMT) training and certification, creating a national registry for EMTs, and developing models for community EMS systems. In addition, the American Trauma Society was created. These events helped to set the framework for EMS systems development. By 1971, money was allocated for formalized medical training, paramedic courses were offered, and the National Registry of Emergency Medical Technicians was created.[1,2,4,8,11]

Over the last few decades significant advances in prehospital trauma care have also been accomplished. There are now trauma courses available to field providers that specialize in trauma care, such as Prehospital Life Support (PHTLS) and Basic Trauma Life Support (BTLS). These courses are designed to help the EMT, paramedic, or nurse improve their trauma assessment and management skills. These types of courses have been shown to help reduce prehospital morbidity and mortality.[8] Physicians attend an Advanced Trauma Life Support course that focuses on trauma assessment and management. In addition, trauma scoring systems (e.g., Injury Severity Scale, Glasgow Coma Scale, and Triage Index) are also available.[4,8,16]

Another tool adapted from the military, and utilized on a daily basis in both the field and hospital setting, is triage. It is an important component because it is used not only to separate the critically injured from the stable patients, but is also used as a transfer guideline. Triage identifies what level of care in what time frame a patient will require, thereby influencing transport destination decisions with the goal of improved patient outcomes.[2,4,12]

EMS is fundamental to any trauma system. Consider the following supporting concepts: For effective trauma care to be provided, it should be initiated as soon as possible or as soon as EMS arrives on scene. Prehospital care providers are the "eyes and ears" for the trauma team. The field provider can relay information to the trauma center staff regarding the patient's condition. If there are hospital destination questions, physician consultation can be obtained via on-line medical control. Many EMS systems have "standing orders" for the management of trauma patients. In these instances, hospital contact is made after initial patient care is rendered. Overall, the goals of prehospital trauma care are to minimize on-scene times, ensure that appropriate care is provided, and ensure that transport to the appropriate trauma center transpires in a timely fashion.[6,11]

INTERNET ACTIVITIES

Visit the National Center for Injury Prevention and Control Web site at http://www.cdc.gov/ncipc. Choose a topic that interests you, such as abdominal injuries, spinal injuries, or eye injuries. What are the latest publications on these topics? Select some of these articles and find their abstracts on the National Library of Medicine's Grateful Med search engine at http://igm.nlm.nih.gov/. Ask your librarian to help you obtain the full article of the abstracts that interest you.

REGIONAL/STATEWIDE TRAUMA SYSTEMS

The development of statewide trauma systems has been in progress for decades. During the 1950s and 1960s the initial attempts to manage the trauma patient were commonly done in a hospital's "accident room." Treatment varied from hospital to hospital; there were minimal established standards of care in place. This changed following the introduction of civilian trauma care. The earliest civilian trauma care began in 1961 under R. Adams Cowley at the University of Maryland. In 1966, the first civilian trauma unit was established at Cook County Hospital (Chicago) by Robert Freeark. By 1971, Illinois had implemented the first statewide trauma system. Two years later Maryland began using a statewide system. In 1977, R. Adams Cowley established the Maryland Institute for Emergency Medical Services (MIEMSS) in Baltimore; it remains the only facility in the country solely dedicated to treating trauma victims.[2,3,4]

Remarkable advancements have been made in trauma system development. Although multiple trauma system components exist, certain ones are often closely evaluated (see Table 3-4). For example, there must be an appropriate and limited number of trauma centers within each system to ensure that medical personnel treat an adequate number of patients, therefore maintaining optimal skill performance. Of course, financial and political burdens are often involved as well.

Prehospital trauma protocols ensure that patients are delivered to the most appropriate hospital. These

Table 3-4
Components of a Trauma System

Medical direction	Prevention
Communication	Training
Triage	Prehospital care
Transport	Hospital care
Public education	Rehabilitation
Evaluation	

protocols should be available to all providers, and consistently followed. Interfacility transfer agreements (from local hospital to trauma centers) ensure the continuum of patient care within the trauma system. The transfer of patients is supported by the 1986 Consolidated Omnibus Budget Reconciliation Act, which requires that all patients receive care regardless of their ability to pay and that patients be transferred as medically necessary.[2,4,11,12]

Within a trauma system there may be several trauma centers; however, some are better equipped for severe trauma than others. To clarify each hospital's resources in trauma care, "trauma center designations" have been established. There are four categories (I–IV) although some states have expanded this to include five (I–V).[1,4,12] In addition, the American College of Emergency Physicians and the American College of Surgeon's Committee on Trauma have published guidelines outlining regional trauma systems development.[1,14] These guidelines have been designed to ensure that the trauma patient receives the best care possible.

A **level I trauma center** offers the entire spectrum of care, from prevention to rehabilitation. Level I trauma centers are often found in university settings, fostering research, education, and systems planning. **Level II trauma centers** are capable of managing most trauma cases and often offer prevention programs, but research may be limited. **Level III trauma centers** are often located in community-based hospitals. They are commonly located in communities without level I or II centers and offer initial resuscitation and stabilization. The patient is transferred to a level I or level II trauma center if further care is needed. **Level IV trauma centers** have been established for remote or rural areas and may be located in clinic settings that offer advanced life support. The fifth category, a **level V trauma center**, is found in desolate areas of the country. Initial resuscitation is available as arrangements for transfer are prepared. Level V centers are designed to promote the concept of an "inclusive system"; that is, it allows for all components of the trauma system to be included in patient care, regardless of the geography and demographics of the area.[3,12] An inclusive system helps to ensure that comprehensive trauma care is available, despite the fact that less than half of the country has access to statewide trauma care.[1,13,17]

Within the trauma system there may be a Model Trauma Care System Plan. This plan allows for the trauma system to be designed in an inclusive manner. Inclusive systems are willing to accept the most "critical" patients in addition to the more "routine" cases. In contrast, "exclusive" systems are primarily focused on attracting only the most critical patients and may not include all of the services available in the statewide trauma system (see Figure 3-2).[3]

Trauma systems are designed to ensure that all patients have access to trauma care. In essence, "local" or "area" facilities manage most routine trauma cases; however, critical patients benefit from transfer to a "regional" or "specialty" facility.[4]

INTERNET ACTIVITIES

Visit the e-medicine Web site at http://www.emedicine.com/. Click on the Emergency Medicine on-line book and select Emergency Medical Services. Then click on EMS systems. Review the chapter on the structure of modern EMS systems in the United States.

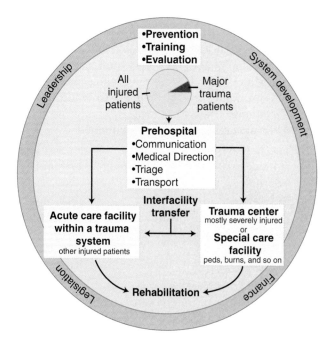

FIGURE 3-2 Model Trauma Care System Plan, Rockville, MD, U.S. Department of Health and Human Services, 1992.

THE GOLDEN HOUR

Reduction of trauma morbidity and mortality means that patients must receive definitive care at a trauma center as early as possible. During the Napoleonic Era it could take 36 hours to get the patient to a "trauma facility"; in the Vietnam War this was reduced to 4 hours[3]; today it is 60 minutes. Developed by R. Adams Cowley, the **Golden Hour** is accepted as a national standard in trauma care. The Golden Hour asserts that the patient has 60 minutes from initial injury to trauma center care for optimal outcome. Meeting the Golden Hour depends on several factors. First, the incident must be reported quickly and EMS dispatched. The patient must be extricated and immobilized within the "Platinum Ten" minutes. During transport, resuscitation must occur. The Golden Hour is difficult to attain in rural areas. In fact, the event itself may go unrecognized for several hours. Statewide trauma systems established in rural communities often reduce morbidity and mortality rates, even though the Golden Hour has been exceeded.[3,4,6]

RURAL COMMUNITIES

Traditionally trauma centers have been located in urban communities, and this accounts for why the death rate following trauma in rural areas of the country (i.e., California, Vermont, Utah) exceeds those of the urban areas. Even though only one-third of the country's population live in rural areas, more than half of MVC fatalities occur in rural areas.[17–20] Of these fatalities, a majority occur on-scene, and many include elderly patients with less severe injuries.[17–20]

Other factors have contributed to the higher mortality in rural areas. These factors include delays in emergency services notification, delays in locating the incident or the victims, the severity of the patients condition once the patients are located, the lack of advanced life support, and the lack of skill retention by the providers.[13,17–19] If modern trauma resources were more accessible to rural areas, rural morbidity and mortality could be reduced—recall that less than half of the country has statewide trauma systems.[17–19]

SUMMARY

Trauma care and emergency medical services have developed considerably since the publication of the White Paper. Today there are trauma system guidelines and EMS system components. Trauma research and education continue despite fluctuating funding. It is imperative to ensure that all patients have access to the appropriate level of care. Continued trauma system progress will help to ensure the availability of trauma care services in the future.

▶ REVIEW QUESTIONS

1. The White Paper was released in:
   a. 1966
   b. 1973
   c. 1990
   d. 1979

2. The Hill Burton Act was designed to:
   a. Establish trauma centers
   b. Create local EMS services
   c. Determine the number of hospitals that existed
   d. Educate the public

3. Prior to the EMSS Act of 1973 most ambulances were:
   a. Operated by fire departments
   b. Hospital based
   c. Privately owned
   d. Modified hearses staffed with morticians

4. The Reconciliation Act of 1981 allowed for:
   a. Unlimited EMS funding
   b. Reimbursement of costs
   c. EMS systems growth
   d. Trauma systems development

5. Inclusive trauma care means that:
   a. All components of the trauma system are involved in patient care.
   b. Only the sickest patient gets treatment.
   c. There is only one trauma center in the system.
   d. Patient transfer agreements are not allowed.

6. Military contributions to the development of civilian trauma include:
   a. The Vietnam War
   b. The Korean War
   c. The Civil War
   d. All of the above

7. Trauma courses (such as BTLS and PHTLS) have:
   a. Improved prehospital trauma outcomes
   b. Decreased EMS providers trauma skills
   c. Met resistance among EMS providers
   d. Not proven to be effective in reducing morbidity or mortality

8. Initial attempts at resuscitation:
   a. Were often done in "accident rooms"
   b. Varied among hospitals
   c. Both a and b
   d. None of the above

9. Level IV and V trauma centers are usually located in:
   a. Urban settings
   b. Suburban settings
   c. Rural or desolate locations
   d. None of the above

10. Rural trauma cases continue to challenge EMS and trauma systems across the country.
    a. True
    b. False

11. The Golden Hour concept promotes the notion that:
    a. Trauma care can be delayed for up to 1 hour.
    b. The patient has 60 minutes after arriving in the hospital to receive care.
    c. The first 60 minutes after initial impact are the most vital.
    d. None of the above.

12. R. Adams Cowley was a pioneer in trauma care and developed:
    a. MIEMSS
    b. The Golden Hour concept
    c. The first trauma unit in Chicago
    d. Both a and b
    e. Both a and c

13. The 15 components of an EMS system were introduced by:
    a. Accident/crashes
    b. The EMSS Act of 1973
    c. The Highway Safety Act of 1966
    d. None of the above

14. The Trauma Care Systems Planning and Development Act of 1990 called for:
    a. Development of only level I trauma centers
    b. EMS to be excluded from trauma care
    c. Continued development of statewide trauma systems
    d. Trauma research to be discontinued

15. The military has contributed to the development of modern-day EMS and trauma care systems.
    a. True
    b. False

16. Early deaths can be reduced by implementing early and aggressive resuscitation.
    a. True
    b. False

17. Trimodal deaths reflect:
    a. The failure of trauma care
    b. The reason why trauma patients die
    c. None of the above
    d. Both a and b

18. Patients who suffer "late death" from trauma:
   a. Tend to die from infection and organ failure
   b. Require aggressive resuscitation
   c. Require extensive and intensive care
   d. Both a and c

▶ CRITICAL THINKING

● List several injuries for each mode of the "Trimodal Distribution of Time of Death." Describe the impact EMS field care has on reducing deaths in each mode. How would you design an EMS system to improve outcomes in each mode?

● If you were designing a regional trauma care system, how would it differ from the existing models of these systems?

● Investigate the trauma care systems of other industrialized nations. (You can find articles describing these systems using Medline or the Internet.) What could the United States learn from these foreign systems?

▶ REFERENCES

1. Eastman AB. Blood in our streets: the status and evolution of trauma care systems. *Arch Surg.* 1992; 127:677.
2. Veise-Berry S, Beachley M. *Evolution of the Trauma Cycle. Trauma Nursing: From Resuscitation Through Rehabilitation.* Philadelphia: W.B. Saunders Co; 1993.
3. Emergency Nurses Association. *Course in Advanced Trauma Nursing: A Conceptual Approach.* Park Ridge, Ill: ENA; 1995.
4. Boyd DR, et al. *Systems Approach to Emergency Medical Care.* Norwalk, Conn: Appleton-Century-Crofts; 1983.
5. Trunkey D. Trauma. *Scie Am.* 1983; 249:2.
6. Campbell J. *Basic Trauma Life Support.* 3rd ed. Englewood Cliffs, NJ: 1995.
7. National Association of Emergency Medical Technicians. *Prehospital Trauma Life Support.* 3rd ed. St. Louis, Mo: Mosby; 1994.
8. Ali J, et al. Effect of the prehospital trauma life support program on prehospital trauma care. *Trauma.* 1997; 42:5.
9. Parr N. EHS Course 200: Introduction to emergency health services. University of Maryland, Baltimore County; 1987.
10. National Research Council: Division of Medical Sciences, et al. *Accidental Death and Disability: The Neglected Disease of Modern Society.* Washington, DC: National Academy of Sciences; 1966.
11. Bazzoli GJ, et al. Progress in the development of trauma systems in the United States. *JAMA.* 1995; 273:5.
12. Task Force of the Committee on Trauma, American College of Surgeons, Resources for Optimal Care of the Injured Patient: An Update. *Bull Am Coll Surg.* 1990; 75(9): 20–9.
13. Caro DH. Toward effective regional trauma networks: Management auditing initiatives in Ontario. *Health Care Manage Rev.* 1997; 22:2.
14. Mulleins RJ, et al. Influence of a statewide trauma system on location of hospitalization and outcome of injured patients. *Trauma.* 1996; 40:4.
15. Ashbeams and Samaritan Air Evac: Timeline of Emergency Air Medical Services. *Air Medical Crew National Standards Curriculum, Advanced Student Model.* 1988.
16. Simmons E, et al. Paramedic injury severity perception can aid trauma triage. *Ann Emerg Med.* 1995; 26:4.
17. Cales RH, Trunkey DD. Preventable trauma deaths: A review of trauma care systems development. *JAMA.* 1985; 254:8.
18. Rogers FB, et al. Trauma deaths in a mature urban vs. rural trauma system. *Arch Surg.* 1997; 132:374.
19. Mann NC, et al. Rural hospital transfer patient before and after implementation of a statewide trauma system. *Acad Emerg Med.* 1997; 4:8.
20. Grossman DC, et al. Urban–rural differences in prehospital care of major trauma. *Trauma.* 1997; 42:4.

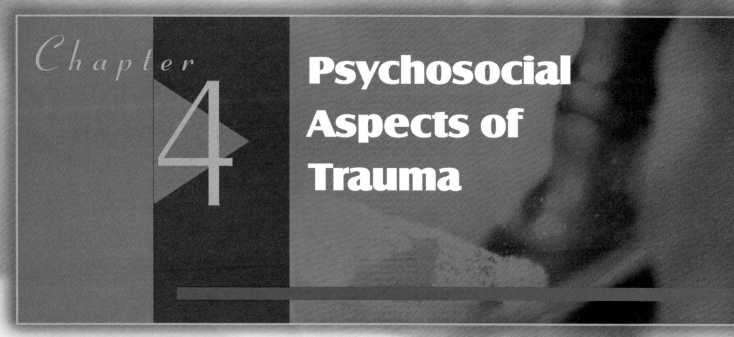

Chapter 4

Psychosocial Aspects of Trauma

OBJECTIVES

Upon completion of this chapter, the reader should be able to:

- Define stress and stressor.
- Identify and define two types of stress.
- Identify the psychological aspects of stress and stress signals.
- Describe posttraumatic stress disorder.
- Identify stress management strategies.
- Define the term *crisis* and describe the crisis reaction.
- Define critical incident stress management (CISM) and differentiate between the various CISM interventions.
- List guidelines for treating the patient's and family members' emotional response to trauma.
- Understand the needs of rape and sexual assault victims and list the special treatment considerations for these patients.
- List special considerations for the dying patient and their family members.
- List guidelines for breaking the news of death to family members.

KEY TERMS

Acute stress disorder
Acute stress reaction
Crisis
Critical incident
Critical incident stress debriefing (CISD)
Critical incident stress management (CISM)
Cumulative stress
Defusing

Demobilization
Fight or flight
On-scene support
Peer counseling
Posttraumatic stress disorder (PTSD)
Stress
Stressor

In this country and around the world there are many traumatic, life-changing events occurring at this very moment. Emergency personnel are receiving calls to respond to these events to help those who are facing danger, devastation, and human tragedy. The physical wounds are apparent: bleeding bodies, dropping blood pressures, and paralyzed limbs. But are these the only wounds that need a paramedic's professional care? What about the emotional trauma incurred by the victim as a result of physical suffering? What impact does this suffering have on paramedics? Can they return home or back to their jobs untouched by their exposure to human agony? This chapter will explore the answers to these questions.

THE STRESS RESPONSE

"I am so stressed out!" "The stress is getting to me." "That was a stressful situation." These statements are examples of how the word *stress* may be used to convey strong emotions. Stress can mean many things to many people. The first attempts to define stress, and the stress response, focused on the physiological aspects. Walter Cannon, an early stress researcher, was the first person to use the term **fight or flight**.[1] This term refers to the body's response to a threat—whether choosing to stand our ground and fight or to run from harm. This fight-or-flight response is an attempt by the various systems of the body to prepare us for protection.

Hans Selye, a pioneer of stress research, defined **stress** as "the nonspecific response of the body to any demand placed on it."[2] Demand on the body is created by any event that evokes the flight-or-fight, or stress, response. These events are called **stressors**. Stressors may include negative events, such as job termination or death, as well as positive events, such as marriage or job promotion. Physiologically, the body does not distinguish between the two types.[3]

PERCEPTION OF STRESS

How an event is perceived plays an important role in whether it is viewed as a stressor. To the brain, a perceived threat is the same as a real threat and is responded to as an actual event. For example, one night, you respond to a single-car collision. Upon arriving at the scene, you discover an unconscious adult and an empty infant car seat. Looking around, you realize that a child may have been thrown from the vehicle. While anxiously searching the surrounding area, you are told that the victim's family has been contacted and that no child was in the car. When you thought there might be an undiscovered child, you were more likely to experience the stress response than afterward, when you realized that no child was present. This example illustrates how each of us perceives or assigns meaning to events that occur in life. A perceived threat is treated as a real threat by the brain.

When a threat is perceived, the stress response usually takes place. The meaning assigned to an event is that person's reality.[4] For example, John and Jack work on the same ambulance crew. Applications are taken for a new supervisory position and both employees apply. When John is informed that he has not been chosen for the new job, he thinks, "I will never be promoted." Interestingly, Jack is not offered the job either. However, Jack tells himself, "There will be other opportunities for advancement." Different cognitive reactions to the same event can strengthen or weaken a stress response.

Imagine that one's thoughts are the steering wheel of a car; where one's thoughts travel determines the direction the body will travel. If thoughts are focused on negative aspects, the stress response is more likely to occur. If thoughts are neutral or positive, the stress response is less likely to occur.

Frequent or unnecessary stress responses are linked to health problems, including ulcers and hypertension.[5] How a person perceives the world plays a role in this process. For emergency medical personnel who experience or witness a traumatic event, the impact of the experience can have long-term effects, including posttraumatic stress disorder, acute stress disorder, and burnout.

EFFECTS OF STRESS

Stress symptoms may manifest in three areas: physiological, emotional, and behavioral. These symptoms are listed in Table 4-1. Stress cues are unique to the individual. One person may experience nausea while another may have headaches. Changes in appetite and sleep patterns are also common responses to stress. Some symptoms require prompt attention from either a medical doctor (i.e., tightness in the chest, increased blood pressure) or a mental health professional (disorientation, flashbacks). It may be beneficial to seek help during a particularly stressful time; seeking help may decrease the risk of experiencing later problems.

TYPES OF STRESS

An **acute stress reaction** occurs during or immediately following an incident, usually within 24 hours. Occasionally, the signals may not occur until much later. Stress signals do not mean a person is weak or ill, but rather indicate a need to take care of one's self in order to limit the impact of an incident.

Table 4-1
Stress Signals

Physiological Signals	Emotional Signals
Increase in heart rate	Irritability
Headaches	Angry outbursts
Elevated blood pressure	Depression
Vomiting	Suspiciousness
Difficulty breathing	Anxiety
Tremors	Feelings of worthlessness
Tightness of the muscles	Lack of interest
Sweaty palms	Sense of panic
Diarrhea	Withdrawing from others
Nausea	Lack of initiative
Loss of appetite	Survivor guilt
Difficulty sleeping	Inappropriate emotional responses
Fatigue	Fear
Chest pain	Emotional numbness
Dry mouth	Anger
Exhaustion	Denial of feelings
Dizziness	Grief
Chills	Identification with the victim
Sleep disturbance	Hopelessness/helplessness
Behavioral Signals	
Preoccupation	Hyperalert
Forgetfulness	Crying spells
Errors in math	Suspiciousness
Inability to concentrate	Smoking more often
Lack of attention to details	Drinking alcohol more often
Decrease in creativity	Quieter than usual
Decrease in productivity	Disoriented
No sense of humor	Nightmares
Decrease in awareness of one's surroundings	

Cumulative stress occurs over time from exposure to numerous stressors related to work or other life experiences. The stressors do not have to be critical incidents. Instead, it is the buildup of stress over time that takes its toll. The signals are the same as those experienced with the acute stress reaction; it is the frequency and duration that differ. The result of cumulative stress can become what is known as "burnout."

POSTTRAUMATIC STRESS DISORDER

Posttraumatic stress disorder (PTSD) may result from a severe traumatic event.[6] The symptoms of PTSD include intrusive thoughts (i.e., thoughts of the event that occur unbidden), nightmares, acting or feeling as though the event is occurring again, and avoiding reminders of the event. A real or imagined cue of the trauma can occur in any of the five senses. For example, the smell of burning leaves may remind a paramedic of a house fire in which small children were trapped, resulting in sleep disturbance, difficulty concentrating, and/or an exaggerated startle response. Posttraumatic stress disorder can occur more than 6 months after the person experiences or witnesses the event. In order for the symptoms to be considered PTSD, the symptoms must be experienced for over a month. **Acute stress disorder** is similar to PTSD, but symptoms must occur within a month after the traumatic event and must last less than a month.[6]

Posttraumatic stress disorder may be experienced by victims, family members, witnesses, or emergency personnel. For example, a young man was waiting to cross a busy intersection and saw a man on a bicycle hit by a car. The cyclist was not wearing a helmet and died on the scene due to a massive head injury. Months after this incident, the witness reported intrusive thoughts and dreams about the incident. This example illustrates that a person does not have to be involved in an incident or have a personal relationship with a victim in order to experience PTSD symptoms. Police, firefighters, and paramedics also may experience symptoms of PTSD. Responding to a certain type of call may be more difficult for a paramedic because it serves as a reminder of an earlier disturbing call. In addition, too many calls or other stressors may create a "pile-up" effect that requires more than the responder can handle individually.

EMERGENCY PERSONNEL AND STRESS

To date, little research on stress has focused primarily on paramedics and the impact of their work. More typically, all emergency personnel are placed in one group and studied. Emergency personnel may include police, firefighters, EMTs, paramedics, and hospital emergency staff. Much of the research has focused on the stress experienced after a large-scale disaster or event.[7–10] The symptoms experienced include those associated with PTSD, intrusion, and avoidance. However, these symptoms can also occur in a person who does not have PTSD. The frequency of these symptoms in emergency workers indicates the great effects of traumatic events, even when individuals are unaware of the impact. Additionally, research has been done on the use of critical incident stress management to deal with the needs of emergency responders.[11]

BASIC STRESS MANAGEMENT

Just as stress responses are unique, each paramedic's way of dealing with stress is also unique. There are methods available to promote coping with stress. Utilizing a range of stress management strategies can make you better prepared to face stressors. These stress management strategies include good nutrition, exercise, deep breathing, relaxation, and biofeedback.

Nutrition and exercise are important stress management tools. In making good choices regarding nutrition and exercise, the body is physically better prepared for stress. Eating a well-balanced diet, and limiting sweets and caffeine helps EMS personnel decrease the stress response. Stress increases the metabolic rate, causing an increase in the levels of sugar, free fatty acids, and lactic acid in the blood. Stress also affects the pituitary gland, leading to changes in water balance, suppression of the immune system, and increases in carbohydrate and protein metabolism.[5] Thus, the stressed body uses energy at a much faster rate. Persons experiencing stress often notice a change in their eating habits. For example, one person may feel too upset to eat while another may overeat. Food can be used as an escape from unpleasant emotions such as boredom, sadness, or anxiety. Any dramatic change in eating habits may be a signal to examine life stressors and to focus on how to deal with the stressors without turning to food.

Exercise provides an outlet from stressors and contributes to overall health, two important factors in stress reduction. If excessive, however, exercise may cause more harm than good. There are many different forms of physical exercise from which to choose. Engaging in an activity that you enjoy will increase the chance that you will maintain a regular exercise program (Figure 4-1). Aerobic exercise for 20 minutes 3 days per week is enough to realize these benefits.[5]

Breathing deeply and slowly is the easiest way to reduce stress immediately. To counteract the stress response, EMS personnel can practice breathing deeply so that the abdomen expands outward, holding the breath for a count of five, then slowly exhaling through the mouth.

There are different methods for achieving relaxation. Progressive muscle relaxation involves systematically relaxing the major muscle groups. Specific instructions may involve tensing and then relaxing the muscles to become accustomed to the sensation of muscle tension versus muscle relaxation. Benefits of relaxation include decreases in heart rate, blood pres-

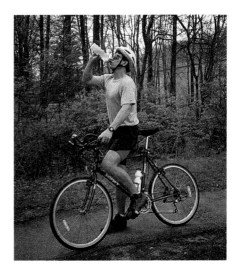

FIGURE 4-1 Regular exercise and proper nutrition help to reduce the effects of stress on the body.

sure, and muscle tension.[5] Another way to evoke the relaxation response is through the use of imagery or creative visualization. Imagine being in a peaceful setting, such as the beach or mountains. Figure 4-2 walks through the technique of guided imagery.

Biofeedback is a specific method of providing feedback on body functions in which one learns to influence these functions to achieve a desired result. The procedures most often used are skin temperature, heart rate, blood pressure, electromyography (EMG), or galvanic skin response (GSR).[12] Once able to influence heart rate and blood pressure, the individual is weaned off the instrument providing the information. The goal is to achieve the desired result without using the biofeedback machine. Biofeedback works, yet the results obtained by this method can also be achieved through relaxation and cognitive restructuring, or focusing on thoughts that lead to a decrease in stress.[12]

In addition to formal methods of stress management, there are many informal strategies as well. These methods include talking to someone about stress or other problems, maintaining enjoyable relationships, developing hobbies, reading, continuing one's education, volunteering, and avoiding procrastination. It is important to participate in high-interest activities as well as frequently interacting with others in a positive manner. In this way, one can find balance between a rewarding career and personal life.

Another important part of stress management is recognizing personal limitations. Sometimes, we are hit with too many stressors in a short period of time to be able to manage life effectively. Other times, the cumulative stress becomes more than can be managed alone. This is the time to seek professional help. Some employers offer an Employee Assistance Program (EAP) that

- Assume a comfortable position in a quiet environment.
- Close your eyes and keep them closed until the exercise is completed.
- Breathe in deeply for a count of 4.
- Hold breath for a count of 4.
- Breathe out for a count of 4.
- Continue to breathe slowly and deeply.
- Think of your favorite place and prepare to take an imaginary journey there. Select a place in which you are relaxed and at peace.
- Picture in your mind's eye your favorite place. Look around you and see all the colors, the light and shadows, and all the pleasant sights.
- Listen to all the sounds. Pay attention to what you hear.
- Feel all the physical sensations...the temperature... the textures...the movement of the air.
- As you take in a deep breath, smell the aromas of your favorite place.
- Taste the foods and drinks you usually consume in your favorite place. Savor each taste fully.
- Focus all your attention totally on your favorite place.
- Breathe in deeply to a count of 4.
- Hold breath for a count of 4.
- Breathe out to a count of 4.
- Resume your usual breathing pattern.
- Slowly open your eyes and stretch, if desired.

This procedure works best when all five senses are used. Like all other relaxation exercises, guided imagery becomes more effective with repetition.

FIGURE 4-2 Guided imagery is a technique often used to reduce stress; it works best with repetition.
From *Fundamentals of Nursing: Standards and Practice,* by S. DeLaune and P. Ladner, 1998, Albany, NY: Delmar Thomson Learning. Copyright 1998 by Delmar Thomson Learning.

provides a resource for workers. Another alternative is to ask your medical doctor, a trusted friend, or clergy for a referral to a mental health professional.

Signs that you need more assistance than your family, friends, or coworkers can provide include thoughts of ending your life, depression, inappropriate emotional responses (i.e., over- or underreacting to an event), increased tardiness or absenteeism, excessive anger, and acts of violence. Seeking help is not a weakness but rather demonstrates the ability to take care of yourself. It is only when we take care of ourselves that we can then care appropriately for others. If you see these signs in someone else, approach them in a non-judgmental manner. Offer support in assisting the person to obtain professional help; this may be the turning point needed to avert a downward spiral. If you talk to someone about seeking help, do not be critical or accusatory. Stick to the facts and your concern for the person. For example, you might say, "I am concerned that you were yelling earlier." This is less likely to make the person defensive than saying, "You're losing it. You have a chip on your shoulder and you need to chill." To stick to the facts, give examples of the person's behavior. Express your concern about the behavior without drawing conclusions that suggest you are labeling the person, such as, "You are depressed." Instead, make statements about direct observations, such as, "I've noticed you withdrawing to your room more often than before," or, "You've raised your voice to me several times today." Always begin with suggestions of ways to help the person. Call your local mental health center or talk with an EAP representative about appropriate referrals for your friend. For example, if your concern is alcohol abuse, get the names and phone numbers of chemical dependency professionals or agencies. Having such information available will speed up the process of getting help. Of course, there is always the chance that the person will not acknowledge that he or she has a problem. At that point, ask a professional to be present when you attempt to approach the topic again. If the threat of suicide is involved, call the local mental health center and get information about how to ensure the person's safety.

INTERNET ACTIVITIES

Take the on-line stress management course at http://www.unl.edu/stress.

CRITICAL INCIDENT STRESS MANAGEMENT

A **critical incident** can be defined as any significant emotional event that has the power to cause unusual psychological distress in healthy, normal people.[13] Critical incidents for emergency services professionals may include (1) serious injury or death of a coworker in the line of duty; (2) suicide of a coworker; (3) a significant event involving children; (4) knowing the victim(s) involved in an event; (5) events that attract unusual attention from the media; (6) multicasualty incident or disaster; (7) any loss associated with extraordinary or prolonged incidents; and (8) any significant or unusually distressing event.

Critical incident stress management (CISM) includes critical incident stress debriefings, traumatic stress defusings, and other stress-related interventions developed to prevent or moderate the psychological effects of distressing events. Examples of these events include acts of physical or sexual violence; acts of nature such as tornados, earthquakes, or hurricanes; acts of terrorism, such as mass destruction from a bomb; or the untimely death of a child. These events have the potential to produce great psychological damage in emergency personnel and cannot be remedied using everyday stress management techniques.[14, 15]

CISM was initially developed by Jeffrey T. Mitchell to facilitate the prevention of posttraumatic stress and related disorders among high-risk occupational groups such as emergency and disaster response personnel.[15] The CISM concept was born during World Wars I and II when military personnel looked for ways to abate the devastating effects of combat on soldiers.[15] The military's goal of returning soldiers to the front line as soon as possible led to rendering "emotional first aid" in field hospitals near combat zones. Quick intervention near the site of the destructive stressor greatly reduced the number of combat stress casualties. These interventions were an informal, one-on-one process. During the 1982 war in Lebanon, the Israeli military employed group-oriented stress interventions and peer groups to support soldiers. As a result, the incidence of psychiatric disturbances was reduced by more than 60%.[16]

Today, much research has been done on the victims of natural and man-made disasters. Until recently, it was not believed that the same devastating psychological effects experienced by the victims of disaster could merge in disaster response workers. It was generally accepted that their training was enough to isolate them from negative and lasting distress.

Two tragic events, the 1978 crash of a Pacific Southwest Airline plane into a San Diego residential area and the 1979 American Airlines flight 191 crash near Chicago, brought to light that emergency personnel are, in fact, vulnerable to the "horrors of human suffering."[15,17] In the days and weeks following these events, psychological counseling of on-scene emergency workers rose significantly. They reported symptoms of sleep and eating disturbances, distressing dreams and flashback memories, personality changes, and extreme emotional reactions. These symptoms are the same symptoms reported by soldiers after experience in combat. It was realized that the men and women who had, until now, suffered in silence against the assumptions of emotional invincibility could indeed become psychological casualties of tragic events.[17] Combining the available information regarding wartime stress reduction techniques, disaster, and work place trauma research, Mitchell developed the concept of critical incident stress debriefing.[17]

Critical incident stress debriefing (CISD) is a structured group process utilizing both crisis intervention and educational techniques to lessen the effects of a traumatic event.[15,16,18] Debriefings are conducted by specially trained mental health professionals and peer support personnel (fellow EMS professionals), ideally 24–72 hours following the incident. The debriefing sessions include any personnel *involved* with the critical incident who wish to attend: paramedics, firefighters, law enforcement, and hospital personnel. *Only* those involved in the incident are allowed to attend. The goal is to decrease the adverse symptoms normally experienced and accelerate normal recovery from traumatic events. Secondary goals include educating those attending about stress, stress reduction, stress prevention, and survival techniques; normalizing stress reactions to abnormal events; predicting and normalizing future or delayed stress reactions (normalizing means emphasizing what the person is experiencing is typical for someone who has been involved in such an incident); educating those present that recovery is a process, not an event, and assuring them that recovery is likely; and screening and referral for those who need further counseling.[15–17]

The CISD team determines which events warrant a CISD. Using the debriefing process for events outside the range of normal experience could greatly reduce the effectiveness of CISD. Other CISM techniques may be more appropriate for the less distressing incidents. Also, a debriefing is a group intervention. If only one or two individuals are involved in the critical incident, then these alternative techniques may be more appropriate for them as well.[15]

CISD is not psychotherapy and should never be a substitute for it. CISD only deals with current critical incidents. The process does not allow for previous events to be discussed. CISD helps the participant handle the stress symptoms related to the event at hand, not stress relating to other events, cumulative stress, interpersonal stress, or stress of any other kind. CISD is not an operational critique of the event nor will CISD solve all issues associated with an incident.

INTERNET ACTIVITIES

Visit the e-medicine Web site at http://www.emedicine.com/. Click on the Emergency Medicine on-line book and select Special Aspects of Emergency Medicine. Then click on critical incident stress management. Review the chapter on managing stress.

OTHER STRESS MANAGEMENT INTERVENTIONS

Although CISD is the most well known and complex of the stress intervention techniques, it is not always the treatment of choice. Other interventions such as defusings, demobilizations, on-scene support services, individual consultations, and peer counseling may be more suited to reduce or prevent the short- and long-term effects associated with involvement in critical events.

Defusings

A **defusing** is a shorter, less formal, less structured version of a CISD. It is a group process managed by trained peers or mental health professionals, similar to a debriefing. However, defusings are designed to eliminate the need for a debriefing or to enhance the debriefing process if one is necessary. Defusings are initiated within 1 to 8 hours after a critical incident. The main goal is to return emergency workers to service as soon as possible, protected from the damaging and harmful effects of traumatic stress. Defusings are generally organized separately for each of the groups of emergency personnel involved and are targeted at the most seriously affected workers (Figure 4-3). In contrast, debriefings usually include all personnel involved in an incident regardless of stress severity or emergency discipline. Defusings are held at neutral locations free from distractions, never at the critical incident scene. The goal of a defusing is to offer rapid stress relief shortly after a traumatic event, normalize reactions to the experience, reestablish group cohesiveness, and determine the need for debriefing or other follow-up services.[15]

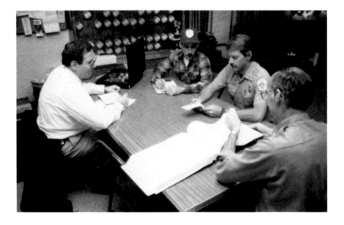

FIGURE 4-3 Defusings are targeted to those workers who are most affected by the critical incident.

Demobilizations

This CISM intervention was developed for use in a large-scale emergency event. **Demobilizations** allow for a transition time for emergency personnel between the major event and return to routine duty or home. Demobilizations are implemented immediately after release from the emergency scene and consist of two main segments. The first segment is a 10–15 minute talk by CISM team members on stress management. The second segment is a 20-minute period to rest and eat. Though difficult to manage, demobilizations can be a very beneficial support service for the hundreds of emergency workers that may be involved in large-scale operations.[17]

On-Scene Support Services

Services provided during the time of a critical incident are referred to as **on-scene support**. Most typically provided by trained peer support personnel, on-scene support includes (1) one-on-one, brief interventions to distressed workers; (2) counsel to operation commanders regarding stress levels and responses of on-scene personnel; and (3) emotional first aid to victims and family members affected by the critical incident.[15]

Individual Consultations

Occasionally, critical incidents may occur where only a few people are affected. An event does not have to be the size or magnitude of a disaster to be considered a critical incident. For instance, two paramedics could be greatly affected after working with a small child that has been maliciously beaten or sexually abused. Though experiencing the same event, some emergency personnel have intense stress reactions while others do not. The intensity of a reaction is contingent not on how "tough" one is but on how "close to home" the event is perceived. Since debriefings, defusings, and demobilizations are group interventions, they are not appropriate for use as an intervention for fewer than three people. Under these circumstances, one-on-one or small-group interventions can be used. Mental health professionals or peer support personnel provide these sessions with the same goals as debriefings and defusings. Many times stress interventions are not provided because only a few people are involved. The rationale is that an event is not critical if the incident or the number affected is small. This can be a grave mistake.[15]

Peer Counseling

Peer counseling is very important and the most often utilized CISM strategy. Peer counseling is friends talking with friends in times of need. Coworkers discussing a call after returning to the ambulance base or informal group discussions after a particularly stressful event or busy shift are examples of peer counseling. Trained peer support personnel can be present during these informal meetings or can be consulted. They can help recognize stress symptoms in coworkers who need stress survival techniques or structured CISM interventions.[15]

Although the concept of peer counseling is not new, it is gaining more attention. Research continues to show the damaging effects of work-related stress. Professionals are seeking more ways to reduce, prevent, or speed recovery from critical incident stress and daily accumulated stress. Peer counseling is proving to be a formidable method for meeting this challenge.

Traditionally, EMS personnel have shown a reluctance to seek professional psychological help. The reasons for this include (1) entering into professional counseling might suggest they are somehow "unfit" to do the job and (2) a belief that someone outside the profession could not understand their plight. These reasons coupled with the closeness experienced among emergency workers favor the development of an effective counseling alliance among peers. People who experience extraordinary events form a bond others can be aware of but never fully understand. This bond offers the opportunity for the kind of trust and open communication that are the hallmarks of a helping relationship.[19]

Specialized training for peer counseling can come from several sources. One option is to attend the 16-hour Basic CISM Training and Instruction course required to become a CISM team member sponsored by the International Critical Incident Stress Foundation. Course topics include an overview of stress (causes, effects, and management), specifics of EMS stress and critical incidents, the basics of CISM team development, all CISM interventions (debriefings, defusings, etc.), and communication and crisis intervention skills.[15]

A second option is to ask local mental health personnel or a private training and consulting service to offer special workshops on peer counseling. These workshops could include how to build an effective peer counseling relationship, enhancement of listening and attending skills, principles of communication and crisis intervention, and recognition and management of EMS stress and problem areas (substance abuse, relationship difficulties, burnout, etc.).[19]

It is important to note that although peer counseling can be a very effective method for helping manage emergency work-related stress, it is not a substitute for professional psychotherapy. Also, a peer counseling workshop is not a substitute for CISM training. No one should attempt the CISM intervention strategies without first being a member of a CISM team and having attended the Basic CISM Training and Instruction course.

Today, there are over 300 CISM teams in the United States and in other parts of the world.[14] This is evidence that the emergency service professions as a whole have come to realize that no matter how extraordinary the job is that they are asked to do, they are ordinary human beings vulnerable to the sometimes harmful psychological effects of their chosen profession.[18]

TREATING THE EMOTIONAL RESPONSE TO TRAUMA

When considering total patient care, it is impossible to ignore the psychological and emotional components of treatment. Physical symptoms such as increased heart and respiratory rates, nausea and vomiting, profuse sweating, or mental confusion could signal the onset of any number of physiological ills. These same symptoms could simply be the body's reaction to an emotional trauma. Many times, physical and emotional reactions are intermixed and indistinguishable. Therefore, attend to both the physical and emotional needs of the patient. To do this, you must understand the emotional needs of the patient in crisis.

WHAT IS A CRISIS?

For most of our lives, we exist in a steady or balanced state. Stressors greet us along the way, but we are armed with a reserve of mental and emotional coping techniques designed to bring us back on course. A **crisis** occurs when the stressors throw us so far outside the normal range of equilibrium that our coping mechanisms fail to return us to a state of balance.[20] A crisis may be precipitated by chronic, developmental, or acute stressors. Chronic stressors occur over and over again, eventually reducing the individual's ability to restore equilibrium. Examples include child abuse, exposure to war or violence, and long-term, difficult working conditions. Developmental crisis may occur as a result of life transitions such as puberty, marriage, parenthood, divorce, or retirement. Most crises, however, are precipitated by acute stressors—sudden and unexpected disruptions such as an automobile crash, heart attack, fire, tornado, robbery, or the death of a loved one.[20] Acute crisis is the type most often encountered by paramedics in the line of duty.

THE CRISIS REACTION

Individual response to crisis is unique and unpredictable, although its course follows a similar pattern in all of us. The following is a description of the phases of crisis response and associated signs and symptoms. Please note that not every person will experience every response described and certainly not necessarily in the order delineated. Phase regression and symptom overlapping will invariably occur.[20–22]

The *first phase* immediately following the onset of the crisis event is characterized by denial, shock, numbness, and disbelief. The person may appear dazed or stunned, saying, "No, this can't be happening." Denial is nature's way of protecting and insulating the individual from the reality of the event. A person in this state will be resistant to outside stimuli. After the crisis has passed, many do not remember what they saw or what was said to them. However, they do remember how others made them feel during their time of tragedy.[21]

A crisis victim in this initial phase may show signs and symptoms of shock. The physiological response may include dizziness and fainting, nausea and vomiting, rapid pulse, sweating, low blood pressure, a dull, blank stare, or cold and clammy skin. The victim may wander about aimlessly or sit frozen, unable to move even in the face of danger. A wide spectrum of "bizarre" behaviors may be observed such as hysterical laughing, outbursts of anger, uncontrollable crying, or frantic overactivity. It is important to expect the unexpected.[22]

The first phase can be seen as the victim attempting to evade the reality of the crisis. The *second phase* begins as the victim undertakes the task of facing the reality of the crisis.[22] This phase is characterized by a deluge of emotions, including anger, rage, fear, terror, anxiety, grief, remorse, emptiness, guilt, blame, confusion, agitation, and frustration. All these emotions and accompanying behaviors stem from the victim's response to feeling helpless and out of control, a desire to restore things to their precrisis state, and the need to make sense of the whole ordeal.

It is impossible for anyone to grasp the full impact of a crisis at once; the process of owning the crisis experience is gradual and oscillates with the denial phase until reconciliation is complete. This could take weeks, months, or years, depending upon the individual and the specific crisis encountered. The *reconciliation phase* is the final dimension of the crisis process. This phase signals a return to normalcy and equilibrium. It involves the victim integrating the new reality and grieving necessary losses incurred by the crisis.[22,23]

Paramedics almost always encounter patients in the first stage of a crisis. Treating the emotional symptoms and managing behavioral responses are crucial. The following are general guidelines for treating a patient in emotional crisis.[19,21,22,24,25] Remember that a patient's family members, although not in need of physical treatment, are experiencing their own crisis and will need your professional consideration as well.

1. *Ensure physical safety.* During the initial stages of crisis, a patient may be disoriented, confused, and inattentive. Thoughts may be clouded or distorted. The patient may fail to assign significant importance to dangerous conditions. Move patients to the safest areas possible and be aware that they might unknowingly place themselves in the path of danger (running back into a burning building, walking into traffic, attempting to rescue another victim).

2. *Look at the situation from the patient's point of view.* No matter how "routine" a stroke, heart attack, or automobile collision may become, it is not an everyday event for the people involved. An empathetic and compassionate approach to what may be a crucial turning point in a person's life is an essential aspect of treatment. However, it is not advisable to swing too far in the other direction, becoming overly involved. This makes the patient's crisis your crisis as well, reducing your ability to be objective and your ability to make decisions.

3. *Create privacy.* Crisis, grief, and the experience of loss are deeply personal and private affairs. Often we open the newspaper to see a profoundly emotional scene (survivors in the aftermath of a tornado, parents at the funeral of their teenager killed by a drunk driver). What is the stance of the victims? Are their hands covering their face or are their heads buried in the safety of a loved one's embrace? Victims instinctively seek privacy. Out of their shame of losing control or their sense of vulnerability, people in crisis need the solace of secluded space.

4. *Remain calm and personally detached.* One way to remain calm in an emergency situation is not to take what happens personally. The patient or family is not angry at you; they are angry because their life just slipped out of their control. Stay compassionate but do not react emotionally to their emotions. Again, do not make an emergency scene your personal crisis. Your patient needs you to be thinking clearly and acting decisively. They may even "borrow" some of your calmness and assurance.

5. *Employ an inviting attitude.* An inviting attitude includes being open, receptive, genuine, caring, respectful, and attentive. This appearance will "invite" cooperation from patients and family members.

6. *Maintain eye contact.* Looking directly at a person allows them to feel you are truly interested and concerned. Eye contact helps build an essential bond of trust. The patient and family must believe that you are being honest and straightforward.

7. *Listen, listen, listen.* Active listening involves attending to what the patient is saying, then reflecting or paraphrasing what you have just heard. You need not agree or even understand what is being expressed. The goal is to validate the person and their experience. Of course, there are many situations when you only have time to get "the facts." But there are other times when active listening can be employed. Also, during a crisis, a person needs to expend great amounts of nervous energy. Letting them "tell their story" is a good way to accomplish this.

8. *Allow and acknowledge feelings.* Never try to control emotions. Allow the tears and the anger. Expressing emotion is the body's way of trying to reconcile the difference between what they want (precrisis condition) and what they have (the crisis event). Validate for the patient what they are experiencing: "I imagine you must be pretty scared (confused, angry, sad, etc.) right now." If their emotion interferes with their medical care, you may need to distract them temporarily. Ask them to tell you about an unrelated event (their family, hobbies, etc.).

9. *Be honest, offer hope.* Be as honest as you can with patients. Do not make promises that may not happen with statements such as "I know everything will turn out all right." You may be wrong and the patient knows this. At the same time it is important to offer reassurance. Act in a confident manner, perhaps stating that "the very best care is being given to you."

10. *Recognize your limitations.* Acknowledge your own feelings of helplessness. Most caregivers, when feeling helpless, compensate by overdoing or overtalking when the patient needs them to listen and be present. Know that you cannot "solve" the crisis or prevent the crisis reaction. Silence is acceptable and often welcomed.

11. *Be willing to repeat.* Remember that during a crisis state, people may block outside stimuli. Their system is overloaded and they cannot process any more information. Therefore, it may be necessary to repeat questions, directions, or explanations.

12. *Use empathy, not sympathy.* Stating to a patient or family member, "I know just how you feel" may elicit a very negative response. You are not experiencing the same crisis and you cannot understand the full implications of how this crisis will change that person's life. Instead, make statements that allow the patient to feel understood, such as "This must be a terrible experience for you" or "I'm very sorry for all that has happened to you today."

13. *Never ask "Why?"* Asking a person "why" ("Why were you driving so fast?") implies that he or she did something wrong. The person may be left feeling blamed or judged. He or she may then decide to take offense, accelerating angry or frantic behaviors.

14. *Avoid an authoritative stance.* Remaining in charge of the emergency scene is important. Placing yourself in charge of a person's choices must be avoided. Do not lecture, preach, or moralize. Do not offer personal advice or constructive criticism. To the extent possible, avoid standing over and "looking down" upon your patient. When dealing with family members, ask for their help instead of issuing orders. And never, ever argue with anyone in crisis. It is a losing proposition for everyone involved.

Rape and Sexual Assault

Responding to a call for a person who has been raped or sexually assaulted can be one of the most difficult and uncomfortable tasks imaginable. In our society, rape is a taboo subject still shrouded in myth and misunderstanding. Rape is an act of violence, not sexual passion. The purpose of the rapist is to inflict control, shame, and humiliation upon the victim. Sexual assault serves as an outlet for the rapist's hatred of self and others, especially women.

According to FBI statistics, 95,769 rapes (male and female) were reported in the United States in 1996.[26] It is thought that only 1 in 10 rapes are actually made known to law enforcement. Unreported episodes of sexual assault may number over 1 million a year.

There are a number of treatment protocols and precautions to consider as you approach any emergency scene. The following are special guidelines for handling rape and sexual assault situations to add to your list.[22,27,28]

1. *Ensure physical safety.* Safety is a number 1 need of sexual assault victims. Keep in mind that the assailant may still be close at hand and could pose a threat.

2. *Remember that this is a crime scene.* Be aware of the need to preserve evidence. Unless the victim needs immediate transport to a hospital for a life-threatening injury, it may be advisable to wait for law enforcement to arrive. Advise the patient not to eat, drink, shower, douche, bathe, urinate, defecate, or change clothes until all evidence is collected. Place a clean sheet on the stretcher; the sheet may hold evidence such as hair or semen (see Chapter 32).

3. *Make no assumptions.* Always believe your patient when he or she tells you he or she has been raped. Do not let an inappropriate effect (i.e., laughter) or no effect lead you to believe nothing happened. This could be an emotional response. Also, do not make assumptions regarding the rapist. The assailant may be the "friend" who met you at the door or the neighbor who comes over to offer "help."

4. *Be extremely respectful of the patient.* Gently introduce yourself and explain your role. Clarify what you are going to do and ask permission before each procedure. Also, do not engage in trivial conversation with anyone at the scene. Do not laugh or make jokes.

5. *Be calm, reassuring, and very patient.* Your patient has just been through a violent experience. Be willing to take your time (medical condition permitting), mirror calmness, and continue to let the patient know that in *this moment* he or she is safe.

6. *Help the patient regain a sense of control.* This can be done in simple ways already discussed. Asking permission and explaining procedures are behaviors that convey to the patient that he or she is in charge. It is important to honor as many patient requests as possible. If he or she is unsure, offer a choice. For instance, "For privacy, would you like to go into the den or living room?" or, "Is there a friend I could call for you or would you rather be alone?" Regaining a sense of control is the first step in healing.

7. *Create a sense of safety and privacy.* Never leave your patient alone once you have initiated contact. Ask all those who are not necessary for the care of the patient to leave the area. If possible, involve a paramedic the same gender as the patient. Avoid touching your patient unless it is necessary for treatment. Do not stand over your patient; it may remind him or her of the dominating act just perpetrated.

8. *Keep the examination brief.* Do not examine the private areas of the body unless hemorrhage is suspected. Only initiate treatment that is absolutely necessary.

9. *Do not ask the patient about the rape.* Your patient will have to answer many questions posed by law enforcement. Do not add to this burden. Do allow your patient to talk about the incident (if he or she initiates) or express any emotion desired.

10. *Document everything.* This incident may go to court and the facts contained in the emergency medical record could help convict a rapist.

11. *Relay pertinent information to law enforcement.* Many times crucial information regarding the rape is given by the victim to the paramedics on the scene. The victim may assume that because the information was given to a person "in uniform" that it does not need to be repeated. These "missing pieces" may prove important.

12. *Be familiar with rape crisis services in your area.* Is there a rape crisis center or hotline? Are there victim advocates that can assist your patient at the hospital? Which hospitals are best suited for evidence collection and treatment of sexual trauma?

Death and Dying

The subject of death is something that you may face each day you go to work. In the EMS profession, talking about death, grief, and other loss seems almost forbidden. And, in general, we are a grief-avoiding society. Two of our best-kept secrets are that everyone suffers and everyone can grow from suffering. As a result of our desire to escape feelings associated with death, dying, loss, mourning, and suffering of any kind, we have created many misconceptions and defenses that limit our contact with this supposed enemy. As a result, we are in the dark when it comes to helping ourselves or others face the inevitability of death.[21]

Before you can give emotional assistance to others, you must first examine your own thoughts and feelings about death. Talk openly to friends, family, clergy, and professional counselors regarding previous losses and losses to come (e.g., the death of your parents), and even the loss of your own life. What are your greatest fears about death and dying? Talking openly to others about death and loss will not only help you to clarify your beliefs but also help you build a support system for a time when it might be needed. A common misconception about the grief experience is that it is something we must "get over" or move away from. True healing comes only when we embrace the grief, then share our thoughts and feelings with others.[29]

INTERNET ACTIVITIES

Visit the e-medicine Web site at http://www.emedicine.com. Click on the emergency medicine e-book, then the psychosocial chapter. Review the material on coping with the death of a child in the emergency department.

The Dying Patient Throughout your paramedic career, you will most likely spend quite a few "last moments" with dying patients and family. Although most of your efforts will be an attempt to save a life, you may be given the opportunity to lend emotional support. Consider the following:

1. Death and the process of dying is a deeply personal and spiritual time.

2. A dying person needs as much dignity, privacy, and safety as is feasible.

3. To the extent possible, honor all requests made by the patient and family.

4. Be familiar with do not resuscitate (DNR) protocols in your area.

5. Remember that death is a natural and inevitable human event.

Sometimes we have to give ourselves permission to let someone go.[19,30]

"Breaking the News" to Family Members
A person's reaction to the loss of a loved one is contingent upon their state of mind at the time of the death. Reaction to the loss of someone who has been ill for quite a while will be different from the reaction following a sudden, unexpected death. Other influencing factors include the nature of the relationship between the deceased and survivor, available support systems, and religious/cultural beliefs.[21]

When relaying the news of a loved one's death, remember that this may trigger a crisis. The issues discussed earlier pertaining to the crisis response relate here as well. The following are special guidelines for "breaking the news" to family members. Go to them quickly, mustering all your sensitivity and compassion. Select a protective environment, perhaps a quiet room or corner with minimal outside stimuli. Look into the eyes of the person(s) to whom you are speaking. Allow for the expression of feelings. Expect the unexpected. Do not take the family's reactions personally. Allow the family as much time with the body as they need. Validate the normalcy of touching and talking with the body. Find out who is a part of their support system. Ask, "Is there anyone I can call for you, a family member, friend, or clergy?" Say things like "I am sorry for your loss." Don't repeat clichés or give advice ("Time heals all wounds" or "He is better off now"). Be an advocate for their grief. Be sensitive to religious and cultural customs.[19,21,30]

SUMMARY

This chapter explored the recognition and treatment of stress reactions in both the paramedic and the patient. It is important for EMS professionals to adopt healthier lifestyles. Stress management techniques that can enhance one's ability to decrease or deflect the impact of stressors were discussed. Stress management involves choice, and each person's successful efforts to manage stress are unique. It takes time to find effective ways to manage stress.

Critical incident stress management (CISM) is vital to EMS. CISM interventions such as debriefings, defusings, demobilizations, on-scene support, and peer counseling were explored here. Also discussed were guidelines for the treatment of an emotional response to crisis. Special emphasis was given to the treatment of rape and sexual assault victims and the dying patient.

Today, the practice of medicine is expanding in a very important way. We are recognizing the value of treating the whole patient and not just apparent physical injuries. We know that paramedics are vulnerable to the stress of their job and suffering of their patients. We are human. It is essential that we treat ourselves and others accordingly.

REVIEW QUESTIONS

1. Define stress.

2. What is a stressor?

3. What role does one's thoughts play in the stress response?

4. Name the three areas in which stress signals can occur. Identify at least one signal in each of these areas.

5. How do an acute stress reaction and cumulative stress differ?

6. Posttraumatic stress disorder (PTSD):
   a. Is found only in individuals who were mentally unstable prior to the onset of PTSD
   b. May develop in a person who has been involved in a traumatic event
   c. Is a disorder that has intrusive and avoidant symptoms
   d. b and c only
   e. None of the above

7. When might you seek professional help or suggest a friend seek professional help?

8. Critical incident stress management was developed for what purpose?

9. Define a "critical incident" and give examples of critical incidents for emergency services professionals.

10. A CISD is conducted by
    a. Mental health professionals
    b. Emergency services supervisors
    c. Specially trained peer counselors
    d. All of the above
    e. a and c only

11. List three CISM interventions.

12. What types of stressors may precipitate a crisis?

13. Which of the following most accurately characterizes the first phase response of an emotional crisis:
   a. Bizarre behaviors
   b. Denial, numbness
   c. Sorrow, remorse, emptiness
   d. Grieving
   e. All of the above
   f. a and b only

14. What is the first step toward emotional healing for any victim of rape or sexual assault?

15. List four factors that might influence a family member's reaction to the loss of a loved one.

CRITICAL THINKING

● Think back to one of your EMS responses in which there was a fatal injury. What grief reactions did you observe in the patient's family? What stress reactions did you notice in yourself or your coworkers?

● What coping mechanisms do you use to deal with the stress of being an EMS worker?

● Think back to the death of someone in your family. What emotional and physical responses did you experience? What responses did your family experience?

REFERENCES

1. Cannon WB. *The Wisdom of the Body*. New York: WW Norton; 1932.
2. Selye H. *Stress without Distress*. Philadelphia: Lippincott; 1974.
3. Fontana D. *Managing Stress*. New York: British Psychological Society; 1989.
4. Burns DD. *The Feeling Good Handbook*. New York: Plume; 1989.
5. Rice PL. *Stress and Health*, 2nd ed. Pacific Grove, Calif: Brooks/Cole; 1992.
6. American Psychiatric Association (APA). *Diagnostic and Statistical Manual of Mental Disorders*. 4th ed. Washington, DC: APA; 1994.
7. Dyregrov A, Mitchell JT. Work with traumatized children—psychological effects and coping strategies. *J Trauma Stress*. 1992; 5:5.
8. Hartsough DM. *Disaster Work and Mental Health: Prevention and Control of Stress among Workers*. Rockville, Md: National Institute of Mental Health; 1987.
9. Hytten K, Hasle A. Fire fighters: a study of stress and coping. *Acta Psychiatr Scand*. 1989; 80:50.
10. McCammon S, et al. Emergency workers' appraisal and coping with traumatic events. *J Trauma Stress*. 1988; 1:353.
11. Mitchell JT, Everly, Jr, GS. The scientific evidence for critical incident stress management services (JEMS) 22(1) 86–93. *J Emerg Med*. 1997; 89.
12. Everly, Jr, GS. *A Clinical Guide to the Treatment of the Human Stress Response*. New York: Plenum; 1989.
13. Mitchell JT. Teaming up against critical incident stress. *Chief Fire Executive*. 1986; 1(1):24.
14. Mitchell JT, Everly, Jr, GS. Critical incident stress debriefing and the prevention of work-related traumatic stress among high-risk occupational groups. In: Everly, Jr, GS, Lating JM, eds. *Psychotraumatology: Key Papers and Core Concepts in Post-Traumatic Stress*. New York: Plenum; 1995.
15. Mitchell JT, Everly, Jr, GS. *Critical Incident Stress Debriefing: An Operations Manual for the Prevention of Traumatic Stress among Emergency Services and Disaster Workers*. Ellicott City, Md: Chevron; 1993.
16. Breznitz S. Stress in Israel. In Selye H. ed. *Selye's Guide to Stress Research*. New York: Van Nostrand Reinhold; 1980.
17. Mitchell, JT. When disaster strikes: the critical incident stress debriefing process. *J Emerg Med Services* (JEMS). 1983; 8(1):36.
18. Mitchell JT, Bray GP. *Emergency Services Stress: Guidelines for Preserving the Health and Careers of Emergency Services Personnel*. Englewood Cliffs, NJ: Prentice-Hall; 1990.
19. Lickel VG. Caring for the caregivers. Presented at the symposium conducted at the meeting of the North Carolina Association of Paramedics; May 1995; Sylva, NC.
20. Young MA. Crisis and stress. Presented at the symposium conducted at the meeting of the National Organization for Victim Assistance; March 1987; Washington, DC.
21. Wolfelt AD. *Death and Grief: A Guide for Clergy*. Muncie, Ind: Accelerated Development; 1988.
22. Mitchell JT, Resnik HL. *Emergency Response to Crisis*. Bowie, Md: JR Brady; 1981.
23. Horowitz MJ, Kaltreider NB. Brief therapy of the stress response syndrome. In: Everly, Jr, GS, Lating JM, eds. *Psychotraumatology: Key Papers and Core Concepts in Post-Traumatic Stress*. New York: Plenum; 1995.
24. Weaver JD. *Disasters: Mental Health Interventions*. Sarasota, Fla: Professional Resource; 1995.
25. SanFilippo CR. Family therapist. Personal communication; July 1996.
26. *Crime in the United States 1996. Uniform Crime Reports*. Washington, DC: Federal Bureau of

Investigation, U.S. Department of Justice; November 19, 1997.

27. Garraputa KM. Victim advocate. Personal communication; July 1996.

28. Gilliland BE, James, RK. *Crisis Intervention Strategies*. Pacific Grove, Calif: Brooks/Cole; 1993.

29. Wolfelt AD. Dispelling five common myths about grief. *Thanatos* 1989; 14:25.

30. Goldstein K. Hospice counselor. Personal communication; July 1996.

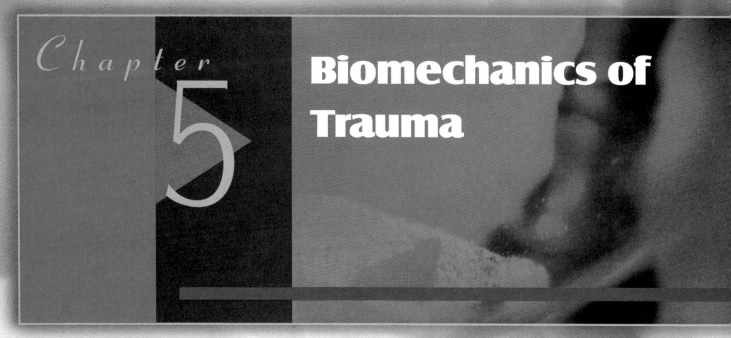

Chapter 5

Biomechanics of Trauma

OBJECTIVES

Upon completion of this chapter, the reader should be able to:

- List the five forms of energy.
- Describe the physical properties of kinetic energy.
- Discuss the role of kinetic energy in producing injury.
- Describe occupant kinematics for the five types of motor vehicle collisions and discuss the clinical implications of each.
- Define the four injury mechanisms of blunt trauma.
- Describe the kinematics of auto-pedestrian collisions.
- Describe the three primary impact configurations of auto-pedestrian collisions and the clinical implications of each.
- Describe the kinematics of motorcycle collisions.
- Describe the four impact configurations of motorcycle collisions and the clinical implications of each.
- Discuss the six components of wound ballistics and their clinical implications.
- List and describe the four types of blast injuries and their clinical implications.
- Define the role of injury biomechanics in the assessment of the trauma patient.

KEY TERMS

Blast wave	Penetrating trauma
Blunt trauma	Permanent cavitation
Compression	Shear strain
Down-and-under pathway	Spalling
Human tolerance	Temporary cavitation
Injury biomechanics	Tensile strain
Kinematics	Torsion
Kinetic energy	Up-and-over pathway

Unexpected traumatic injuries are a significant cause of death in the United States.[1] As with any patient, treatment of the traumatized patient begins with the scene survey and physical assessment. Unlike examining the medical patient where the paramedic has several tools available to assist in the diagnosis, such as blood glucose analyzers and 12-lead electrocardiograms, assessment of the trauma patient relies more on elementary physical examination skills and a suspicion of injury. It is this last assessment skill, suspicion of injury, that requires a thorough understanding of injury biomechanics.

The challenge in managing the trauma patient is pinpointing occult injuries. A patient may suffer from severe and life-threatening injuries, yet exhibit few, if any, external indications of trauma. Consequently, it is incumbent on the paramedic to suspect injuries even in the absence of physical signs. Fortunately, rapidly surveying the scene and obtaining an accurate history will permit the paramedic to predict more than 90% of the patient's injuries *prior* to performing a physical examination.[2]

As discussed in Chapter 2, an injury has three distinct phases: preevent, event, and postevent. A complete history of the trauma patient should include a preevent history. The preevent history includes preexisting medical conditions, alcohol ingestion, or details of events immediately prior to the injury. The information gained from the preevent history may ultimately lead to a definitive diagnosis of injury or prepare those caring for the patient for serious complications. For example, it is easy to see how the treatment of a trauma patient would be altered if the preevent history indicated that the patient suffered from hemophilia. Similarly, if there are no skid marks evident at the scene of a motor vehicle collision (MVC) and the patient has no recall of events immediately prior to the collision, the paramedic should assume that the patient was unconscious prior to the collision. The paramedic should then suspect the patient suffers from medical conditions, such as syncope or hypoglycemia, in addition to any traumatic injuries.

The second phase of injury, and probably the most important in terms of what injuries the patient receives, is the event phase. In the setting of the MVC, this phase begins with the initial contact of the vehicle with some other object. As the vehicle strikes the object, the front of the vehicle begins to deform and decelerate. Simultaneously, the vehicle's occupant is subjected to deceleration forces as he or she impacts the car's interior and sustains injury. Rarely is the paramedic able to witness the collision(s) of occupants with the vehicle's interior. Instead, the paramedic must rely upon the physical evidence that remains after the MVC to suggest specific bodily collisions and the possibility of injury. During the final phase of injury, the postevent, the paramedic observes this evidence and uti-

lizes it in patient management. This process of examining the scene to determine potential injuries that result from the forces of motion is called **kinematics**. Investigations into the physical responses of impact injury are known as injury biomechanics. The principles of kinematics and **injury biomechanics** are the foundations of trauma patient assessment and the focus of this chapter.

ENERGY

The origin of injury is the release of physical energy into human tissue. Healthy human tissue can withstand a certain amount of energy without evidence of injury. This characteristic of human tissue is known as **human tolerance**. Injuries occur when the forces of physical energy exceed human tolerance. The factors that determine whether an injury will occur include the physical condition of the patient, the magnitude of the energy released, and the form of the energy. The five forms of energy that are capable of producing injury are

- Kinetic
- Electrical
- Chemical
- Thermal
- Radiation

Of these, kinetic injury is by far the most common and will be the focus of this chapter. Injuries associated with thermal energy are covered in Chapter 17, and electrical, chemical, and radiation injuries are topics of Chapter 23.

PHYSICAL PROPERTIES

During the scene survey, the paramedic is evaluating physical evidence, such as deformity to the front end of a car involved in an MVC, to identify the injuries that may have resulted from the forces of kinetic energy. Consequently, a working knowledge of the relevant physical laws of motion is helpful.

Newton's Laws of Motion

Sir Isaac Newton, an English physicist and mathematician, formulated the basic concepts and laws of mechanics in the late 1600s. Of his many contributions to science, the most important for injury biomechanics are his laws of motion, of which there are three interrelated physical laws. Newton's first law of motion deals with inertia, or the tendency of objects in motion to remain in motion. Newton's first law is formally stated as follows: An object at rest will remain at rest and an object in motion in a straight line will maintain that motion unless acted upon by some external force. Consider the example of an automobile traveling in a straight line on a highway at 60 miles per hour (mph). Ignoring the influence of friction, this vehicle will continue traveling in a straight line at 60 mph until another force is conveyed to the vehicle. These forces may be the forces of turning, braking, skidding, accelerating, or impacting with another object, which brings the vehicle to a stop. It is also important to note that Newton's first law of motion also applies to the occupants of the vehicle; that is, the occupants will continue traveling in a straight line and at uniform speed until acted upon by some outside force. This concept will be fully explored in a later section.

Newton's second law of motion states: The acceleration of an object is directly proportional to the force acting on it and inversely proportional to its mass. This law formally states what we have all observed in daily living: Ignoring friction, it is more difficult to move large stationary objects than smaller ones. Returning to the example of the automobile striking a stationary object, if the object is relatively small in mass, such as a pedestrian, there will be a great increase in the acceleration of the pedestrian. Conversely, if the struck object is large in mass, such as a truck, there will be little acceleration of the truck.

Newton's second law also relates acceleration of objects to the magnitude of the forces applied. If the mass of an object is held constant, applying more force to the object will increase its acceleration. In the previous example of a motor vehicle–pedestrian collision, the pedestrian struck at higher speeds (i.e., higher force) receives greater acceleration than if struck at lower speeds. Newton's second law, as it applies to trauma, explains why injuries are more likely to occur during collisions involving large objects and/or high speeds.

The example of the vehicle impacting with an object also illustrates another important physical property, Newton's third law of motion, which states: For every action, there is an equal and opposite reaction.

In our example of the vehicle impacting another object, such as a bridge abutment, the forces generated by the vehicle against the bridge abutment are equaled by the forces of the bridge abutment against the vehicle. This law also applies to the unrestrained occupant of the vehicle whose chest collides with the steering wheel at 60 mph. The force of the occupant's chest against the steering wheel is equaled by the force of the steering wheel against the chest.

Force

To acquire an appreciation of the magnitude of the forces that produce injury, a system of measurement is necessary. Force is calculated as $F = ma$, where m is the mass of an object and a is its acceleration. Consider the patient injured in a fall. Ignoring the height of the fall for a moment, the force of the fall can be calculated by multiplying the patient's mass by his or her acceleration. In this example, acceleration is the change in velocity due to gravity, or 9.8 meters per second squared (m/s²). Assuming the patient's mass is 70 kg, the force with which the patient strikes the ground is

$$F = ma$$

$$F = 70 \text{ kg} \times 9.8 \text{ m/s}^2 = 686 \text{ kg/m/s}^2$$

The units of kg/m/s² is also referred to as newtons (N). In the United States, we traditionally refer to forces in terms of gravitational forces, or g forces. Gravitational forces can be approximated by the equation

$$g \text{ forces} = \frac{(\text{mph velocity change})^2}{30 \times (\text{feet of stopping distance})}$$

Velocity is a vector quantity, meaning it has both direction and magnitude. Because we are not concerned with the direction of accelerative forces, we will assume that velocity and speed, a directionless, or scalar, quantity, are equivalent. Later, we will use this equation in calculating the forces to which the human body is exposed during MVCs.

Law of Conservation of Energy

The final physical law that the paramedic should be familiar with is the law of conservation of energy. This principle states that energy is neither created nor destroyed but can only be changed in form. This principle simply states that any form of energy cannot be concocted from anything other than one of the other five forms of energy. In addition, energy is never destroyed, although it can be changed in form or transferred from one body to another. As we will later see, this law accounts for traumatic injuries resulting from the transfer of energy into the human body.

Kinetic Energy

Kinetic energy, or the energy of motion, is the form of energy most often encountered in traumatic injuries. Kinetic energy is a function of an object's mass and velocity and can be calculated by the following equation:

$$\text{Kinetic energy} = 1/2 \times m \times \text{velocity}^2$$

where mass (m) = weight/g = weight/(32.174 ft/s²) and velocity is expressed in feet per second (ft/s). For example, the kinetic energy of a 150-pound occupant of a vehicle traveling at 60 mph is calculated as

$$\text{Kinetic energy} = 1/2 \times \frac{150 \text{ lb}}{32.174 \text{ ft/s}^2} \times (60 \text{ mph} \times 1.467 \text{ ft/s})^2$$

$$= 1/2 \times 4.66 \text{ lb/ft/s}^2 \times (88.02 \text{ ft/s})^2 = 18,060 \text{ ft-lb}$$

As this example portrays, the occupant of a vehicle traveling at 60 mph has 18,060 ft-lb of energy to either convert to another form or transfer when he or she stops. Though kinetic energy is a function of both mass and velocity, velocity has a much more important role in determining total kinetic energy. Table 5-1 illustrates the relationship among kinetic energy, mass, and velocity. If the occupant in our example were 10 pounds lighter (a reduction in weight of 6.67%), his mass is also decreased. The effect of a 6.67% reduction in weight is a 6.67% reduction in kinetic energy if velocity is unchanged. This relationship holds true for a further 10-pound reduction in weight. However, if we hold the occupant's weight constant and alter the velocity, we get a much different result. As shown in Table 5-1, for a 150-pound occupant, increasing velocity from 60 to 70 mph (a 16.67% increase in velocity) increases kinetic energy by 36.11%. The reason for this unequal increase is that the velocity term in the equation is squared. Therefore, we can state that every percentage point increase in mass results in an equivalent increase in kinetic energy, but increases in velocity result in disproportionate increases in kinetic energy. This fact accounts for the increased likelihood of serious injury from high-speed collisions.

ENERGY TRANSFER

As previously stated, energy cannot be destroyed but can only be transferred or changed in form. This concept is readily apparent in trauma. Unrestrained passengers of automobiles undergo the same stopping forces as the vehicle, often resulting in serious injury. Similarly, victims of gunshot wounds receive the kinetic energy of the bullet as it traverses the body. In both of these examples the laws of physics are at work. In neither case is there a destruction of energy. It is changed in form, such as the thermal energy created from the friction of skidding tires or mechanical energy created from the deformity of the colliding vehicle. Alternatively, or in conjunction with changing its form, energy is transferred to the human body by the steering wheel (blunt trauma) or bullet (penetrating trauma).

Any transfer of energy has the potential to produce injury. Whether an injury is produced is dependent on factors such as the magnitude and duration of the forces applied, the areas of the body being subjected to those forces, and the tolerance of the human body. As described in Chapter 2, one goal of injury prevention is to develop methods to avoid the transfer of energy, such as MVCs and gunshot blasts. Despite the success of injury preventionists in reducing the incidence of these events, a certain number of events are inevitable in our present society. Consequently, efforts are also made toward reducing the energy transfer to trauma victims during these inevitable collisions. To that end, much has been accomplished in the field of safety engineering to limit the traumatic forces transferred to occupants during MVCs. Such accomplishments include passive restraints, "crushable" front ends, and padded car interiors. As will be seen in a later section, the intent of these safety features is the same—to limit the transfer of energy to car passengers during a collision to levels within the limits of human tolerance.

BLUNT TRAUMA

Blunt trauma is a nonpenetrating injury that occurs as a result of forces being applied to the body. The most common causes of blunt trauma are MVCs, pedestrian-automobile collisions, motorcycle collisions, falls, and

Table 5-1
Relationship Among Kinetic Energy, Mass, and Velocity

Weight (lb)	% Change in Weight	Velocity (mph)	% Change in Velocity	Kinetic Energy (ft-lb)	% Change in Kinetic Energy
130	−13.33	60	0.00	15,652	−13.33
140	−6.67	60	0.00	16,856	−6.67
150	0.00	60	0.00	18,060	0.00
150	0.00	70	16.67	24,582	36.11
150	0.00	80	33.33	32,107	77.78

assaults. The injuries are the result of the forces of compression and strain that exceed human tolerance.

INJURY MECHANISMS

Injuries are the result of deforming tissues beyond human tolerance. In the setting of trauma, a mechanism of injury is a description of the mechanical and physiological changes that result in anatomical or functional damage of tissue.[3] An understanding of the mechanisms of injury is essential because it forms the basis of assessment and management of the trauma patient. In blunt trauma, there are four primary injury mechanisms: tensile strain, shear strain, torsion, and compression. These injury mechanisms are depicted in Figure 5-1.

Tensile Strain

Strain relates to a change in a dimension of an object divided by the original dimension. **Tensile strain** is the term used when the dimension undergoing change is length. Human tissues, such as muscle, arteries, and organs, are prone to breakage if stretched beyond their tensile strength along their longitudinal axes. This type of injury most commonly results in rupture of vasculature, fractures, lacerations, and avulsions. A common example is fracture of the midshaft femur during MVCs. In frontal collisions of motor vehicles, frequently the occupant strikes his or her knee on the dashboard. The force of this collision flows along the longitudinal axis of the femur, causing an increase in its curvature. The curvature increases tensile strain on the anterior surface of the femur and compression on the posterior surface. A midshaft femur fracture results if the inherent strain tolerance is exceeded. This mechanism is illustrated in Figure 5-2. This type of injury is also common to the ribs where compression of the chest wall exerts tensile strain on the outer surfaces of the rib and compressive forces on the inner surfaces.[3] Compressive forces applied to the chest may also injure the aorta through strain mechanisms. Chest compression may cause the aorta to stretch along its axis at points of attachment. If the elongation exceeds the limits of tensile strain, a transverse laceration of the aorta will result.[4] Also, if the chest compression results in a severe increase of the blood pressure within the aorta, the vessel may dilate, producing tensile strain in both the axial and transverse directions.[3] If the aorta is dilated beyond its limits it may rupture or a traumatic aneurysm may result.

Shear Strain

Shear strain results from the application of forces to a tissue from opposing directions. When the human tolerance to shear strain is reached, the tissue will separate. Many injuries that result from blunt trauma can be explained by the mechanism of shear. During chest impact, for example, the aorta continues forward within the chest cavity even after the patient's body has come to rest. This produces shear strain at the aortic arch where the aorta is fixated by the ligamentum arteriosum. The result is an aortic shear injury resulting in transection or traumatic aneurysm. A similar injury mechanism is responsible for injuries to the liver, brain, and duodenum during frontal MVCs.

Torsion

Torsion strain occurs when one end of some tissue is twisted while the other end remains motionless or is twisted in the opposite direction. For example, the boxer who receives a blow to one side of the mandible will receive torsion forces to the spine as his or her head pivots rapidly in the opposite direction. The result may be torsion injuries to the spinal cord or vertebrae. Approximately 40–50% of all rotation injuries to the cervical spine occur at the C1–C2 level and are often fatal.[5]

Compression

Compression is the term used to describe forces applied to tissue in such a way as to increase the tissue's density or decrease its volume. Examples of injuries due to compression are many, with chest and abdominal injuries representing the more severe injuries. Human tolerance of the chest to blunt frontal impact is 20%, meaning that the chest can be compressed by 20% from its original diameter without injury.[6] Compressions of 20–30% result in primarily skeletal injury, but impacts producing compressions approaching 40% are likely to injure thoracic organs. However, injury tolerance to compression decreases as velocity increases. High-velocity impacts can produce lethal chest injuries at compression levels as low as 20%.

As the chest is compressed, internal organs are squeezed between the chest wall and the spinal column. Examples of compression injuries to the chest include pneumothorax, myocardial contusion, pericardial tamponade, and vascular injuries. Other examples of compression injuries include rupture of abdominal viscera, compression fractures of the spine, and crush injuries to extremities.

MOTOR VEHICLE COLLISIONS

Motor vehicle collisions are the most common form of blunt trauma, followed by pedestrian-MVCs. Because

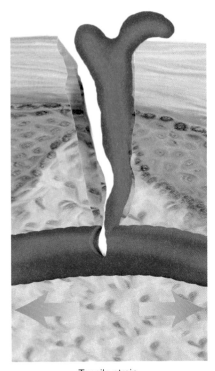

Tensile strain

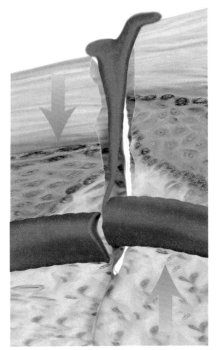

Shear strain

Pseudo-aneurysm   Hemorrhage

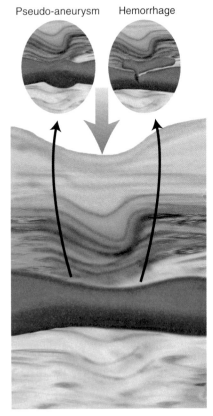

Compression

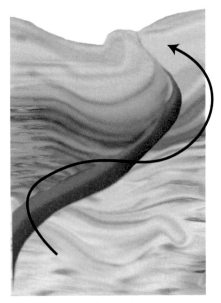

Torsion strain

FIGURE 5-1 Injury mechanisms of blunt trauma.

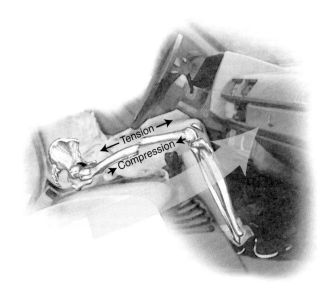

FIGURE 5-2 Midshaft femur fracture resulting from tensile strain and compression.

of the high incidence of MVCs, it is important for the paramedic to be familiar with the injury mechanisms associated with MVCs.

General Crash Statistics

Alcohol is a prominent factor in MVCs. Alcohol is involved in 20% of crashes that result in serious injury, 50% of all fatal crashes, and 60% of all single-vehicle fatal crashes.[7] Not only does alcohol impair the skills of the driver, it also decreases human tolerance to injury and the postinjury immune response.

Other factors play an important role in MVCs, including age, restraint systems, and automotive design. A higher incidence of fatalities from MVCs has been found in certain age groups, particularly in the 15–24-year-old category.[8] The use of alcohol and other drugs, high speed, lack of driving experience, and poor compliance with seat belt laws have been cited as contributing factors to the high fatality rate in this age group.[7] Mortality rates are also higher among older drivers due to the effects of aging that decrease impact tolerance.

Many advances in automotive safety design, such as restraint systems, have reduced the incidence of death and serious injury in MVCs. Fatality rates for MVCs are expected to decline as legislation is enacted mandating the use of these restraints.

Table 5-2 provides the relative frequencies of collision types for collisions in which car occupants are killed. Frontal collisions clearly account for the majority of collisions involving fatalities, with lateral collisions accounting for a significant minority of fatalities. This is important for design considerations of safety systems in cars. Restraints and air bags provide protection primarily for frontal collisions. Only recently have side-impact air bags appeared in vehicles. Even in vehicles equipped with side-impact air bags, it is difficult to provide protection for occupants involved in lateral collisions due to the limited distance between the occupant and the impacting vehicle.

While speed is an important factor in determining kinetic energy and g forces of collisions, significant injuries and even fatalities occur at seemingly low speeds. The majority of MVC fatalities occur with velocity changes of approximately 30 mph.[9] Consequently, automobiles are designed for collisions with velocity changes of 30 mph.

Physics of Motor Vehicle Collisions

Injuries and fatalities resulting from MVCs are due to the transfer of kinetic energy to vehicle occupants. During the collision, kinetic energy is released and converted into heat, sound, and deformity of the vehicle and occupants. The more of this energy converted into deformity of the occupants, the greater the risk of injury.

During a collision, vehicle occupants are subjected to three separate collisions: (1) initial collision of the vehicle, (2) impact of the occupant with the vehicle's interior, and (3) impact of the occupant's organs inside the body. Using the equation for gravitational forces, we can calculate the g force to which the vehicle is subjected (collision 1). During frontal collisions with a velocity change of 30 mph, modern vehicles are designed to provide approximately 2 feet of "crush" in the front end of the vehicle. This 2 feet of crush is essentially 2 feet of

Table 5-2	
Frequency of Collision Types for Car Occupant Fatalities	
Collision Type	**Percentage**
Frontal	48.1%
Lateral	27.5%
Rear	34.0%
Rollover	14.3%
Other	12.0%
Unknown	5.5%

Source: Adapted from "Crash Injury Statistics, Kinematics, and Some History Relating to Impact Biomechanics," by M. M. MacKay, presented at conference, Injury Biomechanics and Emergency Medicine: A Key to Traffic Injury Control, May 10–11, 1992, McLean, VA.

stopping distance for the vehicle. Consequently, the vehicle is subjected to the following *g* force:

$$g \text{ forces} = \frac{(30 \text{ mph velocity change})^2}{30 \times (2 \text{ ft of stopping distance})}$$

$$= \frac{900}{60} = 15g$$

An approximate rule of thumb is that 1 inch of crush equates to 1 mph of impact velocity. In a 30-mph collision with 2 feet of crush, the vehicle undergoes an average deceleration of 15*g*. However, the decelerations are not uniform over the entire stopping distance, and peak values are typically in the 18*g* to 28*g* range.

The human tolerance to injury is about 15*g*. Injury is likely at 30*g* and inevitable at 45*g*. A restrained occupant will undergo the same deceleration force in a 30-mph collision as the vehicle, roughly 15*g*, which is within the range of human tolerance. This is because the restrained occupant is coupled to the vehicle allowing the kinetic energy to be absorbed by the vehicle's front end as it deforms—a concept known as "riding down" the crush of the vehicle.

However, problems arise for the unrestrained occupant. During a frontal collision, for example, the passenger compartment begins to decelerate but the unrestrained driver continues forward at his or her initial 30-mph velocity. Eventually, he or she will impact various structures within the vehicle's interior that are now traveling at much slower velocities than the occupant. Impacts between the occupant and the vehicle's interior constitute the second phase of collision and result in high *g* forces being applied to the occupant. This is because the occupant, by virtue of being unrestrained, is not allowed to ride down the vehicle's crush. Instead, his or her velocity is reduced only by the impact with the vehicle's interior, resulting in a much shorter stopping distance and, consequently, higher *g* forces. Table 5-3 depicts typical *g* forces applied to various body structures during 30-mph collisions. The *g* forces in Table 5-3 do not exactly match

those calculated by the gravitational forces equation. This is because there is some residual forward motion of the vehicle's interior at the instant of collision by the occupant, and the resulting velocity change is not the entire 30-mph initial velocity. As can be seen in Table 5-3, unrestrained occupants are subjected to collisions and *g* forces that are unsurvivable even in crashes with velocity changes of only 30 mph. These same crashes, however, are survivable for occupants wearing safety restraints.

The third phase of collision occurs after the vehicle and the occupant's body have come to rest. Internally, organs continue forward at their initial velocity until tethered by their attachments or until they impact the wall of the cavity within which they reside. This third phase of impact subjects internal organs to the injury mechanisms of shear, compression, torsion, and tensile strain. The brain, lungs, heart, great vessels, and abdominal organs are particularly susceptible to these destructive forces.

Change of Speed Injuries

Differences in speed between a vehicle and its occupants, and differences in speed of tissues within the human body itself, can result in injuries during an MVC. In the next section, specific change of speed injuries are discussed.

Extremity Injuries. During the frontal MVC, the passenger compartment of the vehicle begins to slow and energy is released as the front of the vehicle begins to deform. During this time the passenger compartment begins to decelerate. The occupant, however, continues at his or her initial velocity and begins to sequentially strike portions of the vehicle's interior, beginning with the feet impacting the floor pan followed by the knees impacting the dashboard. These collisions occur early in the crash phase so that their localized contact velocity is relatively low because the floor pan and instrument panel are still moving forward

Table 5-3
Local Deceleration Forces of an Unrestrained Occupant During a 30-mph Collision

	Knee to Dashboard	Chest to Steering Wheel	Head to Windshield	Head to Windshield Header
Contact velocity (ft/s)	34	41	44	44
Local crush (in.)	3	4	5	0.5
Local deceleration (*g*)	72	78	72	721

Source: "Kinematics of Vehicle Crashes," by M. MacKay, 1987, *Advances in Trauma, 2,* p. 21, with permission.

with significant velocity. Consequently, the feet and knees are provided some degree of ride down of the remaining crush of the front of the vehicle. However, if the initial velocity of the vehicle was high, the remaining ride down will not protect the occupant from fractures to the ankles, leg, femur, or pelvic girdle. The force of the knee/dashboard impact is transmitted along the femur, which may result in a midshaft fracture. These forces are also transmitted into the hip, where a posterior hip dislocation may result. The result is the classic triad of the knee-femur-hip injury associated with frontal collisions.

While air bags have prevented many deaths and serious injuries due to chest and head trauma, there has been an increase in serious injuries to the lower extremities. However, it is not likely that air bags are responsible for these injuries. Instead, lower extremity injuries were always a problem but were inconsequential because passengers died of head and chest injuries. Only now that air bags increase the likelihood of surviving crashes are lower extremity injuries of significant concern.

Chest and Abdominal Injuries. The chest contacts the interior of the vehicle later in the crash sequence than do the lower extremities. By this time the vehicle has nearly come to rest, resulting in the loss of ride down and the application of high g forces to the chest. In addition to the forward movement of the patient toward the steering wheel, the steering wheel may be displaced rearward by the collision. Regulations limit the allowable rearward displacement of the steering wheel to 5 inches in the horizontal plane. Even so, chest impacts with the steering wheel are likely even for restrained occupants. If the impact is centered on the anterior chest, the sternum will receive the initial transfer of kinetic energy. The third phase of the collision occurs as the thoracic organs impact the now stationary chest wall or are restrained by their attachments, producing shear injury.

During the impact with the steering wheel, compressive forces are transmitted throughout the chest cavity. With sufficiently high forces, myocardial contusion, pericardial tamponade, or myocardial rupture may result. The lungs are also prone to an injury known as the "paper bag syndrome."[2] As the driver recognizes that a collision is imminent, he or she instinctively takes a deep breath and holds it against a closed glottis, isolating the lungs from the atmosphere. Upon impact, the lungs rupture similar to bursting an inflated paper bag.

The abdominal organs are also subject to the compressive forces of impact with the steering wheel. Once the occupant impacts the steering wheel and comes to rest, the abdominal organs continue forward, causing tears at their points of attachment to the abdominal wall. Organs that shear in this manner are

the intestines, spleen, liver, and kidneys. The liver is particularly susceptible to shear injury at the ligamentum teres where the liver continues forward over the ligament, resulting in a laceration or total bisection.

The abdominal organs are also prone to herniation through the diaphragm. As pressure increases within the abdominal cavity during impact, organs may be herniated through the diaphragm and into the thoracic cavity. The buildup of excessive pressure may also cause retrograde blood flow from the abdomen into the chest, resulting in injury to the aortic valve.

Head Injuries. During a frontal MVC, the head becomes the leading point of the torso. Typically, the head strikes the windshield later in the collision sequence than the impacts of the feet, knees, and chest. Prior to any collision, the head is normally situated 2 feet from the windshield. This means that, upon impact, the vehicle has come to a complete stop by the time the head contacts the windshield or header. The impact of the head, therefore, is at the full initial velocity of the vehicle. If the head strikes the windshield, the local crush will be approximately 5 inches, producing a contact force of 72g. On the other hand, if the trajectory of the head is higher and strikes the windshield header, local crush will be approximately 1/2 inch, producing 721g of force, clearly a nonsurvivable impact.

As the head strikes the windshield or header, compressive forces may result in skull fractures. However, the most severe injuries result during phase 3 of the collision, as the brain continues forward within the cranial vault until it strikes the interior of the skull. This type of injury is referred to as the coup injury and may produce concussion, contusion, diffuse axonal injury, or intracranial hemorrhage as the result of compression and shear injury. Simultaneously, the opposite side of the brain is injured as bridging vessels between the brain and skull are subjected to shear forces. Injury to the brain on the opposite side of impact is referred to as the contrecoup injury.

Neck Injuries. Because of its bony structure, the skull can absorb a significant amount of force as the head collides with the vehicle's interior. The neck, however, has a much lower injury tolerance. The center of gravity of the head is anterior and superior to its point of attachment with the cervical spine. As Figure 5-3 illustrates, lateral collisions force the body from under the head and the head rotates toward the direction of impact. Simultaneously, the neck flexes laterally toward the impact, resulting in torsion injuries of the cervical spine.

The injury mechanisms to the cervical spine during frontal collisions depend upon the angle at which the head impacts the windshield or header. As Figure 5-4 shows, the spine can be compressed along its

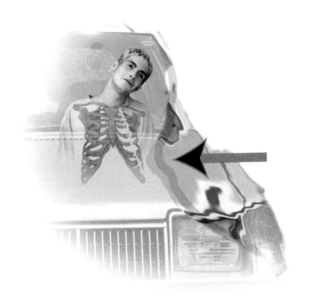

FIGURE 5-3 C-spine injuries resulting from lateral collisions.

Patterns of Injury

Automobile collisions can be divided into five types: (1) frontal impact, (2) rear impact, (3) lateral impact, (4) angular impact, and (5) rollover. Each of these impacts causes different patterns of damage to the vehicle that can be identified during the scene survey. Because the vehicle's occupants are subjected to the same forces as the vehicle, it is possible to look at the vehicle, determine the type of collision, and then predict the likely injuries of the occupants.

INTERNET ACTIVITIES

Review the different types of crash test dummies at http://www.hwysafety.org/safety-facts.

Frontal Impacts. Frontal impacts are the most common type of MVCs. Upon impact, the vehicle rapidly decelerates. As we have seen, the same deceleration forces are applied to the vehicle's unrestrained occupants. There are two possible paths the occupant may take upon impact during a frontal collision: "down and under" or "up and over."[2]

In the **down-and-under pathway**, the occupant continues to move forward as he or she slides under the steering wheel and impacts the floor pan and dashboard with the feet and knees, respectively. This pathway is also referred to as "submarining" and is illustrated in Figure 5-6. As the feet impact the floor pan, the forces generated may exceed human tolerance,

longitudinal axis or forced into hyperextension or hyperflexion, depending on the angle of the windshield and the angle of the head's trajectory. Hyperextension injuries are common in rear collisions, particularly in vehicles with improperly positioned head rests. As Figure 5-5 illustrates, a headrest positioned too low will act as a fulcrum and hyperextend the cervical spine.

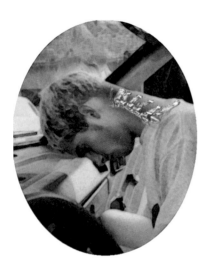

A. Hyperflexion

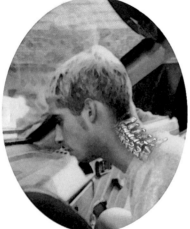

B. Axial Loading

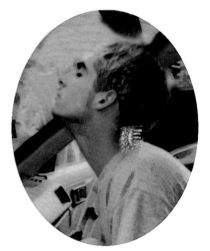

C. Hyperextension

FIGURE 5-4 The angle of head impact determines the mechanism of cervical spine injuries.

femur, resulting in the classic knee-femur-hip injury pattern (Figure 5-7). Therefore, the paramedic should always inspect the vehicle interior for evidence of occupant-vehicle collisions with the dashboard and other structures.

After the occupant collides with the floor pan and dashboard, the upper torso rotates forward into the steering wheel, dashboard, and windshield. This second phase of the down-and-under pathway is the same as the up-and-over sequence.

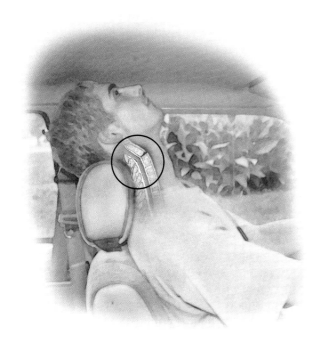

FIGURE 5-5 Improperly positioned headrests function as fulcrums in rear collisions.

resulting in fractures to the ankles, tibia, and fibula. As the knees impact the dashboard, part of the energy will be transmitted to the vehicle in the form of deformity to the dashboard. The energy not absorbed by dashboard deformity will be transmitted to the knee and

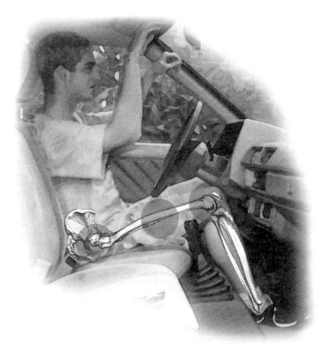

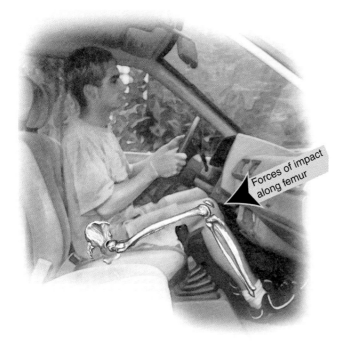

FIGURE 5-6 Down-and-under sequence of frontal collisions.

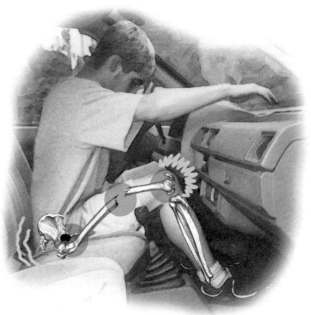

FIGURE 5-7 Classic knee-femur-hip injury of down-and-under collision sequence.

In the **up-and-over pathway**, the occupant's torso continues to move forward, traveling over the steering wheel. The chest and abdomen impact the steering wheel, resulting in compression and shear injuries to the abdominal and thoracic organs. The impact of the torso is followed by the impact of the head with the windshield or header, resulting in head and neck trauma. The up-and-over pathway is shown in Figure 5-8.

Rear Impacts. Rear impacts result in acceleration instead of deceleration. Nonetheless, the physical properties previously described still apply and the energy transfer is the same as frontal collisions when the struck vehicle is stationary. However, when a slow-moving vehicle is struck from behind, the velocity change is the difference in speed between the two vehicles, as opposed to their sum as in frontal collisions. For example, a vehicle moving at 30 mph is struck from behind by a second vehicle moving at 50 mph. The velocity change of the struck vehicle is (50 − 30 = 20 mph). If the collision was a frontal collision, the velocity change would have been 80 mph, the sum of the speed of both cars.

Upon impact, the struck vehicle is accelerated forward. Because of inertia, the vehicle's occupants lag behind in accelerating, loading the back of the seat in which they are sitting. The result is a hyperflexion injury to the neck known as "whiplash." The vehicle may also be accelerated forward into another object, resulting in a secondary frontal collision.

Lateral Impacts. Collisions in which occupants receive injuries from the side structures of the vehicle account for almost 25% of all crashes involving fatalities and serious injury.[7] Occupants on the struck side are subjected to forces applied at the level of the pelvis and chest. In addition to these direct forces, the head may flex laterally and extend through the side window and impact the hood of the striking vehicle, resulting in head and cervical spine injuries.

Because of the limited distance between the occupant and the striking vehicle, there is minimal crush and negligible ride down, and the occupant is subjected to the entire velocity of the striking vehicle. This is the mechanism by which side-impact air bags work; they increase the ride down and, thus, the stopping distance, thereby reducing the g force of the impact.

As the chest receives the impact, lateral compression results in rib and clavicle fractures on the struck side. Injuries to the lungs and abdominal organs are also possible, with splenic injuries more likely in drivers and liver injuries in passengers. Extremity injuries are also possible as forces are applied to the pelvis, leg, and arm. Possible injuries from lateral collisions are illustrated in Figure 5-9.

INTERNET ACTIVITIES

Visit the Insurance Institute for Highway Safety Web site at http://www.hwysafety.org/safety-facts/airbags/airbags.htm. Find the section that discusses side-impact airbags. How effective are side impact airbags in reducing head injury? What safety measures should be taken to protect rescuers from injury when operating in a vehicle equipped with these airbags? How will these airbags affect technical rescue and extrication?

Angular Impacts. Angular impacts occur when off-center forces are applied to the front of a vehicle. The resulting collision causes the vehicle to rotate in the direction of the impact. Consequently, the forces applied to occupants are a combination of those found in frontal and lateral collisions. For example, the driver of a vehicle that is struck at the left quarter panel will move in that direction, likely striking the "A" pillar of the car. The injury patterns will be those of both frontal and lateral collisions.

Rollover. Rollover crashes are the most random in terms of specifying collisions, occupant motion, and injury patterns. Most rollover collisions occur off road with the terrain determining the actual characteristics of the collision. This complicates the process of predicting injury patterns of occupants. Fortunately, provided that

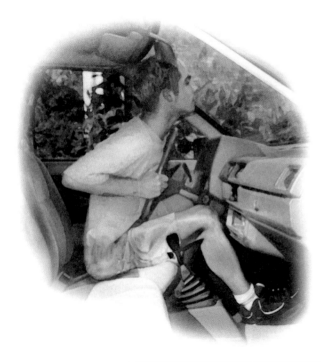

FIGURE 5-8 Up-and-over sequence of frontal collisions.

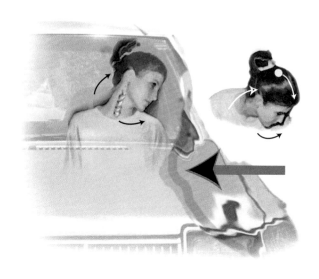

FIGURE 5-9 Injury pattern of lateral collisions.

the occupant remains restrained within the vehicle and is not ejected, rollovers are one of the least injurious crash types. This is because the kinetic energy of the vehicle and its occupants is being dissipated during the many small collisions that occur during the rollover.

Ejection. Ejection from vehicles accounts for 27% of the trauma deaths yearly, and 1 out of 13 ejection victims suffers a spinal injury.[2] While the occupant suffers the same collisions within the vehicle as any other unrestrained occupant, he or she is additionally subjected to the collision with the ground. The collision with the ground may produce injuries more severe than if the victim had remained in the vehicle. This accounts for the fact that ejected occupants are six times more likely to die in an MVC than nonejected occupants.[2]

Restraints

Manufacturers began incorporating safety systems into automobile designs in the early 1960s. Two-point lap belts were required on all new cars in 1966. Unfortunately, seat belt usage was a dismal 20% until the 1980s, when many states enacted mandatory restraint legislation, pushing seat belt compliance to nearly 50%.[7] Passive restraint systems (automatic seat belts or air bags) were mandated later. All 1996 and later models are required to have driver-side air bags, and passenger-side air bags are required in 1998 and later models.

The role of restraints in a frontal collision is to prevent or mitigate the specific contacts between the occupant and the vehicle interior. Upon impact, the vehicle begins to decelerate and the occupant moves forward, loading the seat belt. The seat belt material stretches under this load, allowing the occupant to continue to move forward but, ideally, preventing head and

chest contacts with the vehicle interior. The stretch of the seat belt adds to the occupant's stopping distance so that the occupant's total stopping distance is actually greater than the frontal crush of the vehicle.

In practice, however, most restrained occupants will still impact the dashboard with the knees and the steering wheel with the chest. However, the contacts involve much smaller forces than if the occupant were unrestrained. During the collision, the head of the restrained occupant will also flex forward until the chin impacts the sternum and the head impacts the steering wheel. In vehicles equipped with air bags these secondary collisions are prevented.

Injuries from restraints are also possible, particularly when improperly worn. A properly positioned seat belt is located below the superior iliac spines, above the femur, and is adjusted to fit snugly. When positioned too high, injuries to abdominal organs and upper lumbar and lower thoracic vertebrae are possible. If worn too loosely, the lap belt will not couple the occupant with the vehicle and he or she will be subjected to higher impact forces.

Lap belts should not be worn alone, even when properly positioned. The diagonal shoulder restraint is necessary to prevent head, face, neck, and chest injuries. Air bags, when used in conjunction with lap and shoulder harnesses, provide the best possible protection. However, even when used properly, restraints are still capable of causing injury. The paramedic should assess for fractured clavicles from loads applied by the shoulder harness, evidence of abdominal and chest injury from shoulder and lap belts, and facial injuries resulting from air bag deployment. Occult abdominal injuries have also been reported in passengers protected by air bags.[10] The air bags minimize the typical external signs of abdominal injury, such as bruising and abrasions, even though the passenger has been subjected to severe compression forces to the abdomen. It is possible to identify patients with occult abdominal injuries by lifting the air bag and assessing the steering wheel for damage. A deformed steering wheel should raise the suspicion of occult abdominal injury.

INTERNET ACTIVITIES

Watch the video clips of airbag testing and crash worthiness testing at http://www.hwysafety.org/video/bmwhps.mov.

PEDESTRIAN INJURIES

Injuries from pedestrian collisions with motor vehicles are often fatal.[11] Children are particularly at risk, due to their poorly developed road crossing skills.

One-third of pedestrian fatalities involve children, and the incidence is highest in urban areas.[12]

Pedestrian Kinematics

The laws of motion previously described are equally applicable to pedestrian-motor vehicle collisions (P-MVCs). In addition, two other properties of motion are necessary to fully describe the kinematics of P-MVCs.

Any moving object has the property of momentum. Momentum is the force of continued motion and is defined by an object's mass and velocity:

$$\text{Momentum }(M) = \text{mass }(m) \times \text{velocity }(V)$$

As is apparent in this equation, the momentum of a moving vehicle will be substantially greater than that of a pedestrian because of its larger mass and higher velocity. Upon impact, energy is redistributed between the vehicle and the pedestrian. This change in the momentum of both vehicle and pedestrian is called impulse. Impulse is a function of the energy exchange and the time over which it occurs:

$$\text{Impulse }(I) = \text{force }(F) \times \text{time }(t)$$

During a P-MVC, a very large change in momentum, or impulse, occurs over a very brief period of time. This rapid exchange of momentum explains the magnitude of injuries sustained by pedestrians involved in collisions with motor vehicles.

Injury patterns associated with P-MVC are related to the geometry of the vehicle and the height and position of the pedestrian. The bumper of the vehicle is usually the first point of impact, followed by the grill and hood. Low-speed collisions (less than 12 mph) typically involve a single, primary impact with the pedestrian.[7] Collisions at greater speeds will result in multiple collisions to the pedestrian.

The exact patterns of P-MVC depend on the location of the initial impact relative to the pedestrian's center of gravity (CG). If the initial contact is at the pedestrian's exact CG, he or she will move in the same direction as the striking vehicle (Figure 5-10). This is the pattern seen when adults are struck by large trucks or a small child is struck by a passenger car.

When a pedestrian is struck above the CG, such as a toddler, the pedestrian will rotate in the same direction as travel as the vehicle (Figure 5-11). An additional collision will occur as the child strikes the ground. The child is also at risk for being rolled over by the vehicle's tires or becoming entangled in the vehicle's undercarriage and dragged until the vehicle comes to a stop. In a sense, the child is truly "run over."

In contrast to the small child, taller children and adults are "run under." Because of their heights, these pedestrians are struck below their CG. Following the

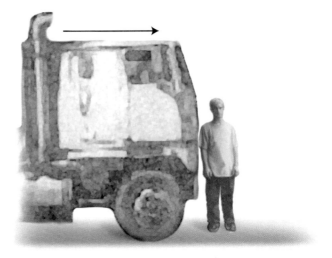

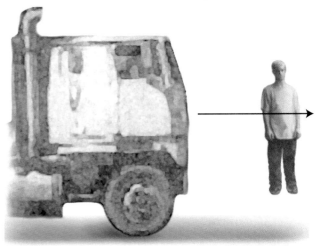

FIGURE 5-10 Initial impact at pedestrian's exact center of gravity.

initial contact, the pedestrian rotates toward the striking vehicle, colliding with other structures of the vehicle such as the hood and windshield. Pedestrians struck below the CG have a more complex sequence of motions that can be described by the sequence of the impacts (Figure 5-12).[7]

Primary Impact. The primary impact is from the vehicle's bumper and strikes the pedestrian at or below the knee. This initial collision starts the pedestrian rotating toward the oncoming vehicle with the head as the leading point.

Secondary Impact. As the pedestrian's head continues to rotate toward the oncoming vehicle, his or her legs are rotating in the opposite direction. The pedestrian's hip collides with the vehicle's grill. The height of the vehicle's bumper and grill along with the angle formed between them is called the "profile" of

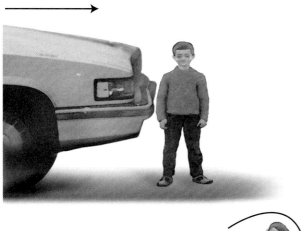

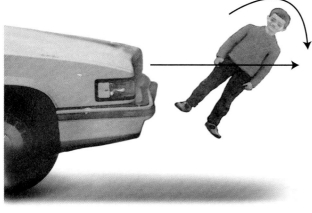

FIGURE 5-11 Initial impact above the pedestrian's center of gravity.

the vehicle. The profile acts as the center of rotation for the pedestrian and determines how he or she will rotate toward other portions of the vehicle.

Tertiary Impact. The pedestrian's head and chest continue to rotate in an arc toward the hood and windshield of the vehicle. Whether the head hits the hood, windshield, or pillars depends upon the height of the pedestrian and the profile of the vehicle. Collisions with these structures are referred to as tertiary impacts.

Quaternary Impact. The final P-MVC impact, the quaternary impact, depends on the speed of the vehicle. At lower speeds, the pedestrian will come to rest on the hood of the vehicle. Typically, the driver of the vehicle has instinctively applied hard braking. As the vehicle comes to a stop, the pedestrian is launched forward, striking the ground.

Alternatively, high-speed collisions will rotate the pedestrian over the hood and roof. The pedestrian will ultimately strike the ground some distance in front of the stopped vehicle. This distance is called the "throw distance" and provides some indication of the impulse sustained by the pedestrian.

Patterns of Injury

As can be seen from the above discussion, the kinematics of the P-MVC is dependent upon the height of the pedestrian. Consequently, the injuries sustained in a P-MVC are determined by pedestrian height. Therefore, injury patterns can be conveniently grouped into age categories, recognizing that the injuries are directly related not to the age of the pedestrian but to his or her height. Children large for their age can be expected to have injury patterns typically associated with older children or adults.

Toddlers. Impacts involving toddlers typically occur above their CG. The anatomical areas most likely incurring the initial blow are the head and chest. Consequently, mortality is high in this age group. In addition to head and chest trauma, toddlers are at risk for injuries resulting from severe impacts with the ground and undercarriage of the vehicle as well as burns from contact with the vehicle's exhaust system. Because of the variation in collisions that may result in this age group, it is difficult to accurately predict injury patterns.

Children. Because of the rapid growth spurts of children, their injury patterns vary between those of toddlers and adults, owing to the large variation in heights. Because children, in general, are shorter than adults, they receive initial impacts higher on the body than adults. Whereas adults are usually struck on the lower extremities, children typically receive initial contact with the femur or pelvis. Depending on the height of the child, he or she may rotate forward, striking the hood similar to an adult, or may rotate under the vehicle. In addition, children are known to turn and face the oncoming vehicle, as opposed to adults who attempt to retreat from the oncoming vehicle. Consequently, collisions with children are usually frontal, with lateral collisions being more common in adults.

Adults. Because most adults are struck below their CG, their injury patterns are much more predictable. The motions of adults following P-MVC are more consistent and well defined than in children. Head, pelvic, and lower extremity injuries are common in adults owing to their initial collisions below the CG. Head injury is responsible for the majority of pedestrian fatalities involving adults. Lower extremity injuries are also quite common. Chest injuries are less common but contribute to higher mortality rates when present.[13]

MOTORCYCLE COLLISIONS

Motorcycle collisions result in fatalities at a rate 20 times greater than passenger cars.[14] Of the collisions

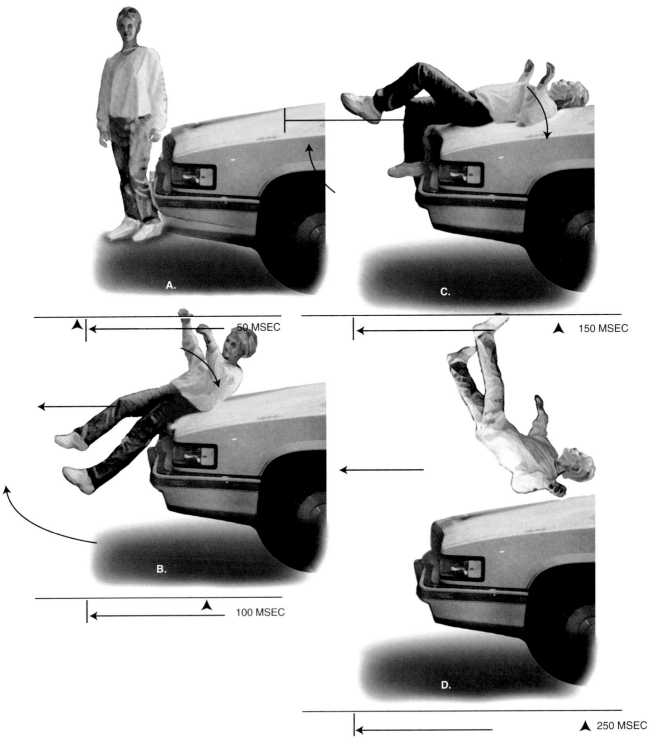

FIGURE 5-12 Initial impact below the pedestrian's center of gravity.

involving motorcycles, 65% involve other vehicles. These troubling statistics come as no surprise given the lack of rider protection during collisions. Aside from helmets, little protection is afforded the rider. Nonetheless, helmet use has a dramatic impact upon reducing motorcyclist mortality. Even so, helmet laws exist in only 26 states.[14]

Rider Kinematics

Unlike the MVC involving a passenger car, the motorcyclist is afforded little protection by his or her bike during a collision. There is no way of coupling the rider to the motorcycle and allowing the motorcycle to absorb the energy of impact. Consequently, the rider is subjected to the full forces of impact, which tend to be quite high.

Upon initial impact of the motorcycle, the rider is ejected over the handlebars, eventually contacting the ground or other object at high velocity. Following these first two phases of the collision, the rider's internal organs strike the walls of the cavity within which they reside or are restrained by their points of attachment. In either case, they are subjected to high forces of compression and strain. The manner in which these forces are applied and the injuries they create vary according to the type of collision.

Frontal Impacts

Upon initial impact with a solid object, such as another vehicle, the motorcycle rapidly decelerates. Because the motorcycle's CG is above and behind the front axle, the front axle acts as a pivot point and the bike rotates forward. As the bike rotates, the rider is pitched forward, sliding across the fuel tank until his or her legs strike the handlebars. During this forward movement, the rider is likely to incur injuries to the groin and pelvis, and fractured femurs. The rider's torso continues forward, up and over the handlebars, eventually striking the head and chest against the other vehicle or ground. With each of these collisions, there are subsequent collisions of organs within the body and the potential for significant injury. If there is a passenger on the motorcycle, the driver is additionally subjected to impacts from behind by the passenger. Using the equation for kinetic energy, it can be seen that a 150-pound passenger would exert over 18,000 ft-lb of energy against the back of the driver in a 60-mph collision.

Angular Impacts

The motorcycle does not decelerate as rapidly during an angular impact as a frontal impact. At angles of less than 60°, the motorcycle and rider "glance off" of the struck object. The rate of deceleration is lower and the bike does not rotate forward. Therefore, the rider tends to remain on the bike longer. However, during the impact the rider's leg is crushed between the bike and the struck object, leading to fractures and crush injuries. Typically, fractures are compound and traumatic amputations are common.

Sliding

Often, the motorcyclist recognizes an impending collision and will attempt to avoid the collision by sliding the bike on its side. The idea is to separate the motorcycle from its rider, preventing the rider from becoming crushed between the bike and another object. This technique also allows the rider to decrease his or her speed over a longer stopping distance and reduce the risk of serious injury. The injuries produced depend on the road surface and the point of contact with the body. These riders typically suffer severe abrasions and fractures but avoid the life-threatening impacts of frontal collisions.

Ejection

Due to the lack of restraints, motorcyclists often are ejected from their bikes and travel over the handlebars at high velocities. Impacts with the ground or other objects occur at relatively high velocities. As in ejection from passenger vehicles, ejection from motorcycles results in serious injuries for the essentially unprotected rider.

FALLS

Victims of falls are subject to the same laws of motion as are victims of MVCs. The height of the fall determines the velocity of the collision, and the landing surface determines the stopping distance. As we have seen in previous sections, velocity and stopping distance determine the energy exchange during a collision and, consequently, the likelihood of injury.

In general, falls are considered severe if they involve heights greater than twice the height of the victim. This is because the victim's impact velocity increases as the height of the fall increases.

In predicting injury patterns, it is important to determine the initial point of impact. Impacts over a larger body surface area tend to disperse the forces of impact. Impacts over smaller anatomical areas, such as the head, concentrate impact forces and are more likely to result in injury. For fall victims who land on their feet, the force of impact is initially transferred to the feet and ankles. Typical injuries include bilateral calcaneus fractures. After the feet stop moving, the force is transmitted up the legs and spinal column, resulting in leg fractures, hip dislocations, and vertebral fractures. Because of the "S" shape of the spine, the lumbar and thoracic vertebrae are particularly susceptible to injury.

If the victim falls onto outstretched arms, posterior shoulder dislocations are likely, as well as Colle's fractures of the radius and ulna, and fractures of the wrist. If the victim lands on the head, as commonly observed in shallow-water diving injuries, the force of the impact travels down the skull and cervical spine. This accounts for the high frequency of skull, brain, and spinal cord injuries associated with diving injuries.

SPORTS INJURIES

Because of the many different sporting activities that may lead to injury, it is difficult to generalize injury patterns. However, the same principles of kinematics apply to sporting injuries. Based upon the survey of the scene, the paramedic should determine what forces were at work, their direction and magnitude, and what areas of the body were contacted. Based upon this initial assessment and a knowledge of kinematics, the paramedic will be able to suspect likely injuries and integrate his or her suspicions into the plan of treatment.

PENETRATING TRAUMA

Injuries that create either a temporary or permanent communication with the atmosphere are referred to as **penetrating trauma**. Blunt trauma is the predominate mechanism of injury across the United States, primarily as a result of MVCs. However, the incidence of penetrating trauma is quickly approaching that of blunt trauma in many urban settings. Three factors account for the increase in deaths resulting from penetrating trauma mechanisms: improvement in motor vehicle safety engineering and adoption of mandatory helmet and seat belt laws, both of which reduce blunt trauma deaths, and the increase in violence (intentional injury) in American society.

The magnitude of the increase in trauma as a result of violence, particularly firearm-related injuries, is astounding.[15] Compared to other developed countries where firearm injuries are much lower, the United States remains the "wild west" of the modern world. Because of the prevalence of intentional injuries, our discussion of penetrating trauma will be limited to knife and gunshot wounds.

GUNSHOT WOUNDS

Firearms are classified as being either low-velocity (projectile velocities of less than 2,000 ft/s) or high-velocity (projectile velocities greater than 2,000 ft/s) weapons. Low-velocity weapons include handguns and some low-powered rifles. High-velocity weapons include higher powered military and hunting rifles.

Firearms are identified by the diameter (caliber) of the bullet they fire. Firearms may be further classified by the projectiles they fire, such as a single projectile (rifles and handguns) or multiple projectiles (shotgun). Figure 5-13 compares the size and shape of projectiles from various calibers of weapons.

Wound Ballistics

Two mechanisms, compression and strain, account for injuries in penetrating trauma. As a bullet impacts the body, the tissue underneath is compressed beyond its tolerance and separates. The severity of the resulting injury is dependent upon the delivered energy, size, and profile of the projectile, and the path of the projectile through the body.

Energy Exchange. Newton's laws of motion apply to penetrating trauma as well as blunt trauma. Once a bullet is fired, its energy is partially transformed into thermal energy due to the friction between the bullet and the surrounding air. The remaining energy is transferred to the gunshot victim upon impact. As the bullet impacts human tissue, kinetic energy is transferred to that tissue. If there is no exit wound, the entire kinetic energy of the bullet was transferred. However, the presence of an exit wound does not mean that less energy was transferred and injuries are less severe. More likely, it indicates that the bullet was fired from a gun with a high muzzle velocity, and consequently, the bullet had enough kinetic energy to pass all the way through its victim. As it did so, it transferred some of its kinetic energy, which may be greater in magnitude than bullets fired from low-powered handguns that do not exit the body.

Weapon Energy The energy of a projectile is related to its mass and velocity upon impact. The bullet of a .357 magnum caliber handgun weighs 140 grains, or 0.02 pound. The muzzle velocity of this weapon is 1,221 ft/s. Assuming the victim is struck at point-blank range, the kinetic energy transferred to the victim is

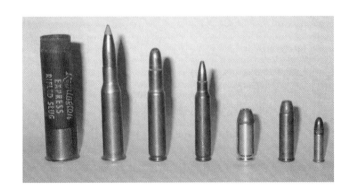

FIGURE 5-13 Comparison of various firearm projectiles.

given by the equation for kinetic energy:

$$\text{Kinetic energy} = 1/2 \times \frac{0.02 \text{ lb}}{32.174 \text{ ft/s}^2} \times (1,221 \text{ ft/s})^2$$
$$= 463 \text{ ft/lb}$$

The caliber and muzzle velocity of weapons, and consequently their kinetic energy, vary considerably. Table 5-4 compares the kinetic energy of various firearms.

Distance Table 5-4 provides the kinetic energy of various weapons at the muzzle. This would be the kinetic energy transferred if the gun were placed directly against the victim. Often, however, the victim is shot from some distance. As it travels through the air, the projectile loses velocity as the result of friction with the surrounding air. Therefore, less kinetic energy is transferred by bullets fired from a distance than those fired at close range.

Tissue Density The amount of energy transfer from a bullet also depends on the density of the tissue that is struck. The more tissue particles struck by the bullet, the greater the energy exchange. Therefore, the density of the tissue determines, in part, the amount of energy transfer. More kinetic energy is transferred by a bullet striking bone, for example, than soft tissue.

Surface Area As previously stated, more energy is exchanged by a bullet when it strikes more tissue particles. In addition to tissue density, the number of particles struck also depends on the surface area struck by the bullet. There are several different ways of increasing the surface area of the impact and, consequently, the energy transfer and potential for injury.

The frontal area, or profile, of a bullet determines the total contact area with tissue upon impact. Bullets made of soft lead tend to expand, or "mushroom," on impact. Some bullets are designed to assume a certain shape upon impact (Figure 5-14). Mushrooming increases the diameter of the bullet and, consequently, its contact area. Larger contact areas mean that more tissue particles are impacted and more energy is transferred to the victim.

Another way to increase the contact area of a bullet is to allow it to tumble as it sails through the air. As seen in Figure 5-15, as the bullet tumbles end over end, its profile is increased, providing a larger contact area upon impact.

The final mechanism for increasing the contact area of a bullet is through fragmentation. To accomplish this, some bullets have hollow centers with a metal jacket around them. These bullets are designed to fragment into numerous smaller projectiles. The effect is that more tissue particles are struck and the damage is spread over a larger area. Shotgun blasts also transfer their destructive force through multiple projectiles. However, many projectiles, or pellets, are fired from a single cartridge and do not fragment on contact. Whether several smaller projectiles are fired at once or a single projectile is fired that fragments into smaller pieces upon impact, the destructive mechanism is the same.

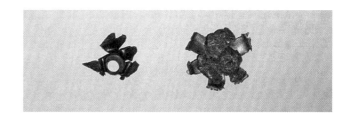

FIGURE 5-14 Some bullets are designed to assume a particular shape on impact.

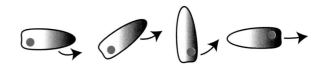

FIGURE 5-15 Bullet tumble increases the contact area of impact.

Table 5-4
Comparison of Kinetic Energy of Various Firearms

	.22 Long Rifle	.38 Special	.30–30	AK-47
Caliber	.22 in.	.358 in.	.30 in.	7.62 mm
Bullet weight (lb)	0.0057	.0200	.0243	.0172
Muzzle velocity (ft/s)	1,280	822	2,017	2,340
Kinetic energy (ft/lb)	145	210	1,536	1,463

Solid bullets may also cause tissue destruction through fragmentation. Instead of the bullet fragmenting, however, structures struck by the bullet, such as bone, may shatter into many pieces and become secondary projectiles.

Cavitation As a bullet passes through human tissue, a large cavity is formed. This cavity is formed of two parts: the temporary cavity and the permanent cavity. **Temporary cavitation** is the result of tissues being stretched by the shock wave produced by the advancing bullet. As the bullet passes by, the tissues recoil but do not return to their original shape. Instead, they leave a smaller residual cavity that is referred to as the **permanent cavity** (Figure 5-16).

The temporary cavity accounts for the serious damage to tissues that lie well out of the path of the bullet. Within the temporary cavity, vascular damage is severe. Smaller leaking vessels allow blood to accumulate within muscle fibers. Larger vessels are usually undamaged due to their elasticity, which allows them to be pushed aside by the expanding shock wave. Nerves, however, sustain extensive damage by the stretching and compression of the temporary cavity. Even though the nerve may not be severed, it will likely be damaged to the point of being rendered nonfunctional.

As the shock wave of the bullet passes, the tissue behind it collapses, leaving the smaller permanent cavity. The size of the permanent cavity is determined by the size of the temporary cavity, which is dependent on the amount of kinetic energy of the bullet. The passing shock wave also creates a negative pressure within the permanent cavity. Because the permanent cavity is connected to the outside atmosphere by the entrance and exit wounds, debris can be pulled into the wound tract by the negative pressure wave, causing contamination.

Ricochet Though entrance and exit wounds provide some indication of the bullet's path, linear relationships do not always exist. It is quite possible for bullets to strike bony structures within the body and ricochet in several directions before actually exiting the body. Furthermore, the bullet may impact a bony structure and fragment, with each fragment in turn striking other bony structures, each assuming a trajectory of its own.

Patterns of Injury

Identifying gunshot injuries as being entrance or exit wounds is quite difficult. While there are medicolegal hazards in identifying entrance and exit wounds in written reports, it is helpful for the paramedic to make an "educated guess" during the patient assessment. With a working assessment of entrance and exit wounds, it is possible for the paramedic to estimate the bullet's trajectory and predict which organs and structures are involved.

An entrance wound lies over tissue that is supported underneath. The entrance wound, therefore, is typically round or oval, owing to the support of the tissue underneath the wound. As the spinning bullet enters the skin, it leaves a small abrasion around the entrance wound. If the bullet was fired at an angle to the tissue it entered, the abrasion will be more pronounced on the side, forming an acute angle with the bullet (Figure 5-17). At close distances, burning gases may produce burns and there may be evidence of "tatooing" from burning cordite.

In contrast, the bullet exits through tissue that lacks any underlying support. Consequently, the wound is much larger and typically takes on a stellate or linear shape.

KNIFE WOUNDS

Knife injuries are considered to be low-energy injuries. However, they can be life threatening. Fortunately, it is easier to predict the underlying organs that are injured in a knife attack by tracing the path of the blade. If the weapon has been removed, examine the width and length of the blade. Also, try to establish the angle of attack, or at least the sex of the assailant. Women tend to stab with downward thrusts, typically inflicting injury to the chest. Men tend to stab with upward thrusts that usually cause abdominal injuries.[2] The paramedic should also consider the movement of the knife within the body. If the blade is twisted after it enters the body, the zone of potential damage is cone shaped (Figure 5-18).

BLAST INJURIES

Blast injuries were first described by Hooker in 1924.[16] Investigation into blast injuries intensified during the 1940s and 1950s, following the increased incidence of blast injuries of World War II. Today, blast injuries remain a threat because of increasing terrorism, military actions, and industrial accidents.

PHYSICS OF BLAST INJURY

Explosions result from the rapid combustion of flammable materials. During the explosion, large amounts of energy are released into the surrounding area in the form of blast waves, blast winds, ground shock, and heat.[17]

The **blast wave** is an impulse of extreme pressure that radiates from the epicenter of the blast. The pressure wave peaks within milliseconds of the blast, followed by a wave of negative pressure. The magnitude of

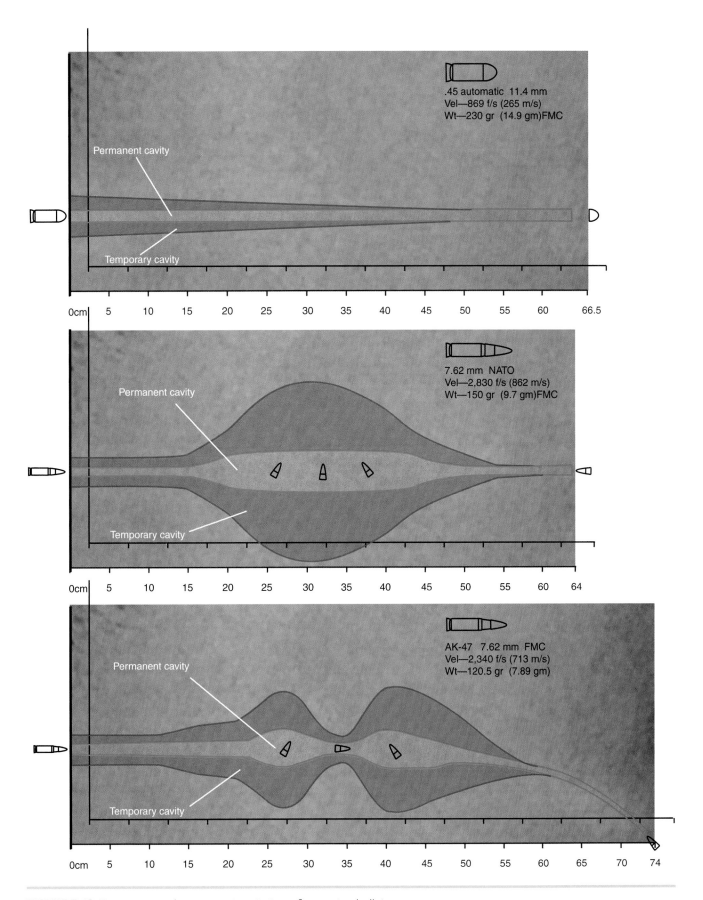

FIGURE 5-16 Temporary and permanent cavitation of a passing bullet.

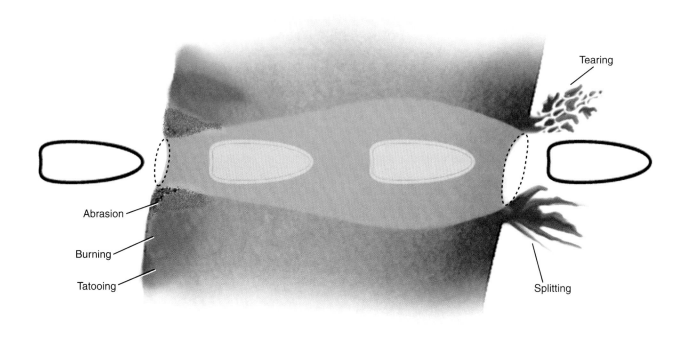

FIGURE 5-17 Identifying entrance and exit wounds. A spinning missile produces a 1 mm to 2 mm abraded edge along the wound if it enters straight. If it enters at an angle, the abraded side is on the bottom of the missile, where there is more contact with the skin, and covers a much wider area.

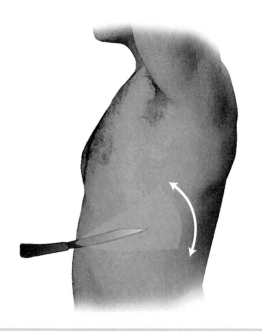

FIGURE 5-18 Twisting of the blade creates a cone-shaped zone of damage.

the pressure wave decreases with distance from the epicenter. Because of its density, water allows blast waves to reach higher peak pressures and be transmitted over greater distances. In both air and water, the initial blast wave and the following wave of negative pressure are implicated in the mechanism of blast injury.

Within the immediate area of an explosion, the pressure of the blast wave is so high that the blast is immediately fatal. Death usually results from disruption of major blood vessels, rupture of major organs, or lethal dysrhythmias secondary to cardiac concussion. Air embolism within coronary or cerebral arteries is also a frequent cause of death.[18] Because of these rapidly fatal injuries near the site of the blast, this area is called the "lethal zone."[17]

The initial explosion produces high-velocity blast winds in the range of 1,000 to 1,500 mph.[19] These winds will cause ground shock capable of producing injury or collapsing buildings that injure the occupants inside.

TYPES OF BLAST INJURIES

There are four types of blast injuries: primary, secondary, tertiary, and blast-associated injury. Primary blast injuries result from the rapid changes in atmospheric pressure from the movement of the blast wave. Hollow organs are much more susceptible to primary blast injury than solid organs. There are two basic mechanisms by which the blast wave causes injury. In the first mechanism, the blast wave rapidly passes through tissues of varying densities. When the wave passes through a tissue of high density that is adjacent to a tissue of lower density, the surface of the tissue of higher density is disrupted. This mechanism of injury is referred to as **spalling**.[19] Spalling is responsible for injuries to hollow organs, such as the lungs. As the wave traverses the walls of the alveoli (high density), they rupture as the wave encounters the air within the alveoli (low density). The result is massive destruction of alveoli and diffuse hemorrhage within the lung.

Implosion is the second mechanism of injury of the blast wave. As the pressure wave passes through the lung, it forces blood out of the vascular space and into the alveoli. The wave of high pressure is then followed by a wave of negative pressure allowing the alveoli to expand rapidly with further tearing of the lung parenchyma, atelectasis, and hemorrhage.

Secondary blast injury results from flying debris created by the explosion and carried by the blast winds. Injuries are typically penetrating in nature and severe due to the high kinetic energy of the projectiles. Small fragments created by an explosion commonly attain speeds of several hundred feet per second. Skin lacerations occur at 50 ft/s and body cavities are penetrated at 400 ft/s.[19]

Tertiary blast injuries occur when the blast winds are of sufficient force that the victim becomes a human missile. Injuries occur when the victim strikes the ground. In addition, the organs within the body undergo another impact within the chest or abdominal cavity. This impact is analogous to the third phase of an MVC.

The final category of injury includes the injuries resulting from the changes within the environment as a consequence of the explosion. These environmental changes include fire, combustion of toxic products, and leaks of toxic chemicals. Injuries, therefore, are diverse and include burns, poisoning, and asphyxiation.

INTERNET ACTIVITIES

Visit the e-medicine Web site at http://www.emedicine.com/. Click on the Emergency Medicine on-line book and select Trauma and Orthopedics. Then, under the heading "penetrating," click on blast injuries. Review the chapter on the kinematics and management of blast injuries.

SUMMARY

Much of the challenge in treating the traumatized patient centers around the difficulty in identifying what are often occult injuries. Seemingly "uninjured" patients may suddenly deteriorate as a result of unrecognized internal injuries. Consequently, it is the responsibility of the paramedic to survey the scene and identify possible mechanisms of injury. Based upon a thorough understanding of the biomechanics of injury, the paramedic will then be able to make the clinical correlation between the scene survey and the potential for injury.

REVIEW QUESTIONS

1. List the five forms of energy.
2. List the five types of motor vehicle collisions.
3. Define human tolerance.
4. State Newton's first, second, and third laws of motion.
5. What is the *g* force of a 45-mph collision with a 36-inch stopping distance?
6. What is the kinetic energy of a 150-pound occupant travelling at 50 mph?
   a. 18,060 ft-lb
   b. 12,536 ft-lb
   c. 11,343 ft-lb
   d. 15,235 ft-lb
7. Energy is neither created nor destroyed but can only be changed in form. This is known as the:
   a. Law of conservation of mass
   b. Law of conservation of momentum
   c. Law of conservation of energy
   d. Law of kinetics
8. Which variable has the greatest effect on kinetic energy?
   a. Velocity
   b. Mass
   c. Stopping distance
   d. Momentum
9. The four mechanisms of injury in blunt trauma are:
   a. Shear, tensile, stretch, twist
   b. Shear, tensile, compression, torsion
   c. Compression, blunt, penetrating, tolerance
   d. Stretch, compression, torsion, strain
10. Collisions of organs within bodily cavities constitute the _____ of an MVC.
    a. First collision
    b. Second collision

c. Third collision
d. Fourth collision

11. Modern vehicles are designed to produce _____ of crush during a 30-mph collision.
a. 18 inches
b. 24 inches
c. 36 inches
d. 48 inches

12. The "paper bag syndrome" refers to a:
a. Pneumothorax
b. Hemothorax
c. Pericardial tamponade
d. Traumatic asphyxia

13. Because of their _____, toddlers are "run over."
a. Small mass
b. High density
c. High center of gravity relative to the vehicle
d. Low center of gravity relative to the vehicle

14. The zone of destruction created by a bullet passing through human tissue is called:
a. Cavitation
b. Fragmentation
c. Tumble
d. Spalling

15. Tissue destruction from an explosion is the result of:
a. High pressure
b. Negative pressure
c. Both a and b
d. Neither a nor b

16. Spalling is an injury mechanism associated with:
a. Primary blast injury
b. Secondary blast injury
c. Tertiary blast injury
d. Blast-associated injury

17. The classic knee-femur-hip injury is associated with:
a. Rear collisions
b. Lateral collisions
c. Up and over
d. Down and under

18. The primary purpose of the crush zone of an automobile is to provide:
a. Ride down
b. Rigid structural protection
c. Both a and b
d. Neither a nor b

19. The path of tissue damage inflicted by a knife assumes the shape of a:
a. Tunnel
b. Sphere
c. Linear wound
d. Cone

20. A typical shear injury of the aorta occurs at the:
a. Ligamentum teres
b. Ligamentum arteriosum
c. Ligament of Treitz
d. Ascending aorta

CRITICAL THINKING

● Using your knowledge of impact biomechanics, describe additional safety features that could be incorporated into automobile design to reduce injury.

● Passenger automobiles are designed to withstand collisions with velocity changes of 30 mph with minimal risk of injury to its occupants. What would be the effect on occupant safety if automobiles were designed to withstand velocity changes of 60 mph?

● Think back to your last response to an MVC in which the automobile sustained a high-speed impact. What was the estimated velocity change? What was the direction of the impact(s)? Were any safety restraints used? Correlate the patient's injuries with the impacts between the patient and the interior of the vehicle.

REFERENCES

1. Centers for Disease Control and Injury Prevention/National Center for Injury Prevention and Control. Top 10 leading causes of death in 1992. Internet: www.cdc.gov/ncipc/osp/10lc92c.html; September 1996.

2. McSwain NE, Paturas JL, Wertz E, eds. *Prehospital Trauma Life Support*. St. Louis, Mo: Mosby Lifeline; 1994.

3. Viano DC, et al. Injury biomechanics research: an essential element in the prevention of trauma. *J Biomech*. 1989; 22:403.

4. Mohan D, Melvin JW: Failure properties of passive human aortic tissue. II-Biaxial tension tests. *J Biomech*. 1983; 16:31.

5. Huelke DF. Anatomy, injury and biomechanics of the cervical spine. Presented at Injury Biomechanics and Emergency Medicine: A Key to Traffic Injury Control; May 10–11, 1992; McLean, Va.

6. Viano DC. Chest: anatomy, types and mechanisms of injury, tolerance criteria and limits, and injury factors. Presented at Injury Biomechanics and Emergency Medicine: A Key to Traffic Injury Control; May 10–11, 1992; McLean, Va.

7. Martinez R, ed. *Applying an Injury Control Model to the Treatment of Motor Vehicle-Related Injuries*.

Dallas, Tex: American College of Emergency Physicians; 1994.

8. U.S. Department of Transportation/National Highway Traffic Safety Administration. Traffic safety facts 1995. Internet: www.nhtsa.dot.gov/ people/ncsa/factshet.html; October 1996.

9. MacKay MM. Biomechanics and the regulation of vehicle crash performance. Presented at Injury Biomechanics and Emergency Medicine: A Key to Traffic Injury Control; May 10–11, 1992; Mclean, Va.

10. Augenstein JS, et al. Occult abdominal injuries to airbag-protected crash victims: a challenge to trauma systems. *J of Trauma.* 1995; 38:502.

11. National Highway Traffic Safety Administration. *Traffic Safety Facts 1992—Pedestrians.* Washington, DC: National Center for Statistics and Analysis, U.S. Department of Transportation; 1993.

12. Malek M, Gayer B, Lescohier I. The epidemiology and prevention of child pedestrian injury. *Accident Analysis and Prevention.* 1990; 22:301.

13. Derlet RW, Silva J, Holcroft J. Pedestrian accidents: adult and pediatric injuries. *J of Emerg Med.* 1989; 7(1):5.

14. U.S. Department of Transportation/National Highway Traffic Safety Administration. Traffic safety facts 1992. Internet: www.nhtsa.dot.gov/ people/injury/pedbimot/rd000028.html; October 1996.

15. Coalition to Stop Gun Violence. The extent of gun violence. Internet: www.gunfree.org; October 1996.

16. Hooker DR. Physiological effects of air concussion. *Am J Physiol.* 1924; 2:219.

17. Magnusson AR, Schriver JA. Mechanisms of injury: pathophysiology of blunt, blast, and penetrating injury of the chest. *Topics Emerg Med.* 1988; 10:1.

18. Benzinger T. Physiological effects of blast in air and water. In: *German Aviation Medicine, World War II.* Washington, DC: U.S. Government Printing Office; 1950.

19. Stapczynski JS. Blast injuries. *Ann Emerg Med.* 1982; 11(12): 687.

Chapter 6

Assessment of the Trauma Patient

OBJECTIVES

Upon completion of this chapter, the reader should be able to:

● Identify the components involved in the scene size up.

● Differentiate between the golden hour and the platinum ten minutes and discuss the importance of each in providing care to the multisystem trauma patient.

● Apply the trauma triage protocols, based on mechanism of injury and physical assessment findings.

● Identify the components of the initial assessment using the acronym ABCDE.

● Acquire systematic approach to performing a physical assessment of the trauma patient.

● Differentiate singular system trauma from multisystem trauma.

● Identify load-and-go patients based on assessment findings.

● Identify conditions requiring immediate definitive field treatment from those requiring treatment once en route to the most appropriate facility.

● Identify and discuss the essential equipment required to handle multisystem trauma patients.

● Identify the components of the focused assessment.

KEY TERMS

CUPS classification system
Decerebrate
Decorticate
Golden hour
Load and go

Multisystem trauma
Platinum ten minutes
Singular system trauma
Stick-em-up position

In the late 1960s, ambulance personnel began to actually treat seriously injured patients in the prehospital setting, and the era of "scoop and swoop" began to disappear. However, many critically injured, multisystem trauma patients received care for injuries that were obvious, but minor, while they died from severe hypoxemia or shock prior to arrival at a medical facility. With the indoctrination of the Advanced Trauma Life Support (ATLS) course for emergency physicians, the scoop-and-swoop form of prehospital care reemerged, but with a new focus: the rapid identification and resuscitation of life-threatening conditions prior to transport that result in compromised airway, breathing, circulation, and neurological status. No longer are these patients "grounded" for long periods of time with field personnel trying to stabilize these injuries prior to transport. The old credo, "stabilize the patient before leaving the scene," which had replaced "scoop and swoop," has been replaced by the battle cry **"load and go."**[1] It is no longer acceptable for the paramedic to delay transportation while attempting to start IVs, auscultate a blood pressure, bandage simple soft tissue wounds, or splint minor fractures when the patient's airway, breathing, circulatory, or neurological status are severely compromised. Our load-and-go patients are those who present with decreased level of consciousness (LOC), compromised airway or difficulty breathing, sucking chest wounds, large flail segments, tension pneumothorax, signs or symptoms of shock, head injury with altered LOC or unequal pupils, indications of abdominal trauma, unstable pelvis, bilateral femur fractures, or a combination of these criteria. In managing load-and-go patients appropriately, we have realized that these patients must be transported to the "most appropriate" medical facility, which may not be the closest medical facility, in order to decrease mortality and morbidity. A fact of considerable significance to emergency medical service providers is that 70% of trauma deaths occur in remote or rural areas where patients are treated at medical facilities unable to appropriately manage their multiplicity of trauma injuries.[1] The paramedic must be able to rapidly, systematically, and correctly identify load-and-go patients and initiate transport to the most appropriate medical facility if survival rates are to increase.

SCENE SIZE UP

The initial observation during the approach to the scene will provide early clues regarding the potential for multisystem trauma. Prearrival information provided by the emergency medical dispatcher (EMD) will often provide patient information that will enable the paramedic to predict what injuries may exist upon arrival. Unfortunately, initial dispatch information is often sketchy due to inadequate information from the person reporting the incident. In any event, try to obtain as much information regarding the scene from the dispatcher as possible so that some prearrival decisions can be made regarding equipment and other backup assistance.

Upon arrival make a quick assessment of the scene. Ascertain if it is safe to proceed into the scene. Determine if there are hazards that will require specialized equipment (e.g., fire apparatus, HAZ-MAT specialists, rescue tools). Call for law enforcement to contain the area prior to entry if needed. Ask the following questions:

- Is there a fire or imminent danger of fire or explosion?
- Are any vehicles carrying hazardous materials?

- Is there danger from oncoming vehicles?
- Are all disabled vehicles out of the way ?
- What is the mood of the bystanders? Do they appear to be hostile or calm and approachable?
- Is the vehicle or structure unstable, requiring special stabilizing equipment prior to approaching the injured patient(s)?[1]

Once the scene has been deemed safe to enter, determine the mechanisms of injury and the kinematics involved in producing the injury (see Chapter 5). Based on the mechanism, determine the injuries that may exist from the appearance of the scene, the patient's position or location, and bystander information obtained. Ask the following questions:

- Are there obvious signs of injury that suggest life-threatening injuries may exist?
- How many patients appear to be involved and are additional personnel, resources, and EMS units needed?
- Do you need to employ triage?

Upon arrival, the paramedic must gather the equipment necessary to provide initial field care to life-threatening injuries. With critically injured patients, precious time is wasted returning to the ambulance several times for equipment. Essential equipment that should be carried to each scene includes:

1. Personal protective equipment (PPE)
2. Long spine board, straps, head-immobilizing device, and cervical-immobilizing device
3. Oxygen (O_2) and airway management equipment [O_2 delivery devices, bag valve mask (BVM), suction device, decompression supplies, intubation equipment]
4. Trauma kit that contains dressing-bandage material, blood pressure cuff, stethoscope, IV equipment and other supplies for trauma care
5. Pneumatic antishock garment (PASG) per local protocol

ASSESSMENT AND MANAGEMENT PRIORITIES

The majority of trauma patients have **singular system trauma**, that is, trauma that does not systemically compromise the patient. Less than 10% of all trauma patients are considered **multisystem trauma**, and therefore, the paramedic must be able to quickly identify these load-and-go patients from those with minor trauma.[2] According to Donald D. Trunkey, the time of death from trauma has a trimodal distribution:[3]

1. Within seconds to minutes

2. Within minutes to hours (golden hour)

3. Within several days or weeks after the initial injury

Therefore, in dealing with multisystem trauma patients, the paramedic identifies and manages life-threatening conditions under specific time constraints. This requires that assessment, diagnosis, stabilization, management, and reassessment be performed rapidly and systematically.

Time is the vital link to patient survival when dealing with a multisystem trauma patient. The **golden hour**, as publicized by the Maryland Institute for Emergency Medical Services, is the accepted standard for these patients. R. Adams Cowley discovered that when the critically injured, multisystem trauma patient is received into surgery within an hour of injury, approximately 85% survive.[4] On-scene time, including assessment, critical interventions, and packaging, should not exceed the **platinum ten minutes**, unless special circumstances dictate otherwise. These special situations include extended disentanglement time and unexpected dangers or hazard occurrence. The average response time from the onset of the incident to the arrival of EMS is 8–9 minutes.[2] Therefore, EMS systems strive for an on-scene time of 5 minutes or less. Response times in rural areas often exceed the 8–9 minute average, which eats deeply into the golden hour. Therefore, the shorter the on-scene time, the sooner the patient receives critical definitive care.

As trauma care has evolved, it has become evident that each patient must be transported to the most appropriate medical facility capable of providing the treatment required, rather than the closest facility. Table 6-1 identifies the mechanisms of injury and physical findings that should prompt the paramedic to apply triage protocols that will meet the objectives of the golden hour and platinum ten minutes.

Therefore, the initial approach is directed toward rapid identification and correction of the following four major areas: airway, breathing, perfusion, and presence or absence of significant external and internal hemorrhage.[6] Trauma patients are not assessed as thoroughly as are medical patients; therefore, the key words are "stabilization" of the most immediate airway, breathing and circulatory problems, and "rapid" transportation.[6]

INTERNET ACTIVITIES

Visit the Electronic Medicine Web site at http://www.medicine.com. Click on the Emergency Medicine folder. Then click on the Trauma and Orthopedics on-line book. Review the chapter on Hemorrhagic Shock.

Table 6-1
Indicators of Multisystem Trauma

Mechanism of injury

Falls greater than 20 feet for adults, greater than 10 feet for infants or children, or three times the patient's body height

Death of any car occupant

Struck by a vehicle traveling greater than 20 mph

Ejection from a vehicle

Severe vehicle deformity

Rollover with signs of severe impact

Penetrating injuries to the head, chest, or abdomen

Physical findings

Pulse greater than 120 beats per minute (bpm) or less than 50 bpm

Systolic blood pressure (BP) less than 90 millimeters of mercury (mm Hg)

Respiratory rate less than 10 or greater than 30 breaths per minute

Glasgow Coma Score less than 13

Penetrating trauma, excluding extremities

Flail chest

More than two proximal long-bone fractures

Burns greater than 15% total body surface area (TBSA)

Facial and airway burns

ASSESSMENT

The initial assessment addresses life-threatening conditions and employs the following sequential five-step approach:[2]

A—Airway management and cervical spine control

B—Breathing (ventilation)

C—Circulation and hemorrhage

D—Disability

E—Expose, examine, and evaluate

This assessment approach provides a systematic and organized evaluation of the patient's initial status and allows for detection and stabilization of solely life-threatening problems on-scene. The components of the initial assessment must be internalized, not just memorized. Once internalized, the initial assessment should immediately surface into an automatic response, without hesitating to recall what step of the assessment should be performed next. The focus must be on what the assessment data reveal in relation to the patient's overall physiological status, and how the patterns of injuries and conditions are affecting overall aerobic metabolism and homeostatic well-being. The paramedic must be able to analyze assessment data and, based on that data, anticipate, predict, and appropriately manage the patient in order to prevent further detrimental effects. The paramedic should follow, as closely as possible, the order of the initial assessment, keeping in mind there are circumstances that require deviation from the survey format (e.g., severe external hemorrhage requiring immediate treatment when the patient is obviously breathing upon initial approach). When the paramedic must deviate from the order of the survey, vital organ system assessment may be omitted; therefore, it is important to go back to the previous steps if they were omitted initially.

Multisystem trauma patients quickly deteriorate into anaerobic metabolism as a result of inadequate tissue perfusion. This is described as a four-component deterioration:

1. Inadequate oxygenation of the red blood cells (RBCs) in the lungs

2. Inadequate delivery of the RBCs to the tissue cells

3. Inadequate distribution of the oxygen to the tissues

4. Inadequate availability of RBCs necessary to deliver oxygen to tissue cells

The paramedic is able to appropriately and adequately manage the first two phases of deterioration during the first steps of the initial assessment by rapidly evaluating and resuscitating those conditions that are physiologically linked to this deterioration. A clinically competent paramedic, who has developed a consistent approach to the assessment of every patient, will be able to determine whether or not the problem is immediately life threatening and if it involves singular or multisystem trauma in less than 2 minutes.[4]

The initial assessment begins upon arrival and includes scene size up and a global evaluation of the patient's respiratory, circulatory, and neurological status.[2] Upon approaching the scene, the paramedic answers the following: Does the patient appear to be conscious? What is the patient's position? Is the patient moving or does he or she appear to be unresponsive?[2] A sweeping glance over the patient may detect gross external hemorrhage or deformity or extreme use of accessory or neck muscles, possibly indicating severe airway compromise. The paramedic may see that the patient is extremely pale, exhibiting restlessness and agitation, indicative of early signs of shock. A patient with an injury around cervical spine vertebrae number 6 (C-6) often lies with forearms flexed across his or her chest and hands half closed. Another position often

assumed with spinal injury is the arms flexed and extended above the head, termed the **stick-em-up position**[1] (see Figure 6-1). Movement of the patient out of this position should not be attempted, unless the airway is compromised, until adequate personnel are available to move the patient as a unit.[1]

While comparing the initial global assessment findings with scene size up, mechanism of injury (MOI), and kinematic findings, begin formulating an initial impression of whether the patient is a singular or a multisystem trauma patient. This global assessment takes about 15 seconds and provides a rapid gross evaluation of the patient's respiratory, circulatory, and neurological functions.[7]

It is a fundamental instinct to reach the injured patient(s) as quickly as possible. However, if possible, it is best to approach the patient from the front. If responsive to verbal stimuli, the patient may turn his or her head or body toward the sounds of approaching personnel. This excessive or sudden body movement could produce further injury to the C-spine or other internal organ structures if injury is already present. If unable to assume a frontal approach, the paramedic should avoid startling or stimulating the patient during the approach. Often a simple statement, such as "please don't move, we are here to help," will prevent unnecessary patient movement.

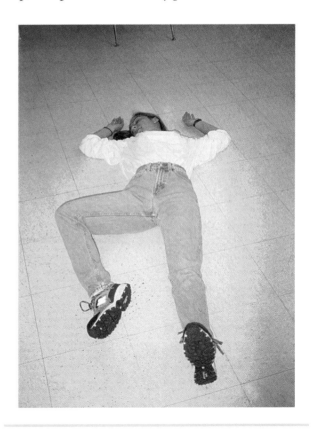

FIGURE 6-1 Stick-em-up position often assumed by the patient with a spinal injury.

It is important to repeat the phrase "please remain still" as you approach and once you arrive at the patient's side. The lead paramedic should direct his or her partner or first responder to obtain manual stabilization of the patient's head and neck, using a trauma jaw thrust procedure to open the airway. It is assumed that all trauma patients have the potential for spinal injury and, therefore, all suspected trauma patients should be manually stabilized in this manner (see Figure 6-2). Care must be taken not to intentionally stimulate the patient who appears to be unconscious until manual stabilization has been obtained, because the patient may turn his or her head laterally or rotate his or her body in an attempt to locate voice or touch. If manual stabilization is obtained before the LOC is assessed, the paramedic may avoid a disastrous outcome for the patient.

Airway

Airway management and control are two of the most important priorities of care when confronted with a multisystem trauma patient. The airway can be opened using a trauma jaw thrust maneuver. If the patient's head is not in a neutral position, the paramedic must gently move it into a neutral position unless resistance is met with movement or the patient develops intolerable pain. If the patient is in a seated position or lying on the ground, someone may need to take frontal or lateral stabilization of the head and neck until another responder can assume a posterior, kneeling, or on-ground position (see Figures 6-3 and 6-4). When manual stabilization is obtained, the paramedic places his or her fingers on the mandibular curve, gently pushing forward to create an open airway without hyperextension of the head.

Assessment begins with evaluation of the patient's LOC. If the patient is not verbally responding, the paramedic must gently tap while verbally stimulating a response from the patient. It is important *not* to shake the patient because doing so could aggravate existing injuries. A verbally responsive or moaning patient indicates an open airway. Any patient with a decreased LOC is considered a load-and-go patient and should receive immediate oxygenation with 100% oxygen delivered by a nonrebreathing mask or, if respirations are inadequate, by BVM assist. Paramedics should be

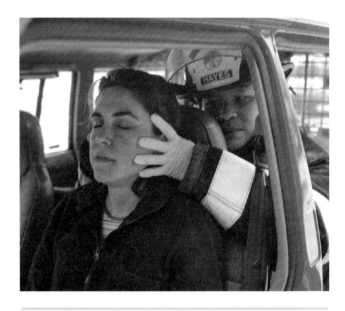

FIGURE 6-3 Manual stabilization of the head from behind the seated patient.

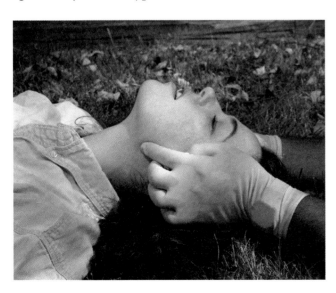

FIGURE 6-2 Manual stabilization of the head and neck using a trauma jaw thrust to manage the patient's airway.

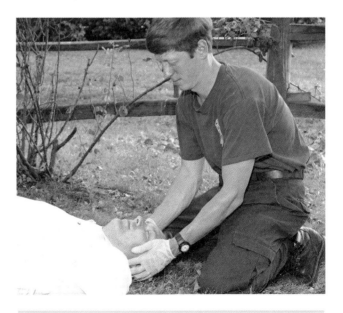

FIGURE 6-4 Manual stabilization of a supine patient's head and neck.

very attentive to the airway of a patient with an altered mental status. These patients may have difficulty managing oral secretions. Once opened, the airway should be immediately suctioned to clear blood, debris, and secretions, if present.

The paramedic must gather further information regarding the patient's perfusion status if there is a verbal response elicited with the initial LOC assessment. This assessment can occur simultaneously as the paramedic continues to assess the patency of the patient's airway by asking how the incident occurred, the general time of day, general location, and the patient's name. If the patient is alert but confused, this is indicative of early inadequate tissue perfusion. Again, immediate resuscitation with 100% oxygen with a nonrebreathing mask should be initiated.

During this initial assessment, the paramedic must *listen* for signs indicative of airway compromise. Are there silent, snoring, gurgling, or stridorous sounds present that may require immediate action such as repositioning the airway, removing a foreign body airway obstruction, suctioning, or immediate intubation? Any delay in recognizing and resuscitating these conditions will lead to increased hypoxemia, anaerobic metabolism, acidosis, and possibly death. Figure 6-5 provides an algorithm for assessment of the airway.

Breathing

Trauma patients revert to anaerobic metabolism primarily due to hypoxemia. Simultaneous assessment of the patient's breathing status is conducted while the patient's airway is being opened and during the initial LOC evaluation. This initial evaluation focuses on the patient's relative respiratory rate (normal, fast, or slow) and quality of ventilations, and employs the *look, listen, and feel* method of evaluation.

First, the paramedic must determine if the patient has spontaneous respirations. This is accomplished by looking, listening, and feeling for breathing and chest excursion. Noisy or windy environments may interfere with hearing or feeling the patient's exhaled air. Under such conditions it may be necessary to auscultate breathing by placing the head of the stethoscope over the trachea at the suprasternal notch. This will provide clear, audible air movement sounds upon inspiration and expiration in breathing patients.[7] Immediate resuscitation is required if there are no spontaneous respirations or if the patient has agonal respirations. Initially, this should be accomplished by insertion of an oropharyngeal or nasopharyngeal airway and use of a BVM with 100% oxygen. If this method of airway control and ventilation is effectively oxygenating the patient, it is not necessary to immediately intubate.

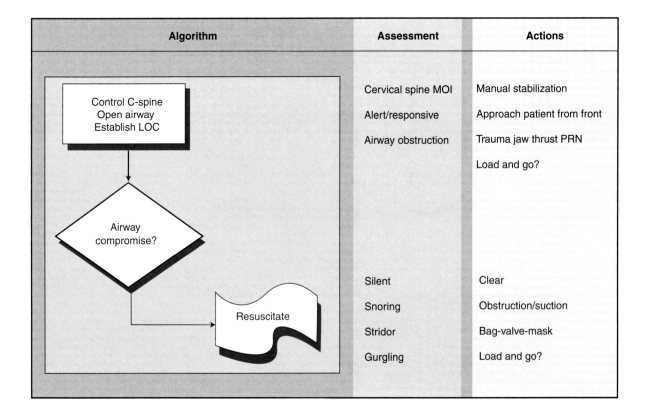

Algorithm	Assessment	Actions
Control C-spine / Open airway / Establish LOC → Airway compromise? → Resuscitate	Cervical spine MOI	Manual stabilization
	Alert/responsive	Approach patient from front
	Airway obstruction	Trauma jaw thrust PRN
		Load and go?
	Silent	Clear
	Snoring	Obstruction/suction
	Stridor	Bag-valve-mask
	Gurgling	Load and go?

FIGURE 6-5 Airway assessment algorithm.

Intubation can be delayed until there are adequate personnel on-scene to quickly accomplish this procedure or until the patient is loaded into the ambulance.

Patients with spontaneous respirations should be evaluated for breathing difficulty. First, the paramedic determines if the patient is experiencing an irregular breathing pattern, apnea, bradypnea, hypopnea, tachypnea, or dyspnea. Look for signs of respiratory distress or compromise, which include pallor, cyanosis, nasal flaring, tracheal tugging, use of accessory muscles, intercostal muscle retractions, and diaphragmatic breathing. With a C-6 injury, intercostal muscles will be paralyzed, severely compromising respiratory efforts. An injury at C-4 will paralyze the diaphragm, making breathing virtually impossible, and the patient will be using accessory muscles in the neck to breathe.[1] If any of these signs are present, immediate resuscitative efforts must be initiated. The patient will quickly deteriorate if allowed to continue this inadequate ventilatory process. An apneic, bradypneic, or hypopneic patient must receive assisted ventilation with 100% oxygen using a BVM. The tachypneic or dyspneic patient may need assisted ventilation, or may only need to be placed on 100% oxygen by a nonrebreathing mask. The paramedic determines which oxygen delivery device is going to be the most beneficial to the patient's current ventilatory pattern and which device the patient will tolerate. This determination is based on the general rules of airway and breathing management found in Table 6-2.

The initial goal of breathing assessment is to detect life-threatening conditions. Therefore, the next step in the assessment process should be to seek out the etiology of the respiratory compromise, especially if tachypnea is present. Remember, tachypnea is indicative of hypoxia, acidosis, and anaerobic metabolism. The paramedic should quickly expose and assess the patient's chest for symmetry, paradoxical movement, sucking chest wounds, impalements, ecchymosis, hueing, deformity, or obvious signs of blunt trauma to the chest wall. If the patient has an injury to the lower cervical or upper thoracic spinal cord, there may be paralysis of the intercostal muscles. These types of injuries may present with abdominal breathing, which may be detected during the assessment for symmetrical movement of the chest wall.

Bilateral breath sounds should be auscultated to determine if the breath sounds are clear, equal, diminished, or absent. This auscultation should be quick, using a two-point midaxillary assessment (see Figure 6-6). Percussion can detect hyporesonance or hyperresonance but is often difficult to perform in the prehospital setting due to ambient noise. Pneumothorax, tension pneumothorax, hemothorax, hemo-pneumothorax, and flail chest are conditions often responsible for inadequate ventilation.

Table 6-2
General Rules of Airway and Breathing Management

Adult respiratory rates

Less than 12 is considered slow and may be associated with central nervous system (CNS) trauma.

Less than 10 is inadequate.

Twelve to 20 is considered a normal range but may have inadequate tidal volume.

Greater than 20 and up to 24 is considered possible early warning sign of developing respiratory/circulatory compromise.

Greater than 24 and up to 30 indicates developing respiratory and systemic compromise associated with hypovolemia.

Greater than 30 indicates hypoxemia, acidosis, or hypoperfusion.

Resuscitation rules of management

Respiratory rates less than 12 require assisted or total ventilatory control with a fraction of inspired oxygen (FiO_2) of 0.85 or greater.

Respiratory rates of 12–20 may need supplemental 100% O_2 by nonrebreather or assisted ventilations if the tidal volume is very shallow or the LOC is depressed.

Respiratory rates of greater than 20 and up to 30 require supplemental O_2 or assisted ventilation.

Respiratory rates of greater than 30 should receive assisted ventilation with 100% O_2 and early intubation may be required to maintain full ventilatory control.

Source: Adapted from *PHTLS Basic and Advanced Prehospital Trauma and Life Support.* (4th ed.), by N.E. McSwain, J.L. Paturas, E.M. Wertz, 1999, Mosby: St. Louis.

The final step of the breathing assessment involves palpating the anterior neck for jugular venous distention (JVD) or flatness and assessing the trachea for deviation (see Figure 6-7). Jugular venous distention is associated with a building tension pneumothorax, or pericardial tamponade, whereas flat neck veins can indicate hemorrhage and hypovolemia. However, it must be remembered that approximately 3–4 cm of venous engorgement is normal in patients lying supine. Venous engorgement in excess of this amount signifies JVD while flat neck veins in a supine patient may indicate hypovolemia.

If JVD or tracheal deviation is present, the patient is severely compromised and must be transported as soon as possible. Positive JVD associated with a tension pneumothorax must be definitively resuscitated with

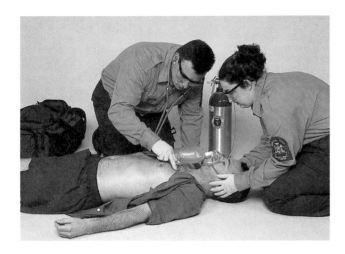

FIGURE 6-6 Auscultation of bilateral breath sounds utilizing a two-point midaxillary assessment.

needle decompression and assisted ventilation with 100% oxygen. The paramedic must also decide whether intubation can be delayed until the patient is en route to the medical facility. Any patient who is unable to maintain an airway, has a high risk of aspiration, displays a large flail segment, presents with airway injuries or midface trauma, or has a Glasgow Coma Score of less than 9 requires a definitively secured airway as soon as possible.[2]

If the patient must be assist ventilated or hyperventilated, the paramedic stabilizing the head and neck can provide this treatment by placing his or her knees on either side of the patient's head. It will be important that someone obtain manual stabilization frontally while the paramedic assumes this position. This allows all other treatment personnel to focus on completion of the assessment process and preparation of the patient for packaging and transport. Figure 6-8 presents an algorithm for assessment of breathing.

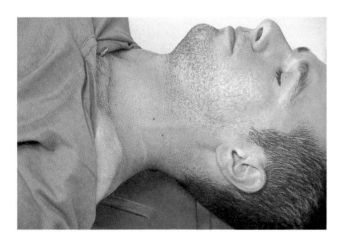

FIGURE 6-7 Jugular venous distention.

Circulation and Hemorrhage

Circulatory assessment is divided into three components: assessment of cardiac output, exsanguinating hemorrhage, and, if internal hemorrhage is suspected, PASG survey.[9] Failure of the circulatory system results in inadequate delivery of oxygen to the target tissue cells, which leads to the signs and symptoms associated with inadequate tissue perfusion. Initial assessment of cardiac output, cardiovascular status, and perfusion status can be rapidly obtained during the initial assessment of central and peripheral pulses, skin color, skin temperature, and capillary refill time. Quantitative vital signs may be included during this phase of the initial assessment only if adequate personnel are available to perform this assessment without interruption of the focused assessment process.

Assessment of Pulses The patient's carotid and radial pulse should be evaluated simultaneously for presence, quality, equality, and regularity. At this time only a relative rate and quality will be obtained. If a radial pulse is palpable, this establishes an initial baseline estimate that the patient's systolic blood pressure is at least 80–90 mm Hg depending on the strength of the pulse (see Table 6-3 for a comparative analysis of peripheral pulses and systolic blood pressure). A radial pulse that is tachycardic and weak or weakening may be the first indicator that the patient is experiencing circulatory system failure or shock. Unexplained tachycardia may be indicative of internal hemorrhage, especially intra-abdominal hemorrhage. An absent radial pulse indicates the patient's blood pressure is below 80 mm Hg and that the patient is profoundly hypovolemic. A radial pulse that is full, bounding, and bradycardic may be suggestive of increasing intracranial pressure (ICP). Refer to Chapter 11 for an in-depth discussion of increased intracranial pressure and Cushing's reflex. The presence of a bounding radial pulse suggests the systolic blood pressure (BP) is significantly above 100 mm Hg. A normocardic or bradycardic pulse rate could

Table 6-3 Estimating Systolic Blood Pressure Based on Pulses	
Pulse Palpable at	**Systolic Blood Pressure of at Least:**
Radial	80–90 mm Hg
Brachial	70–80 mm Hg
Femoral	70–80 mm Hg
Carotid	60–70 mm Hg

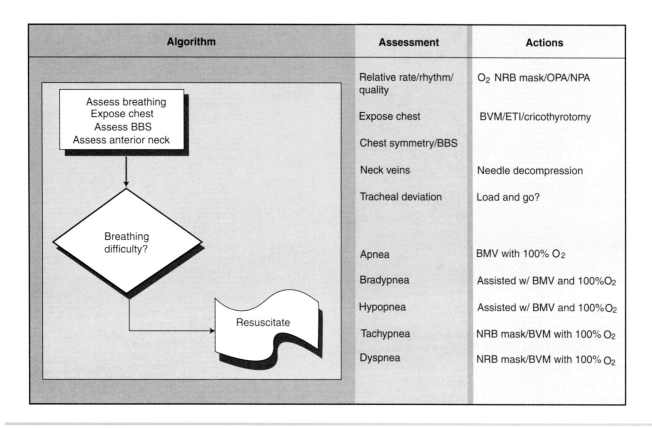

Algorithm	Assessment	Actions
	Relative rate/rhythm/quality	O$_2$ NRB mask/OPA/NPA
	Expose chest	BVM/ETI/cricothyrotomy
	Chest symmetry/BBS	
	Neck veins	Needle decompression
	Tracheal deviation	Load and go?
	Apnea	BMV with 100% O$_2$
	Bradypnea	Assisted w/ BMV and 100%O$_2$
	Hypopnea	Assisted w/ BMV and 100%O$_2$
	Tachypnea	NRB mask/BVM with 100% O$_2$
	Dyspnea	NRB mask/BVM with 100% O$_2$

FIGURE 6-8 Breathing algorithm.

be suggestive of neurogenic shock associated with spinal cord injury. The paramedic must begin to associate the mechanism of injury (MOI) with assessment findings and analyze how these findings are directly related to the physiological response the patient is exhibiting. Definitive field treatment relates directly to the ability to recognize and differentiate normal from abnormal physiological responses and how these responses relate to load-and-go patients.

Assessment of Skin Color and Skin Temperature   Skin color and temperature will provide a rapid initial assessment of peripheral perfusion status. This assessment can be simultaneously performed during the carotid and radial pulse check. A hypovolemic patient will normally present with pale, cool or cold, clammy, and diaphoretic skin, whereas patients with neurogenic shock may present with normal to pink, warm, and dry skin below the level of spinal cord injury and pale, cool, clammy, and diaphoretic skin above the level of cord injury. A patient with head injury may present with warm, sometimes hot skin temperature, and skin color can be normal to flushed in appearance due to the increased systolic BP.

Assessment of Capillary Refill   The paramedic can quickly assess capillary refill time (CRT),

once the radial pulse check is completed, by exerting pressure to the nail beds or hypothenar eminence causing the underlying tissue to blanche (see Figure 6-9). If the patient is normovolemic, color will return within 2 seconds. However, if the sympathetic nervous system has caused a sympathomimetic response due to hypovolemia, return of color will be greater than 2 seconds. The paramedic must keep in mind that capillary refill delay, without the presence of other associated signs and symptoms, may be unreliable. Changes can be caused by age, hypothermia, or simple fractures. Normal CRT may occur in the presence of neurogenic shock, isolated head trauma with increasing ICP, and pharmacological vasodilatory medications.

Assessment of Hemorrhage   External exsanguinating hemorrhage must be rapidly detected and controlled to prevent deterioration of the patient's cardiac output and perfusion status. Severe external hemorrhage may be detected and corrected by application of direct pressure, prior to any other assessment, if the patient is breathing or if there are adequate personnel present to begin hemorrhage control. There are circumstances that prevent the paramedic from detecting life-threatening hemorrhage until a quick body sweep is performed (e.g., patient's size or position or inadequate lighting). This body sweep generally occurs once initial airway,

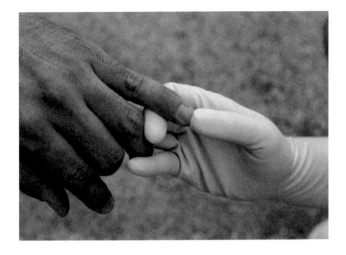

FIGURE 6-9 Assessment of CRT by exerting pressure to the nail beds or hypothenar eminence.

breathing, and circulatory status have been assessed. It consists of running the hands, beginning at the head, down the patient, paying particular attention to areas where blood can pool (e.g., posterior scapular area, lateral axillary area, lumbar-sacral area, medial/inner thigh area) (see Figure 6-10). As the quick sweep is performed, the paramedic is looking at his or her gloved hands for evidence of significant venous or arterial bleeding and feeling for sudden warmth. If significant bleeding is found, the area must be quickly exposed and the patient positioned for visual examination of the area. Control methods must be initiated if significant hemorrhage is detected. Use of pressure bandages, PASG, or even air splints may provide adequate control, freeing the paramedic to perform other critical interventions or to continue assessing the patient. Significant internal hemorrhage can occur in four body areas: the chest, the abdomen, the retroperitoneal/pelvic cavity, and the thigh. If internal hemorrhage is suspected, based on the presenting MOI, unexplained restlessness, tachypnea, and tachycardia, the paramedic must deviate from the strict ABCDE assessment format and perform the PASG survey by exposing the abdomen, pelvis, and legs. He or she must look for hueing or ecchymosis, edema, or signs of blunt trauma and *palpate* for rigidity, swelling, or deformity. A quick palpation of the pelvic region should be performed since pelvic fractures have a high percentage of associated intra-abdominal hemorrhage. If internal hemorrhage is detected, rapid immobilization onto a long spine board with PASG in place, rapid transportation, and resuscitation with warmed IV fluids should be initiated. The paramedic quickly completes the initial assessment while the patient is being readied for transport, searching for any other life-threatening injuries that may be present. Movement of the patient prior to completion of the assessment could aggravate undetected injuries.

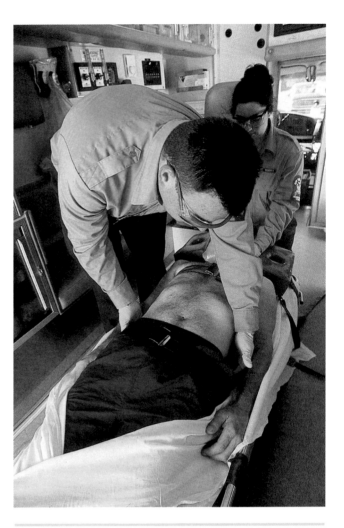

FIGURE 6-10 A quick sweep of the lumbar-sacral area for gross exsanguinating hemorrhage.

Assessment of Vital Signs Quantitative vital signs (heart rate, respiratory rate, and blood pressure) provide necessary baseline data, especially when the patient is rapidly deteriorating. Therefore, quantitative vital signs should be obtained as soon as possible but should not take precedence over essential steps of assessment, resuscitation, stabilization, and transport. Continual reevaluation of relative rate and quality of respirations and core versus peripheral pulses can provide adequate baseline data until the patient is en route or adequate personnel are available to obtain quantitative vital signs. Figure 6-11 presents an algorithm for assessment of circulation.

Disability

Rapid neurological evaluation is a very important part of the initial assessment. It measures cerebral function and indirectly measures cerebral oxygenation based on the patient's response to external stimuli and other assessment data. This evaluation establishes the patient's level of consciousness, pupillary size and reaction, and motor and sensory response in upper and lower extremities.

Assessment of Level of Consciousness   The patient's initial LOC is assessed by gently tapping or verbally stimulating, *not shaking*, the patient to elicit a response at the beginning of the initial assessment. At that time a general idea of responsiveness is ascertained. Now the paramedic must perform a more definitive assessment using the AVPU scale (see Table 6-4). If the patient is able to verbally respond, determine if he or she is appropriately oriented by asking questions

Table 6-4
Scale Used to Determine a Patient's LOC
AVPU SCALE
A—Alert (to person, place, time, event)
V—Verbal stimuli (appropriate or inappropriate response)
P—Painful stimuli (appropriate or inappropriate response)
U—Unresponsive

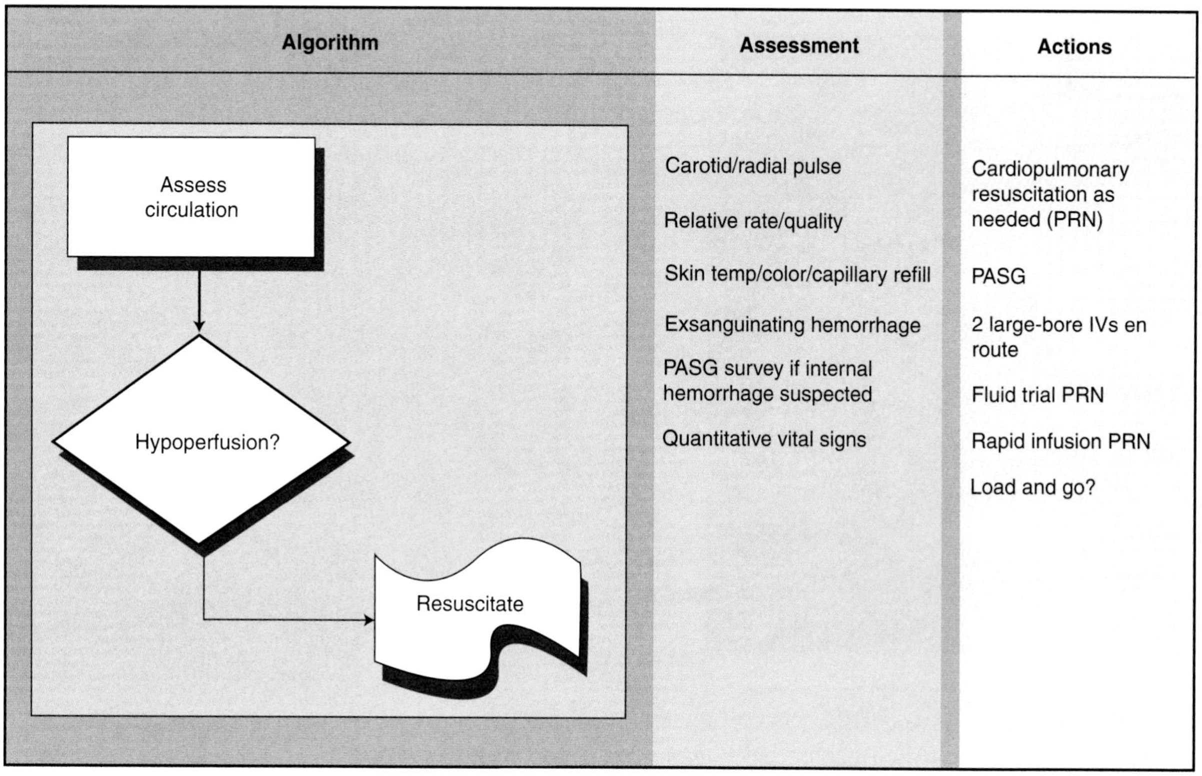

related to time, place, person, and event. As cerebral function declines, the patient will begin to lose orientation to place and events prior to the injury. As the patient worsens, orientation to person will decline, not just to family members, but to self as well. At this point the patient is moving toward unconsciousness. The patient will respond to verbal stimuli by opening his eyes and moving body parts when spoken to but is unable to coherently communicate. Verbal responses are not intelligible and sound garbled or moaned.

When the patient is no longer responsive to verbal stimuli, the paramedic must determine the depth of unresponsiveness by eliciting a purposeful response to pain. Several methods are discussed in the literature that may be more appropriately used on medical patients (e.g., sternal rub or ear lobe pinch).[7] However, these methods may produce unwanted movement in the trauma patient. A sternal rub may cause the patient to move the torso in an attempt to avoid/escape the painful stimuli. This movement may aggravate chest, spine, abdominal, and pelvic injuries. Pinching the ear lobe could produce a severe lateral or twisting rotation of the head in an attempt to move away from the pain. Obviously, if there is cervical spine injury, this type of movement could be disastrous, especially if the person manually stabilizing the head and neck is not ready for

Algorithm	Assessment	Actions
Assess circulation → Hypoperfusion? → Resuscitate	Carotid/radial pulse Relative rate/quality Skin temp/color/capillary refill Exsanguinating hemorrhage PASG survey if internal hemorrhage suspected Quantitative vital signs	Cardiopulmonary resuscitation as needed (PRN) PASG 2 large-bore IVs en route Fluid trial PRN Rapid infusion PRN Load and go?

FIGURE 6-11 Circulation algorithm.

this type of movement. For these reasons, the sternal rub and ear lobe pinch are not recommended.

There are two methods that can be employed to elicit a painful response with minimal risk for further injury:

1. Pinch the patient's upper arm, on the medial aspect, mid-way between the antecubital space and axilla in the softest portion of the skin (see Figure 6-12).
2. Take the fleshy region between the patient's thumb and forefinger, preferably in an uninjured extremity, and pinch or squeeze it forcefully (see Figure 6-13).

Purposeful response to this painful stimuli is indicated by patient movement away from the pain. A twitch, or slight movement of the hand or forearm, indicates severe cerebral dysfunction. Look for abnormal movements such as **decorticate** (rigid flexion of the arms and extension of the legs) and **decerebrate** (rigid extension of the arms and legs; the back and neck may be arched) posturing with and without this stimuli (see Figures 6-14 and 6-15).

A patient who does not exhibit any response to painful stimuli is considered unresponsive. This is an ominous sign and indicates profound hypoxemia, acidosis, total patient decompensation, and severe inadequate tissue perfusion, especially cerebral hypo-

perfusion. Obtaining initial baseline data regarding the patient's LOC with frequent reevaluation establishes a fairly clear picture of how rapidly the patient is deteriorating. As the patient slips down the AVPU scale, he or she may become combative, display irrational responses, exhibit uncooperative and belligerent behavior, and refuse medical help. The paramedic must try not to antagonize the patient, knowing that the patient's behavior may be the result of head injury, hypoxemia, and hypoperfusion. This type of behavior requires immediate or continued treatment with 100% oxygen.[2]

During this evaluation it is very important to determine the history of the event. Specific questions would include: Did the patient lose and regain consciousness prior to EMS arrival or since the injury occurred? Does the patient have any preexisting medical conditions that might be responsible for altered LOC (e.g., diabetes, epilepsy, heart problems)? Could there be toxic substances involved (e.g., drugs, alcohol, or other chemical substances)? The paramedic must gather this history from the patient, family members, or bystanders, without interrupting the initial assessment.

Assessment of Pupils   The pupils, controlled by higher cranial nerves, are a direct link to the brain and provide invaluable information concerning cerebral perfusion. Under normal conditions pupils react quickly and consensually to changes in light intensity. A quick pupil evaluation to determine if the pupils are equal, round, and reactive to light (PERRL) will provide important baseline information regarding intracranial

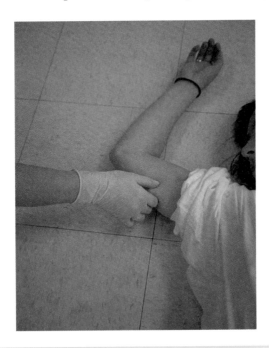

FIGURE 6-12 Painful stimuli applied by pinching the medial aspect of the upper arm midway between the antecubital space and axilla.

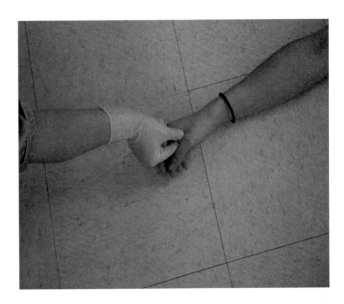

FIGURE 6-13 Painful stimuli applied by pinching or squeezing the fleshy region between the patient's thumb and forefinger.

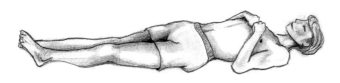

FIGURE 6-14 Decorticate posturing.

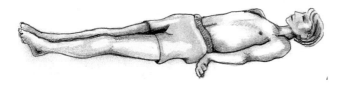

FIGURE 6-15 Decerebrate posturing.

pathology and cerebral perfusion. A sluggish pupil reaction may reflect CNS depression from hypoxia, hypercarbia, injury, or the effects of drugs. Unequal pupils (anisocoria) may indicate eye trauma, head trauma, or cerebrovascular accident (CVA). Dilated or fixed pupils are indicative of hypoxia, severe ICP, or CNS injury.[2] Pupils are usually equal to within 1 mm, remain equal, and constrict equally when exposed to light. Abnormal or sluggish reactions to light, significantly unequal pupils, or lack of consensual reaction usually results from insult to the brain or one of the oculomotor nerves in the absence of direct eye injury.[7]

Assessment of Pulse, Motor, and Sensation
The paramedic should quickly perform a pulse, motor, and sensation (PMS) assessment of the upper and lower body extremities (PMS × 4) during the disability assessment. (*Note:* The lower extremity PMS evaluation can be integrated into the "expose, examine, and evaluate" component of the lower extremities to save time.) This is not an in-depth evaluation, but rather a quick determination of neurological intactness prior to moving the patient to a long spine board (LSB). This will establish baseline assessment data for motor or sensory deficits in the extremities of a responsive patient, which may indicate brain injury, spinal cord injury, or injury to a limb. A deficit in distal circulation may reflect a reduction in systemic circulation or compromised circulation in that limb.[7] Evaluation in a verbally responsive patient consists of:

1. Having the patient unilaterally, then bilaterally, squeeze one of your fingers, to compare the presence and equality of strength in the other extremities (see Figure 6-16). This detects paralysis or paresis (weakness) in one or both upper extremities.

2. Having the patient unilaterally, then bilaterally, push and pull back on your hands with the feet as you compare the strength and quality of the movement (see Figure 6-17). Impairment may indicate a spinal cord injury.

3. Having the patient wiggle the fingers and toes, which indicates the motor nerves are intact.

4. Asking the patient if he or she feels you touching his or her fingers and toes to rule out numbness, tingling, or decreased sensation.

Evaluation of the unresponsive patient consists of:

1. Pinching the fingers and toes or running a blunt object along the palms and soles of the feet to determine if the patient withdraws or localizes the pain. Intact motor and sensation usually indicates normal or minimally impaired cortical function, whereas a positive Babinski response indicates spine injury. A positive Babinski is present if the big toe turns upward when a blunt object is introduced to the sole of the foot (see Figure 6-18). Normally the big toe will turn downward.

2. Exerting pressure with your thumb into the patient's palm, which should produce curling, withdrawal, or flexion.

During this evaluation the paramedic should note any posturing displayed when painful stimuli are initiated. If there is no movement produced with painful stimuli, the paramedic should assess for flaccid paralysis by lifting the patient's forearm slightly, if there is no sign of extremity injury, and then let it fall. Absence of any muscle tone usually denotes spinal cord injury.

Distal pulses should be assessed in each extremity and should be compared. Simultaneous assessment of the radial pulses and then pedal pulses can provide invaluable assessment data regarding circulatory function. The paramedic is able to determine the presence, absence, equality, and relative pulse rate, which may indicate hypovolemia, undetected fractures, cardiac tamponade, or aortic aneurysm. Remember, lower extremity PMS assessment can be carried out with the lower extremity quick initial assessment.

Assessment of Cervical Spine   The paramedic will want to apply a cervical collar (C-collar) at this point. Prior to application, assessment of the posterior neck must be performed to determine if there is tenderness, deformity, edema, muscle spasms, palpable vertebral "step-offs" or gaps, impaled objects, or soft tissue injury. One should assume a cervical spine fracture in any patient with an injury above the clavicle

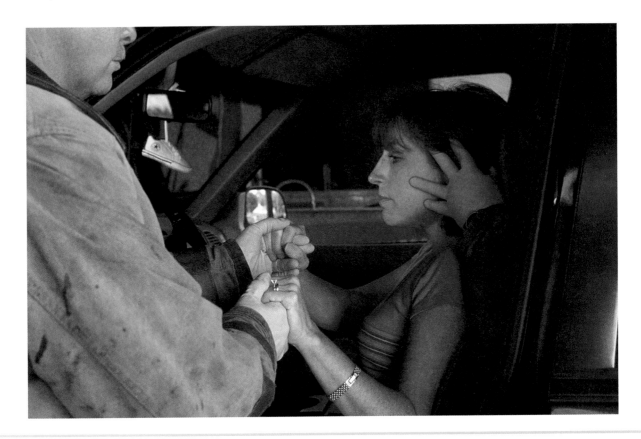

FIGURE 6-16 Assessment for paralysis or paresis by having the patient squeeze two to three of your fingers.

as 10% of all patients with head injuries will have cervical spine fracture.[9] If the paramedic suspects chest trauma, a quick reevaluation of the anterior neck for JVD and tracheal deviation should be performed before applying the C-collar. Application of the C-collar can be delayed if continued reevaluation of the anterior neck is warranted. For more complete stabil-

ization of the head and neck the C-collar should always be applied prior to movement of the patient onto the LSB. Once the cervical collar has been applied, the paramedic manually stabilizing the head and neck must continue this stabilization until the patient is fully strapped to an LSB with head-immobilizing devices in place.

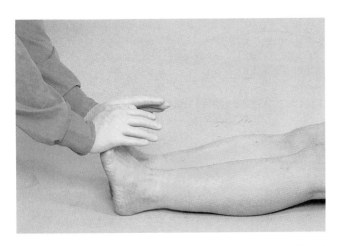

FIGURE 6-17 Assessment for lower extremity paralysis or paresis by having the patient push, then pull back on your hands.

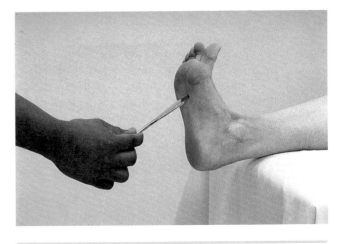

FIGURE 6-18 A positive Babinski; the big toe turns upward when a blunt stimulus is applied to the sole of the foot.

Glasgow Coma Score   The paramedic should obtain a Glasgow Coma Score (GCS) on all trauma patients. This scale provides a numerical measure based on an assessment of the patient's eye opening and verbal and motor responses. If the score is less than 9, this implies severe neurological insult, which requires airway support with hyperventilation and rapid transport. Do not stop the evaluation process to score the patient; instead, obtain baseline assessment data and record these data as soon as possible, usually after the patient is in transit. The GCS is usually used in conjunction with the revised trauma score, which measures on the severity of trauma. For a detailed discussion of these trauma-scoring systems, refer to Chapter 7. Figure 6-19 presents an algorithm for checking disability.

Expose, Examine, and Evaluate

The last step in the expanded initial assessment involves a quick assessment of all systems not previously exposed. It is important to expose the patient when assessing each system for severe soft tissue injury, open and closed fractures, and undetected hemorrhage, especially when the patient is wearing bulky clothing. It is very important to keep in mind that a patient experiencing anaerobic metabolism becomes hypothermic quickly. Preserve body heat by covering the patient once body parts are exposed and examined or expose only what is necessary, especially if the outside temperature is cold. If the patient is not fully exposed prior to movement, complete exposure and examination must take place once in the EMS unit.

Usually this assessment involves the chest, if not previously evaluated, abdomen, flanks, pelvis, lower extremities, and back. All injuries should be located prior to PASG application and, hopefully, prior to patient movement since movement can aggravate existing injuries (e.g., pelvic, femur, and lower leg fractures). Based on assessment findings, conventional movement strategies may have to be modified to accommodate the type of injury detected (e.g., utilizing a scoop stretcher instead of the log roll to place a patient with an unstable pelvic fracture onto an LSB).

Chest and Thorax Evaluation   If the paramedic has not exposed and examined the chest during the breathing assessment or if there is reason to quickly reevaluate the chest, this quick evaluation should be performed at this time. As the chest is exposed, look for signs of injury such as hueing, ecchymosis, deformity, impalements, asymmetrical movement, soft tissue injuries, and intercostal retractions. Quickly feel for symmetrical expansion and movement of the chest wall (see Figure 6-20), paradoxical movement, crepitus, and instability. Finally, listen for bilateral breath sounds and reevaluate endotracheal tube placement if the patient has already been intubated. If this assessment has been performed as part of the breathing assessment, the evaluator can proceed on to the abdominal evaluation.

Abdominal Evaluation   Rapidly expose the abdominal area and look for evidence of internal hemorrhage in the form of abrasions, hueing, ecchymosis, edema, swelling, lacerations, penetrating wounds, and eviscerations. The abdominal area superior and inferior

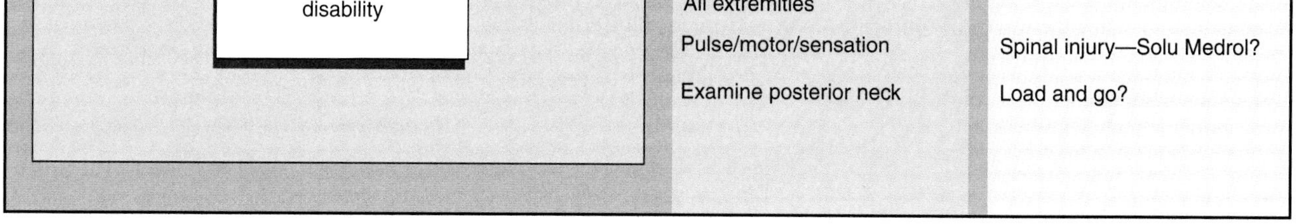

Algorithm	Assessment	Actions
Assess disability	AVPU	Apply cervical collar
	Pupils	Unequal—hyperventilate?
	All extremities	
	Pulse/motor/sensation	Spinal injury—Solu Medrol?
	Examine posterior neck	Load and go?

FIGURE 6-19 Disability algorithm.

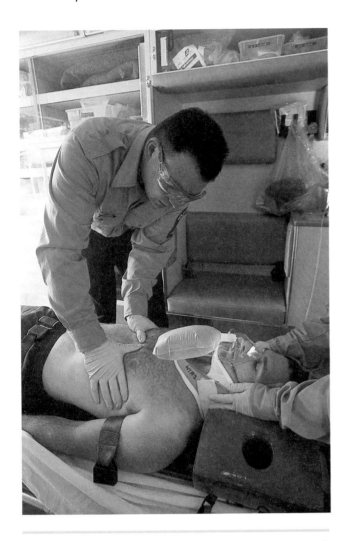

FIGURE 6-20 Assessment for expansion and movement of the chest wall.

Remember that unexplained tachycardia may be the first indicator of intra-abdominal hemorrhage.

Management priorities include consideration of PASG application, especially if intra-abdominal hemorrhage is suspected. This treatment may help tamponade significant hemorrhage long enough for the patient to be received into surgery. Initiation of 100% oxygen should occur immediately if not already initiated. Two large-bore IVs should be established once the patient is en route, unless an extended extrication time is anticipated, which may warrant initiation of IV therapy prior to loading the patient. It is important to keep in mind that this patient needs definitive surgical treatment as soon as possible, and time spent trying to initiate IVs prior to loading the patient for transport may unnecessarily delay this definitive treatment.

Pelvic Evaluation   Pelvic fracture is most commonly caused by motor vehicle trauma, crush injury, or a fall. Internal hemorrhage is the major cause of death in patients with pelvic fractures. Thirty percent of the total blood volume may be lost into the surrounding soft tissue of the pelvic cavity and retroperitoneally.[1] Initial scene evaluation, MOI, and patient position can often provide early clues that there might be an underlying pelvic fracture or dislocation present, such as when the patient's knees have impacted the vehicle's dashboard.[1]

The paramedic may notice, with a patient lying on the ground, lateral or medial rotation of one leg suggestive of hip dislocation. Once the patient is exposed, the paramedic may observe ecchymosis, swelling, or deformity. The patient may complain of pain in that area. Palpation of the pelvic region begins with compression of the iliac wings laterally and inwardly. If there is no crepitus heard or felt and the pelvis feels stable, exert gentle downward pressure on the iliac crests, again noting any crepitus, instability, or painful response from the patient. If this assessment is negative, then place gentle downward pressure on the pubis, feeling for instability on crepitus (see Figure 6-21). If evidence suggestive of pelvic fracture is present, do not palpate any further. Movement of the patient onto an LSB can often produce further injury, and therefore, the patient may need to be moved onto the LSB by use of a "scoop stretcher." Patients with an unstable pelvis should not be log rolled except when an alternative method would result in a life-threatening delay. The paramedic must assume that any patient with an unstable pelvis has a high potential for intra-abdominal or retroperitoneal hemorrhage. Therefore, the LSB should already have PASG in place for immediate stabilization of the fracture as well as control of internal hemorrhage (see Figure 6-22). Spinal immobilization must be provided because an unstable pelvis

to the umbilicus should be carefully evaluated for signs of contusion, often initially showing as a hued area about 4 cm wide lying transversely across the abdomen. This is indicative of an incorrectly worn seat belt and may result in hollow viscus injury in the abdomen or a lumbar spine fracture.[2]

Assessment includes palpation of all four quadrants of the abdomen. Observe any painful response or guarding reaction. Feel for rigidity, spasms, edema, local warmth, coolness, or masses. If a painful response is elicited, such as voluntary or involuntary guarding, do not continue to palpate that area because further injury can occur to the patient. The paramedic should not be concerned with auscultating the abdomen for bowel sounds since this is not a reliable or easily performed prehospital evaluation. During the abdominal examination remember to quickly feel laterally around the patients's flank area to check for deformity, edema, impalements, or undetected hemorrhage that may be pooling in the curvature of the lumbar-sacral area.

often presents with associated spinal injuries, especially to the lumbar and lower thoracic spine.

Lower Extremity Evaluation Evaluation of the lower extremities begins with the initial assessment of the MOI. Any patient who has been involved in a motor vehicle crash (MVC) or fall may have sustained hip, femur, knee, or lower leg injury, which must be detected prior to movement and prior to application of the PASG. Hands-on assessment begins with palpation of the hip area to determine if there is an anterior or posterior hip dislocation. Dislocations frequently occur in MVCs, especially when the knees hit the dashboard, resulting in the femur being forced back into the hip joint. This may result in disruption of the blood supply to the femoral head and/or sciatic nerve damage. Basic assessment includes looking for hip flexion, adduction and internal rotation, shortening of the leg, and palpating for a bony prominence posteriorly. Noticeable prominence in the inguinal area is indicative of an anterior hip dislocation. The patient is often positioned with the leg and foot laterally rotated (see Figure 6-23). If

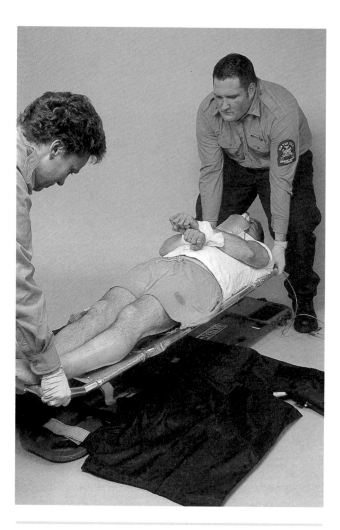

FIGURE 6-22 Utilization of a scoop stretcher with an unstable pelvic fracture to place the patient onto an LSB. The PASG should be placed and secured on the LSB prior to placement of the patient on the board.

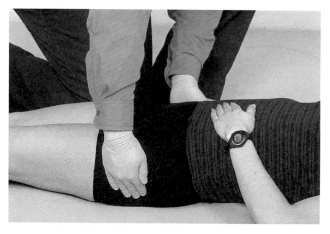

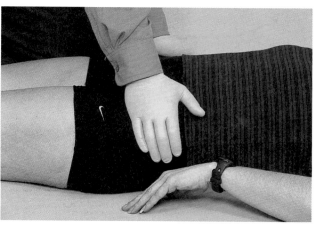

FIGURE 6-21 Assessment for pelvic injury by compression of the iliac wings.

the head of the femur has dislocated posteriorly, the paramedic may palpate a bony prominence in the buttocks area and the patient's leg may be rotated medially. This injury is an orthopedic emergency because the blood supply to the femur may be obstructed, leading to avascular necrosis of the femoral head.[1] The patient may have his or her leg flexed in order to relieve the pressure and pain. The paramedic must assess distal pulse, motor, and sensation with this injury by checking the dorsalis pedus pulse and having the patient dorsiflex and plantar flex the foot if conscious. In an unresponsive patient, provide a painful stimuli with a blunt object to the sole of the foot to elicit a reflex response. This type of injury does not take precedence over airway, breathing, or circulatory problems. It may be necessary to stabilize the hip in the position found, but with a multisystem trauma patient requiring rapid transportation this is not always possible.

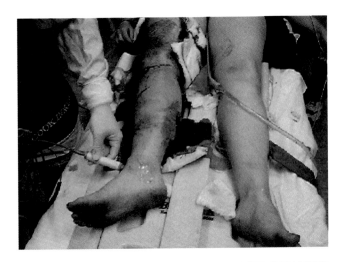

FIGURE 6-23 Foot and leg rotation indicative of a hip dislocation. Courtesy of Deborah Funk, MD. Albany Medical Center, Albany, NY.

Femur fractures can be life threatening and therefore must be detected during the initial assessment. Assessment begins with exposure of the area. Once the area is exposed, the paramedic looks for hueing or ecchymosis, shortening of the leg, deformity, and swelling. Palpation should be gently applied, and if crepitus or shifting of the bone is felt, measures to stabilize the extremity should be initiated. In the multisystem trauma patient, this can be accomplished by application of PASG for femoral stabilization. Prior to application of the PASG, assessment of distal PMS for neurovascular impairment must be performed. If the paramedic elects to utilize a traction splint for stabilization along with application of PASG, the traction splint must be placed over the PASG after inflation. During inflation of the PASG, traction should be applied to the fractured femur to prevent spiraling or twisting of the femur.

The knee must be quickly palpated for dislocation or fracture. A dislocation can be an orthopedic emergency, especially if the popliteal artery or peroneal nerve is damaged. Assessment findings include the presence of ecchymosis, swelling, deformity, crepitus with palpation, and decreased or absent distal PMS in that extremity. Again, this injury must not take precedence over ABCD problems, but the paramedic must detect and report this injury to the receiving facility.

Direct and indirect forces produce fractures to the tibial and fibular area and the paramedic must again relate this injury with the MOI. Any direct blow is likely to result in open fractures requiring hemorrhage control. Closed fractures can develop into compartment syndrome, and the paramedic must quickly assess for the "5 P's of ischemia": pain, pallor, paresthesia, paresis, and puffiness.[1] See Chapter 16 for further discussion.

Often, especially in multisystem trauma patients, the paramedic will take short cuts and fail to expose and evaluate the lower extremities. Because these injuries often produce orthopedic emergencies, they must be detected. During this quick examination it is very important to assess for and detect deformity, shortening, swelling, ecchymosis, tenderness, grating, crepitus, and exposed bone ends prior to placing the patient on an LSB. It is also important to note skin temperature, presence or absence of distal pulses, CRT, and motor and sensory function and to compare the extremity findings. Remember, it may not be possible to perform a complete focused assessment en route to the medical facility. These injuries may not be treated for several hours, or even days, once the patient has arrived at the receiving facility, but the paramedic must report his or her findings to the receiving nurse or physician. If the PASG is applied, the paramedic will not be able to assess the lower extremities after application; therefore, it is essential that assessment be quickly performed during the PASG survey segment and prior to movement of the patient. Failure to assess the lower extremities could result in further injury during movement of the patient onto the LSB. Alternative packaging techniques may be necessary to prevent further patient compromise. Figure 6-24 provides an algorithm for exposure assessment.

Remember: If you have not assessed distal PMS in the lower extremities, quickly perform this evaluation prior to movement of the patient. Movement of the patient could produce further injury and result in decreased or absent PMS once the movement is completed. The paramedic should be able to report to medical control any changes noted in neurological and circulatory function after patient movement.

RAPID PATIENT PACKAGING AND TRANSPORT

The paramedic is now ready to package the patient for transport. This involves placement of the patient onto an LSB with complete cervical immobilization. If your system uses PASG, this device should already be placed on the LSB. Movement of a supine patient will require log rolling the patient onto the side and lowering the patient onto the board, unless there exists an unstable pelvic fracture, which will require a scoop stretcher for placement onto the board. Refer to Chapter 19, for a complete description of immobilizing devices and techniques. As the patient is log rolled, assessment of the entire back must be performed to detect any injuries. The paramedic should palpate from the occipital area down to the lower leg area. At this time removal of clothing should be completed if it has not already been

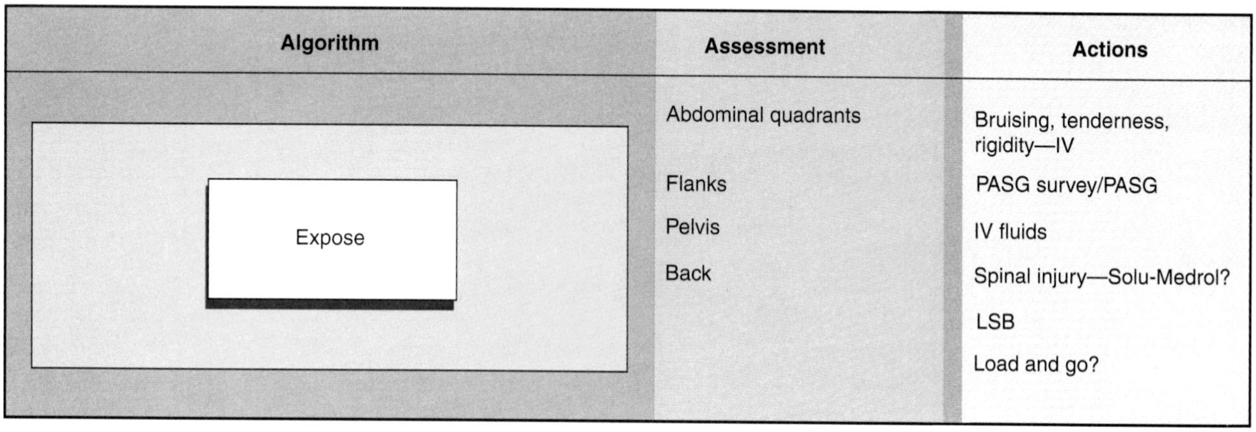

Algorithm	Assessment	Actions
Expose	Abdominal quadrants Flanks Pelvis Back	Bruising, tenderness, rigidity—IV PASG survey/PASG IV fluids Spinal injury—Solu-Medrol? LSB Load and go?

FIGURE 6-24 Expose, examine, and evaluate algorithm.

removed. If the patient is extricated from a sitting position, the back should be quickly assessed prior to lowering the patient onto the LSB. Paramedics often forget this important assessment step and miss injuries that may be life threatening. Steps involved in rapid extrication techniques are found in Chapter 19.

With multisystem trauma patients time should not be spent splinting/stabilizing fractures or dressing and bandaging soft tissue injuries. The initial goal is to stabilize only what is necessary to prevent further injury. Once the patient has been placed on the LSB, treatment team members must secure the patient to the board and secure the PASG around the patient. The patient's body is secured to the board first and the head is secured last. During this time the lead paramedic should reassess the patient's LOC, airway, breathing, circulatory, and neurological status. As soon as the patient is fully secured onto the backboard, he or she is quickly transferred into the ambulance or helicopter for immediate transportation.

Paramedics must remember they are working against the clock with a patient who has sustained critical injuries. Therefore, transport to the "most appropriate" definitive care facility is imperative. This may involve an actual increase in overall initial transport time, but the patient will be received by a facility with a trauma and surgical team.

ON-SCENE RESUSCITATION VERSUS EN ROUTE RESUSCITATION

Critical trauma patients rapidly decompensate and die due to hypoxemia and shock. Therefore, prioritize patients using the **"CUPS" classification system** (Table 6-5). Patients who fall into the urgent category have injuries or conditions that, regardless of interventions provided in the field, continue to be life threaten-

ing and require definitive care such as blood replacement or surgical intervention.[7] The elapsed time between onset and definitive care is a paramount factor affecting these patients' morbidity and survival.[7] Nonurgent patients have no life-threatening injuries or conditions, and therefore, further examination can be done prior to packaging and transport.[7]

The paramedic's initial goal is to provide early airway management, oxygenation, and ventilatory support as soon as the problem is identified. A suction unit should always be part of the initial equipment taken to the patient's side in case there are immediate and ongoing problems with secretions, debris, vomit, or blood in the airway. Early resuscitation consists of applying 100% oxygen by a nonrebreathing mask, BVM, or early intubation if the patient's condition warrants field intubation. If the paramedic detects a tension pneumothorax, immediate pleural decompression should be performed and intubation should follow as soon as possible. The paramedic must reevaluate the patient's airway and breathing status frequently during the initial assessment and patient packaging, constantly assessing for compliance problems if the patient is being assist ventilated with a BVM. Compliance problems may indicate the need to decompress the pleura, reposition the patient's airway, or perform immediate oral or nasal intubation. If the patient's airway and breathing can be managed effectively with assisted ventilation until he or she is loaded into the ambulance or helicopter, intubation can be delayed. It is often easier to intubate once the patient is in a more controlled environment and in a better position for visualization of anatomical landmarks. If the patient does not require immediate intubation to secure the airway but requires assisted ventilation or hyperventilation, do not forget to use an oropharyngeal or nasopharyngeal airway. Use of these adjunctive devices is often forgotten, resulting in an inadequately opened and maintained airway.

Table 6-5
Classification System for Determining Patient Priority for Transport Decisions

Category	Action	Examples of Patient Condition
C—Critical	Airway and spinal control, treat only immediate threats to life, then rapid transport	Cardiac or respiratory arrest
U—Unstable	Same as above	Respiratory distress and/or shock
P—Potentially unstable	Rapid assessment, treatment of potential threats to life, airway and spinal control, then expedient transport	Marginal vital signs
S—Stable	Continue with focused assessment	Normal vital signs, no apparent distress, no major mechanism of injury

Severe exsanguinating hemorrhage should be immediately controlled using basic techniques of direct pressure, pressure dressings, or pressure points. Volume resuscitation may be delayed until the patient is en route to the hospital unless a prolonged disentanglement is in progress. When there are adequate personnel on scene, someone can prepare two large-bore, 14–16-gauge IVs of normal saline or lactated Ringer's in the ambulance or helicopter. As soon as the patient is loaded, resuscitation can be initiated. The IV fluid should be warmed, if possible, to prevent hypothermia. It is no longer acceptable to delay transport to initiate fluid resuscitation in the field, for the critical trauma patient generally requires blood transfusion to restore the cardiovascular system and maintain adequate perfusion status.

The use of PASG should be considered when the patient's systolic blood pressure is 60–80 mm Hg, especially if there are abdominal or pelvic injuries.[2] Specific criteria for inflation will be based on local medical protocols. The PASG is an excellent immobilizing device for stabilization of femur and pelvic fractures. Refer to Chapters 15 and 21 for further discussion regarding use and application of this device with these injuries.

As soon as the patient is loaded for transport, reevaluation of the ABCs begins, intubation is performed if the airway is unstable, two large-bore IVs are initiated preferably with trauma tubing, quantitative vital signs are obtained, and the patient is completely stripped of all clothing and covered to prevent hypothermia. All multisystem trauma patients are placed on a cardiac monitor as soon as possible to monitor for dysrhythmias that often accompany head and thoracic trauma. Some EMS systems require a nasogastric (NG) tube to be placed to reduce the incidence of aspiration. Nasogastric tube placement is contraindicated in patients with cribriform fractures and cerebrospinal fluid (CSF) drainage.[9]

INTERNET ACTIVITIES

Visit the British Trauma Society Web site and review the material on the organization of the trauma team at http://www.trauma.org/resus/traumateam.html. How is this system of trauma resuscitation similar to that of the field resuscitation team? How does it differ?

FOCUSED ASSESSMENT

Once definitive treatment has been provided for all initial problems, the paramedic can begin to perform a detailed physical examination. The purpose of the focused assessment is to detect other potentially life-threatening injuries missed in the initial assessment, to obtain a more detailed analysis of existing injuries, and to detect other non-life-threatening minor injuries. Often this survey is performed en route to the emergency department or sometimes it is not completed at all while all energies and time are spent managing life-threatening injuries.

When the focused assessment is performed, the paramedic obtains quantitative assessment information and a patient history and performs a complete physical examination. The focused assessment consists of the criteria found in Table 6-6. Begin this survey by obtaining, if possible, information regarding the patient's history, using the acronym AMPLE (Table 6-7). During the "head-to-toe survey," look for medic alert necklaces or bracelets that could provide some of the AMPLE information. Quantitative vital signs, if not obtained soon after the patient was loaded for transport, should be performed and recorded now, and every 3–5 minutes throughout transport.

Table 6-6
Criteria for Performing a Focused Assessment

See	Inspect-look-observe for contusions, abrasions, lacerations, ecchymosis, edema, hemorrhage, deformity (angulation shortening, abnormal position)
Listen	Auscultate for breath sounds, heart sounds
Feel	Palpate for tenderness, deformities, crepitus, masses, edema, subcutaneous air, instability, rigidity

Source: Adapted from *The Paramedic Manual,* by J. Greenwald, 1988, Englewood, CO: Morton Publishing Co.

Table 6-7
Use of the Acronym AMPLE in Gathering Pertinent Patient Information

A—Allergies

M—Medications

P—Past and present pertinent history

L—Last meal

E—Events leading up to the incident

Using the look, listen, and feel methods of assessment, perform the focused assessment, region by region, as found in Table 6-8. If PASG has been applied, the survey will examine down to the diaphragm level. If PASG has not been applied, the survey will include the entire anterior and lateral body. Look for signs of ecchymosis, deformity, hemorrhage, masses, swelling, abnormal indentations, or abnormal skin color that would indicate injury or underlying medical problems. Listen for abnormal breath sounds or abnormal heart sounds (e.g., muffled heart tones). Feel all areas of the body for the presence of pulses in all extremities; for skin temperature; and for abnormal findings such as the presence of abnormal pulsations, crepitus, abnormal movement of long bones or joints, deformity, subcutaneous emphysema, depressions in the skull, abdominal rigidity, or impaled fragments of glass or metal. Reassessment of the patient's previous ABCD vitals will be performed during this assessment phase. Reassess the patient's respiratory status, ECG, vital signs, neurological status, skin color, and temperature at least every 3–5 minutes while en route. It is equally important to closely monitor fluid replacement by frequently reassessing the patient's pulse strength, LOC, and lung sounds.

Table 6-8
Algorithm for Performing Focused Assessment

Region	Assessment
Head	Soft tissue injuries,* raccoon's eyes, Battle's sign, cerebrospinal fluid or blood from nose and/or ears, skull deformity, eye orbits, stability of nasal and facial bones, foreign bodies or blood in the oral cavity, stability of mandible, pupillary response, extraocular movements
Neck	Soft tissue injuries,* jugular venous distention, tracheal deviation, carotid pulse, subcutaneous emphysema, cervical spine deformity or tenderness
Chest	Soft tissue injuries,* stability of ribs, sternum, and clavicles, chest symmetry and expansion, bilateral breath sounds, open pneumothorax, subcutaneous emphysema, flail segments, heart sounds, electrocardiogram
Abdomen and pelvis	Soft tissue injuries,* distention, tenderness, guarding, pulsatile masses, rigidity, bowel sounds, rebound tenderness, pelvic stability, priapism
Extremities	Soft tissue injuries,* bony instability, pulses, motor, sensation, range of motion, tenderness, crepitus, deformity, malrotation, shortening, lengthening, open fractures
Back	Soft tissue injuries,* vertebral deformity or tenderness, stability of ribs, stability of sacrum, buttocks

*Soft tissue injuries include lacerations, contusions, abrasions, incisions, penetrating injuries, burns, edema, hematoma, hueing, and amputations.

RADIO AND REPORT COMMUNICATION

As soon as the paramedic can establish radio communication with the emergency department, vital patient information should be communicated. It will be very important to communicate specific information regarding the patient's MOI and the kinematics involved, ventilatory, circulatory, and neurological status, treatment and response to treatment, and estimated time of arrival (ETA). Be as short and concise as possible. Try to paint a realistic picture of the patient's overall status. This will allow emergency department personnel time to prepare for the patient's arrival and alert the surgical team. Upon arrival at the medical facility, verbally transfer the patient to the receiving physician or nurse, providing a detailed account of the patient's injuries and treatment.

Finally, provide a written ambulance call report to the receiving hospital. This report is important because it gives the hospital staff a thorough understanding of the events surrounding the incident and a progressive account of the patient's condition and response (or lack of response) to treatment initiated on scene and en route to the hospital.

▶ SUMMARY

The multisystem trauma patient must be rapidly, systematically, and thoroughly evaluated. Paramedics must develop an organized and consistent approach to the trauma patient that outlines priorities of care (refer to Figure 6-25 for a complete patient assessment algorithm). These priorities are found during the initial survey, which evaluates the MOI and kinematics of the injuries, airway and C-spine control, breathing, and circulatory and neurological status and includes completely exposing the patient. Definitive field treatment revolves around rapid recognition and treatment of hypoxemia and shock resulting from inadequate airways, compromised ventilatory and circulatory status, and inadequate cerebral perfusion.

The paramedic must be able to systematically evaluate and constantly reevaluate the patient every 3–5 minutes, providing immediate definitive treatment for airway, breathing, and circulatory problems as they are encountered. Needlessly delaying transportation of the trauma patient may increase the patient's morbidity and severely decrease his or her chances for survival. Finally, initiate transportation to the most appropriate medical facility with treatment teams trained to manage the critically injured trauma patient.

▶ INTERNET ACTIVITIES

Review the prehospital trauma resuscitation protocols of the North Central Texas Trauma Regional Advisory Council at http://www.dfwhc. org/ncttrac/protocols.htm. To review the protocols, you will need Acrobat Reader, which can be downloaded free of charge from http://www. adobe.com/.

▶ REVIEW QUESTIONS

1. Which of the following represents a "load and go" patient?
   a. A patient with an isolated radius/ulna fracture
   b. A patient with a large flail segment
   c. A patient with venous bleeding that is controlled by direct pressure
   d. A patient with a dislocated shoulder

2. It is acceptable to bypass the local hospital in favor of transporting a critically injured patient directly to a trauma center.
   a. True
   b. False

3. List several questions that should be incorporated into the scene size up.

4. List several questions that should be incorporated into the global assessment upon approach of the scene.

5. Overall, what percentage of patients are truly "load and go"?
   a. 5
   b. 10
   c. 15
   d. 20

6. Compare and contrast the golden hour and platinum ten minutes.

7. List five mechanisms of injury that suggest major trauma.

8. List five physical findings that suggest major trauma.

9. Which oxygen delivery device is most appropriate for a patient with a C-4 spinal injury?
   a. Nasal cannula
   b. Nonrebreather mask
   c. BVM
   d. Simple mask

10. Bulging neck veins may indicate which of the following pathologies?
    i. Simple pneumothorax
    ii. Tension pneumothorax
    iii. Cardiac tamponade
    iv. Myocardial contusion
       a. i and ii
       b. ii and iii
       c. iii and iv
       d. ii and iv

11. If a radial pulse is palpable, a crude estimate of systolic blood pressure is:
    a. At least 50 mm Hg
    b. At least 60 mm Hg
    c. At least 70 mm Hg
    d. At least 80 mm Hg

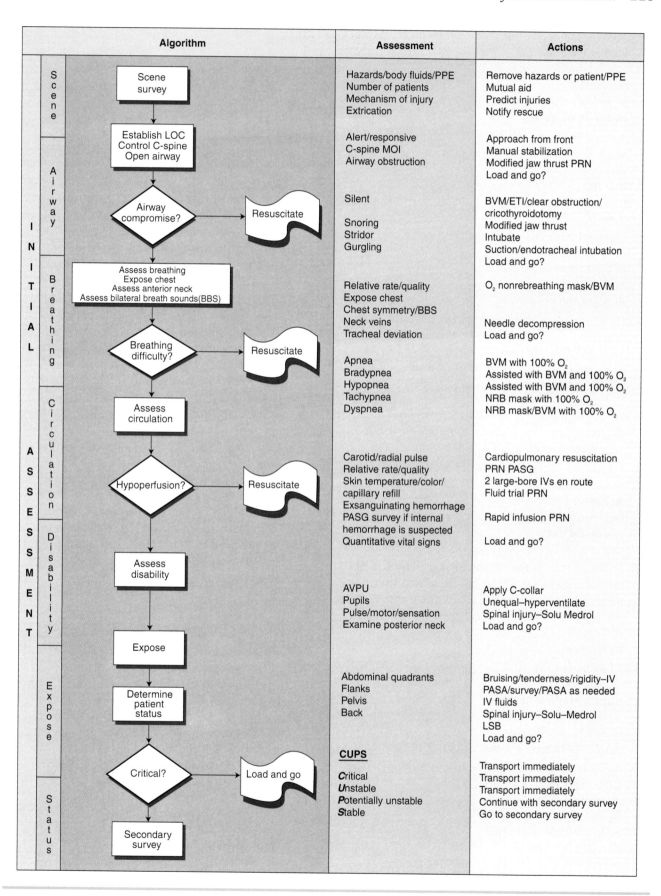

FIGURE 6-25 Patient assessment algorithm.

12. The most likely source of unexplained internal hemorrhage is the:
   a. Abdomen
   b. Chest
   c. Retroperitoneal space
   d. Epidural space

13. Normal capillary refill time is less than or equal to:
   a. 1 sec
   b. 2 sec
   c. 3 sec
   d. 4 sec

14. Unequal pupils may indicate:
   a. Head trauma
   b. Cerebrovascular accident
   c. Eye trauma
   d. All of the above

15. Upon applying lateral and inward pressure on the iliac wings, crepitus and instability are noted. The paramedic should next:
   a. Palpate the iliac wings in a downward and posterior direction
   b. Palpate the symphysis pubis
   c. "Rock" the pelvis to confirm instability
   d. Recognize the pelvic fracture and discontinue further palpation of the pelvis

16. The most immediate life threat from bilateral femur fractures is:
   a. Fat emboli
   b. Deep vein thrombus
   c. Hemorrhage
   d. Femoral nerve injury

17. Following the initial examination at the scene, the critical patient should be packaged and transport initiated with continued assessment conducted while en route to the trauma center.
   a. True
   b. False

18. The letter M of the pneumonic AMPLE represents:
   a. past Medical history
   b. last Meal
   c. Medicine allergies
   d. Medications the patient is currently taking

19. Subcutaneous emphysema may indicate which of the following?
   a. Pneumothorax
   b. Tracheal disruption
   c. Bronchiole disruption
   d. Any of the above

20. Quantitative vital signs must be obtained during the initial assessment even if it is necessary to delay airway and hemorrhage control.
   a. True
   b. False

CRITICAL THINKING

- Correlate the etiologies of death in the trimodal distribution of time of death (Chapter 3) with the rapid trauma assessment. Why do you think the assessment sequence is A–B–C–D–E as opposed to some other priority? How do the treatment priorities of the rapid trauma assessment impact each mode of the distribution?

- Think back to your last EMS response to a multi-system trauma patient. Was an organized assessment plan implemented? Were the on-scene treatments properly prioritized? Based upon your understanding of rapid trauma assessment, what would you now do differently if faced with a similar scenario? Why?

- For the following scenario, describe your assessment plan and treatment priorities: You are called to the scene of an MVC. A single car left the roadway at a high rate of speed and struck a tree. There are no skid marks on the road, and there is approximately 36 inches of crush to the front of the vehicle. The driver is slumped over the steering wheel and appears unconscious. There is obvious deformity to the steering wheel and windshield. No restraints were worn and the car was not equipped with airbags.

REFERENCES

1. Caroline NL. *Emergency Care in the Streets*. 5th ed. Philadelphia, Pa: Lippincott Williams and Wilkins, 1995.
2. Paturas JL, Wertz EM, McSwain NE Jr. *PHTLS Basic and Advanced Prehospital Trauma and Life Support*. 4th ed. St. Louis: Mosby-Year Book, 1999.
3. Trunkey, DD. Trauma. *Sci Am*. 1983; 249:28.
4. Campbell, JE. *Basic Trauma Life Support*. Englewood Cliffs, NJ: Prentice-Hall, 1998.
5. Bledsoe BE, Porter RS, Shade BR. *Paramedic Emergency Care*, 3rd ed. Englewood Cliffs, NJ: Prentice-Hall, 1997.

6. Miller RH, Wilson JK. *Manual of Prehospital Emergency Medicine*. St. Louis: Mosby-Year Book, 1992.

7. Butman AM, et al. *Comprehensive Guide to Pre-Hospital Skills: A Skills Manual*. Akron, Ohio: Emergency Training, 1995.

8. Pons P, Cason D, eds. *ACEP Paramedic Field Care*. St. Louis: Mosby, 1997.

9. Trauma: Review of Initial Management, Initial Assessment and Management Priorities. Internet: http://www.mc.vanderbilt.edu/surgery/backup/trauma.html, 1997.

10. Cleveland Clinic Foundation: Spine and Spinal Cord Trauma, Department of General Anesthesiology. Internet: http://www.anes.ccf.org.8080/PILOT/NEURO/SCI.html, 1997.

11. Campbell JE. *Basic Trauma Life Support*, 3rd ed. Englewood Cliffs, NJ: Prentice-Hall, 1995.

12. Greenwald J. *The Paramedic Manual*. Englewood, Col.: Morton Publishing, 1988.

Chapter 7

Trauma Scoring Systems

OBJECTIVES

Upon completion of this chapter, the reader should be able to:

● Discuss the functions and components of trauma assessment tools.

● Describe the application of trauma assessment tools in evaluating and determining the severity of injuries in the trauma patient.

● Define physiological changes that determine the severity of traumatic injuries.

● List assessment tools that evaluate injuries based on anatomic criteria.

● Explain the utility of identifying and classifying the mechanism of injury in evaluating traumatic injuries.

● Discuss the use of retrospective analysis and classification of injuries and their impact on EMS field management.

● Describe the trauma score, Glasgow Coma Scale, CRAMS score, abbreviated injury scale, injury severity score, and prehospital index.

● Describe the pediatric trauma score.

● Explain trauma outcome evaluation using the TRISS methodology.

KEY TERMS

Abbreviated injury scale (AIS)
CRAMS score
Glasgow Coma Scale (GCS)
Injury severity score (ISS)
Pediatric trauma score (PTS)
Penetrating abdominal trauma index (PATI)
Prehospital index (PHI)

Revised trauma score (RTS)
Trauma score (TS)
Trauma systems
TRISS method
W-statistic
Z-statistic

Before the 1970s little work was done in the field of stratification of injuries, or triage. Patients were transported to the nearest hospital for care, regardless of the severity of their injuries. Data collected by the National Research Council in the 1960s provided feedback on the treatment of trauma and concluded that changes were needed.[1,2] The results of this study gave birth to trauma care systems or trauma centers. **Trauma systems** are an interconnected source of services and providers with the resources and expertise to manage

119

life-threatening, traumatic injuries. These systems require a great deal of administrative, capital, and medical staff support, which increases operating expenses and demands on limited resources. The high cost of operating trauma centers, coupled with the low incidence of major trauma, limited the development of trauma centers to certain strategic locations throughout each state or region. With the development of a limited number of trauma centers, decisions on patient delivery had to be considered. Through the development of an integrated trauma care system, it was suggested that patients no longer be transported to the closest facility, but to the most appropriate facility to manage their injuries. Discussion focused on who would make these transport decisions, what mechanism should be used to aid in the decision, and how health care systems would evaluate the decision. It was quickly decided that the scope of treatment begins at the scene with EMS and continues until discharge from the hospital or death. Every decision made about patient care needed evaluation in an attempt to conserve resources for the most severely injured.

DEVELOPMENT OF TRAUMA SCORING SYSTEMS

In an attempt to evaluate and direct treatment decisions, health care facilities and trauma experts created assessment tools to quantify the traumatic injuries suffered by patients. Assessments designed to evaluate patients' risk of mortality from injuries needed to provide an encompassing approach, yet remain applicable to field providers.

Initial assessment tools developed in the early 1970s focused on the evaluation and recording of physiological criteria. These tools collected data that could be observed and assimilated in the field, such as blood pressure and level of consciousness. In the early development of trauma scoring systems, it was believed that injuries could be classified by injury focus, indicators of severity, the individuals assessing the injuries or locus of application, and the underlying concepts of physiological, anatomical, and mechanism of injury indicators.[1] Based on analysis and review of available evaluation tools, the National Center for Health Services Research and the American Trauma Society developed basic criteria for assessment tools: (1) scales for evaluation should be simple and the data for assessment readily available, (2) the tool should have predictive validity (i.e., it should correlate with measured outcomes), (3) tools should be intuitively reasonable (i.e., high face validity for multidisciplined health care providers), and (4) data collection methods should be clear, reliable, and subject to review.[1]

The models developed evaluate the injuries at the scene, emergency department, or both. Evaluation models, or severity scores, serve multitask functions, assisting in prehospital triage and transport determinations, clinical management, and outcome evaluation.[1] Scoring systems are generally evaluated on their sensitivity and specificity in identifing critically injured patients.

PURPOSE OF TRAUMA SCORING SYSTEMS

Trauma scoring systems augment the judgment and resources of EMS personnel. Trauma scoring assists in identifying needed resources, including treatment and transport priorities, transporting source, and appropriate receiving facilities.

Outcome Evaluation

Trauma scoring systems allow hospitals and trauma centers to compare the performance of their system against a standard.[3] A common **Z-statistic** can be utilized to compare the actual number of survivors within the trauma center with the number of expected survivors (with the same injuries). An important addition to the Z-statistic, the **W-statistic**, compares the sample population treated at that facility with other facility patient populations. The W-statistic was introduced to evaluate the statistical significance of small, and seemingly indiscernible, differences—differences that are statistically significant solely from the use of large samples. Figure 7-1 outlines the Z- and W-statistics used to examine outcomes given a specific patient population.

Z-Statistic: $Z = (A - E)/s$

This statistic compares the actual number of survivors (A) in the facility with the number of expected survivors (E), based on current industry data. Statistical variation is measured by s. The power to detect statistically significant, yet small differences between survivors and expected survivors increases with sample size. With large sample populations (>150 patients), Z-values between -1.96 and $+1.96$ indicate no significant statistical difference between industry expectations and the facility's performance.

W-Value: $W = (A - E)/(N/100)$

The W-statistic, where N is the number of patients analyzed, provides a perspective on the clinical significance of the Z-statistics. Positive W-values indicate the number of successful clinical outcomes beyond the industry trends per 100 patients treated.

FIGURE 7-1 *Z*-statistic and *W*-value.

These statistics are important in evaluating programs across a varied field of providers. Hospitals may treat a varied population of trauma patients. Discerning how an institution's program performs would be impossible without these statistical analyses. These analyses also allow a facility to compare its services over a period of time. For example, a facility may treat 291 severe trauma patients in 1999 with a mortality value of 3.62, and in 2000 the facility receives 234 patients with a value of 2.05. Did the facility's service improve over the past year? With the use of the *W*-value and Z-statistic investigators can determine trends in the quality of care as well as the impact of new programs on patient outcomes.

Quality Assessment

In outcome performance analysis, facilities examine the process of managing trauma services. Processes are reviewed for consistency, pattern, and compliance with local and national standards. Often, regulatory agencies provide detailed and elaborate treatment standards. The American College of Surgeons (ACS) Committee on Trauma offers audit criteria to assess care standards. The committee suggests criteria to examine quality-of-care measures. Similarly, the Joint Commission on Accreditation of Healthcare Organizations (JCAHO) has identified quality indicators to ensure the continuity of care among facilities.[3]

Those participating in the JACHO accreditation process must demonstrate the utilization of outcome measurements and mechanisms for evaluating the process of care. The quality assessment program evaluates the process of care by focusing efforts on treatment protocols, institutional guidelines, and communications.

TRAUMA ASSESSMENT TOOLS

Physiological and anatomic assessment, the mechanism of injury, and solid clinical judgment affect the triage process.[1,2] Physiological assessments are often time dependent, diminishing their usefulness in the prehospital setting. Traumatic derangements may develop over time. There are critically injured patients whose initial evaluation demonstrates normal or stable physiological scores.[1] Anatomic criteria define injuries of specific organ systems, thus requiring definitive diagnosis, making some injuries impossible to evaluate in the prehospital setting. In addition, because mechanism-of-injury criteria are collected through second-hand accounts, challenges exist in collecting accurate data. Collecting information and assessing traumatic injuries in the field pose significant challenges for the prehospital provider. Understanding these challenges and combining sound clinical evaluations with sensitive assessment tools provides valuable information and enhance decision making.

PHYSIOLOGICAL VARIABLES

Instruments designed to systematically survey and evaluate physiological findings in the trauma patient generally require serial evaluations to rank the severity of injuries. These findings may be tallied to increase the sensitivity of the evaluation tool.

Glasgow Coma Scale

A very popular physiological tool for prehospital use is the **Glasgow Coma Scale** (Table 7-1). This tool evaluates and provides a quantitative analysis of consciousness. Older assessment tools relied on the subjective differentiation of the patient's presentation using broadly defined terms such as *semiconscious* and *lethargic*. In 1974, Teasdale and Jennette published the Glasgow Coma Scale (GCS) based on objective physiological criteria.[4] Teasdale's coma score also evaluates the entire brain's ability to function, not a particular portion or section of the brain.[5] Studies of blunt head trauma patients suggest that the GCS is the best neurological assessment in the prehospital environment in determining the depth of coma.[6]

Table 7-1
Glasgow Coma Scale

Eye opening	Spontaneous	4
	To voice	3
	To pain	2
	None	1
Verbal response	Oriented	5
	Confused	4
	Inappropriate	3
	Incomprehensible	2
	None	1
Motor response	Obeys command	6
	Localizes pain	5
	Withdraws from pain	4
	Flexion to pain	3
	Extension to pain	2
	None	1
Total GCS:	3–15	

The coma score evaluates three major activities to assess cerebral function: (1) eye opening, (2) verbal response, and (3) motor response. These criteria are reliable, simple to use, and easily communicated between health care providers of varying backgrounds and expertise. Note that the evaluator is responsible for eliciting the best response for each of the categories.

Each criterion is graded on a numerical scale and provides information about cerebral function. Eye opening is scored on a scale from 1 to 4. It evaluates arousal mechanisms within the brainstem and provides an insight to the functioning capabilities within the brain.[5]

Verbal response correlates with higher levels of central nervous system function. The scale for verbal response ranges from 1 to 5. The evaluator must use clinical judgment to assess the patient's ability to recognize the surroundings. Caution should be used when speaking with the patient prior to the evaluation because the patient may memorize responses gleaned during treatment.

The motor response component of the GCS evaluates the functioning of the central nervous system. Patients are observed for their response to simple motor skill testing. It has been suggested that this category alone accounts for the reliability of the GCS.[5,6] Table 7-1 outlines the GCS and each of its monitors. The score is also used as the framework for other trauma evaluations in prehospital and in-hospital settings.

Research suggests that prehospital treatment may occur so rapidly that early physiological signs of deterioration in the trauma patient are masked. One study showed that although rapid field treatment did not allow for a complete physical assessment, it did allow for a baseline assessment. This baseline allowed hospital providers to determine the patient's net change.[6] The significance of this net change is that it points out transient neurological deficits that may account for the high degree of "overtriage" to trauma centers. Overtriage is inappropriately transporting patients to trauma centers when care could have been adequately provided at a local hospital. Overtriage has been reported to be as high as 80% in some trauma systems.

Trauma Score

Another reliable evaluation tool is the **trauma score (TS)** (Table 7-2) or **revised trauma score (RTS)** (Table 7-3). This evaluation tool relies on the combination of the GCS and other evaluation criteria to assign a numeric value to represent the extent of injury. The TS evaluates respiratory rate and expansion, capillary refill, and blood pressure ranges, defining each by numeric values. The lower the numeric value, the more severe the injury. The TS has demonstrated high interuser

reliability for predicting survival/death outcomes for blunt and penetrating trauma.[7] EMS agencies often combine the TS with anatomic findings and mechanism-of-injury indicators to increase triage reliability.

The original design of the TS assessed capillary refill and respiratory expansion. However, darkness and other environmental conditions can make evaluation of these factors difficult in the field. The Major Trauma Outcome Study (MTOS) reports that the TS in its original design made accurate determination of head trauma difficult, often underestimating the severity of the injury.[7] Concerns for the application of the TS to field triage led to revisions that used the GCS and the patient's blood pressure and respiratory rate instead of respiratory expansion (Table 7-3). Studies demonstrate that the RTS is more sensitive in evaluating head trauma, easier to apply to field triage, and possesses a higher degree of reliability in directing the care of the patient.[7]

Table 7-2
Trauma Score

Respirations/min	>36	2
	25–35	3
	10–24	4
	1–9	1
	None	0
Respiratory expansion	Normal	1
	Shallow	0
	Retractive	0
Systolic blood pressure (mm Hg)	>90	4
	70–89	3
	50–69	2
	0–49	1
	No pulse	0
Capillary return	Normal	2
	Delayed	1
	None	0
Glasgow Coma Scale contribution	14–15	5
	11–13	4
	8–10	3
	5–7	2
	3–4	1
Total trauma score: 1–16		

Table 7-3
Revised Trauma Score

Respirations/min	10–29	4
	>29	3
	6–9	2
	1–5	1
	None	0
Systolic blood pressure (mm Hg)	>89	4
	76–89	3
	50–75	2
	1–49	1
	No pulse	0
Glasgow Coma Scale contribution	13–15	4
	9–12	3
	6–8	2
	4–5	1
	3	0

Total revised trauma score: 1–12

Other research reveals that not all physiological findings must be combined into a scoring mechanism. Data suggest that specific portions of the RTS, utilized independently, offer a high degree of sensitivity.[7] Triage criteria evaluating systolic blood pressure and respiratory rate independently or combined are independent parameters that can identify or suggest major trauma.

INTERNET ACTIVITIES

Visit the British Trauma Society Web page and review the section on the Revised Trauma Score at http://www.trauma.org/scores/rts.html. Notice the chart showing the relationship between RTS and the probability of survival. Insert your own values for systolic blood pressure (BP), respiratory rate, and GCS into the regression equation and calculate your own RTS. Check your answer by inserting these values into the RTS calculator on the Web page.

CRAMS

The **CRAMS** (circulation, respiration, abdomen, motor, and speech) **score** is a triage instrument combining the scores of physiological, anatomic, and historic variables to pinpoint the severity of injuries.[5,8,9]

Including previously cited physiological variables, the CRAMS score also incorporates assessment criteria for abdominal and thoracic injuries.

The CRAMS score provides a broad spectrum of patient presentations. Researchers using this scoring system note that the wide criteria make the score poorly suited for patient care decisions.[5,9] For example, under the CRAMS method a patient receives a score of zero if their systolic BP is less than 85 and/or they have delayed capillary refill. There is no provision for patients to receive a higher score if they present with normal vital signs but with capillary refill delays due to environmental conditions or other unrelated medical situations. Because CRAMS does not analyze specific patient injuries, it is considered to have little practical clinical application in predicting outcomes. However, application of the scoring mechanism provides researchers some definable means to describe traumatic injuries in a group of patients.

ANATOMIC CRITERIA

Assessment tools that evaluate the severity of injuries in relation to organs injured or site of injury are classified as anatomic criteria.[1,8] Anatomic findings categorize injuries into two types: (1) blunt or (2) penetrating. In addition, the site of injury will identify anatomic groups, such as thoracic, neuromuscular, vascular, abdominal, or cardiovascular, to assist in the evaluation.

Although the site of injury offers clues to possible major organ injuries, it is difficult to use the anatomic site as the sole determining factor in judging the severity of the injury. Researchers have found that the site of injury is of great importance in identifying major trauma patients but is not able to clarify what prehospital factors are useful in the diagnosis of anatomic injuries.[8] One study used penetrating anatomic injuries as the absolute criteria for identifying major trauma. The penetrating criteria reduced the amount of undertriage conducted in the field but increased the number of overtriage or false-positive patients by 143%.[10]

Abbreviated Injury Scale

The **abbreviated injury scale (AIS)** is the worldwide accepted threat-to-life scale used for evaluating injuries of road-related trauma.[11] The scale was first developed by the American Medical Association, the American Association for Automotive Medicine, and the Society of Automotive Engineers to stratify injuries sustained by automobile crash victims.

The AIS formulates an injury scale through assessing seven body regions: (1) head and face, (2) neck, (3) chest, (4) spine, (5) abdomen and pelvic contents,

(6) extremities and pelvic girdle, and (7) integument. The AIS assigns severity on a numeric value from 1 (minor) to 6 (unsurvivable).[10] The scale has been revised over time to broaden its scope and increase its sensitivity and specificity in injury identification. To assist researchers, injuries are grouped by mechanism of injury: blunt and penetrating. Initially, the AIS had 73 injury definitions; the latest revision includes greater than 1,300 different injuries, and each injury definition assigns severity of injury. An example of this specificity can be found with the scoring mechanism AIS-90, the latest edition, which has 13 different injury definitions for a femur fracture and severity of injury for eight abdominal organs. To achieve a severity scoring, the scale compares the likelihood of the injury resulting in a fatal outcome; however, extended intensive care, extent of disability, or total cost of the recovery process can also be considered.[9] Researchers depend on the AIS injury definitions to ensure injuries are scored consistently.

It is difficult to evaluate the severity of trauma with the AIS since most patients suffer multiple injuries. Because the AIS groups injuries into single-system groupings, multiple injuries within the area are defined only by the most serious injury.[9] Injuries that cause death in these cases are usually not considered fatal if occurring independently. The AIS scores can compare individual injury patterns and anatomic injuries but cannot compare injury groups or patient groupings requiring a more complex approach. Additionally, the complexity of the AIS makes it difficult to apply in the field setting. However, the AIS represents a compromise between the clinical demands for detail and pragmatic application.[9]

Injury Severity Score

A popular evaluation tool based on anatomic criteria is the **injury severity score (ISS)**. The ISS is derived from summing the squares of the highest of the seven AIS scores.[12] Summary scoring based on this calculation results in numerical scoring from 1 to 75. Patients receiving an AIS score of 6, a nearly unsurvivable injury, receive an ISS of 75.

Research demonstrates that the use of the ISS explains 49% of the variance in mortality, an increase from the 25% explained using the (AIS) single worst injury method.[7] The scoring system is widely and predominantly used in trauma research and is collected retrospectively. Originally, the ISS was designed to capture blunt trauma; it demonstrated limitations in evaluating penetrating trauma mortality. The challenge in predicting penetrating trauma mortality is grounded in the fact that these injuries tend to concentrate all injuries into one body region, leading the evaluator to score only the most severe and underscore the ISS.[9,12]

To address this issue, researchers and physicians developed the **penetrating abdominal trauma index (PATI)** to accompany the ISS.[9] This scale assigns a numeric risk factor to each organ in the abdominal cavity (bladder = 1, pancreas = 5) and provides a numeric assignment, 1–5, based on the intensity of the injury or amount of surgical intervention required.[9] The PATI score provides a thorough evaluation of penetrating abdominal injuries but does not address penetrating injuries to other body regions.

MECHANISM OF INJURY

The very nature of the injury event has been identified as contributing information for determining the most appropriate transport facility. The injury delivery mechanism is suggestive of the amount of energy transferred to the patient during impact and is used to predict the destructive capabilities of the event.[13] Events suggesting significant injury transfer are ejection, prolonged extrication, occupancy death, and a high-velocity change.[13,14] Other mechanisms suggestive of high energy transfer include falls greater than 15 feet, pedestrians struck by vehicles, motorcycle crashes, and vehicular roll-overs.[13,14]

The trauma mechanism offers prehospital providers the ability to quickly collect information associated with the event. Often EMS providers collect important information about the transfer of energy simply by surveying the scene. The ability to rapidly collect and impart information is important. Paramedics face stringent time constraints and must accurately relay descriptive information to other health care providers who never view the injury scene.

When used as a sole identifier for patients needing immediate treatment at a trauma center, research shows that mechanistic criteria produce a comparatively high false-positive ratio; that is, they often overestimate the severity of injuries. The mechanism of injury aids in the identification of injury severity but must be used carefully as a triage tool for transport to a trauma center.

FIELD ASSESSMENT

In the field, triage and transport sector decisions should be reached after careful utilization of a trauma scoring mechanism. The scoring system utilized should allow for accurate and rapid prediction of major injuries requiring a trauma center.[2] The most common scoring system utilized in the field is the GCS. The popularity of this score is due to its ability to collect physical findings during the initial assessment, with relatively few items required to reach a reliable summary. Although the GCS is popular in EMS, some systems choose to use a combination of several assessment tools to reach a final decision on the severity of a patient's injuries (Table 7-4).

PREHOSPITAL INDEX

In an attempt to better define field triage and identify patients needing trauma center surgical intervention, researchers developed the **prehospital index (PHI)** by combining four triage tools. The PHI was designed and tested using trauma criteria and identifies patients requiring emergency surgery within 24 hours or patients who will die as a result of injuries within 72 hours.

The four components of the PHI are outlined in Table 7-5 and include systolic blood pressure, pulse, respiratory status, and level of consciousness. Each are assigned a score between 0 and 5; abdominal and/or chest injuries are given additional numerical assignments. Patients receiving a PHI of 3 or less are considered minor injuries and should be treated at a community hospital. The PHI assignments of 4–20 are major traumas and should be triaged to a trauma center.

This index is designed to provide an objective, accurate, and reliable method for field personnel to evaluate trauma patients quickly and effectively in the field. The PHI has demonstrated limited clinical success in field tests. Concern surrounds the index's definition of broad trauma criteria, specifically, trauma patients that have sustained injuries that do not require emergency surgery within 24 hours but need definitive treatment offered only at a trauma center. The continued testing and evaluation of the PHI should focus on local resources and the effective organization of these limited resources for the best utilization in aggregate patient care.

Table 7-4
Clinical Variables for EMS Evaluation

Anatomic	Penetrating wound to head, neck, chest, abdomen, back, or groin
	Traumatic amputation above elbow or knee
	Traumatic neurological deficit
	Two or more proximal long-bone fractures
Physiological	Pulse
	Systolic blood pressure
	Respiration
	Glasgow Coma Scale score
Mechanism of injury	Death of occupant in same vehicle
	Long extrication time
	Automobile versus pedestrian > than 20 mph
	Vehicle rollover without restraints
	Falls greater than 15 feet
	Submersion with trauma

Table 7-5
Prehospital Index

Systolic blood pressure (mm Hg)	>100	0
	86–100	1
	75–85	2
	0–74	5
Pulse	>120	3
	51–119	0
	<50	5
Respiratory expansion	Normal	0
	Labored/shallow	3
	>10 min intubated	5
Consciousness	Normal	0
	Confused/combative	3
	Unconsciousness	5
Total PHI: 0–20*		

*Penetrating abdominal or chest injuries receive 4 points in addition to the calculated PHI.

Source: Adapted from "Prehospital Index: A Scoring System for Field Triage of Trauma Victims," by J. Koehler et al., 1986, *Annals of Emergency Medicine, 15*(2), p. 51.

PEDIATRIC TRAUMA PATIENTS

In ideal situations prehospital providers are able to assess patient injuries objectively utilizing a trauma assessment tool that accurately determines the severity of patient injuries. This evaluation allows providers to allocate the appropriate health care delivery system resources for each patient. Pediatric patients are not "small adults"; they have special needs, different physiological findings, and different injury processes.

Pediatric patients present challenges for prehospital providers from the infrequency of contact and the differences in physiology compared with adults. Because of the vast differences, the trauma score is often not valid for the pediatric patient population.[15–17] Using the TS, paramedics are required to evaluate pediatric patients based on adult criteria, such as blood pressure, pulse rate, and verbal response. Often, physiological assessment tools using verbal responses to determine patients' cerebral function are not appropriate since developmental skills may not be mature enough to allow for an objective evaluation.

In order to more accurately assess this unique patient population, the pediatric trauma score was developed (Table 7-6).[16,17] The **pediatric trauma score (PTS)** is similar in design to the APGAR system in that it assigns a numeric +2, +1, and –1 to each criterion.[15–17] The scoring system evaluates six parameters to determine injury severity: (1) size, (2) airway, (3) blood pressure, (4) level of consciousness, (5) skeletal assessment, and (6) cutaneous evaluation. The PTS combines physiological and anatomic indexes to evaluate the patient's injuries.

Size, the first parameter, recognizes the limited physiological reserves and the greater surface area of infants and toddlers. Multisystem trauma in these young patients is the rule instead of the exception due to the dispersion of energy throughout the entire body.[17]

Airway is evaluated on the amount of management that is required to provide an adequate airway. Because of the patient's large cranium in comparison to body size, the normal developmental process of the trachea, and a relative small airway, pediatric airways are susceptible to life-threatening injuries requiring extensive intervention. The scoring system evaluates the amount of management needed and assigns a sliding numeric value to airways that require maintenance with oral airways and invasive mechanics.

Normal blood pressure varies with age. Paramedics often must estimate the patient's age, making identifying a normal systolic blood pressure difficult. The PTS aids in identifying the child in evolving shock.[17] The scoring system compensates for the inability to acquire a systolic blood pressure due to size, equipment, or other extenuating factors. Evaluating a pulse, its quality and location, allows for an objective evaluation. A higher score (+2) is assigned if a distal pulse is available, +1 for femoral or brachial pulses, and –1 for no pulse attainable.

In the adult patient, the level of consciousness in the field is often evaluated through verbal criteria. This is often difficult to do in a very young patient. The PTS allows the provider to evaluate the neurological status by categorizing the patient as awake, obtunded, or comatose.

Skeletal and cutaneous evaluations attempt to provide a profile of injury patterns, which can be suggestive of more serious internal injuries. A child's skeletal structure is more flexible than an adult's, and certain fractures, such as rib fractures, may indicate possible underlying organ injury and potentially serious transfers of energy occurring during the accident.

The PTS has proven to be an easy and sensitive assessment tool for evaluating traumatic injuries in pediatrics. The individual assessment criteria are totaled and scores of 8 and less have demonstrated that patients need greater airway management, intensive care, or surgery and require transport to a trauma center capable of managing severly injured pediatric patients.[17]

OUTCOME EVALUATIONS

Initiated in 1982, the MTOS refined trauma scoring systems and established national expected outcomes for trauma. In addition, the MTOS provided trauma systems with data and methods for evaluating their own effectiveness in terms of patient outcomes. Between 1982 and 1989, the MTOS compiled data on more than 170,000 seriously injured patients treated at over 160

Table 7-6
Pediatric Trauma Score

Category	+2	+1	–1
Size	>20 kg	10–20 kg	<10 kg
Airway	Normal	Maintained	Unmaintained
Systolic blood pressure	>90 mm Hg	50–90 mm Hg	<50 mm Hg
Central nervous system	Awake	Obtunded	Coma
Skeletal	Intact	Closed fracture	Open fracture
Cutaneous	None	Minor	Major

hospitals, nearly 85% of which were U.S. Level I and II trauma centers. Based on these data, the TRISS methodology (discussed below) can be used to estimate the probability of survival for each patient treated at a trauma center. Applied retrospectively, TRISS provides a means of comparing an individual trauma center's patient outcomes against the outcomes of patients with similar injuries treated at other trauma centers.

TRISS

Methods have been developed to address the injury severity score's limitations and integrate an evaluation for a cluster of injuries. The ISS is often combined with the RTS to formulate a relative severity of the injury. This is a combined score known as the **trauma score, injury severity score, age combination index (TRISS) method.**[8] Figure 7-2 outlines the formula for the TRISS evaluation. While this calculation is impractical for EMS field use, it provides a valid criterion for evaluating patients sustaining multisystem trauma.

TRISS is used in the MTOS and most trauma registries to estimate the probabilities of survival for trauma patients. In essence, TRISS allows trauma centers to compare their patient outcomes with those of a baseline norm while controlling for patient injury severity.

$$P_s = 1/(1 + e^{-b})$$

In this formula $b = b_0 + b_1(\text{TS}) + b_2(\text{ISS}) + b_3(\text{Age})$ and b_0, b_1, b_2, b_3 are coefficients derived from the Major Trauma Outcome Study (MTOS),[7] and RTS, ISS, and Age are the patient's revised trauma score, injury severity score, and age, respectively. The age variable equals 1 if the patient is greater than 54 years of age, 0 otherwise. Current TRISS norms were developed in 1986 and validated in 1992.

TRISS Regression Weights

	b_0	b_1	b_2	b_3
Blunt trauma	−1.2470	0.9544	−0.0768	−1.9052
Penetrating trauma	−0.6029	1.1430	−0.1516	−2.6676

Sample calculation:

Patient data: Blunt trauma, RTS = 6, ISS = 26, Age = 67

$$b = b_0 + b_1(\text{TS}) + b_2(\text{ISS}) + b_3(\text{Age})$$

$$b = -1.2470 + 0.9544(6) - 0.0768(26) - 1.9052(1)$$

$$b = 0.5774$$

$$P_s = 1/(1 + e^{-b}) = 1/(1 + e^{-0.5774}) = 0.63$$

(63% probability of survival)

FIGURE 7-2 TRISS formula used to evaluate survival probabilities.

INTERNET ACTIVITIES

Visit the British Trauma Society Web page and review the section on the revised trauma score at http://www.trauma.org/scores/triss.html. Review the material on the TRISS method. Calculate the probability of survival using data from your last major trauma patient using the TRISS equations. Next, check your answer by inserting your values into the TRISS calculator. You may also copy the TRISS calculator onto your computer's desktop.

CONTRIBUTION OF PREHOSPITAL CARE

An extension of TRISS, PARTITION estimates the prehospital contribution to a patient's potential for survival. PARTITION separates the effects on survival of prehospital care from the care received in the hospital. The system estimates the potential for survival based on the RTS at the scene, the patient's age, and the ISS at the time of admission. By separating the effects of prehospital and hospital care, the impact of prehospital care on patient survival can be quantified.

SUMMARY

Health care experts, challenged to define the financial impact of patients treated at trauma centers whose injuries could be handled at a community facility, developed evaluation tools to examine the impact transport decisions had on the expenditure of trauma care resources. The development of early scoring systems utilized physiological presentations to evaluate patients' injuries. As physicians and researchers began to search for an in-depth evaluation of injury processes, the development of broader, more sensitive tools evolved.

Instruments for quantifying trauma were developed to provide a basis for evaluating prehospital decision making regarding traumatic injuries. Also, trauma systems have attempted to define traumatic injuries using scoring systems that classify the severity of injuries based on the MTOS. These scoring systems are designed to provide a norm against which the quality of trauma care of an individual trauma center can be evaluated. These tools have been extended into prehospital care where the impact of field treatment on patient outcome can be evaluated.

REVIEW QUESTIONS

1. Traumatic injuries require one of the greatest expenditures of resources for any medical center and affects all patients served.
   a. True
   b. False

2. The reasons that trauma centers were located only in limited, strategic locations include all of the following except:
   a. Administrative support required
   b. Capital needs of these centers
   c. Research findings that did not support the need for change in the existing system
   d. Extensive medical staff requirements

3. Initial assessment tools developed in the early 1970s focused on the evaluation of this criterion to base decisions on the severity of injuries.
   a. Anatomic
   b. Physiological
   c. Paramedic discretion
   d. Mechanism of injury

4. To properly identify critically injured patients, scoring systems are generally evaluated on their:
   a. Sensitivity and specificity
   b. Specificity and reliability
   c. Sensitivity and ease of use
   d. Clinical and field application

5. One of the most common scoring systems utilized in the field is the:
   a. Anatomic injury scale
   b. CRAMS
   c. TRISS method
   d. Glasgow Coma Scale

6. To determine injury severity, anatomic findings divide the type of assault into:
   a. Blunt and site of injury
   b. Blunt and penetrating
   c. Speed and location of accident
   d. Penetrating and type of weapon

7. The abbreviated injury scale groups injuries into multiple-system groupings, where each injury within a grouping is evaluated for severity.
   a. True
   b. False

8. The Glasgow Coma Scale evaluates which three major activities to assess cerebral function?
   a. Eye opening, verbal response, and motor response
   b. Motor response, pupil response, and systolic blood pressure
   c. Verbal response, motor response, and capillary refill
   d. Capillary refill, pupil response, and systolic blood pressure

9. The trauma score relies on the combination of the Glasgow Coma Scale, the patient's respiratory rate and expansion, and patient's capillary refill to make an evaluation of injury.
   a. True
   b. False

10. The mechanism of injury is suggestive of the amount of energy transferred during the collision.
   a. True
   b. False

CRITICAL THINKING

1. For any given ISS, TS, and patient age, the probability of survival (P_s) of penetrating trauma is higher than for blunt trauma. Why do you think this is so?

2. Determine which trauma scoring systems are used in your EMS system. Evaluate their accuracy, ease of calculation, and purpose.

3. From your answer to Question 2 above, develop a plan for how your EMS system could use these values to monitor its clinical performance.

REFERENCES

1. Maslanka AM. Scoring systems and triage from the field. *Emerg Med Clin North Am.* 1993; 11(1):15.
2. Fries G, McCalla G, Levitt MA, Cordova R. A prospective comparison of paramedic judgment and the trauma triage rule in the prehospital setting. *Ann Emerg Med.* 1994; 24(5):885.
3. Champion HR, Sacco WJ, Copes WS. Trauma scoring. In: Feliciano D, Moore EE, Mattox KL, eds. *Trauma.* 3rd ed. Stamford, Conn: Appleton & Lange; 1996.
4. Teasdale G, Jennett B. Assessment of coma and impaired consciousness: A practical scale. *Lancet.* 1974; 2:81.
5. Knight RL. The Glasgow Coma Scale: Ten years after. *Crit Care Nurse.* 1988; 6(3):65.
6. Winkler JV, Rosen P, Alfrey EJ. Prehospital use of the Glasgow Coma Scale in severe head injury. *J Emerg Med.* 1984; 42(2):1.
7. Champion H, Sacco WJ, Copes WS, Gann DS, Gennarelli TA, Flanagan ME. A revision of the trauma score. *J Trauma.* 1989; 29(5):623.
8. Cottington E, Young JC, Shufflebarger CM, Kyes F, Peterson FV Jr., Diamond DL. The utility of physiologic status, injury site, and injury mechanism in

identifying patients with major trauma. *J Trauma*. 1988; 28(3):305.

9. Osler T. Injury severity scoring: Perspectives in development and future directions. *Am J Surg*. 1993; 165(2A):43S.

10. Knopp R, Yangai A, Kallser G, Geide A, Duehring L. Mechanism of injury as criteria for prehospital trauma triage. *Ann Emerg Med*. 1988; 17(9):55.

11. Rowles JM, Kirsh G, Macey AC, Colton CL. The use of injury scoring in the evaluation of the Kegworth M1aircrash. *J Trauma*. 1992; 32(4):441.

12. Rutledge R, Fakhry S, Baker C, Oller D. Injury severity grading in trauma patients: A simplified technique based upon ICD-9 coding. *J Trauma*. 1993; 35(94):497.

13. Cooper ME, Yarborough DR, Zone-Smith L, Byme TK, Noreross ED. Application of field triage guide-lines by prehospital personnel: Is mechanism of injury a valid guideline for patient triage. *Am Surg*. 1995; 4:61.

14. O'Rourke B, Bade RH, Drezner T. Trauma triage: A nine-year experience. *Ann Emerg Med*. 1991; 21:6.

15. Yurt RW. Triage, initial assessment, and early treatment of the pediatric trauma patient. *Pediatr Clin North Am*. 1992; 39:5.

16. Tepas J, Mollit D, Talbert JL, Bryant M. The pediatric trauma score as a predictor of injury severity in the injured child. *J Pediatr Surg*. 1987; 22:14.

17. Reynolds EA. Trauma scoring and pediatric patients: Issues and controversies. *J Emerg Nurs*. 1992; 18(3):205.

Chapter 8

PRINCIPLES OF TRIAGE

OBJECTIVES

Upon completion of this chapter, the reader should be able to:

● Define the term *triage*.
● Discuss the functions and principles of triage.
● Explain the purpose of field triage.
● Define the incident command system (ICS).
● Discuss the importance of staff development and system education to the effective utilization of triage.
● Explain how an integrated triage sector within a system's response protocol enhances the service's ability to manage treatment decisions and the needs of the patient.
● Describe the following triage classification systems: four-tier system, five-tier system, and START system.
● Describe the importance of preparation and triage drills to an emergency medical service.

KEY TERMS

Incident command system (ICS)
Simple triage and rapid treatment (START)
Triage

Triage is the allocation of resources based on the number and severity of patient injuries in relation to the health care system's ability to manage a given incident.[1] Triage methods were originally developed and implemented to improve the survivability of soldiers wounded on the battlefield. The large number of traumatic injuries and deaths in wartime forced military medical personnel to make decisions about which soldiers would receive immediate, delayed, or no medical care. These decisions were made to achieve the goal of saving the lives of as many soldiers as possible with the available medical resources. Civilians have enhanced and adapted these field triage methods to improve the allocation of resources for patients sustaining traumatic injuries.

Civilian triage principles have developed largely from transportation incidents such as motor vehicle crashes and airline disasters. Research into motor vehicle crash deaths and injuries shows that 70% of deaths occur at the scene or within hours after the incident due to multisystem bodily injury. The remaining 30% of severely injured patients at the scene can be offered a positive outcome if swift, skillful intervention and assessment are provided.[2] This 30% of patients can have significantly improved outcomes with EMS triage and intervention.

The first function of triage is to assist health care providers in ensuring that limited resources are best used for the greatest good of the patients involved. The second function of triage is to minimize the time from injury to definitive surgical intervention. If used properly, triage systems should allow for expedient field treatment and rapid transport of critically injured patients to the appropriate medical facility. Consequently, differentiation of critical and noncritical injuries is paramount. Overburdening a trauma center with noncritical patients that could be effectively managed at a community hospital is just as detrimental as sending critically injured patients to community facilities incapable of providing definitive surgical care.

Approaching triage management from a field perspective, the triage system relies on two principles: (1) the ability of prehospital providers to correctly evaluate and categorize injuries and (2) correct use of an objective protocol evaluating patients based on anatomic, physiological, and incident characteristics (see Chapter 7).[1]

INITIAL EVALUATION

Triage is intended to identify events with the potential for high-energy transfers that are likely to produce life-threatening injuries.[1] The difficulty in this process is determining the relatively small number of patients who have sustained significant trauma.[2] The extent of overtriage—that is, noncritical patients sent to trauma centers or critical patients not directed to trauma centers (undertriage)—affects morbidity and the financial cost associated with treatment. The American College of Surgeons, Committee on Trauma has established triage guidelines that combine physiological measures with certain anatomic factors and mechanisms of injury. The criteria identify patients who have an estimated 10% or greater chance of dying. However, the committee acknowledges that overtriage rates as high as 50% may be experienced.[3] Although levels of acceptance for overtriage are disputed among experts, it is agreed that some degree of overtriage of patients to trauma centers is necessary to ensure that severely injured patients are not excluded from appropriate treatment. Each system must individually assess available resources, transport facilities, and in-field resources and examine the feasibility of physician-directed triage and the developmental maturity of the operating trauma system.

The development of an integrated system includes coordination of health care resources away from the scene; but for EMS the development of an integrated system must begin prior to patients reaching the best facility to manage their injuries. EMS agencies must strive to develop an integrated prehospital trauma management system that best utilizes the resources on the scene. This prehospital development is initiated through staff development, response system design (a tiered response), and defining the roles and expectations of each responding agency. The initial approach to any traumatic event that stresses the response limitations of the emergency system and requires a coordinated, expedient effort is best initiated through the use of an incident command system.

INCIDENT COMMAND SYSTEM

An **incident command system (ICS)** is the coordinated and controlled management of responding resources, so that limited expenditure of those resources can produce the greatest positive effect. Within an ICS is the provision for triage to be directed and managed by assigning one person or group, depending on the size of the incident, responsibility for triage and the determination of the treatment needs of the patients. Figure 8-1 depicts a simple ICS design matrix. Triage is considered a mandatory sector of all ICS and is a major component within the command structure.

Initial evaluation should occur by the first arriving agency, and should involve a structured scene examination with emphasis on establishment of the triage sector. The triage system in place should allow prehospital personnel to perform the initial evaluation and determine injury severity.

Triage Sector

Triage sectors are usually supervised by the senior or highest medically trained personnel on the scene. In most incidents, an experienced paramedic assumes responsibility for the direction of patients through triage. In special situations or large events, a physician who has expertise in prehospital triage should facilitate the management of the triage sector.

Establishing and managing a triage sector extend beyond the direct responsibility to determine patient treatment needs. The sector chief or manager must effectively organize and direct recovery efforts and gain access to injured patients so that the triage plan can be implemented. An effective triage plan loses its ability to affect patient outcome if the sector cannot organize patient access and egress through the triage process. Figure 8-2 depicts an example of triage sector organization; each system and, in part, each incident will dictate the physical attributes of the triage sector, but the principles of the sector remain unchanged.

Physicians or any health care provider who has not received specialized training in the management of a major sector within ICS may be best utilized in a consultant role. The triage and decision making are best coordinated, if possible, with a physician. A system's plan may

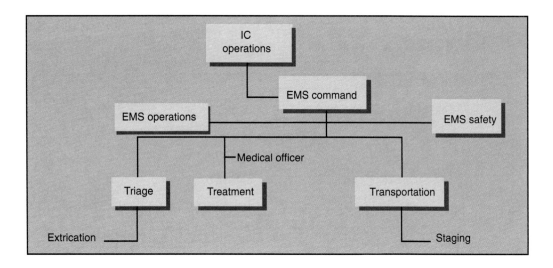

FIGURE 8-1 EMS command structure within an ICS.

include on-line radio contact with an emergency department physician to assist in patient triage decision or, with physician involvement, detailed decision-making criteria are developed to assist prehospital personnel in evaluating the injured. Triage decisions are made by using three essential criteria: anatomical, physiological, and mechanism of injury (see Chapter 7).[1,4]

TRIAGE PRINCIPLES

Health care delivery systems, including prehospital services, must explore triage systems or instruments that are effective within their local delivery system. To be effective, a triage instrument must be implemented into the entire delivery system, be transferable among incident types, and be understood and practical for each system member. Implementation depends on acceptance by the in-house medical community and the prehospital community and by demonstration of the tool's sensitivity in identifying the severity of injuries.[4] Sensitivity is determined by a tool's ability to accurately score or evaluate the severity of the injuries. Other important aspects of any triage instrument are that it must be practical for field use and be transferable among various prehospital providers. Through evaluating different triage procedures, an EMS system can determine which procedure best meets their needs.

TRIAGE CLASSIFICATION SYSTEMS

There is no universally accepted system for categorizing a patient's injuries. Injury classifications are defined by the triage instrument in use by the local system and, therefore, vary by locale. Many systems use color codes, numbers, or symbols to denote injury classifications and severity.

Classifications are used to denote the level of injury, medical attention required, and priority for transport. These injury classifications are arbitrary unless everyone within the system understands their significance and meaning. Each triage classification system has its own advantages and disadvantages. Classification systems limited to two categories are simple to remember but do not offer the precision of systems using four or five categories. The trade-off, then, is one of simplicity versus accuracy, and while no one system is universally accepted, the more popular systems are reviewed below.

Four-Tier System

The most commonly accepted and utilized tools to categorize injuries use four classifications to prioritize treatment and transport. Table 8-1 outlines the classifications used under this triage system. This classification system allows responders to divide patients into critical, immediate, nonemergent, and dead.

This tool allows the delivery system to offer precise triage categories for the trauma system without becoming cumbersome and complicated. The four-tier system is the most used of all classification systems because of its ability to place patients into broad ranges and still provide descriptive patient classes. Many commercial triage tags and triage principles utilize a four-tier injury classification.

Five-Tier System

Some EMS systems attempt to more precisely define patient injury categories and have adopted a five-tier triage system. The primary difference between the four- and five-tier systems is that the latter further divides

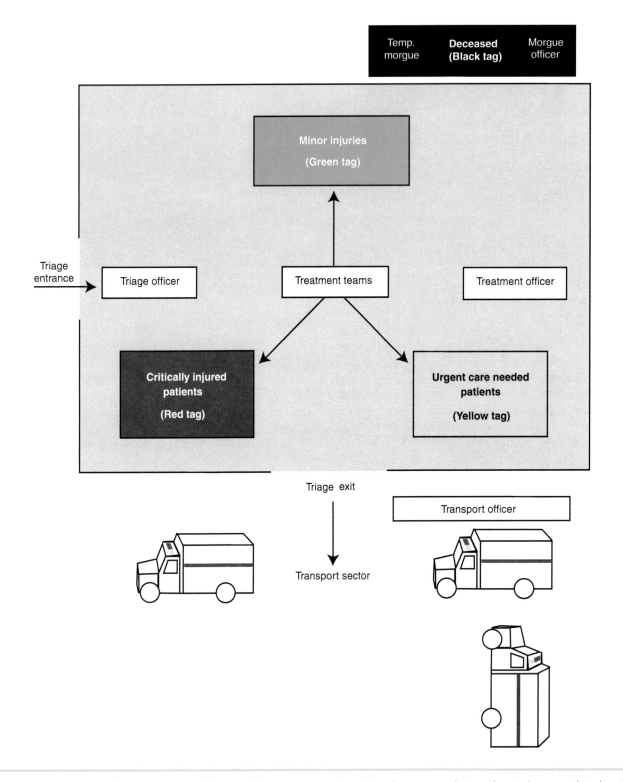

FIGURE 8-2 Example of the organizational layout of a triage sector. Note the other sectors that are located near or that directly impact the triage sector.

critically injured patients into those who are likely to survive and those who are unlikely to survive even with major medical intervention (Table 8-2). Otherwise, the five-tier system is similar to the four-tier system in that patients with injuries impeding or affecting the airway are generally given highest priority, while patients with uncomplicated extremity fractures and minor injuries are given the lowest transport priority.

Table 8-1
Color Categories Used to Identify Patient Medical Needs

Color	Priority	Patient Condition
Green	Third	Minor: first aid only, transport can be delayed
Yellow	Second	Urgent: nonurgent, but hospital care is needed.
Red	First	Critical: urgent care needed to ensure survival; hospital care required
Black	None	Dead

Table 8-2
Five-Tier Patient Triage Category

Color	Priority	Patient Condition
Green	Fourth	Minor: transport can be delayed; patient likely to survive even if care is delayed for hours or days
Yellow	Third	Urgent: likely to survive if care initiated within few hours
Blue	Second	Catastrophic: unlikely to survive and/or complicated medical care needed within minutes
Red	First	Critical: urgent care needed to ensure survival; likely to survive if care initiated
Black	None	Dead

START System

A method designed to allow agencies to provide a quick assessment of patients involved in mass casualty incidents is the assessment principle "**simple triage and rapid treatment (START)**."[5] This process is widely used in fire departments, ambulance services, and first-responder agencies. The system can triage patients based on a flow chart that leads the evaluator through easily assessed anatomic criteria.

The criteria evaluated are patients' ability to walk, breathing, perfusion, and mental status.[5] Figure 8-3 demonstrates the four criteria used to place the patient into the three transport categories: (1) immediate, (2) delayed, or (3) need for further evaluation. This classification allows EMS to quickly organize a transport plan and place patients into large, general treatment areas. The ability to quickly assess and sort large numbers of patients is accomplished by not conducting a detailed physical exam. Quantitative assessments are required only for breathing and capillary refill.

The lack of a detailed assessment does not preclude large numbers of patients from being "overtriaged." Preventing overtriage is the responsibility of the first agency conducting the assessment by organizing patients for the triage sector. Once patients are introduced into the triage sector, a triage officer must direct personnel in conducting continuous patient assessment. Triage personnel can continue to update the condition of patients in the triage area using more in-depth and detailed triage tools (see Chapter 7).

Triage Tags

Many EMS triage tools utilize a tagging system to prioritize the medical needs of patients. The tag system prevents patients from being "retriaged" by different providers. In addition, the tags allow EMS providers to identify patients and track their movements through the system.

The tags commonly used are color coded to represent the medical condition of the patient. Most systems use four to five colors to identify patient needs (Table 8-1). A commonly used triage tag on the market is the METTAG (Figure 8-4), which allows reclassification of the medical need if the patient deteriorates during the incident and provides identification numbers to assist in tracking patient movements.

INTERNET ACTIVITIES

Review the trauma triage criteria, hospital bypass protocols, and air evacuation protocols of the North Central Texas Trauma Regional Advisory Council at http://www.dfwhc.org/ncttrac/protocols.htm. To review the protocols, you will need Acrobat Reader, which can be downloaded free of charge from http://www.adobe.com/prodindex/acrobat/readstep.html.

TRAUMA SYSTEM DEVELOPMENT

An advantage of field triage is the proper allocation of resources. The principles and tools of triage cannot be implemented properly if an integrated trauma system has not been established. Without an integrated trauma system, the ability of emergency medical services to

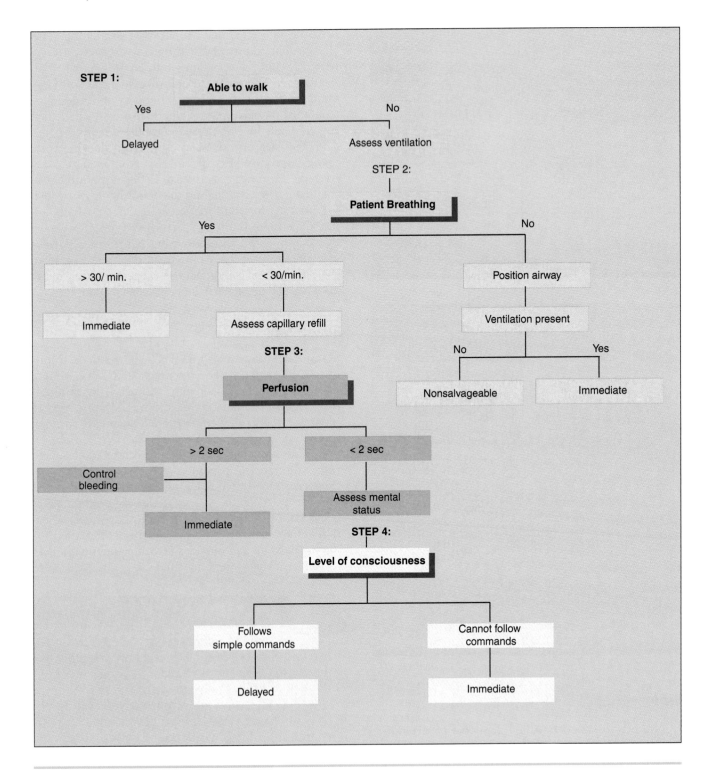

FIGURE 8-3 The START flow diagram enables first responders to quickly organize patients into treatment and transport groups

respond and provide for the needs of the community is greatly diminished.[6]

In meeting this challenge EMS must examine and explore an integrated trauma management system that incorporates the principles of the ICS (see Chapter 30). An ICS provides an integrated network of

services allowing field personnel to effectively utilize time and resources on the scene.

The development of a local trauma management system requires close evaluation of the capabilities of the local health care system. Services that must be examined include not only the prehospital components,

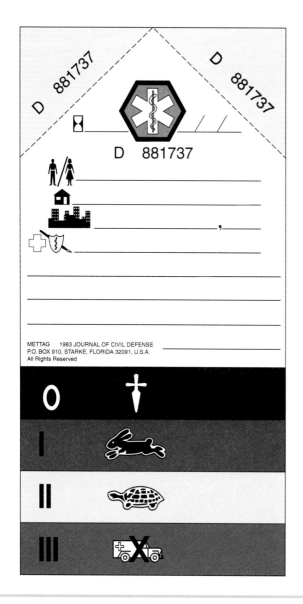

GREEN: (Bottom strip)
   Symbol: Ambulance–crossed-out
   Meaning: No hospital treatment needed; first aid only
YELLOW: (second strip from bottom)
   Symbol: Turtle
   Meaning: Non-urgent; hospital care
RED; (Third strip from bottom)
   Symbol: Rabbit
   Meaning: Urgent; hospital care
Black: (Fourth strip from bottom)
   Symbol: Cross/dagger
   Meaning: Dead or unsalvageable; no CPR

(Adapted from: METTAG literature, Starke, FL)

FIGURE 8-4 Example of a commonly used triage tag.

including first responders, but also hospital services (emergency departments, blood banks, diagnostic testing, and surgical services) and communication capabilities. Close attention must be given to developing each component of the trauma management system that includes various health care delivery services. Each group must also have knowledge of local trauma patterns and must possess expertise in meeting patient care for each traumatic event. Exclusion of any member or component during the planning and implementation of the system fails to deliver the best care available to the critically injured trauma patient.

Each service will be expected to contribute its skills and expertise to the overall development of the area's trauma delivery system. Ideally, EMS provides an orderly response, rapid identification of the injured, determination of injury severity, appropriate treatment, and swift transport of the injured to an appropriate treatment facility. Accomplishing these goals depends on an effective triage system.

Developing proficient triage skills among all individuals and providers within the local trauma system is also extremely important. Policies, education, and drills permit the members of the trauma system to examine problems with triage protocols and to develop proficient triage skills. Triage protocols should be tailored to meet the needs of the local trauma system and should reflect the type, number, and frequency of local trauma-producing events. In tiered systems, first responders and other members of the prehospital team cannot be overlooked in triage education and training.

Triage principles alone are not sufficient to ensure optimal patient outcomes. Triage is one facet of the larger trauma system, but it is necessary to achieve improved survival rates among the injured.

INTERNET ACTIVITIES

Review the following examples of trauma triage protocols:

- New Jersey Pediatric Trauma Triage: http://www.state.nj.us/health/ems/pedtrig.htm
- Florida Adult Trauma Triage: http://www.ufhscj.edu/traumaone/docs/FLADTR.html
- Alberta, Canada Pediatric Triage: http://www.ualberta.ca/~pediatri/clinical/trauma.htm
- Sacramento, California Triage: http://www.co.sacramento.ca.us/ems/5053.html
- Victoria, Australia, Field Criteria: http://hna.ffh.vic.gov.au/ahs/trauma2/apps/append7b.htm
- Victoria, Australia, Destination Criteria: http://hna.ffh.vic.gov.au/ahs/trauma2/apps/append7c.htm
- Victoria, Australia, Transfer Criteria: http://hna.ffh.vic.gov.au/ahs/trauma2/apps/append7d.htm

---

SUMMARY

The development of effective triage tools requires a careful, deliberate approach. Individual services and delivery systems must examine local needs and resources and the level of sophistication of all responders.

The objective of each delivery system is to establish guidelines and criteria for triage that allow field personnel at various levels to manage patient treatment and transport decisions quickly, accurately, and effectively. Emergency services must strive to develop integrated incident command systems that utilize triage sectors to manage patient access and egress into the treatment sequence. Integration of triage sectors into a structured response of emergency services allows the system to provide a framework for all responders, and a familiar operational framework provides a consistent approach to incident management.

The development of a linked group of triage principles depends on local emergency service input, combined with close internal evaluation of triage needs for the system. Coordinated guidelines involving community hospitals, trauma centers, responding agencies, physicians, and surgeons can establish evaluation criteria that ensure appropriate allocation of patients. The combination of triage tools used to evaluate and triage patients must be determined at the local level. Regardless of the triage system adopted, the triage decision is an extension of medical treatment, saddled by political, socioeconomic, and medical issues.[6] A service that can avoid these biases, which adversely affect field performance, can successfully establish the groundwork for a strong response structure.

REVIEW QUESTIONS

1. Seventy percent of deaths caused by automobile collisions occur at the scene or within hours after the incident due to multisystem failure.
   a. True
   b. False

2. Triage principles were originally designed to:
   a. Improve EMS operations
   b. Increase the effectiveness of the National Fire Services operations
   c. Improve the survivability of soldiers wounded on the battlefield
   d. Better evaluate patients' injuries and illnesses

3. The advantage of field triage is:
   a. The assurance of proper resource allocation to match patient needs
   b. Notifying hospitals which patients they are receiving
   c. Closely evaluating the performance of field personnel
   d. Evaluating new field techniques and treatments

4. The second function of triage is to:
   a. Increase field time
   b. Minimize field time to definitive intervention
   c. Allow field personnel to practice their decision-making skills
   d. Increase patient treatment skills performed by field personnel

5. Overtriaged patients can be as detrimental to patient care as undertriaged patients.
   a. True
   b. False

6. Trauma should not be managed as a disease process.
   a. True
   b. False

7. Field triage systems rely on two principles:
   a. Judgment ability of field personnel and objective evaluating criteria
   b. Judgment of physician and subjective evaluating criteria
   c. Calling several physicians to consult on the best treatment and a dynamic evaluating tool
   d. Committee consensus and subjective evaluating criteria

8. Trauma system development should involve only the lead agency responsible for the ultimate patient care.
   a. True
   b. False

9. The START system stands for:
   a. Simple treatment and rapid transport
   b. Simple triage and rapid treatment
   c. Start talking and run treatment
   d. Simply triaging and right treatment

10. Experts in the medical field suggest that a certain amount of overtriage of patients to trauma centers is necessary to ensure critically injured patients are not overlooked.
   a. True
   b. False

CRITICAL THINKING

- The "catastrophic" category is the primary feature that distinguishes the four-tier from the five-tier triage system. If you were to respond to a major incident involving large numbers of patients, what types of injuries would you place into the "catastrophic" category? If you were using only the four-tier system, how would you categorize the same patients? Why the difference?

- You have been dispatched to a motor vehicle crash involving a school bus and a large truck. Additional resources are en route. Five ambulances and one helicopter are available. The helicopter can transport only one patient and each ambulance can transport two. There are six first responders on the scene with EMT level training. The nearest hospital is 30 minutes away. You are faced with the following patients, all of whom are between the ages of 12 and 19:

Patient initial assessment findings

   1. Walking at scene; minor laceration to the right arm; bleeding is controlled.
   2. Open femur fracture; vital signs are stable; no other injuries.
   3. Tension pneumothorax; obvious decompensation.
   4. Severe head injury; agonal respirations; fixed and dilated pupils.
   5. Amputated left arm; bleeding controlled; no other injuries.

   6. Unconscious; hematoma to left temporal area; snoring respirations; vital signs stable.
   7. Conscious patient complaining of abdominal pain; abdomen tender with contusion in right upper quadrant.
   8. Walking at scene; left humerus fracture.
   9. Running around the scene; appears confused.
   10. Lying on ground; no obvious signs of trauma; continuously repeats "I'm diabetic."
   11. Pulseless and apneic; no external signs of trauma; CPR being performed by first responder.
   12. Entrapped in truck; bilateral femur fractures and unstable pelvis; conscious and alert.
   13. Open pneumothorax; vital signs stable; states "I can't breathe."
   14. Abdominal evisceration with profound hemorrhage.
   15. Fractured clavicle; no other injuries.
   16. Head injury with decerebrate posturing.

Prioritize these patients for transport.

- Using the same scenario, prioritize your patients for transport if only four ambulances are available and no helicopter is available. Which patients change? Justify your decision.

REFERENCES

1. Wesson DE, Scorpio R. *Symposium Trauma Update: Field Triage Guidelines and Aspects of Early Resuscitation—What's New?* Toronto: Canadian Association of Emergency Physicians; 1990.
2. Schmidt J, Moore GP. Management of multiple trauma. *Emerg Med Clin North Am.* 1993; 11(1):29.
3. Knudson P, Frecceri CA, DeLateur SA. Improving the field triage of major trauma victims. *J Trauma.* 1988; 28(5):435.
4. Emerman CL, Shade B, Kubincanek J. A comparison of EMT judgment and prehospital trauma triage instruments. *J Trauma.* 1991; 31(10):1369.
5. Heide EA. *Disaster Response: Principles of Preparation and Coordination.* St. Louis: CV Mosby Company; 1989.
6. Kane G, Engelhardt R, Celentano J, et al. Empirical development and evaluation of prehospital trauma triage instruments. *J Trauma.* 1985; 25(6):482.

Chapter 9

Pathophysiology of Shock

OBJECTIVES

Upon completion of this chapter, the reader should be able to:

● Describe the anatomy and physiology of the heart and explain its autonomic innervation.

● Describe the formulas for cardiac output and blood pressure.

● Explain how preload, afterload, and contractility affect cardiac stroke volume.

● Discuss the factors that determine oxygen delivery.

● Explain the three phases of cellular metabolism: glycolysis, the TCA cycle, and electron transport.

● Discuss the pathophysiology of shock due to respiratory failure, hypovolemia, vascular failure, and cardiac failure.

● Describe the compensatory mechanisms of respiratory compensation, sympathetic nervous system response, neuroendocrine response, and transcapillary refill.

● Understand the role of systemic inflammation in the pathophysiology of shock and the cascade of events culminating in death.

● Describe interventions that improve oxygen delivery.

● Explain the common complications of shock.

KEY TERMS

Afterload
Arterial blood pressure (BP)
Cardiac output (CO)
Contractility
Electron transport
Fick principle
Glycolysis

Hydrostatic pressure
Oncotic pressure
Preload
Shock
Starling's law of the heart
Stroke volume (SV)
TCA (Krebs) cycle

Shock, a condition resulting from serious injury, received increasing attention by the medical community in the latter half of the 1800s, but only after breakthroughs in anesthesia and surgical infection had occurred. The following quote, written by the preeminent American surgeon of the mid nineteenth century, Samuel Gross, embodies the understanding of shock at that point in time:

"But a more careful examination soon serves to show that deep mischief is lurking in the system; that the machinery of life has been rudely unhinged, and the whole system profoundly shocked; in a word, that the nervous fluid has been exhausted" (A System of Surgery, 1859).[1]

The question challenging surgeons of the 1800s—how an injury to one part of the body produced deleterious, and often fatal, effects on the body as a whole—could only be explained by a disturbance of the nervous system. Somehow, they postulated, the wounding object "jarred" (*shocked*) the nervous system, leading to the typical signs and symptoms of shock: weak, rapid pulse; pale, cool skin; and listlessness.

Astley Cooper, another physician who accepted this theory, believed treatment for shock should be aimed at stimulating the nervous system. He opted to administer strychnine, which in small doses induced convulsions, believing this would stimulate the nervous system. Others employed alcohol; a few even applied electrical current to patients in shock. Such therapies failed to achieve clinical success and shock carried a tremendously high mortality rate.

George W. Crile, a Cleveland surgeon, was one of the earliest to study shock in an experimental manner. Utilizing the recently invented sphygmomanometer, he realized in 1899 that a fall in blood pressure could account for all the symptoms manifested by a patient in shock. He later theorized that "shock was not a process of dying, but rather a marshaling of the bodily defenses in a struggle to live."[2]

Our current understanding of shock is derived from this notion. We now understand **shock** to represent a generalized failure of the body to deliver sufficient amounts of oxygen to its tissues. Many of the easily recognizable signs and symptoms represent compensatory measures utilized by the body to maintain the delivery of oxygen (O_2) to its most vital organs: the brain, heart, and lungs. If appropriate therapy is delayed, a cascade of events may ensue that results in damage to crucial organs and, eventually, death of the patient.

Despite the work of countless physicians and scientists who have advanced our understanding of the clinical presentation of shock and unraveled the pathophysiology of this potentially fatal condition, the effort remains unfinished. Despite earlier and more aggressive therapies aimed at restoring and maintaining crucial oxygen delivery, some patients fail to respond to appropriate, standard therapy and eventually succumb to complications of their injuries. We have also learned in recent years that some of the complications of shock result from an overactivation of the body's defense mechanisms.[3]

In this chapter, the focus will be on the normal delivery of O_2 to the tissues of the body, methods for improving O_2 delivery, and the complications of shock. We will discuss those conditions that interfere with O_2 delivery and how the body attempts to compensate for these problems. Despite the many etiologies of the shock state, it is clear that the cascade of deleterious events initiated by insufficient O_2 delivery are common to all forms of shock.

The prehospital assessment of shock is limited, in large part, by current training and technology. The three most important aspects in the prehospital management of shock are (1) recognition of shock in the early stages, (2) appropriate airway management and administration of O_2, and (3) transportation of the patient to a center where appropriate resuscitation can be continued. Despite the fact that many interventions described herein cannot be delivered in the prehospital setting, their consideration is fundamental to a comprehensive understanding of the pathophysiology of shock.

CARDIOVASCULAR PHYSIOLOGY

The cardiovascular system provides three essential roles in the human body: (1) the delivery of nutrients, including O_2, to the tissues and cells of the body; (2) the transportation of waste products, produced by normal metabolism, to the liver and kidneys for detoxification and excretion; and (3) delivery of carbon dioxide (CO_2) to the lungs for exhalation. The circulatory system is composed of three primary components: the heart (a pump), the blood vessels (the pipes), and the blood (the perfusate).

THE HEART

The heart is a four-chambered organ composed of two smaller atria and two larger ventricles, which circulate the blood throughout the vascular network. Consider the circulatory system to be two separate circuits, the lower pressure pulmonary circulation, driven by contraction of the right heart, and the systemic circulation, propelled by the thicker-walled left heart. Four valves ensure unidirectional flow. Two atrioventricular valves separate the atria from the ventricles, with the tricuspid valve located on the right and the mitral valve on the left. The pulmonic and aortic valves separate the right and left ventricles, respectively, from their more distal vascular network.

An intrinsic pacemaker, the sinoatrial (SA) node, initiates the cardiac contraction, normally 60–100 beats per minute. Its electrical stimulus is sent through the atrioventricular (AV) node and then along the bundles to the Purkinje fibers so that the ventricular contraction begins at the apex and compresses the blood upward toward the pulmonic and aortic valves.

Autonomic Innervation

Despite the presence of the intrinsic pacemaker, the central nervous system influences heart rate and contractility through the two opposing divisions of the autonomic nervous system: the *sympathetic* and the *parasympathetic* nervous systems. Nerves from the sympathetic nervous system exit from the thoracic and lumbar portions of the spinal cord and synapse in the sympathetic chain ganglia, which lie along the vertebral column. Branches off these ganglia then innervate the heart, releasing norepinephrine as their primary neurotransmitter when stimulated. Norepinephrine possesses both alpha (α) and beta (β) adrenergic activity. The beta receptors on the heart are primarily β_1, which, when activated, increase both the heart rate (chronotropic activity) and the contractility (inotropic activity).

Parasympathetic innervation to the heart is primarily carried through the right and left 10th cranial (vagus) nerves. When stimulated, these nerves release acetylcholine as the neurotransmitter, resulting in a slowing of the heart rate and decrease in contractility.

Cardiac Output and Blood Pressure

The **cardiac output (CO)** represents the volume of blood pumped by the heart within 1 minute. It is calculated as the product of the heart rate (HR) in beats per minute multiplied by the **stroke volume (SV)**, which is the amount of blood ejected from the left ventricle with each contraction:

$$CO \text{ (L/min)} = HR \times SV$$

where HR is in beats per minute (bpm) and SV is liters of blood ejected per contraction. Typically, the CO of the average adult is about 5 liters. Assuming a normal heart rate of 70 bpm, one can calculate the average stroke volume to be about 70 mL (0.07 liter) per beat. If there is no change in the stroke volume, an increase or decrease in the heart rate results in an increase or decrease, respectively, in the CO. Similarly, in the face of a decreased stroke volume, the heart can maintain the same CO by correspondingly increasing its heart rate.

The **arterial blood pressure (BP)** indicates the pressure of the fluid found within the arterial side of the circulation. Mathematically, it is directly proportional to the product of the cardiac output multiplied by the systemic vascular resistance (SVR):

$$BP \approx CO \times SVR$$

or

$$BP \approx HR \times SV \times SVR$$

The SVR is the resistance to flow in the system and corresponds to the relative size of the blood vessels; namely, vasoconstriction represents an increased SVR and vasodilation relates to a decreased SVR. The units for measuring BP are millimeters of mercury (mm Hg), while SVR is reported as dynes/sec/cm.[5] As seen above with the CO, an increase in HR, SV, or SVR leads to a an increase in blood pressure, unless one or both of the other parameters decreases. These compensatory mechanisms will be considered in greater detail below.

Factors Affecting Stroke Volume

Cardiovascular physiologists generally identify three factors that affect the stroke volume: *preload, afterload,* and *contractility.* Preload is a term adopted from the study of muscle contraction. Early physiologists realized that, up to a point, increasing amounts of weight (tension) on a segment of skeletal muscle resulted in contractions of increasing strength (force) when a stimulus was applied.

The English scientist Ernest Starling applied this concept to cardiac physiology, proposing what is known as **Starling's law of the heart**. This law states that, over a physiological range, increased filling of the heart ventricle (which increases tension on the cardiac muscle fibers) results in better emptying (a larger stroke volume). However, a point is reached where added filling (or tension) fails to increase the stroke volume and, in fact, continued overfilling of the heart is associated with a decreased stroke volume, as is the case in heart failure (Figure 9-1). Therefore, **preload** represents the filling of the ventricle and is dependent upon venous return.

Afterload is the term applied to the amount of resistance the heart has to overcome in order to eject fluid from the ventricle. This term can also be represented by the SVR, with an increased SVR corresponding to increased afterload. As the SVR decreases, so does the afterload but the SV, therefore, increases.

Contractility refers to the heart's inherent ability to forcibly contract and eject blood. Contractility can be diminished by scar tissue in the ventricular wall, which develops following a myocardial infarction, or medications that have a negative inotropic activity, such as beta-adrenergic or calcium channel blocking agents. Beta-adrenergic agonists, drugs that stimulate β_1 receptors, increase contractility.

BLOOD VESSELS

Blood vessels comprise the second of the three essential components of the cardiovascular system. The systemic arteries carry oxygenated blood away from the heart to the peripheral tissues. As they travel distally,

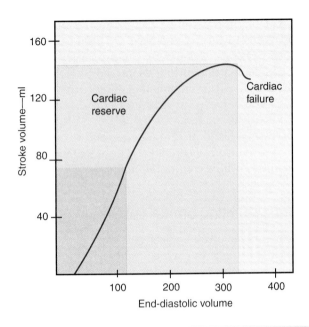

FIGURE 9-1 Starling's curve of the left ventricle. Increasing left ventricle filling pressures (left ventricle end-diastolic pressure) results in increased stroke volume until the heart begins to fail and stroke volume falls off. From *Critical Care Nursing: A Holistic Approach*, 2nd ed., by C. Hudak, B. Gallo, and P. Morton, 1998, Philadelphia: Lippincott Publishing, p. 351.

the arteries branch into smaller arterioles. Compared to their venous counterparts, arteries and arterioles have a thicker layer of smooth muscle. The muscular layer is under the control of the sympathetic nervous system, which provides a baseline "vascular tone." Should this sympathetic innervation be disrupted, the vessels will vasodilate and the SVR will decrease. Because of the vascular tone, which creates the SVR, arterioles are referred to as "resistance vessels."

Vessels emerging from the capillary beds and returning blood to the heart are known as venules and, as they coalesce into larger structures, veins. During normal circulation, about two-thirds of the blood volume is located in the systemic veins and venules, leading them to be referred to as capacitance vessels. Venoconstriction increases venous return to the heart and is also influenced by sympathetic innervation, however to a lesser extent than are the arterioles.

Between the systemic arterioles and venules lie the many capillary beds, networks of tiny vessels in which the exchange of nutrients and waste products occurs. Flow through individual capillaries is controlled by precapillary sphincters that relax and allow perfusion of the bed in response to several local factors, including hypoxemia. Only a relatively small percentage of the many capillary beds of the body's tissues are being perfused at a given point in time, and we know

that only about 5% of the total blood volume is found in the capillaries during normal circulation[4] (Table 9-1).

Hydrostatic pressure and oncotic pressure are the two primary opposing forces that control the net flow of nutrients and fluid out of the proximal capillaries and net flow of waste products and fluid into the distal capillaries. The **hydrostatic pressure** is the pressure of the fluid (i.e., blood pressure) and serves to drive fluid out of the capillary and into the interstitial space. The **oncotic pressure** is the force exerted by the large protein molecules in the blood that draw fluid into the vascular system. In the proximal capillary, the hydrostatic pressure prevails, allowing intravascular fluid and nutrients to diffuse out of the capillaries. In the distal capillary, the hydrostatic pressure is lower and the oncotic pressure predominates, drawing interstitial fluid and waste products of cellular metabolism back into the capillaries.

Blood exiting the right ventricle travels through pulmonary arteries and arterioles to the pulmonary capillaries that surround the alveoli of the lungs. In these beds oxygen readily diffuses into the blood stream while CO_2 diffuses into the alveoli for exhalation. This oxygenated blood enters the pulmonary venules, which join to form pulmonary veins. These vessels then empty their blood into the left atrium.

BLOOD

Blood serves two crucial functions. First, it delivers oxygen and nutrients to the tissues of the body and transports wastes to the liver and kidney for detoxification and excretion. An equally important function is its role in the human immune system, laboring to rid the body of invading microorganisms. Total blood volume represents about 7% of the weight of an adult (about 4,900 mL or 5 liters) but accounts for about 8%–9% of a child's weight.

TABLE 9-1
Distribution of Blood Volume in Various Vascular Beds

Structure	Percent of Blood Volume
Heart	9
Systemic arteries/arterioles	15
Capillaries	5
Systemic veins/venules	59
Pulmonary circulation	12

Blood is composed of two primary components: the formed elements, namely the cells, and the liquid portion, known as the plasma. The percentage of formed elements is known as the hematocrit and accounts for about 35%–45% percent of the blood volume. The formed elements include the erythrocytes, or red blood cells; the leukocytes (white blood cells); and the platelets.

Each erythrocyte contains many hemoglobin molecules, which bind O_2 for transport to the tissues. More than 98% of O_2 is transported bound to hemoglobin, with only a small fraction dissolved in the blood plasma. In environments with a high partial pressure of O_2 (PO_2), such as the normal lung, hemoglobin avidly binds oxygen. In the peripheral tissues, the PO_2 is much lower and the hemoglobin molecule unloads its O_2. This unique binding and release of O_2 by hemoglobin is represented by the oxyhemoglobin dissociation curve (Figure 9-2).

Various factors can shift this curve to the right or to the left, affecting the affinity of hemoglobin for oxygen. Acidosis causes a shift to the right, meaning that, for a given PaO_2, the affinity for oxygen will not be as great and the oxyhemoglobin saturation will be lower. That is, for a given PaO_2, hemoglobin will release more oxygen into an acidotic tissue. Alkalosis results in a shift of the curve to the left, causing hemoglobin to have a higher affinity for oxygen and decreasing the amount of oxygen released in alkalotic tissues.

Leukocytes and platelets play important roles in immune functioning and blood clotting, respectively. Numerous types of leukocytes have been identified, but such classification is beyond the scope of our present attention. These cells play significant roles in fighting infection, recognizing foreign cells, and rejecting transplanted tissues. Some of these cells produce molecules that are necessary for the inflammatory response, but, in excess, they contribute to the pathophysiology of shock. Platelets are fragments of larger cells, called megakaryocytes, and are essential for blood clotting. Therefore, they play a fundamental role in hemostasis.

The blood plasma contains essential electrolytes and components necessary for humoral immunity and blood clotting. Antibodies are found in large numbers in the blood and serve to identify invading microorganisms for leukocytes to destroy. They also play a role in allergic reactions. Many different proteins comprise the coagulation cascade, but their activation leads to the production of a fibrin matrix that traps the platelets, resulting in a blood clot.

FACTORS AFFECTING OXYGEN DELIVERY

So far, we have considered the interrelationships of the heart, blood vessels, and blood in the transport of O_2 to the cells of the body. Some authors have used the term **Fick principle** to describe the factors necessary for systemic O_2 delivery, namely: (1) ability of O_2 to diffuse across the alveolar membrane into the blood stream, (2) adequate numbers of red blood cells present for O_2 transport, (3) adequate blood flow to transport red blood cells to the systemic tissues, and (4) ability of red blood cells to off-load O_2 in the peripheral capillaries. More correctly, the Fick principle refers to the fact that the amount of a substance (i.e., O_2) taken up by an organ is the product of the blood flow to the organ and the difference in concentrations of the substance in the precapillary and postcapillary beds. This principle is often used to calculate cardiac output.[5]

We will now focus on the specific components that govern the delivery of O_2 to the tissues. Though several of these factors cannot be quantified in the prehospital setting, consideration of their roles permits a thorough comprehension of the pathophysiology of shock. As shock is a widespread failure of O_2 delivery to the body's tissues, understanding how an alteration in each factor may result in a decrease in O_2 delivery will establish a foundation for both identifying etiologies of shock as well as creating a logical approach for appropriate intervention.

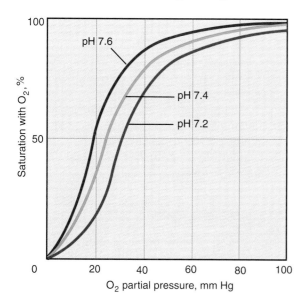

FIGURE 9-2 Oxyhemoglobin dissociation curve. At physiological pH (7.4), increasing partial pressure of oxygen (PO_2) leads to increased binding of oxygen to hemoglobin. Acidotic tissues (pH 7.2) permit a greater unloading of oxygen, as demonstrated by a rightward shift of the curve. An alkalotic environment (pH 7.6) causes the hemoglobin to unload less oxygen. From *Principles of Biochemistry*, by A. L. Lehninger, 1983, New York: Worth Publishers, p. 189.

ARTERIAL OXYGEN CONTENT

The oxygen content of arterial blood (CaO_2) can be calculated from the following equation:

$$CaO_2 = (1.34 \times Hgb)SaO_2 + 0.0031(PaO_2)$$

The variables are as follows: Hgb represents the hemoglobin concentration in grams per deciliter (g/dL), obtained from a complete blood count or arterial blood gas sample; SaO_2 is the percent saturation of arterial blood, represented as a fraction (97% = 0.97); and the PaO_2 is the partial pressure of oxygen, also obtained from an arterial blood gas analysis. The 1.34 represents the number of milliliters of oxygen carried by 1 gram of fully saturated hemoglobin. Many intensive care experts ignore the contribution of the PaO_2, as so little O_2 is carried dissolved in blood plasma and it is often a minuscule number. Therefore, the CaO_2 for a patient with a hemoglobin of 12 and an arterial saturation of 96% is $1.34 \times 12 \times 0.96$ or 15.4 g/dL. Thus, the CaO_2 is increased by raising the hemoglobin (via blood transfusion) or by increasing the O_2 saturation, while it is decreased by the presence of anemia or hypoxemia.

OXYGEN DELIVERY

Oxygen delivery (DO_2) is calculated utilizing the following formula:

$$DO_2 = CO \times CaO_2 \times 10$$

By substituting the equations for cardiac output and for arterial oxygen content, DO_2 can be rewritten as:

$$DO_2 = HR \times SV \times (1.34 \times Hgb)SaO_2 \times 10$$

The factors that contribute to **oxygen delivery** can now be identified: the *heart rate* (HR), the *stroke volume* (SV), the *hemoglobin concentration* (Hgb), and the *arterial oxygen saturation* (SaO_2). Clearly, any disease process that affects any of these variables will lead to a fall in oxygen delivery to the body's tissues and, therefore, shock.

Under normal circumstances, the body only extracts about 20% of the O_2 delivered to the tissues (extraction ratio, ER), and 80% of it returns to the heart for reoxygenation in the lungs and recirculation. Thus, the normal ratio of O_2 delivered to O_2 consumed (VO_2) is about 5:1. In shock, O_2 demands are greatly increased and the tissues may increase the extraction up to 50%, with the ratio of O_2 delivery (DO_2) to O_2 consumption (VO_2) falling to 2:1. This relationship may be plotted as a graph of O_2 consumption (VO_2) versus O_2 delivery (DO_2) (Figure 9-3).

The oxygen consumption graph contains two portions. The first part of the graph is quite steep. Here, increases in oxygen delivery are rewarded with

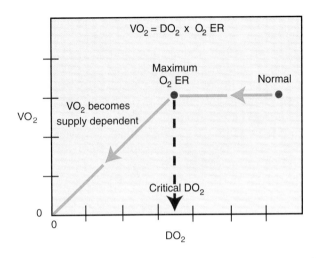

FIGURE 9-3 Oxygen consumption plotted versus oxygen delivery. The initial steep portion of the curve corresponds to the flow-dependent oxygen consumption. Here, increases in oxygen delivery produce increases in oxygen consumption. A point is reached where the curve flattens into a plateau phase where oxygen consumption becomes independent of oxygen delivery. From *The ICU Book*, 2nd ed., by P. L. Marino, 1998, Baltimore: Williams and Wilkins, p. 24.

increases in oxygen consumption. This portion of the curve is referred to as "flow dependent oxygen consumption," as increases in flow (i.e., oxygen delivery) result in increased oxygen consumption. A point is reached, however, where oxygen consumption becomes flow independent and further increases in oxygen delivery no longer lead to corresponding increases in oxygen consumption. Once this point is achieved, the cells are believed to be utilizing oxygen at the maximum rate possible and further increases in oxygen delivery are unnecessary.

CELLULAR METABOLISM

Why is oxygen so crucial to the normal functioning of cells? The individual cells of the body utilize carbohydrates (sugars), amino acids (proteins), and lipids (fats) in order to produce energy necessary for cellular functioning and create new macromolecules (proteins and lipids) required for dividing cells; but these processes are dependent upon aerobic conditions, wherein oxygen is readily available to the cells.

Our examination of cellular metabolism will focus on the breakdown of simple sugars (monosaccharides); however, fatty acids and amino acids can also be used to produce cellular energy. Cellular metabolism is broken down into three components, each occurring at a specific site within the cell: glycolysis, tricarboxylic acid (TCA or Krebs) cycle, and electron transport.

GLYCOLYSIS

The first part of cellular metabolism, **glycolysis**, occurs in the liquid matrix of the cell, the cytoplasm. In this stage, monosaccharides containing six-carbon atoms, such as glucose, are converted through a number of enzyme-catalyzed reactions into two three-carbon molecules, pyruvic acid. Only two high-energy molecules (adenosine triphosphate, or ATP) are created in this stage. If oxygen is present, further aerobic metabolism progresses. If oxygen is not present, as in hypoperfused tissues in a shock state, the pyruvic acid is converted to lactic acid. The liver can convert some of this lactic acid back into monosaccharides, but if generalized shock exists, the amount of lactate produced by anaerobic metabolism soon surpasses the liver's ability to metabolize it. While some tissues of the body (such as skeletal muscle and skin) are capable of functioning under anaerobic conditions for relatively brief periods of time, most body tissues have little reserve of oxygen and energy compounds and cannot tolerate significant periods of shock. Brain tissue is the most sensitive to hypoxemia. Thus, in anaerobic conditions, glucose metabolism is extremely inefficient at producing ATP for cellular functioning.

TCA (KREBS) CYCLE

Under aerobic conditions, the pyruvic acid molecules enter mitochondria, intracellular structures known as the "powerhouse of the cell," because of their role in producing energy. In the liquid matrix of the mitochondria, each pyruvic acid molecule travels through a number of reactions, collectively known as the **TCA (Krebs) cycle**, again catalyzed by specific enzymes. The TCA cycle can be subdivided into two parts. In the first step, pyruvic acid is converted to a two-carbon molecule, an acetyl group, with the production of one molecule of CO_2. Each acetyl group then travels along the TCA cycle, producing two additional CO_2 molecules and a single ATP molecule. Also produced are a number of electron-acceptor molecules [nicotinamide adenine dinucleotide (NAD) and flavin adenine dinucleotide (FAD)], which will be utilized in electron transport, to create additional ATP. Thus, up to this point, each glucose molecule has produced six CO_2 molecules and four ATP molecules, plus a number of electron-acceptor molecules.

ELECTRON TRANSPORT

Electron transport occurs in a series of proteins bound to the membrane of the mitochondria. In this phase, all of the electron-acceptor molecules produced during glycolysis and the TCA cycle are converted through a series of reactions with O_2 molecules into an additional 32 ATP molecules. Thus, electron transport is the primary site of O_2 utilization within the cell and, under anaerobic conditions, energy production is very inefficient. However, in the presence of O_2, each glucose molecule is converted into 6 CO_2 molecules, 36 ATP molecules, and 44 H_2O (water) molecules. Without O_2, little ATP is produced for vital cellular processes and the cells eventually die if oxygen delivery is not restored within an appropriate amount of time.

CLASSIFICATIONS OF SHOCK

Shock may be classified into four primary etiologies, each of which results from a failure of one component necessary for oxygen delivery to the tissues (Table 9-2): (1) *respiratory failure*, wherein oxygen is prevented from reaching the alveoli or is inhibited from diffusing across the alveolar membrane into the bloodstream; (2) *perfusate failure*, due to a loss of blood or plasma; (3) *vascular failure* with resultant vasodilation or vascular permeability; and (4) *cardiac failure* leading to impaired heart function. Though considered separate entities, these processes often overlap and the exact etiology is blurred. Many trauma patients may have shock with multiple causes, resulting from a combination of these etiologies. And, though blood loss accounts for most shock seen in the prehospital care of trauma patients, each of these types of shock may be encountered while caring for trauma patients.

RESPIRATORY FAILURE

Though not generally included by most authors as a common etiology for shock, respiratory failure can result in decreased oxygen delivery to tissues and, therefore, shock. Perhaps this is because some of the processes that may result in respiratory failure can be highly malignant, rapidly resulting in death. Foreign body airway obstruction exemplifies one such process, in that anoxia rapidly develops and, if untreated, brain and cardiac cells quickly die. Death under these circumstances is more commonly referred to as asphyxia, rather than shock; however a failure of oxygen delivery to these tissues produces the tragic result.

Other causes of respiratory failure may cause hypoxia, rather than anoxia, and can clearly interfere with normal O_2 delivery. These causes fall into three main groups: first, processes interfering with pulmonary mechanics; second, processes interfering with O_2 diffusion across the alveolar membrane; and, finally, exposures to toxic materials that impair the utilization of O_2.

TABLE 9-2
Classifications of Shock

Etiology	Names	Subtypes and Examples
Respiratory failure	Hypoxia	Airway obstruction: foreign body Mechanical failure: open pneumothorax, massive flail chest Diffusion failure: pulmonary contusion, pulmonary burns, pneumonia Toxic: carbon monoxide, cyanide
Perfusate failure	Hypovolemic shock	Hemorrhage: internal or external blood loss Plasma loss: thermal burns, severe crush injury, diabetes insipidus, dehydration
Vascular failure	Distributive shock	Sepsis: systemic inflammation, severe infection Neurogenic: high spinal cord injury, brain stem injury Anaphylaxis: severe allergic reaction
Cardiac failure	Cardiogenic shock	Intrinsic: valvular disruption, myocardial infarction, dysrhythmias Extrinsic: pericardial tamponade, tension pneumothorax

Mechanical Failure

Normal inspiration occurs by contraction of the diaphragm and intercostal muscles, which enlarge the size of the thoracic cavity. The intrathoracic pressure then falls below normal atmospheric pressure and air enters the lungs. Numerous processes may interfere with this "bellows" action of the lungs, such as open pneumothorax and flail chest. These injuries are topics of Chapter 13.

Diffusion Failure

Despite adequate concentrations of oxygen in the alveoli, numerous processes can impede the passive diffusion of O_2 across the alveolar membrane into the bloodstream. This membrane may become thickened by interstitial blood, as occurs in a pulmonary contusion, or serous fluid, as accumulates in pneumonia, congestive heart failure, inhalation injuries associated with thermal burns, and the acute respiratory distress syndrome (ARDS). Though ARDS is a complication of shock to be considered in greater detail in Chapter 29, once it develops, it may further impair O_2 delivery. In general, these failures of diffusion can be overcome with mechanical ventilation.

Toxic Exposures

Two toxic exposures that interfere with oxygen delivery and utilization may be encountered in trauma patients, though most often seen in victims of burn injury. These include carbon monoxide and cyanide poisoning. Carbon monoxide, when bound to hemoglobin, actually increases the affinity of hemoglobin for oxygen.

Therein lies the problem—carboxyhemoglobin binds oxygen so tightly that it does not release the oxygen in the tissues where it is needed. Thus, while there is adequate arterial oxygen saturation, the peripheral tissues are starved for oxygen as little is released by carboxyhemoglobin. In contrast, cyanide interferes with the electron transport aspect of cellular metabolism. The mitochondria are unable to utilize the available oxygen for production of ATP and energy production proceeds in an inefficient manner. The cells soon lose their ability to function because of the depletion of ATP required for vital processes.

PERFUSATE FAILURE

Loss of blood or plasma results in hypovolemic shock. Hemorrhage may be either external, that is, blood lost outside the body by injury to a major vessel, or internal. Internal hemorrhage can be separated into three categories: intracavitary, intraluminal, and interstitial. Life-threatening internal hemorrhage in most trauma patients involves bleeding into one of the body cavities. Injury to a solid organ, such as the liver or spleen, or to a major abdominal vessel results in a hemoperitoneum, while injury to the heart, lungs, or thoracic vessels may lead to a hemopericardium or hemothorax. Intraluminal hemorrhage involves bleeding into the lumen of the gastrointestinal tract, as may occur from stress ulceration following shock or severe head injury. Though often overlooked, significant hemorrhage can occur into the interstitial spaces surrounding fractures. Each long-bone fracture (humerus, radius, ulna, tibia, and fibula) can result in as much as 500 mL of hemorrhage, while a femoral fracture can be associated with 1 liter or more of blood loss. A rib fracture can involve several hundred milliliters of hemorrhage. In the case of multiple fractures with their potential interstitial blood loss, it becomes obvious that shock may develop despite the lack of external hemorrhage or injuries to intra-abdominal organs.

▶ INTERNET ACTIVITIES

Visit the SpringNet continuing education Web site at http://www.springnet.com/ce/ p509a.htm. Review the case and presentation of the hypovolemic trauma patient.

The amount of blood loss may be estimated after performing an adequate assessment (Table 9-3). Healthy adults tolerate blood loss of up to 750 mL, about 15% of their blood volume, without significant side effects. This amount of hemorrhage, similar to donating a unit of blood, falls well within the normal body's ability to compensate. Slight anxiety and an increased pulse pressure (difference between the arterial systolic and diastolic pressures) may be the only notable signs. Loss of up to 30% of one's blood volume requires more sophisticated compensation. Hemorrhage of this amount generally results in tachycardia, tachypnea, mild anxiety, a narrowed pulse pressure, and slight oliguria. Significantly, hypotension usually only appears once a patient has lost more than 30% (greater than 1,500 mL) of their blood volume. At this point, compensatory mechanisms are failing and blood pressure can no longer be maintained. More pronounced tachycardia, tachypnea, and oliguria occur, and the patient may be confused. Patients with loss of greater than 40% of their blood volume (Class IV shock) are truly "minutes away from death" if proper care is not immediately initiated. These patients have marked tachycardia, tachypnea, and hypotension and are often lethargic.

Plasma loss resulting in shock can occur from several types of trauma. Intravascular fluid may be lost due to thermal injury, severe crush injuries, and diabetes insipidus. Burn injury results in significant dehydration. When skin is damaged by full-thickness burns, fluid loss becomes a life-threatening problem. Fluid moves from the intravascular compartment into the interstitial and intracellular compartments. Crush injury, like burn injury, is associated with damage to the cells and blood vessels resulting in fluid being lost into the interstitial space from the intravascular and intracellular spaces. One potential complication of severe head injury is diabetes insipidus. In this condition, inadequate amounts of vasopressin (antidiuretic hormone) are produced, limiting the kidneys' ability to resorb free water. The net result is a tremendous diuresis; the body can actually urinate itself into hypovolemic shock.

TABLE 9-3
Classes of Hemorrhagic Shock

	Class I	Class II	Class III	Class IV
Percent blood volume loss*	<15	15–30	30–40	>40
Blood loss* (mL)-	<750	750–1,500	1,500–2,000	>2,000
Pulse (beats/min)	<100	>100	>120	>140
Pulse pressure	Normal or increased	Narrowed	Narrowed	Narrowed
Respiratory rate (breaths/min)	14–20	20–30	30–40	>35
Mental status	Normal or slightly anxious	Mildly anxious	Anxious or confused	Very confused or lethargic
Blood pressure	Normal	Normal	Decreased	Markedly decreased
Urine output (mL/hr)	>30	20–30	5–15	Minimal

*Represents estimated blood loss and assumes an average 70-kg adult.

Adapted from *Advanced Trauma Life Support Instructor Manual*, by the American College of Surgeons Committee on Trauma, Chicago, 1997, American College of Surgeons, p. 98.

The primary mechanism of shock associated with hypovolemia is inadequate venous return (preload). Decreased filling of the ventricles results in a decreased SV and CO (Starling's law). Hypovolemic shock resulting from blood loss produces acute anemia, which contributes to inadequate O_2 delivery. Note that hemoglobin and hematocrit levels are notoriously inaccurate in assessing for the presence of shock in the actively bleeding patient. Damaged vessels bleed whole blood; that is, both erythrocytes and blood plasma are lost. Thus, the hemoglobin and hematocrit levels often do not change acutely. Thus, while the concentration of blood cells in the circulating blood may appear normal, the total volume of blood cells is diminished, and this relative anemia significantly impairs the delivery of oxygen to vital tissues.

INTERNET ACTIVITIES

Visit the e-medicine Web site at http:// www.emedicine.com/. Click on the Emergency Medicine on-line book and select Trauma and Orthopedics. Then click on Shock. Review the chapter on the management of hemorrhagic shock.

VASCULAR FAILURE

Injury to the central nervous system, sepsis, and anaphylaxis may all cause shock by disrupting the normal functioning of blood vessels. Neurogenic shock may result from either a brain stem injury or vertebral injury with spinal cord damage. Injuries at these levels may interrupt the sympathetic innervation to peripheral blood vessels. Without this innervation, the baseline vascular tone is lost, the vessels dilate, and the SVR falls. This creates a state of "relative hypovolemia." While no blood volume may have been lost, the normal blood volume no longer adequately fills the enlarged vascular space. One may view this as 5 liters of blood in a 6- or 7-liter vascular container; therefore, volume resuscitation generally restores adequate perfusion.

Upon assessing the patient with neurogenic shock, the classic signs of shock may be absent due to the body's impaired ability to compensate for this injury. Without sympathetic innervation to the heart, compensatory tachycardia does not occur. In fact, bradycardia is often found due to the unopposed effect of the vagus nerves on the heart. Similarly, the cool, clammy skin seen in shock, a result of α_1 innervation to the cutaneous vessels leading to vasoconstriction and shunting of blood to the vital organs, is usually seen above the level of the spinal cord injury. In the skin

below the injury the vessels dilate and skin is initially pink and warm. These victims lose their ability to maintain body heat due to this vasodilation and are prone to hypothermia. Oxygen delivery is impaired because of the decreased preload causing a fall in cardiac output and because of the inability of the sympathetic nervous system to stimulate the heart to compensate.

Patients with sepsis, usually resulting from severe infection, may suffer shock from several etiologies. Toxins associated with bacterial infections may cause widespread vasodilation and a state of relative hypovolemia similar to neurogenic shock. Additionally, products released by the leukocytes fighting the infection cause an increase in vascular permeability. Fluid "leaks" out of the intravascular space into the interstitial space, contributing to the hypovolemia. A severe allergic reaction, anaphylaxis, results in shock by similar mechanisms. Products released by the cells involved in the reaction lead to both widespread vasodilation and a similar "capillary leak" phenomena. This capillary leak explains the edema found in these patients. In sepsis and anaphylaxis, both the vasodilation and intravascular volume loss greatly decrease cardiac preload and thereby diminish cardiac output and impair oxygen delivery.

CARDIAC FAILURE

Causes of cardiac failure may be separated into *intrinsic* and *extrinsic* etiologies. Intrinsic causes, while uncommon in trauma victims, do occasionally occur. These include acute valvular disruption, myocardial infarction, and dysrhythmias. Severe blunt chest trauma, such as a deceleration impact on a steering wheel, can disrupt cardiac valves and result in acute valvular insufficiency. This is often rapidly followed by cardiac failure because the heart is no longer capable of adequately ejecting its stroke volume. Severe myocardial infarction may be associated with the inability of the heart to adequately pump and deliver oxygen to the body.

Dysrhythmias may also cause cardiac failure. Bradycardias less than 50 bpm may not generate an adequate cardiac output and blood pressure. Similarly, tachycardias with rates in excess of about 150–160 bpm may not allow for adequate cardiac filling and similarly may impair oxygen delivery. Disordered rhythms, such as atrial fibrillation, may also be associated with shock. The atrial contraction, or "kick," provides about 25% of ordinary cardiac output, and therefore, atrial fibrillation or atrioventricular dissociation (third-degree heart block) can rapidly lead to impaired oxygen delivery.

The prehospital care provider must keep in mind that a medical problem, such as an acute myocardial infarction, may cause the injury, such as a motor vehicle collision or fall. Also, while hypovolemic shock is the most common type of shock found in trauma victims, the possibility that another type of shock, such as cardiac failure, may be involved should not be overlooked.

Examples of extrinsic causes of cardiac failure found in trauma patients include both pericardial tamponade and tension pneumothorax. While pericardial tamponade is more frequently associated with penetrating chest trauma, victims with traumatic cardiac rupture rarely survive to reach the hospital. Blood in the pericardium impairs adequate cardiac filling, and stroke volume and cardiac output decrease. A tension pneumothorax impairs venous return by kinking the vena cavae as they enter the right atrium, decreasing SV and CO and O_2 delivery.

INTERNET ACTIVITIES

Visit the e-medicine Web site at http://www.emedicine.com/. Click on the Emergency Medicine on-line book and select Cardiovascular. Then click on Shock. Review the chapter on the management of cardiogenic shock.

COMPENSATORY MECHANISMS

Evolution has provided the human body with numerous mechanisms to compensate for impaired oxygen delivery. Two of these, respiratory compensation and the sympathetic nervous system, respond almost immediately. The other two compensatory mechanisms, the neuroendocrine response and transcapillary refill, take a number of hours to produce their effects.

RESPIRATORY COMPENSATION

Chemoreceptors located in the carotid body (in the carotid artery) and in the aortic arch communicate to the respiratory center of the brain via cranial nerves IX and X, respectively. These receptors constantly monitor the blood and send messages to the brain when they detect hypoxemia (PaO_2 less than 50 mm Hg), hypercarbia (increased $PaCO_2$), or acidosis. Stimulation to the respiratory center results in increases in the rate and depth of respiration. Mild tachypnea is probably the earliest sign of inadequate oxygen delivery.

SYMPATHETIC NERVOUS SYSTEM ACTIVATION

Baroreceptors that monitor the blood pressure are found in the carotid sinus, which communicates with the brain through cranial nerve IX, and the aortic arch, which communicates via cranial nerve X. When decreases in blood pressure are detected, these nerves increase the activity of the sympathetic nervous system and correspondingly decrease vagal activity. Activation of this part of the autonomic nervous system accounts for many of the signs and symptoms classically associated with shock; however, many are mechanisms that compensate for inadequate oxygen delivery. In essence, the sympathetic nervous system strives to maintain adequate oxygen delivery to the vital organs (brain, heart, and lungs), often at the expense of oxygen delivery to less vital structures [i.e., gastrointestinal (GI) tract, skin, uterus].

The activation of α_1 receptors causes vasoconstriction, which is probably the single most important compensatory mechanism. Blood is shunted away from the gastrointestinal tract and the peripheral tissues, which better tolerate ischemia (skin and fat), to the vital visceral organs. The shunting of blood away from the GI tract accounts for the nausea and vomiting occasionally seen in shock victims, while the peripheral vasoconstriction causes the cold, clammy skin. Venoconstriction makes initiating peripheral intravenous lines a challenge.

Of somewhat lesser importance is the stimulation of the beta-adrenergic receptors. Activation of the β_1 receptors leads to increased heart rate and contractility. These actions help maintain blood pressure. Assume that hemorrhage causes a fall in venous return, with a corresponding decrease in blood pressure. The baroreceptors stimulate adrenergic activity, resulting in an increased heart rate and SVR and improved cardiac contractility (SV). Blood pressure is thus maintained. When β_2 receptors are stimulated, bronchodilation occurs in an effort to improve oxygenation of the blood.

NEUROENDOCRINE RESPONSE

When the body recognizes such problems as injury, fluid loss, or infection, it responds by secreting a number of hormones with complex functions. Adrenocorticotropic hormone (ACTH), released by the pituitary, stimulates the adrenal cortex to produce aldosterone and cortisol. Aldosterone causes increased reabsorption of sodium and water in the kidney and, therefore, production of highly concentrated urine. Another stimulus for the release of aldosterone begins in the kidney. When cells comprising the juxtaglomerular apparatus (JGA) experience decreased perfusion, they release renin. In the blood plasma, renin accelerates the conversion of angiotensinogen to angiotensin I. Lung tissue converts angiotensin I to angiotensin II, which is a very potent vasoconstrictor agent and a potent stimulus to aldosterone secretion.

Cortisol stimulates many aspects of metabolism, including protein synthesis. Epinephrine and norepinephrine may be secreted by the adrenal medulla, contributing to the sympathetic response. Vasopressin (antidiuretic hormone, ADH) is released by the posterior pituitary in response to increases in serum osmolality. This hormone causes the distal renal tubules to increase the absorption of water. These complex hormones help compensate for hypovolemia but take hours to achieve their maximum effects.

TRANSCAPILLARY REFILL

Following hypovolemia, osmosis allows for the passive movement of fluid from the intracellular and interstitial spaces into the intravascular space. This process, which may take several hours to complete, is believed to be self-limited and probably accounts for the movement of less than 2 liters of fluid. Hemoglobin and hematocrit values are of little use in the actively bleeding patient, as whole blood is lost. It is only after transcapillary refill occurs or intravenous fluid resuscitation is performed that the anemia becomes apparent as the blood is diluted.

DECOMPENSATION

Compensatory mechanisms function quite well, provided the initiating cause of the shock quickly resolves. But if there is ongoing hemorrhage or fluid loss, continued hypoxia, or continued infection, the body's compensatory mechanisms may be overwhelmed and the oxygen delivery may once again begin to fall. In this section, we shall examine the host factors that may limit compensation and the consequences of continued shock.

HOST FACTORS AFFECTING COMPENSATION

Host factors, those inherent to the injured person, may dramatically limit the ability to compensate for even mild shock and include age, medications, alcohol intoxication, and physical conditioning. Shock is poorly tolerated by those at the extremes of life: the very young (neonates and infants) and geriatric patients. In neonates, compensatory mechanisms are not well developed, while in the old, underlying diseases of the heart, lungs, and blood vessels may prevent appropriate compensation. Certain medications, such as beta-adrenergic blocking agents or calcium channel blocking agents, may prevent the compensatory tachycardia necessary to maintain blood pressure following hypovolemia. Alcohol intoxication leads to peripheral vasodilation, which may not be overcome by alpha-adrenergic stim-

ulation. This can also contribute to the development of hypothermia. In contrast, young healthy adults and well-conditioned athletes can compensate exceedingly well with normal blood pressures and pulse rates. They may appear to be minimally injured right up until the time they suffer cardiovascular collapse and cardiac arrest.

SYSTEMIC INFLAMMATION

Numerous inflammatory mediators are released from various body cells in response to severe injury or infection.[3] While many of these have a beneficial role in fighting infection and tissue repair, shock may "prime" the immune system, contributing to the overproduction of these active molecules. The result is an ongoing inflammatory response, further impairing O_2 delivery. Once this becomes cyclical, continued inflammation resulting in further impairment in O_2 delivery, resulting in continued inflammation, and so on, it becomes almost impossible to control. Some of these inflammatory mediators are found in the blood plasma, such as the complement cascade, while many others are produced by leukocytes, including free radicals, eicosanoids, and cytokines.

Complement is a complex series of enzymatic proteins found in blood plasma that have a role in normal immune response. When activated, several of these proteins cause damage to the endothelial cells that line blood vessels, leading to increased vascular permeability and intravascular fluid loss. Free radicals, such as superoxide, hydrogen peroxide, and hydroxyl molecules, are believed to be released by injured or ischemic tissues once perfusion is reestablished. These compounds also cause endothelial damage and can disrupt intracellular enzymes and destroy cell membranes.

The eicosanoids are a relatively diverse group of molecules derived from the fat arachidonic acid. Arachidonic acid may be converted by the enzyme lipoxygenase to one of a number of leukotrienes, which cause the bronchoconstriction and vascular permeability seen in anaphylaxis. It may also follow a cyclooxygenase pathway to become one of many types of thromboxanes, causing platelet aggregation and vasoconstriction; prostaglandins, causing vasodilation and immunomodulation; or prostacyclins, causing vasodilation and inhibiting platelet aggregation. Cytokines are a group of small protein molecules produced by leukocytes. Many cytokines have very potent effects, although most are degraded within seconds. Though these agents are beneficial to the immune response, their harmful effects include endothelial injury and increased vascular permeability.

A common side effect of many of the inflammatory mediators is vascular permeability. All these agents contribute to the "capillary leak" syndrome seen in severe shock and the development of interstitial edema. This intravascular fluid loss further impairs O_2 delivery by decreasing venous return. Thus, these patients often do not develop interstitial edema because of fluid resuscitation, but require the fluid resuscitation because of the ongoing intravascular fluid loss.

STAGED DEATH

Shock is an insidious killer. From animal experiments, Wiggers[6] realized that shock can become irreversible. Most animals, when bled into hypotension, survived if the shed blood was transfused within 2 or 3 hours. If the shock state was permitted to persist for a longer period of time, retransfusion of the shed blood often returned vital signs to normal; however many of these animals eventually died.[6] In the five decades following Wigger's publication, many investigators have studied this issue, yet many questions remain unanswered.

The systemic inflammation and reperfusion injury discussed above clearly plays a central role in cell injury and death. Anaerobic metabolism is only tolerated for a brief period of time. If it persists, ATP production falls to only 5%–10% of normal. Lactic acid accumulates and the bicarbonate buffer system of the blood is overwhelmed. Inflammatory mediators are released, leading to additional intravascular fluid losses. As noted above, this may establish a vicious cycle of worsening oxygen delivery leading to more inflammation (Figure 9-4).

Those tissues from which oxygen delivery is first compromised are at highest risk for becoming ischemic. If adequate oxygen delivery is not promptly reestablished, these ischemic cells may suffer permanent damage and eventually die. Free radicals may disrupt cell membranes and damage vital enzymes, while a lack of ATP may prevent the cell from maintaining its homeostasis, resulting in derangements in intracellular electrolyte composition. Some researchers believe that an influx of calcium molecules into the cell may activate enzymes that destroy mitochondria and the cytoskeleton, creating an irreparable situation.[7]

Thus, shock may be seen as "staged death." As significant numbers of cells die, the damaged tissues containing these cells may succumb. This, in turn, leads to dysfunction of the organs containing these tissues. Virtually all tissues are vulnerable to injury from shock, but pulmonary and renal dysfunction occur most frequently. As inflammation and impaired oxygen delivery continue, poorly functioning organs often fail, requiring therapies such as mechanical ventilation or dialysis. All this can result in death of the organism that suffered the shock.

IMPROVING OXYGEN DELIVERY

As shock represents a failure of adequate oxygen delivery, proper therapy to treat shock must focus on improving oxygen delivery. Specifics of prehospital care for shock are discussed elsewhere in this text; however, an overall approach for resuscitation will be outlined. This approach is particularly useful because, when the principles are followed, it may be used to treat any type of shock, regardless of the etiology. While some of this discussion includes interventions performed in the emergency department or intensive care unit (ICU), their inclusion is crucial to a comprehensive understanding of shock therapy. The formula for oxygen delivery is

$$DO_2 = HR \times SV \times (1.34 \times Hgb)SaO_2 \times 10$$

With this in mind, our approach to resuscitation should focus on the following factors: (1) ensuring an adequate arterial oxyhemoglobin saturation; (2) ensuring an adequate heart rate; (3) ensuring an adequate hemoglobin concentration; and (4) maximizing stroke volume.

ARTERIAL OXYHEMOGLOBIN SATURATION

Initial interventions for a victim of shock should be focused on achieving and maintaining an adequate arterial oxygen saturation (SaO_2). Should the patient be apneic or unable to control his or her airway, endotracheal intubation should be performed. All patients with hypoxemia should be at least considered for intubation. Once an adequate airway is assured, ventilatory support, if needed, should be provided. Oxygen should be delivered to maintain the SaO_2 greater than 90% or 92%, providing a buffer for desaturation. Maintaining the SaO_2 higher than this level contributes little to further improvements in oxygen delivery, as can be seen by calculating out the following DO_2: Given a CO of 7.0 liters/m and Hgb concentration of 12 g/dL, the DO_2 for a saturation of 92% is 1,035, compared to the DO_2 of 1,103 for an SaO_2 of 98%. Improving the SaO_2 by 6 percentage points only improved the oxygen delivery by 6.5%. Recalling the oxyhemoglobin dissociation curve, note that below a saturation of about 90%, small decreases in PaO_2 result in significant drops in SaO_2, as this portion of the curve is quite steep.

A trauma patient with impaired arterial oxygen saturation must also be carefully assessed for the presence of a pneumothorax or tension pneumothorax. A tension pneumothorax can frequently be identified with clinical assessment alone (diminished or absent breath sounds, increasing respiratory distress or difficulty ventilating a patient, and arterial hypotension), though a chest X-ray

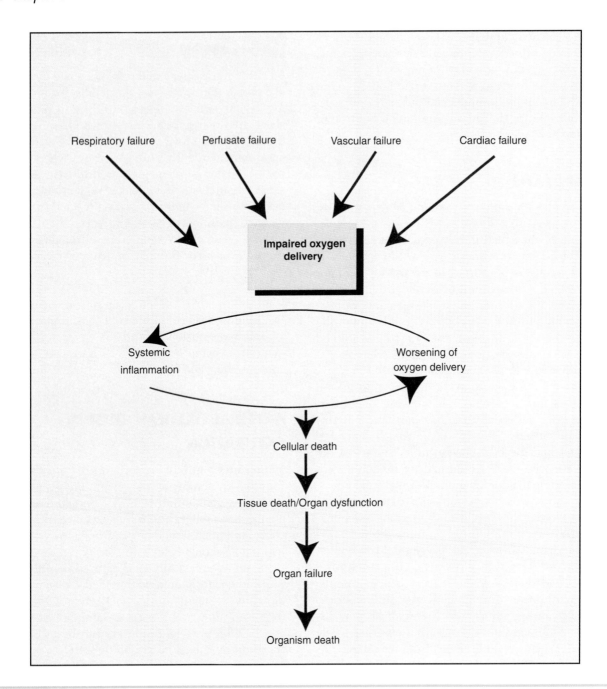

FIGURE 9-4 Shock, widespread impairment in oxygen delivery, may establish a cycle of systemic inflammation that further worsens oxygen delivery. Eventually, ischemic cells die. This may then be followed by organ dysfunction, organ failure, and death.

may be necessary to identify a developing tension pneumothorax.

HEART RATE

Once an adequate SaO_2 is achieved, an adequate heart rate must be assured. Patients who are considered acceptable candidates for resuscitation but are pulseless should undergo cardiopulmonary resuscitation. As noted above, the heart can maintain a normal cardiac output over quite a broad range; however, severe bradycardias and tachycardias may impair cardiac output and oxygen delivery. Patients with heart rates less than 55 bpm associated with shock should receive atropine and transcutaneous pacing should be considered. Severe tachycardias, especially those with rates in excess of 160 bpm, may cause shock due to inadequate ventricular filling times. These patients may benefit from emergent cardioversion or, if time permits, the administration of either a calcium channel antagonist or beta-blocking agent. However, caution must be exercised as these agents may aggravate hypotension. Few trauma patients present with heart rates outside of this 55–160 bpm range and, therefore, will not need manipulation of their heart rate in order to improve oxygen delivery.

HEMOGLOBIN CONCENTRATION

Because of the oxygen-carrying capacity of erythrocytes, blood transfusion can dramatically increase oxygen delivery in anemic patients with shock. Most critical care surgeons will strive to maintain the hemoglobin in the range of 10–12 g/dL in critically injured patients who demonstrate evidence of impaired oxygen delivery. Most patients with anemia have associated hypovolemia. Blood has the advantage of both restoring blood volume and providing oxygen-carrying capacity. Increasing the hemoglobin concentration from 8 to 12 g/dL will increase oxygen delivery by 50%. Higher levels may, in fact, impair oxygen delivery by increasing the viscosity of the blood. Autotransfusion of lost blood provides a useful technique in patients with massive blood loss. Blood drained from a hemothorax can be filtered and returned to the circulation, providing a rapid method of delivering compatible blood.

At the present time, blood is extremely cumbersome to use in the prehospital setting. No good blood substitutes are yet available. In the field, attention should be given to controlling external and internal hemorrhage. Direct pressure and pressure dressings often adequately handle external hemorrhage. Splinting fractures limits interstitial hemorrhage, and virtually all extremity fractures can be rapidly and adequately immobilized with the use of a long spine board. The pneumatic antishock garment may help tamponade intra-abdominal bleeding and hemorrhage from pelvic fractures.[8] Excessive delays at the scene may worsen shock when internal hemorrhage cannot be controlled. The need for blood transfusion remains an important reason why trauma patients with shock should be rapidly transported to a facility fully capable of caring for them.

A cautionary note about blood transfusion—all anemia does not require transfusion. In general, young healthy individuals can tolerate Hgb levels as low as 6 g/dL (Hct 18%–20%). Most experts will withhold transfusion in these individuals, *provided they have evidence of good tissue perfusion and are asymptomatic*, as blood transfusion does carry the small but important risks of transfusion reactions and infectious disease. Patients should be capable of producing their own replacement cells. Should evidence of compromised oxygen delivery be noted, or should the patients have serious underlying medical problems, such as heart disease or chronic lung disease, most physicians will opt to transfuse, believing that the benefits of improved oxygen delivery should outweigh the minimal risks of reaction or transfusion-associated illness.

MANIPULATING STROKE VOLUME

Once the SaO_2, heart rate, and hemoglobin concentration are addressed, improvements in O_2 delivery can only be accomplished by improving the stroke volume. Attention should first be focused on ensuring an adequate cardiac preload. Only when this fails to adequately improve O_2 delivery should pharmacological intervention be initiated to adjust afterload or cardiac contractility.

Preload

As we have noted, most shock associated with injury results from hypovolemia due to blood loss. Because of this, the initial step aimed at improving stroke volume should be a rapid fluid challenge. This improves cardiac filling and, correspondingly, cardiac output. Children should receive 20 mL/kg of crystalloid solution, while adults should receive 30 mL/kg (about 2 liters for the average adult). Poiseuille's law states that fluid flow through a pipe is directly proportional to the fourth power of the radius of the conduit, while flow is inversely proportional to the length of the pipe. Based upon this, emergency workers should opt for large-diameter (16-gauge or larger), short-intravenous catheters. Central lines, especially multilumen catheters, will not deliver fluid as rapidly as a peripheral IV due to the length of the tubing.

The response of the patient's vital signs to this fluid bolus provides an indication of the presence of ongoing hemorrhage. If the vital signs return to normal and O_2 delivery dramatically improves, the bleeding has probably ceased. In contrast, if the vital signs transiently improve (such as the pulse slowing), then begin to deteriorate again, the patient is experiencing ongoing blood loss. If there is no improvement to the initial fluid challenge, blood loss has probably been massive and is continuing. This patient needs emergent surgical intervention in order to survive.

INTERNET ACTIVITIES

Visit the British Trauma Society Web site and review the material on shock and fluid resuscitation at http://www.trauma.org/eates/ectc/ectc-shock.html.

Fluid Choice

Controversy has centered around the type of fluid to administer. Some believe that colloid solutions such as dextran, plasma protein, or albumin are better than crystalloid solutions such as lactated Ringer's or normal saline. It is true that a larger volume of crystalloid is required to achieve the same hemodynamic effects when compared to colloids. Proponents of colloids argue that the crystalloids rapidly leave the intravascular compartment and that colloids remain in this space longer, producing less interstitial edema. However, in patients with severe shock, the endothelial injury creates openings in the capillaries through which even larger molecules such as albumin readily leak out.

Opponents of colloid solutions argue that albumin in the interstitial space increases the oncotic pressure there and prolongs the presence of interstitial fluid. In the absence of studies to conclusively show that colloid solutions are superior to crystalloids, most trauma surgeons opt for the more cost-effective choice—crystalloids. As long as liver perfusion is maintained, the lactate in lactated Ringer's does not contribute to a metabolic acidosis as it is rapidly metabolized to CO_2 and water. A more detailed comparison of intravenous fluids is provided in Chapter 21.

INTERNET ACTIVITIES

Visit the National Library of Medicine Web site at http://www.ncbi.nlm.nih.gov/PubMed/. Conduct a literature search on the use of blood substitutes in the setting of hemorrhagic shock. Review the abstracts of the search results. Ask your librarian to assist you in obtaining the journals with the five most relevant articles. Review these articles and summarize their findings.

Invasive Monitoring

Invasive monitoring techniques, generally employed in the ICU, permit more accurate assessment of cardiac preload. The two types of pressure monitoring traditionally utilized involve insertion of catheters into the superior vena cava to assess central venous pressure (CVP) or into the pulmonary artery for monitoring left heart pressures. The CVP lines can be inserted through the internal jugular, external jugular, or subclavian vein and are advanced to a position just proximal to the right atrium. For many situations, the right atrial pressures provide a general idea of the filling pressures for the left heart. Many factors, including mechanical ventilation, heart disease, lung disease, and sepsis, can interfere with the usefulness of CVP monitoring.

A pulmonary artery (PA) catheter (or Swan-Ganz catheter) is inserted through the internal jugular or subclavian vein and advanced into the superior vena cava. At this point, a small balloon on the tip of the catheter is inflated, allowing the catheter to "float" through the right atrium and right ventricle and into the pulmonary artery. The balloon permits blood flow to direct the catheter, much like a sail directs a boat. The catheter is advanced until the balloon wedges in a distal pulmonary artery. A pressure transducer at the tip of the artery then transduces the pulmonary capillary wedge pressure (PCWP). This "wedge" pressure corresponds to the left atrial pressure, as a solid fluid column exists between the transducer and the left atrium, through the pulmonary artery, pulmonary capillary, and pulmonary vein (Figure 9-5). The left atrial pressure, in most circumstances, provides useful information about left ventricular filling pressure and is a helpful, but not completely reliable, indicator of left ventricular preload. Sepsis, processes of the lung parenchyma such as ARDS, and aortic or mitral valvular disease can all interfere with the interpretation of data obtained from a PA catheter.

In general, PCWP varies from about 6 to 12 mm Hg and pulmonary edema from congestive heart failure is believed to develop when the PCWP is between 18 and 24 mm Hg. For many patients, preload can be considered to be maximized between 15 and 18 mm Hg. A cardiac output can also be determined using this catheter. Therefore, a Starling's curve can actually be plotted for each patient. Fluid boluses are administrated, and PCWP and CO measurements are then obtained. As long as the CO continues to increase with a fluid bolus, the patient may be viewed as still climbing the curve. Should the CO only minimally improve and the PCWP increase, the plateau of the curve is being attained. Once the CO begins to fall following fluid administration, the left ventricle is beginning to fail.

Optimal filling pressures vary between patients and may even vary in a single patient as the disease process resolves or worsens. For example, in severe sepsis, the ventricle becomes much less compliant. This stiff ventricle requires higher than normal filling pressures for maximum contractility.

No prospective research studies have yielded conclusive evidence that patients in whom PA catheters were inserted had improved clinical outcomes. Some argue that the presence of a PA catheter may lead to a more aggressive approach to critically ill patients, and this may increase their mortality rate. Supporters of PA catheter monitoring often espouse that the PA catheter provides clinicians with information about heart function and oxygen delivery and consumption not obtainable by less invasive means. This information, they believe, results in decreased mortality rates. Despite

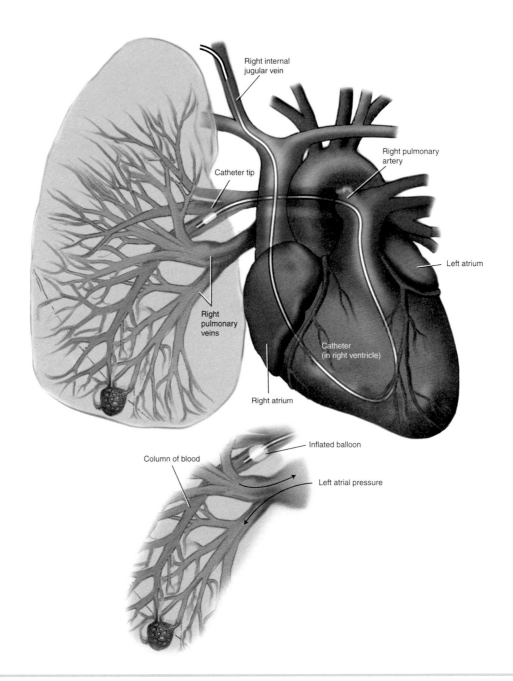

FIGURE 9-5 Pulmonary arterial catheter measures pressure in the pulmonary artery when the balloon is deflated. Because flow in the vascular system generates a pressure drop as the blood passes through the microvasculature, the pressure from the pulmonary artery to the left atrium gradually falls. When the balloon is inflated, flow in the vasculature distal to the tip is eliminated; therefore, there is no pressure drop. Because there is no pressure drop and because there are no valves between the left atrium and the pulmonary artery, the pressure in the pulmonary artery distal to the point of occlusion must equal the pressure in the left atrium, provided that there is an open column of blood between the end of the catheter and the left atrium. That is, pulmonary arterial wedge pressure will equal left atrial pressure as long as the catheter is in a dependent portion of the lung with a vasculature that remains open during ventilation. Because the catheter is flow directed, it usually will end up in such a dependent, well-perfused area. This is not a certainty, however. If inflated alveoli occlude the microvasculature, wedge pressure will equal alveolar pressure. This inaccuracy cannot be easily detected. Verification that the catheter is in the dependent portion of the lung requires a cross-table lateral chest X-ray. We do not routinely obtain these X-rays unless the wedge pressures are absolutely critical for treatment and unless the reliability of the wedge pressure tracing is suspect. Suspicion usually arises when excessively wide pressure swings are evident as the lungs are inflated and deflated.

this controversy, the PA catheter is thought by many intensivists to be an invaluable tool for managing volume resuscitation in patients with severe shock.

Complications of PA catheter monitoring are numerous, but in critically ill patients, the benefits of additional information about the heart and oxygen utilization outweigh the uncommon, but significant, complications associated with its use. Many complications are associated with catheter insertion and are common to the insertion of central intravenous lines, including hemorrhage, pneumothorax, catheter embolus, and infection. Complications most commonly associated with PA catheters as opposed to CVP lines include cardiac dysrhythmias, injury to heart valves, and pulmonary hemorrhage or infarction from prolonged inflation of the balloon.

Afterload

Once preload is maximized, manipulation of the afterload should be considered. The systemic vascular resistance can be calculated from data obtained from the PA catheter using the following formula:

$$SVR = \frac{MAP - CVP}{CO} \times 80$$

where SVR is systemic vascular resistance, MAP is mean arterial pressure, CVP is central venous pressure, and CO is cardiac output. The normal SVR ranges between 800 and 1,200 dynes/sec/cm.[5] While most hypotensive shock patients initially have a high SVR, the SVR generally normalizes once preload has been maximized. A low SVR corresponds to peripheral vasodilation. Patients with cardiogenic shock (intrinsic pump failure) generally present with a low cardiac output, high PCWP, and high SVR (Table 9-4). In these patients, the judicious administration of an agent that will decrease the SVR often improves cardiac functioning and CO by decreasing the afterload. Arteriole vasodilators employed for this purpose include infusions of sodium nitroprusside and nicardipine. Nitroglycerine has more venodilating effects than these two agents and is generally not used in this manner.

If a vasodilating agent is required to return the SVR to the normal range, preload should again be assessed. Often the arteriolar dilation increases the size of the intravascular container and additional volume resuscitation may be necessary to optimize preload once again.

Contractility

The final manner in which stroke volume may be increased is with the administration of an inotropic agent to increase cardiac contractility. Beta-adrenergic

TABLE 9-4
Cardiovascular Parameters in Various Types of Shock

Type Of Shock	Cardiac Output	PCWP	SVR
Hypovolemic	Low	Low	High
Septic	High	Low	Low
Neurogenic	Low	Low	Low
Cardiogenic	Low	High	High

agents are the first-line drugs for this purpose; the most commonly used are dobutamine and dopamine. Dobutamine is a synthetic beta agonist with strong β_1 effects. Dopamine also causes beta-adrenergic stimulating effects; however, at higher doses, α_1 (vasoconstriction) predominates. The potent inotropes amrinone and milrinone may be used for failing hearts if dobutamine is not effective. All inotropes increase myocardial oxygen demand and, in the setting of myocardial ischemia, may promote myocardial infarction. This is why these agents are the last to be utilized in an effort to improve O_2 delivery.

Vasopressors

Agents that raise blood pressure through vasoconstriction virtually have no use in shock. Blood pressure does not equate with blood flow and oxygen delivery. If our goal in shock was to increase blood pressure, the use of vasopressors (α_1 agents such as epinephrine, norepinephrine, neosynephrine, phenylephrine, and high-dose dopamine) could help us achieve this goal. Impaired oxygen delivery, not hypotension, is the fundamental defect in shock. Vasopressors may improve blood pressure, *but at the cost of further decreasing blood flow and oxygen delivery*. Peripheral vasoconstriction equates to increased afterload with which the heart must contend, and the vasoconstriction may worsen metabolic acidosis by further decreasing peripheral oxygen delivery. Therefore, these agents should be used only if all other measures are not working.

Bicarbonate Therapy

The acidosis found most often in victims of shock is a metabolic acidosis resulting from lactic acid production from anaerobic metabolism. The administration of an alkalinizing agent, such as bicarbonate, does nothing to improve oxygen delivery. In the setting of lactic acidosis, intravenous bicarbonate results in increased CO_2 production. This CO_2 readily diffuses into the cells, producing an intracellular acidosis, unless the patient's minute ventilation is increased for the CO_2 to be blown off. Overzealous use of bicarbonate can create a metabolic alkalosis, causing a shift of the oxyhemoglobin dissociation curve to the left. As noted, this further impairs oxygen delivery to the tissue. Most physicians now withhold bicarbonate administration unless the pH is less than 7.2. Continued resuscitation should be associated with improvements in the arterial pH, crucial details that are masked by the injudicious administration of bicarbonate.

Trendelenburg and Shock Positions

For years, emergency workers have placed patients in either the Trendelenburg position (entire body on a tilt with legs higher than head) or, more recently, the shock position (head and torso supine, with legs elevated). It was believed that these positions improved venous return to the heart and improved cardiac output for hypovolemic shock. These positions are no longer recommended as the venous capacitance vessels in most trauma victims with hypovolemia are already depleted of blood volume and raising the legs simply increases the afterload on the heart.[9]

COMPLICATIONS OF SHOCK

As discussed previously, virtually any organ system can suffer injury from prolonged or profound shock. Two of the more common complications of shock involve the lungs (ARDS) and the kidneys (acute renal failure). As these organs fail, so, too, can the entire body, resulting in multiple organ system failure (MOSF). Only through early recognition of shock and aggressive therapy can these complications be prevented.

ACUTE RESPIRATORY DISTRESS SYNDROME

Though currently known as ARDS, this syndrome was originally known as shock lung or Da Nang lung, as it was first described in the Vietnam conflict. It is the most common complication of shock currently seen in ICUs. ARDS involves the extravasation of intravascular fluid into the pulmonary interstitial and alveolar spaces, resulting in a defect in O_2 diffusion. In general, it presents 24–48 hours following the shock episode. Upon auscultation, crackles may be heard through the lung fields. On chest X-ray, both lung fields have diffuse white hazy infiltrates, consistent with pulmonary edema; this pulmonary edema is noncardiogenic. That is, it is not the result of cardiac failure and increased pulmonary hydrostatic pressure. It results from the sys-temic inflammation and the subsequent capillary leak seen in severe shock. A pulmonary artery catheter can be used to differentiate ARDS from cardiogenic pulmonary edema (congestive heart failure). Patients with ARDS develop acute respiratory failure and require mechanical ventilation for days to months. ARDS involves a mismatch of perfusion to poorly ventilated (oxygenated) alveoli. This is best treated with positive end-expiratory pressure (PEEP) as increased levels of PEEP help open up collapsed alveoli and improve the ventilation/perfusion mismatch. Despite modern critical care, the mortality associated with ARDS ranges from 50% to 65%, with most patients dying from MOSF.

ACUTE RENAL FAILURE

Hypoperfusion to the renal tissue may lead to injury of the distal renal tubules, found in the renal cortex. When these tubular cells die, they slough off into the lumen of the tubules. Though the exact nature of the renal injury is not fully understood, the kidneys lose their ability to excrete nitrogenous waste products and often water and potassium. Most patients who develop shock-induced renal damage will eventually require some form of renal dialysis. Indications for dialysis in trauma patients include volume overload in the face of oliguria, hyperkalemia, profound metabolic acidosis, and uremia (elevated blood urea nitrogen). Patients who develop oliguric renal failure (less than 500 mL of urine per day) have a higher mortality rate, often approaching 90%, compared to a mortality rate of about 50% for those who maintain their urine output.

MULTIPLE ORGAN FAILURE SYNDROME

Should the systemic inflammatory response continue or the patient receive repeated bouts of shock and impaired oxygen delivery, injury to the many vital organs of the body may lead to MOSF. In addition to renal and pulmonary failure, these patients may develop severe coagulopathies, hepatic failure, gastrointestinal tract ulceration with hemorrhage, and profound immune dysfunction. Eventually, the heart is no longer able to compensate for the systemic derangement and cardiac failure soon progresses to death. Of patients with failure of more than two organ systems, about 90% will not survive their hospitalization.

▶ SUMMARY

Shock is a life-threatening condition in which defects in either or both of the respiratory and circulatory systems result in insufficient quantifies of oxygen delivered to the systemic tissues. The presence of oxygen is crucial to the effective production of energy in the cell. Several physiological equations help to illustrate the mechanics of oxygen delivery. Blood pressure is related to heart rate, stroke volume, and systemic vascular resistance. Cardiac stroke volume is determined by preload (Starling's curve), afterload, and contractility. Oxygen delivery, in turn, is a product of heart rate, stroke volume, arterial oxygen saturation, and hemoglobin concentration.

Shock may result from respiratory failure, hypovolemia (perfusate failure), vascular failure, and cardiac failure. The body attempts to compensate for hypoperfusion in several manners, including increasing respiration; activating the sympathetic nervous system; releasing hormones that retain salt and water; and refilling the intravascular space from interstitial and intracellular fluid. If it is prolonged, shock results in systemic inflammation, involving a number of different biological mediators. Shock kills its victims in stages, by depriving cells of oxygen, vital to cellular metabolism.

Initial intervention to improve oxygen delivery includes assuring an adequate arterial oxyhemoglobin saturation and optimizing the heart rate and hemoglobin level. Stroke volume is maximized by optimizing cardiac filling (preload), decreasing afterload, and, finally, the use of inotropic agents. Complications of shock include ARDS, acute renal failure, and MOSF. Potential complications of shock should be minimized by early recognition of the presence of shock combined with aggressive therapy aimed at improving oxygen delivery.

REVIEW QUESTIONS

1. The American surgeon who was one of the earliest to study shock in an experimental manner was:
   a. Samuel Gross
   b. George W. Crile
   c. Sir Joseph Lister
   d. Louis Pasteur

2. The chamber of the heart with the thickest wall and responsible for pumping blood to the systemic circulation is the:
   a. Right atrium
   b. Right ventricle
   c. Left atrium
   d. Left ventricle

3. The mitral valve is located between the:
   a. Right atrium and right ventricle
   b. Right atrium and left atrium
   c. Left atrium and left ventricle
   d. Right ventricle and left ventricle

4. Select the normal pathway taken by a normal electrical impulse in the heart:
   a. SA node, AV node, bundle branches, Purkinje fibers
   b. AV node, SA node, bundle branches, Purkinje fibers
   c. SA node, bundle branches, AV node, Purkinje fibers
   d. AV node, Purkinje fibers, SA node, bundle branches

5. Activation of a β_1 receptor results in:
   a. Increase in both heart rate and cardiac contractility
   b. Decrease in both heart rate and cardiac contractility
   c. Increase in contractility and cutaneous arteriolar vasoconstriction
   d. Increase in heart rate, decrease in cardiac contractility

6. Cardiac output is the product of:
   a. Heart rate times systemic vascular resistance
   b. Stroke volume times systemic vascular resistance
   c. Heart rate times stroke volume
   d. Systemic vascular resistance times blood pressure

7. In the normal skeletal muscle capillary:
   a. Both oxygen and carbon dioxide diffuse out of the capillary.
   b. Oxygen diffuses out of the capillary while carbon dioxide diffuses in.
   c. Oxygen diffuses into the capillary while carbon dioxide diffuses out.
   d. Both oxygen and carbon dioxide diffuse into the capillary.

8. To maintain a normal blood pressure in the face of hypovolemia, the body can compensate by:
   a. Increasing heart rate while decreasing systemic vascular resistance
   b. Decreasing heart rate while increasing systemic vascular resistance
   c. Increasing stroke volume while decreasing systemic vascular resistance
   d. Increasing heart rate while increasing systemic vascular resistance

9. In the normal adult, total blood volume represents what percentage of body weight?
   a. 5%
   b. 7%
   c. 9%
   d. 15%

10. Cardiogenic shock in trauma victims can result from each of the following except:
    a. Pericardial tamponade
    b. Acute blood loss
    c. Blunt cardiac injury (myocardial contusion)
    d. Valvular disruption

11. In general, hypotension occurs only when blood loss amounts to what percentage of total blood volume?
    a. Less than 15%
    b. 15–30%
    c. 30–40%
    d. Greater than 40%

12. All of the following conditions may produce vascular failure leading to shock except:
    a. Anaphylaxis
    b. Myocardial infarction
    c. High spinal cord injury
    d. Severe infection (sepsis)

13. Initial attempts to treat shock, regardless of the etiology, should be focused on:
    a. Volume resuscitation with blood or crystalloid to ensure adequate preload
    b. Decreasing afterload with sodium nitroprusside infusion
    c. Increasing contractility with dobutamine
    d. Airway management, support of respiration, and oxygen administration

14. Starling's law of the heart states:
    a. Increased ventricular filling always results in increased cardiac output.
    b. Excessive filling of the ventricle may diminish cardiac output.
    c. The heart pumps better when ventricular filling is minimized.
    d. When high concentrations of oxygen are present, the heart utilizes little oxygen.

15. Pulmonary artery wedge pressure is measured in order to gain an understanding of:
    a. Left atrial pressures
    b. Right ventricular filling pressures
    c. Peripheral capillary pressures
    d. Cardiac output

16. Which of the following is the most correct early treatment of shock
    a. Dopamine infusion for an arterial blood pressure of 78/50 resulting from hemorrhage
    b. Fluid bolus of crystalloid solution for neurogenic shock
    c. Elevating the legs of a patient in septic shock
    d. Administration of sodium bicarbonate for an initial arterial pH of 7.26

17. What is shock?

18. What are the three primary components of the cardiovascular system and what is its function in oxygen delivery?

19. What is Starling's law of the heart? How does heart failure relate to this law?

20. What is the equation for calculating oxygen delivery and what does each term represent?

21. What are the four primary etiologies of shock?

▶ CRITICAL THINKING

- In treating a multisystem trauma patient with profound hemorrhage, you draw a blood sample while starting the first IV. The I-stat analysis returns the following values: Hgb, 14.8; Hct, 44; PaO_2, 110; PCO_2, 36. Comment on your evaluation of these values.

- Dobutamine infusion and high-flow crystalloid infusion are temporary methods of treating cardiac tamponade until pericardiocentesis is available. Using your knowledge of Starling's law and the autonomic nervous system, explain why these treatments are thought to be beneficial, if only temporary.

- The standard of care for the field management of patients in hemorrhagic shock is airway control, high-flow oxygen, control of hemorrhage, and circulatory support with crystalloid fluids. What are the benefits of this therapy? What are the limitations, especially in the setting of active hemorrhage? What other technologies might possibly improve the field treatment of patients in hemorrhagic shock?

▶ REFERENCES

1. Gross SD. *A System of Surgery: Pathological, Diagnostic, Therapeutic, and Operative.* Philadelphia: Blanchard and Lea; 1859:434 (reprinted by Classics of Surgery Library, Birmingham, Ala, 1991).
2. English PC. *Shock, Physiological Surgery and George Washington Crile: Medical Innovation in the Progressive Era.* Westport, Conn: Greenwood Press, 1980:213.
3. Baue AE. The horror autotoxicus and multiple-organ failure. *Arch Surg.* 1992; 127:1451.
4. Guyton AC. *Basic Human Physiology: Normal Function and Mechanisms of Disease.* Philadelphia: W. B. Saunders; 1977:196.
5. Little RC. *Physiology of the Heart and Circulation.* Chicago, Ill: Year Book Medical Publishers; 1977:148.

6. Wiggers CJ. *Physiology of Shock*. New York: Commonwealth Fund Publishers; 1950.
7. Gann DS, Wright PA. Shock—the final common pathway? In: Maull KI, et al, eds. *Advances in Trauma and Critical Care*. St. Louis: Mosby-Year Book; 1995:53.
8. McSwain NE. Pneumatic anti-shock garment: State of the art 1988. *Ann Emerg Med*. 1988; 17:506.
9. Marino PL. *The ICU Book*. 2nd ed. Baltimore: Williams and Wilkins; 1998:217.

▶ BIBLIOGRAPHY

Abrams JH, Cerra F, Holcroft JW. Cardiopulmonary monitoring. In: Wilmore DW, et al, eds. *Scientific American Surgery*. Vol. 1. New York: Scientific American; 1995.

Committee on Trauma. Shock. In: Committee on Trauma, American College of Surgeons. *Advanced Trauma Life Support for Doctors*. Chicago, Ill: American College of Surgeons, 1997.

Holcroft JW, Robinson MK. Shock. In: Wilmore DW, et al, eds. *Scientific American Surgery*. Vol. 1. New York: Scientific American; 1992: 266–271.

Lehninger AL. *Principles of Biochemistry*. New York: Worth Publishers; 1982.

Little RC. *Physiology of the Heart and Circulation*. Chicago, Ill: Year Book Medical Publishers; 1977.

Mullins RJ. Management of shock. In: Feliciano DV, Moore EE, Mattox KL, eds. *Trauma*. 3rd ed. Stamford, Conn: Appleton and Lange; 1996.

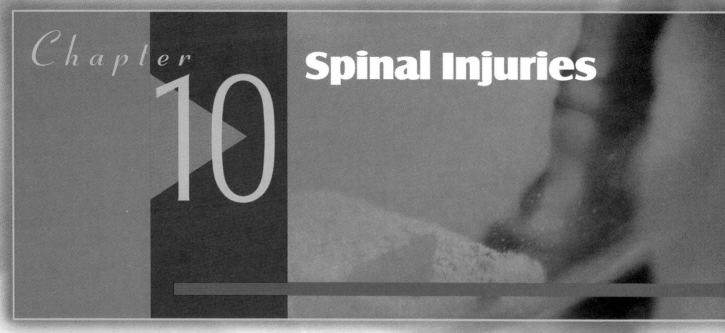

Chapter 10

Spinal Injuries

OBJECTIVES

Upon completion of this chapter, the reader should be able to:

- Describe the anatomy of the vertebrae from the cervical, thoracic, lumbar, sacral, and coccyx regions.
- List the major functions of the spinal cord.
- List the general functions of the ascending and descending tracts.
- List the specific functions of the major ascending tracts.
- List the specific functions of the major descending tracts.
- Identify the components of the reflex arc.
- Describe the function of the reflex arc.
- Identify the location of the spinal nerves.
- Describe the anatomy of a spinal nerve.
- Describe the function of the individual components of a spinal nerve.
- Identify the location and describe the function of the major spinal plexuses.
- Identify the four most common mechanisms of spinal injury.
- Describe the syndromes associated with partial cord lesions.
- Describe the clinical presentation of spinal cord transection.
- Describe the pathophysiology of neurogenic shock.
- Discuss the management of neurogenic shock.
- Discuss the role of anti-inflammatory agents used in the management of patients with suspected spinal cord injuries.

KEY TERMS

Anterior branch	Cauda equina	Dorsal root	Pedicles
Anterior cord syndrome	Central cord syndrome	Incomplete lesion	Pelvic sacral foramina
Ascending tract	Cervical vertebrae	Interneurons	Plexus
Atlas	Coccyx	Intervertebral disks	Poikilothermy
Axial loading	Complete lesion	Lumbar vertebrae	Posterior branch
Axis	Dermatomes	Meningeal branch	Priapism
Brown-Séquard's syndrome	Descending tract	Neurogenic shock	Proprioception

(continues)

(continued)

Reflexes	Spinal cord	Transverse process	Vertebral column
Sacrum	Spinal nerves	Ventral root	Visceral branch
Spinal column	Thoracic vertebrae	Vertebrae	

Superman, the man of steel—able to leap tall buildings in a single bound, able to see with X-ray vision, stronger than 10 men . . . now confined to a wheelchair and paralyzed from the neck down. Christopher Reeve, Superman in the movies, suffered one of the most devastating injuries that can result from trauma: spinal cord injury (SCI). Spinal cord injuries can affect anyone at any age and cause a drastic lifestyle change as well as a financial burden for the victim and family.

Spinal cord injury affects approximately 13,000 Americans per year and costs in excess of $1,250,000 in health care costs per victim per year.[1–3] With increased research and advances in prehospital equipment, education, and training, both the number and the severity of SCI patients have decreased.[4] The key to managing the SCI patient begins with an understanding of the normal anatomy and physiology of the spinal cord and associated structures and continues with pathophysiology and kinematics, as discussed in Chapter 5.

ANATOMY

The axial skeleton consists of bones that form the axis of the body: bones of the skull, auditory ossicles, hyoid bone, vertebral column, and bones that form the thoracic cage. This chapter will concentrate on the structures of the vertebral column. It is essential that the spinal cord be separated from the spinal column for discussion purposes.

The **vertebral column** extends from the base of the skull to the pelvis (Figure 10-1). It consists of 33 vertebrae separated by tough cartilaginous disks called

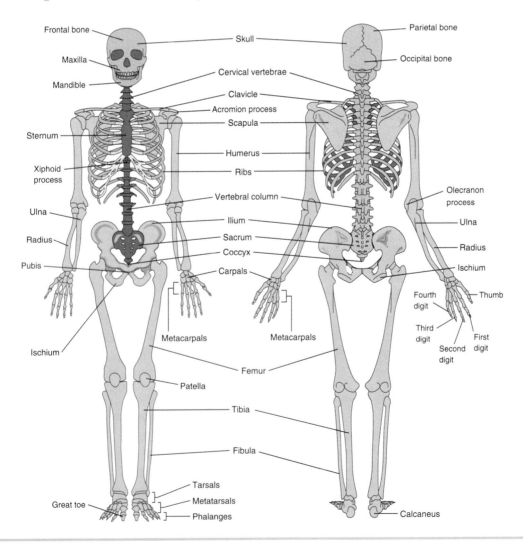

FIGURE 10-1 The vertebral column extends from the base of the skull to the pelvis.

intervertebral **disks**. The vertebrae are connected to each other by ligaments. The vertebral column supports the head and the trunk; however, its flexibility allows for bending forward, backward, and laterally. It protects the spinal cord which passes through the vertebral canal formed by openings in the vertebrae.

The **spinal column** is divided into five regions: cervical, thoracic, lumbar, sacral, and coccygeal. There are four curvatures in the spinal column, named for the regions in which the curves occur: The thoracic and pelvic curvatures are concave anteriorly and are the primary curves; the cervical and lumbar curves are convex anteriorly and are referred to as secondary curves. The cervical curve develops when a baby begins to hold up its head; the lumbar curve develops when the child begins to stand (Figure 10-2).

VERTEBRAE

All **vertebrae** have some common characteristics as well as unique characteristics. A typical vertebra has a body that forms the thick anterior portion of the bone. Superior and inferior vertebrae are attached by ligaments: anterior ligaments attach anterior portions of the bodies and posterior ligaments attach posterior portions of the bodies (Figure 10-3).

Pedicles arise from the posterior portion of the body and form the sides of the vertebral foramen. The spinous process is formed by two fused plates that originate from the pedicles. The spinal cord passes through the vertebral foramen, which is created by the pedicles, laminae, and spinous process (Figure 10-4).

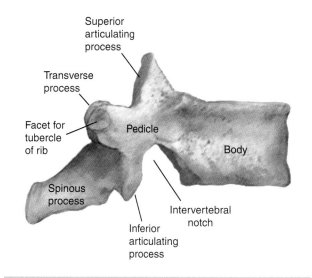

FIGURE 10-3 Lateral view of vertebra.

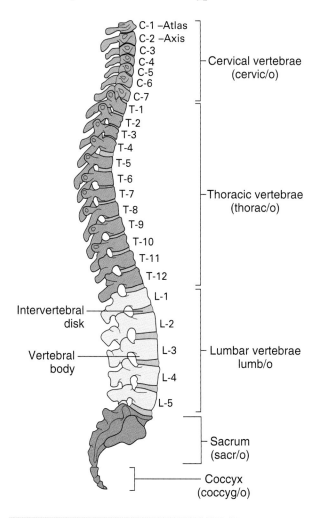

FIGURE 10-2 The spinal column is divided into five regions: cervical, thoracic, lumbar, sacral, and coccyx.

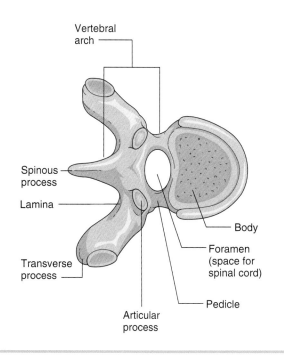

FIGURE 10-4 Superior view of vertebra.

The **transverse process** originates between the pedicle and the laminae and extends laterally and posteriorly. Muscles and ligaments attach to the dorsal spinous process and the transverse processes. Vertebrae are joined to one another by articulating processes. Superior and inferior articulating arches are found on the vertebral arch (Figure 10-5).

Intervertebral foramina are created by notches found on the lower surfaces of the pedicles. These openings provide a pathway for the spinal nerves that proceed between conjoining vertebrae and connect to the spinal cord.

The cervical region is comprised of seven vertebrae and makes up the axis of the neck. The bones in this region are more dense than any other region of the vertebral column. The spinous processes of the second through fifth cervical vertebrae are forked, allowing for attachments for various muscles. Also, the spinous process of the seventh vertebra is much longer than any of the other vertebrae and can be felt through the skin. This is called the vertebra prominens and can be used as a landmark for locating other vertebral parts.

Two **cervical vertebrae** are of special interest (Figure 10-6). They are the only vertebrae that are named: the **atlas** (C-1) and **axis** (C-2). The atlas supports and balances the head. It has the appearance of a bony ring with two transverse processes and has virtually no body. There are two kidney-shaped facets on the superior surface articulating with the occipital condyles of the skull. The axis (C-2) has a rounded toothlike projection referred to as a dens or odontoid

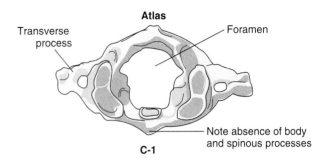

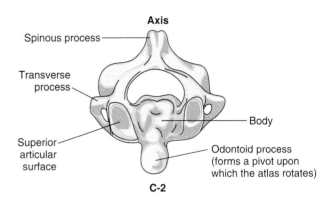

FIGURE 10-6 The atlas (C-1) and axis (C-2) cervical vertebrae.

process on its body. This projection points upward into the ring of the atlas. When the head turns from side to side, the atlas pivots around the dens.

The 12 **thoracic vertebrae** are considerably larger than those found in the cervical region because they bear substantial weight. All of the vertebrae in this region have a long and pointed spinous process. The spinous processes slope downward and have facets on each side of the body, which articulate with a rib. Progressing inferiorly from the third thoracic vertebra (T-3), the size of each body increases, allowing for the increased stress they bear (Figure 10-7).

The five **lumbar vertebrae** support more weight than the superior vertebrae and have much larger and stronger bodies. The transverse processes of the lumbar region project posteriorly at sharp angles; the spinous processes are almost horizontal (Figure 10-8).

At the base of the vertebral column is a triangular shaped structure called the **sacrum**. The sacrum consists of five vertebrae, which are fused gradually between ages 18 and 30. The spinous processes of these fused bones form a ridge of tubercles, the median sacral crest. Nerves and blood vessels pass through openings called the dorsal sacral foramina, found on the lateral aspect of the tubercles. The sacrum is located between the coxal bones of the pelvis and is attached to them by fibrocartilage of the sacroiliac joints (Figure 10-9). The body's weight is

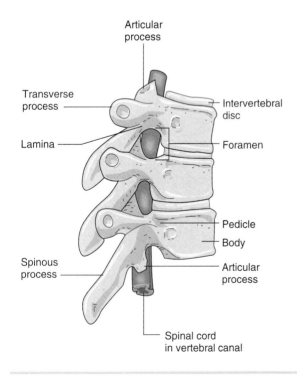

FIGURE 10-5 Vertebrae are joined by articulating processes.

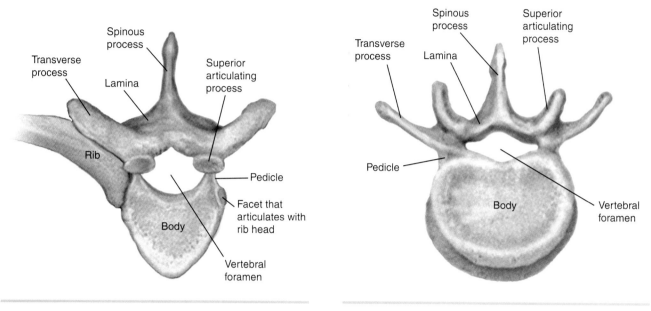

FIGURE 10-7 Superior view of thoracic vertebra.

FIGURE 10-8 Superior view of lumbar vertebra.

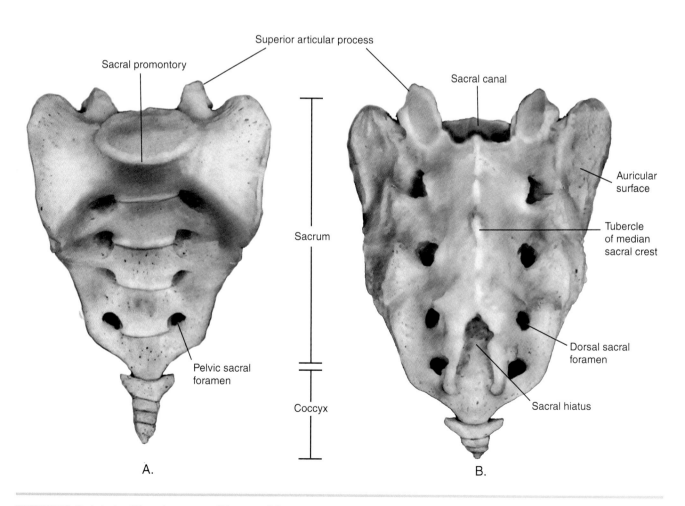

FIGURE 10-9 Anterior (A) and posterior (B) view of the sacrum and coccyx.

transmitted to the legs at these joints. The sacrum also forms the posterior wall of the pelvic cavity.

The sacral canal, formed by the vertebral foramina of the sacral vertebrae, continues through the sacrum to an opening called the sacral hiatus. The foramina exist because the laminae of the last sacral vertebra are not fused. The **pelvic sacral foramina**, found on the ventral surface of the sacrum, provide pathways for nerves and blood vessels.

The **coccyx** is the lowest part of the vertebral column. It is usually comprised of four vertebrae, fused by age 25, and attaches to the sacral hiatus by ligaments.

SPINAL CORD

The **spinal cord**, which is found within the spinal cavity, extends from the foramen magnum to the lower border of the first lumbar vertebra. The cord is approximately 17–18 inches long in the average human body (Figure 10-10).

An oval-shaped cylinder, the spinal cord tapers slightly downward and has two bulges, one in the cervical region and one in the lumbar region. There are two deep grooves—the anterior median fissure and the posterior sulcus—that almost divide the cord in two symmetrical halves (Figure 10-11). A cross-sectional view reveals that the cord consists of gray and white matter. The gray matter is surrounded by the white matter and has a pattern that resembles a butterfly or the letter H. The upper portion of the gray matter is called the posterior horns while the lower portion is referred to as the anterior horns. The gray matter between the posterior and anterior horns is called the lateral horn. Motor fibers pass out through spinal nerves to the skeletal muscles and originate from large neuronal cell bodies in the anterior horn (anterior horn cells).

The horizontal bar of gray matter, the portion between the two vertical lines of the H, is called the gray commissure and connects the right and left sides. The gray commissure surrounds the central canal, which is uninterrupted from the ventricles of the brain and contains cerebrospinal fluid. The white matter of the spinal cord is divided into three regions by the gray matter. These regions are the anterior, lateral, and posterior

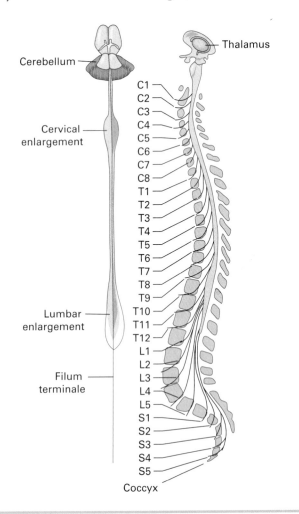

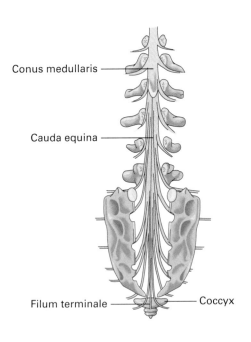

FIGURE 10-10 The spinal cord begins at the level of the foramen magnum and is approximately 17–18 inches in length.

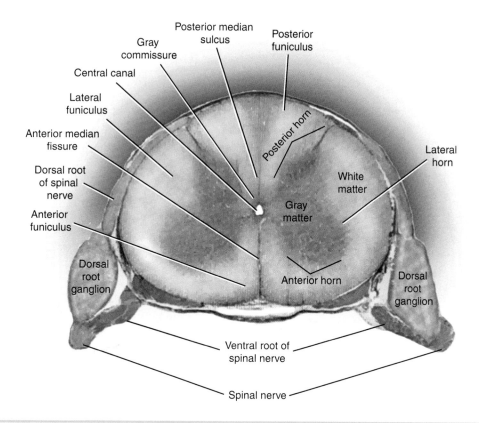

Posterior median sulcus
Gray commissure
Posterior funiculus
Central canal
Posterior horn
Lateral funiculus
Lateral horn
Anterior median fissure
White matter
Dorsal root of spinal nerve
Gray matter
Anterior funiculus
Dorsal root ganglion
Anterior horn
Dorsal root ganglion
Ventral root of spinal nerve
Spinal nerve

FIGURE 10-11 Cross section of the spinal cord.

funiculi. These regions consist of longitudinal bundles of myelinated nerve fibers that make up the major nerve pathways called nerve tracts (Figure 10-12).

PHYSIOLOGY

There are two major functions of the spinal cord: conduction of nerve impulses and spinal reflexes. The two-way communication pathway between the brain and body consists of the spinal cord and the spinal nerves. **Ascending tracts** conduct sensory information to the brain (Figure 10-13). **Descending tracts** conduct motor impulses to motor neurons that extend to the muscles and glands (Figure 10-14).

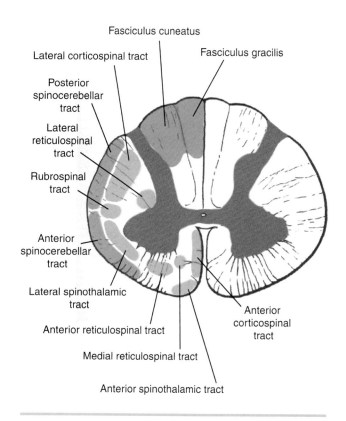

Fasciculus cuneatus
Lateral corticospinal tract
Fasciculus gracilis
Posterior spinocerebellar tract
Lateral reticulospinal tract
Rubrospinal tract
Anterior spinocerebellar tract
Lateral spinothalamic tract
Anterior corticospinal tract
Anterior reticulospinal tract
Medial reticulospinal tract
Anterior spinothalamic tract

FIGURE 10-12 Major ascending and descending nerve tracts of the spinal cord.

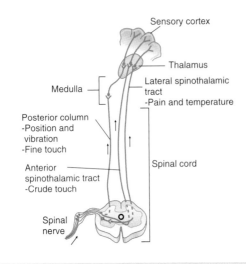

FIGURE 10-13 Ascending tracts of the spinal cord.

Nerve fibers within these tracts are called axons. For the most part, all axons in a given tract arise from neuron cell bodies located in the same part of the nervous system and end together in another part. Names used to identify tracts reflect the common origins and termination. For example, the spinothalamic tract begins in the spinal cord and carries impulses associated with the sensations of pain and touch to the thalamus gland in the brain.

ASCENDING TRACTS

Because there are a multitude of ascending tracts of the spinal cord, discussion will be limited to the three major ascending tracts of the spinal cord:

1. *Fasciculus gracilis* and *fasciculus cuneatus.* These fibers transmit sensory impulses from the skin, muscles, tendons, and joints to the brain, where they are recognized as sensations of touch, pressure, and movement. These tracts are located in the posterior funiculi of the spinal cord. As they ascend, they cross over in the medulla oblongata from one side to the other. Because of this crossover, impulses originating from the left side of the body reach the right side of the brain.

2. *Spinothalamic tracts.* These tracts are located in the lateral and anterior funiculi. Impulses from various regions of the body are transmitted to the brain via the lateral tracts and are recognized as sensations of pain and temperature. The anterior tracts carry sensations interpreted as touch and pressure. These tracts cross over in the medulla as well.

3. *Spinocerebellar tracts.* Located near the surface in the lateral funiculi of the spinal cord, the fibers of the posterior tract are uncrossed, while fibers of the anterior tract cross in the medulla.

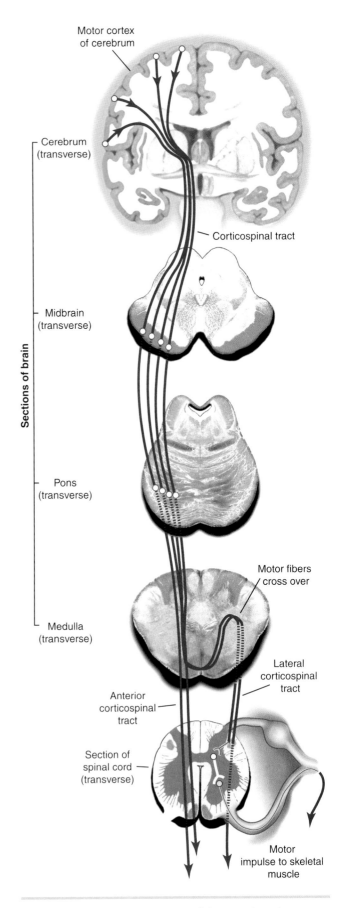

FIGURE 10-14 Descending tracts of the spinal cord.

Impulses originate in the lower limbs and the trunk and travel to the cerebellum. These impulses aid in the coordination of muscular movement.

DESCENDING TRACTS

As with ascending tracts, there are many descending tracts. Discussion will be limited to the major descending tracts:

1. *Corticospinal tracts.* Also referred to as pyramidal tracts, after the pyramid-shaped regions in the medulla through which they pass, these tracts assist in the control of voluntary movements. The fibers are found in the lateral and anterior funiculi. The majority of the lateral tracts cross over in the medulla. The anterior tract fibers descend uncrossed. Both the anterior and posterior tracts transmit motor impulses from the brain to the spinal nerves, which are then conducted to the skeletal muscles.

2. *Reticulospinal tracts.* These tracts are responsible for the control of muscular tone and sweat gland activity. The anterior and medial reticulospinal tracts, located in the anterior funiculi, descend uncrossed. Some of the fibers of lateral reticulospinal tracts, found in the lateral funiculi, cross over in the medulla.

3. *Rubrospinal tracts.* These fibers cross over in the brain and pass through the lateral funiculi. Motor

impulses originate in the brain and are passed to the skeletal muscles. These impulses help to coordinate muscles and control posture.

Table 10-1 summarizes the location and function of the major ascending and descending tracts.

Of its many communication functions, the spinal cord is responsible for many **reflexes**. A reflex, or a response to a stimulus, results from an impulse conducted over a reflex arc. Reflex center refers to the center of a reflex arc, the place in the arc where incoming sensory information becomes outgoing motor impulses. The nuclei in spinal cord gray matter act as reflex centers for all spinal reflexes. These centers switch impulses from afferent neurons to efferent neurons. Reflex centers of two-neuron arcs are synapses between sensory and motor neurons. Reflex centers of all other arcs are interneuron interceded amid sensory and motor neurons (Figure 10-15).

SPINAL NERVES

Thirty-one pairs of **spinal nerves** arise from the spinal cord (Figure 10-16). Spinal nerves are numbered according to the level at which they emerge from the spinal cavity. There are 8 cervical, 12 thoracic, 5 lumbar, 5 sacral, and 1 coccygeal pairs of spinal nerves. The first cervical pair arises from the cord in the space above the first cervical vertebra, between the occipital bone and C-1. The remaining cervical and all thoracic spinal nerves emerge horizontally through the intervertebral foramina of their respective vertebrae.

Table 10-1
Major Nerve Tracts of the Spinal Cord

Ascending Tracts	Location	Function
Fasciculus gracilis Fasciculus cuneatus	Posterior funiculi	Conduct sensory impulses of touch, pressure, and body movement from skin, muscles, tendons, and joints to the brain
Spinothalamic	Lateral and anterior funiculi	Conduct sensory impulses of pain, temperature, touch, and pressure from various regions of the body
Spinocerebellar	Lateral funiculi	Conduct sensory impulses for coordination of muscle movements from muscles of the lower limbs and trunk to the cerebellum
Descending Tracts		
Corticospinal	Lateral and anterior funiculi	Conduct motor impulses of voluntary movement from the brain to various skeletal muscles
Reticulospinal	Lateral and anterior funiculi	Conduct motor impulses to maintain muscle tone and control sweat glands from the brain
Rubrospinal	Lateral funiculi	Conduct motor impulses responsible for muscular coordination and maintenance of posture from the brain

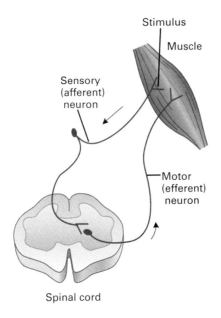

FIGURE 10-15 Reflex arc.

Spinal nerves arising from the superior portion of the spinal cord exit outward almost horizontally; spinal nerves originating from the inferior portion of the spinal cord condescend at sharp angles. This orchestration is a result of the growth process. In early years, the spinal cord extends the length of the spinal column; however, with age, the column grows faster than the cord. Because of this, the spinal cord of an adult ends at the level between the first and second lumbar vertebrae; therefore, the lumbar, sacral, and coccygeal nerves descend to their exits beyond the end of the cord. The **cauda equina**, or horse's tail, is formed by these descending nerves.

The spinal nerves emanate from the cord by two short branches referred to as roots. The posterior, or sensory, or **dorsal root** is identified by an enlargement called the dorsal root ganglion. The dorsal root is responsible for sensory information (Figure 10-17). The dorsal root ganglion contains cell bodies of the sensory neurons that conduct impulses inward from peripheral body parts. Axons of these neurons attenuate through the dorsal root and into the spinal cord. It is here that these neurons form synapses with dendrites of other neurons. **Dermatomes** are areas of the skin in which sensory nerve fibers of a particular spinal nerve innervate. These are highly organized but vary in size and shape. Knowledge of the dermatomes is useful in localizing the site(s) of injury to the spinal cord (Figure 10-18). The anterior, or motor, or **ventral root** of the spinal nerves consists of axons from motor neurons of which the cell bodies are located in the gray matter of the spinal cord. The ventral root is responsible for motor function (Figure 10-19).

A spinal nerve is comprised of a dorsal root and a ventral root (Figure 10-20). The spinal nerve extends outward from the vertebral canal through an intervertebral foramen. The spinal nerve branches just beyond its respective foramen. Of these branches, a small portion called the **meningeal branch** reenters the vertebral canal through the intervertebral foramen to supply the meninges and blood vessels of the cord, including the intervertebral ligaments and the vertebrae. The posterior ramus, or **posterior branch**, of each spinal nerve innervates the muscles and skin of the back. The **anterior branch**, which is the main portion of the spinal nerve, proceeds forward to supply the front and sides of the trunk and limbs. Spinal nerves of the thoracic and lumbar region have an additional branch. The fourth branch, referred to as the **visceral branch**, of the thoracic and lumbar region is part of the autonomic nervous system.

SPINAL PLEXUSES

Anterior branches of the spinal nerves, with the exception of the thoracic region, combine to form complex networks called **plexuses**, in lieu of continuing directly to the peripheral body parts (Figure 10-21). The fibers in plexuses are of various spinal nerves that are sorted and recombined, so fibers associated with a particular body part reach it in the same nerve, although the fibers embark from different spinal nerves.

Formed by the anterior branches of the first four cervical nerves, the cervical plexuses are found deep on either side of the neck. Fibers from these plexuses supply the muscles and skin of the neck. Nerve fibers from the third, fourth, and fifth cervical nerves pass into the right and left phrenic nerves; phrenic nerves conduct motor impulses to the muscle fibers of the diaphragm.

The brachial plexuses are formed by the last four cervical nerves and the first thoracic nerve. These fibers can be found deep within the shoulders between the neck and the axillae.

The lumbosacral plexuses are formed by the last thoracic nerve and the lumbar, sacral, and coccygeal nerves. Extending from the lumbar region and into the pelvic cavity, these nerve fibers give rise to a number of motor and sensory fibers associated with the lower abdominal wall, external genitalia, buttocks, thighs, legs, and feet.

Anterior branches of the thoracic spinal nerves do not enter a plexus. However, they travel into the intercostal spaces and become the intercostal nerves. Motor impulses to the intercostal muscles and upper abdominal wall are carried by these nerves. Sensory impulses from the skin of the thorax and abdomen are received by these nerves as well. Table 10-2 summarizes the spinal plexuses.

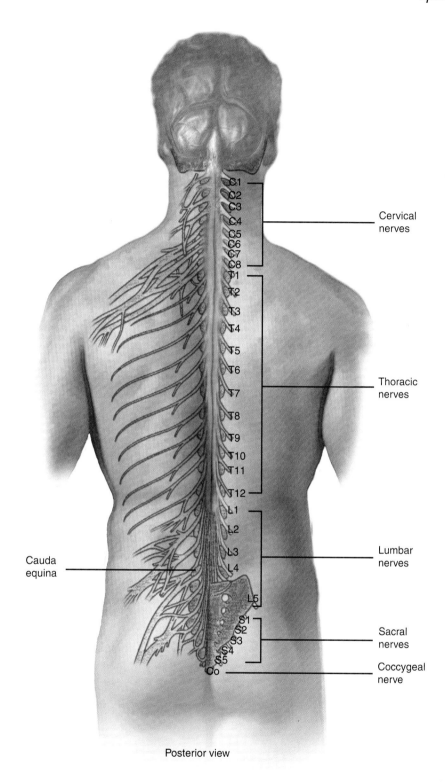

Cervical
nerves

Thoracic
nerves

Lumbar
nerves

Cauda
equina

Sacral
nerves

Coccygeal
nerve

Posterior view

FIGURE 10-16 Thirty-one pairs of spinal nerves arise from the spinal cord.

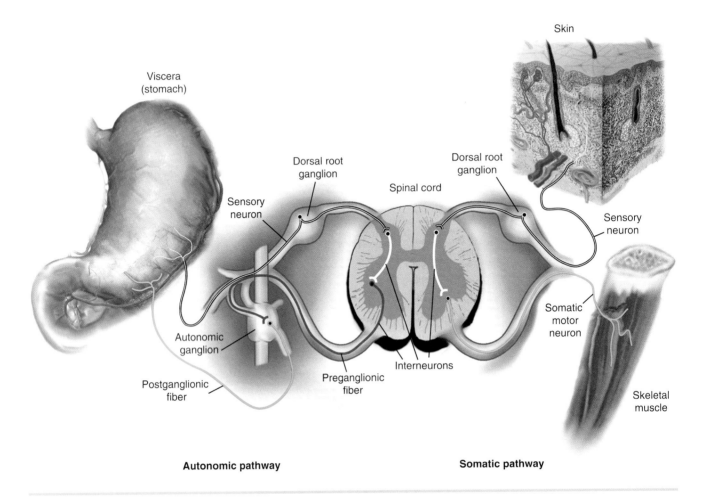

Skin

Viscera
(stomach)

Dorsal root
ganglion

Dorsal root
ganglion

Spinal cord

Sensory
neuron

Sensory
neuron

Autonomic
ganglion

Somatic
motor
neuron

Postganglionic
fiber

Preganglionic
fiber

Interneurons

Skeletal
muscle

Autonomic pathway

Somatic pathway

FIGURE 10-17 Spinal nerves emerge from the cord via the ventral and dorsal roots: (A) autonomic pathway; (B) somatic pathway.

MECHANISM OF INJURY

The spinal column, like any other joint in the body, has a certain range of motion. When stressed beyond this range, injury can occur. Injuries can include damage to the ligaments, bone, intervertebral disk, and/or spinal cord. The mechanism of injury (MOI) plays an important role in patient assessment and determining treatment options. The four most common MOIs are axial loading; extremes of flexion, hyperextension, or hyperrotation; excessive lateral bending; and distraction.

AXIAL LOADING

Axial loading, or spinal compression, occurs when forces are transmitted directly through the spinal column. This causes compression of the vertebrae and can result in the narrowing of the intervertebral spaces, shifting of interveterbral disks, or fractures to a vertebral body or posterior process. Due to the forces applied, injuries of this type can cause encroachment on nerve roots or blood vessels or result in partial or total cord lesion. These forces are generated when a blow is received directly to the top or bottom of the spinal column. Examples include shallow-water diving injuries, diving head first from great heights, or "up-and-over" pathway windshield strikes (see Chapter 5). This can also occur during falls if the patient lands directly on their feet or buttocks. The patient may exhibit signs and symptoms of paralysis, numbness, tingling, or pain as a result of nerve compression or partial cord lesion. As with all trauma-related injuries, the extent of injury is in direct correlation to the force of the blow. Figure 10-22 is an example of a spinal compression injury.

FLEXION, HYPEREXTENSION, OR HYPERROTATION

Flexion, hyperextension, or hyperrotation injuries often involve the ligaments and surrounding musculature of the spinal column. Fractures and interveterbral disk displacement may also be present. This type of injury can be the result of a subluxation or rotation of the vertebrae, dislodging or rupturing the intervertebral disk, swelling of the soft tissues around the column, or

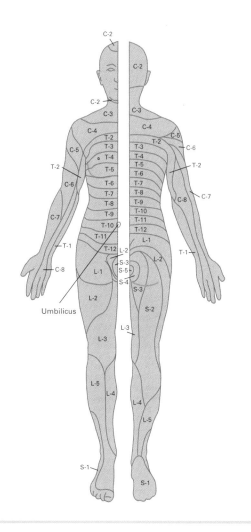

FIGURE 10-18 Dermatomes of the anterior and posterior surfaces.

hemorrhage of the vessels inside the cord. Displaced bone or intervertebral disk that encroaches into the spinal canal can result in complete or incomplete spinal cord lesions, narrowing of the intervertebral spaces and pinching of the nerve roots, or reduction of blood supply to the cord or can lead to development of central cord syndrome.

Flexion, hyperextension, or hyperrotation injuries most often result from rapid deceleration or acceleration mechanisms found in motor vehicle crashes (MVCs). Figure 10-23 illustrates this type of MOI. The spine is often subjected to an abrupt forward motion as the vehicle comes to a sudden stop. The body is then propelled back toward or past its original position due to equal and opposite forces. The type of restraint device worn by the patient must also be considered. Persons wearing the shoulder harness and lap belt combination may undergo hyperextension or rotation, while the patient wearing only a lap belt can suffer injuries to both lumbar and cervical regions of the spine.

Another indicator the patient has sustained flexion, hyperextension, or hyperrotation injuries is trauma to the midface region. Blows to the midfacial region produce sudden hyperextension of the cervical spine followed by rotation. This is a typical deceleration pattern. The hyperextension, combined with the weight of the head, can cause significant cervical injury.

INTERNET ACTIVITIES

Visit the trauma Web site sponsored by the British Medical Society and the Australian Medical Society at http://www.trauma.org/resus/moulage four/Dcspine.html. Work through this scenario for treating a patient with a spinal cord injury.

LATERAL BENDING

Lateral injuries require less motion than flexion or extension; this is due to the limited range of lateral motion of the spinal column. Cervical and thoracic injuries resulting from this mechanism include fractures and soft tissue edema. The body mechanics involved in lateral injuries first moves the body sideways, leaving the upper torso and head to follow. This movement results in damage to the ligaments and muscles as well as the other supporting structures of the head. Mechanisms resulting in these types of injuries include MVCs with side impacts, pedestrians struck by motor vehicles, and injuries from contact sports. Figure 10-24 illustrates this MOI.

INTERNET ACTIVITIES

Visit the trauma Web site sponsored by the British Medical Society and the Australian Medical Society at http://www.trauma.org/spine/lateral cspine.html. This tutorial will guide you through the process of evaluating a lateral cervical spine film.

DISTRACTION

Distraction results when the head is suddenly stopped and the body continues to move away. This causes stretching or shearing of cervical region ligaments. This motion results in soft tissue swelling, laceration or tearing of ligaments, fractures of the vertebral processes, and severing of the spinal cord. Common events resulting in the distraction injury pattern are intentional or unintentional hangings. In the vast majority of these incidents, the weight of the individual causes a fracture

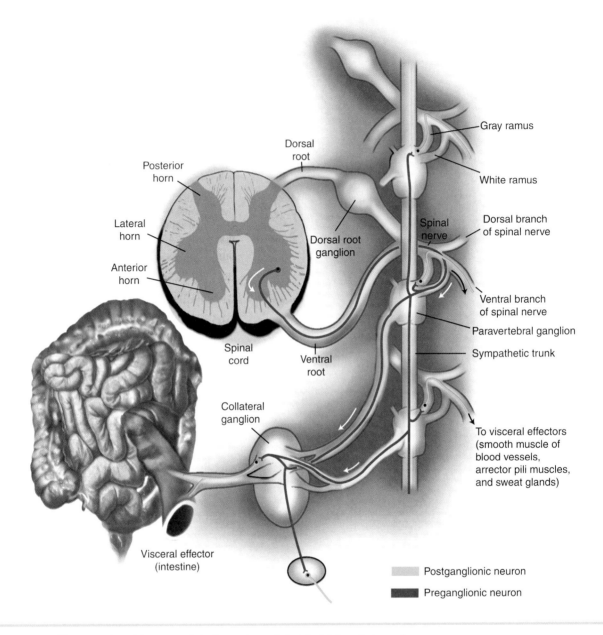

FIGURE 10-19 The ventral root is responsible for motor activity (skeletal and visceral).

of C-2, creating an unstable cervical spine. This is often referred to as a "hangman's fracture." Patients surviving this type of injury with some intact function must be handled carefully; failure to do so will result in further injury or complete paralysis.

The majority of the mechanisms associated with detrimental spinal cord injuries are high-speed MVCs, injuries above the level of the clavicles, or falls from distances greater than three times the patient's height.[2,5] Patients suffering ground-level falls or falls from a standing height rarely suffer spinal injury. However, the chronically ill or the elderly should receive proper evaluation and management based on

the possibility of degeneration or osteoporotic changes. These changes place the patient at high risk for spinal injury from relatively insignificant trauma.

Anytime a patient presents with antegrade amnesia, the paramedic must maintain a high index of suspicion for an MOI capable of producing spinal cord injuries. Any patient who has lost consciousness or admits to a loss of consciousness combined with alcohol or drug use should be suspected of having a spinal cord injury when a mechanism of spinal cord injury is present.

The MOI is a fundamental instrument, in conjunction with signs and symptoms, in the evaluation of any patient. The MOI can help predict injuries and

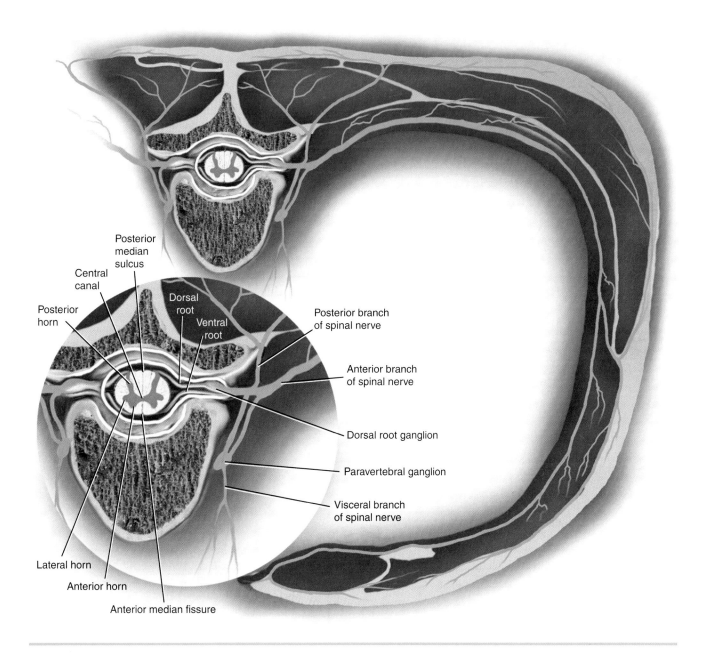

Posterior
median
sulcus

Central
canal

Dorsal
root

Ventral
root

Posterior
horn

Posterior branch
of spinal nerve

Anterior branch
of spinal nerve

Dorsal root ganglion

Paravertebral ganglion

Visceral branch
of spinal nerve

Lateral horn

Anterior horn

Anterior median fissure

FIGURE 10-20 Branches of a spinal nerve.

assist with management options. Each patient responds to traumatic injuries differently. The possibility of spinal cord injury can never be ruled out based solely on the MOI or the lack of symptoms on initial assessment.

SPECIFIC INJURIES

Lesions to the spinal cord are referred to as complete or incomplete. **Complete lesions** fully transect the spinal cord and are often associated with spinal fractures or dislocations. **Incomplete lesions** involve only a portion of the spinal cord and may actually leave the spinal cord intact. The paramedic should be familiar with the signs and symptoms of these spinal injuries.

As a review, the central core of gray matter is surrounded by a myelin sheath. This collection of nerve cells is an extension of the gray matter found within the cranial vault, coupling motor and sensory impulses with the brain. Motor or efferent neurons originate in the anterior portion of the gray matter, and sensory or afferent neurons originate in the posterior portion of the gray matter. The **interneurons** in the gray matter allow for connection of efferent and afferent impulses creating the reflex arc. Anterior and posterior positioning of neuron pairs makes it possible to injure one type of neuron without affecting the other. This results in an incomplete or partial cord lesion. There are three types of syndromes in which

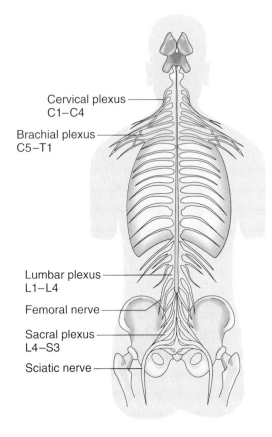

Cervical plexus
C1–C4

Brachial plexus
C5–T1

Lumbar plexus
L1–L4

Femoral nerve

Sacral plexus
L4–S3

Sciatic nerve

Cervical plexus
Nerve supply to muscles of neck and shoulder
Includes phrenic nerve which stimulates the
diaphragm

Brachial Plexus
Includes Axillary, Radial, Median, Musculocutaneous,
Ulnar

Lumbar Plexus
Includes Femoral, Obturator

Sacral Plexus
Includes Sciatic (largest nerve in the body),
Common Peroneal, Tibial

FIGURE 10-21 Spinal plexuses.

this occurs: Brown-Séquard's syndrome, anterior cord syndrome, and central cord syndrome.

COMPLETE CORD LESIONS

Complete lesions are often associated with spinal fractures or dislocations. To prevent a partial lesion from becoming a complete lesion, the paramedic gives particular attention to the MOI. Patients suffering a complete lesion will generally present with total absence of pain, pressure, and point sensation and complete motor paralysis below the level of injury. Depending on the level of involvement, patients may also suffer from autonomic nervous system dysfunction. Autonomic nervous system dysfunction can be identified by the following signs: bradycardia from loss of sympathetic autonomic activity; hypotension from loss of vascular tone and peripheral vascular resistance, **priapism** (sustained erection of the penis), decreased sweating and shivering below the level of injury, **poikilo-thermy** (body temperature assumes that of the environment), and incontinence of bowel and bladder. The inability of the autonomic nervous system to respond to hypotension will often result in neurogenic shock.

PARTIAL CORD LESIONS

Brown-Séquard's syndrome is a rarely occurring partial cord lesion that involves only half of the spinal cord. This syndrome most often results from penetrating trauma to the spine or from bony fragments or intervertebral intrusion into the spinal canal. Patients will present with paralysis or paresis and loss of **proprioception** (sense of position) on the side of injury and a loss of pain and temperature sensation on the opposite side.

Pressure on the anterior portion of the spinal cord or damage to the main anterior artery from either a bone fragment or a ruptured intervertebral disk results in **anterior cord syndrome**. This syndrome is typically the result of hyperflexion injuries. Patients suffering from anterior cord syndrome will be paralyzed below the level of the lesion and exhibit decreased pain response and difficulty regulating temperature below the level of the lesion. Because only the anterior portion of the cord is affected, response to light touch and proprioception is not affected.

Central cord syndrome is a direct result of contusion within the spinal cord. This type of injury often occurs as a result of hyperextension or flexion mechanisms. Rapid flexion or extension can damage

Table 10-2
Spinal Plexuses and Their Innervation

Number of Spinal Nerves in Each Plexus		Spinal Nerve Branched from Plexuses	Anatomical Regions Innervated
Cervical nerves 1–4	Cervical Plexuses Formed from Anterior Rami	Lesser occipital, greater auricular, cutaneous nerve of neck, anterior supraclavicular, middle supra-clavicular, posterior supraclavicular, branches to numerous neck muscles	Sensory to back of head, front of neck, and upper part of shoulder; motor to numerous neck muscles
Cervical 5–8 Thoracic 1	Brachial Plexuses Formed from Anterior Rami	Phrenic (branches from cervical nerves before formation of plexuses; most fibers from fourth cervical nerve)	Diaphragm
		Suprascapular and dorsoscapular	Superficial muscles* of scapula
		Thoracic nerves, medial and lateral branches	Pectoralis major and minor
		Long thoracic nerve	Serratus anterior
		Thoracodorsal	Latissimus dorsi
		Subscapular	Subscapular and teres major
		Axillary (circumflex)	Deltoid and teres minor and skin over deltoid
		Musculocutaneous	Muscles of front of arm and skin on outer side of forearm
Lumbar 1–5, sacral 1–5, coccygeal 1	Lumbosacral Plexuses formed from Anterior Rami	Iliohypogastric, Ilioinguinal (often fused)	Sensory to anterior abdominal wall; sensory to anterior wall and external genitalia; motor to muscles of abdominal wall
		Genitofemoral	Sensory to skin of external genitalia and inguinal region
		Lateral cutaneous of thigh	Sensory to outer thigh
		Femoral	Motor to quadriceps, sartorius, and iliacus muscles; sensory to front of thigh and medial side of lower leg (saphenous nerve)
		Tibial (medial popliteal)†	Motor to muscles of calf of leg; sensory to skin of calf of leg and sole of foot
		Common peroneal (lateral popliteal)	Motor to evertors and dorsiflexors of foot; sensory to lateral surface of leg and dorsal surface of foot
		Nerves of hamstring muscles	Motor to muscles of back of thigh
		Gluteal nerves, superior and inferior	Motor to buttock muscles and tensor fasciae latae
		Posterior cutaneous nerve	Sensory to skin of buttocks, posterior surface of thigh and leg
		Pudendal nerve	Motor to perineal muscles; sensory to skin of perineum

*Although nerves to muscles are considered motor, they do contain some sensory fibers that transmit proprioceptive impulses.
†Sensory fibers from the tibial and peroneal nerves unite to form the medial cutaneous (sural) nerve that supplies the calf of the leg and lateral surface of the foot. In the thigh, the tibial and common peroneal nerves are usually enclosed in a single sheath to form the sciatic nerve, the largest nerve in the body, approximately three-quarters of an inch wide. About two-thirds of the way down the posterior part of the thigh, it divides into its components. Branches of the sciatic nerve extend into the hamstring muscles.

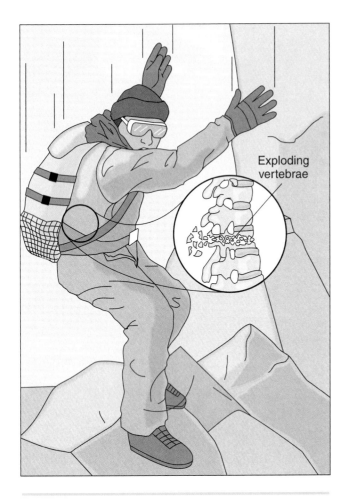

Exploding
vertebrae

FIGURE 10-22 Axial loading.

blood vessels within the spinal column. These small tears and/or weaknesses of the blood vessels lead to hemorrhage, which builds pressure and compromises the function of the cord. As a result of the loss of oxygen and nutrients, the central nervous system can be damaged. Because the corticospinal tract, central portions of the posterior columns, and the lateral spinothalamic tracts contain fibers from the upper extremities, symptoms are more pronounced in the arms. Patients often present with loss of sensation and function in the upper extremities, while sensation and function remain intact in the lower extremities.

Partial cord injuries are not always a result of damage to the spinal column's integrity. Soft tissue swelling or vasculature damage can also cause partial cord syndromes. Musculature or ligamental injuries resulting in edema that impinges on blood vessels supplying the cord with oxygen may also result in partial cord syndromes. Initial neurological exams may be normal, while subsequent exams may show signs of deterioration. This deterioration can be related to changes in blood flow to the area. This progressive change is an important finding and should be relayed to the receiving physician. Table 10-3 summarizes these spinal cord lesions.

Table 10-4 indicates other areas of interest to the prehospital provider. The phrenic nerve, branching from the brachial plexus, controls the diaphragm. A patient with a partial or complete lesion at the level of C-3 or C-4 has little or no respiratory function. With injuries to C-5 to C-8, the patient has intercostal paralysis and paralysis below the shoulder and upper arms; sensory loss includes the arms, hands, chest, abdomen, and lower extremities. Injuries to T-1 to T-6 cause paralysis below the midchest with sensory loss below the midchest. Injuries to T-7 to T-12 affect both motor and sensory function below the waist. Injuries to the lumbar spine at levels L-1 to L-3 produce motor loss in most leg muscles and in the pelvis; sensory dysfunction can be observed in the lower abdomen and legs. Injuries to L-4 and L-5 produce paralysis in the lower legs, ankles, and feet with a sensory loss to parts of the lower legs and feet. Sacral injuries cause paralysis of the bladder, rectum, feet, and ankles. Sensory loss from sacral injuries can be seen in the posterior inner thigh, lateral foot, and perineum.

INTERNET ACTIVITIES

Visit the e-medicine Web site at http://www.emedicine.com. Click on the Emergency Medicine on-line book and select Neurology. Then click on Brown-Séquard syndrome. Review the chapter on the management of this partial cord lesion.

NEUROGENIC SHOCK

Often referred to as spinal shock, **neurogenic shock** is an interruption of nervous system control between the brain and the rest of the body. Injury to the spinal cord results in dilation of the blood vessels served by nerves that branch from the spinal cord below the area of injury. Although the patient may not have lost actual blood volume, the size of the vascular container has increased. The increased size of the container with no actual increase in blood volume results in a decreased stroke volume, and decreased stroke volume results in decreased cardiac output.

Baroreceptors, which note a drop in blood pressure and decreased blood flow, relay this information to the brain by way of the nervous system. Normally the brain responds by sending information to the sympathetic nervous system, causing a release of norepinephrine. Norepinephrine, released from the adrenal medulla, is responsible for vasoconstriction as well as increased chronotropic and inotropic activities of the heart. Because of the interruption in the nervous system, normal sympathetic responses to shock do not occur.

The normal response of the parasympathetic nervous system is to decrease the heart rate and cause

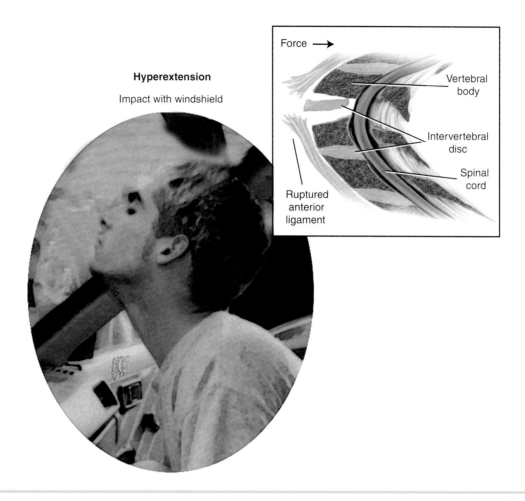

Hyperextension

Impact with windshield

Force →

Vertebral body

Intervertebral disc

Spinal cord

Ruptured anterior ligament

FIGURE 10-23 Hyperextension.

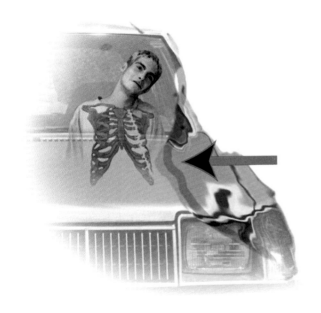

FIGURE 10-24 Lateral bending.

vasodilation. Without the balance of the sympathetic nervous system, the parasympathetic nervous system continues unrestricted. Below the level of spinal cord injury, parasympathetic vasodilation results in blood pooling in the extremities, causing the skin to be warm, pink, and dry. Because of the vasodilation and blood pooling in the extremities, the patient is at risk for developing hypothermia. The patient loses heat via radiation; precautions are taken to keep the patient warm. Due to a loss of peristalsis in the digestive system, paralytic ileus and vomiting may occur, especially if the patient has food in the stomach.

SECONDARY INJURIES

Primary injuries are not the only cause of permanent spinal cord injury. The possibility of secondary injury was first theorized in 1911 by Allen.[6] Allen hypothesized that a noxious agent present in necrotic material caused further damage to the spinal cord and was a "biochemical" agent.[6] Many pathophysiological mechanisms have been thought to explain posttraumatic injuries to spinal cord tissue. Secondary injuries are the

Table 10-3
Summary of Spinal Cord Injuries

Cord Lesion	Area of Cord Injury	Signs and Symptoms	Anatomical Area of Involvement
Complete cord transection		Loss of sensory and motor function below the level of the lesion May result in neurogenic shock Loss of bowel and bladder control	
Anterior cord syndrome		Typically the result of hyperflexion injuries Loss of voluntary and reflex motor activity Loss of pain and temperature sensation Preservation of proprioception, vibratory sense, and ability to sense light pressure	
Central cord syndrome		Typically the result of hyperextension injuries Damage to central spinal tracts which mainly affect the upper extremities Paralysis or paresis in upper extremities with possible preservation of function in lower extremities Paresis often denser distally in upper extremities than proximal Variable sensory impairment and bladder dysfunction	
Brown-Séquard's syndrome		Cord damage limited to one hemisphere. Usually the result of penetrating trauma Ipsilateral motor loss Ipsilateral loss of proprioception Contralateral loss of pain and temperature sensation	

Table 10-4
Signs and Symptoms for Spinal Cord Lesions at Various Levels

Level of Injury	Nerve Root	Motor Loss	Sensory Loss
C-1 to C-4	Cervical	Diaphragm weakness or paralysis; intercostal paralysis; total skeletal muscle paralysis below the neck	Neck and below
C-5 to C-8	Cervical	Intercostal paralysis; paralysis below shoulders and upper arms	Arms and hands, chest, abdomen, and legs
T-1 to T-6	Thoracic	Paralysis below midchest	Below midchest
T-7 to T-12	Thoracic	Paralysis below waist	Below the waist
L-1 to L-3	Lumbar	Paralysis in majority of leg muscles and pelvis	Lower abdomen and legs
L-4 to L-5	Lumbar	Paralysis in lower legs, ankles, and feet	Parts of lower legs and feet
S-1 to S-5	Sacral	Paralysis of bladder and rectum, feet, and ankles	Posterior inner thigh, lateral foot, and perineum

cause of long-term complications that follow primary injuries. There is a biochemical deluge leading to the production and release of chemicals thought to be responsible for secondary injuries.

Following mechanical injury to the spinal cord, the cord undergoes a sequence of pathological changes. These changes include hemorrhage, edema, axonal and neuronal necrosis, and demyelination. The process occurs early after the initial injury; it begins with localized hemorrhage and edema within the microcirculation of the spinal cord. This is followed by a release of amino acids and a large influx of calcium, causing phospholipase enzymatic activity. This phospholipase enzymatic activity results in the production of prostaglandins. A portion of these prostaglandins cause cerebral vasoconstriction, platelet aggregation, and cerebral hypoxemia. This cascade of events leads to lipid peroxidation that causes permanent damage.

INTERNET ACTIVITIES

Visit the National Spinal Cord Injury Association Resource Center Web site's fact sheet on autonomic dysreflexia at http://www.eskimo.com/~jlubin/disabled/nscia/fact17.html. What is the cause of this serious complication of spinal cord injury? How can it be recognized? How is it treated?

INTERNET ACTIVITIES

Visit the trauma Web site sponsored by the British Medical Society and the Australian Medical Society at http://www.trauma.org/spine/index.html. Click on case presentations and read the online article "Vertebral Artery Injuries Associated with Cervical Spine Trauma." You may first have to register with MEDSCAPE to view this article. Registration is free and takes about 2 minutes.

MANAGEMENT AND INTERVENTIONS

The importance of correct spinal immobilization techniques cannot be overemphasized to the prehospital provider and are discussed in Chapter 19. This chapter will discuss the pharmacological interventions in the management of neurogenic shock and anti-inflammatory therapies of the spinal cord.

The management of neurogenic shock begins with "the basics." Spinal immobilization should be followed by airway management. In the unconscious patient with suspected spinal cord injury, the airway should be opened using the trauma jaw thrust. During the initial assessment of the patient, the airway should be maintained, if necessary, with an oropharyngeal airway until advanced life support measures can be taken.

Next assess breathing; it may be necessary to assist ventilations with a bag-valve-mask (BVM) device. This should be accomplished with the head in the in-line neutral position. It is recommended that, if possible, this be accomplished with one provider maintaining cervical stabilization while an additional provider ventilates the patient. Patients requiring assisted ventilations should have supplemental oxygen supplied to the BVM to ensure high oxygen concentrations. Those patients with adequate respiratory function should receive supplemental oxygen with a nonrebreather mask. Patients with spinal cord injuries have hypoxic nervous tissue, and any attempt at improving hypoxia will benefit the SCI patient. Pulse oximetry cannot be relied on to determine the oxygen delivery device used, as it does not accurately reflect oxygenation of nervous tissue.

After life-threatening breathing problems receive appropriate management, circulatory status is evaluated. This begins with the pulse comparison between carotid and radial arteries. Patients with spinal cord injury may exhibit the following circulatory findings: bradycardia; full and regular pulse in the absence of cardiac arrhythmias; warm, pink, dry skin below the lesion; regular to slightly delayed capillary refill; and hypotension (less than 90 mm Hg). Above the level of the lesion patients will have normal physiological responses to this hypotension.

The initial assessment of disability is limited to evaluation of the pupils and reevaluation of the level of responsiveness using the A-V-P-U (alert-verbal-pain-unresponsive) scale. Patients should be exposed and areas that will be covered by pneumatic antishock garments (PASGs) should be examined and evaluated.

Resuscitation of the circulatory system should be accomplished en route to the receiving facility. Due to the controversies surrounding the application and inflation of the PASGs, these devices should only be used on the basis of local protocols. Patients should receive intravenous fluid by large-bore catheters and large-bore trauma tubing. Patients should receive an initial bolus of 250–500 mL of solution and be reevaluated for hemodynamic status. Vasopressors, such as dopamine or dobutamine, may be ordered by medical control. Blood pressure should be maintained between 110 and 120 mm Hg systolic to ensure adequate perfusion of ischemic tissue.

ANTI-INFLAMMATORIES

There is evidence suggesting that large doses of glucocorticoid steroids improve posttraumatic microvascular perfusion.[7–9] Methylprednisolone (solu medrol) is one such steroid. It is a synthetic glucocorticoid thought to limit secondary injury to the spinal cord by preventing lipid peroxidation and limiting the formation of other biochemical mediators (arachidonic acid, prostaglandins, eicosanoids). Thus, blood flow within the spinal cord is maintained, decreasing nerve degeneration and enhancing nerve excitability.

Glucocorticoids such as methylprednisolone have been used since the early 1960s in the management of SCIs. Primary use focuses on the drug's effect for reducing spinal cord edema. Investigators from the Second National Acute Spinal Cord Injury Study (NASCIS-II) used high-dose intravenous methylprednisolone shortly after injury and found that muscle function and sensation were dramatically improved at 6 weeks, 6 months, and 1 year follow-up compared with those patients not receiving methylprednisolone.[8] Major adverse reactions in the NASCIS-II trials included increased wound and urinary tract infections. Other adverse reactions of high-dose therapy included severe arrhythmias and cardiac arrest in patients suffering from multiple sclerosis and concomitant kidney dysfunction, probably due to severe electrolyte shifts. Normal dose side effects include hyperglycemia, hypokalemia, hypocalcemia, hyponatremia, fluid retention, edema throughout the body, hypertension, and psychosis.

The dosage of methylprednisolone can be difficult and should be reviewed for accuracy. Methylprednisolone is supplied as 40-, 125-, 500-, and 1000-mg injections. It is supplied with its own diluent because it is incompatible with most IV solutions. The initial dose of 30 mg/kg can be initiated in the prehospital setting, administered as a direct IV infusion over 15 minutes. This should be followed in 45 minutes by a 5.4-mg/kg/hr infusion for the next 23 hours. This infusion is better prepared in the clinical environment, as special tubing is required.

EMERGING THERAPIES

New pharmacological agents are being studied for use with SCIs. Many are aimed at preventing the secondary injuries of lipid peroxidation. Lazaroids are one such group under investigation. These are a group of nonglucocorticoid agents designed to inhibit lipid peroxidation by binding to iron and removing it from the cascade. Iron is thought to be a catalyst for lipid peroxidation. Lazaroids may also have fewer side effects than glucocorticoids.

Gangliosides such as GM-1 are complex acidic glycolipids present in high concentrations in central nervous system cells. Because these are a major component of cell membranes, studies are currently underway for the possibility of improving outcomes by stimulating growth of nerve cells. A pilot program has suggested favorable outcomes when these agents are administered within 72 hours after injury.[10]

INTERNET ACTIVITIES

Visit the e-medicine Web site at http://www.emedicine.com. Click on the Emergency Medicine on-line book and select Neurology. Then click on spinal cord injuries. Review the chapter on the management of spinal cord injuries.

SUMMARY

Understanding the normal anatomy and physiology of the nervous system will help in the evaluation of abnormal findings. The prehospital provider must evaluate the mechanism of injury, conduct a thorough physical assessment, and obtain an accurate history to properly evaluate the SCI patient. The paramedic should also possess extensive knowledge of the varied signs and symptoms of SCI.

Successful management of SCI requires an index of suspicion, effective immobilization, and prevention of secondary injury. Secondary injury involves a complex cascade of biochemical events. The paramedic can limit the devastating effects of secondary injury through attention to the ABCs, proper oxygenation, and early administration of methylprednisolone.

REVIEW QUESTIONS

1. Which of the following are ascending spinal tracts?
   a. Spinothalamic
   b. Spinocerebellar
   c. Fasciculus gracilis
   d. All of the above

2. Ascending spinal tracts primarily
   a. Conduct motor impulses from the brain to target organs and muscles
   b. Conduct sensory impulses from the body to the brain
   c. Form a portion of the reflex arc
   d. Both b and c

3. The area of the spinal cord where incoming sensory information becomes outgoing motor impulses is called a:
   a. Spinal nerve
   b. Synapse
   c. Reflex arc
   d. Plexus

4. The distal portion of the spinal cord is called the:
   a. Cauda equina
   b. Dorsal root
   c. Distal root
   d. Dermatome

5. The phrenic nerves are formed from fibers originating from the:
   a. Cervical plexus
   b. Thoracic plexus
   c. Brachial plexus
   d. Lumbar plexus

6. Which of the following mechanisms of spinal injury are likely to result from a shallow-water diving injury?
   a. Flexion
   b. Extension
   c. Axial loading
   d. Hyperrotation

7. Which of the following mechanisms of spinal injury are likely to result from an accidental hanging?
   a. Axial loading
   b. Distraction
   c. Flexion
   d. Hyperextension

8. A spinal injury resulting in total absence of pain, pressure, and point sensation and complete motor paralysis below the level of the injury is called:
   a. Anterior cord syndrome
   b. Brown-Séquard's syndrome
   c. Spinal cord transection
   d. Central cord syndrome

9. Loss of autonomic nervous system response due to spinal cord injury is called:
   a. Cord shock
   b. Neurogenic shock
   c. Central nervous system paralysis
   d. Spinal cord concussion

10. Patients who present with paralysis or paresis and loss of proprioception on the side of injury and loss of pain and temperature sensation on the opposite side of spinal cord injury suffer from:
    a. Central cord syndrome
    b. Anterior cord syndrome
    c. Brown-Séquard's syndrome
    d. Spinal cord transection

11. Patients exhibiting paralysis and decreased pain response below the level of the lesion but still responding to light touch and proprioception suffer from:
    a. Central cord syndrome
    b. Anterior cord syndrome
    c. Brown-Séquard's syndrome
    d. Spinal cord transection

12. Patients exhibiting decreased motor and sensory function in the arms while the legs are affected to a lesser extent most likely suffer from:
    a. Central cord syndrome
    b. Anterior cord syndrome
    c. Brown-Séquard's syndrome
    d. Spinal cord transection

13. Loss of function of the diaphragm indicates a spinal cord injury at the level of:
    a. C-2
    b. C-8
    c. T-2
    d. T-6

14. Paralysis and loss of motor function from the nipple line down indicate a cord lesion at the level of:
    a. C-2
    b. C-8
    c. T-4
    d. T-8

15. The lack of tachycardia in the setting of neurogenic shock is due to:
    a. Lack of catecholamine secretion
    b. Loss of nervous control to the heart
    c. Hyperactivation of the parasympathetic system
    d. Pooling of blood in the extremities

16. BVM-assisted ventilation is most likely needed in patients with injury to which of the following levels of cord injury?
    a. T-12
    b. T-4
    c. C-6
    d. C-4

17. Which of the following drugs may be needed in the treatment of spinal cord injury and neurogenic shock?
    a. Dobutamine
    b. Dopamine
    c. Methylprednisolone
    d. All of the above

18. Methylprednisolone is used in the management of what kind of cord injury?
    a. Primary
    b. Secondary
    c. Tertiary
    d. Quaternary

19. The loading dose of methylprednisolone is:
    a. 30 mg/kg over 15 minutes
    b. 30 mg/kg over 23 hours
    c. 5.4 mg/kg over 15 minutes
    d. 5.4 mg/kg/hr over 23 hours

20. Side effects of methylprednisolone include:
    a. Electrolyte imbalance
    b. Edema
    c. Increased wound infections
    d. All of the above

CRITICAL THINKING

- Testing for meningitis involves collecting a sample of cerebrospinal fluid. This is usually done through a procedure known as a lumbar puncture, or spinal tap, in which a needle is inserted into the fourth lumbar intervertebral space. Why do you think this space is chosen above all other possible sites in the spinal column?

- Why should a nasogastric tube be placed in a patient with a spinal cord injury?

- Immediately following a cord transection, there is loss of sensation, motor function, and reflex arc activity. Hours to days later, reflex activity returns. How is this different from a lower motor neuron injury? Why?

REFERENCES

1. Committee on Trauma Research, Commission on Life Sciences, and the Institute of Medicine. *Injury in America: A Continuing Public Health Problem.* Washington DC: National Academy Press; 1985.

2. Rice DP, Mackenzie EJ, Associates. *Cost of Injury in the United States: A Report to Congress.* San Francisco, Ca: Institute for Health and Aging, University of California and Injury Prevention Center, The John Hopkins University; 1989.

3. University of Alabama. *Spinal Cord Facts and Figures,* Birmingham, Ala: University of Alabama; 1986.

4. Meyer PR, ed. *Annual Progress Report of the Midwest Regional Spinal Cord Injury Care System.* Chicago, Ill: Northwestern University–McGaw Medical Center, Northwestern Memorial Hospital, Rehabilitation Institute of Chicago; 1988.

5. Allen AR. Remarks on the histopathological changes in the spinal cord due to impact: an experimental study. *J Ner Ment Dis.* 1914; 41:141.

6. Bresnahan JC, King JS, Martin GF, Yashon D. A neuroanatomical analysis of spinal cord injury in the Rhesus monkey (*Macaca mulatta*). *J Neurol Sci.* 1976; 28:521.

7. Bracken MB, Shepard MJ, Collins WF. A randomized, controlled trial of methylprednisolone or naloxone in the treatment of acute spinal cord injury. Results of the Second National Acute Spinal Cord Injury Study. *N Engl J Med.* 1990; 322:1405.

8. Bracken MB, et al. Methylprednisolone or naloxone treatment after acute spinal cord injury: 1-year follow-up data. *J Neurosurg.* 1992; 76:23.

9. Marwick C. Administering methylprednisolone promptly appears to mitigate cord-injury paralysis. *JAMA.* 1990; 263(16):2150.

10. Geisler FH, Dorsey FC, Coleman WP. Recovery of motor function after spinal cord injury: a randomized placebo-controlled trial with GM-1 ganglioside. *N Engl J Med.* 1991; 324:1829.

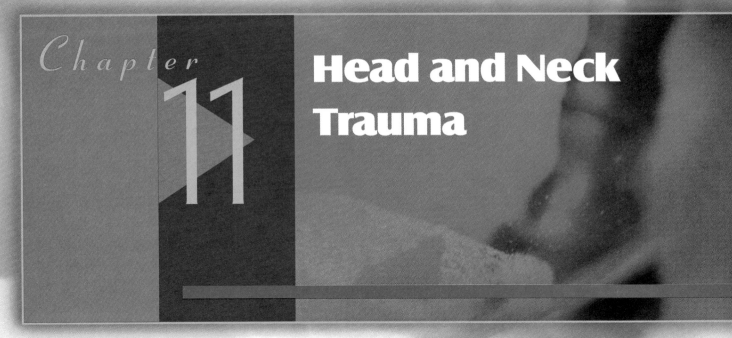

Chapter 11
Head and Neck Trauma

OBJECTIVES

Upon completion of this chapter, the reader should be able to:

- Describe the basic epidemiology of head and neck trauma.
- Describe the concept of primary and secondary brain injury.
- Discuss the role of initial patient management in reducing secondary brain injury.
- Discuss the relevant anatomy and pathophysiology of (a) increased intracranial pressure, (b) loss of consciousness, (c) Cushing's response, and (d) coup/contrecoup injuries.
- Describe the anatomical zones of the neck.
- Describe the major injuries and trauma considerations by zone.
- List and describe the pathology and clinical presentations of the major types of intracranial hematomas.
- Contrast concussion and contusion in terms of pathology, clinical presentation, and outcome.
- Discuss the focused assessment of the patient with head and neck injury.
- Describe the Glasgow Coma Scale and its implications in patient care.
- Describe the airway considerations for the initial management of patients with head and neck injury.
- Briefly describe the major research and experimental treatment issues for (a) hyperventilation, (b) volume replacement, (c) hypothermia, and (d) neuroprotective agents.

KEY TERMS

Anisocoria
Basilar skull fracture
Brain
Brain stem
Central herniation syndrome
Cerebellum
Cerebral laceration
Cerebral perfusion pressure
Cerebrum
Coma

Concussion
Contusion
Coup/contrecoup
Cushing's triad
Deep cervical fascia
Depressed skull fracture
Diffuse axonal injury
Dural sinuses
Epidural hematoma
Epidural space

Falx cerebri
Galea aponeurotica
Glasgow Coma Scale (GCS)
Gray matter
Hypercapnia
Intracerebral hematoma
Linear fracture
Meninges
Monro-Kellie principle
Open skull fracture

(continues)

(continued)

Platysma muscle	Secondary brain injury	Subdural space
Primary brain injury	Skull	Superficial cervical fascia
Reticular activating system	Subarachnoid hemorrhage	Tentorium cerebelli
(RAS)	Subarachnoid space	Uncal herniation
Scalp	Subdural hematoma	White matter

Head and neck injuries are among the most frequently encountered and serious threats to life. The ability to recognize and manage these injuries efficiently and effectively is fundamental to managing trauma. The care of head and neck injuries has become one of the most rapidly evolving areas of trauma care. Major new advances in the understanding of the pathophysiology and treatment of brain injury are on the horizon. This chapter will present the topic of head and neck trauma with emphasis on prehospital management of this complex and challenging problem and will discuss some of the current research areas and the controversies surrounding them.

EPIDEMIOLOGY AND ETIOLOGY

Approximately 200 head injuries occur each year per 100,000 people in the United States.[1,2] Of these, half are significant enough to require medical attention, and the majority can be expected to utilize EMS transport to the medical facility. While the peak incidence of head trauma occurs in males ages 15–30 years, the wide range of potential mechanisms of injury guarantees that head trauma occurs in all age groups and genders.[2,3] Head trauma is most commonly associated with motor vehicle collisions, falls, and penetrating injuries.

Head and neck injuries are a significant component of trauma mortality and morbidity. In a population of 100,000 there are 17–25 deaths from head injury each year.[4] Overall, 50% of all trauma deaths are associated with head injury.[5] In motor vehicle deaths, 60–75% are connected with some component of head injury.[6] Of the 120,000 people with head injuries classified as severe each year, about half will die in the prehospital setting with few treatments that can be rendered after the injury to alter patient outcome.[2] However, if these patients with severe head injury arrive at the emergency department alive, most have or will soon develop airway compromise and increased intracranial pressure (ICP).[2] For these patients, appropriate and aggressive prehospital care can make a significant difference in mortality and long-term morbidity.[7,8]

Less than 10% of all traumatic injuries involve serious injury to the neck.[9] Although neck injuries are relatively infrequent, they carry a high risk for morbidity and mortality. Penetrating neck injuries are the most common and tend to be the most severe form of neck trauma.[9] Most penetrating neck trauma results from gun or knife wounds, with fatality rates of 1–2% for stab wounds, 5–12% for gunshot wounds, and 50% for rifle and shotgun wounds.[9–11] Blunt neck trauma is less common but carries a tremendous risk for airway compromise. Early and aggressive care for neck trauma is critical. It is estimated that up to half of neck trauma deaths may be preventable with appropriate early medical treatment.[9,12]

INTERNET ACTIVITIES

Visit the National Center for Injury Prevention and Control Web site at http://www. cdc.gov/ncipc/dacrrdp/tbi.htm. What are the latest estimates of traumatic brain injury (TBI) incidence and prevalence? What is the cost of treating this injury? What are the risk factors of TBI?

ANATOMY

The **scalp** is composed of five highly vascular, superficial layers: (1) skin, (2) subcutaneous tissue, (3) galea aponeurotica, (4) loose areolar tissue, and (5) periosteum. The scalp's subcutaneous layer contains most of the larger blood vessels and nerves. The **galea aponeurotica** is a tough fibrous sheet spanning the cranium and connecting the frontalis muscles over the forehead with the occipital muscles at the back of the skull. The loose connective tissue between the galea and the periosteum of the skull contains the emissary veins.

The skeleton of the **skull** can be divided into the cranium and the face. The eight bones of the cranium are the frontal, occipital, ethmoid, sphenoid, parietal (two), and temporal (two) (Figure 11-1). In the adult, the cranial bones form a rigid, inflexible, and closed container with a volume of about 1900 cc. This container, or vault, is completely filled by the brain, spinal fluid, and blood. All eight bones contribute to form the uneven, jagged cranial floor. This floor is divided into the anterior, middle, and posterior fossa and contains many openings, or foramina, through which blood vessels and nerves traverse. With the exception of the foramen magnum, most of these openings are small and completely filled by their passing structures. The foramen magnum is the conspicuously large opening in

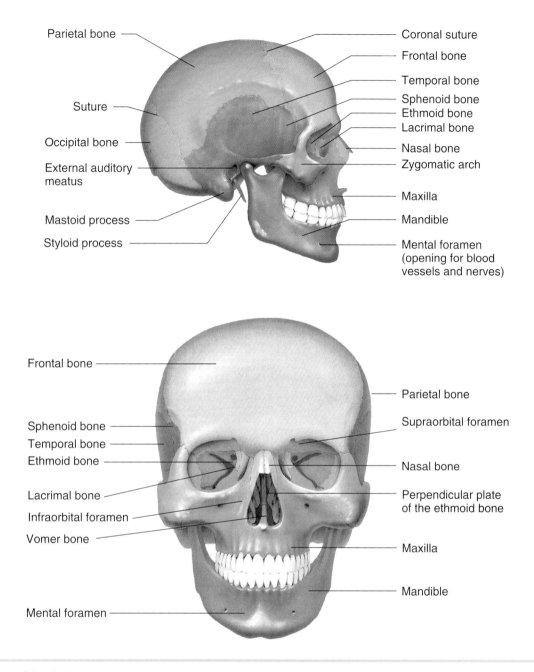

FIGURE 11-1 Bones of the skull.

the occipital bone in the posterior fossa and functions as the passageway for the spinal cord, vertebral vessels, and associated structures.

The **meninges** are the connective tissue elements that cover the external surface of the brain and are composed of three layers: (1) dura mater , (2) pia mater, and (3) arachnoid mater (Figure 11-2). The dura mater is the outermost layer and is relatively thick, tough, and fibrous. Although the dura is tightly adhered to the inside of the skull, a potential space exists between these two structures called the **epidural space**. The epidural space contains the middle meningeal arteries.

The dura has two main projections into the cranial vault: the falx cerebri and the tentorium cerebelli. The **falx cerebri** is a double-layered vertical projection of dura from the superior portion of the skull that separates the two cerebral hemispheres of the brain. The **tentorium cerebelli** is a horizontal projection of the dura arising from the posterior wall of the skull to form a shelf separating the occipital lobes of the cerebrum from the posterior cranial fossa and the cerebellum. The **dural sinuses** are collecting areas for venous blood from the brain and are found in the folds of the dura as it makes these two projections in the cranial vault.

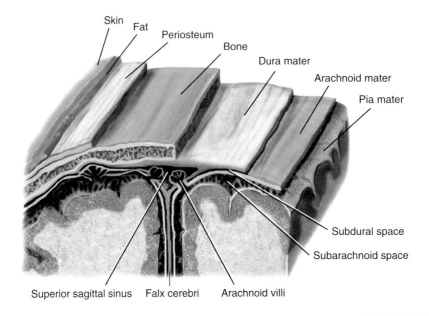

Skin Fat Periosteum Bone Dura mater Arachnoid mater Pia mater Subdural space Subarachnoid space Superior sagittal sinus Falx cerebri Arachnoid villi

FIGURE 11-2 Cranial meninges.

Beneath the dura is the thin, filmy arachnoid layer. The **subdural space** separates the arachnoid layer and dura mater and is crossed by the small venous vessels that empty into the dural sinuses. Weblike trabeculations connect the arachnoid layer to the pia mater. The innermost layer, the pia mater, is a thin and delicate structure and is, essentially, the outermost layer of the brain. It is invested with many small arterial blood vessels. The **subarachnoid space** separates the arachnoid layer and pia mater and is filled with cerebral spinal fluid (CSF), which is produced by the choroid plexus, located in ventricles deep inside the brain. The CSF circulates through the brain's ventricular system before exiting into the subarachnoid space through three small channels at the level of the brain stem. Specialized projections of the arachnoid layer, called arachnoid villi, reabsorb CSF into the dural venous sinuses.

The three primary structural elements of the **brain** are the cerebrum, cerebellum, and brain stem. The **cerebrum** is structurally divided into the diencephalon and the two cerebral hemispheres. The diencephalon is located in the center of the cerebrum and acts as a connecting and processing point for information entering and leaving the cerebral hemispheres. Each cerebral hemisphere has four lobes: frontal, occipital, temporal, and parietal, each bearing the name of its overlying bone (Figure 11-3). At the skull floor, the base of the frontal lobe is located in the anterior fossa, the temporal lobe sits in the middle fossa, and the occipital lobe rests on the shelf formed by the tentorium cerebelli. An important consideration is that part of the temporal lobe, called the uncus, is located at the edge of the tentorium cerebelli. The uncus can be forced to herniate over the edge of the tentorium cerebelli in the setting of a large superior intracranial mass lesion.

The two broad categories of brain tissue are the **white matter** and the **gray matter**. The gray matter, located in the outer layer of the cerebral hemispheres or cortexis, is composed mainly of nerve cell bodies. The white matter is composed mainly of myelinated nerve axons that act as insulated pathways for nerve conduction. The cerebrum is responsible for higher brain activities, including voluntary motor control, behavior, and most modalities of sensation and speech.

The **cerebellum** is located in the posterior fossa and is separated from the cerebrum by the falx cerebelli. This structure is primarily responsible for subconscious fine tuning of skeletal musculature—for equilibrium, locomotion, and coordination.

The main structural components of the **brain stem** are the midbrain, pons, and medulla oblongata. These structures are located below the tentorium cerebelli and rest on the clivus, the smooth area of the sphenoid and occipital bones that slopes down into the foramen magnum. These structures contain multiple motor and sensory pathways that act to unite the brain stem, cerebellum, and cerebrum. In addition, the brain stem is responsible for most lower brain functions such as cardiac and respiratory regulation (Figure 11-4).

The neck is an extremely complex and compact anatomical region containing multiple vital structures. It includes airway structures, great vessels to the brain, major neurological structures, and the esophagus. Because these critical structures are relatively unprotected by bone or muscle, they are particularly vulnerable to trauma. The neck is divided into the

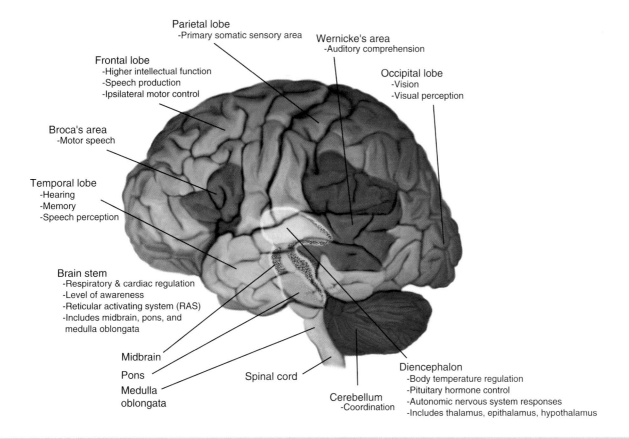

Parietal lobe
-Primary somatic sensory area

Wernicke's area
-Auditory comprehension

Frontal lobe
-Higher intellectual function
-Speech production
-Ipsilateral motor control

Occipital lobe
-Vision
-Visual perception

Broca's area
-Motor speech

Temporal lobe
-Hearing
-Memory
-Speech perception

Brain stem
-Respiratory & cardiac regulation
-Level of awareness
-Reticular activating system (RAS)
-Includes midbrain, pons, and
 medulla oblongata

Midbrain
Pons
Medulla
oblongata

Spinal cord

Cerebellum
-Coordination

Diencephalon
-Body temperature regulation
-Pituitary hormone control
-Autonomic nervous system responses
-Includes thalamus, epithalamus, hypothalamus

FIGURE 11-3 Lobes of the brain.

anterior and posterior triangles by the sternocleidomastoid muscle (see Figure 11-5). A suboccipital triangle is also located in the upper posterior neck. The anterior triangle is bound by the sternocleidomastoid muscle posteriorly, the mandible superiorly, and the midline of the neck anteriorly.

The neck contains two main cervical fascial layers. The **superficial cervical fascia** is the thin layer of connective tissue that lies immediately beneath the skin. This fascial layer contains the **platysma muscle**, which is a major landmark in trauma management. The platysma is a thin, superficial muscle that originates in the deep fascia of the upper chest, inserts on the mandible and angle of the mouth, and functions to pull the angle of the mouth downward. The **deep cervical fascia** supports the major anatomical structures of the neck. This fascia layer is further divided into multiple planes, one of which is the carotid sheath. The carotid sheath contains the carotid artery, internal jugular vein, and vagus nerve.

For trauma considerations, the anterior neck is divided into three zones (Figure 11-5). Zone I is bound by the sternal notch inferiorly and the cricoid cartilage superiorly. Zone II is bound inferiorly by the cricoid cartilage and superiorly by the mandible, and zone III contains neck structures above the angle of the mandible. Table 11-1 lists the anatomical contents by zone.

PHYSIOLOGY

Physiologically, the brain is an extremely demanding and delicate organ. In the resting adult the brain consumes 20% of all the oxygen used by the body. To meet these demands, the brain has both an exceptionally high blood flow, approximately 700 mL/min, and a high oxygen extraction ratio. Limited in its capacity to store energy, the brain is very vulnerable to ischemia. Even a brief interruption of normal blood flow for 5–10 seconds can cause loss of consciousness. The carotid and vertebral arteries are the major vessels that supply the

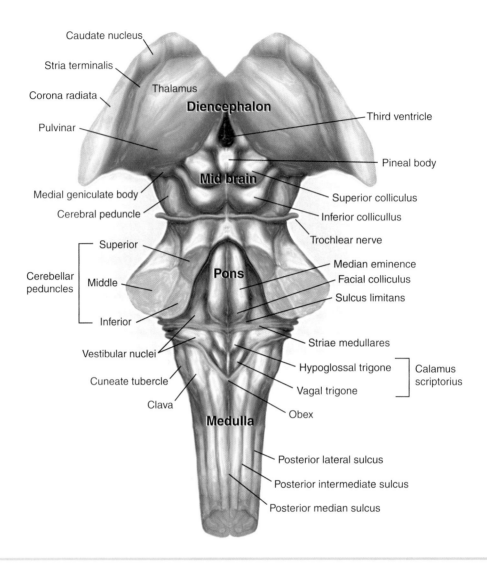

FIGURE 11-4 Cross section of the brain showing relationship of brain stem to other structures.

brain. The carotid arteries monitor arterial pressure via the carotid sinuses. Through reflex arcs that are able to alter cardiac function, the carotid sinus maintains adequate arterial pressure to the brain. In addition, there are local cerebral autoregulatory mechanisms to maintain cerebral blood flow. These autoregulatory mechanisms alter blood vessel diameter and are highly effective at maintaining adequate cerebral blood flow over arterial pressures from 80 to 180 mm Hg.

The principal trigger to increase or decrease cerebral blood flow in the brain is carbon dioxide (CO_2). **Hypercapnia**, or elevated $PaCO_2$, can increase cerebral blood flow and hypocapnia can likewise decrease cerebral blood flow. For every decrease in $PaCO_2$ of 1 mm Hg the cerebral blood flow decreases by 2–4%.[13] If $PaCO_2$ is decreased to 15–20 mm Hg, cerebral blood flow can be diminished to the point of causing dangerous cerebral hypoxia. A secondary mechanism for cerebral blood flow regulation is

oxygen (O_2) level. High $PaCO_2$ levels tend to cause cerebral vasoconstriction and low PaO_2 levels cause cerebral vasodilation.

Cerebral perfusion pressure (CPP) can be approximated by subtracting the mean ICP from the mean arterial pressure (MAP):

$$CPP = MAP - ICP$$

The MAP is estimated by adding one-third of the pulse pressure to the diastolic blood pressure (BP):

$$MAP = (systolic\ BP - diastolic\ BP)/3 + diastolic\ BP$$

The normal mean ICP is 2–12 mm Hg and the normal CPP is 90 mm Hg. The CPP must be maintained above 50–60 mm Hg to prevent cerebral ischemia. As can be seen from the first equation, management of the head-injured patient requires both an adequate MAP and control of ICP.

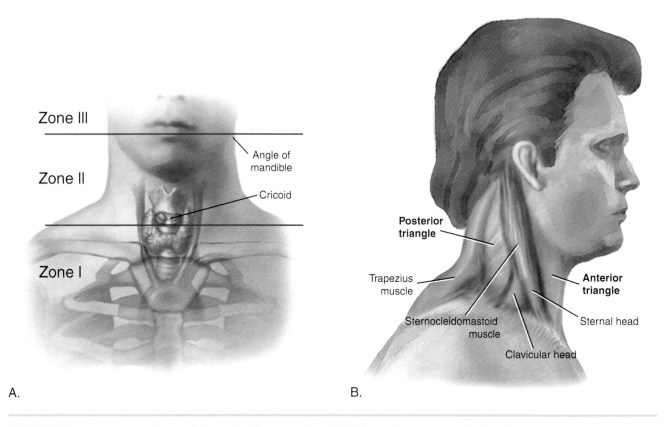

Zone III

Zone II

Zone I

Angle of mandible

Cricoid

A.

Posterior triangle

Trapezius muscle

Sternocleidomastoid muscle

Clavicular head

Anterior triangle

Sternal head

B.

FIGURE 11-5 Anatomical divisions of the neck: (A) zones I, II, and III; (B) anterior and posterior triangles.

Table 11-1
Major Anatomical Contents of the Neck by Zone

Zone I	Zone II	Zone III
Subclavian vessels	Larynx	Internal carotid artery
Pulmonary pleura	Pharynx, base of tongue	External carotid artery
Great vessels of neck	Carotid artery	Vertebral artery
Recurrent laryngeal nerve	Jugular vein	Cranial nerves
Trachea	Phrenic and vagus nerve	
	Thyroid gland	

PUPIL RESPONSE

The eye, with its extraordinary abilities, is controlled by an equally complex nervous system. There are two principal pathways providing motor control for pupil size. The sympathetic nervous system provides the motor control to dilate the pupil. These neurons originate in the hypothalamus and travel down into the spinal cord, exiting at the first thoracic vertebra, on the way to the iris. These nerve fibers return to the cranium by following the internal carotid artery. The parasympathetic nervous system provides the motor

control to constrict the pupil. These neurons originate in the brain stem and travel within the oculomotor nerve (CN III) to reach the iris. The size of the pupil is determined by the balance between these two competing systems.

There are many disease processes that cause dysfunction of pupillary response or alterations of pupil size. In head trauma, **anisocoria**, or unequal pupils, can be caused by increased ICP. The oculomotor nerve exits the midbrain at the level of the tentorium cerebelli. In a mass effect, an expanding lesion forces the brain toward the foramen magnum, and the oculomotor nerve becomes vulnerable to compression by the herniating brain tissue. Pressure on the oculomotor nerve can result in loss of the parasympathetic motor signal to constrict the pupil. The competing sympathetic nerve follows a much different path to reach the iris and is not subjected to the same pressures during this pathological process. The unchecked sympathetic signal dilates the pupil, usually on the same side as the injury that is causing the increased intracranial pressure.

MOTOR AND SENSORY PATHWAYS

The efferent neural pathways that transmit voluntary motor commands to skeletal muscle originate in the lateral aspects of the cerebrum. Each cerebral hemisphere provides the voluntary motor control for the opposite side of the body. After leaving the cerebral cortex, the motor neurons travel in the corticospinal tract to reach the anterior aspect of the medulla in the brain stem. At this point the corticospinal fibers cross over to the opposite side. The anatomical structure where this crossover occurs in the brain stem is called the pyramids, named because of their shape on dissection. The corticospinal fibers then travel down the anterior aspect of the spinal cord on the side of the body that they control.

The sensory fibers that carry information concerning pain, temperature, and touch originate at innumerable points in the body. These sensory nerve fibers enter the posterior aspect of the spinal cord and immediately cross to the opposite side to form the spinothalamic tract. These afferent neurons travel the spinothalamic pathway on the opposite side of the body from their origination to eventually reach the cerebral cortex. Similar to the voluntary motor control system, each cerebral hemisphere provides the sensory control for the opposite side of the body.

Knowing this anatomical configuration can be extremely useful in locating a lesion or defect in the pathway. Head-injured patients can present with loss of sensory and motor function on the side of the body contralateral to the brain injury. This loss of function can be caused by direct injury to the cerebral hemisphere or from compression of the nerve pathways as they travel trough the brain stem. In contrast, some spinal cord injuries can present with loss of motor control on the side of injury and loss of sensory function on the side opposite to the injury.

PATHOPHYSIOLOGY OF BRAIN INJURY

Most trauma to the head results from acceleration-deceleration forces or penetrating injuries. Acceleration-deceleration force trauma typically occurs secondary to motor vehicle collisions, falls, and blows to the head. When the head strikes an object and stops, the dissipation of energy causes trauma to the underlying structures. Because the brain is mobile inside the cranium, it may recoil to strike the cranial wall opposite to the initial impact point. This type of injury, called **coup/contrecoup**, can lead to significant tissue destruction in areas far from the point of contact. The classic example of penetrating force trauma is the gunshot wound. The cavitation effects of high-speed projectiles can lead to tissue injury that extends far beyond the path of the projectile.

PRIMARY BRAIN INJURY

Injuries to the brain can be divided into two broad categories, primary and secondary injury. **Primary brain injury** results from the transfer of kinetic energy at the moment of impact. These injuries occur instantaneously at the scene and are caused by mechanical damage to anatomical structures. Unfortunately, these injuries frequently result in problems that must be managed surgically, as little else is effective. Initial management for this type of trauma tends to be supportive, directed by the presenting complaints; it rarely corrects the underlying pathology.

SECONDARY BRAIN INJURY

In contrast, **secondary brain injury** typically occurs minutes, hours, or even days later. These injuries are the result of other pathological processes that impair cerebral perfusion, oxygenation, and nutrition. Common mechanisms that lead to additional tissue infarction and destruction include hypoxia, systemic hypotension, intracranial hypertension, infection, and seizures. The management goal for secondary injuries is to prevent or minimize their occurrence. Unlike primary injuries, initial care can significantly alter the course of this pathophysiological process.

LOSS OF CONSCIOUSNESS

A loss of consciousness is the hallmark of significant brain injury. The **reticular activating system (RAS)** is the primary structural element that regulates arousal and consciousness. The RAS is located in the brain stem and has widespread neuronal projections into the cerebral hemispheres. A wide variety of sensory stimuli can activate the RAS, which in turn activates the higher brain centers, resulting in arousal and consciousness.

The initial loss of consciousness in the head trauma patient is usually secondary to disruption of the RAS as the head dissipates the mechanical energy of the injury. These patients typically become lucid again after a brief period if no anatomical damage has been done to the brain. However, continued loss of consciousness represents a much more ominous sign. To remain unconscious, the patient must have widespread dysfunction of both cerebral hemispheres or dysfunction of the brain stem. A **coma**, which is a failure of arousal, is seen in about 8% of head injury patients and is associated with a 30–50% mortality rate.[6] Up to 50% of head injury patients arriving at the hospital unconscious will have elevated ICP.[1]

When the dysfunction is less severe, a wide range of altered levels of consciousness and confusional states are possible. Clinicians often describe these patients as having a "clouded consciousness," which may mean disoriented, inattentive, heightened or depressed alertness, or drowsy. In addition to trauma, the pathways that control consciousness can be disrupted by hypoxia, metabolic disorders, drugs, toxins, and infection.

Patients with significant neurological dysfunction and unconsciousness may demonstrate involuntary posturing. Decerebrate posturing, which is extension of extremities and flexion at the wrist, is seen in the unconscious patients with midbrain dysfunction (see Chapter 6). Decorticate posturing, which is flexion at the elbows and wrist and extension of lower extremities, is seen in the unconscious patient with hemispheric central nervous system (CNS) dysfunction. Unconscious patients that present with involuntary posturing have a 60–70% mortality.[6]

INCREASED INTRACRANIAL PRESSURE

The **Monro-Kellie principle** provides a helpful model for understanding ICP. In this model, the cranium is viewed as a closed, rigid container with a limited volume and is completely filled with its three main elements: the brain, blood, and CSF. An increase in the volume of one element must be compensated for by a decrease in the volume of the other elements, or the pressure in the system will rise. For example, the brain volume could be increased by cerebral edema, the blood volume by an intracranial hematoma, and the CSF volume by a traumatic obstruction of the ventricular system. The minimum volume of the brain is relatively fixed and unyielding. For that reason, initial compensation for volume increase is movement of CSF and venous blood out of the vault. This compensatory mechanism is limited and typically fails with increases beyond a critical volume of 30–50 mL. After this critical point, small increases in volume result in much larger changes in ICP. The normal ICP is 2 to 12 mm Hg, and sustained pressures greater than 20–30 mm Hg are associated with increased risk of secondary brain injury and poor outcome.[3,14–16]

Recalling that CPP = MAP – ICP, as mean ICP rises, CPP will decrease unless the body compensates by increasing MAP. This compensatory mechanism presents as **Cushing's triad** and is described as increased blood pressure, decreased pulse, and irregular respirations in the face of increased ICP. The decrease in pulse is caused by the carotid sinus reflex arch as blood pressure rises. Because the brain has such high metabolic demands and limited reserves, cerebral ischemia will occur once CPP falls below 40–60 mm Hg. Compounding the problem of maintaining cerebral perfusion, the normal compensatory mechanisms are frequently compromised by systemic hypoxia and hypotension. A hypotensive patient with even mildly elevated ICP is nearly certain to have inadequate cerebral perfusion. Dysfunction of the normal cerebral autoregulatory mechanisms that maintain cerebral blood flow also occurs secondary to brain tissue injury, further jeopardizing brain tissue perfusion.

BRAIN HERNIATION

Ultimately, continued increases in ICP will compress the brain stem and result in the patient's death. As discussed earlier, the cranium is divided into multiple compartments by the dural projections. In the setting of an expanding mass lesion, elevated compartment pressure can force brain tissue to herniate toward compartments of lower pressure. In addition, the shape of the cranium and dural projections form a funnel-like pathway toward the brain stem and foramen magnum. Multiple herniation syndromes and patterns of brain stem compression have been well described.[13] The herniation syndromes are summarized in Figure 11-6.

An **uncal herniation** occurs when there is a space-occupying lesion displacing one of the cerebral hemispheres. As the lesion expands, it forces a portion of the temporal lobe, the uncus, to herniate over the edge of the tentorium cerebelli. In this type of transtentorial herniation, the displaced tissue is usually on the same side as the expanding lesion. As the uncus is displaced, it compresses the motor tracts of the cerebral peduncles above their point of the crossover, resulting in contralateral muscle weakness and paralysis. The oculomotor nerve is also in this area; compression of the oculomotor nerve results in ipsilateral pupil dilation. Eventually, unchecked elevation of ICP in any herniation syndrome and pressure on the brain stem will lead to Cushing's triad of elevated systemic blood pressure, decreased pulse, and irregular respiration.

A **central herniation syndrome** can occur when a space-occupying lesion displaces both of the cerebral hemispheres downward toward the tentorial notch. The bilateral tentorial herniation of cerebral tissue results in bilateral motor weakness and paralysis.

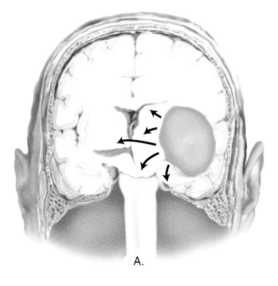

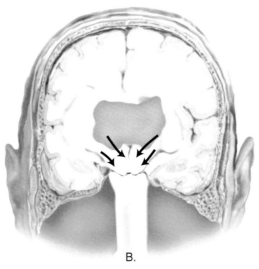

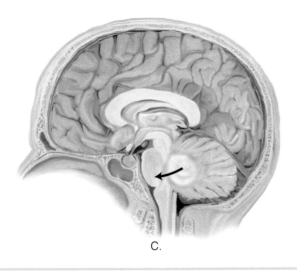

FIGURE 11-6 An expanding cerebellar mass forces cerebellar tonsils into foramen magnum. Pupillary response is spared, but patient presents with flaccid quadriplegia, apnea, and circulatory collapse.

Central herniation syndrome is associated with progressive loss of neurological function and late bilateral pupil dilation. This syndrome is also associated with Cheyne-Stokes respirations and decorticate posturing.

In **cerebellar herniation** the cerebellum and other structures in the posterior fossa can be forced to herniate out of their compartment. In this syndrome, herniation can be upward over the tentorium or downward toward the foramen magnum. Because of the early vulnerability of the brain stem to compression, loss of consciousness, respiratory dysfunction, and cardiac dysfunction occur early in the course of posterior fossa herniation.

BRAIN STEM COMPRESSION

Increasing ICP ultimately compresses the brain stem. Brain stem compression interferes with the normal function of pupillary control, respirations, and consciousness and may produce abnormal motor responses. The progression of clinical signs associated with brain stem involvement varies depending upon whether the source of compression is an uncal or central herniation. Table 11-2 summarizes the findings associated with brain stem compression, and Figure 11-7 details the respiratory patterns associated with varying levels of brain stem involvement.

SCALP INJURIES

The principal scalp injuries are lacerations, avulsions, and hematomas. Because of the rich vascularity of the scalp, these injuries can result in significant blood loss. A common pitfall is to underestimate blood loss from these typically nonlethal injuries. It is possible for a patient to have significant enough blood loss from a scalp injury to cause hypovolemic shock. The subcutaneous tissue, which contains larger blood vessels, tends to separate when lacerated, causing gaping wounds. These wounds hamper hemostasis by preventing the blood vessels from contracting. The loose connective tissue between the tough galea and the rigid periosteum offers little resistance to dissection, so large hematomas can form in this space. Because the tissue planes above and below the galea are relatively easy to dissect, avulsion or flaplike injuries are also common. These injuries should be handled with delicacy and respect; it is often impossible to determine if they are associated with an underlying skull fracture or communication into the cranium.

SKULL FRACTURES

The four types of skull fractures are linear, depressed, open, and basilar. In general, a skull fracture of any type represents a significant application of traumatic

Table 11-2
Summary of Clinical Findings of Brain Stem Compression

		Uncal Herniation Syndrome			
Clinical Assessment	**Local Early Signs**	**Diencephalon–Midbrain**	**Midbrain–Upper Pons**	**Lower Pons–Upper Medulla**	**Medulla**
Pupils	Unilateral, dilated pupil; sluggish, nonreactive	Unilateral, dilated, and fixed	Bilateral, dilated, fixed	→	→
Level of consciousness	Little effect on consciousness; may notice restlessness. Once deterioration begins, can proceed to deep coma quickly.	Stupor; coma	Deep coma	→	→
Motor		Hemiparesis on side of lesion or contralateral hemiparesis to hemiplegia; decerebration	Bilateral decerebration	Flaccidity with occasional decerebration	→
Sensory	Progressive deterioration	→	→	→	→
Babinski sign		Bilateral positive	→	No reflexes	→
Respirations		Cheyne-Stokes	Central Neurogenic Hyperventilation (CNH)	Apneustic or cluster breathing	Biots breathing, then apnea
Other			Bradycardia Elevated systolic BP Widening pulse pressure Wide variations in temperature	Deterioration of vital signs Elevated temperature	No vital signs Elevated temperature

		Central Herniation Syndrome			
Clinical Assessment	**Early Diencephalon**	**Later Diencephalon**	**Midbrain–Upper Pons**	**Lower Pons–Upper Medulla**	**Medulla**
Pupils	Both small and reactive	→	Unequal, midpoint and nonreactive	→	Dilated and fixed
Level of consciousness	Difficulty with concentration and becomes agitated or drowsy, then stuporous	Stuporous; coma	Deep coma	→	→
Motor	Contralateral hemiparesis to hemiplegia	Paratonic rigidity on ipsilateral side, becoming decorticate	Bilateral decerebration	Flaccidity with occasional decerebration	→

(continued)

Table 11-2 (continues)
Summary of Clinical Findings of Brain Stem Compression

	Central Herniation Syndrome *(continues)*				
Clinical Assessment	Early Diencephalon	Later Diencephalon	Midbrain– Upper Pons	Lower Pons– Upper Medulla	Medulla
Sensory	Progressive deterioration	→	→	→	→
Babinski sign	None	Bilateral positive Babinski	→	→	→
Respirations	Cheyne-Stokes	→	Cheyne-Stokes and CNH	Apneustic or cluster breathing	Biots breathing, then apnea
Other			Wide variations in temperature, often very high May develop diabetes insipidus Bradycardia Elevated systolic BP Widening of pulse pressure	Elevated temperature Erratic pulse Hypotension	→ No vital signs

Source: Adapted from *The Clinical Practice of Neurological and Neurosurgical Nursing,* (3rd ed., p. 264), by J. Hickey, 1992, Philadelphia: J.B. Lippincott Publishing. Used with permission.

forces to the head and should raise the index of suspicion for cervical spine injury and underlying brain tissue trauma. Of the skull fractures, the **linear fracture** is typically the most benign. The presence or absence of a linear fracture does not significantly alter long-term prognosis or treatment for most patients. The main concern with a linear skull fracture is the degree of underlying brain tissue trauma. There are no specific physical signs for linear fractures; this is typically a radiographic diagnosis.

Other types of skull fractures are far more concerning. **Depressed skull fractures** are associated with underlying intracranial hematoma in about 7% of cases. Unlike linear fractures, these patients are far more likely to have long-term neurological deficits. **Open skull fractures** expose the brain and meninges to bacteria and put the patient at great risk for infection. **Basilar skull fractures** are seen in 24% of severe head traumas and frequently have a communication into the cranial vault, making them an open skull fracture.[17] Fractures involving the temporal bone can present with blood or CSF in the external auditory canal, hemotympanum, and facial (CN VII) or vestibular nerve (CN VIII) dysfunction. A later sign of temporal bone fracture is Battle's sign, or ecchymosis over the mastoid process. Basilar skull fractures involving the anterior cranial floor bones, such as the frontal, ethmoid, or sphenoid bones, can present with CSF from the nose or olfactory nerve dysfunction. A later sign of a basilar skull fracture involving the frontal bones is raccoon eyes, which is bilateral periorbital ecchymosis.

Normal CSF is a golden straw-colored fluid. When leaking into the external auditory canal or nose, it is easily obscured by mucous secretions, tears, or blood. One technique for detecting CSF that is mixed with blood is the halo sign. When a drop of fluid is allowed to fall onto a bed sheet or gauze, the CSF will diffuse from blood and form a halo ring around the blood. A technique for detecting CSF within a mixture of clear fluids, like tears or mucous secretions, is to measure the glucose concentration. Cerebrospinal fluid contains a concentration of glucose that is similar to serum. Since nasal mucous discharge and tears are relatively glucose free, simple glucose reagent strips can be used to detect the presence of CSF. This technique of using glucose reagent strips is obviously not helpful if the fluid mixture contains blood or serum. Both techniques for detecting CSF are fraught with potential for error and should not be considered diagnostic.

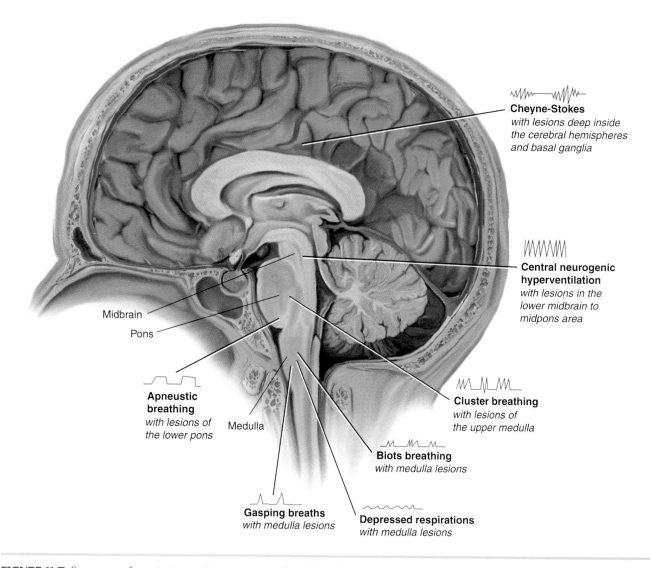

Cheyne-Stokes
*with lesions deep inside
the cerebral hemispheres
and basal ganglia*

**Central neurogenic
hyperventilation**
*with lesions in the
lower midbrain to
midpons area*

Midbrain

Pons

Cluster breathing
*with lesions of
the upper medulla*

**Apneustic
breathing**
*with lesions of
the lower pons*

Medulla

Biots breathing
with medulla lesions

Gasping breaths
with medulla lesions

Depressed respirations
with medulla lesions

FIGURE 11-7 Summary of respiratory patterns associated with head injury.

DIFFUSE BRAIN INJURIES

The principal diffuse brain injuries are concussion and diffuse axonal injury. A **concussion** represents the mildest form of brain trauma. In a concussion, the pathology is principally the temporary disruption of normal neurological function without structural damage to the brain. The anatomy will appear normal by computerized tomography (CT). If a structural change exists, it is usually minimal diffuse edema without an identifiable focal lesion (Figure 11-8). The dissipation of energy from the mechanism of injury disrupts the RAS, resulting in a brief period of unconsciousness with rapid recovery. The patient often has postconcussion mental clouding that can present as impaired judgment, unsteady gait, and motor dysfunction. A postconcussion syndrome of headache, photophobia, personality changes, sleep disturbances, and short-term memory impairment is also recognized with this type of

injury. The prognosis is good for this injury with postconcussion mental clouding, typically clearing in minutes to hours. Postconcussion syndromes persisting for longer periods may require rehabilitation services. If not recognized, this syndrome can have significant social and family consequences. Although there is no specific treatment for concussion, these patients must be transported and evaluated in the emergency department. Other more severe injuries may have similar initial presentations and cannot be ruled out in the field.

Diffuse axonal injury represents a more severe and potentially life-threatening injury. The mechanism of injury is almost exclusively caused by an acceleration-deceleration force secondary to vehicular crashes.[18] However, the pathogenesis of this injury is incompletely understood. The traditional theories postulate that tensile forces tear the axons at the moment of trauma as a primary injury.[19–21] These theories are based on the histological differences between gray and

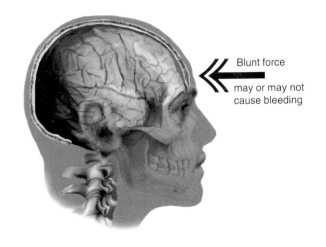

FIGURE 11-8 Concussion.

white matter tissue types. The white matter of the brain, or axons, has a high fatty acid content. The gray matter, or neuron cell body, has a high water content. It is believed that rapid deceleration can cause diffuse axonal injury throughout the brain when these two structures with different densities attempt to separate from each other at or near the moment of initial trauma.

Newer theories with convincing evidence have demonstrated that diffuse axonal injury does not necessarily occur immediately at the initial moment of trauma but at a later point as a secondary injury.[19,20,22,23] It is thought that the neurons dismantle their internal cytoskeletal structures, resulting in axonal separation, as part of a complex metabolic process in response to the trauma. It is likely that hypoxia and other potentially preventable metabolic derangements significantly contribute to this process. Much of the current research and many of the experimental treatments for head injury are targeted toward halting this pathophysiological process. It has been speculated that some traditional treatments for head injury, like barbiturate-induced comas, were effective because they blunted this metabolic response. Regardless of the exact pathophysiological process, it is known that these injuries are associated with progressive axonal swelling with ultimate axonal destruction. The prognosis and clinical presentation can vary widely and are dependent on the location and amount of tissue damage.

FOCAL BRAIN INJURIES

The principal focal brain injuries are contusions, lacerations, and intracranial hematomas. The four intracranial hematomas are epidural hematoma, subdural hematoma, subarachnoid hemorrhage, and intracerebral hematoma. In addition to location, the intracranial hematomas are distinguishable by their pathophysiology and clinical presentation.

A **contusion** represents the mildest form of focal brain injury. From a practical point of view, it is essentially impossible to distinguish a contusion from a concussion in the field. Concussions and contusions can have identical mechanisms of injury and initial clinical presentations. However, a contusion represents a more severe insult. Unlike a concussion, the brain parenchyma in a contusion can show microhemorrhages and focal areas of trauma (Figure 11-9). Like concussion, there is no specific treatment. In most cases these patients are admitted for conservative management and observation. Patients with contusions are at greater risk for long-term neurological sequela; microhemorrhages associated with this injury can progress to form an intracranial hematoma.

Cerebral lacerations are commonly caused by rotational forces. They are typically seen on the brain surfaces that contact the orbital roof and sphenoid wing of the skull. Foreign bodies and bone fragments can cause frank rupture of brain tissue. Overall, cerebral lacerations have a 40% mortality rate; when combined with a subdural clot the death rate can reach 75%.[24]

An **epidural hematoma** is a collection of blood between the skull and the dura mater (Figure 11-10). This potentially life-threatening injury occurs in about 1% of all head injuries. Classically, these patients will have a blow to the relatively thin portion of the temporal bone on the side of the skull above the middle meningeal artery. The resulting skull fracture, which is seen in 90% of epidural hematomas, lacerates the underlying artery. The initial blow disrupts the

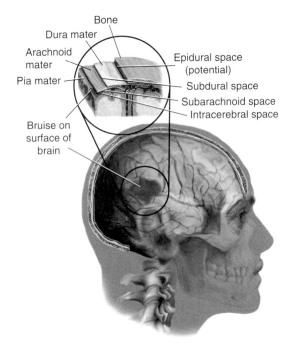

FIGURE 11-9 Contusion.

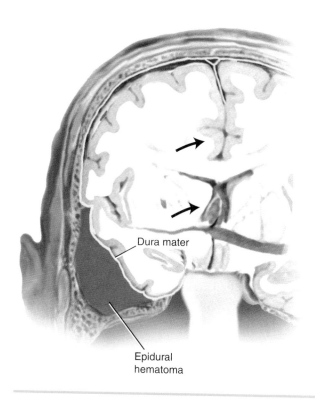

FIGURE 11-10 Epidural hematoma. Note the shift of midline structures (small arrows).

RAS, causing a temporary loss of consciousness. As the hematoma expands and ICP elevates, the level of consciousness begins to deteriorate. The expanding lesion can result in an uncal herniation syndrome with contralateral muscle weakness and paralysis and ipsilateral pupil dilation. This pathological scenario can occur with startling speed and precipitous deterioration and death of the patient. Children are especially at risk for extensive hematoma formation because the dura is less adherent to the skull and offers less resistance to hematoma formation.

The classic presentation of a loss of consciousness followed by mental clearing and subsequent deterioration is only seen in about one-third of all patients with epidural hematomas. Another one-third of the patients will never lose consciousness, and the remaining third will never regain consciousness. Unequal pupils, or anisocoria, is also an unreliable sign of epidural hematoma, especially in the setting of systemic hypotension, and is only seen in 30–50% of cases.[13,24,25] If the pupils are unequal, 80–90% will have a dilated pupil on the same side as the lesion.[24] Hemiparesis is more common and is seen in 50–70% of the cases.[24,26] If hemiparesis is present, 95% experience hemiparesis on the side contralateral to the injury. Bradycardia is a late sign, more common in children, and only seen in 25% of the cases.[24]

In this type of hematoma very little acute accumulation of blood is necessary to cause a life-threatening

emergency. A hematoma estimated to contain more than 15 mL of blood is an indication for emergent surgical intervention to evacuate the lesion and ligate the bleeding vessel. A craniotomy or emergently placed burr hole is used to relieve life-threatening increased ICP. In the interim, care is largely supportive and directed at reducing ICP through moderate hyperventilation, hyperosmotic intravenous fluids, and steroids. Early diagnosis and neurosurgical intervention can reduce mortality to about 8%. Those receiving prompt treatment usually recover with minimal long-term neurological deficits. Without early treatment death is common.

INTERNET ACTIVITIES

Visit the e-medicine Web site at http://www.emedicine.com. Click on the Emergency Medicine on-line book and select Trauma and Orthopedics. Then click on Epidural Hematoma. Review the chapter on the management of epidural hematoma.

A **subdural hematoma** is a collection of blood in the space between the dura mater and the arachnoid membrane (Figure 11-11). This hematoma is caused by shear forces that tear surface blood vessels as the brain moves within the skull. Typically the injured vessels are bridging veins as they cross the subdural space to empty blood from the brain into the dural sinus. Atrophy of the brain, which can be seen in alcoholism and the elderly, stresses these bridging vessels, allows for more movement within the skull, and increases the risk for this type of hematoma.

Since the injured vessels, typically venous, are under low pressure, hematomas large enough to cause a

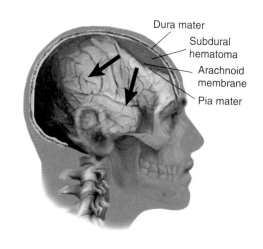

FIGURE 11-11 Subdural hematoma. Note the shift of midline structures.

mass effect may take days to weeks to develop. The complications of this injury are slow to develop, so the patient or family may not associate the traumatic event that caused the initial injury with the present complaint. However, not all subdural hematomas form slowly. Patients with rapidly developing lesions can present with an enlarged pupil and hemiparesis similar to the symptoms of an epidural hematoma. An enlarged pupil is seen in 50–80% of cases and is typically on the side of injury. Focal neurological signs, posturing, and hemiparesis contralateral to the side of injury are found in 50% of cases.

Subdural lesions are seen in 1% of all head trauma and in 26–36% of severe head trauma associated with a Glasgow Coma Score of 8 or less.[24] Subdural hematomas are associated with high mortality. In simple subdural hematomas, without a significant underlying contusion or brain parenchyma laceration, mortality is 21%. In complicated subdural hematomas, with significant contusion or parenchyma laceration, mortality is 53%. The mortality rate is 12% in patients who become conscious after the initial trauma, 27% in patients that remain unconscious, and 78% in patients with abnormal posturing.

INTERNET ACTIVITIES

Visit the e-medicine Web site at http:// www.emedicine.com. Click on the Emergency Medicine on-line book and select Trauma and Orthopedics. Then click on Subdural Hematoma. Review the chapter on the management of subdural hematoma.

Subarachnoid hemorrhages typically occur secondary to damage to the small arterial vessels that invest the outermost surface of the brain. These injuries occur as the brain moves across the uneven and jagged internal surface of the cranial vault. Subarachnoid hemorrhages are the most common type of intracranial hematoma, but fortunately they also tend to be the least significant.[2]

Subarachnoid hemorrhages are the only intracranial hemorrhages that are not focal in nature. Bleeding in the subarachnoid space diffuses throughout the cerebral spinal fluid. The bleeding causes signs and symptoms generally associated with meningeal irritation such as headache, decreased mentation, nuchal rigidity, confusion, stupor, hemiparesis, and posturing.

Intracerebral hematomas are seen in 1–7% of all head injuries.[27,28] These injuries are a potentially surgically correctable cause of secondary brain injury if recognized and treated early.[29] However, the initial identification of these lesions is difficult, and they may

INTERNET ACTIVITIES

Visit the e-medicine Web site at http:// www.emedicine.com. Click on the Emergency Medicine on-line book and select Trauma and Orthopedics. Then click on Subarachnoid Hemorrhage. Review the chapter on the management of subarachnoid hemorrhage.

not clinically declare themselves for days, making the diagnosis even more elusive. Severe intracerebral hemorrhages can produce a mass effect, especially when combined with underlying cerebral contusions and edema. Patients with intracerebral hematomas in the temporal or parietal areas near the temporal lobe are at greatest risk for tentorial herniation and poor outcome.[30] These injuries have a mortality rate of approximately 55%.[27]

PENETRATING TRAUMA

Approximately 12 penetrating head injuries occur each year per 100,000 people in the United States, the highest incidence in the world.[31] Gunshot wounds and other injuries of violence are the most common causes of penetrating head trauma.[2,31] These injuries can cause tissue destruction that extends well beyond their initial path. Because of the potential for massive tissue destruction, mortality rates are high. Patient outcome is dependent upon the amount of direct and indirect tissue destruction and the presenting neurological status. Injuries that have bilateral cerebral hemisphere involvement are commonly fatal.[27,31] Patients that present with unconsciousness have mortality rates as high as 93%.[31] The management issues for these injuries are the same as for other types of head injury.

COMPLICATIONS OF HEAD TRAUMA

In addition to the cardiovascular and respiratory systems, head injury is also associated with complications involving other organ systems. The genitourinary system can be affected by multiple mechanisms. The pituitary gland, located in the cranial floor, can be damaged in head injury, resulting in diabetes insipidus with massive renal diuresis. Dysfunction of the autonomic control of the urinary system predisposes the patient to increased risk of urinary tract infection. In the musculoskeletal system and the skin, head injury patients are at risk for decubitus ulcers and contractures of the extremities as a result of immobility from paralysis or coma. In the gastrointestinal system, the digestive tract is at increased risk for stress erosions.

Following injury, thromboplastic and fibrinolysis activity increase in the brain tissue and can detrimentally affect coagulation. In 40% of patients with severe head injury, coagulation parameters will be elevated and 8% will develop disseminated intravascular coagulation.[32] These patients are treated with fresh frozen plasma, cryoprecipitate, and platelet transfusions.

PATHOPHYSIOLOGY OF NECK INJURY

It is useful to classify neck injuries by anatomical triangle and zone (Figure 11-5). Injuries to the anterior triangle may involve the airway, esophagus, or vascular or neurological structures. Zone I injuries carry the highest mortality and can involve major vascular and intrathoracic structures. These injuries can be particularly problematic because they are hidden in the chest and difficult to assess. Zone I and posterior triangle trauma is associated with thoracic injuries that may compromise ventilation and breathing. Zone II injuries are the most common and typically least fatal neck injuries. Because zone II is relatively well exposed, the injuries tend to be more obvious. Carotid artery injuries and airway problems are common in zone II trauma. Zone III injuries typically involve vascular structures and cranial nerves. Zone III offers another difficult exposure problem for evaluation and surgical repair. Clinical signs of significant injury in neck trauma are provided in Table 11-3.

VASCULAR INJURIES

Blood vessels are the most commonly injured structures in neck trauma. These injuries are immediately life threatening for most neck trauma patients. In one series of patients with penetrating neck trauma, 18% had major arterial injuries and 26% had major venous injury.[9,33] In addition to the risk of hemorrhage, major vascular injuries can decrease blood flow to the brain, causing cerebral ischemia, and expanding hematomas in the neck can compromise the airway. While less common, blunt trauma is also associated with significant vascular injuries. In particular, cervical spine hyperextension can cause carotid or vertebral artery injury.

TRACHEA AND LARYNX INJURIES

Significant airway injuries are commonly seen in blunt trauma. These injuries are less dramatic than penetrating trauma and can easily be overlooked. Mechanisms of injury that produce maxillofacial trauma, first rib fractures, or sternum fractures should trigger a high index of suspicion for blunt occult airway injury. A typical mechanism of injury is an anterior impact that crushes the larynx or trachea against the cervical vertebrae. These patients are at high risk for development of complete airway obstruction that may necessitate a surgical airway.

Table 11-3
Clinical Signs of Significant Injury in Penetrating Neck Trauma

Vascular	Airway
Shock	Dyspnea
Active bleeding	Stridor
Large or expanding hematoma	Hemoptysis
Pulse deficit	Hoarseness, dysphonia/voice change
Thrills and bruits	Subcutaneous emphysema, crepitus
Neurological	**Digestive tract**
CNS deficit	Hemoptysis
Cranial nerve deficit	Dysphagia/odynophagia
Lateralized neurological deficit	Hematemesis
Hoarseness	Subcutaneous emphysema, crepitus

Source: Adapted from Jurkovich GJ: Definitive Care Phase: Neck Injuries. In Greenfield LZ, (ed): *Surgery: Scientific Principle and Practice.* JB Lippincott, Philadelphia, 1993.

PHARYNX AND ESOPHAGUS INJURIES

Penetrating neck injuries are the most likely cause of esophagus and pharyngeal injuries. Injuries to these structures are seen in about 5% of penetrating neck trauma patients.[9] While an esophageal injury may seem benign, these injuries are difficult to detect and are easily overlooked. Missed esophageal injuries are a common cause of late mortality with a near 100% fatality rate if surgery is significantly delayed.

NEUROLOGICAL INJURIES

Neurological deficits in neck trauma involving structures outside of the spinal cord are most commonly caused by direct injury to nerves. The most common nerve injuries involve the brachial plexus, deep cervical plexus, phrenic nerve, recurrent laryngeal nerve, and cranial nerves. Two of these nerve injuries are life threatening. The recurrent laryngeal nerve provides the only motor control to open the vocal cords, and injury can paralyze the cords in a closed position resulting in airway obstruction. The phrenic nerve provides motor function to the diaphragm, and injury dramatically compromises breathing. In addition to direct nerve injury, neurological deficits can occur secondary to cerebral ischemia. Blunt and penetrating vascular injuries can impair cerebral blood flow, causing ischemic strokes and transient ischemic attacks.

THYROID INJURIES

The thyroid gland is located in the anterior neck below the thyroid cartilage. In its unprotected position, the gland is vulnerable to injury. While rare, trauma can result in development of goiter, or even thyrotoxicosis.

INITIAL ASSESSMENT

The initial priorities of resuscitation in the patient with head or neck injury are identical to other patients with multiple trauma. The immediate threats to life from head or neck injury are from compromise of the airway, breathing, and circulation. In addition, these patients have a high probability for having other potentially life-threatening injuries that must be addressed in the primary survey. It has been reported that 75% of civilian neck trauma patients have serious multisystem trauma.[34] Even in the absence of multisystem trauma, the complications of head and neck injuries may create problems that should be immediately identified and corrected as part of the standardized trauma initial assessment.

AIRWAY AND CERVICAL SPINE

The mechanisms of injury that lead to head and neck trauma are so commonly associated with cervical spine (C-spine) injuries that it should be routinely presumed that a C-spine injury is present. In one series, trauma patients with clinically significant head injuries were 4 times more likely to have C-spine injury as compared to those without head trauma.[35] In this same series, the presence of unconsciousness nearly doubled the incidence of C-spine trauma.[35] All assessments and manipulation of the airway should be performed with appropriate C-spine stabilization. Patients should be assessed for adequacy of airway and presence of air movement. Two common complications of head injury that place the airway at risk are altered levels of consciousness and vomiting. While a detailed neurological exam is inappropriate at this point, the patient's level of consciousness must be taken into consideration when assessing their ability to protect the airway.

In neck trauma, airway compromise secondary to hemorrhage is common. Bleeding directly into the airway can result in aspiration and obstruction. Bleeding into the soft tissues of the neck can create a hematoma large enough to cause airway obstruction. Airway obstruction can also occur secondary to soft tissue edema or from disruption of anatomical structures like the larynx. Hoarseness, voice change, and stridor are potential signs of impending airway obstruction from edema or structural disruption. Injuries to the trachea, esophagus, or lung can produce crepitus and subcutaneous emphysema as air under pressure is forced into the surrounding soft tissues. Unfortunately, there may be little warning before a precipitous decompensation in airway status and development of acute obstruction. Frequent reassessment is imperative.

BREATHING

Assessment of breathing includes determination of the quality and quantity of respiratory efforts. In severe head injury, CNS dysfunction can produce pathological respiratory patterns with inadequate oxygenation. In neck trauma, and especially in zone I and posterior triangle trauma, concomitant thoracic injuries are common. Assessment of breathing must include determination of breath sounds, chest wall excursion, and percussion resonance to exclude pneumothorax, hemothorax, and tension pneumothorax.

CIRCULATION

The patient should be assessed for hemorrhage and shock. The most likely cause of shock in a trauma patient is from hypovolemia; thus, it is never assumed that head injury alone is the cause of shock or hypotension. Autonomic instability is an unlikely source of initial hypotension. Hemorrhage from a major scalp laceration can be the source of hypovolemia. In infants, intracranial blood loss can be of sufficient volume to cause hypovolemia. In neck trauma, massive hemorrhage is the most likely initial threat to life. The absence of visible bleeding does not rule out major vascular injury. Patients may have occult blood loss in the chest and mediastinum from neck injuries.

DISABILITY AND EXPOSURE

The initial assessment of level of consciousness and pupil response should be performed early after establishing patient contact. The mnemonic AVPU is widely advocated as a rapid and simple qualitative method to assess level of consciousness (see Chapter 6).

A more thorough neurological evaluation is performed as part of the focused assessment. The Glasgow Coma Scale evaluation is performed as part of the initial assessment and will be discussed in detail later. As in all trauma patients, clothing is removed to facilitate examination. Environmental controls to protect body temperature should not be overlooked. The head injury patient should be protected against hypothermia.

FOCUSED ASSESSMENT

The more detailed head-to-toe examination is conducted after the initial assessment has been completed, the ABC's (Airway, Breathing, Circulation) are controlled, and resuscitation measures are under way. It can not be overemphasized that the major and most immediate threats to life in head and neck trauma are addressed by the initial assessment and resuscitation. The special considerations for head and neck injury patients are discussed below.

HISTORY

As with any trauma, it is important to assess the scene and determine the mechanism of injury. The head-injured patient may be unable to provide a history or may prove to be an unreliable or misleading historian. Often clues at the scene, bystanders, and family members are valuable sources of information.

The history should include information regarding loss of consciousness. It should be determined if the patient lost consciousness and, if so, for how long. Simply asking a patient if he or she "passed out" may not yield accurate information. Patients often confuse dizziness, lightheadedness, or other temporary alterations of consciousness as unconsciousness. If the patient did lose consciousness, he or she is generally not in a good position to estimate the duration. Patients with true loss of consciousness will frequently have some degree of associated amnesia or poor recall of the details immediately proximal to the traumatic event.

Preexisting and precipitating medical disorders must be considered when evaluating head injury patients. Medical conditions, such as hypoglycemia, syncope, or cardiac disease, can be contributing factors to how the injury occurred, complicating patient evaluation. The "AMPLE" history provides a structure to organize a brief past medical history in the trauma patient. An AMPLE history includes allergies, medications, past medical history, last meal, and event related to the injury.

VITAL SIGNS

Serial vital signs at frequent intervals are indicated in the management of head and neck trauma. Prevention of secondary brain injury is foremost and is dependent upon maintaining adequate oxygenation and perfusion. Vital signs provide valuable information about resuscitation efforts and the status of intracranial lesions. Patients should be monitored for the development of pathological patterns in vital functions, such as Cheyne-Stokes respirations or Cushing's triad.

NEUROLOGICAL EXAM

The neurological exam assumes special importance in the evaluation of a head and neck trauma patient. These patients often present with deficits that can be difficult to communicate without using a common evaluation scheme. The neurological exam can be organized into the following categories: (1) level of consciousness and mental status, (2) pupillary function and cranial nerves, (3) peripheral sensory and motor function, and (4) reflexes. Like vital signs, serial evaluations of level of consciousness and neurological function are indicated at frequent intervals.

Level of Consciousness and Mental Status
The most fundamental and important element of the neurological evaluation is level of consciousness. While not specific, level of consciousness can provide some insight into ICP. If a patient is awake and able to provide intelligible verbal responses, increased ICP is unlikely. There are many terms commonly used to describe alterations in level of consciousness, such as stupor or lethargy. However, the use of this terminology is not sufficiently standardized and can lead to miscommunication. When describing alterations in level of consciousness, it is best to simply describe the actual deficit or to employ a standardized evaluation scale.

The **Glasgow Coma Scale (GCS)** is an evaluation tool that is widely accepted in evaluation of the level of consciousness. It is simple to use, reproducible, and accurate. While the GCS has demonstrated a high correlation with the severity of brain injury, it is considered by some to have poor prognostic value. Its simplicity also causes some limitations: It is a global assessment, not the equivalent of a mental status exam; it does not assess for more subtle changes, such as memory loss or amnesia; and it is less useful in children and those unable to respond to commands secondary to chemical sedation or paralysis. It is important to obtain an accurate initial GCS because the rapid treatment of severe head injury patients in the field, which often includes sedation and paralysis, can be a major barrier to later assessment if not obtained initially.[36]

The GCS range is 3–15 and is based on three areas of responsiveness: (1) eye opening, (2) verbal response, and (3) motor response. (See Table 11-4.) The ability to open the eyes requires an intact reticular activating system but does not imply awareness. If the eyes are swollen shut, this test is invalid. Speech requires a relatively intact CNS. The verbal response is actually an assessment of orientation. This test is invalid if the patient is unable to speak, such as in endotracheal intubation. The motor response score is based on the best response obtained. This test is primarily intended to assess CNS function. A patient may have complete paralysis in three out of four extremities secondary to peripheral nerve injury but still obtain the maximum score if he or she can move the remaining limb upon command.

In addition to the GCS, a more detailed assessment of mental status should be conducted. The patient should be assessed for orientation, to include evaluation of awareness to person, place, time, and event. Amnesia and memory loss are common findings in head trauma and should be documented. Subtle changes in short-term memory may be detected by testing the patient with a simple three-object recall.

Pupil Function and Cranial Nerves   The pupils should be assessed for symmetry, shape, reactivity, and size in millimeters. In a patient with decreasing level of consciousness, anisocoria may provide a late warning of increasing ICP and impending cerebral herniation as cranial nerve III is compressed. Pupil diameter differences of 1 mm or greater are considered abnormal. However, up to 5% of the normal population may have unequal pupils. Irregularly shaped and unequal pupils are also commonly seen in elderly patients who have had cataract surgery. It is important to recall that 50% of the patients with significant intracranial mass lesion may have equal pupils and that pupil response can also be altered by drugs, local trauma, and hypotension. An ophthalmic exam of the fundus and posterior structures of

Table 11-4
The Glasgow Coma Scale

Eye-opening response	
Spontaneous	4
To voice	3
To pain	2
None	1
Best verbal response	
Oriented	5
Confused	4
Inappropriate words	3
Incomprehensible sounds	2
None	1
Best motor response	
Obeys commands	6
Localizes (pain)	5
Withdraws (pain)	4
Flexion (pain)	3
Extension (pain)	2
None	1
Total GCS points (3–15)	_____

the eye may demonstrate changes earlier in the course of increasing ICP. The loss of a sharp margin to the optic disk edge and engorgement of retinal vessels are seen in increased ICP.

Assessment of the remaining cranial nerves is an important component of a complete neurological evaluation. Although this takes a secondary priority during the resuscitation of trauma patients, assessment of cranial nerve function may be particularly helpful when evaluating neck trauma. Cranial nerves V, VII, and IX–XII have prominent pathways outside the skull and are at higher risk for injury in maxillofacial and neck trauma. (See Table 11-5.)

INTERNET ACTIVITIES

Visit the University of North Carolina School of Medicine Web site at http://oisvideo2.med. unc.edu/ga/crannerves.ram and view the video on cranial nerve examination. This 20-minute video will play on your computer screen. You must have the RealPlayer media application installed on your computer. If you do not have this program, it is available free of charge from http://www.real.com.

Table 11-5
Cranial Nerve Assessment

Nerve	Name	Assessment
CN I	Olfactory	Ability to smell soap, tobacco, etc.
CN II	Optic	Visual acuity, visual fields, ophthalmoscopic
CN III	Oculomotor	Pupillary reaction, extraocular movement
CN IV	Trochlear	Extraocular movement
CN V	Trigeminal	Sensory—corneal reflex, light touch to face Motor—forced opening of mouth to resistance
CN VI	Abducens	Extraocular movement
CN VII	Facial	Raise eyebrow, forced eyelid closing, puff out cheeks
CN VIII	Vestibulo-cochlear	Audio acuity, balance, Romberg
CN IX	Glosso pharyngeal	Say "Ah," elevate palate
CN X	Vagus	Swallow, phonation
CN XI	Spinal accessory	Raise shoulders against resistance
CN XII	Hypoglossal	Stick out tongue, say "la-la-la"

Peripheral Sensory and Motor Function The sensory and gross motor function of each limb should be assessed for symmetry and strength. Unilateral deficits, also known as lateralizing, can be caused by central lesions or peripheral trauma. Abnormal posturing is seen in severe neurological dysfunction and in increased ICP.

Reflexes Assessment of reflexes can provide information to isolate lesions in trauma. The central motor pathways that connect the cerebral cortex to the anterior horn of the spinal cord are termed upper motor neurons (UMNs). The peripheral motor pathways distal to this point connect the spinal cord to the muscle and are termed lower motor neurons (LMNs). Injuries to either pathway can produce muscle paralysis. However, injuries to UMNs result in spastic muscle paralysis and hyperreflexia and can result in a positive Babinski reflex. In this abnormal reflex the great toe moves upward and the remaining toes fan outward when the bottom of the foot is briskly stroked. In contrast, LMN injuries result in flaccid muscle paralysis, hyporeflexia, and no Babinski reflex.

Other optic and vestibular reflexes (such as doll's eyes and cold calorics) are occasionally discussed as potential diagnostic tools for the evaluation of head trauma (Figures 11-12 and 11-13). While these tests may allow for a more specific diagnosis and isolation of the lesion, they are considered potentially harmful, difficult to interpret, and of little immediate diagnostic value.[37] The general recommendation is that they are best left to the neurologist and neurosurgeon.[37]

TREATMENT

The key prehospital priorities in head and neck trauma are the stabilization of the ABCs and the prevention of secondary brain injury. Despite major advances in the care of head and neck injury patients, the relatively basic measures of maintaining adequate oxygenation, perfusion, and support for other organ systems are the principal mechanisms for preventing secondary brain injury.[38] The frequent occurrence of hypoxemia and hypotension at the scene and during transport in head injury has been recognized as a widespread problem of international scale.[38–40]

AIRWAY CONTROL

Frequently, the most critical decision in airway management is whether the patient should be intubated. Endotracheal intubation may be required to manage the airway and to ensure adequate ventilation. In severe head trauma, early endotracheal intubation and aggressive airway control result in improved patient

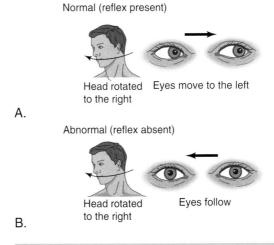

FIGURE 11-12 Test for oculocephalic reflex response (doll's eyes phenomenon): (A) normal response: eyes turn together toward opposite side of head turn; (B) abnormal response: eyes do not turn in conjugate manner. This test is best left for a physician.

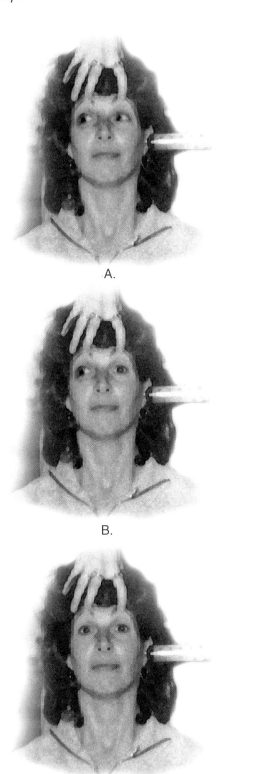

A.

B.

C.

FIGURE 11-13 Test for oculovestibular reflex (cold caloric test): (A) normal response: conjugate eye movements; (B) abnormal response: dysconjugate eye movement; (C) absent response: no eye movement. This test is best left for a neurosurgeon or neurologist.

outcome, and inappropriate airway care is frequently a major contributor to preventable trauma death.[41–43] Patients with GCS scores of less than 8 usually require immediate endotracheal intubation.[24] Oral endotracheal intubation is generally preferred in the prehospital setting; nasotracheal intubation should be avoided in any patient with a suspected basilar skull fracture and in children.[41,44] Cervical spine injury should be presumed and all manipulations of the airway must employ appropriate stabilization of the C-spine.

The most common indication for the use of neuromuscular blocking agents outside of the hospital setting is for airway management in the multiple-trauma victim with head injury. In one study, 68% of the patients that received neuromuscular blocking agents during transport had an associated head injury.[45] Rapid-sequence intubation (RSI) and use of neuromuscular blocking agents are safe and effective methods to facilitate oral intubation in these patients.[45–47] Indications for their use in head trauma include (1) to prevent elevated ICP during the process of intubation, gagging, and "bucking the tube"; (2) to reduce the risk of vomiting and aspiration during intubation; and (3) to reduce adverse effects of patient combativeness. The most common agents used for RSI in the head-injured patient are succinylcholine, fentanyl citrate (Sublimaze), and midazolam hydrochloride (Versed). While controversial, lidocaine (1 mg/kg) administered prior to RSI has demonstrated the ability to limit the increase in ICP associated with the intubation process.[48] For continued neuromuscular paralysis, the long-acting agents such as vecuronium are employed. However, it has been suggested that initial management of severe head trauma can be accomplished by using sedation alone and that early, routine, and long-term use of neuromuscular blocking agents is unnecessary and potentially harmful.[49]

The airway management of severe neck trauma is more complicated and controversial. Unfortunately, emergent airways are frequently needed in neck trauma. In determining the need for airway interventions in penetrating neck trauma, one series reported that emergent airways were necessary in over 50% of the patients, and a second series reported that intubation was emergently necessary in 23% and ultimately required for 60% of the patients.[50,51] In the hospital setting mortality can clearly be minimized by aggressive airway management, but airway procedures are not without risk in this patient group.[50] The straightforward task of routine airway control with endotracheal intubation can be technically difficult, if not impossible. For that reason, paralytics and RSI must be used with extreme caution. Although it has been shown that endotracheal intubation with RSI can be accomplished safely in selected neck trauma patients in the hospital setting, their safety and effectiveness in the prehospital setting remain largely unproved.[50] The airway control issue is further complicated by the potential to dramatically worsen laryngeal and tracheal injuries during airway manipulations and attempts at intubation. A misdirected attempt at intubation can convert a marginal airway into complete airway obstruction and death of the patient.[52] A conservative recommendation is to attempt elective intubations only with a surgical team present. The risks of blind intubations can be avoided with the use of fiber-optic bronchoscopy.[53] In general, elective intubations, especially blind nasotracheal intubations in the breathing patient, should be avoided in the prehospital setting. When the airway must be controlled and oral endotracheal intubation is not possible, a surgical airway may be necessary.

The most common indications for a prehospital surgical airway are massive facial trauma and failed oral intubation.[54] The principal prehospital surgical airway options are percutaneous transtracheal jet insufflation (TJI) and cricothyrotomy. These techniques are effective methods for rapid airway access during acute emergencies when standard airway techniques fail or are contraindicated.[55–60] While these temporizing measures can be life saving and have been associated with low complication rates, there are potential limitations.[57,58] Cricothyroidotomy is unlikely to work in the setting of cricothyroid separation and has been associated with thyroid cartilage lacerations, significant hemorrhage, displacement, and failure to obtain an airway.[59] Transtracheal jet insufflation is associated with total expiratory obstruction, pneumothorax, subcutaneous emphysema, and failure to obtain an airway.[55,61] The gold standard for a surgical airway in the setting of neck trauma is a tracheotomy placed by a surgical team.

BREATHING AND HYPERVENTILATION

Patients should be ventilated using high-flow supplemental oxygen to maintain a minimum PaO_2 greater than 90 mm Hg and monitored with continuous pulse oximetry. Untreated hypoxia and hypoventilation are common pitfalls to be avoided. The patient must be treated for any concomitant thoracic injuries, such as a tension pneumothorax, that may compromise breathing.

Although coming under increasing controversy, most trauma centers continue to hyperventilate severe head injury patients. A 1995 survey of trauma centers showed that 83% commonly use hyperventilation to reduce ICP with 29% of the centers aiming for $PaCO_2$ values of less than 25 mm Hg.[62] The physiological rationale for hyperventilation is that induced hypocapnia causes cerebral vasoconstriction, decreases cerebral blood flow, and results in reduced ICP. There is mounting evidence that hyperventilation in head injury may not

be as effective as previously thought, that it can potentially exacerbate neurological injury, and that it exposes the patient to potential side effects.[63–75] The clinical implication is that while aggressive hyperventilation, especially to achieve $PaCO_2$ levels below 30 mm Hg, will decrease ICP, it is not a benign therapy and its potential adverse effects must be taken into consideration.

CIRCULATION AND FLUID RESUSCITATION

In the multitrauma patient, systemic hypotension secondary to hypovolemia poses one of the greatest risks to cerebral perfusion. While controversy exists over the appropriate role of fluid resuscitation in trauma patients, fluid resuscitation is indicated in the head injury patient with hypovolemia and hypotension.[76–78] For head-injured patients, the goal is to maintain an adequate cerebral blood flow and perfusion while keeping the patient as normovolemic as possible. Fluid overload can contribute to cerebral edema and should be avoided. Isotonic crystalloids are the most commonly used fluids for initial resuscitation.

Head-injured patients can also present with hypertension. This condition is mainly seen in euvolemic patients with increased ICP. Because the increased systemic pressure may be a protective response to maintain cerebral perfusion in the face of increased ICP, antihypertensives are rarely appropriate or indicated in the prehospital setting.[79]

Hemorrhaging from neck injuries is treated with direct pressure. Attempting to control bleeding vessels by applying clamps or other instruments is not recommended. Major vessels, nerves, and the esophagus can be damaged by misplaced instruments. When establishing IV access for fluid resuscitation in neck trauma, avoid placing the IV in the arm on the same side as possible subclavian or zone I injuries. When these injuries are suspected, it is ideal to establish IV access above and below the diaphragm.

DIURETICS

Diuretics are commonly used by most trauma centers in severe head injury to reduce ICP.[62] Mannitol, an osmotic diuretic, is the principal diuretic agent employed to decrease ICP in the cardiovascularly stable head injury patient.[80] Its benefit is likely related to its ability to remain in the intravascular space and to increase serum osmolality. This agent produces an osmotic gradient between the brain and the intravascular space, causing a net movement of water across the blood-brain barrier. The movement of water into the intravascular space results in decreased brain parenchyma volume and reduced ICP. Mannitol is given as a bolus IV, over 10–30 minutes, in doses ranging from 0.25 to 1.0 g/kg body weight.[50] Although mannitol has not been associated with significant systolic blood pressure changes in the head injury patient, osmotic diuretics should be used with caution in patients with hypovolemia and multiple trauma.[80,81] Loop diuretics, like furosemide, have been used in conjunction with mannitol. However, loop diuretics by themselves have no effect on ICP. Patients receiving diuretics should have a Foley catheter and must be monitored for fluid and electrolyte imbalances.

PATIENT POSITION

Patient position during transport can theoretically affect ICP. It is a universally recommended practice that the head should be elevated to 30 degrees to decrease ICP and be maintained in a midline position to prevent jugular venous flow obstruction.[3,82,83] However, investigators have demonstrated that the decrease in ICP from head elevation may not be associated with an improvement in CPP.[82,84–86] Ideally, the degree of head elevation should be guided by monitoring ICP and CPP. In the prehospital setting and during acute resuscitation, the potential benefit of head elevation is of secondary importance and should never compromise immobilization of the C-spine. It has also been suggested that acceleration and deceleration forces generated during transport could affect ICP, but there is little evidence to support changing standard patient packaging or positioning practices.[3]

SEIZURES AND RESTLESSNESS

Patients with moderate or severe head injuries are at increased risk for seizures.[87] Early seizure disorders, which occur in less than 7 days postinjury, are seen in approximately 3%–5% of head injury patients.[88] However, seizures that occur early after injury are not a good prognostic indicator for chronic seizure disorders. Open head injuries and penetrating trauma carry the highest risk for late posttraumatic seizures, with about 4% of closed head injury and 50% of penetrating head-injury patients developing a long-term seizure disorder.[88,89] In pediatric head trauma, loss of consciousness, a GCS of 8 or less, and diffuse cerebral edema have also been associated with posttraumatic seizures.[90,91]

Patients who have been pharmacologically paralyzed may not present with a "typical" seizure. Cases of "invisible" or "subclinical" seizures without clinical motor convulsions have been identified in head-trauma patients by electroencephalogram (EEG).[92,93]

However, simply removing the motor component of the seizure does not protect the patient from the detrimental effects of the increased neurological activity of a seizure. In these patients, a seizure may present as increased pulse, hypertension, and pupillary change. Unrecognized seizures in head injury can result in increased secondary brain injury from increased ICP and cerebral hypoxia.

While it remains controversial to provide seizure prophylaxis, it should be considered in patients with open head injuries or depressed skull fractures. Phenytoin is commonly used at a loading dose of 10–20 mg/kg IV bolus (50 mg/min) and a maintenance of 300–400 mg/day in divided doses. Rapid administration can cause hypotension and should be avoided. Seizures can be treated in the prehospital setting with a short-acting benzodiazepine such as diazepam.

EMERGENCY DEPARTMENT

Initial hospital-based care will focus on the same goals as prehospital care: stabilization of the ABCs, decreasing ICP, and preventing secondary brain injury. The standard trauma resuscitation will typically begin with a reassessment of the ABCs and evaluation of prehospital interventions. If airway control remains an issue, it will be top priority. The hospital environment provides additional airway control options. In particular, the fiber-optic bronchoscope has been advocated for use in endotracheal intubation in neck trauma. This device allows for intubation under direct visualization of the airway structures below the vocal cords. The device can prevent the blind passage of an endotracheal tube into false channels created by trauma. It also allows the operator to confirm that the tube cuff is positioned below any tracheal or laryngeal injury.

Cardiac monitoring is standard. Hemodynamic monitoring, which may include arterial pressure lines and Swan-Ganz catheters, is typically indicated. A urinary catheter is placed to monitor renal output. Pharmacological therapies and fluid resuscitation, guided by hemodynamic monitoring, are administered to maintain high normal cardiac output and systolic blood pressures. An orogastric tube is typically preferred in the setting of head trauma in place of a nasogastric tube. Routine trauma laboratory studies, such as arterial blood gases, serum chemistries, blood counts, blood type and crossmatch, blood alcohol, and drug screens, are typically performed.

The standard initial radiographic studies conducted in the resuscitation of a multiple-trauma patient are of the C-spine, chest, and pelvis. This routine series provides an excellent starting point for head and neck trauma. The C-spine X-rays are typically conducted to evaluate for cervical skeletal trauma. Soft tissue films of the neck are indicated in the setting of neck trauma to rule out occult injury, which includes retropharyngeal hematomas, tracheal narrowing, foreign bodies, subcutaneous air, or retropharyngeal air. For evaluation of the larynx, CT is used.

Computerized tomography is the radiographic study of choice in the evaluation of acute head injury. Most patients with a GCS score of less than 15, focal neurological findings, or abnormal mental status will receive CT studies. The role of plain film skull radiographs and magnetic resonance imaging is limited in the initial evaluation of head trauma.

Additional special studies are commonly needed in the evaluation of head and neck trauma. When vascular injury is suspected, arteriography is the gold standard diagnostic study. Cerebral angiography is indicated in blunt neck trauma patients that present with neurological findings to rule out vascular injury-induced cerebral hypoxia and ischemia. Esophagoscopy, bronchoscopy, and laryngoscopy are additional studies employed to evaluate neck trauma.

Surgical consultation should be obtained early in the care of the trauma patient. Emergent neurosurgical evaluation and possible intervention is required for patients with (1) presence of coma; (2) altered mental status resulting from nonvehicular trauma; (3) focal neurological findings or unequal motor strength; (4) massive, depressed, or open skull fractures; or (5) large focal lesions on CT scan.[94] Emergent surgical consultation for neck trauma is clearly indicated in patients with (1) zone II injuries that penetrate the platysma, (2) subcutaneous or retropharyngeal airseal on neck radiograph, (3) active bleeding, (4) absent pulse or bruit, and (5) neurological deficit. In actual practice, most significantly injured trauma patients are admitted to surgical services. Because of the need for specialized surgical and support services, these patients are frequently transferred to tertiary care facilities.

Intracranial pressure monitoring is routinely performed for severe head injury patients in many institutions and is most commonly used for patients with a GCS score of 8 or less, patients with GCS scores of 9–12 that require nonneurosurgical interventions under general anesthesia, and all patients that require a neurosurgical procedure.[62] Head-injured patients that are unable to follow simple commands are candidates for ICP monitoring and close, frequent neurological evaluation. The subarachnoid screw, or bolt, and the intraventricular catheter are the two most common devices used to monitor ICP. Both devices require drilling a small hole into the skull. After placement, the device is attached to a transducer for continuous pressure monitoring. The subarachnoid bolt is threaded into the subarachnoid space, carries less risk of infec-

tion, and is often easier to place. The ventriculostomy catheter is positioned into the lateral ventricle, and is advantageous because of its ability to drain CSF. Because of this advantage, one survey showed that 72% of the trauma centers use this device, and of those, 44% commonly employed therapeutic CSF drainage to reduce ICP.[62] Other options for ICP monitoring include the intraparenchymal fiber-optic catheter and epidural monitor (Figure 11-14).

INTERNET ACTIVITIES

Visit the e-medicine Web site at http://www.emedicine.com/. Click on the Emergency Medicine on-line book and select Trauma and Orthopedics. Then click on Neck Trauma. Review the chapter on the management of neck trauma.

CURRENT RESEARCH AND EXPERIMENTAL TREATMENTS

Hyperventilation, once a traditional cornerstone of prehospital and hospital care for the head-injured patient, has come under considerable controversy.[63–75,82] More recent research using xenon-enhanced CT (Xe-CT) has demonstrated that the effects of CO_2 on cerebral blood flow are not uniform throughout the brain.[63,69,72,95,96] These studies show that normal patterns of autoregulation are impaired by injury, and decreasing CO_2 causes vasoconstriction and decreased cerebral blood flow in some regions and paradoxical vasodilation in other regions. Xenon-enhanced CT has shown that the tissue within and around a cerebral trauma is relatively hypoperfused and hypersensitive to the effects of hyperventilation therapy.[69,72,75,96] The Xe-CT studies show that hyperventilation causes a highly variable response in and around injured brain tissue, including increased blood flow into the lesion, ischemic blood flow in previously normal areas, and worsening of existing ischemia.[69,75] The implications are that aggressive hyperventilation can worsen secondary brain injury by a complex and variable mechanism. Current research has consistently reported that routine and indiscriminate use of hyperventilation negatively affects head-injured patient outcomes; one of the few randomized clinical trials looking at the issue was discontinued because of poor outcomes in the group treated with hyperventilation.[75,97] This leads to the recommendation that unless specifically attempting to decrease ICP in the face of a pending cerebral herniation, aggressive hyperventilation should be avoided in patients without appropriate

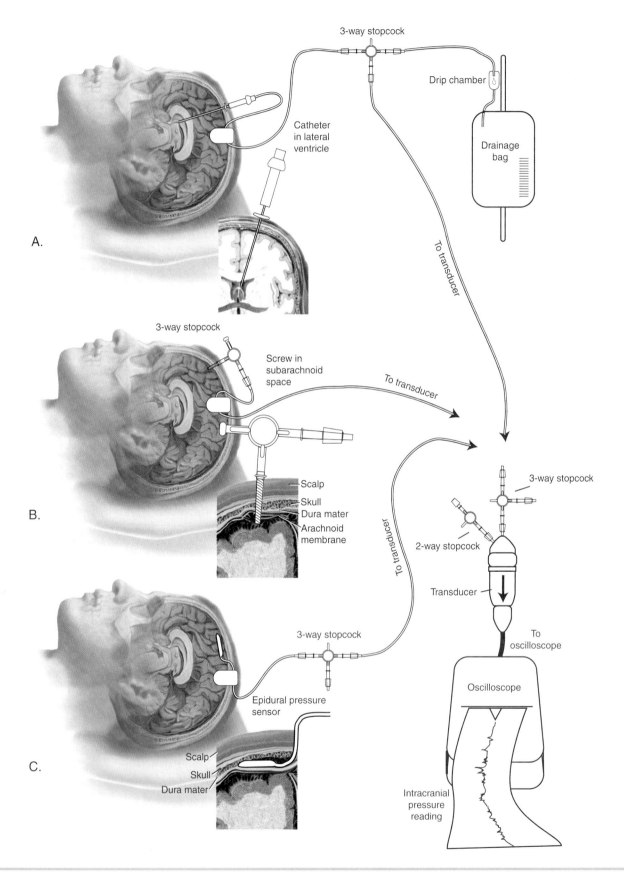

FIGURE 11-14 Intracranial pressure monitoring techniques: (A) intraventricular catheter; (B) subarachnoid screw; (C) epidural pressure sensor.

physiological monitoring.[71,75,97,98] While not universally accepted as the standard of care, authorities are beginning to recommend that prophylactic hyperventilation not be a part of routine prehospital care for head injury and that most head injury patients should be ventilated to achieve adequate oxygenation and normocapnia.[71,75,97,98] In the hospital setting, routine ventilation for head injury should be adjusted to achieve a measured $PaCO_2$ of about 35 mm Hg.[98]

Head injury is associated with elevated CSF lactate and cerebral acidosis, which can be a contributing cause of cerebral edema and increased ICP.[99,100] Hyperventilation to produce systemic alkalosis has been advocated in head injury to counter these effects. However, it is now known that the effects of hyperventilation on buffering CSF acidosis are short lived and the resulting cerebral vasoconstrictive effects of aggressive hyperventilation may worsen cerebral acidosis.[97,101] As an alternative and adjunct to hyperventilation, the use of trishydroxymethyl aminomethane (THAM) has been advocated. An intravenously administered buffering solution, THAM can cross the blood-brain barrier and alkalize the CSF. Initial studies have shown that when THAM is given by constant infusion for 5 days, patients have improved control of ICP, less requirement for barbiturate coma, and improved 3- and 6-month outcomes.[97,101,102]

VOLUME REPLACEMENT

Researchers are attempting to define the optimal volume status for severe head injury patients.[82] The traditional biases toward fluid restriction and diuresis to reduce ICP in the setting of severe head injury have come under question. While the normal adult CPP is 80–100 mm Hg, the targeted CPP during treatment is often significantly lower and typically near 60 mm Hg.[82,83] A higher CPP of 70–80 mm Hg has demonstrated lower mortality and morbidity.[84,103] Some centers have shifted focus of management from reducing ICP to maintaining CPP.[103] To maintain this higher CPP, patients often require complex management with volume expansion, systemic vasopressors (phenylephrine or norepinephrine), CSF drainage via ventriculostomy, and mannitol.[103] Patients treated with volume restriction and diuresis have shown worse outcomes. It is clear that hypotension continues to be a common problem in the management of head trauma and that it is associated with worse patient outcomes.[104] In one series, hypotension as defined by a systolic blood pressure of less that 90 mm Hg in the setting of head injury is associated with a 150% increase in mortality.[105] There is no evidence that fluid administration to achieve normovolemia in the trauma patient has an adverse effect on ICP.[105] However, vigorous volume expansion in hemorrhagic hypovolemia with crystalloid, to the point of elevated central venous pressure (CVP) in experimental animal models with traumatic brain injury results in increased intracranial hypertension.[106] Current researchers are recommending aggressive initial fluid therapy in the face of hypotension, fluid volume resuscitation to achieve normovolemia, and avoiding diuresis.[98,105] Ideally, volume replacement should be guided by hemodynamic monitoring to achieve a CVP of 6–8 mm Hg and a CPP of 70 mm Hg.[82,105]

HYPOTHERMIA

It is known that hypothermia decreases cerebral metabolic rate and improves ICP in the head injury patient. Initial studies investigating the effects of moderate hypothermia of 32°C–34°C in head injury have shown improved ICP control, decreased O_2 consumption, reduced cerebral ischemia, and improved outcomes.[107–113] Hypothermia is induced by cooling the patient's body surface area with water-circulating cooling blankets; other methods such as peritoneal dialysis and cold saline gastric lavage have also been used.[108,114] However, potentially hazardous cardiac, renal, coagulation, and pancreatic side effects may be associated with hypothermia.[111]

NEUROPROTECTIVE AGENTS

Investigators continue to implicate secondary brain injury as a much more important cause of head trauma morbidity and mortality than previously believed. While we know the prevention of hypoxia and hypotension is the primary means to reduce secondary brain injury, much of the current research is focused on understanding the pathophysiology of this process. It is thought that the traumatic event of a head injury activates a "neurotoxic cascade." This biochemical process exacerbates the neuronal destruction and may also cause damage to surrounding uninjured brain cells. The two pathways that have received the most attention are the excitatory amino acids and free radicals.

Following injury, the brain releases a large quantity of excitatory neurotransmitters. In particular, the release of amino acid glutamate stimulates cell membrane receptors that allow an influx of calcium into the cell. The increased intracellular calcium is thought to cause enzyme dysfunction, increased acidosis, cellular edema, and cell death. Ischemia within the cell results in the production of highly reactive oxygen-free radicals. The oxygen-free radicals react with the lipids in the cell membrane, resulting in damage that contributes to the cellular edema and death of the cell. There are numerous novel pharmacological agents under investigation to alter this biochemical process.[98,115–117] Examples of these neuroprotective agents are listed in Table 11-6. It is also speculated that the "success" of certain traditional therapies, like mannitol and glucocorticoids, can be attributed to their effect on this neurotoxic pathway and not their traditionally accepted mechanisms of action.[115]

STEROIDS

Although commonly employed by many trauma centers, the use of steroids to treat increased ICP is controversial.[62] Dexamethasone and other agents have been used, but their effectiveness has been questioned. Critics of steroid therapy cite multiple studies that have failed to prove that high-dose steroids can improve ICP or long-term patient outcome.[118] While more research is needed, evidence is emerging that triamcinolone, a relatively new synthetic corticosteroid, started within 4 hours of trauma improves outcome in severe head trauma.[119] Methylprednisolone, a glucocorticoid steroid, has been used to enhance recovery in spinal cord injury.[120] This steroid is thought to have some neuroprotective effects through inhibition of oxygen-free radicals, but its use in head trauma is largely unresolved.[121] Other agents, such as the 21-amino steroids, are under investigation and may play a role in the management of head trauma in the future.[122]

▶ SUMMARY

Regardless of the practice environment, head and neck injuries are frequently encountered. Because these injuries represent some of the most serious threats to life in the trauma patient, the skills to manage these problems must be mastered. A major advance has been our new understanding of the critical role that secondary brain injury plays in the destruction of neurological tissue. This has reinforced the view that the management priorities in head and neck trauma are the stabilization of the ABCs. Despite the development of novel pharmacological agents and the potential of other experimental treatment, the relatively basic measures of maintaining adequate oxygenation, perfusion, and support for other organ systems are the principal mechanisms for preventing secondary brain injury.

Table 11-6
Investigational Pharmacology for Head Injury

Group	Example Drugs	Action
Glutamate antagonist	MK801 D-CPP-ene Cholinergic agents (citacholine, scopolamine, PCP) Magnesium Dextromethorphan	Inhibit neurotoxic effect of excitatory amino acids. Some specifically block glutamate effect on NMDA cell membrane receptor and prevent calcium influx.
Calcium antagonist	Nimodipine	Block calcium channel to reduce influx of calcium.
Oxygen radical scavenger	PEG-SOD Dimethyl sulfoxide Mannitol Tirilazad mesylate Vitamin E	Inhibit lipid peroxidation of cell membrane by oxygen-free radicals. Stabilize cell membrane.

Other
  Anti-inflammatory
 	
  Narcotic antagonist
 	
  Growth factors
	
	Ibuprofen
	Indomethacin
	Naloxone
	
	Gangliosides
	NGF, BDGF
		
		Reduce ICP and improve CPP by blocking effects of cyclooxygenase.
		Block endogenous opiate release following percussion head injury leading to decreased cerebral blood flow.
		Neuroregenerative action and possible reduction of neuronal damage by blocking "neurotoxic cascade"

▶ REVIEW QUESTIONS

1. Approximately what percentage of trauma deaths are associated with head injury?
   a. 25%
   b. 50%
   c. 75%
   d. None of the above

2. Cerebral perfusion pressure can be approximated by:
   a. Mean intracranial pressure minus mean systolic blood pressure (ICP – SBP)
   b. Mean systolic blood pressure minus mean intracranial pressure (SBP – ICP)
   c. Mean intracranial pressure minus mean arterial pressure (ICP – MAP)
   d. Mean arterial pressure minus mean intracranial pressure (MAP – ICP)

3. Which of the following statements are correct?
   a. The right cerebral hemisphere provides motor function to the left side of the body.
   b. The right cerebral hemisphere provides sensory function for the right side of the body.
   c. Both a and b
   d. Neither a nor b

4. Which statement about secondary brain injury is correct?
   a. It results from the transfer of kinetic energy at the moment of impact.
   b. It is defined and described by the Monro-Kellie principle.
   c. An example is the contrecoup component of a coup/contrecoup injury.
   d. Common mechanisms include hypoxia, systemic hypotension, or increased ICP.

5. Cushing's triad is described as:
   a. Increased blood pressure, increased pulse, and increased respirations
   b. Increased pulse pressure, decreased respirations, and irregular pulse
   c. Increased blood pressure, decreased pulse, and irregular respirations
   d. Increased pulse pressure, dilated pupil, and unresponsiveness

6. Which is *not* a theory about the mechanism of diffuse axonal injury?
   a. That it represents one of the mildest and most benign forms of brain injury
   b. That it is a primary injury seen in rapid deceleration caused by the separation of tissues with different densities
   c. That it is a secondary injury that can be exacerbated by hypoxia and hypotension

   d. That it represents a potentially lethal form of brain injury

7. Which statement concerning an epidural hematoma is correct?
   a. The "classic" presentation involves a brief initial loss of consciousness, followed by mental clearing, then subsequent deterioration.
   b. About one-third never lose consciousness and about one-third never regain consciousness after injury.
   c. Both a and b
   d. Neither a nor b

8. Which statement concerning a subdural hematoma is *incorrect*?
   a. It involves a collection of blood between the dura mater and the arachnoid mater.
   b. Typically the injured vessel is a bridging vein.
   c. Signs in over 50% of the cases include ipsilateral dilated pupil, focal neurological deficits, and contralateral hemiparesis.
   d. This type of hematoma is 10 times more common than an epidural hematoma.

9. The most fundamental and important element of the neurological evaluation is:
   a. Pupil size and reaction
   b. Level of consciousness
   c. Glasgow Coma Scale
   d. Focal neurological findings

10. While establishing an IV in the right arm of a head injury patient, you note the following: no movement of the right arm with painful stimulation but reaches with the left arm toward the right side, no eye opening, and makes incomprehensible sounds. What is this patient's GCS score?
    a. 6
    b. 7
    c. 8
    d. None of the above

11. Which of the following statements are true about the oculomotor nerve?
    a. It contains the parasympathetic fibers that innervate the pupil to constrict.
    b. If compromised by an acute mass lesion, the lesion is typically on the opposite side of the skull in about 90% of the cases.
    c. Both a and b
    d. Neither a nor b

12. The primary priority in severe head injury with suspected mass lesion is:
    a. Airway control
    b. Decreasing ICP
    c. Maintaining CBF (cerebral blood flow)
    d. Preventing systemic hypotension

13. Hypotension in the setting of severe head injury:
  a. Is almost never due to intracranial hemorrhage in an adult
  b. Is frequently secondary to compression of the cardiovascular centers from massive intracranial bleeding in adults
  c. Should not be treated with rapid fluid resuscitation because of the risk of increased ICP
  d. May develop from hypovolemia secondary to intracranial bleeding or subgaleal hematoma in infants with isolated head injury

14. Head injury patients with a GCS score of 8 will typically require:
  a. Endotracheal intubation with careful cervical spinal stabilization
  b. Nasotracheal intubation if under age 16
  c. Surgical airway because they have high incidence of cervical spine injuries
  d. Rapid-sequence induction in nearly all cases

15. In the prehospital setting, hypertensive head injury patients with suspected mass lesion and increased ICP should receive immediate treatment with:
  a. Antihypertensive agents
  b. Prophylactic use of anticonvulsant agent
  c. Both a and b
  d. Neither a nor b

16. Emergent neurosurgical evaluation of a head injury patient is indicated with:
  a. Coma
  b. Focal neurological findings
  c. Depressed skull fracture
  d. All of the above

▶ CRITICAL THINKING

● In neurotrauma intensive care units, patients are frequently placed on norepinephrine drips to maintain relatively high blood pressures, so high in fact that patients sometimes require amputation of digits due to profound vasoconstriction and ischemia. Why are such high doses of vasoconstrictors sometimes necessary?

● Using your knowledge of the mechanisms of hyperventilation to treat elevated intracranial pressure, explain why "paper bag" therapy should never be employed in the treatment of simple hyperventilation syndrome.

● You are called to the scene to treat a patient who was injured during a softball game. Upon arrival you find a 27-year-old male who was struck in the left temporal area by a line drive. There was an initial loss of consciousness of approximately 3 minutes, after which the patient regained consciousness and returned to the dugout complaining of a headache. About an hour later the patient was found unconscious. Physical examination reveals a hematoma over the left temple, a dilated left pupil, and flaccid paralysis on the right side. What is your assessment of this patient? At what level has brain stem compression progressed? What is the pathophysiology of the history of the present illness and presenting signs and symptoms?

▶ REFERENCES

1. Borel C, Handley D, Diringer MN, Rogers MC. Intensive management of severe head injury. *Chest*. 1990; 98:180.
2. Olshaker JS, Whye DW. Head trauma. *Emerg Med Clin North Am*. 1992; 11(1):165.
3. Vernon D, Woodard G, Skjonsberg A. Management of the patient with head injury during transport. *Crit Care Clin*. 1992; 8:619.
4. Buterworth J, Dewitt D. Severe head trauma: pathophysiology and management. *Crit Care Clin*. 1989; 5:807.
5. Rockswald GL. Head injury. In: Tintinalli JE, Raize, Kromer, et al, eds. *Emergency Medicine: A Comprehensive Study Guide*. 4th ed. New York: McGraw-Hill; 1996: 1139.
6. Cooper PR. Epidemiology of head injury. In: Cooper PR, ed. *Head Injury*. Baltimore, Md: Williams & Wilkins; 1982.
7. Gentleman D, Jennett B. Hazard of interhospital transfer of comatose head injured patients. *Lancet*. 1981; II:853.
8. Grande C. Critical care transport: a trauma perspective. *Crit Care Clin*. 1990; 6(1):165.
9. Jurkovich GJ. Definitive care phase: neck injuries. In: Greenfield LZ, et al, eds. *Surgery: Scientific Principle and Practice*. Philadelphia: JB Lippincott; 1993.
10. Saletta J, Lowe RJ, Lim LT, Thornton J, Delk S, Moss GS. Penetrating neck trauma. *J Trauma*. 1976; 16:579.
11. Sankaran S, Walt A. Penetrating wounds of the neck: principles and some controversies. *Surg Clin North Am*. 1977; 57:139.
12. Pfenninger J, Kaiser G, Lutschg J, Slutter M. Treatment and outcome of the severely head injured child. *Intens Care Med*. 1983; 9:13.
13. Plum B, Posner J. *The Diagnosis of Stupor and Coma*. 3rd ed. Philadelphia: FA Davis; 1982.
14. Bruce DA, Schut L, Bruno, LA: Outcome following severe head injuries in children. *J Neurosurg*. 1978; 48:679.

15. Miller JD, Becker DP, Ward JD, Sullivan HG, Adams WE, Rosner MJ. Significance of intracranial hypertension in severe head injury. *J Neurosurg.* 1977; 47:503.

16. Marmarou A, Anderson R, Ward J, et al. Impact of ICP instability and hypotension on outcome in patients with severe head trauma. *J Neurosurg.* 1991; 75:S59.

17. Esinhorn A, Mizrahi EM. Basilar skull fracture in children: the incidence of CNS infection and the use of antibiotics. *Am J Dis Child.* 1978; 132:1121.

18. Gennarelli TA. Mechanisms of brain injury. *J Emerg Med.* 1993; 11:5.

19. Povlishock JT. Pathobiology of traumatically induced axonal injury in animals and man. *Ann Emerg Med.* 1993; 22(6):980.

20. Strich SJ. Diffuse degeneration of the cerebral white matter in severe dementia following head injury. *J Neurol Neurosurg Psychiatry.* 1956; 19:163.

21. Strich SJ. Shearing nerve fibers as a cause of brain damage due to head injury. *Lancet.* 1961; 2:443.

22. Adams JH, Graham DI, Gennarelli TA, Maxwell WL. Diffuse axonal injury in non-missile head injury. *J Neurol Neurosurg Psychiatry.* 1991; 54:481.

23. Polishock JT, Cristman CW. The pathobiology of traumatically induced axonal injury in animals and humans: a review of current thought. *J Neurotrauma.* 1995; 12:555.

24. Salcman M, Geiser F. Emergency: head trauma. *Hosp Med.* 1993; 29(4)78.

25. Andrews BT, Levy ML, Pitts LH. Implications of systemic hypotension for the neurological examination in patients with severe head injury. *Surg Neurol.* 1987; 28(6):419.

26. Jamieson KG, Yllland JDN. Extradural hematoma: report of 167 cases. *J Neurosurg.* 1968; 29:13.

27. Pons PT. Head trauma. In: Rosen P, Baker J, Barker R, eds. *Emergency Medicine: Concepts and Clinical Practice.* St Louis, Mo: Mosby Year Book; 1992.

28. Elsner H, Rigamonti D, Corradino G, Schlegel R Jr., Joslyn J. Delayed traumatic intracerebral hematomas: "Spat-Apoplexie." *J Neurotrauma.* 1990; 72:(5):813.

29. Robertson CS, Gopinath SP, Chance B. A new application for near-infrared spectroscopy: detection of delayed intracranial hematomas after head injury. *J Neurotrauma.* 1995; 12(4):591.

30. Andrews BT, Chiles BW 3rd, Olsen WL, Pitts LH. The effect of intracerebral hematoma location on the risk of brain stem compression and on clinical outcome. *J Neurosurg.* 1988; 69(4):518.

31. Ward JD, Chisholm AH, Prince VT, Gilman CB, Hawkins AM. Penetrating head injury. *Crit Care Nurs Q.* 1994; 17(1):70.

32. Kaufman H, Moake JL, Olson J, et al. Delayed and recurrent intracranial hematomas related to dissem-inate intravascular clotting and fibrinolysis in head injury. *J Neurosurg.* 1980; 7:445.

33. Golueke P, Sclafani S, Phillips T, Goldstein A, Scalia T, Duncan A. Vertebral artery injury: diagnosis and management. *J Trauma.* 1987; 27:856.

34. Angood PB, Attia EL, Brow BA, Mulder DS. Extrinsic civilian trauma to larynx and cervical trachea: important predictors of long-term morbidity. *J Trauma.* 1986; 26:869.

35. Hills MW, Deane SA. Head injury and facial injury: is there an increased risk of cervical spine injury? *J Trauma.* 1993; 34(4):549.

36. Marion DW, Carter PM. Problems with initial Glasgow Coma Scale assessment caused by prehospital treatment of patients with head injuries: results of a national survey. *J Trauma.* 1994; 36(1):89.

37. American College of Surgeons (ACS). *Advanced Trauma Life Support Student Manual.* Chicago, Ill: ACS; 1993.

38. Chesnut RM. Secondary brain insults after head injury: clinical perspectives. *New Horizons.* 1995; 3(3):366.

39. Stocchetti N, Furlan A, Volta F. Hypoxemia and arterial hypotension at the accident scene in head injury. *J Trauma.* 1996; 40(5):764.

40. Wald SL, Shackford SR, Fenwick J. The effect of secondary insults on mortality and long-term disability after severe head injury in a rural region without a trauma system. *J Trauma.* 1993; 34(3):377.

41. Pepe P, Stewar R, Copass M. Prehospital management of trauma: a tale of three cities. *Ann Emerg Med.* 1986; 15(12):1484.

42. Ampel L, Hott KA, Sielaff GW, Sloan TB. An approach to airway management in the acutely head-injured patient. *J Emerg Med.* 1988; 6(1):7.

43. Esposito TJ, Sandal ND, Hansen JD, Reynolds S. Analysis of preventable trauma deaths and inappropriate trauma care in a rural state. *J Trauma.* 1995; 39(5):955.

44. O'brien DJ, Danzl DF, Sowers MB, Hooker EA. Airway management of aeromedically transported trauma patients. *J Emerg Med.* 1988; 6:49.

45. Murphy-Macabobby M, Marshall WJ, Schneider C, Dries D. Neuromuscular blockade in aeromedical airway management. *Ann Emerg Med.* 1992; 21(6):664.

46. Norwood S, Myers MB, Butler TJ. The safety of emergency neuromuscular blockade and orotracheal intubation in the acutely head injured trauma patient. *J Am Coll Surg.* 1994; 179(6):646.

47. Redan JA, Livingston DH, Tortella BJ, Rush BF Jr. The value of intubating and paralyzing patients with suspected head injury in the emergency department. *J Trauma.* 1991; 31(3):371.

48. Walls R. Rapid-sequence intubation in head trauma. *Ann Emerg Med.* 1993; 22:1008.

49. Hsiang JK, Chestnut RM, Crisp CB, Klauber MR, Blint BA, Marshall LF. Early routine paralysis for intracranial pressure control in severe head injury: is it necessary? *Crit Care Med.* 1993; 22(9):1471.

50. Grewal H, Roa PM, Mukerji S, Ivatury R. Management of penetrating laryngotracheal injuries. *Head & Neck.* 1995; 17(6):494.

51. Eggen JT, Jorden RC. Airway management, penetrating neck trauma. *J Emerg Med.* 1993; 11(4):381.

52. Shearer VE, Giesecke AH. Airway management for patients with penetrating neck trauma: a retrospective study. *Anesthesia & Analgesia.* 1993; 77(6):1135.

53. Cicala RS, Kudsk KA, Butts A, Nguyen H, Fabian TC. Initial evaluation and management of upper airway injuries in trauma patients. *J Clin Anesthesia.* 1991; 3(2):91.

54. Spaite DW, Joseph M. Prehospital cricothyrotomy: an investigation of indications, technique, and patient outcome. *Ann Emerg Med.* 1990; 19(3):279.

55. Weymuller EA Jr, Pavlin EG, Paugh D, Cummings CW. Management of difficult airway problems with percutaneous transtracheal ventilation. *Ann Otol Rhinol Laryngol.* 1987; 96(1):34.

56. Xeropotamos NS, Coats TJ, Wilson AW. Prehospital surgical airway management: one year's experience from the Helicopter Emergency Medical Service. *Injury.* 1993; 24(4):222.

57. Salvino CK, Dries D, Gamelli R, Murphy-Macabobby M, Marshall W. Emergency cricothyroidotomy in trauma victims. *J Trauma.* 1993; 34(4):503.

58. Jacobson LE, Gomez GA, Sobieray RJ, Rodman GH, Solotkin KC, Misinski ME. Surgical cricothyroidotomy in trauma patients: analysis of its use by paramedics in the field. *J Trauma.* 1996; 41(1):15.

59. Hawkins ML, Shapiro MO, Cue H, Wiggins SS. Emergency cricothyroidotomy: A reassessment. *Amer Surg.* 1995; 61(1):52.

60. Delaurier GA. Acute airway management: role of cricothyroidotomy. *Am Surg.* 1990; 56(1):12.

61. Metz S, Parmet JL, Levitt JD. Failed emergency transtracheal ventilation through a 14-gauge intravenous catheter. *J Clin Anesthesia.* 1996; 8(1):58.

62. Ghajar J, Hariri RJ, Narayan RK, Iacono LA, Firlik K, Patterson RH. Survey of critical care management of comatose, head-injured patients in the United States. *Crit Care Med.* 1995; 239(3):560.

63. Stringer W, Hasso AN, Thompson JR, Hinshaw DB, Jordan KG. Hyperventilation-induced cerebral ischemia in patient with acute brain lesion: demonstrated by xenon enhanced CT. *Am J Neuroradiol.* 1993; 14:475.

64. Muizelaar J, Marmarou A, Ward JD, et al. Adverse effects of prolonged hyperventilation in patients with severe head injury: a randomized clinical trial. *J Neurosurg.* 1991; 75:731.

65. Buoma GJ. Blood pressure and intracranial pressure-volume dynamics in severe head injury: relationship with cerebral blood flow. *J Neurosurg.* 1992; 77(1):15.

66. Cold GE. Does acute hyperventilation provoke cerebral oligaemia in comatose patients after acute head injury? *Acta Neurchir.* 1989; 98:153.

67. Crosby LJ, Parsons LC. Cerebrovascular response of closed head injury patients to a standardized endotracheal tube suctioning and manual hyperventilation procedure. *J Neurosci Nurs.* 1992; 24(1):40.

68. Cruz J, Miner ME, Allen SJ, Alves WM, Gennarelli TA. Continuous monitoring of cerebral oxygenation in acute brain injury: injection of mannitol during hyperventilation. *J Neurosurg.* 1990; 73:725.

69. Darby JM, Yonas H, Marion DW, Latchaw RE. Local "inverse steal" induced by hyperventilation in head injury. *J Neurosurg.* 1988; 23:84.

70. Elias-Jones AC, Punt JA, Turnbull AE, Jaspan T. Management and outcome of severe head injury in Trent region 1985–90. *Arch Dis Child.* 1992; 67:1430.

71. Kerr ME, Brucia J. Hyperventilation in the head-injured patient: an effective treatment modality? *Heart Lung.* 1993; 22:516.

72. Marion DW, Darby J, Yonas H. Acute regional cerebral blood flow changes caused by severe head injuries. *J Neurosurg.* 1991; 74(3):407.

73. Obrist WD, et al. Cerebral blood flow and metabolism in comatose patients with acute head injury. *J Neurosurg.* 1984; 61:241.

74. von Helden, Schneider C, Unterberg A, Lanicsa W. Monitoring of jugular venous oxygen saturation in comatose patients with subarachnoid hemorrhages and intracerebral hematomas. *Acta Neurchir.* 1993; 59:102.

75. Geraci E, Geraci T. A look at recent hyperventilation studies: outcomes and recommendations for early use in the head injured patient. *J Neurosci Nurs.* 1996; 28(4):222.

76. Pollack CV Jr. Prehospital fluid resuscitation of the trauma patient: an update on the controversies. *Emerg Med Clin North Am.* 1993; 11(1):61.

77. Bickell WH, Wall MJ Jr., Pepe PE, et al. Immediate versus delayed fluid resuscitation for hypotensive patients with penetrating torso injuries. *N Engl J Med.* 1994; 331(17):1105.

78. Capone AC, Safar P, Stezoski W, Tisherman S, Peitzman AB. Improved outcome with fluid resuscitation in treatment of uncontrolled hemorrhagic shock. *J Am Coll Surg.* 1995; 180(1):49.

79. Cottrell J, Patel K, Turndorf H, Ransohoff J. Intracranial pressure changes induced by sodium

nitroprusside in patients with intracranial mass lesions. *J Neurosurg*. 1978; 48:329.

80. Bullock R. Mannitol and other diuretics in severe neurotrauma. *New Horizons*. 1995; 3(3):448.

81. Sayre MR, Daily SW, Stern SA, Storer DL, van Loveren HR, Hurst JM. Out-of-hospital administration of mannitol to head-injured patients does not change systolic blood pressure. *Academic Emerg Med*. 1996; 3(9):840.

82. Eisenhart K. New perspectives in the management of adults with severe head injury. *Crit Care Nurs Q*. 1994; 17:2.

83. Marshall SB, et al. *Neuroscience Critical Care: Pathophysiology and Patient Management*. Philadelphia: WB Saunders; 1990.

84. Rosner MJ, Daughton S. Cerebral perfusion management in head injury. *J Trauma*. 1990; 30:933.

85. March K, Mitchell P, Grady S, Winn R. Effect of backrest position on intracranial and cerebral perfusion pressures. *J Neurosci Nurs*. 1990; 22:375.

86. Rosner MJ, Coley I. Cerebral profusion pressure, the ICP and head elevation. *J Neurosurg Nurs*. 1986; 65:636.

87. Annegers JF, Grabow JD, Groover RV, Laws ER Jr, Elveback LR, Kurkland, LT. Seizures after head trauma: a population study. *Neurology*. 1980; 30:683.

88. Kuhl DA, Boucher BA, Muhlbauer MS. Prophylaxis of post-traumatic seizures. *DICP*. 1990; 24(3):277.

89. Jennett B, Miller J, Braakman R. Epilepsy after nonmissile depressed skull fracture. *J Neurosurg*. 1974; 41:2008.

90. Lewis RJ, Yee L, Inkelis SH, Gilmore D. Clinical predictors of post-traumatic seizures in children. *J Neurosurg*. 1988; 22(5):864.

91. Hahn, YS, Hahny, Fuehs S, Flannery A, Barthel M, McLone D, et al: Factors influencing post-traumatic seizures in children with head trauma. *Ann Emergmed*. 1988; 22(5)864.

92. Beni L, Constantiini S, Matoth I, Pomeranz S. Subclinical status epilepticus in a child after closed head injury. *J Trauma*. 1996; 40(3):449.

93. Ryan C, Edmonds J. Seizure activity mimicking brain stem herniation in children following head injuries. *Crit Care Med*. 1988; 16:812.

94. Pousada L, Osborn H, Levy D. *Emergency Medicine (House Officer Series)*, 2 ed. Baltimore: Williams & Wilkins; 1966: 144.

95. Marion D, Buoma G. The use of stable xenon-enhanced computer tomographic studies of cerebral blood flow to define changes in cerebral carbon dioxide vasoresponsivity caused by severe head injury. *J Neurosurg*. 1991; 29:869.

96. McLaughlin MR, Marion DW. Cerebral blood flow and vasoresponsivity within and around cerebral contusions. *J Neurosurg*. 1996; 85(5):871.

97. Muizelaar JP, Schroder ML. Overview of monitoring cerebral blood flow and metabolism after severe head injury. *Can J Neurol Sci*. 1994; 21:S6.

98. Mayer TA. Frontiers in the management of traumatic brain injury. Presented at the 1996 ACEP Scientific Assembly; 1996; New Orleans, La.

99. DeSalles AA, Kontos HA, Becker DP, et al. Prognostic significance of ventricular CSF lactate acidosis in severe head injury. *J Neurosurg*. 1986; 65:615.

100. Envoldsen EM, Jensen FT. Cerebrospinal fluid lactate and pH in patients with acute severe head injury. *Clin Neurol Neurosurg*. 1977; 80:213.

101. Wolf A, Levi L, Marmarou A, et al. Effect of THAM upon outcome in severe head injury: a randomized prospective clinical trial. *J Neurosurg*. 1993; 78:54.

102. Rosner MJ, Elias KG, Coley I. Prospective, randomized trial of THAM therapy in severe brain injury: preliminary results. In: Hoff JT, Betz AL, eds. *Intracranial Pressure*. Vol VII. Berlin: Springer-Verlag; 1989.

103. Rosner MJ, Rosner SD, Johnson AH. Cerebral perfusion pressure: management protocol and clinical results. *J Neurosurg*. 1995; 83(6):949.

104. Winchell RJ, Simmons RK, Hoyt DB. Transient systolic hypotension: a serious problem in the management of head injury. *Arch Surg*. 1996; 131(5):533.

105. Chestnut RM, Marshall LF, Klauber MR, et al. The role of secondary brain injury in determining outcome from severe head injury. *J Trauma*. 1993; 34(2):216.

106. Hariri RJ, Firlick AD, Shepard SR, et al. Traumatic brain injury, hemorrhagic shock, and fluid resuscitation: effects on intracranial pressure and brain compliance. *J Neurosurg*. 1993; 79(3):421.

107. Miller JD, Butterworth JF, Gudeman SK, et al. Further experience in the management of severe head injury. *J Neurosurg*. 1981; 54:289.

108. Marion D, Obrist WD, Carlier PM, Penrod LE, Darby JM. The use of moderate therapeutic hypothermia for patients with severe head injury. *J Neurosurg*. 1993; 79:354.

109. Shiozaki T, Sugimoto H, Taneda M, et al. Effect of mild hypothermia on uncontrollable intracranial hypertension after severe head injury. *J Neurosurg*. 1993; 79:363.

110. Smith SL, Hall ED. Mild pre- and post-traumatic hypothermia attenuates blood-brain barrier damage following controlled cortical impact injury in the rat. *J Neurotrauma*. 1996; 13(1):1.

111. Metz C, Holzschuh M, Bein T, et al. Moderate hypothermia in patients with severe head injury: Cerebral and extracerebral effects. *J Neurosurg*. 1996; 85(4):532.

112. Clifton GL. Hypothermia and hyperbaric oxygen as treatment modalities for severe head injury. *New Horizons*. 1995; 3(3):474.

113. Clifton GL, Allen S, Barrodale P, et al. A phase II study of moderate hypothermia in severe brain injury. *J Neurotrauma*. 1993; 10(3):263.

114. Cancio LC, Wortham WG, Zimba F. Peritoneal dialysis to induce hypothermia in a head injury patient: case report. *Surg Neurol*. 1994; 429(4):30.

115. Wald S. Advances in the early management of patients with head injury. *Horizons in Trauma Surgery*. 1995; 75:2, 225.

116. Hall ED. The role of oxygen radical in traumatic injury: clinical implications. *J Emerg Med*. 1993; 11:31.

117. Bullock R. Opportunities for neuroprotective drugs in clinical management of head injury. *J Emerg Med*. 1993; 11:23.

118. Kelly DF. Steroids in head injury. *New Horizons*. 1995; 3(3):453.

119. Grumme T, Baethmann A, Kolodziejczyk D, et al. Treatment of patients with severe head injury by triamcinolone: a prospective controlled multicenter clinical trial of 306 cases. *Res Exper Med*. 1995; 195(4):217.

120. Hall ED. The neuroprotective pharmacology of methylprednisolone. *J Neurosurg*. 1992; 76(1):13.

121. Braakman R, Schouten HJ, Blaauw-van Dishoecki M, Minderhoud JM. Megadose steroids in severe head injury: results of a prospective double-blind clinical trial. *J Neurosurg*. 1993; 58:326.

122. Mcintosh TK, Thomas M, Smith D, Banbury M. The novel 21-amino steroid U74006F attenuates cerebral edema and improves survival after brain injury in the rat. *J Neurotrauma*. 1992; 9:33.

12 Facial and Ocular Trauma

OBJECTIVES

Upon completion of this chapter, the reader should be able to:

● Describe basic maxillofacial and ocular anatomy.

● Discuss the etiology and epidemiology of facial and ocular injuries.

● Discuss the pathophysiology of facial soft tissue injuries, impaled objects and penetrating trauma, facial fractures, epistaxis, dental injuries, temporomandibular joint dislocation, and tympanic membrane perforation.

● Describe the assessment and management of the patient with facial or ocular trauma.

● Discuss the pathophysiology of conjunctival injuries, corneal injuries, eyelid lacerations, ocular burns, hyphema, iris and ciliary body injuries, retinopathies, penetrating eye injuries, and ocular avulsions.

● Describe the assessment and management of the patient with facial or ocular trauma.

KEY TERMS

Ciliary body	Iris	Sublingual gland
Cornea	Lacrimal gland	Submandibular gland
Diplopia	Le Fort I fracture	Traumatic iridocyclitis
Enophthalmos	Le Fort II fracture	Traumatic iritis
Epistaxis	Le Fort III fracture	Traumatic miosis
Facial nerve	Parotid gland	Traumatic mydriasis
Glossoptosis	Retina	Trigeminal nerve
Iridodialysis	Sclera	Vestibulocochlear nerve

This chapter will provide an overview of injuries to the maxillofacial region and ocular structures. While many of the injuries presented in this chapter are not immediately life threatening, maxillofacial and ocular injuries still remain a worrisome and challenging trauma management problem. These injuries are frequently associated with other potentially life-threatening problems, including airway obstruction, head injury, and cervical spine injury. They also have the potential to be debilitating and disfiguring. For unprepared health care providers, the dramatic and psychologically distressing nature of these injuries can be a formidable barrier to providing appropriate care. For the patient, the functional and aesthetic implications of these injuries can lead to long-term psychological and physical disability.

MAXILLOFACIAL TRAUMA

Maxillofacial trauma is a frequently encountered problem in all age groups. The mechanism of injury is typically a blunt force to the face. The exact etiology varies considerably with age, sex, and geographic location. The most common causes are assault, motor vehicle crashes (MVCs), sports-related injuries, and falls.[1–3] Men are involved in more penetrating trauma and assaults, while women sustain the majority of their injuries during MVCs and falls.[1] Penetrating facial trauma is rare.[4] Maxillofacial trauma is commonly associated with other serious injuries. In one series, 25% of patients with facial fractures also had basilar skull fractures.[5] The incidence of skull base fractures was directly related to the number of facial fractures. Patients with one, two, or three facial fractures had incidences of basilar skull fractures of 21%, 30.4%, and 33.3%, respectively.[5] In another series, patients with facial fractures had a 17.5% incidence of closed head injury.[6] In the same series, closed head injuries occurred four times more often in males, most commonly resulting from MVCs (61%), with the most severe injuries resulting from motorcycle crashes.[6] Of the patients in the 16- to 30-year-old age group, the cause of injury was MVCs 61%, and the most severe injuries were from motorcycle crashes.[6] In a similar study, patients with facial fractures had a 4.4% incidence of cranial fractures. These patients were also predominately male between the ages of 16 and 30, with the injury most often resulting from an MVC. Other common causes of injury were assaults and sports injuries.[6]

The etiology of dental trauma varies with age. In children three years of age and under, falls are the most common cause of dental trauma. In older children, MVCs, falls, bicycle crashes, projectiles, fight injuries, and sports injuries are important causes of injury.[7] Oral trauma may also be the result of child abuse. In adults, oral trauma most often occurs during an MVC. Injuries associated with assault, including those associated with alcohol abuse and partner violence, are also frequently cited causes of oral trauma.[8]

NORMAL ANATOMY AND PHYSIOLOGY

Maxillofacial anatomy is a complex topic. A fundamental understanding of the bony structures, great vessels and major branches, and vital nerves in the region is essential in the identification and treatment of maxillofacial injuries.

Soft Tissue Structures

The soft tissues of the maxillofacial region are significantly vascularized. Injury may result in profound bleeding that will serve to disguise normal landmarks in the trauma victim.

The tongue is an important soft tissue structure that attaches to the base of the mandible, hyoid bone, styloid process, and palate. Injury of these structures, as in mandibular fracture, can result in **glossoptosis** (downward displacement of the tongue) and airway compromise.

The skin of the maxillofacial region is tightly adherent to a layer of multiple facial muscles that govern facial expression. This heavily vascularized and innervated strata provides only a thin layer of protection for major tributaries of the external carotid artery. Fortunately, serious hemorrhage is rare and superficial vessels are easily accessible for compression.

Salivation   Multiple glands for salivation are located in the maxillofacial region (Figure 12-1). The **parotid gland** is a paired serous gland that lies anterior to the auditory canal and just inferior to the zygomatic arch. The main parotid duct exits the gland, passes superficially over the masseter muscle, and pierces the buccinator just lateral to the second molar. Due to its superficial course, the main parotid duct can easily be damaged in facial lacerations. The **submandibular gland**, also a paired gland, lies medial to the mandibular ramus just inferior to the angle of the mandible. The **sublingual gland**, yet another paired gland, lies at the base of the tongue. Strategically located, the sublingual and submandibular glands are less frequently injured.

Lacrimation   The lacrimal system consists of paired **lacrimal glands** found in the anterosuperolateral aspects of the orbits (Figure 12-2). These glands provide lubrication for the eye; lubricant flows in a superolateral to inferomedial direction. The eye is drained by superior and inferior lacrimal puncta just lateral to the medial canthus. The puncta empty medially into the lacrimal sac, which drains via the nasolacrimal duct to just beneath the inferior turbinate. This is why rhinorrhea accompanies excessive tear production.

Bony Structures

The bony structure of the face is composed of multiple bones anchored centrally by the maxilla (Figure 12-3). The superior aspects of the orbits are formed by the inferior margin of the frontal bone. The zygomatic bone forms the lateral border of the orbit and part of the infraorbital ridge. It is consistent with the maxilla anteriorly. The posterior orbit is formed by the maxilla and the orbital surfaces of the zygomatic, ethmoid, and sphenoid bones. The orbital floor is formed by a paper-thin layer of bone that separates the orbit from the maxillary sinus. Disruption of the orbital floor, as in the orbital blow-out fracture, will allow herniation of the

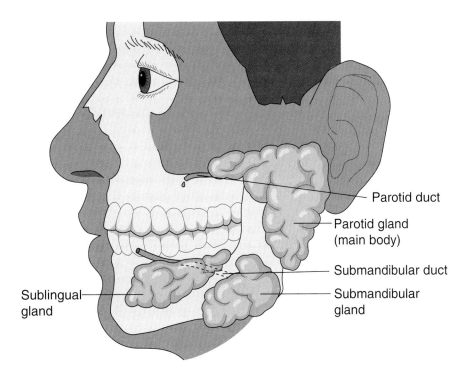

FIGURE 12-1 Location of salivary glands.

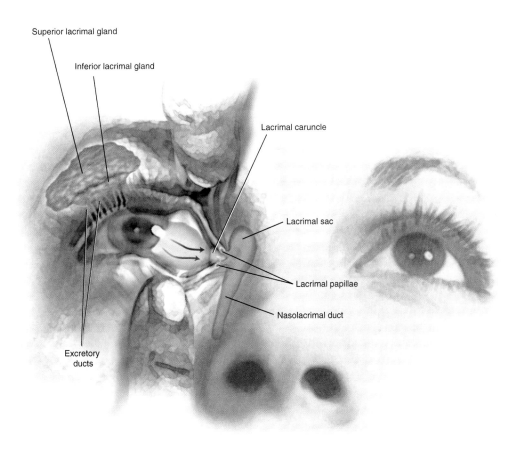

FIGURE 12-2 Lacrimal apparatus. Arrows indicate direction of drainage from the excretory ducts of the lacrimal glands across the eye to the nasolacrimal ducts.

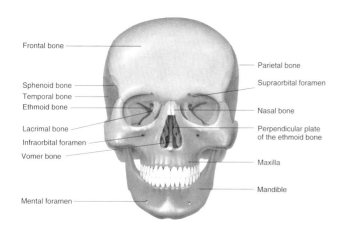

FIGURE 12-3 Bony structure of the face.

orbital contents into the maxillary sinus, possibly trapping the muscles of ocular motion.

The bony nose is formed by the perpendicular plate of the ethmoid bone and the vomer bone internally. The bridge of the nose is formed by the paired nasal bones superiorly. The major factor in determining the shape of the nose in the sagittal plane is the septal cartilage, which is consistent with both the ethmoid and vomer bones. The lateral aspects of the nose are shaped by two sets of paired cartilage, the upper and lower lateral nasal cartilage. The nares are bordered medially by the columella and the nasal septum and extend in a semicircular arch to include the lateral aspect of the nose.

The mandibular condyle articulates with the maxilla at the glenoid fossa forming the temporomandibular joint. Inferior alveolar vessels and nerves course through the body of the mandible after entering the mandibular foramen on the medial aspect of the bone. These are vulnerable to injury in mandibular fractures.

INTERNET ACTIVITIES

Visit the University of North Carolina School of Medicine Web site at http://oisvideo2.med.unc.edu/ga/bonesoface.ram and view the video on the bony anatomy of the face. This 6-minute video will play on your computer screen. You must have the RealPlayer media application installed on your computer. If you do not have this program, it is available free of charge from http://www.real.com.

Oral Cavity and Dentition

Normal adult dentition consists of 32 teeth (Figure 12-4). Each upper and lower dental arch contains 2 central incisors, 2 lateral incisors, 2 canines, 4 premolars, and 6 molars. All degrees of malocclusion are

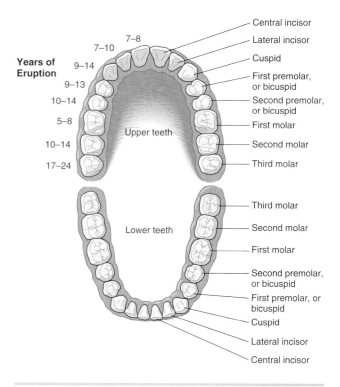

FIGURE 12-4 The 32 permanent teeth and their age of eruption.

found in the normal population. However, any degree of malocclusion found in the trauma patient is significant until proven otherwise.

INTERNET ACTIVITIES

Visit the University of Geneva School of Dentistry, Department of Orthodontics and Pedodontics Web site at http://www.unige.ch/smd/ordent.html. Review the material on traumatic intrusions and luxations.

Cranial Nerves

Most of the innervation to the face is derived from cranial nerves V and VII. The **trigeminal nerve** (CN V) controls the muscles of mastication and provides sensory function to the face. The trigeminal nerve is divided into three main branches, each responsible for sensation in a well-delineated topographic segment of the face.

The **facial nerve** (CN VII) controls the facial musculature and controls lacrimation and salivation. After exiting the cranium through the stylomastoid foramen at the lateral skull base, this nerve passes through the parotid gland and divides into multiple branches. Major branches include a zygomaticofacial and a cervicofacial branch.

Vascular Structures

Vital vascular structures of the maxillofacial anatomy are normally safely housed within the bony matrix of the skull, or shielded by the mandible. The close juxtaposition of these bony structures to vital soft tissues sets the stage for disaster when a traumatic injury to the maxillofacial region is sustained. Multiple collateral vessels exist in the head and neck, accounting for its notable vascularity. Multiple lymphatic channels also exist within the head and face.

The common carotid artery is a muscular vessel found in the carotid sheath, where it is joined by the internal jugular vein and cranial nerves IX, X, and XII, the glossopharyngeal, vagus, and hypoglossal nerves, respectively (Figure 12-5). It splits into the internal and external carotid branches at the carotid bifurcation

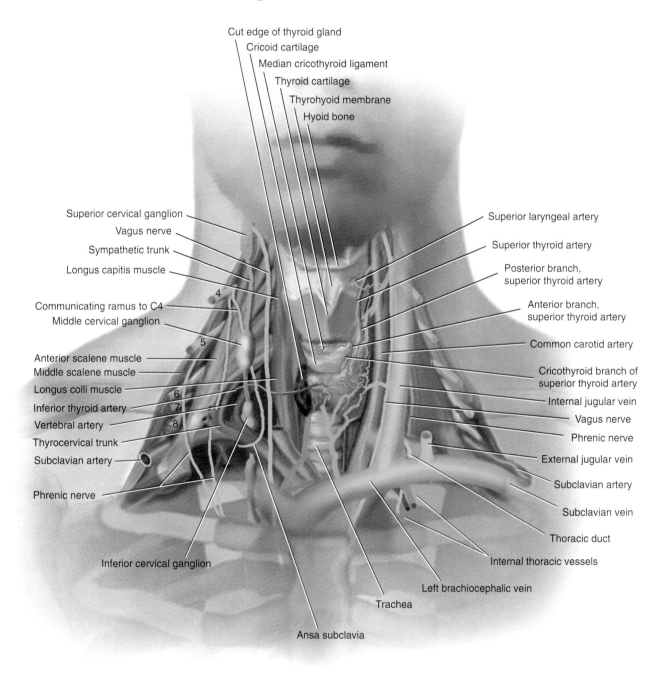

FIGURE 12-5 Vasculature and nervous structures of the neck.

in the neck. The external carotid artery branches extensively to provide blood supply to the superior pole of the thyroid gland, pharynx, tongue, face, scalp, and all maxillary structures inferior to the orbit. The internal carotid artery enters the carotid canal at the base of the skull and courses intracranially. It sends branches to the ocular structures and branches to form the cerebral vessels that supply the brain.

The internal jugular vein is a thin-walled structure that exits the jugular foramen at the base of the skull. This vessel is formed by a confluence of dural venous sinuses that drains the entire cranial vault. The external jugular vein is a superficial vein of the neck that drains the face and scalp. It is not a deep structure and is easily transected.

These vascular structures can be damaged by penetrating injuries that transect the vessels or by blunt injuries that compromise vessel integrity. Blunt forces may compromise flow through these conduits as a result of trauma-induced occlusions, vasospasm, or confinement between displaced bony structures.

The nasal cavity has a complex and rich vascular supply (Figure 12-6). Anterior arterial blood supply is provided by the anterior and posterior ethmoidal arteries. These arteries converge to form Kiesselbach's plexus in the anterior nose. The posterior nasal cavity receives blood supply from the sphenopalatine artery.

Ear and Auditory

Sound waves enter the ear at the auricle, a cartilaginous structure whose funnel-shaped center continues one-third of the distance of the external auditory canal. The remainder of the canal is bony and lined with skin (Figure 12-7). The tympanic membrane, or ear drum, is a delicate structure protected by the length and slight tortuosity of the external auditory canal. Tightly adhered to the tympanic membrane is the bony ossicular chain, which links with the vestibulocochlear

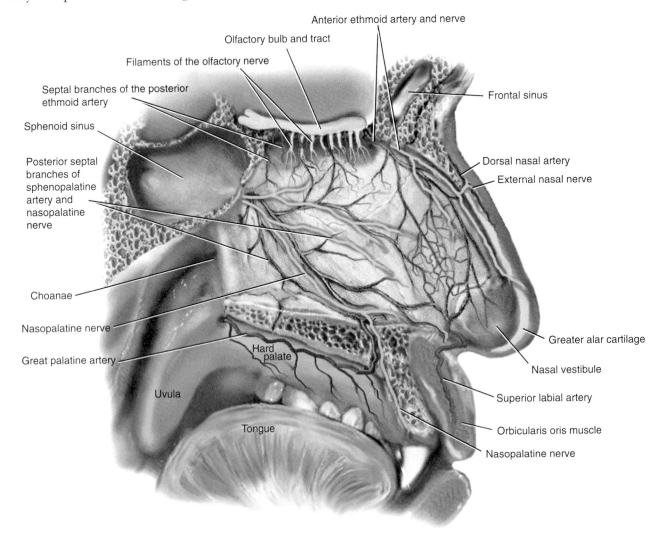

FIGURE 12-6 Vasculature and nervous structures of the nasal cavity.

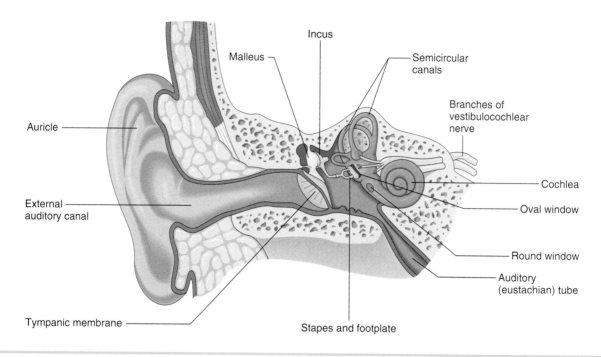

FIGURE 12-7 Structure of the internal ear.

apparatus, the organ responsible for hearing and coordination. Housed within the temporal bone, it receives innervation from cranial nerve VIII, the **vestibulocochlear nerve**. Temporal bone fractures may either injure the sense organs or disrupt their innervation.

PATHOPHYSIOLOGY

Soft Tissue Injuries

A simple facial laceration is the most commonly encountered facial emergency in the field. Bleeding can be extensive due to the rich blood supply in the head and face. This vascularity also enables lacerations and other injuries to heal quickly with a low propensity for infection. Occasionally, severe hemorrhage can occur secondary to transection of a major branch of the facial blood supply. Fortunately, severe bleeding of this nature is rare, as is hemorrhagic shock secondary to maxillofacial injury.[9] Shock with maxillofacial injury mandates a search for a second site of hemorrhage. Facial lacerations can result in injury to the glands of salivation and lacrimation. Injury to the facial nerve and its branches is also commonly seen in facial lacerations.

In addition to facial lacerations, other soft tissue injuries are frequently seen. Contusions are common and generally benign. However, they can indicate the presence of more extensive underlying injuries, such as fractures. Hematomas, or subcutaneous collections of blood, can be identified as edematous and discolored areas of soft tissue. While these injuries are usually self-limited, treatment and evaluation are indicated. Without treatment, large hematomas can undergo subsequent clot organization with fibrotic encapsulation that will lead to permanent deformity.

Human and animal bites of the face can be quite severe. In addition to the interruption in skin integrity, a crush injury may coexist and not be recognized immediately. These wounds are also of concern due to the introduction of multiple pathogens from the mouth. The risk of infection is high, especially with human bites. When the injury is less severe, it is far too easy to underestimate the potential for complications. Without proper treatment, death or severe disability can result from apparently minor injuries secondary to animal or human bites.

Occasionally, the pediatric patient will sustain a traumatic electrical injury to the face after biting through a live electrical cord or placing a live extension cord such as a "zip cord" into the mouth. The severity of soft tissue injury is increased as the saliva in contact with the tissues is heated to an extremely high temperature. Thermal energy destroys the labial, lingual, and oral tissues.[9] These patients are also at risk for airway compromise.

Impaled Objects and Penetrating Trauma

Foreign objects are frequently found in association with traumatic injuries. Occasionally, these become impaled in soft tissues or bone. Foreign objects may compromise the airway or impinge on major vessels and nerves. It is difficult to visualize which structures are involved, but large branches of the external carotid artery can be injured. Secondary massive bleeding associated with cheek injuries may obstruct the airway.

While penetrating trauma to the face is rare, it is more commonly associated with life-threatening airway compromise and hemorrhage than are traumatic blunt injuries. The most common cause of penetrating injury to the face is a gunshot wound. High-velocity projectiles and shotgun-type weapons can result in extensive tissue destruction.

Facial Fractures

The facial bones most susceptible to fracture are the nasal bones, zygoma, and mandibular condyle. Relatively less force is required to fracture these bones; they can occur as isolated injuries or components of multiple trauma. The bones least susceptible to fracture are the parasymphyseal region of the mandible and the supraorbital ridge.[4] Fracturing these bones requires considerable force, so other life-threatening injuries are common in these patients.

Fractures of the nasal bones are common and are often seen following MVCs.[10] These injuries occasionally cause deformity. More often, it is a fracture of the cartilaginous septum that results in a gross deformity of the nose, requiring careful reduction and surgical reconstruction depending on the extent of tissue destruction.

Mandibular fractures occur most often as the result of an assault.[11] The most common mandibular fracture is the angle fracture, but the most worrisome is the symphyseal fracture. The symphyseal fracture may result in glossoptosis, which may threaten the airway. Surgical reduction and internal fixation techniques are used in mandibular fracture repair.

Zygomatic fractures occur most commonly in the zygomaticomaxillary complex. Other fractures include the orbital rim fracture and the zygomatic arch fracture. Concomitant ocular injury is common. These fractures are surgically reduced and reconstructed with metal plates.

Maxillary fractures are classified by the Le Fort system.[12] These represent the fracture planes noted by Le Fort when he subjected fresh cadaver skulls to blunt forces. These are the same fractures that are encountered in daily practice. Unexpected fracture lines have been reported in patients subjected to blast injuries.[13] The Le Fort system divides maxillary fractures into three categories (Figure 12-8). The **Le Fort I fracture** separates the hard palate and lower maxilla from the remainder of the skull. The **Le Fort II fracture** separates the nasal skull and lower maxilla from the facial skull and remainder of the cranial bones. The **Le Fort III fracture** is also known as craniofacial disjunction; it effectively separates the entire midface from the cranium. These fractures are typically repaired by internal screw fixation.

The orbital blow-out fracture is seen following a direct blow to the globe. The force transmitted through the globe shatters the thin orbital floor dislocating the orbital contents posteroinferiorly (Figure 12-9). The necessity of repair depends on the symptoms produced. Many do not require repair, while others require orbital floor reconstruction with a synthetic material. It should be noted that all aspects of the orbit are susceptible to fracture.

Epistaxis

Epistaxis (nosebleed) without fracture is one of the most commonly encountered emergencies.[14] It is rarely massive unless associated with concurrent fracture.[15] Epistaxis is usually associated with disruption of Kiesselbach's plexus in the anterior nose. Less frequently, posterior epistaxis is associated with disruption of the sphenopalatine artery. Posterior bleeding is more difficult to control because it is impossible to achieve direct pressure without posterior nasal packing. Unilateral epistaxis in children and young adults is known to occur secondary to disruption of the anterior nasopharyngeal blood supply, often without any antecedent injury.[15] In most circumstances direct pressure by pinching the nares together will arrest the bleed.

Severe epistaxis is more likely to be seen in the elderly and is often associated with hypertension. This type of bleed is most likely to originate in the posterior nasopharynx and may or may not emanate through the nares. Meticulous inspection of the posterior oropharynx may reveal a posterior bleed. A massive posterior bleed constitutes a life-threatening emergency.

Dental Injuries

Mechanisms of injury resulting in tooth avulsion include MVCs, assault, projectiles (e.g., baseball), or other direct force to the dentition or mandible. Suspicion of tooth avulsion mandates a search for the missing tooth and, if not found, is assumed to be aspirated until proven otherwise.

Temporomandibular Joint Dislocation

During a dislocation of the temporomandibular joint (TMJ), the mandibular condyle slips out of the glenoid fossa. Dislocation of the TMJ is suspected in the patient who cannot close the mouth. These patients are often in distress, with a wide-open mouth, and uttering imperceptible sounds. Pain may be severe due to secondary spasm of the pterygoid muscles following dislocation of the jaw.

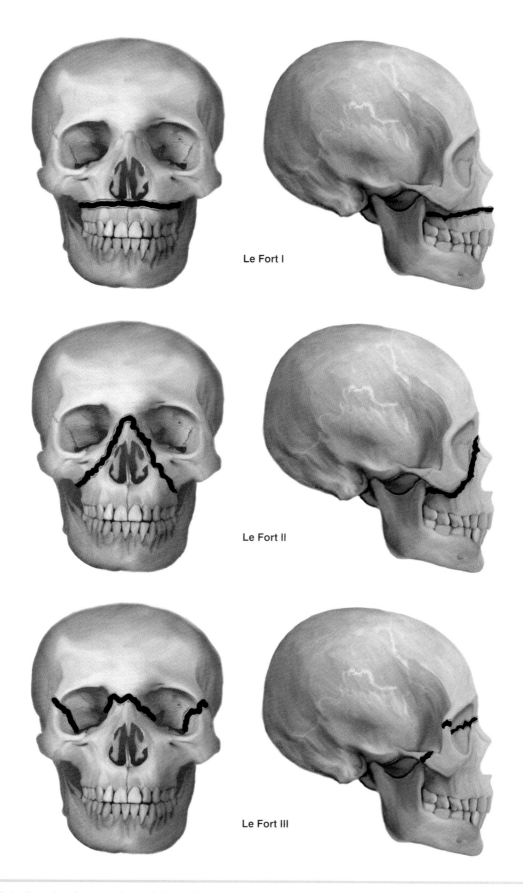

Le Fort I

Le Fort II

Le Fort III

FIGURE 12-8 Le Fort classification of maxillofacial fractures.

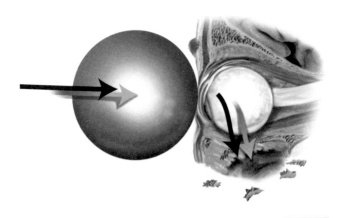

FIGURE 12-9 Blunt trauma to the eye may result in an orbital blow-out fracture.

Patients receiving a blow to the jaw may have a TMJ dislocation. Other injuries may be present, however, and attempts at reduction should not be undertaken in the field. These patients require radiographic evaluation in the emergency department prior to appropriate intervention.

Tympanic Membrane Perforation

Traumatic injury can perforate the tympanic membrane (TM) (Figure 12-10). Patients commonly complain of hemorrhagic otorrhea. Causes of TM perforations include diving or water-skiing injuries,

direct blows to the auricle, exposure to an explosion, or barotrauma.[9] These injuries are induced by exposure to pressures exceeding the structural integrity of the TM. Ossicular involvement may be present, causing a conductive hearing loss. Immediate otorrhea suggests compromise of deeper structures. More frequently, the cause of TM rupture is passing a foreign object into the external ear canal causing direct trauma to the drum. Following any head trauma with resultant otorrhea, patients are assumed to have a skull base fracture with resultant cerebrospinal fluid (CSF) leak until proven otherwise.

FOCUSED ASSESSMENT

The dramatic nature of maxillofacial injuries can be extremely distracting; however, most of these injuries are not life threatening. Prior to any assessment of maxillofacial injuries, all life-threatening injuries must be addressed.

Airway and Breathing

Massive maxillofacial trauma places the airway in jeopardy. Airway considerations with regard to dental injuries involve the possible aspiration of dental fragments. If it is determined that loss of airway is imminent, immediately proceed with intubation. It cannot be overemphasized that airway control and ventilation must take priority over all other interventions.

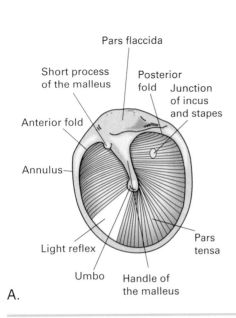

A.

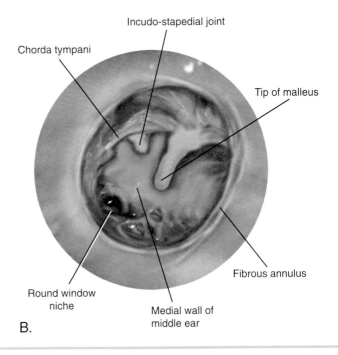

B.

FIGURE 12-10 A. Normal anatomy and appearance of the tympanic membrane. B. Large tympanic membrane perforation, permits visualization of deeper structures.

Circulation and Hemorrhage Control

The presence of shock in the trauma victim with maxillofacial injuries must not be presumed to result from the maxillofacial injuries. Resuscitation from shock must take place as with any other trauma patient, and a source should be sought prior to attending to the maxillofacial injuries. Once the patient is stabilized, the focused assessment concentrates on the patient's maxillofacial injuries. Hemorrhage should be controlled by direct pressure to the injured area. At no time should vessels be clamped because this may compromise later surgical repair.

Maxillofacial Assessment

The mouth must be inspected for evidence of tooth fragments or dentures that may have been aspirated. Fragments must be removed, and any blood present in the oropharynx suctioned. The entire oral cavity should be inspected for laceration or significant hemorrhage.

Mandibular fractures are recognized by instability, immobility, malocclusion, and occasionally a laceration in the buccal membranes. They are usually apparent by visualization or gentle palpation. In the event of inferior alveolar nerve compromise, anesthesia in the ipsilateral lower lip will be noted. Severe pain will usually be reported by the conscious patient.

Assess the supraorbital ridges, frontal sinus walls, orbits, and globes for symmetry. The orbits can be assessed for symmetry by noting if a normal horizontal plane exists between the two pupils. Orbital fractures may present as **enophthalmos** (recession of the globe into the orbit), diplopia, or restriction of extraocular movement.

Palpation for tenderness is particularly helpful in the assessment for zygomatic fractures. Tenderness in the infraorbital rim and lateral rim are common. Damage to the infraorbital nerve will result in numbness to the cheek and lip.

The nose is best examined by observation. Epistaxis or laceration increases the possibility that a nasal fracture exists. Asymmetry of the nose or obvious disfigurement is indicative of either a bony or a cartilaginous fracture.

Patients should be questioned concerning loss of hearing, tinnitus, or vertigo (dizziness that gives the sensation of a rotating external environment). This provides clues to the severity of damage to deeper structures. The eyes should be observed for nystagmus. A positive response to any of these increases the likelihood that the ossicular chain has been involved in the injury.[16] A slight conductive hearing loss is expected with any tympanic perforation.

MANAGEMENT

Securing the airway, ventilation, and perfusion take precedence over all other aspects of emergency management. Once these elementary aspects of life support have been adequately addressed, other injuries can be assessed and approached.

Airway

The principal cause of death from maxillofacial injuries is obstruction of the upper airway; the tongue is the most common airway obstruction in the unconscious or conscious patient.[17,18] Evolving airway compromise should be suspected when any of the following are noted: wheezing, dyspnea, hoarseness, subcutaneous emphysema, difficulty swallowing, choking, agitation, labored breathing, tachypnea, tachycardia, cyanosis, nostril flaring, lethargy, or rhonchi to auscultation.

The critical decision in airway management is whether the patient should be intubated. Endotracheal intubation may be required to manage the airway and to ensure adequate ventilation. In severe head trauma, early endotracheal intubation and aggressive airway control has demonstrated improved patient outcome.[19,20] Inappropriate airway care is frequently a major contributor to preventable trauma death.[21] Oral endotracheal intubation is generally preferred in the prehospital setting and nasotracheal intubation should be avoided in children and any patient with a suspected basilar skull fracture.[22] Cervical spine injury should be presumed and all manipulations of the airway must employ appropriate stabilization of the cervical spine.

The most common indications for a prehospital surgical airway are massive facial trauma or failed oral intubation.[23] The principal prehospital surgical airway options are percutaneous transtracheal jet insufflation (TJI) and cricothyrotomy. These techniques are effective methods for rapid airway access during acute emergencies when standard airway techniques fail or are contraindicated.[24] While these temporizing measures can be life saving and have been associated with low complication rates, there are potential limitations with these techniques.[25] Cricothyroidotomy is unlikely to work in the setting of cricothyroid separation and has been associated with thyroid cartilage lacerations, significant hemorrhage, displacement, and failure to obtain an airway.[26] Transtracheal jet insufflation is associated with total expiratory obstruction, pneumothorax, subcutaneous emphysema, and failure to obtain an airway.[27] The gold standard surgical airway in the setting of neck trauma is a tracheotomy placed by a surgical team.

Bleeding

Facial lacerations should be treated the same as any other laceration, with primary attention given to arresting hemorrhage with direct pressure and sterile dressing.

Epistaxis is usually managed quite easily. The first attempt at arresting the bleed should consist of pinching the nares together at the level of the alar and upper lateral nasal cartilage. Rarely is there an indication for insertion of a nasal pack for an anterior bleed. Vital signs are frequently reevaluated. The conscious, stable patient should undergo placement of a bite block. The patient should be placed in a sitting position holding an emesis basin for collection of blood. This facilitates an estimate of blood loss to guide rehydration and serves to prevent emesis from swallowed blood. Patients are instructed to breathe through the mouth and are encouraged not to swallow blood, as this leads to vomiting, which further complicates the situation.

Impaled Objects

Foreign objects occasionally become impaled in the face. In general, the impaled object should be stabilized and the patient transported with the object in place. Impaled objects are typically removed in the controlled environment of an operating room. One notable exception is the object impaled in the cheek. Removal is justified in this case, particularly during hemorrhage from an unidentifiable source. Removal will facilitate hemostasis by enhancing exposure to the traumatized tissues. If it is possible to remove the object safely, it should be removed. Other exceptions relate to objects impinging on and threatening the airway and respiration. An emergency airway such as a cricothyrotomy may need to be established in these instances.

The cheek should be gently palpated to determine the depth of penetration. The object should be removed from the side from which it entered. If resistance to attempts to gently remove the object is encountered, the object should be left in place. Attempts to remove it may result in further trauma. If removal has been successful, the inside of the oral cavity must be packed, with special attention given to the area between the teeth and cheek. Counterpressure must be maintained by a dressing and bandage secured firmly over the external aspect of the wound. A bandage can be wrapped around the patient's head in order to stabilize the external dressing and keep the internal pack in place by stabilizing the jaw in a closed position.

Dental Emergencies

An intact tooth that has been found should be handled only at the crown; the root should not be manipulated in any way. The tooth should be transported, cushioned by gauze, in a container of physiologically balanced solution, such as Ringer's lactate or normal saline. Refrigerated whole milk may serve as a reasonable alternative.[7] If the estimated time of arrival at the emergency department will approach or exceed 20 minutes and other more critical problems do not take precedence, EMS personnel may make an attempt at reimplantation. First, the tooth and the socket should be flushed with sterile saline. The tooth should then be properly aligned, with visual comparison made with its anatomical correlate on the opposite side, if possible. Once assured of proper placement, the tooth should be gently, yet firmly inserted, allowing fluid to seep out of the socket as the tooth is advanced. Once the tooth is in the socket, the patient should be instructed to bite down on a gauze roll for a period of no less than 20 minutes. Do not attempt replacement in the unconscious patient as aspiration may occur.[7] The success of reimplantation is a function of the amount of time that a tooth has remained avulsed.[7] In the event of a fracture to the crown of the tooth, without accompanying pulp exposure, emergency treatment is not warranted.[7]

TMJ Dislocation

No attempt at reduction of a TMJ dislocation should be made in the trauma patient. In the field, an attempt to relocate the mandible into its anatomically correct position is considered only if it can be determined with certainty that the dislocation occurred spontaneously. Reduction becomes increasingly more difficult with worsening pterygoid muscle spasm. Reduction procedure instructions can be found in maxillofacial textbooks.

Auditory Injuries

Disturbances in auditory function must be further investigated. Definitive treatment will follow a complete evaluation. When auditory injuries are suspected, a cold pack may be applied in order to slow any hemorrhage and lessen patient discomfort.

OCULAR TRAUMA

Trauma is the second leading cause of blindness in the United States, with 40,000 new cases of visual impairment occurring each year.[28] In one large survey, the lifetime prevalence of ocular injury was 14.4% and was nearly twice as common in men.[29] Common causes include MVCs, assaults, sports, work-related injuries, and consumer products. Sports are responsible for more than 48,000 eye injuries each year, with basketball, baseball, and aquatic activities as the most common causes.[30] The workplace accounts for about 15% of all severe ocular trauma, with men at greatest risk.[31] Intentional violence is also a common cause of ocular injury. In urban settings, one series reported that 35% of all ocular trauma was related to assaults.[32] In this study the most common motive for assault was theft and the most common injuries were to the globe and retina. In the emergency department, ocular injuries are a common presenting complaint of battered women; unfortunately, this etiology often goes unrecognized.[33] In child abuse where infants are intentionally shaken, ocular and retinal hemorrhages are commonly seen, even when no other evidence of trauma exists.[34]

Motor vehicle crashes are a common source for ocular trauma, especially in the multiple-trauma patient. The incidence of blunt globe rupture is high, legal blindness is a common outcome, and the overall prognosis tends to be poor.[35] A relatively new source for ocular injury is automobile airbags. While these devices have reduced mortality, a wide range of ocular injuries ranging from corneal abrasions to retinal detachments have been reported with airbag deployment, even in relatively minor collisions.[36,37] Patients wearing glasses are at highest risk for serious ocular injury.[38]

In pediatric patients most injuries occur while at home or at play.[39] Injuries commonly result from toys and sports. Injuries involving bicycles and BB guns are particularly common.[40] Pediatric ocular injuries occur four times more often in males than in females.

Ocular injury is frequently associated with other injuries. At one trauma center, ocular injury was seen in 13.5% of all admitted multiple-trauma patients.[41]

The cause of injury was an MVC in 52% and an assault in 8%. In patients that present with facial fracture, ocular injuries occurred in 29% and, of these, complete blindness occurred in 6%.[42] Patients with thermal facial burns frequently have ocular involvement, with one series reporting that 15% of patients admitted to the burn unit had significant globe or eyelid involvement.[43]

NORMAL ANATOMY AND PHYSIOLOGY

The anatomy of the eye is extremely intricate (Figure 12-11). The main parts of the globe of the eyeball can be divided into three coats: (1) fibrous, (2) vascular pigmented, and (3) nervous. The outer fibrous coat is made of an opaque white material called the **sclera**. The outer coat also contains a thin, transparent material over the anterior surface, called the **cornea**. The vascular pigmented coat contains the iris and the ciliary body. The **iris** is a thin sheet of pigmented tissue that provides "eye color." The central opening in the iris is the pupil. The iris has contractile properties that alter pupil diameter to adjust the amount of light that enters the eye. Deep to the iris is the **ciliary body**, which is an intricate structure of ligaments and muscles that attach to the lens within the eye. The ciliary body focuses images onto the back of the eye by altering lens shape. The innermost layer is the nervous coat, or **retina**. This structure contains a pigmented tissue layer and nervous tissue that acts as the photoreceptive organ of the eye. An important landmark on the retina is the optic disk, which is the area of convergence for the vascular supply to the inner surfaces of the eye and optic nerve (Figure 12-12).

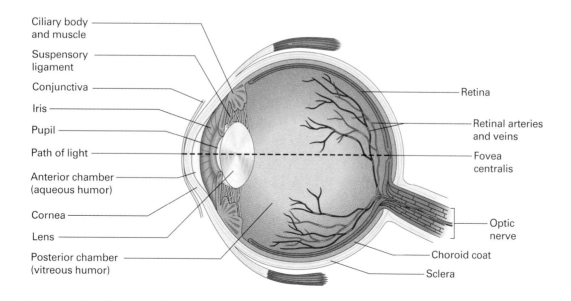

FIGURE 12-11 Normal anatomy of the eye.

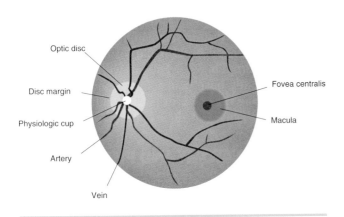

FIGURE 12-12 Retinal structures of the left eye.

The eye is separated into two chambers by the lens. The anterior chamber is the space between the cornea and the lens and is filled with aqueous humor. The posterior chamber is located behind the lens and is filled with vitreous humor. The entire globe has a diameter of approximately 1 cm and is securely housed within the orbit. Six extraocular muscles attach to the external surface of the eye and control eye movement (Figure 12-13).

Multiple cranial nerves are involved in the function of the eye. The optic nerve, cranial nerve II, carries photoreceptive information from the retina to the brain. The oculomotor nerve, the trochlear nerve, and the abducens nerve (cranial nerves III, IV, and VI, respectively) control the extraocular muscles. The trigeminal nerve, cranial nerve V, provides sensory innervation to the cornea. The facial nerve, cranial nerve VII, provides motor innervation to the orbicularis oculi muscle to close the eyelid.

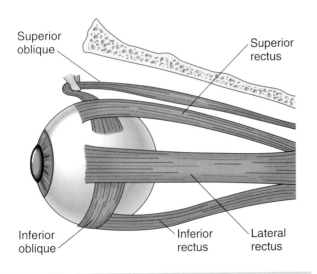

FIGURE 12-13 Extraocular muscles of the eye.

The pupil diameter is controlled by a competitive balance of sympathetic and parasympathetic innervation. The oculomotor nerve, cranial nerve III, contains parasympathetic fibers that innervate the iris to constrict the pupil. The cervical ganglia in the neck supply the sympathetic innervation to the iris to dilate the pupil.

INTERNET ACTIVITIES

Visit the University of North Carolina School of Medicine Web site at http://oisvideo2.med.unc.edu/ga/bonesoforbit.ram and view the video on the bony anatomy of the orbit of the eye. This 12-minute video will play on your computer screen. You must have the RealPlayer media application installed on your computer. If you do not have this program, it is available free of charge from http://www.real.com.

PATHOPHYSIOLOGY

Conjunctival Injuries

Blunt trauma to the eye can rupture blood vessels within the conjunctiva. Normally the conjunctiva is clear, and the presence of hemorrhage within this structure may appear quite dramatic. Fortunately, this is a relatively minor injury when it occurs alone and will resolve spontaneously. However, the presence of a subconjunctival hemorrhage should prompt a search for further injury, such as globe rupture.

Corneal Injuries

Corneal abrasions are one of the most common ocular injuries. Corneal abrasions can occur in an unconscious patient when contact lenses are left in place. Trauma to the corneal surface by direct contact results in epithelial denudation. Patients complain of pain, foreign body sensation, excessive lacrimation, photophobia, blurred vision, and blepharospasm (involuntary contraction of the eyelids). Motion of the eye underneath a closed eyelid will further exacerbate the pain, and the patient will report a feeling that "something is in the eye." Severe discomfort may make visualization of the eye impossible. Foreign bodies in the cornea or conjunctiva can produce symptoms similar to a corneal abrasion. Glass fragments, rust particles, dust, dirt, and vegetable matter small enough to remain suspended in the air are frequent culprits. These patients require emergency department evaluation where topical anesthesia will facilitate the examination.

Eyelid Lacerations

Lacerations to the eyelid and surrounding soft tissue may involve ocular and lacrimal structures. In general, these injuries are more complex than they appear and will require evaluation and repair by an ophthalmologist. Lacerations that pierce the lid and lacerations that involve the muscles for opening the eyelid are evaluated and repaired in the operating room.

Thermal, Chemical, and Radiation Injuries

Thermal injuries to the eye are commonly seen in patients with facial burns. Isolated injuries are frequently seen in patients that have direct contact to the eye from heat sources such as cigarette ash, charcoal particles, or industrial metal slag. Molten material can cause serious damage to the ocular structures because of their high melting point. Compounds with the highest melting points, such as glass and iron, are often greater than 1200° centigrade and have the potential to cause the most damage. Magnesium hydroxide burns that result from injuries involving sparklers should be managed as chemical burns rather than thermal burns.

Chemical burns of the eye require immediate attention and aggressive irrigation in order to prevent permanent damage to the eye. Permanence of the injury is a function of chemical concentration and duration of exposure prior to lavage. The two broad classifications of chemical burns of the eye are alkali injuries and acid injuries. Alkali burns are often more serious injuries and can rapidly lead to total blindness if not immediately attended. Alkaline chemicals can easily penetrate into the tissue by diffusely disrupting cell membranes.[44] Common alkali agents include ammonia, lime, and lye. Mace and pepper spray burns are treated as alkali burns.[45] Acid burns tend to precipitate tissue proteins and thus remain localized at their point of initial contact. Thus, they tend to be less penetrating than alkali burns but can still result in intraocular scarring, especially when the exposure is from heavy metals or hydrofluoric acid.

Most burns secondary to radiation exposure are from an ultraviolet or infrared source. Such sources include solar rays, welding arcs, and artificial sources of solar radiation. Ultraviolet keratitis, one of the most commonly seen injuries, is damage to the corneal epithelium after excessive sun exposure. Patients with light injuries to the eye will usually have a suggestive history and symptoms of photophobia, lacrimation, blepharospasm, and pain. Examination is frequently unremarkable, with lid edema and erythema occasionally noted. Fortunately, radiation does not penetrate into the deep structures of the eye and deep damage is not expected.

Hyphema

A hyphema is a gross collection of blood in the anterior chamber of the eye, typically the result of blunt trauma (Figure 12-14). The bleeding is usually from torn peripheral vessels of the iris but can also follow a tear of the sphincter muscles of the pupil, lens dislocation, vitreous or retinal hemorrhage, or retinal detachment. When the patient's upper body is erect, the red blood cells will settle inferiorly in the chamber. Otherwise, they may circulate diffusely, making the identification of hyphema difficult. When the collection of blood is small, the injury may go unappreciated in the field. A severe hyphema may preclude visualization of any of the posterior structures of the eye. Once a hyphema has been identified, global rupture must be ruled out.

Most complications of hyphema are associated with rebleeding. Between 20% and 30% of hyphemas may rebleed, with the more severe hyphemas at greatest risk.[9] Microscopic hyphemas rarely rebleed. Total hyphemas, either primary or due to rebleed, often result in a diminution of visual acuity. Hyphemas are associated with glaucoma, optic atrophy, peripheral anterior synechiae formation (adhesion of iris to the cornea), dislocation of the lens, vitreous hemorrhage, and retinal hemorrhages.[45]

Iris and Ciliary Body Injuries

Blunt trauma can result in multiple problems with the iris, ciliary body, and their related structures. **Traumatic iritis** or **traumatic iridocyclitis**, which is inflammation of the iris or iris and ciliary body, is commonly seen after blunt trauma. These patients will

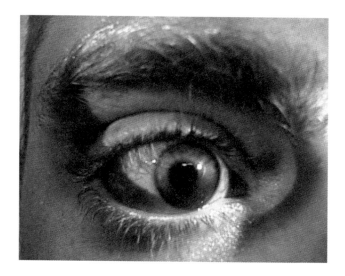

FIGURE 12-14 Hyphema. Courtesy of Kevin Reilly, Albany Medical Center, Albany, NY.

complain of pain and photophobia with no specific gross physical finding. Following trauma, the ciliary body may dilate, called **traumatic mydriasis**, or constrict, called **traumatic miosis**. More severe injuries include damage to the muscles of the ciliary body and tearing of the iris from the ciliary body, called **iridodialysis**. Iridodialysis may present as an accessory pupil and hyphema.

Traumatic Retinopathies

The retina is a frequently injured ocular structure. Most often, these injuries result from blunt trauma and include retinal detachments, commotio retinae (retinal concussion), and retinal hemorrhages. These injuries generally require advanced ophthalmic examinations for diagnosis and may have minimal gross physical findings. In the field, the mechanism of injury and patient symptoms are the primary clues to the underlying pathology. In a retinal detachment, there is a separation between the retinal sensory layer and the retinal pigmented epithelium layer by a collection of fluid. The fluid can gain access to this potential space by (1) escaping from the vitreous cavity through a retinal defect, (2) escaping from damaged vessels, or (3) tractional retinal detachment from intraocular foreign bodies or perforating injuries. Patients often complain of painless flashes of light alternating with black spots, dimmed vision or a filmy sensation, and visual field defects such as a "curtain." Retinal detachments are a surgical emergency.

In commotio retinae, the advanced ophthalmic examination reveals retinal edema following blunt trauma. In retinal and vitreous hemorrhages there is bleeding into the posterior chamber. The bleeding can occur secondary to disrupted retinal capillaries or from a more severe problem such as a retinal tear. With retinal tears, the bleed is often more significant.

Penetrating Injuries and Globe Rupture

A ruptured globe is a serious ocular injury and carries a high risk for blindness. When aqueous humor is lost from the anterior chamber secondary to a penetrating injury of the eye, the prognosis is guarded but vision may be spared because the fluid is gradually replaced. In contrast, vitreous humor from the posterior chamber cannot be replenished, and once lost, blindness is likely. A high index of suspicion for globe rupture should be maintained when the patient describes a loss of vision following a blow to the eye or penetrating ocular trauma. Common penetrating agents include pens, pencils, knives, needles, fish hooks, and darts. Industrial injuries in which projectiles cause global rupture or penetration are common. A history of using a hammer and chisel, other metal-to-metal contact, or industrial machinery is a frequent cause of intraocular foreign bodies. Extrusion of intraocular contents makes the diagnosis obvious but physical findings may also be minimal. Perforation may exist in the apparently normal eye with no immediate gross visual defect. More commonly, patients will have decreased visual acuity, decreased intraocular pressure, a flattened anterior chamber, chemosis (edema of conjunctiva about the cornea), subconjunctival hemorrhage or laceration, grossly irregular pupil with changes in shape and color, hyphema, and obvious irregularity, in comparison with contralateral ocular structures. Globe rupture, corneal laceration, and other penetrations are surgical emergencies.

Ocular Avulsions

Partial avulsions or traumatic enucleations can be seen in severe maxillofacial trauma. The potential for visual recovery is dependent upon the extent of the injury and initial care. However, complete avulsion of the globe signifies permanent loss of vision, and the avulsed eye is not replantable. The rich vascular supply of the eye can be a source of significant hemorrhage in these type of injuries. The optic nerve may become avulsed following a direct blow to the eye. This diagnosis is suspected based on history, a denial of light perception, and pupillary signs.

FOCUSED ASSESSMENT

Field assessment and stabilization of life-threatening injuries take priority over ocular trauma. It may not be possible or practical to complete the full ocular assessment. The patient's other injuries, the time available, and the equipment at hand determine the extent of the field ocular assessment.

Ophthalmologic History

The history is crucial in the evaluation of the ocular trauma patient. Often the patient's symptoms and history will point toward the diagnosis more than observable signs. The four cardinal areas to assess are (1) the nature of the trauma and mechanism of injury; (2) change in vision; (3) change in appearance of the eye, such as redness or discharge; and (4) pain and discomfort.[44] It is important to determine when the injury occurred and the time line of the symptoms. The complete ocular history should include (1) use of corrective lens; (2) ophthalmological diseases and disorders, such as cataracts or glaucoma; (3) ophthalmological medications; (4) ophthalmological surgery; (5) systemic diseases with ophthalmic manifestations, such as diabetes; and (6) systemic symptoms of ophthalmic diseases, such as headache or nausea.[44]

Visual Acuity

The initial ocular evaluation should begin with a visual acuity screen of central vision. This is the most important element of the ocular physical examination and should be performed prior to all ocular treatments, with one exception. The visual acuity examination should never delay the emergency treatment of chemical burns to the eye. As with all ocular examination elements, both eyes should be examined thoroughly and it should never be assumed that a reportedly uninjured eye is normal.

Commonly used standardized assessment tools for visual acuity testing include the Snellen chart for far visual acuity (20 feet) (Figure 12-15) and the Rosenbaum card for near visual acuity (about 13–15 inches). The patient should be assessed for the smallest

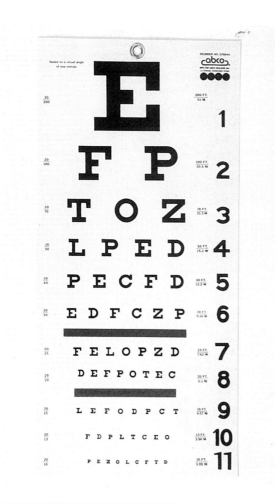

FIGURE 12-15 Snellen visual acuity chart for assessing distance vision.

line readable for each eye. If no standardized chart is available, any printed material, such as a package label, can be used. General assessment includes having the patient completely cover the eye not being tested, testing the injured eye first, and testing uncorrected vision before corrected vision. Ideally, corrected vision should be assessed with the patient's prescription glasses. If the patient's corrective lenses are unavailable, the patient can look through a pinhole placed in a notecard. This simple technique will provide considerable correction of refractory error. The scoring for these systems is recorded as a fraction, with the numerator as the patient's distance from the chart (standardized to 20 feet) and the denominator as the line that the patient could see clearly. For example, a score of 20/40 would indicate that at a distance of 20 feet from the chart, the patient could see as well as a normal eye could at 40 feet.

If the patient is unable to read the top line on the standardized acuity tool, the patient should be assessed for more rudimentary visual functions, including the ability to count fingers, the ability to perceive hand movement, and the perception of light. These values should be accurately and thoroughly documented to establish a baseline for future evaluations.

Pupillary Reactions

The pupils should be examined for shape, size in millimeters, and reactivity to light and accommodation. The normal pupil will be black, round, and equal in size to the contralateral pupil and react by constriction to light and accommodation. The normal constrictive response to light stimulation of one pupil causes consensual constriction of the other pupil. Normal variance in size between the two pupils is usually less than 1 mm.

External Examination

Next a visual inspection of the external anatomy of the eye should be performed. If a ruptured globe is suspected, it is important not to attempt to separate the eyelids, palpate the globe, or apply any type of external pressure to the eye. A protruding globe may indicate posterior orbital hematoma, or a sunken globe may indicate orbital fracture or ruptured globe.[44] The orbit, lids, and conjunctiva should be inspected for any ecchymosis, edema, foreign bodies, lacerations, or other trauma. The globe should be examined for infection, hemorrhage, shape, laceration, and penetrating objects. Small penetrating objects may not be apparent upon gross visual inspection. The anterior chamber can be grossly visualized for signs of trauma and hyphema.

The upper eyelid can be inverted for visualizing the underlying conjunctiva (Figure 12-16). The

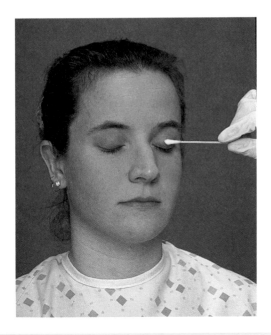 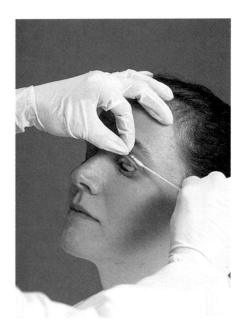

FIGURE 12-16 Procedure for inverting the eyelid.

technique involves placing a rigid object such as the shaft of a cotton tip applicator on the eyelid about 1 cm above the eyelash. As the patient gazes downward, the examiner grasps the eyelid. The eyelid is then gently inverted over the rigid object and held in place by the examiner. Upon completion of the exam, the eyelid is repositioned by gently pulling the lash forward.

Ocular Motility

Extraocular movement should be assessed by having the patient move their eyes through all six positions of gaze (Figure 12-17). Any deficits or dysconjugate gaze should be noted. **Diplopia**, or double vision, suggests involvement of the extraocular muscles and is a com-

mon finding in orbital fractures. With diplopia, the patient should be asked to cover one eye to determine if the diplopia disappears, which would support the suspicion of extraocular muscle involvement. Diplopia that persists after closing one eye is suspicious for lens injury, corneal injury, or a malingering patient.[44] Presence of nystagmus should be noted and may suggest related injuries.

Visual Field Testing

The pattern of visual field loss is used to isolate the location of a lesion along the pathway from the eye to the brain. The visual fields for each eye can be thought of as a circle divided into four quadrants. For visual

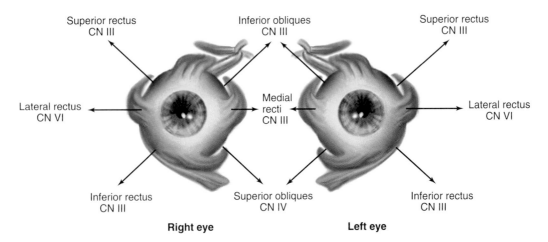

FIGURE 12-17 Extraocular movements and their muscular and nervous control.

field testing of peripheral vision, the examiner faces the patient at a distance of about 2 feet. The patient covers one eye and looks directly at the examiner. The examiner then moves an object, such as a finger or ink pen, into the peripheral vision of the patient until the patient indicates they can see the object. The patient must continue to look straight ahead during the test. The visual field is tested from eight directions, starting at the top of the visual field circle and incrementing 45 degrees around the circle (Figure 12-18). The normal visual fields are slightly restricted at the top by the brow and medially by the nose (Figure 12-19).

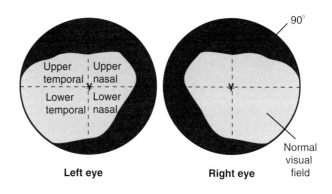

FIGURE 12-19 Normal visual fields are restricted superiorly by the brow, inferiorly by the cheeks, and medially by the nose (shaded areas).

Advanced Assessments

Funduscopic examination with an ophthalmoscope is used to magnify and visualize the anterior and posterior structures of the eye. The first entity seen on funduscopy is the red reflex of light off the retina. The presence of this reflex indicates that there is no pathologic obstruction between the observer and the retina. The cornea and anterior chamber are visualized for evidence of corneal abrasion or hyphema. Posteriorly, the optic nerve is inspected for evidence of atrophy, cupping, edema, or hemorrhage. All vessels converging at the optic disc are followed to the periphery. The normal optic disk edge is sharp and distinct.

Slit-lamp biomicroscopy is typically employed in the emergency department for detailed visualization of the anterior segment of the eye. This examination provides a well-illuminated, highly magnified view of the anterior structures. The name "slit" lamp describes the fact that the light is attenuated from a scattered beam to a slit of light. This allows the examiner to determine the thickness of anterior ocular structures. To facilitate the slit-lamp examination, the pupil is frequently pharmacologically dilated and the corneal surface is marked with special stains.

Fluorescein is one of the stains commonly employed in the evaluation of the cornea. In a fluorescein examination, the stain is topically applied to the cornea by optic drops or by optic strips. Any damaged area of corneal epithelium, such as an abrasion, will act as a well for the stain and will "fluoresce" yellowish-green when examined with a cobalt blue lamp.

Intraocular pressure can be easily measured in the emergency department with devices such as a Schiötz tonometer or an electronic tonometry pen. These devices measure intraocular pressure by determining the amount of force necessary to indent the cornea. The normal intraocular pressure is 14–17 mm Hg. Intraocular pressure can be altered by trauma or disease.

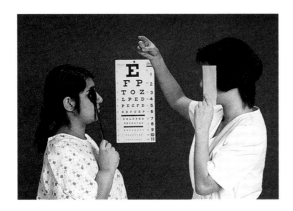

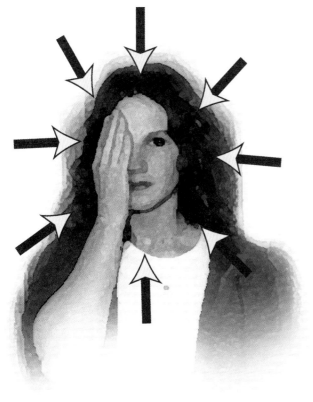

FIGURE 12-18 Visual field assessment is performed in 45 degree segments about each eye.

MANAGEMENT

Shielding and Stabilization of Foreign Bodies

After addressing life-threatening injuries, objects penetrating the globe can be stabilized. This is accomplished by cutting several 4 × 4 gauze pads so that they pass easily around the object. Once the gauze is in place, a cup with the bottom punched out is placed over the entire apparatus and anchored in place using a bandage (Figure 12-20). This technique can also be used to stabilize an enucleated globe. Both eyes should be covered to prevent paired motion when the "good eye" moves. Any foreign body whose depth is suspect is assumed to be a penetrating injury, especially if the foreign body overlies the anterior chamber. Removal of a penetrating foreign body can result in a loss of vitreous or aqueous humor with resulting blindness.

When a globe or cornea disruption is suspected, the eye must be rigidly shielded to protect it from external pressure of any type. Failure to observe this simple rule may result in further compromise of the

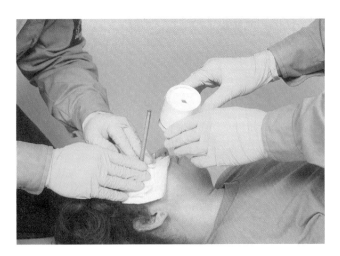

FIGURE 12-20 Stabilization of a penetrating object in the eye.

organ. Extrusion of global contents will result in irreversibly damaging the eye. A rigid aluminum shield is placed over the orbital rims and must not contact the globe. The eyelid should not be taped or obstructed in an attempt to keep it from moving. Both eyes are covered in order to prevent conjugate motion when the "good eye" moves. If such devices are unavailable, a similar shield can be constructed from plastic or paper cups or other available resources.

Soft patching with bulky dressing that contacts the eyelid is commonly used as an adjunctive treatment for corneal abrasions and other injuries where movement of the eyelid from blinking can further injure the cornea. The patches should apply enough gentle pressure to hold the lid in place. Patients with one eye patched will have greatly impaired depth perception and are at risk for falls or other injury. Soft patching is contraindicated in patients with globe injuries, globe laceration, or suspected intraocular foreign bodies.

Contact Lens Removal

Contact lenses must be removed in all patients who suffer chemical burns to the eye, and removal should be considered in unconscious patients with prolonged transport times. A contraindication to contact lens removal is suspected ruptured globe. If field removal is not possible or if it is feared that further injury may result, the eyelids should be taped shut. Both verbal and written reports should clearly indicate that contact lenses are in place.

Contact lenses can be removed by several methods. The general procedure involves gently sliding the lens off the cornea and onto the inferior sclera, where it can be safely removed. For soft lens a gloved finger can be used to move the lens and for "pinching" it off the eye with the thumb and index finger. Hard lenses require gently breaking the seal by pushing on one edge prior to removal. Lenses can be irrigated loose but are easily lost in the irrigation runoff. Commercial contact removal kits that have a plungerlike device are available. Once the lens is removed, it should be stored in a container and labeled as coming from the left or right eye.

Irrigation

Irrigation is indicated for chemical burns and foreign body removal. Irrigation of chemical burns should never be delayed for physical examination, visual acuity test, or any other non-life-saving procedure. In the field, immediate irrigation with normal saline solution through intravenous tubing is the best option, performed by manually opening the eye and directing the stream of fluid at the sclera on the nasal side, not at the cornea. The patient should be positioned to allow the stream to flow across the cornea and off the eye on the temporal side. Good exposure of the entire globe while irrigating is necessary to prevent residual chemical from collecting in the deep orbit adjacent to the eye. Spasm of the orbicularis oculi muscle may make this a difficult task. The eyes should be irrigated for a minimum of 30 minutes for most chemical burns, and transport should not delay or interrupt irrigation. Alkali burns require extensive irrigation. Following several minutes of ocular lavage, the lavage area should be expanded to include the periorbital skin so that residual chemical will not find its way back into the eye.

Devices are available for irrigation, such as a Morgan lens. These devices are placed directly on the globe and require topical anesthesia. If used improperly, these devices have increased risk for corneal abrasions and exacerbating existing injuries.

CURRENT RESEARCH AND EXPERIMENTAL TREATMENTS

Recent advances in maxillofacial trauma include the use of three-dimensional computed tomography to visualize bony defects, the evolution of new materials for bony defect repair, and new osseointegrated implants for dental and facial rehabilitation.[46,47] The use of computer-generated three-dimensional images provides the most accurate morphologic diagnosis obtainable.[48] Physicians are able to determine the best surgical approach for reconstruction and are able to establish a reliable prognosis.

Bony defects can be filled with a hydroxyapatite matrix that has a porosity similar to bone. This prosthetic material will provide a matrix that will promote angioneogenesis and new tissue formation, stabilizing the dynamic healing process. This is particularly important in midface defects, which exhibit the most noticeable cosmetic deformity. Osseointegrated implants can be used to facilitate retention stability and support for facial and intraoral prostheses used to restore head and neck defects.[47] Current research is based on results in head and neck cancers.

Visual recovery following ocular trauma has become more likely over the past 20 years due to the more widespread use of microsurgery involving vitreoretinal techniques.[49] By 1983, 70% of patients with penetrating ocular injuries achieved at least 20/40 vision.[50]

SUMMARY

Injuries to the maxillofacial region and ocular structures, while rarely life threatening, may complicate the resuscitation and management of the trauma victim. A sound understanding of the anatomy, coupled with a knowledge of the etiology of maxillofacial and ocular injuries, will enable the rescuer to respond appropriately. It must be appreciated that these injuries often occur in conjunction with other life-threatening injuries. As such, recognition of these problems will prompt the search for more devastating injuries.

Trauma is the second leading cause of blindness in the United States. The immediate recognition of traumatic ocular injuries will ensure that the patient will have the best prognosis for recovery. It cannot be overstated that these patients must be initially managed as all other victims of trauma, with attention focused on threats to life prior to addressing any other injuries.

▶ REVIEW QUESTIONS

1. The most common cause(s) of maxillofacial trauma in all age groups is (are):
   a. Gunshot wounds
   b. Other penetrating trauma such as knife wounds
   c. Assault, motor vehicle crashes, sports-related injuries, and falls
   d. Motorcycle accidents in which the operator was not wearing a helmet

2. Mandibular fractures may result in:
   a. Glossoptosis
   b. Damage to the inferior alveolar vessels and nerves
   c. Malocclusion
   d. All of the above

3. Soft tissue injuries are of concern primarily because:
   a. They are usually extremely disfiguring.
   b. They may cause significant hemorrhage and compromise the airway.
   c. They are extremely painful.
   d. They usually result in systemic symptoms of shock.

4. The Le Fort III maxillary facial fracture describes:
   a. A separation of the hard palate and lower maxilla from the remainder of the skull
   b. A separation of the nasal skull and lower maxilla from the facial skull
   c. Craniofacial disjunction
   d. A facial fracture that combines a mandibular fracture with a fracture of the zygoma

5. Which of the following constitutes a life-threatening emergency?
   a. The orbital blow-out fracture
   b. A complex midface fracture

c. A mandibular fracture with inferior alveolar nerve involvement

d. A massive posterior nosebleed

6. Which of the following impaled objects should be removed in the field?
a. A knife in the anterior chest
b. A dart that has penetrated the globe of the eye
c. A large fragment of plastic impaled in the cheek
d. A fishhook impaled in the wrist

7. When should a traumatic TMJ dislocation be reduced?
a. Never
b. Immediately, before pterygoid muscle spasm worsens
c. Once the patient has been intubated
d. Before the initial survey

8. An avulsed tooth should:
a. Be transported in a bag of ice
b. Kept at body temperature
c. Be transported in a glass of refrigerated milk
d. Be transported in vinegar

9. An eyelid laceration that extends laterally to involve the superolateral aspect of the eyelid may involve which structure?
a. The lacrimal gland
b. The superior oscillatory ductule
c. The lacrimal caruncle
d. The nasolacrimal duct

10. Which of the following is true?
a. Acid burns tend to precipitate proteins and remain localized.
b. Acid burns are more penetrating than alkali burns.
c. Alkali burns are usually minimal and require no therapy.
d. Radiation injuries typically penetrate into the deep structures of the eye.

11. Retinal detachments:
a. Constitute a surgical emergency
b. Will usually heal spontaneously
c. Bleed profusely, causing intraocular pressures greater than 150 mm Hg
d. Involve the anterior structures of the eye

12. Ocular avulsions:
a. Have the best prognosis if the eye is packed in normal saline prior to reimplantation by the ophthalmological surgeon
b. Signifies permanent loss of vision
c. Are best managed by replanting the eye at the scene
d. Require the placement of a free tissue graft prior to replanting the eye

13. What should be done if a pencil has penetrated the globe of the left eye in a young adult?
a. The pencil should be removed immediately, an ice pack should be placed, and the patient prepared for transfer.
b. First threats to life should be attended to, followed by gently removing the pencil and placing an ice pack on the eye.
c. The pencil should be stabilized while still in the eye, then both eyes covered so that the patient cannot "see" at all.
d. This injury is not addressed as nothing further can be done.

14. Contact lenses:
a. Should be removed in the field in an unconscious patient with prolonged transport times
b. Should only be removed if the patient has not suffered an acid or alkali burn
c. Should be left in place
d. Should be immediately removed and discarded

CRITICAL THINKING

- You are dispatched to the scene of a sporting event injury. Upon arrival, you find a 22-year-old-male holding an ice pack to the right side of his face. You are greeted by the coach who informs you that the patient was struck in the eye with a hockey puck. The patient complains of pain around the orbit and a "curtain" partially obstructing his vision. You also note that the eye is fixed in a downward gaze and the pupil is reactive. The patient also complains of numbness of the right cheek. Describe the pathophysiology present in this patient. How will you treat this injury?

- What is the mechanism by which a neck laceration may produce a constricted pupil?

- What airway procedures are likely to be required in the setting of massive facial fractures? What are the possible hazards of nasally intubating a patient with facial fractures?

REFERENCES

1. Beck RA, Blakeslee DB. The changing picture of facial fractures. *Arch Otolaryngol Head Neck Surg.* 1989; 115:826.
2. Nakamura T, Gross CW. Facial fractures—analysis of five year experience. Arch Otolaryngol. 1973; 97:288.
3. Schultz RC. Facial injuries from automobile accidents: study of 400 consecutive cases. *Plast Reconstr Surg.* 1967; 40:415.

4. Barot LR. Maxillofacial trauma. *Top Emerg Med.* 1991; 13(4):17.

5. Slupchynskyj OS, Berkower AS, Byrne DW, Cayten CG. Association of skull base and facial fractures. *Laryngoscope.* 1992; 102(11):1247.

6. Haug RH, Savage JD, Likavec MJ, Conforti PJ. A review of 100 closed head injuries associated with facial fractures. *J Oral Maxillofac Surg.* 1992; 50(3):218.

7. Bringhurst C, Herr RD, Aldous JA. Oral trauma in the emergency department. *Am J Emerg Med.* 1993; 11(5):486.

8. Andreasen J. *Traumatic Injuries of the Teeth.* 2nd ed. Philadelphia: Saunders, 1981.

9. Kravis TC, Warner CG, Jacobs LM. *Emergency Medicine: A Comprehensive Review.* 3rd ed. Philadelphia: Lippincott-Raven; 1993.

10. Rogers S, Hill JR, Mackay GM. Maxillofacial injuries following steering wheel contact by drivers using seat belts. *Brit J Oral Maxillofac Surg.* 1992; 30(1):24.

11. Fridrich KL, Pena-Velasco G, Olson RA. Changing trends with mandibular fractures: a review of 1,067 cases. *J Oral Maxillofac Surg.* 1992; 50:586.

12. Le Fort R. Etude experimentale sur les fractures de le machoire superieure. *Rav Chir.* 1901; 23:208.

13. Shuker ST. Maxillofacial blast injuries. *J Craniomaxillofac Surg.* 1995; 23(2):91.

14. Committee on Trauma. *Advanced Trauma Life Support Student Manual.* Chicago, Ill: American College of Surgeons; 1993.

15. Pollack RA. Nasal trauma: pathomechanics and surgical management of acute injuries. *Clin Plast Surg.* 1992; 19(1):133.

16. Furgurson JE, Meislin HW. *Airway Problems in the Trauma Victim: Priorities in Multiple Trauma.* Germantown, Pa: Aspen Corp; 1980.

17. Cicala RS, Kudsk KA, Butts A, Nguyen H, Fabian TC. Initial evaluation and management of upper airway injuries in trauma patients. *J Clin Anesthesiol.* 1991; 3:91.

18. Kovac AL. Upper airway trauma and obstruction: a review of causes, evaluation and management. *Respir Care.* 1993; 38(4):356.

19. Pepe P, Stewart R, Copass M. Prehospital management of trauma: a tale of three cities. *Ann Emerg Med.* 1986; 15(12):1484.

20. Ampel L, Hott KA, Sielaff GW, Sloan TB. An approach to airway management in the acutely head injured patient. *J Emerg Med.* 1988; 6:1.

21. Esposito TJ, Sanddal ND, Hansen JD, Reynolds S. Analysis of preventable trauma deaths and inappropriate trauma care in a rural state. *J Trauma.* 1995; 39(5):955.

22. O'Brien D, Danzl DF, Sowers MB, Hooker EA. Airway management of aeromedically transported trauma patients. *J Emerg Med.* 1988; 6:49.

23. Spaite DW, Joseph M. Prehospital cricothyrotomy: an investigation of indications, technique, complications, and patient outcome. *Ann Emerg Med.* 1990; 19(3):279.

24. Weymuller EA, Jr., Pavlin EG, Paugh D, Cummings CN. Management of difficult airway problems with percutaneous transtracheal ventilation. *Ann Otol Rhinol Laryngol.* 1987; 96(1):34.

25. Salvino CK, Dries D, Garnelli R, Murphy-Macobobby M, Marshall W. Emergency cricothyroidotomy in trauma victims. *J Trauma.* 1993; 34(4):503.

26. Hawkins ML, Shapiro MD, Cue JI, Wiggins SS. Emergency cricothyrotomy: a reassessment. *Am Surg.* 1995; 61(1):52.

27. Metz S, Parmet JL, Levitt JD. Failed emergency transtracheal ventilation through a 14 gauge intravenous catheter. *J Clin Anesth.* 1996; 8(1):58.

28. *Fact Sheet.* New York: National Society for the Prevention of Blindness; 1980.

29. Katz J, Tielsch JM. Lifetime prevalence of ocular injuries from the Baltimore Eye Survey. *Arch Ophthalmol.* 1993; 111(11):1564.

30. Ready R. Commentary on sports related eye trauma. *ENA Nursing Scan Emerg Care.* 1994; 4(2):10.

31. Baker RS, Wilson MR, Flowers CW Jr., Lee DA, Wheeler NC. Demographic factors in a population-based survey of hospitalized, work-related ocular injury. *Am J Ophthalmol.* 1996; 122(2):213.

32. Hemady RK. Ocular injuries from violence at an inner-city hospital. *J Trauma.* 1994; 37(1):5.

33. Beck SR, Freitag SL, Singer N. Ocular injuries in battered women. *Ophthalmology.* 1996; 103(1):148.

34. Gilliland MG, Folberg R. Shaken babies—some have no impact injuries. *J Forensic Sci.* 1996; 41(1):114.

35. Kuhn F, Collins P, Morris R, Witherspoon CD. Epidemiology of motor vehicle crash–related serious eye injuries. *Accid Anal Prev.* 1994; 26(3):385.

36. Duma SM, Kress TA, Porta DJ, et al. Airbag-induced eye injuries: A report of 25 cases. *J Trauma.* 1996; 41(1):114.

37. Vichnin MC, Jaeger EA, Gault JA, Jeffers JB. Ocular injuries related to airbag inflation. *Ophthalm Surg Lasers.* 1995; 26(6):542.

38. Gault JA, Vinchin MC, Jaeger EA, Jeffers JB. Ocular injuries associated with eyeglass wear and airbag inflation. *J Trauma.* 1995; 38(4):494.

39. Luff AJ, Hodgkins PR, Baxter RJ, Morrell AJ, Calder I. Etiology of perforating eye injury. *Arch Dis Child.* 1993; 68(5):682.

40. Kutschke PJ. Ocular trauma in children. *Ophthalm Nursing Technol*. 1994; 13(3):117.

41. Sastry SM, Paul BIL, Bain L, Champion HR. Ocular trauma among major trauma victims in a regional trauma center. *J Trauma*. 1993; 34(2):223.

42. Jabaley ME, Lerman M, Sanders HJ. Ocular injuries in orbital fractures: a review of 119 cases. *Plast Reconstr Surg*. 1975; 56:410.

43. Stern JD, Goldfarb IW, Slater H. Ophthalmological complications as a manifestation of burn injury. *Burns*. 1996; 22(2):135.

44. Handler JA, Ghezzi KT. General opthamalogical examination. *Emerg Clin North Am*. 1995; 13(3):521.

45. Pavan-Langston D. *Manual of Ocular Diagnosis and Therapy*. 4th ed. New York: Little, Brown and Company; 1996.

46. Fabbri M, Celotti GC, Ravaglioli A. Hydroxyapatite-based porous aggregates: physico-chemical nature, structure, texture and architecture. *Biomaterials*. 1995; 16(3):225.

47. Beumer J, Roumanas E, Nishimura R. Advances in osseointegrated implants for dental and facial rehabilitation following major head and neck surgery. *Sem Surg Oncol*. 1995; 11(3):200.

48. Mole C, Gerard H, Mallet JL, Chassagne JF, Miller N. A new three dimensional treatment algorithm for complex surfaces: applications in surgery. *J Oral Maxillofac Surg*. 1995; 53(2):158.

49. Gossman MD, Roberts DM, Barr CC. Ophthalmic aspects of orbital injury: a comprehensive diagnostic and management approach. *Clin Plast Surg*. 1992; 19(1):71.

50. DeJuan E, Steinberg P, Michaels RG. Penetrating ocular injuries: types of injuries and visual results. *Ophthalmology*. 1983; 90:1318.

Chapter 13

Chest Trauma

OBJECTIVES

Upon completion of this chapter, the reader should be able to:

- Describe the incidence, morbidity, and mortality of thoracic injuries.
- Provide an overview of the normal anatomy and physiology of the thorax.
- Discuss the pathophysiology, assessment findings, and treatment of chest wall injuries.
- Discuss the pathophysiology, assessment findings, and treatment of lung injuries.
- Discuss the pathophysiology, assessment findings, and treatment of myocardial injuries.
- Discuss the pathophysiology, assessment findings, and treatment of vascular injuries.
- Discuss the pathophysiology, assessment findings, and treatment of diaphragmatic injuries.
- Discuss the pathophysiology, assessment findings, and treatment of tracheal, bronchiolar, and esophageal injuries.
- Discuss the pathophysiology, assessment findings, and treatment of traumatic asphyxia.
- Acquire a systematic approach to the patient with chest trauma, taking into consideration the anatomy, pathophysiology, and possible life-threatening injuries that can occur.
- Describe the invasive procedures of pericardiocentesis, needle thoracentesis, and chest tube insertion.

KEY TERMS

Aortic disruption
Beck's triad
Cardiac tamponade
Flail chest
Hamman's sign
Kussmaul's sign
Massive hemothorax
Mediastinum
Minute ventilation (MV)
Myocardial concussion

Myocardial contusion
Myocardial rupture
Needle thoracentesis
Open pneumothorax
Parietal pleura
Pendelluft
Pericardiocentesis
Pericardium
Physiological dead space
Pneumothorax

Pseudocoarctation syndrome
Pulmonary contusion
Pulsus paradoxus
Tension pneumothorax
Tidal volume (TV)
Tube thoracostomy
Ventilation-perfusion (V/Q) matching
Visceral pleura

Chest trauma is one of the most life-threatening injuries encountered by paramedics. Isolated chest injuries account for 25% of all trauma deaths in North America (second only to head trauma) and contribute to another 25% of multiply-injured fatalities.[1] The major causes of blunt chest trauma are automobile steering wheels and bicycle handlebars, while gunshot wounds and stabbings account for the majority of penetrating injuries. However, life-threatening thoracic injuries can result from even seemingly insignificant causes such as a BB shot or a blow from a baseball. Less than 10% of patients with blunt chest injuries ultimately require surgery and only 15%–30% of patients with penetrating chest trauma require open thoracotomy. Many deaths are preventable with prompt diagnosis and treatment.[2–5]

Most patients sustaining either blunt or penetrating chest trauma are managed with relatively simple procedures provided the proper diagnoses are made. To make the proper diagnosis, the paramedic must pay careful attention to the details of the history, physical assessment, and mechanisms of injury. It is essential that the paramedic possess a sound knowledge of the pathophysiology of chest trauma in order to effectively treat the injured patient.

ANATOMY AND PHYSIOLOGY

When evaluating injured patients, always consider the anatomy of the affected region in a systematic fashion. For the thoracic region, an outside-to-inside approach works well, beginning with the skin and advancing into the lungs and mediastinum.

The outermost layer of the thorax consists of skin and subcutaneous tissues, including the pectoral and upper back muscles. The chest wall is an elastic structure supported by 12 pairs of ribs that articulate with the sternum and the thoracic spine. Between the ribs, there are two to three layers of intercostal muscles. Along the inferior and internal surface of the ribs lies the costal groove, where the intercostal vein, artery, and nerve can be found. The intercostal vein is the most superior and the nerve is the most inferior neurovascular structure within the groove.

The chest wall serves many functions. First, it supports and protects the lungs and heart. Second, movement of the chest wall facilitates ventilation by expansion and contraction. Depending on anatomic location, the intercostal muscles have two to three layers that assist both inspiration and expiration. The intercostal muscles work with the diaphragm and accessory muscles to facilitate breathing. Expansion of the rib cage combined with contraction (flattening) of the diaphragm increases the thoracic volume and

therefore decreases intrathoracic pressure, causing air to enter the lungs. Conversely, relaxation (or active contraction of the inner layer) of the intercostal muscles and the diaphragm decreases thoracic volume and increases intrathoracic pressure, forcing air out of the lungs.

The intercostal muscles are innervated by the intercostal nerves. These nerves branch from the spinal cord at the level where the ribs articulate with the thoracic vertebrae. The diaphragm is innervated primarily by the right and left phrenic nerves, which originate from the spinal cord at the level of the C3–C5 cervical vertebrae. The diaphragm also receives limited innervation from the intercostal nerves.

The lungs are elastic structures that occupy the right and left pleural cavities. The chest wall is lined with a thin, tough membrane called the **parietal pleura**. The outer surface of each lung is covered by a separate **visceral pleura**. Normally, there is just a small amount of fluid between the parietal and visceral pleural surfaces to provide lubrication and to keep the lung adhered to the chest wall by high surface tension. In adults, either pleural cavity could potentially contain 3 liters of blood or air within the space between the visceral and parietal pleura.[6]

The volume of air inhaled and exhaled is referred to as **tidal volume (TV)**. **Minute ventilation (MV)** is a calculated or measured volume of air exchanged by the lung in 1 minute and is the product of TV and respiratory rate (RR). In the normal adult, TV is approximately 500 mL and the average RR is 14 breaths per minute. Therefore, the average adult MV is 7,000 mL/min. Not all of this volume, however, is used for gas exchange. For example, the trachea and bronchi are thick structures and cannot exchange oxygen and carbon dioxide. The volume of air in these areas is referred to as **physiological dead space** and is usually about 100 mL. Therefore, the volume of air reaching alveoli would be the tidal volume minus the physiological dead space, or 400 mL in the average breath. Consequently, average alveolar ventilation is approximately 5,600 mL/min in the average adult. However, patients with chest trauma often take rapid and shallow breaths due to pain. If the breath is only 200 mL, only 100 mL is actually getting to the alveoli for gas exchange, less if there is pulmonary injury (e.g., pathological dead space from pneumothorax).

The most basic functional unit of the lung is the alveolus. Alveoli are mildly resistant to collapse due to surfactants produced that decrease their surface tension. The exchange of oxygen and carbon dioxide occurs at the interface of the alveolar-pulmonary capillary membrane. Normally pulmonary blood flow (perfusion) is directed to areas of the lung that are well ventilated. This is referred to as **ventilation-perfusion (V/Q)**

matching. When V/Q mismatching occurs, blood enters systemic circulation without being adequately oxygenated. In trauma patients, there are many injuries that may result in V/Q mismatching, such as shock, pneumothorax, and hemothorax. Ventilation-perfusion mismatching is discussed in detail in Chapter 18.

Oxygen and carbon dioxide diffuse at different rates between the alveoli and bloodstream because of their chemical properties. Carbon dioxide diffuses rapidly from the blood to the alveoli. As a result, the concentration of carbon dioxide in the blood is dependent on alveolar ventilation. As alveolar ventilation increases, carbon dioxide levels will decrease. However, oxygen does not diffuse as quickly from the alveoli to the bloodstream. Therefore, the delivery of oxygen is dependent on the number of open alveoli in order to have maximal surface area for diffusion into the bloodstream. There are two ways to improve oxygenation: increase the inspired oxygen concentration and/or increase the number of open alveoli (alveolar recruitment). Increasing the number of open alveoli can be achieved by adequate pain control, which allows adequate expansion of the lung.[2] If the patient is intubated and on a ventilator, positive end-expiratory pressure (PEEP) will keep more alveoli open and improve oxygenation. However, higher levels of PEEP (greater than 15 cm H_2O) can decrease venous return to the heart and can elevate pressures within the lung (see Chapter 18).

The central region of the thorax is the **mediastinum**, which contains the heart, great vessels, esophagus, lymphatic channels, trachea, mainstem bronchi, and paired vagus and phrenic nerves. The heart is contained within a tough fibrous sac called the **pericardium**. Much like the pleura, the pericardium has two surfaces: the inner visceral layer, which adheres to the heart and forms the epicardium, and the outer, parietal layer, which is considered the sac itself. The parietal pericardium is a fibrous layer and acutely nondistensible, yet diseases that cause slow accumulations of fluid can distend the sac by as much as 1,000–1,500 mL.[7] Normally there are 30–50 mL of lubricating fluid secreted by the visceral pericardium and contained within the space between the heart and pericardial sac.[7] The pericardium that covers the inferior aspect of the heart is directly attached to the diaphragm. The heart is positioned so that the most anterior portion is the right ventricle, which has relatively thin chamber walls. The pressure within the right ventricle is approximately one-fourth of that within the left ventricle. Most of the heart is protected anteriorly by the sternum. With each beat the apex of the heart can be felt in the fifth intercostal space along the midclavicular line. This is referred to as the cardiac impulse. The average cardiac output for an adult (heart rate times stroke volume) is 4–8 liters/min; the exact amount depends on the patient's size.

The trachea, superior vena cava, aortic arch, recurrent laryngeal nerves, and esophagus are found in the superior mediastinum. The recurrent laryngeal nerves are branches of the vagus nerves that innervate the muscles of the larynx. The left recurrent nerve travels around the inferior aspect of the aortic arch before it ascends along the trachea to the larynx. The posterior mediastinum contains the descending aorta, esophagus, and lymphatic channels. The descending aorta is firmly attached to the thoracic vertebrae and is tethered to the heart by the tough ligamentum arteriosum, which is a remnant of fetal circulation.[6] Compared to the other vessels, the aorta is thicker and more elastic. The aorta is made up of several layers: the tunica intima, tunica media, and tunica adventitia. The tunica intima is a relatively thin layer of cells lining the lumen of the aorta. The tunica media is a thick elastic muscular layer and the tunica adventitia is a tough fibrous outer layer.

PATHOPHYSIOLOGY

Systemic hypoxia, hypercarbia, and acidosis often result from chest injuries. Acutely, hypoxia is the most important to treat.[2] With severe injury and stress, the oxygen requirements of the body increase significantly. Systemic hypoxia results from inadequate oxygen delivery secondary to hypovolemia, pulmonary V/Q mismatches, changes in intrathoracic pressure relationships, and direct trauma to the heart. Pulmonary V/Q mismatches can result from damage to lung tissue, altering the ability of oxygen to diffuse into the pulmonary capillaries. Ventilation-perfusion mismatches can also occur if the alveoli are collapsed or filled with blood.[8] Examples of changes of intrathoracic pressure are **pneumothorax** or hemothorax. When air enters the pleural space, adhesion by surface tension to the chest wall is lost wherever the visceral and parietal pleura lose contact. Without enough adhesion, adequate expansion of the lung is not possible, compromising ventilation. In contrast, if there is too much blood or other fluid in the pleural space, compression of the lungs will cause alveolar collapse, resulting in hypercarbia and respiratory acidosis.

Both blunt and penetrating trauma to the heart and pericardium can decrease the ability to provide adequate systemic perfusion. Cardiac tamponade or tension pneumothorax will cause compression of the heart. This can result in **pulsus paradoxus**, which is a decrease in the systolic blood pressure by greater than 10 mm Hg with inspiration. During inspiration the lung volume increases, as well as the volume within the pulmonary vessels. If the right ventricle is compressed, the ejected volume may not be adequate to fill the pulmonary vasculature. This will reduce the preload of the left side of the heart and decrease cardiac output.[6] Advanced cases of pulsus paradoxus may result in loss of the radial pulse during inspiration, resulting in a waxing and waning of the radial pulse that is synchronized with breathing.[9]

INITIAL ASSESSMENT AND STABILIZATION

The approach to the patient with a chest injury should consist of initial assessment, resuscitation, further assessment, and definitive care.[2] To effectively manage chest trauma, the paramedic must know what life-threatening injuries are possible and how to identify them.

As with all patients, the first considerations are airway, breathing, and circulation. When evaluating the patient's airway, check first for patency and evaluate the quality of air exchange. Look for retractions, stridor, hoarseness, subcutaneous emphysema, and potential foreign bodies. Early protection of the patient's airway and adequate oxygenation are essential for survival.[9]

Breathing should be evaluated by exposing the patient's chest. Assess the patient's respiratory rate, effort, pattern, and skin color. Cyanosis is a late finding that should be treated as rapidly as possible. However, the absence of cyanosis does not necessarily indicate adequate systemic oxygenation.[9] Carefully examine the chest wall for contusions and open wounds. Excessive abdominal movement during respiration may indicate that only the diaphragm is controlling ventilation.[2] This could occur if there is lower cervical or thoracic spinal trauma with loss of innervation to the intercostal muscles. Systematic auscultation should be performed to assess heart sounds, bowel sounds, and symmetry and adequacy of respirations.

The thorax should be palpated, starting with the trachea to ensure normal position. Crepitus associated with subcutaneous emphysema is a sign of injury to the lungs or lower airway. In addition, the ribs should be palpated for crepitus, tenderness, or deformity.

Circulation should be evaluated by checking the quality, rate, and regularity of the patient's pulses, followed by assessment of the blood pressure. Auscultation of the heart may reveal muffled heart tones or rubs, indicating excess fluid in the pericardium. The skin should be checked for color and temperature, and the neck veins should be examined for signs of distention. However, hypovolemic patients may not have adequate volume to produce distended neck veins, even in the presence of cardiac tamponade or tension pneumothorax.

The chest should be palpated to locate the cardiac impulse. A dull cardiac impulse, especially in a slender young adult, could indicate excessive pericardial fluid. Likewise, a shifted cardiac impulse could indicate a tension pneumothorax. Patients should be placed on a cardiac monitor to evaluate for dysrhythmias that could result from myocardial trauma. Frequent premature ventricular contractions are treated with a lidocaine bolus of 1 mg/kg, followed by an infusion of 2–4 mg/min.[2] Pulseless electrical activity (PEA) may be present from cardiac tamponade, tension pneumothorax, hypovolemia, or cardiac rupture.

STABILIZATION OF THE PATIENT

Essential elements of stabilization of chest trauma patients are airway control and large-bore intravenous access with close physiological monitoring. Airway control does not necessarily mean intubation. As long as easy ventilation occurs with spontaneous breathing or bag valve mask (BVM) ventilation, intubation is not an immediate priority. High concentrations of oxygen should be administered to maximize systemic oxygen delivery to meet the increased metabolic demands of the trauma patient and should be monitored by pulse oximetry. Intravenous fluids should be given judiciously for reasons described later in this chapter. Clearly, if the patient is in shock, fluids should be given rapidly to improve systemic perfusion. Persistent hypotension despite large amounts of intravenous fluids should raise the concern of continuing hemorrhage, cardiac tamponade, or tension pneumothorax.

Patients with penetrating chest trauma have been reported to arrest during or soon after intubation. Such arrests are caused by several factors, including inadequate preintubation oxygenation, esophageal intubation, mainstem bronchial intubation, vasovagal response, excessive respiratory alkalosis, and excessive positive pressure ventilation.[10] Excessive positive pressure ventilation decreases venous return to the heart and can cause a tension pneumothorax quickly, either of which will diminish cardiac output.[10]

Tension pneumothorax, open pneumothorax, massive hemothorax, flail chest, cardiac tamponade, and dysrhythmias are life-threatening injuries that require correction when found in the initial assessment. Each will be discussed in turn.

TENSION PNEUMOTHORAX

Tension pneumothorax results from the formation of a one-way valve. Air enters the pleural space from either a defect in the lungs or the chest wall and cannot leave, resulting in almost complete collapse of the affected lung and compression of the mediastinum (Figure 13-1). It is not, however, the collapse of the lung that is life threatening. Rather, it is the compression and shift of the mediastinal structures to the contralateral side due to the accumulation of air and increased intrathoracic pressure. Shifting of the mediastinum will cause the great veins within the mediastinum to kink, hindering venous blood return to the heart and decreasing cardiac output. The decrease in cardiac output may result in cardiogenic shock and death. The most common causes of tension pneumothorax are mechanical ventilation, spontaneous pneumothorax caused by rupture of emphysematous alveoli, blunt trauma [including cardiopulmonary resuscitation (CPR)] that shears the bronchi, and penetrating chest injuries.

The clinical picture of a tension pneumothorax is that of respiratory distress, jugular venous distention (absent with concomitant hypovolemia), deviation of the trachea (a late and often preterminal event) and

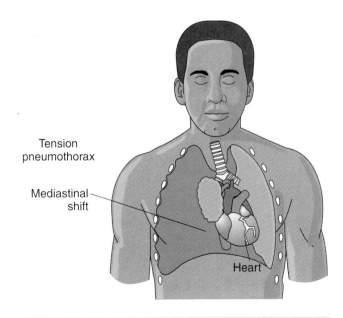

Tension pneumothorax

Mediastinal shift

Heart

FIGURE 13-1 Tension pneumothorax. Note the deviated mediastinum.

cardiac impulse away from the affected side, tachycardia, narrowed pulse pressure, and unilateral absent or decreased breath sounds on the affected side. Chest rise with ventilation is often asymmetric; only the uninjured side will rise and fall with ventilation.[6] If the affected side of the chest is percussed, an increase in resonance will be noticed when compared to the other side. Pulsus paradoxus may be present and, when severe, may result in loss of the radial pulse during inspiration.[9]

Tension pneumothorax requires immediate decompression. Temporizing maneuvers can be either needle decompression or, in the case of penetrating trauma, reopening the wound.[2] A rush of air should be heard and hemodynamic improvement will hopefully result. In patients with a thick chest wall, standard needle decompression may not provide adequate decompression.[11]

Definitive treatment of tension pneumothorax requires placement of a chest tube. The chest tube can be relatively small (24 French) and can be placed either in the second intercostal space in the midclavicular line or in the fourth intercostal space in the midaxillary line (Figure 13-2).[2] If the chest tube is placed in the midaxillary line, it should be directed anteriorly toward the apex of the thoracic cavity in order to maximize air drainage.[9] The techniques of needle thoracostomy and tube thoracostomy are discussed later.

INTERNET ACTIVITIES

Visit the e-medicine Web site at http://www. emedicine.com/. Click on the Emergency Medicine on-line book and select Trauma and Orthopedics. Then click on Pneumothorax. Review the chapter on the management of tension pneumothorax.

OPEN PNEUMOTHORAX

An **open pneumothorax** is the result of a defect in the chest wall that allows air to enter the thoracic space. These injuries are often the result of penetrating injuries, such as impaled objects and gunshot and knife wounds, but may also result from blunt trauma, such as falls and motor vehicle collisions (MVCs).[6] The most common mechanism of injury is a shotgun blast.[12] Some open pneumothoraces, such as small knife wounds, are self-sealing and do not allow entrainment of atmospheric air. In contrast, gunshot wounds, especially from shotgun or large-caliber weapons, produce large defects in the chest wall that allow intrathoracic and atmospheric pressures to equilibrate, markedly decreasing the effectiveness of ventilation. The size of the defect does not need to be large to compromise

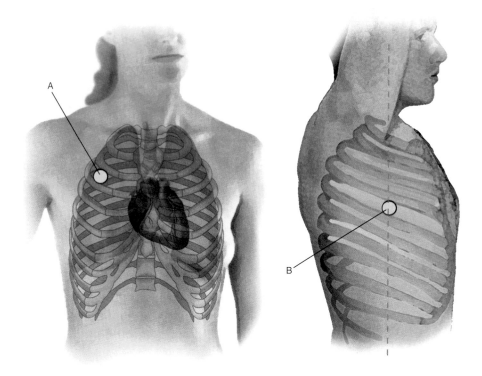

FIGURE 13-2 Locations for (A) needle thoracostomy and (B) tube thoracostomy.

ventilation.[1] Airflow follows the path of least resistance. Resistance to flow through an opening is directly proportional to the length of the opening and inversely proportional to the radius elevated to the third power. Consequently, if a defect in the chest wall is greater than two-thirds of the diameter of the trachea, air will preferentially flow into the chest through the defect because of its decreased resistance to airflow relative to the upper airway, creating the pathognomonic "sucking" sound.[1]

Treatment is aimed at oxygenation and closure of the chest wall defect. Most authorities agree that these injuries need prompt treatment by covering the defect with an occlusive dressing, such as petroleum-based gauze, taped on three sides to allow air to escape and effectively converting the open pneumothorax to a closed pneumothorax.[8] The patient must then be monitored carefully for signs of a developing tension pneumothorax, such as hypotension, respiratory difficulty, decreased pulse pressure, hypoxia, and jugular venous distention. If these occur, then the dressing should be temporarily removed and the wound may even need to be opened to allow the intrapleural air to escape.[6] However, some believe the risk of developing a life-threatening tension pneumothorax outweighs the potential benefit of the occlusive dressing and recommend leaving the chest wall open to air, while others believe that an occlusive dressing should be used only

when the defect in the chest wall is greater than two-thirds the diameter of the trachea, especially if the patient is intubated.[3]

Definitive treatment of an open pneumothorax depends on the size of the injury. Placement of a chest tube combined with an occlusive dressing may be adequate or, if not, surgical repair is necessary.[1] Chest tubes should not be inserted into open wounds because (1) the tube is likely to follow a tear in a lung or the tract of a penetrating wound further into the lungs and mediastinum, (2) the defects in the chest wall are usually contaminated, (3) surgical closure of the chest wall defect is usually required, and (4) the chest wall defect is usually larger than the diameter of the chest tube, making it impossible to obtain an adequate seal around the tube.[9,13,14]

MASSIVE HEMOTHORAX

Massive hemothorax results from a collection of approximately 1,500 mL of blood in the pleural space.[2] Hemothorax occurs in roughly 25% of patients with chest trauma and is most commonly caused by tears of the lung parenchyma but may also result from penetrating wounds that puncture the heart or major vessels within the mediastinum or from blunt trauma with deceleration shearing of major vessels.[1,15] Hemorrhage from injured lung parenchyma tends to be self-limiting but can be substantial if there is a major laceration. Specific vessel injuries are less often the source of hemorrhage, but when present, the intercostal and internal mammary arteries are more likely to be injured than hilar or great vessels.[16–18] Hemothorax due to tears in the lung parenchyma requires thoracotomy in only 5%–15% of patients admitted with chest trauma, due to the compressing effect of the shed blood, the high concentration of thromboplastin in the lungs, and the relatively low pulmonary arterial pressure.[1] In severe cases of lung parenchymal injury or injury to the heart or major vessels, the severe hypovolemia that can result is often further complicated by the reduced pulmonary capacity and compromised ventilation, resulting in severe hypoxia. In addition, the presence of greater than 300 mL of blood in the pleural cavity may form large clots that act as a local anticoagulant by releasing fibrinolysins and fibrinogenolysins from their surface, resulting in continued bleeding.[1]

The clinical presentation of hemothorax is usually that of shock, tachycardia, absent or decreased breath sounds, and/or dullness to percussion on the affected side.[2] Neck veins may be flat or distended depending on the degree of hypovolemia and intrathoracic pressure. Blood in the pleural space does not hinder ventilation as much as air because blood has adequate surface tension to expand the lungs when the chest wall is expanded. However, the combination of hypovolemia and V/Q mismatching decreases systemic oxygen delivery and signs of air hunger are usually present. A differential diagnosis between this condition, pericardial tamponade, and tension pneumothorax is given in Table 13-1.

The initial management of these patients is establishing a secure airway with delivery of 100% oxygen and large-bore IV access with rapid infusion of crystalloid fluid. The pneumatic antishock garment may also be used, although this is controversial. Needle decompression is of little value but may be needed to differentiate between tension pneumothorax and massive hemothorax. Once needle decompression has been performed, the catheter should remain in place until a chest tube is placed to drain any air that may have been introduced or that may also be present. Blood products should be administered as soon as possible. A large-bore (38 French or larger) chest tube should be placed in patients with hemothorax to allow adequate drainage.[2] The chest tube should be placed in the midaxillary line at the level of the fourth intercostal space and directed posteriorly to maximize blood drainage. Because of its decompressing effect, the chest tube may actually increase the rate of hemorrhage, potentially allowing the patient to exsanguinate through the chest tube. Consequently, if the chest tube is placed in the field and greater than 1,500 mL of blood returns or the patient's vital signs deteriorate, the chest tube should be clamped to prevent further blood loss until the patient can reach the hospital where open thoracotomies or definitive thoracic surgery can be performed.

Autotransfusion is occasionally performed as a temporizing measure until surgical correction of bleeding can be performed. Blood from the chest cavity is ideal for autotransfusion because of the lack of contaminants.[1] If adequate type-specific blood is not available, shed blood is carefully collected and treated with citrate or heparin to reduce clotting. The blood is then filtered and washed with saline before being returned to the body. Unfortunately, autotransfusion is time consuming and often leads to coagulation problems, especially if large volumes of blood are transfused. In most cases, it is much easier and faster to use blood from the blood bank.[9]

Table 13-1
Differential Diagnosis of Massive Hemothorax, Tension Pneumothorax, and Cardiac Tamponade

Assessment	Massive Hemothorax	Tension Pneumothorax	Cardiac Tamponade
Pulse	Rapid	Rapid	Rapid
Blood pressure	Low	Low	Low
Pulsus paradoxus	No	Yes	Possibly
Heart sounds	Audible	Audible	Muffled
Neck veins	Flat	Distended	Distended
Percussion	Dull	Hyperresonant	Normal
Trachea	Midline/deviated	Deviated	Midline
Chest symmetry	Normal/asymmetrical	Asymmetrical	Normal
Breath sounds	Absent/rhonchi/rales	Absent	Present

FLAIL CHEST

Flail chest is a common major injury to the chest wall, occurring in up to 20% of admitted trauma patients.[19] The associated mortality rates range as high as 50% in some series, even higher in patients over 60 years of age, and is directly related to the underlying and associated injuries.[20–23] The underlying lung is injured in most cases of flail chest, with pulmonary contusion and/or hemothorax occurring in greater than 50% of cases.[19] Flail chest typically results from direct impacts, such as striking the steering wheel during a MVC, or compression, such as that encountered in pedestrian injuries where the patient is run over by the vehicle. Because of the pliability of their ribs, children rarely experience flail injuries.[19]

Flail chest results when a segment of the chest wall loses bony contact with the rest of the thoracic cage. Usually two or more adjacent ribs are fractured in two or more locations. Flailing may be located anteriorly, laterally, or posteriorly (Figure 13-3). Anterior flail areas, also called flailed sternum, result from direct impacts resulting in sternal fracture and multiple costochondral dislocations.[19] Lateral flails frequently occur as a result of crushing injuries involving fractures or dislocations of ribs anteriorly, with another row of fractures in the lateral or posterior chest wall.[19] Posterior flail areas usually result from fractures at approximately the midaxillary line with associated fractures or dislocations near the costovertebral junction.

The classic presentation of flail chest is one of paradoxical chest wall motion, where the flail segment appears to move in the opposite direction of the chest wall during the respiratory cycle. Because the flail segment has lost its bony structure, the negative intrathoracic pressure created during inspiration allows the unstable flail segment to be retracted. In contrast, the increased intrathoracic pressure of expiration causes the flail segment to bulge outward.

Often flail chest may not be initially apparent due to marked intercostal muscle spasm and splinting of the chest following injury. Paradoxical movement becomes apparent only later, when the muscles fatigue, lung compliance decreases, and respiratory work increases. This may be a contributing factor in the failure to identify flail chest within the first 6 hours in up to 30% of patients with this injury.[24] Consequently, the paramedic should not expect to see the classic paradoxical motion but a patient demonstrating splinting of the affected region, with somewhat asymmetric chest wall movement, tachypnea, and complaints of significant pain.[2] In addition, patients requiring intubation will not present with paradoxical motion due to the internal splinting effect of positive pressure ventilation.[25] However, paradoxical motion will be exaggerated by increases in inspiratory intrathoracic pressure, such as occurs in airway obstruction, or expiratory intrathoracic pressure, such as that associated with expiratory grunting. Correction of these will decrease the magnitude of flailing and improve ventilation.[19]

Although the paradoxical motion of the unstable flail can greatly increase the work of breathing, the main cause of hypoxemia of flail chest is the underlying pulmonary contusion. In the past, **pendelluft** (movement of air between the injured and uninjured lung with each breath) was thought to be an important cause of hypoxemia. However, pendelluft is probably significant only when flail chest is accompanied by partial upper airway obstruction.[1] Nonetheless, paradoxical movement prevents full expansion of the underlying lung, decreasing minute ventilation. In addition, pain will prevent the patient from making full expansion of the chest. Thus, the major problems associated with flail chest are the underlying pulmonary complications.

Pulmonary contusion usually accompanies flail chest, resulting in the affected sections of lung becoming filled with fluid. The affected lung sections impair oxygenation of the blood and become less compliant. Decreased lung compliance will increase the labor of breathing, resulting in fatigue of the intercostal muscles, allowing the flail segment to move more easily. This perpetuates a vicious cycle of increased respiratory effort with less effective ventilation, further increasing respiratory effort. The patient can fatigue rapidly at this point, and sudden respiratory failure can occur. Respiratory failure can occur anywhere from minutes to 24 hours, depending on the extent of the injury and the health of the patient.[9]

For patients with flail chest it is crucial to treat hypoxia and pain. Pain control minimizes patient splinting, allowing better ventilation.[2] If the flail segment is unstable, it should be stabilized using a pressure dressing. Sandbags add unnecessary resistance to respiratory efforts and should be avoided.[9] Ventilatory support should be provided early to prevent significant fatigue. Not all patients with flail chest will require intubation, but all should receive supplemental oxygen.

Indications for early ventilatory support include shock, labored breathing, head injury, three or more associated injuries, fracture of more than eight ribs, preexisting pulmonary disease, and age greater than 65.[9] If intubation and positive pressure ventilation become necessary, the patient should be monitored closely for the development of tension pneumothorax.

In contrast to the standard treatment of most trauma patients, fluids should be used cautiously in the setting of flail chest. In the absence of hypotension, limit fluid resuscitation due to the likelihood of pulmonary contusion. Excessive IV fluids will contribute to edema of the injured area of the lung, further decreasing oxygen exchange and lung compliance.

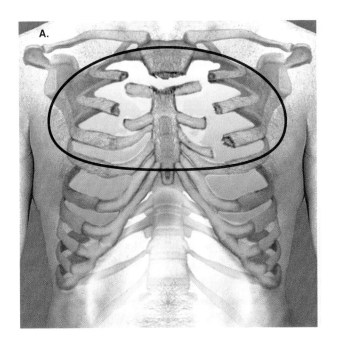

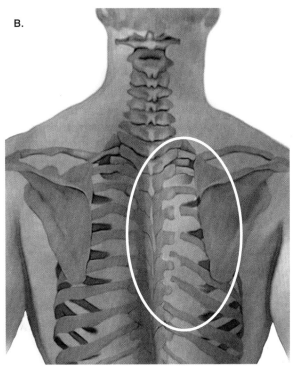

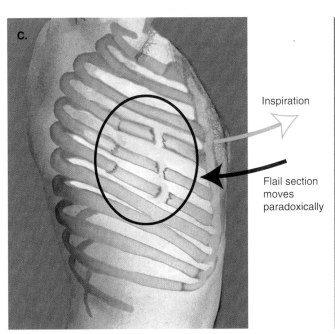

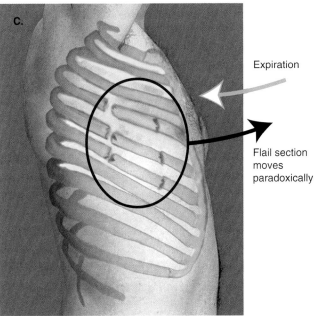

FIGURE 13-3 Areas of flail segments: (A) anterior, (B) posterior, and (C) lateral.

CARDIAC TAMPONADE

Penetrating injuries to the heart appear to be rising, presumably because of an increase in civilian violence.[26,27] **Cardiac tamponade** occurs in about 2% of patients with penetrating trauma to the chest and lower abdomen, and rarely occurs in the setting of blunt chest trauma.[28,29] In a collective review of 1,802 patients, the most common site of cardiac penetration was the right ventricle (42.5%), owing to its maximal anterior exposure, followed by the left ventricle (33%). The right atrium (15.4%) and the left atrium (5.8%) were much less frequently involved. The intrapericardial great vessels were injured in only 3.3% of patients, and injury to the coronary vasculature was rare.[30] Because it is difficult to predict the trajectory of a bullet or the length and direction of a knife wound, the paramedic must suspect cardiac tamponade with any penetrating injury to the thorax, especially wounds that lie over the precordium or epigastrium.

Cardiac tamponade is defined as excessive fluid in the pericardial sac, causing compression of the heart and decreased cardiac output. The hemodynamic effects of cardiac tamponade are determined by the size of the perforation in the pericardium, the rate of hemorrhage from the cardiac wound, and the chamber of the heart involved.[31] Pericardial lacerations secondary to knife wounds may be sealed rapidly by adjacent fatty tissue or by the formation of clots, setting the stage for accumulation of blood within the pericardium and cardiac tamponade.[27,32] Consequently, 80%–90% of patients with stab wounds of the heart develop tamponade.[31] In contrast to stab wounds, gunshot wounds of the pericardium and cardiac chambers are relatively large, favoring massive hemorrhage over developing a tamponade.[31] Pericardial tamponade develops in only 20% of gunshot wounds of the heart and pericardium.[30]

Once the pericardial laceration seals, continued hemorrhage fills the pericardial space. Because the pericardium is inelastic, small changes in volume can have significant effects on the pressure within the pericardium; as little as 50 cc of blood can compromise cardiac output. Compression of the heart prevents adequate filling during diastole and will increase diastolic pressure. This can be seen with central venous pressure (CVP) monitoring. The CVP will be elevated (greater than 15 cm H_2O) and will lose the characteristic drops in the waveform during diastole, resulting in a dampened appearance.[10] In the field, elevated CVP can be recognized as jugular venous distention, increased diastolic pressure, and a narrowed pulse pressure. In addition to reducing cardiac output, cardiac tamponade decreases perfusion of the myocardium by compressing the coronary arteries,

which can further the vicious cycle of shock by reducing myocardial perfusion.[33]

Blunt trauma can cause tamponade, but it usually results from parasternal stab wounds. Cardiac injury should be suspected with any penetrating trauma between the nipples and the inferior edge of the rib cage. Severe cardiac lacerations are usually immediately fatal. However, patients with penetrating wounds to the chest can often be successfully resuscitated from a recent (less than 5 minutes) cardiac arrest by emergent thoracotomy.[10] Small wounds, especially those on the right side of the heart, often bleed minimally or result in tamponade. Ironically, in some cases, cardiac tamponade may prolong life by controlling bleeding but will ultimately be fatal if allowed to progress.

The classic presentation of tamponade is **Beck's triad**: increased venous pressure, decreased arterial pressure, and muffled heart tones. The latter sign, muffled heart tones, is an unreliable sign. Notwithstanding the difficulty of assessing heart tones in a noisy field environment, heart tones are usually fairly audible even in the presence of large pericardial tamponade.[1] Overall, the classic Beck's triad was present in less than 10% of cases in one series and in less than 40% of several other reports.[31,34]

A "pericardial knock" is seen in about 40% of cases of constrictive pericarditis with effusion but may or may not be present in traumatic cardiac tamponade.[6,35] If present, it is an early diastolic, short and clicking sound, caused by the rapid flow of blood into a ventricle with limited distensibility.[7]

Venous pressure increases because cardiac output is diminished. This can be seen as distention of the neck veins. **Kussmaul's sign** (increased jugular venous distention with spontaneous inspirations) is a fairly reliable sign that can be used at the scene or in the emergency department.[2] However, if the patient is hypovolemic from other injuries, neck vein distention will not be present. Pulsus paradoxus may also be present.

Many EKG changes can be seen with cardiac tamponade, but most are nondiagnostic.[36–38] Electrical alternans, however, has been reported to be a highly specific marker of cardiac tamponade but is more commonly seen in chronic pericardial effusions that develop into tamponade rather than acute tamponade secondary to trauma.[39–41] Electrical alternans is an alternating amplitude of the P, QRS, and T waves in any single lead occurring in every other beat and is thought to be caused by the heart swinging back and forth within the excessive pericardial fluid (Figure 13-4). The additional fluid may also act as an insulator, decreasing the overall voltage of the EKG. In addition, ST- and T-wave changes can be indicators of tamponade or injury, and PEA and sudden bradycardia have been shown to precede cardiac arrest.[10,36] Although the

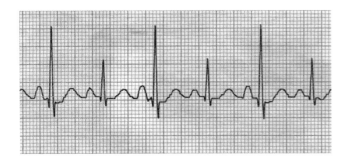

FIGURE 13-4 Electrical alternans of cardiac tamponade.

prognosis for pulseless electrical activity in trauma is usually poor, the survival rate of patients with PEA secondary to cardiac tamponade who receive proper treatment is much improved.

Treatment of cardiac tamponade hinges on aggressive airway control, oxygenation, circulatory support, and rapid transport for definitive treatment. Rapid infusion of IV fluids will increase venous pressure and improve cardiac output. Pericardiocentesis, the aspiration of blood from the pericardial sac, should be limited to those patients who do not respond to the usual measures for hemorrhagic shock and who have the potential for tamponade. Withdrawal of even 15–20 cc from the pericardial space can significantly improve hemodynamics.[2] However, the procedure is not benign and may not be therapeutic or diagnostic because blood may be clotted in the pericardial sac. Potential complications of pericardiocentesis include injury to a coronary artery, induced dysrhythmias, right ventricular puncture or laceration, and further (or new) pericardial bleeding.[2] Trauma patients who undergo a pericardiocentesis will require surgical inspection and possible repair of the heart.

INTERNET ACTIVITIES

Visit the e-medicine Web site at http://www.emedicine.com. Click on the Emergency Medicine on-line book and select Cardiovascular. Then click on Pericarditis and Cardiac Tamponade. Review the chapter on the management of cardiac tamponade.

MYOCARDIAL RUPTURE

Myocardial rupture is an acute traumatic perforation of the ventricles, atria, intraventricular septum, intraatrial septum, chordae, papillary muscles, or valves. Myocardial rupture is almost universally immediately fatal and accounts for 15% of fatal chest injuries.[42] It

has been estimated that 5% of deaths from motor vehicle collisions are the result of blunt cardiac rupture.[43] The overall incidence of myocardial rupture among blunt chest trauma patients ranges from 0.5% to 2%.[44-47]

Rupture of the heart from blunt trauma most commonly results from motor vehicle collisions and, less commonly, from falls.[43,45] However, the forces necessary to rupture a cardiac chamber need not be as great as those involved in motor vehicle collisions. Blunt cardiac rupture has been reported following CPR and when a playmate accidentally fell on a 12-year-old boy who was sledding in a prone position.[48,49]

Myocardial rupture occurs when blood-filled chambers are compressed with sufficient force to produce a rent in the chamber wall or septum or to rupture a cardiac valve. The ventricles are more prone to this type of injury during diastole or early systole when they are maximally distended with blood. In contrast, the atria are most susceptible to rupture in late systole, when they are maximally distended and the atrioventricular valves are closed.[50,51] Laceration of the pericardium accompanies blunt cardiac rupture in 10%–33% of cases.[46,52]

The clinical presentation of myocardial rupture is that of cardiac tamponade or severe hemorrhage. A patient with blunt cardiac rupture and a developing tamponade typically displays the usual signs of cardiac tamponade described above, most notably shock and signs of an elevated CVP. On physical inspection, the chest may reveal little more than a precordial contusion or lack any sign of injury, but more often other signs of chest injury are present.[51] Common signs and symptoms and associated injuries found in victims of myocardial rupture include sternal fracture, first rib fracture, multiple rib fractures (greater than 7), diaphragmatic rupture, hypotension unresponsive to fluid resuscitation, elevated CVP, jugular venous distention (JVD), muffled heart sounds, tachycardia, unresponsiveness, hemothorax, and cyanosis of the head, neck, arms, and upper chest.[53-55] Patients with septal defects will have profound hypoxemia if there is mixing of blood from a right-to-left shunt. A harsh holosystolic murmur may be present, but often does not appear until 2–4 hours after the injury.[10]

One-third of patients with cardiac rupture have associated rents in the pericardial sac and promptly exsanguinate.[51] The remaining two-thirds of patients with myocardial rupture have an intact pericardium that protects them from immediate exsanguination.[52] Consequently, the only survivors of blunt cardiac rupture likely to be encountered by paramedics are those with cardiac tamponade. Therefore, field treatment should concentrate on identifying patients likely to have sustained blunt cardiac rupture based on their mechanism of injury, immediate stabilization, treatment of cardiac tamponade as described above, and rapid transport to a trauma center.

DYSRHYTHMIAS

Blunt and penetrating trauma to the heart can cause dysrhythmias, making continuous cardiac monitoring a necessity for all patients with chest trauma. Injured heart tissue can be electrically unstable, making it the origin of ectopic foci of contractions. Dysrhythmias that can include unexplained sinus tachycardia, premature ventricular contractions, atrial fibrillation, atrioventricular blocks, ventricular tachycardia, and ventricular fibrillation. All symptomatic rhythms should be treated as per Advanced Cardiac Life Support protocol. Premature ventricular contractions that are more frequent than six per minute are treated with oxygen, and then a lidocaine bolus of 1 mg/kg, followed by an infusion of 2–4 mg/min, if still present.[2]

CONTINUED ASSESSMENT

Once the initial assessment and immediate stabilization maneuvers have been performed, efforts should be directed toward rapid trauma examination and definitive care. Continued assessment, meticulous observation, and monitoring of vital signs are essential. At this point, potentially life-threatening injuries that are not obviously apparent may be detected or should be suspected. Life-threatening injuries to consider in the continued assessment include aortic disruption, pulmonary contusion, myocardial contusion, cardiac injuries, traumatic diaphragmatic rupture, tracheobronchial disruption, pneumothorax, and esophageal disruption.

AORTIC DISRUPTION

Aortic disruption is a common cause of sudden death after an automobile collision or fall from a great height. Each year at least 5,000–8,000 people in the United States die as a result of aortic or great vessel rupture.[1] Rapid deceleration from high speed will cause shearing forces on the aorta and other great vessels. Depending on the magnitude, shear forces can cause either partial or complete tears of the vessels. If the tear is complete, it is usually fatal at the scene because the patient exsanguinates into the left pleural cavity. It is estimated that this occurs in 80%–90% of patients with trauma to the great vessels.[56] Patients who survive the initial injury have a high likelihood of salvage if aortic rupture is identified and treated rapidly. If the injury is not identified, one-third will die within the first 6 hours. Another third of these patients will die within the first day, and from then on, half of the survivors will die each day if not treated.[1] Seventy percent of patients sustaining aortic disruption are male and the average age is 33 years. Because of the relatively young age of these patients, many patients sustaining this injury are otherwise healthy and, if the diagnosis is made promptly and followed by rapid surgical intervention, they can be salvaged from an otherwise fatal injury.[57]

In deceleration injuries, the descending aorta, which is fixed to the vertebrae, will decelerate at the same rate as the body. The heart and aortic arch will often continue to move laterally and inferiorly into the left hemithorax even after the patient has come to rest. The force that results is a combination of shearing, torsion, and bending that produce maximal stress on the descending aorta at the ligamentum arteriosum, starting at the inner surface.[1] Most injuries are the result of high-speed deceleration such as MVCs. Although rare, other mechanisms of aortic disruption have been documented, including CPR, kicks by animals, and crush injuries.[58–60] Falls may also result in rupture of the ascending aorta by producing an acute lengthening of the aorta.[61]

The most common site of rupture is the descending aorta at the isthmus, just distal to the left subclavian artery, occurring in 80%–90% of cases (Figure 13-5).[60,62] Other, less common sites of disruption are the ascending aorta, the distal descending aorta at the level of the diaphragm, the midthoracic descending aorta, and the origin of the left subclavian artery.[51,60,62] Although less common than disruptions of the descending aorta, ruptures of the ascending aorta do occur and have a 70%–80% incidence of associated fatal cardiac injury.[60]

The injury tends to progress from the tunica intima out to the tunica adventitia. Because the adventitia is fibrous, it can withstand more force and will often be the only layer keeping the aorta intact in a partial aortic tear. Blood under pressure can cause the aortic layers to separate and create a dissection that can travel distally and proximally along the aorta. Although much less common, tears of the ascending aorta may dissect down to the coronary arteries, resulting in myocardial ischemia.[33,63]

Despite the severe nature of the injury, the clinical signs of aortic rupture are often occult and easily missed.[51] Up to 50% of patients will have no external signs of chest trauma.[64] Consequently, the single most important factor in establishing the diagnosis is a high index of suspicion, based on the mechanism of injury. The diagnosis of aortic disruption should be considered in any patient sustaining a severe deceleration injury, especially in automobile collisions with speeds in excess of 45 mph, or if there is evidence of severe blunt forces

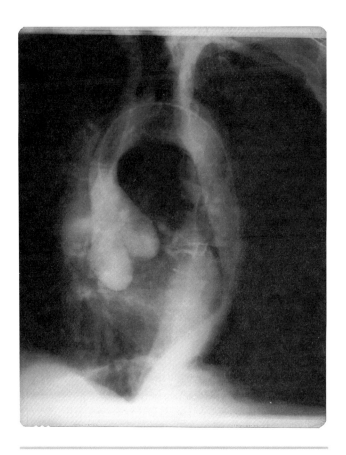

FIGURE 13-5 Chest X-ray demonstrating aortic disruption.

to the chest, such as deformity to the steering wheel.[51] Frontal or lateral impact patients with aortic rupture usually complain about other associated injuries. The most common symptom is retrosternal or subscapular tearing pain from dissection of the adventitial layers of the aorta, especially when blood pressure increases, but this symptom is present in only 25% of patients with aortic injury.[1,64]

On physical exam, there may be no findings to indicate rupture. Findings that should raise the concern for possible rupture include chest wall trauma, upper extremity hypertension, lower extremity paralysis, or cardiac irritability from myocardial contusion.[10] If the tear causes partial or complete obstruction of the aorta, there may be upper extremity hypertension or asymmetry of blood pressures in the upper extremities. **Pseudocoarctation syndrome**, characterized by acute upper extremity hypertension along with absent or diminished femoral pulses, has been reported in up to 33% of patients.[64,65]

An expanding aortic hematoma may cause compression of the esophagus or the left recurrent laryngeal nerve, resulting in dysphagia, hoarseness, stridor, or dyspnea. A harsh systolic murmur over the precordium or posterior interscapular area has been reported in up to 31% of patients and is thought to result from turbulent flow across the transected area.[51,64] Persistent or recurrent hypotension should also indicate the possibility of partial aortic rupture. Occasionally, swelling of the base of the neck or a pulsatile neck mass may appear, caused by the extravasation of blood from the mediastinum into the soft tissues of the neck.[51]

Definitive diagnosis of aortic rupture can only be made by angiography. Radiographic findings that are suggestive of aortic disruption include a widened (greater than 8 cm) superior mediastinum, loss of the aortic knob, an apical pleural cap, and deviation of the esophagus (visualized with nasogastric tube in place) to the right.[1]

Blunt injuries occur much less frequently to the innominate or subclavian arteries. Innominate vessel injuries may present with diminished right upper extremity pulses but rarely cause limb ischemia.[1] Severe deceleration can cause avulsion of the subclavian artery at its origin, but this is uncommon.[1] Damage to the subclavian artery is often associated with clavicular fractures and first-rib fractures. These fractures combined with other blunt forces can cause intimal damage and occlusion, resulting in distal limb ischemia. Because of the proximity of the brachial plexus, there will often be distal neurological deficits as well.

Management consists of administration of a high concentration of oxygen, careful transport, and cautious hydration. To limit shear forces on the aorta and great vessels, patients who are not hypovolemic should not be overhydrated. Pressor medications should also be avoided if possible.[2] Definitive treatment is operative repair. Occasionally, if operative repair will be delayed, maintaining the blood pressure between 100 and 120 mm Hg with intravenous nitroprusside, esmolol, or propranolol may be necessary to minimize the shearing effect on the remaining intact layers of the aorta.[57,66]

INTERNET ACTIVITIES

Visit the e-medicine Web site at http:// www.emedicine.com/. Click on the Emergency Medicine on-line book and select Cardiovascular. Then click on Aortic Dissection. Review the chapter on the presentation and management of aortic dissection.

PULMONARY CONTUSION

Pulmonary contusion is the most common potentially lethal chest injury seen in North America, with an incidence of 30%–70% among patients sustaining blunt chest trauma.[2,67] In a review of 86 patients with pulmonary contusions, the most common mechanism of injury was MVCs (76%), followed by farming injuries (10%) and falls (9%).[68] Up to 87% of patients with pulmonary contusions have at least one other associated chest injury, including rib fracture (70%), pneumothorax (57%), hemothorax (40%), subcutaneous emphysema (30%), and clavicle fracture (11%).[69] The finding of a flail chest almost invariably is associated with a pulmonary contusion.[70,71] The mortality rate for pulmonary contusions ranges between 14% and 20%.[16,23]

Blunt trauma to the chest may cause pulmonary contusions with or without broken ribs. Pulmonary interstitial edema and capillary leakage of blood into the alveoli can result after contusion. The increased capillary membrane permeability and alveolar damage can be local and relatively minor or extensive.[68] The increased pulmonary fluid decreases the compliance of the lung and prevents adequate gas exchange between the alveoli and bloodstream. Even small amounts of blood (20–30 mL) in the bronchi and alveoli can cause significant hypoxia.[9] Decreased lung compliance will increase the effort required for ventilation, thus increasing the patient's oxygen requirement. Ventilation-perfusion mismatches at the affected region of the lung will shunt blood to the left side of the heart without oxygenation, thus decreasing systemic oxygen delivery. The cycle of increasing oxygen requirement and decreased oxygen delivery can result in respiratory failure. This is often a slow process in a healthy individual, so continuous monitoring is essential.

The clinical presentation of pulmonary contusion includes a range of respiratory symptoms from asymptomatic to frank respiratory failure.[70] Tachypnea, dyspnea, tachycardia, hemoptysis, chest pain, cough, bloody mucous secretions, rales or rhonchi, and signs and symptoms of hypoxia may all be seen depending on the severity of the contusion and the magnitude of the resulting loss in ventilatory function. None of these signs or symptoms are specific for pulmonary contusion, though hemoptysis has been reported in up to 50% of patients.[25,72] Because the radiographic changes associated with pulmonary contusion do not become apparent until 4–6 hours following the injury, they lag behind the patient's physiological condition.[68] Consequently, the cornerstone of diagnosis is clinical suspicion based on the history and mechanism of injury.

Management of these patients is the same in the field and in the hospital. Initial management is to ensure adequate ventilation and oxygenation. Supplemental oxygen should be given because these patients can be seriously hypoxic. The decision to intubate should revolve around the arterial PaO_2. Consequently, arterial blood gas (ABG) analysis in the field is beneficial in determining management strategies (see Chapter 18 for ABG analysis techniques). If the patient cannot maintain a minimum PaO_2 of 60 mm Hg with an FiO_2 of 0.5, then intubation should be undertaken.[70] In addition, the PaO_2/FiO_2 ratio may be used to determine the need for intubation. The normal ratio is 500, with intubation being indicated for patients with ratios below 300.[73]

Because pulmonary contusion leads to a capillary membrane leak, judicious fluid management is essential to minimize the formation of edema in the injured region of the lung. Fluids should only be given at a fast rate with signs of hypovolemia. Good bronchial toilet should be maintained through nasotracheal suction, analgesia for chest wall pain, and chest physiotherapy. If ventilatory assistance is necessary, ventilation with intermittent mandatory ventilation (IMV) and PEEP usually provides better results (see Chapter 18).[1] Patients who develop frank respiratory failure do poorly, even with intubation and positive pressure support because of the severe hypoxemia and stress placed on the body. Therefore, patients with signs of tachypnea, hypoxia, and labored breathing should be placed on ventilatory support sooner rather than later.[9]

Pneumonia is the most common complication of pulmonary contusion and, when present, worsens the prognosis.[74,75] Nonetheless, prophylactic antibiotics are not recommended and should be reserved for cases in which pneumonia develops. If atelectasis and pneumonia can be prevented through aggressive treatment, the clinical condition of the patient rapidly improves over the next 2–6 days postinjury.[1]

MYOCARDIAL CONCUSSION AND CONTUSION

The reported incidence of myocardial contusion ranges between 3% and 76% in studies of blunt chest trauma, reflecting the variability in diagnostic criteria and the distinction between the terms *concussion* and *contusion*.[76–78] In general, **myocardial concussion** is used to describe a sharp blow to the midanterior chest, resulting in a brief dysrhythmia, hypotension, or loss of consciousness. Similar to a brain concussion in the setting of head trauma, a concussion injury to the myocardium results in a "stunned" myocardium without any histological evidence of cellular injury.[51] However, cellular dysfunction may persist resulting in dysrhythmias and/or a decrease in cardiac output, which may explain cases of sudden death following a blow to the chest without histopathological changes in the myocardium at autopsy.[51,76]

In contrast to myocardial concussion, a **myocardial contusion** results in histopathological changes.

Cellular injury occurs with extravasation of erythrocytes into the muscle wall, along with necrotic areas of myocardial fibers, focal myocardial edema, interstitial hemorrhage, and subendocardial hemorrhage.[1,51] Damage may include the conduction system or coronary arteries. Coronary artery damage may result in frank myocardial infarction.[2] The areas of the heart most frequently involved are the anterior wall of the right ventricle, the anterior ventricular septum, and the apex of the left ventricle.[1] Myocardial contusion can significantly impair contractility of the heart. The significance of the injury depends on the extent of injury and health of the patient.

Although high-speed deceleration collisions are the most common cause of myocardial contusion, speeds of only 20–35 mph have been implicated in this injury.[79,80] Consequently, myocardial contusion should be suspected in all patients involved in MVCs of 20 mph or greater, especially if there is damage to the steering wheel or anginalike chest pain. It is estimated that at least 20% of patients with steering wheel impacts sustain myocardial contusions, 16% of which are fatal.[80,81] The clinical significance of cardiac contusion is directly related to its complications and associated injuries, including dysrhythmias, valvular lesions, thromboembolus, reduced left ventricular ejection fraction and cardiac output, congestive failure, ventricular aneurysm, pericardial effusion, coronary artery laceration, cardiac rupture, traumatic myocardial infarction, and constrictive pericarditis.[26,31,51] Without complications or associated injuries, there is complete recovery with minimal residual scarring within 3–6 weeks.[1]

Although myocardial contusion is usually well tolerated, the possibility of life-threatening sequelae necessitates a careful examination of all blunt chest trauma victims for this injury.[51] Unfortunately, the clinical presentation of myocardial contusion is variable and the physical examination provides information of only limited diagnostic value, increasing the importance of suspicion of injury based on the history and mechanism of injury.[51,82] Symptoms of myocardial contusion may be minor, transient, masked by other injuries, or totally absent. The clinical picture is further complicated by the fact that 25% of patients will have no external signs of injury.[31,82] When signs and symptoms are present, tachycardia is the most common and is present in 70% of patients with documented myocardial contusion, though it lacks diagnostic specificity.[83] Cardiac examination is usually normal but may reveal a friction rub or the murmur of valvular damage, septal rupture, or papillary muscle dysfunction.[78] Examination of the chest wall may or may not reveal contusions, abrasions, tenderness, or crepitus.

Chest pain, when present, is typically retrosternal in location, nonpleuritic, and anginal in character, mimicking the pain of myocardial infarction.[51,82] It may occur immediately, but often is delayed 24 hours to 3 days after the initial injury.[51] The pain may be alleviated by oxygen administration but will not be relieved by nitroglycerin, making differentiation from an acute myocardial infarction problematic, particularly in older patients.[1,82]

The ECG is probably the single best predictor of myocardial contusion, but the ECG alone is nonspecific.[84–87] Also, the right ventricle is the most frequently injured, but the ECG receives most of its voltage potentials from the more massive left ventricle, thus limiting the sensitivity of the ECG. Consequently, up to 50% of patients with abnormal ECG findings do not have a myocardial contusion, but other problems (hypoxia, electrolyte disturbances, hypotension, and head injuries) that can cause ECG changes, and up to 30% of patients with elevated enzymes have a normal ECG.[78,82,88]

Sinus tachycardia and nonspecific ST-T wave changes are the most common findings in myocardial contusion, but virtually any abnormality may be seen.[82] Conduction disturbances encountered include right and left bundle branch blocks, left anterior hemiblock, first- and second-degree heart block, sinus bradycardia, intraventricular conduction delay, and prolonged QT interval. Dysrhythmias include sinus tachycardia, premature atrial and ventricular contractions, atrial fibrillation, paroxysmal supraventricular tachycardia, and ventricular tachycardia. Nonspecific ST-T wave changes have been reported in 84% of patients with documented myocardial contusion, and axis deviation occurs in 16%–18% of patients.[89]

The type of cardiac dysrhythmia is thought to be dependent on the site of the chest injury.[90] Because of the heart's position in the thorax, the right atrium and ventricle are more susceptible to injury. Thus the sinoatriol node, atrioventricular junction, bundle of His, and bundle branches are prone to injury. A blow to the right chest presumably affects the right atrium and conduction system, resulting in atrial dysrhythmia, sinoatrial block, and a high degree of atrioventricular block.[51] In comparison, blows to the left chest result in predominantly ventricular dysrhythmias, including premature ventricular contractions and bundle branch block.

Because of the difficulty in identifying myocardial contusion clinically, definitive diagnosis is often made by ultrasound to demonstrate wall motion abnormalities. Serum enzymes have also been used to diagnose myocardial contusion, but their use remains controversial. Serum glutamic-oxaloacetic transaminase (SGOT or AST), lactic dehydrogenase (LDH), and total creatine kinase (CK) levels are often elevated in the setting of blunt chest trauma because of associated injuries to the liver, brain, lung, or skeletal muscle. Consequently, they are of little value in diagnosing myocardial contusion. However, myocardial CK (CK-MB or CK-2) levels will usually be markedly elevated and are considered more accurate.[1] Other investigators, however, have questioned their reliability.[10,76,91]

As with any other victim of multiple trauma, the priorities of treating the patient sustaining a myocardial contusion are airway, oxygenation, and circulatory support. The single most important treatment for these patients is supplemental oxygen.[2] Patients should be transported with supplemental oxygen, continuous ECG monitoring, and an established intravenous line. Dysrhythmias should be managed with the same pharmacological interventions used in nontraumatic situations. In patients demonstrating depressed cardiac output and hypotension secondary to cardiac contusion, judicious fluid administration is required, and if ineffective, inotropic support with dobutamine may be required. Pressor medications should be used cautiously to minimize myocardial stress and oxygen requirements.[2] Coronary vasodilators should not be used unless preexisting coronary artery disease is suspected.[1] Patients with myocardial contusions are usually admitted for telemetry monitoring if they have had dysrhythmias or if they have preexisting disease. Because sternal fractures are highly associated with myocardial contusion, these patients are frequently admitted, even if they have been asymptomatic.

VALVULAR INJURY

Injuries to the heart valves should be considered in any patient with blunt heart trauma. Although they occur much less commonly than other cardiac injuries, their exact incidence is unknown.[92,93] Valve rupture may involve the chordae tendineae, leaflets, or papillary muscles. The most commonly affected valve is the aortic valve, followed by laceration of a papillary muscle or chordae tendineae of the mitral valve.[1,10]

The clinical presentation and prognosis of these patients depend on which valve is involved and the severity of any associated injuries. Complete rupture of the aortic or mitral valve is usually immediately fatal.[51] Incomplete rupture of the aortic valve produces a loud, harsh diastolic murmur heard at the right parasternal border of the second intercostal space, with frank left heart failure and cardiogenic shock (Figure 13-6). However, if the patient is in a low-output state, the associated thrills and murmurs of aortic insufficiency may not be appreciated.[51]

Mitral valve or papillary muscle rupture carries a grave prognosis and is usually fatal within a few days after the injury if not repaired.[2] Mitral valve injuries

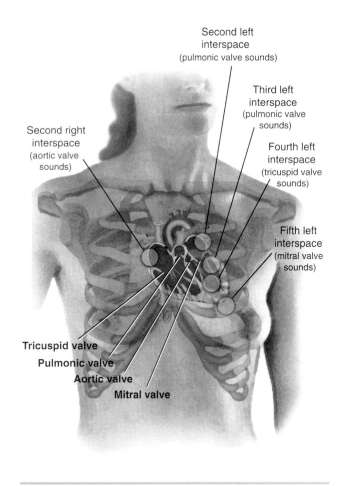

FIGURE 13-6 Locations for auscultating the valves of the heart.

are poorly tolerated because of the high pressures of the left ventricle, producing signs of acute pulmonary edema and acute mitral insufficiency (harsh apical systolic murmur, S_3 and S_4 heart sounds, palpable thrill at the apex, JVD, and tachycardia). Patients may quickly deteriorate to cardiogenic shock or arrest.[94]

The tricuspid valve is rarely involved in blunt trauma, and tricuspid insufficiency is usually well tolerated unless the patient has pulmonary hypertension.[1] The clinical presentation of this injury is minimal and the physical examination may reveal only a diastolic murmur and prominent jugular venous pulsations.[95]

Field treatment of these injuries is generally supportive. Medical therapy commonly relieves the symptoms of congestive failure. If the patient survives the initial insult and tolerates the sequelae, many years may elapse before operative repair is required.

DIAPHRAGMATIC RUPTURE

Diaphragm injuries occur in 1%–3% of patients with blunt chest trauma and are usually the result of

MVCs.[96–98] In one series of thoracic penetrating injuries, 15% of patients with lower thoracic knife wounds had diaphragm injuries, as did 46% of patients with gunshot wounds to the same area.[99] Fifty-three percent of traumatic diaphragmatic herniations (TDHs) are the result of penetrating trauma, of which 55% are knife wounds and 45% are gunshot wounds.[100] Traumatic diaphragmatic herniation is nine times more likely to appear on the left because of the protective effect of the liver, but the distribution is more equal in more severe trauma.[101–104] Comorbidity among these patients is high; almost all patients have associated injuries, including liver, spleen, bowel, pancreas, and duodenal injuries, as well as pulmonary contusion and pelvic, rib, and long-bone fractures.[100,105,106] The mortality rate ranges between 17% and 28% and is related to the severity of the comorbidity.[106,107]

The mechanism of injury in penetrating trauma is direct violation of the diaphragm by the invading object, usually a knife or bullet. In blunt trauma, increased intra-abdominal and/or intrathoracic pressure is transmitted to the diaphragm. These pressures seek the path of least resistance. Because the abdomen is bounded posteriorly by the ribs and vertebral column, anteriorly by the abdominal muscles, laterally by ribs and intercostal and abdominal muscles, and inferiorly by the viscera and bony pelvis, the least resistive path is upward through the diaphragm. During severe abdominal trauma, a 10-fold increase in pressure can be produced within the abdomen and transmitted through the domes of the hemidiaphragm.[108] If the tolerance of the diaphragm is exceeded, a tear is created. The size of the tear varies somewhat with the mechanism of injury. In one series of patients, stab wounds produced defects in the diaphragm that were smaller than 6 cm, while blunt trauma produced tears averaging 11 cm and defects secondary to gunshot wounds averaged 18 cm.[105] In penetrating trauma the location of the defect can involve any portion of the diaphragm, while blunt trauma typically produces a radial tear in the posterolateral area of the left side of the diaphragm, an embryologic point of weakness.[109–111]

There is a positive pressure gradient between intraperitoneal and intrapleural pressure of 7–20 cm H_2O, which can exceed 100 cm H_2O during maximal respiratory effort. This positive pressure gradient encourages transdiaphragmatic herniation of abdominal viscera through the defect in the diaphragm.[104,112] The organs most often herniated through the diaphragm include the colon (43%), spleen (20%), stomach (17%), omentum (8%), liver (6%), and ileum (6%).[105] However, in patients requiring intubation, the intraperitoneal-intrapleural pressure gradient is negated by the effects of positive pressure ventilation and may prevent herniation of intra-abdominal organs.[106]

The clinical presentation of TDH progresses through three phases: acute, latent, and obstructive.[109] The acute phase begins at injury and continues until recovery of the primary injuries. In the acute phase, the injury is frequently overshadowed by other injuries. The cardiovascular signs of TDH result from the mechanical effects of herniation. Gross herniation may produce mediastinal shift and may decrease cardiac output by interfering with ventricular filling, resulting in tachycardia, hypotension, dysrhythmias, and elevated jugular venous pressure.[105] Rarely, herniation extends into the pericardial sac, resulting in cardiac tamponade. Other signs and symptoms include chest pain radiating to the left shoulder, asymmetric chest wall motion, dyspnea, tachypnea, cough, hiccough, abdominal pain, scaphoid abdomen, and cyanosis. Up to 50% of patients with TDH present with hypotension due to associated injuries.[104,107] Frequently, bowel sounds in the chest have been promoted as a classic sign of diaphragm rupture. However, ileus usually occurs after the injury and ipsilateral diminished lung sounds are a more common finding.[96]

Radiographic findings of TDH include abdominal viscera or bowel gas in the thorax, elevated diaphragm, small shift of the mediastinum, or the tip of a properly inserted nasogastric tube positioned above the diaphragm. Diagnostic peritoneal lavage (DPL) is often performed in these patients but carries a 25% false-negative rate.[96,113]

If the diaphragm rupture is not diagnosed in the acute phase, the patient enters the latent phase, which may last for months to years before complications ensue. This phase is characterized by intermittent herniation of abdominal contents, vague abdominal complaints, dyspnea, and cough. The obstructive phase produces the complications caused by the vascular compromise of the abdominal viscera that are now incarcerated and strangulated. Signs of this stage include abdominal pain, obstipation, nausea, vomiting, and abdominal distention that are often profound and unrelenting.[100] Mortality has been reported as high as 20% with incarcerated viscera and may be as high as 80% following strangulation.[109,114,115]

Patients with TDH are at increased risk for a condition known as "tension viscerothorax" or "tension gastrothorax." This condition is physiologically similar to tension pneumothorax except that the increased intrapleural pressure is caused by herniated bowel and abdominal viscera rather than extrapulmonary air. The elevated intrapleural pressure results in mediastinal shift, decreased ventricular filling, and compression of the contralateral lung. The clinical picture is similar to that of tension pneumothorax. Consequently, caution must be exercised when performing a needle thoracostomy or inserting a chest tube prior to obtaining a chest radiograph due to the risk of perforating abdominal viscera lying within the thoracic cavity. Moreover, chest tubes should never be placed using a trocar, and internal palpation of the chest structures is indicated prior to placement of the tube.[116]

The definitive treatment of TDH is surgical, yet the paramedic plays an important role in assisting the emergency physician in making the diagnosis. Herniated diaphragm is a frequently missed or delayed diagnosis following blunt or penetrating injury.[117] Paramedics can improve the accuracy of diagnosing ruptured diaphragm by suspecting this injury based on the mechanism of injury and reporting this to the emergency physician.

Initial management is aimed at supporting airway, ventilatory, and circulatory functions. Assisted positive pressure ventilations with 100% oxygen will help provide adequate ventilation. Placement of a nasogastric tube with suction will empty the stomach, decreasing the volume of bowel contents in the hemithorax and improving ventilation. Because most patients are hypotensive, aggressive fluid resuscitation is indicated. However, the pneumatic antishock garment (PASG) is contraindicated in the setting of TDH. The PASG has been shown to increase intra-abdominal pressure and, in the setting of TDH, increase respiratory compromise, decrease cardiac output and blood pressure, and result in deterioration of ABGs.[118] Moreover, patients who suddenly deteriorate following inflation of the PASG should be suspected of having sustained a TDH and the PASG should be immediately deflated.[118] Definitive care is by laparotomy and direct hernia repair.

INTERNET ACTIVITIES

Visit the e-medicine Web site at http://www. emedicine.com. Click on the Emergency Medicine on-line book and select Trauma and Orthopedics. Then click on Diaphragmatic Injuries. Review the chapter on the management of tears and herniation of the diaphragm.

TRACHEOBRONCHIAL DISRUPTION

Injuries to the lower trachea and bronchi are rare and often fatal. The incidence of tracheobronchial injuries is 3% among patients with significant chest injury, with a mortality rate of 30%, 50% of whom die within the first hour.[119-123] Those who survive tracheobronchial injuries usually have cervical trachea injuries and no associated injuries. Injuries to the lower trachea are associated with at least two other major injuries and survival is rare.[1] Approximately 25% of patients with penetrating tracheobronchial injury also have an esophageal injury.[1]

The majority of tracheobronchial injuries are due to sudden deceleration with shearing between the trachea and bronchi. Several other mechanisms have been proposed as the cause of this injury, including traction, crush of the airway between an object and the vertebral column, and increased intrabronchial pressure resulting from compression of the chest against a closed glottis.[82,124,125] Regardless of the mechanism, 80% of tears occur within 2 cm of the carina or at the point where the bronchus divides into lobar bronchi.[121] Penetrating injuries of the lower trachea or bronchi are less common.[2] Because of the magnitude of the force to produce these injuries, patients will often succumb to other associated injuries.

Patients with tracheobronchial disruption that survive the initial injury may present with dyspnea, cough, hemoptysis, subcutaneous emphysema, sternal tenderness, noisy breathing, and hoarseness.[1] However, approximately 10% of patients are asymptomatic.[1] Auscultation of the heart may reveal a **Hamman's sign**, which is a "crunching" sound heard during systole. This sign usually indicates air within the mediastinum. The distal trachea and proximal main stem bronchi are extrapleural; injuries to these structures will result in mediastinal or cervical emphysema.[82] The distal main stem bronchi and smaller airways are intrapleural and when injured will cause pneumothorax or a persistent air leak. Ventilation of these patients may be difficult because of the air loss. These patients can also easily develop a tension pneumothorax. If a chest tube is placed to correct the pneumothorax, these patients will often have a persistent air leak if the chest tube is placed to suction. Definitive diagnosis is made in the hospital by bronchoscopy.

Management in the field should be focused on adequate oxygenation of the patient. It is preferable not to intubate a patient with a tracheal injury, if possible. This will allow for endoscopic evaluation in the emergency department or operating room. However, if the patient is not breathing adequately, then the endotracheal tube should be placed with the balloon extending beyond the injury to prevent aspiration of blood. If a pneumothorax is discovered, it should be decompressed or a chest tube placed if the patient begins to deteriorate. Persistent air leak from the chest tube may require intubation of the uninvolved bronchus.[126] There are several different approaches for hospital treatment of these patients depending on the severity of the injury. These patients may require operative repair, either emergent or elective. Smaller air leaks may seal spontaneously, requiring only observation in a hospital for several days.

SIMPLE PNEUMOTHORAX/ PNEUMOMEDIASTINUM

Pneumothorax results from air entering the pleural space. The most common cause of pneumothorax is lung laceration from penetrating or blunt trauma with a resultant air leak. In blunt trauma, rapid compression of an inflated lung may tear the lung parenchyma in the same manner that an inflated paper bag explodes when sudden force is exerted on it. People that have underlying lung disease, such as asthma and chronic obstructive pulmonary disease (COPD), are especially prone to pneumothorax. Air in the pleural space will prevent the underlying lung from expanding and filling the alveoli. A V/Q mismatch occurs in the nonventilated region, preventing oxygenation of the blood returning to the heart. In a partial pneumothorax, the defect is usually at the apex. Pneumomediastinum can be the result of perforation of the lungs or of the esophagus.

The presentation of patients with pneumothorax will vary according to the size of the defect. Patients may be asymptomatic or they may complain of pleuritic chest pain. The classic sign is decreased or absent breath sounds on the affected side. Careful attention should be given to auscultation of the apices of the lungs. Asymmetry of breath sounds may be difficult to hear in the field or even the emergency department. The affected side may be more resonant to percussion when compared to the other side. Patients may also have tachypnea or subcutaneous emphysema. Hamman's sign may also be present, especially with a pneumomediastinum.[1]

Management of these patients includes administration of high concentration of oxygen and careful ventilatory support if needed. Patients with pneumomediastinum rarely require treatment. Positive pressure ventilation will usually exacerbate a pneumothorax, possibly causing a tension pneumothorax, and should be done with caution. Needle decompression or chest tube placement in the field is not necessary if the patient is stable. It is preferable to obtain an X-ray to confirm the diagnosis if possible. Treatment in the hospital depends on the size of the pneumothorax. Generally, if the pneumothorax is confined to the upper one-third of the lung, a chest tube is not required and the patient will be observed for at least 6 hours for further enlargement.[1] Outpatient follow-up is all that is necessary because the pneumothorax will slowly resolve. However, if the patient with a pneumothorax is to undergo surgery or prolonged transport (especially with positive pressure ventilation), then a chest tube should be placed.[9]

ESOPHAGEAL DISRUPTION

Perforation of the esophagus has been described as the most rapidly fatal perforation of the gastrointestinal system.[127,128] When diagnosis is delayed, death is almost assured. With prompt diagnosis and treatment (within 12 hours) the mortality rate is lowered to around 30%.[129] Mortality from sepsis can be high (up to 66%) if the proper diagnosis is not made within 24 hours.[1,2]

Esophageal disruption is usually the result of penetrating trauma, with an incidence of 5%–10%.[130] Injury of the cervical esophagus is more common than of the thoracic esophagus, and esophageal injuries secondary to blunt trauma are almost always cervical and usually associated with tracheal or laryngeal trauma.[131–133] However, disruption can result from blunt trauma if gastric contents are rapidly forced up into the esophagus.[2] The high mortality and prolonged morbidity is related to the anatomy of the esophagus. The esophagus has no serosal covering and any perforation allows direct access to the mediastinum. Drainage from the gastrointestinal tract frequently erodes the pleura, permitting the contaminated material to be pulled into the pleural space by negative intrathoracic pressure. The time course to enter the pleural space can be either immediate or delayed and will result in a collection of inflammatory and infectious fluid, referred to as an empyema.[2]

Initial symptoms of esophageal injury are subtle, vague, and frequently missed in the setting of multiple trauma.[82] The most common symptom is substernal pleuritic chest pain with radiation to the neck or shoulders. Patients may also complain of pain along the course of the esophagus that is exacerbated by swallowing and by neck flexion.[100] Other signs and symptoms include heartburn-type pain over the epigastrium, abdominal pain, dyspnea, dysphagia, change in voice pitch, subcutaneous emphysema, fever, pneumothorax, mediastinal air, and Hamman's crunch. These patients may have pain that is out of proportion to the findings on physical examination. Esophageal disruption is often seen in conjunction with hemothorax and pneumothorax and should be suspected if there are signs of hemothorax without associated broken ribs or penetrating injuries. Definitive diagnosis is made by fiber-optic exam of the esophagus.

Treatment of esophageal injury in the field is supportive. Attention to airway, ventilation, oxygenation, and circulatory support takes precedence. The patient should be given nothing by mouth and a nasogastric tube should be carefully passed to decompress the stomach. A large-bore intravenous catheter is required for volume replacement and should be followed with broad-spectrum antibiotic therapy. Operative repair is the definitive treatment, consisting of bypassing the affected region and drainage of the pleural space.

TRAUMATIC ASPHYXIA

The term *traumatic asphyxia* is a misnomer. Although these patients appear to have been strangled, the mechanism is quite different. Sudden severe crushing of the chest causes retrograde blood flow from the right heart into the veins of the head and neck. The vena cava and the large veins of the head and neck lack valves, allowing the neck and facial capillaries to become engorged with blood.[25] The patient presents with facial and upper extremity cyanosis, edema, swollen tongue, subconjunctival hemorrhage or petechiae, and vascular engorgement. Venous congestion results and cranial blood flow becomes sluggish. Transient hypoxia, seizures, cerebral edema, and even small strokes can result.[2] Intracranial hemorrhage is rare, probably because of the shock-absorbing characteristics of the venous sinuses.[134] The initial neurological impairment is usually temporary, but visual impairment may be permanent if the cause is retinal hemorrhage rather than retinal engorgement and edema.[25] Treatment both in the field and in the hospital is supportive only. Careful examination for other concomitant injuries is essential. Despite the dramatic appearance of traumatic asphyxia, the condition itself is usually benign and self-limiting, and in the absence of other injuries the long-term prognosis is good.[135]

CHEST WALL INJURIES

SOFT TISSUE INJURIES

Wounds of the chest wall should receive standard dressings if there is no evidence of obvious air movement through the wound.[7] Bleeding from muscular injury can be significant and should be controlled with pressure dressings. Penetrating chest wounds should not be probed in the field or in the emergency department. Probing to assess depth could further damage underlying tissues and precipitate an air leak or brisk recurrent bleeding.[2] Sucking chest wounds should be dressed with a sterile occlusive dressing secured along three of four edges.

Management in the emergency department for soft tissue injuries of the chest wall consists of cautious local wound care and observation. If there is the possibility of penetration into the pleural cavity, a chest X-ray is obtained. If there is no evidence of pneumothorax, the patient is observed for an additional 6 hours and the chest X-ray is repeated. If no pneumothorax is evident, the patient is discharged with follow-up.[1] Surgical consultation is obtained for large soft tissue or muscular defects.

BONY INJURIES

Isolated fractures of the clavicle are commonly seen and are relatively harmless. However, occasionally fracture ends may injure the adjacent subclavian vessels and brachial plexus, resulting in hemorrhage, thrombosis, or neurological deficits in the ipsilateral extremity.[19] Claviculosternal dislocations deserve particular attention. These injuries are frequently associated with manubrial fracture and the clavicular heads or the manubrium may be displaced posteriorly, injuring the trachea or innominate vessels. Careful history is obtained to assess the risk of other associated injuries from the force causing the fracture. The affected extremity should be examined for compromise of the blood supply and innervation. Treatment consists of pain control and splinting with either a sling or figure-eight shoulder strap.

Scapular fractures are significant because the amount of force required to cause such a fracture could also cause severe thoracic trauma. Treatment for scapular fractures is pain control and a sling, unless there is significant displacement of the bony fragments or joint involvement.[1]

Sternal fractures are usually the result of a direct blow to the chest by the steering wheel of an automobile. The most common sites of sternal fracture are transversely throughout the sternal body and at the juncture of the body with the manubrium.[19] These injuries are frequently associated with costochondral dislocations of multiple ribs and, therefore, with flail chest as well as significant damage to the heart, including myocardial contusions and damage to the coronary arteries. These injuries are frequently associated with rib fractures, aortic injuries, and anterior myocardial contusions.[9] Sternal fractures have long been considered serious and life-threatening injuries; however, recent studies have demonstrated that the mortality is much lower than initially thought. One study found that in patients with sternal fracture, the incidence of dysrhythmias requiring treatment was 1.5% and mortality was 0.7%.[136] Diagnosis of sternal fracture is made primarily by physical examination because the sternum is easily palpated and the fracture or "step-off" can usually be felt. Treatment of sternal fracture is generally not required in the field unless there is a flail segment. However, the paramedic should evaluate the patient carefully for associated injuries. Definitive treatment is operative fixation by direct wiring.

Rib fractures are the most common injuries of the thoracic cage and should be assumed to be present when localized pain is present on the rib(s) after trauma. The fourth through ninth ribs are most commonly involved; ribs 1–3 are relatively protected and ribs 9–12 are more mobile at the anterior end and resistant to fracture.[25] Pain on motion will cause the patient to splint the affected area, compromising ventilation and the ability to cough up secretions. Isolated rib fractures are usually benign but in rare incidences may cause pneumothorax or hemothorax. Localized pain, point tenderness, bony crepitus, ecchymosis, palpable discontinuity of the rib outline, and possibly deformity are present. Chest X-rays are obtained to assess for pneumothorax or hemothorax. Rib fractures are identified only about half of the time on chest X-ray.[1] Rib X-rays are not frequently obtained because they will not change management of the patient. Splinting of the chest wall is usually not recommended because of possible interference with respiratory function, especially in older adults. The mainstay of treatment is pain control and incentive spirometry if indicated to prevent atelectasis. If patients cannot cough and clear secretions adequately, admission should be considered.

Multiple rib fractures occur most commonly in rib numbers 4–9 as the result of significant anteroposterior compression.[7] The ribs will bow out with this force and fracture in the middle of the shafts. Fractures of two or more ribs at any level is associated with a higher incidence of internal injuries, and 50% of patients with fractures of seven or more ribs will have an intrathoracic injury.[137] Fractures of ribs 9, 10, or 11 suggest an associated intra-abdominal injury.[1] Older adults have ribs that are more likely to fracture, compared to children and younger adults. Consequently, these injuries should always be considered significant.

The greatest risk of rib fractures is not the fracture itself, but the sequelae and associated injuries. Respiratory splinting of the fracture by the patient leads to inhibition of cough and retained secretions, carbon dioxide retention, atelectasis, increased work of breathing, poor pulmonary toilet, hypoxia, pneumonia, and empyema.[19] Older adults poorly tolerate the resulting ventilatory compromise.[2] Patients with multiple rib fractures at risk for respiratory compromise are often admitted for pain control and apnea monitoring. Pain control is best achieved with intercostal nerve block or epidural anesthesia due to the risk of apnea with narcotic analgesics.

Special consideration should be given to fractures of the first and second ribs. It takes great force to fracture these ribs from blunt trauma. These fractures by themselves will not cause significant problems, but they are associated with myocardial contusion, tracheobronchial disruption, major vascular injury, and severe head injuries.[2] The injuries associated with first or second rib fractures have a 27% mortality.[138] Tenderness of the rib cage inferior to the clavicles without evidence of clavicular fracture should raise concern for fractures of the first or second ribs. Because of the force required to fracture these ribs, injury to adjacent structures, such as the brachial plexus, thoracic inlet, and subclavian vessels should be suspected, particularly in the setting of neurovascular compromise in the ipsilateral extremity, hematoma at the base of the neck or upper chest, or marked displacement of the first rib segment.

PROCEDURES

PERICARDIOCENTESIS

Pericardiocentesis is a procedure that is rarely performed in the field but, when indicated, can be life saving. However, pericardiocentesis has a high complication rate and temporizing measures should be tried prior to attempting the procedure. In patients with suspected tamponade and without JVD, the administration of intravenous crystalloid fluids may improve hemodynamics.[139] Inotropic and pressor agents have also been recommended as temporizing measures in cardiac tamponade. Both dopamine and dobutamine have demonstrated improvements in hemodynamics.[140,141] Either agent is acceptable, but dobutamine may be preferable because of its greater beta activity.[141]

In preparation for pericardiocentesis, all equipment should be assembled, including a 10-mL syringe with a long 18-gauge spinal needle, sterile wire with alligator clips, three-way stopcock, and local anesthetic. Complete sets containing the equipment are commercially available (Cook, Bloomington, IN). One end of the wire is connected to the needle syringe assembly and the other to any of the precordial leads (V leads) (Figure 13-7). Generally lead V_1 is used because it permits continuous monitoring during the procedure. If

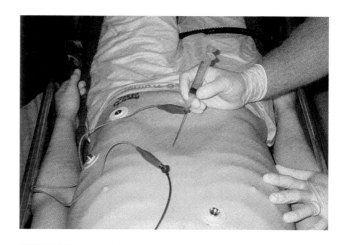

FIGURE 13-7 ECG lead and needle setup for pericardiocentesis.

the patient's condition permits, the torso should be elevated at a 45-degree angle to bring the heart closer to the anterior chest wall.[142] A nasogastric tube should be inserted to decompress the stomach if the abdomen is distended because of gastric contents or positive pressure ventilation.[142] The entire lower xiphoid and epigastric area should be prepared with 10% povidone-iodine solution and the injection site anesthetized with 1% lidocaine.

The needle is inserted between the xiphoid process and the left costal margin at a 45-degree angle to the skin (Figure 13-8 A and B). Approaches at angles greater than 45 degrees risk injury to intra-abdominal organs. The needle is directed toward the left shoulder and advanced slowly while gently aspirating. The pericardium is about 6–8 cm below the skin in adults and is particularly sensitive; patients will experience a sharp pain as it is entered. However, penetration of the pericardium is not palpable through the needle by the clinician.

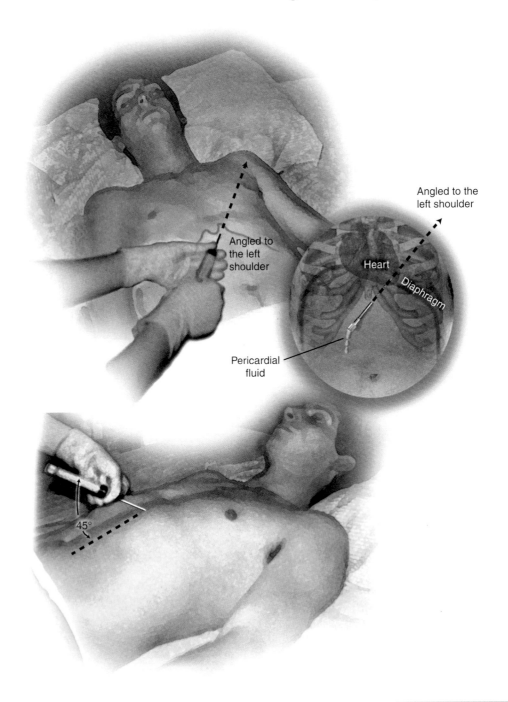

FIGURE 13-8 (A) Anterior and lateral views of the chest indicating insertion routes for the pericardial needle.

As the needle is advanced, the ECG should be continuously monitored to gauge the position of the needle and avoid ventricular puncture. When the needle touches the epicardium, ST-segment elevation or current-of-injury pattern is noted on the ECG (Figure 13-9). Contact with the ventricle may produce premature contractions or ventricular dysrhythmias, while contact with the atrium can cause atrial dysrhythmias, elevation of the PR segment, or atrioventricular dissociation.[143] If the current-of-injury pattern is noted, the

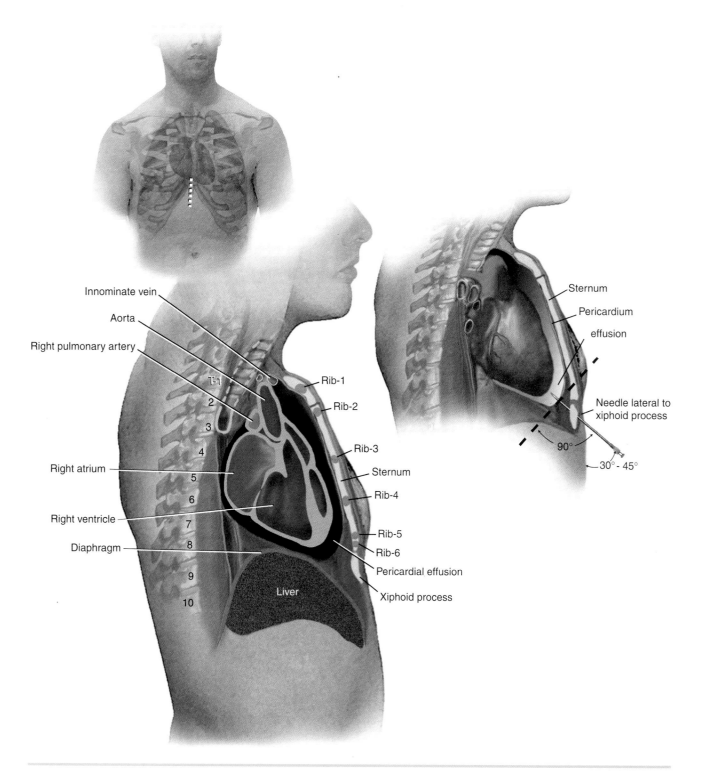

FIGURE 13-8 (B) Sagittal view of the thorax indicating the orientation of the pericardial needle. Note that the needle enters the pericardium at a right angle.

Needle Slightly Withdrawn

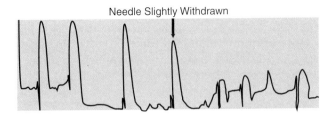

FIGURE 13-9 Current-of-injury pattern noting needle contact with epicardium. There is an obvious change in the ECG when the pericardiocentesis needle touches the epicardium. Following slight withdrawal (arrow), the ST-segment elevation diminishes.

needle is touching the epicardium and can easily lacerate the myocardium or coronary vessels and should be withdrawn a few millimeters until the ECG pattern disappears. An attempt is then made to drain blood from the pericardial space. Aspiration of as little as 50 mL of blood may result in marked clinical improvement. In addition to improved hemodynamics, analysis of the aspirate can distinguish circulatory blood from hemorrhagic pericardial fluid. The latter will have a substantially lower hematocrit than venous blood and is usually about 0.10 pH unit more acidic than simultaneously obtained arterial blood.[144] Bloody pericardial fluid will clot, especially when bleeding is brisk. Consequently, clotting of aspirated blood does not necessarily mean it was obtained from a cardiac chamber. However, nonclotting blood is indicative of defibrinated pericardial blood.[142]

Obviously, given the invasive nature of the procedure, pericardiocentesis is not without complications. Lacerations of the myocardium, lung, or coronary artery have been reported, as well as pneumothorax, new hemopericardium, dysrhythmias, pneumopericardium, vasovagal hypotension, and cardiac arrest.[145-150]

NEEDLE THORACENTESIS

Needle thoracentesis is a temporizing, yet life-saving procedure in the setting of tension pneumothorax. The goal of needle thoracentesis is not to reexpand a collapsed lung, but to relieve the intrathoracic pressure that impedes cardiac output and threatens to collapse the opposite lung. High intrapleural pressure can be evacuated using a standard IV catheter and will suffice until a chest tube can be placed.

There are two acceptable sites for performing needle thoracentesis: the second or third intercostal space in the midclavicular line and the fourth or fifth intercostal space in the midaxillary line (Figure 13-2).

In pregnant patients the second or third intercostal space is preferred due to elevation of the diaphragm by the gravid uterus. When identifying the appropriate site, it is helpful to remember that the sternal prominence, or angle of Louis, is at the same level as the second rib, and the nipple line is roughly the fourth intercostal space in most patients.

At either location, insert a large-bore (10- to 14-gauge) over-the-needle catheter in the middle of the intercostal space perpendicular to the chest wall. While most paramedic texts recommend inserting the needle in the bottom of the space because the neurovascular bundle lies under the rib margin, this is true only in the intercostal spaces posterior to the midaxillary line (Figure 13-10). There are two neurovascular bundles in each intercostal space anterior to the midaxillary line where needle thoracentesis is performed. Advance the needle until you hear the sound of escaping air. At this point remove the rigid stylet and secure the catheter in place. Once the tension has been relieved, it is important to provide a one-way valve to prevent introducing air into the pleural space through the catheter. The

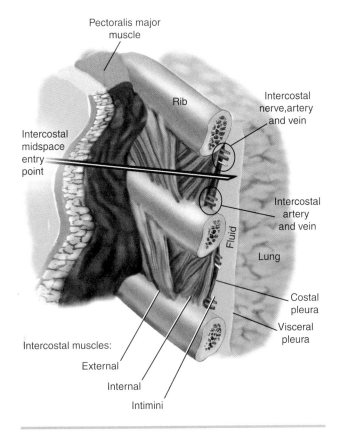

FIGURE 13-10 Location of neurovascular bundle. (A) Anterior thoracentesis is performed through the middle of the interspace as there are two neurovascular bundles in each intercostal space. One bundle lies posteriocaudad to the rib and one lies anteriocephalad to the rib.

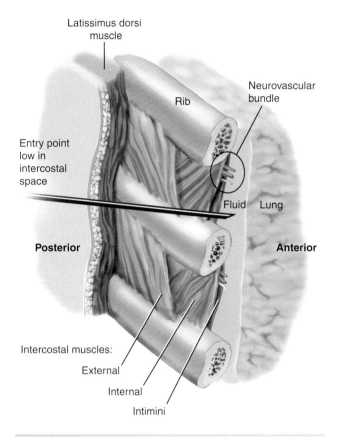

Latissimus dorsi muscle

Rib

Neurovascular bundle

Entry point low in intercostal space

Fluid

Lung

Posterior

Anterior

Intercostal muscles:

External

Internal

Intimini

FIGURE 13-10 Location of neurovascular bundle. (B) Posterior thoracentesis is used more often for draining a pleural effusion than for pleural decompression. When performed, the needle is inserted at the inferior aspect of the interspace as there is only one neurovascular bundle at the inferior edge of each rib.

most popular technique advocated has been the flutter valve formed by securing the finger of a latex glove around the hub of the catheter (Figure 13-11).[151] However, this method does not always produce a functional valve.[152] A better technique is to connect a length of IV extension tubing to the catheter and place the opposite end under a water seal. The water seal will allow intrapleural air under pressure to escape while preventing the introduction of air into the pleural space via the catheter. The water seal can easily be assembled by partially filling a urinal with sterile water or IV solution. The urinal can then be hung on the side rail of the stretcher for easy transport (Figure 13-12).

Needle thoracentesis, while potentially life saving, is not without complications. Once the catheter has penetrated the pleural cavity, the tension pneumothorax is converted to a simple pneumothorax. Moreover, if the diagnosis of tension pneumothorax was wrong, a new simple pneumothorax has been created. In either instance, the patient will require a chest tube at the hospital. Other hazards of needle thoracentesis include laceration of the intercostal artery or vein, hemorrhage, pericardial tamponade, myocardial laceration, pleural infection and empyema, and laceration of intra-abdominal organs if anatomical landmarks are misidentified.

TUBE THORACOSTOMY

Tube thoracostomy refers to the insertion of a large-bore plastic drainage tube into the pleural cavity and is used in the treatment of numerous maladies, including tension pneumothorax, moderate to large simple pneumothorax, hemothorax, and empyema. Some EMS systems and many air medical programs routinely perform tube thoracostomies.[153] However, all paramedics should be familiar with the technique of chest tube insertion and maintenance of drainage systems as they are frequently encountered during interfacility transports. This section will discuss chest tube insertion, while maintenance of chest drainage systems is covered in Chapter 18.

The equipment necessary to perform a tube thoracostomy is listed in Table 13-2. Once the equipment is assembled, the skin over the insertion site is prepared with antiseptic solution and draped. The proce-

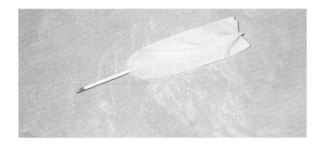

FIGURE 13-11 Latex glove around catheter hub used to form a flutter valve.

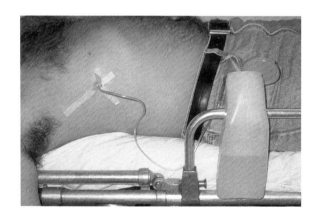

FIGURE 13-12 Creating a water seal using a urinal and sterile water. (Courtesy of Dr. Michael W. Hubble.)

Table 13-2
Equipment Needed for Tube Thoracostomy

Antiseptic solution and drapes	
1% lidocaine	Kelly clamp
10-mL syringe	Appropriate size thoracostomy tube
25-gauge and 22-gauge needles	Chest drainage unit
No. 10 scalpel	Suture kit

dure is most commonly performed at the fourth or fifth intercostal space anterior to or at the midaxillary line. The size of the thoracostomy tube depends on the reason for insertion and the size of the patient. Pneumothoraces can be evacuated with 24–32 French thoracostomy tubes in adults, while hemothoraces are best drained with a 36 French thoracostomy tube. A 32 French thoracostomy tube is used for evacuating a hemothorax in a small adult.

The actual skin incision will be made approximately 1 inch inferior to the interspace chosen for the insertion site. This provides an oblique tract through the chest wall, which reduces the risk of infection or creating a pneumothorax on removal of the tube.[154] In the conscious patient when time permits, the skin at the incision site is anesthetized with 1% lidocaine injected with a 25-gauge needle over a 2–3-cm area. A 22-gauge needle is substituted and the subcutaneous tissue, muscle, periosteum, and anterior rib margin to the pleura are anesthetized (Figure 13-13). A minimum of 20 cc of lidocaine is required for anesthesia in a 70-kg adult.

Estimate the length of the tube that must be intrathoracic and mark that length with a hemostat. A 2–3-cm horizontal incision is then made with the scalpel at the area previously anesthetized. The subcutaneous tissue is bluntly dissected using a Kelly clamp until the upper border of the chosen rib is reached. The parietal pleura is penetrated with the closed tip of the clamp, after which a sudden rush of air or blood escapes, indicating that the pleural cavity has been entered (Figure 13-14). The clamp is removed and the operator inserts a gloved finger through the opening to confirm entry into the pleural space and dislodge any pleural adhesions (Figure 13-15). The tip of the thoracostomy tube is clamped with a Kelly clamp and inserted into the incision as the operator's finger is removed (Figure 13-16). An intrapleural position is confirmed by "fogging" of the tube as the patient breathes. The tube is then directed posteriorly for hemothorax or anteriorly for pneumothorax and inserted until it meets resistance from the apex of the pleural cavity or until the last hole in the tube is clearly

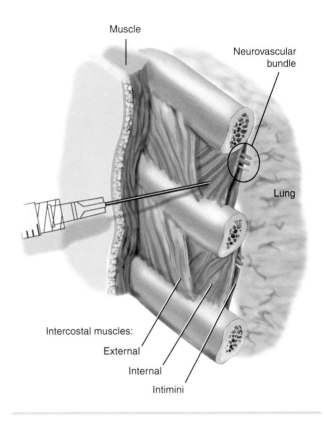

FIGURE 13-13 Anesthetizing the skin, subcutaneous tissue, muscle, and periosteum in preparation for tube thoracostomy.

within the pleural cavity. The tube is then connected to an underwater seal and the distal end of the tube is unclamped. Placement is confirmed by the return of air or blood into the chest drainage system. The tube can then be secured in place with sutures (Figure 13-17) or taped in place if time is not available for suturing. The insertion point is then dressed and taped. Tube placement should be confirmed radiographically upon arrival at the hospital.

► SUMMARY

Chest trauma contributes to 25%–50% of all trauma deaths in the United States. Early diagnosis and resuscitation are the keys to improving the survival in patients with chest trauma. An accurate history coupled with a thorough physical exam is essential for making the proper diagnoses and treatment.

Many injuries of the chest can be managed with minimally invasive procedures. In a patient that has pulseless electrical activity in the setting of chest trauma, the procedure should be to oxygenate, fluid resuscitate, and needle decompress both the left and right sides of the chest, followed by pericardiocentesis if the patient shows no sign of improving. Following blunt thoracic trauma, hypoxemia is frequently caused by pulmonary contusions.

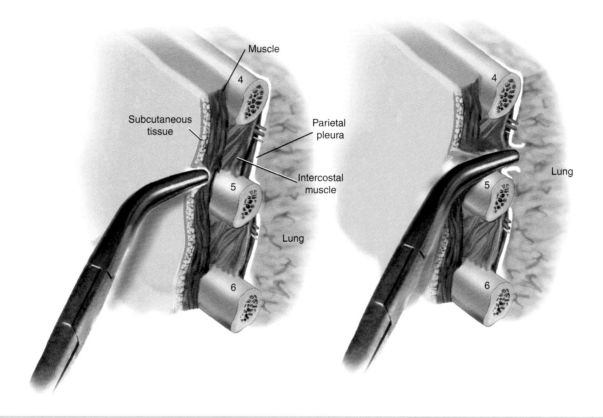

FIGURE 13-14 Blunt dissection of the pleura with a Kelly clamp.

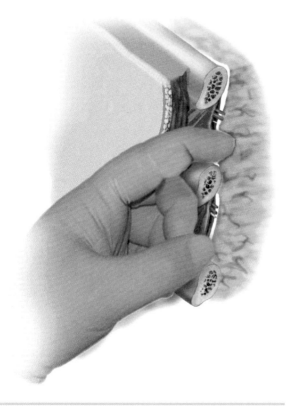

FIGURE 13-15 Performing a "finger thoracostomy" to dislodge pleural adhesions and ensure an intrapleural position.

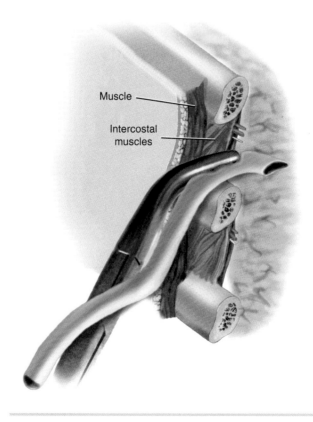

FIGURE 13-16 Inserting the tube using the Kelly clamp.

Method I

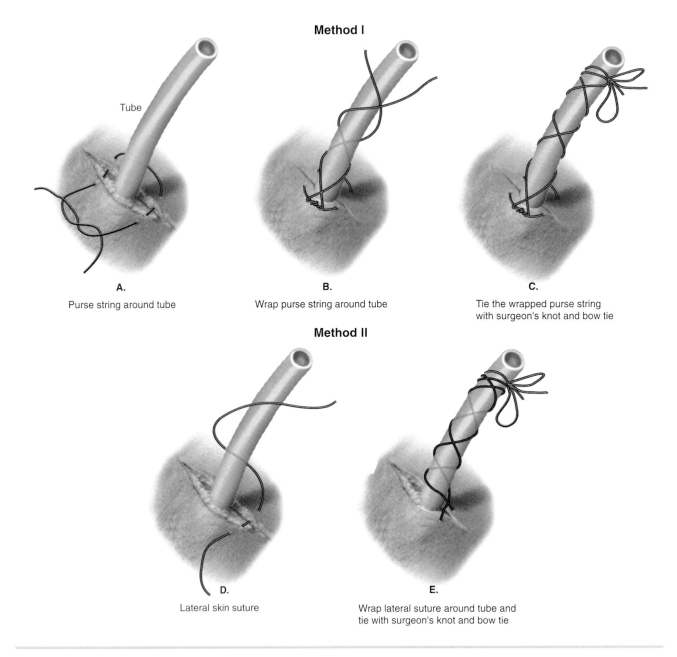

A.

Purse string around tube

B.

Wrap purse string around tube

C.

Tie the wrapped purse string
with surgeon's knot and bow tie

Method II

D.

Lateral skin suture

E.

Wrap lateral suture around tube and
tie with surgeon's knot and bow tie

FIGURE 13-17 Two methods of suturing the tube in place.

Compression of the heart by tension pneumothorax or cardiac tamponade will cause distended neck veins and pulsus paradoxus. Hypovolemic patients will not necessarily have distended neck veins. Patients with labored breathing with chest wall injuries can eventually have respiratory failure. A small amount of blood within the alveoli can cause significant hypoxia. Fractures of the scapula or first two ribs are indicators of a significant mechanism of injury and should prompt further evaluation of the patient for severe injuries.

Hemodynamically unstable patients need volume resuscitation. Hemodynamically stable patients with blunt chest trauma should receive only minimal IV

hydration to minimize edema from pulmonary contusions or strain on partially torn large vessels.

Any patient with significant blunt trauma to the chest should be suspected of having a myocardial contusion and great vessel injuries. Valvular or septal damage should be suspected in a patient that has significant heart failure after blunt injury to the chest. The most common valve injured is the aortic valve.

After penetrating injury to the heart, patients can often be successfully resuscitated from a recent (less than 5 minutes) cardiac arrest. Patients with respiratory distress and diminished breath sounds on the left may have a large diaphragmatic hernia. Hamman's sign may indicate pneumomediastinum, air in the pericardium, pneumothorax, or tracheobronchial disruption. A patient with heartburn-type pain after blunt trauma to the chest may have an esophageal disruption.

Treatment of rib fractures consists of pain control and ensuring adequate oxygenation. Chest tubes should not be placed in open chest wounds because of the possibility of causing further damage.

▶ REVIEW QUESTIONS

1. What percentage of trauma deaths are the result of isolated chest trauma?
   a. 10
   b. 15
   c. 20
   d. 25

2. What percentage of blunt chest injuries ultimately require surgery?
   a. 10
   b. 15
   c. 20
   d. 25

3. Contraction of the diaphragm is responsible for exhalation.
   a. True
   b. False

4. How many liters of blood can be accommodated in each pleural cavity?
   a. 1
   b. 2
   c. 3
   d. 4

5. What is the normal tidal volume for an adult?
   a. 100 cc
   b. 300 cc
   c. 500 cc
   d. 700 cc

6. Pulsus paradoxus is defined as a(n) _____ in _____ blood pressure by greater than 10 mm Hg during _____.
   a. Increase, systolic, inspiration
   b. Increase, diastolic, exhalation
   c. Decrease, diastolic, inspiration
   d. Decrease, systolic, exhalation

7. The goal of decompressing a tension pneumothorax is to reinflate the collapsed lung.
   a. True
   b. False

8. Tracheal deviation is an early sign of tension pneumothorax.
   a. True
   b. False

9. Hypotension in the setting of tension pneumothorax is due to:
   a. Hypovolemia
   b. Venous pooling
   c. Kinking of the vena cava
   d. Hydraulic brake effect on the heart

10. Air will preferentially enter through a chest wall defect if the size of the defect is _____ the diameter of the trachea.
    a. One-third
    b. Two-thirds
    c. One-half
    d. Three-fourths

11. Treatment of an open pneumothorax includes:
    a. Occlusive dressing sealed on three sides
    b. Manually reopening the wound if a tension pneumothorax develops
    c. Inserting a chest tube
    d. All of the above

12. If a chest tube is placed to drain a massive hemothorax and greater than 1500 mL of blood returns, the paramedic should:
    a. Place a second chest tube.
    b. Remove the chest tube.
    c. Clamp the chest tube.
    d. Increase the suction setting on the chest drainage system.

13. The mortality rate of flail chest can be as high as 50% and is mostly due to:
    a. Hemorrhage from rib fractures
    b. Paradoxical chest wall movement
    c. Sternal fracture
    d. Underlying lung injury

14. Paradoxical chest wall movement is universally seen immediately following a flail injury.
    a. True
    b. False

15. Cardiac tamponade usually results from penetrating trauma.
    a. True
    b. False

16. The most common location of cardiac penetration is the left ventricle.
    a. True
    b. False

17. Elevated CVP in the setting of cardiac tamponade is evidenced by:
    a. Hypotension
    b. Jugular venous distention
    c. Elevated diastolic pressure
    d. Both b and c

18. Beck's triad consists of:
    a. Increased venous pressure, hypotension, muffled heart tones

b. Elevated CVP, pulsus paradoxus, hypotension

c. Pulsus paradoxus, muffled heart tones, elevated CVP

d. Hypotension, elevated CVP, jugular vein distention

19. Electrical alternans is highly specific for cardiac tamponade.
    a. True
    b. False

20. Cardiac tamponade is a possible cause of PEA.
    a. True
    b. False

21. Myocardial rupture is almost universally immediately fatal.
    a. True
    b. False

22. The most common site of aortic rupture is:
    a. Ascending aorta
    b. Bifurcation of the aorta into the common iliac arteries
    c. Proximal aortic arch
    d. Ligamentum arteriosum

23. Signs and symptoms of aortic disruption include:
    a. Upper extremity hypertension
    b. Asymmetrical blood pressures in the arms
    c. Diminished femoral pulses
    d. All of the above

24. Signs and symptoms of pulmonary contusion include:
    a. Respiratory distress
    b. Hemoptysis
    c. Rales
    d. All of the above

25. Intubation is indicated when the PaO_2/FiO_2 ratio falls below:
    a. 300
    b. 400
    c. 500
    d. 600

26. Pain from myocardial contusion usually responds to nitroglycerine.
    a. True
    b. False

27. Blows to the left chest typically result in:
    a. AV blocks
    b. Bundle branch block
    c. Junctional rhythms
    d. Ventricular ectopy

28. Rupture of the aortic or mitral valves are usually well tolerated.
    a. True
    b. False

29. Blunt traumatic diaphragmatic rupture is most likely to occur:
    a. On the right side
    b. On the left side
    c. In the midline
    d. Equally likely on either side

30. The PASG is contraindicated in the setting of traumatic diaphragmatic herniation.
    a. True
    b. False

31. It is preferable not to intubate patients with tracheal injuries, if possible.
    a. True
    b. False

32. Esophageal injuries are usually minor and rarely require treatment.
    a. True
    b. False

33. The mechanism responsible for the appearance of patients suffering from traumatic asphyxia is:
    a. Pulmonary compression
    b. Chest compression with cardiac tamponade
    c. Chest compression with retrograde blood flow
    d. Tension pneumothorax accompanied by cardiac tamponade

34. Circumferential splinting is the preferred treatment of multiple rib fractures.
    a. True
    b. False

35. Pericardiocentesis is the definitive management of cardiac tamponade, although _____ and _____ may be used as temporizing measures.
    a. Norepinephrine, epinephrine
    b. Calcium chloride, epinephrine
    c. Dobutamine, dopamine
    d. Dopamine, calcium chloride

▶ **CRITICAL THINKING**

● Compare and contrast the pathophysiology and clinical presentations of hemothorax, tension pneumothorax, cardiac tamponade, and tension viscerothorax.

● Positive pressure ventilation is frequently used to treat massive flail segments with underlying pulmonary contusion. What other options exist for providing positive pressure ventilation without the need for intubation?

● Why is a flutter valve not needed following a needle thoracentesis in a patient receiving positive pressure ventilation?

● You have been dispatched to the scene of a MVC. Your patient was the unrestrained driver of an automobile involved in a high-speed frontal collision. Upon arrival the patient has been extricated from the vehicle by rescue personnel and is immobilized on the spine board. Inspection of the vehicle notes approximately 30 inches of crush to the hood and a grossly deformed steering wheel. Physical examination of the patient reveals an 18-year-old male who is conscious, alert, oriented x 3, and complaining of chest pain and dyspnea. He also complains of difficulty swallowing and hoarseness. A pulsatile mass is noted in the area of the suprasternal notch. Vital signs are blood pressure 130/P, heart rate 110, respirations 28. What is your impression of this patient? What is your most immediate concern? What treatments will you render?

REFERENCES

1. Wilson RF. Thoracic trauma. In: Tintinalli JE, Ruiz E, Krome RL, eds. *Emergency Medicine: A Comprehensive Study Guide*. 2nd ed. New York: McGraw-Hill; 1996.
2. American College of Surgeons. *Advanced Trauma Life Support: Course for Physicians*. 5th ed. Chicago: American College of Surgeons; 1993.
3. Sheehy SB. Chest trauma. In: Sheehy SB, ed. *Emergency Nursing: Principles and Practice*. 3rd ed. St. Louis: Mosby; 1992.
4. Bond SJ, Schnier GC, Miller FB. Air-powered guns: too much firepower to be a toy. *J Trauma*. 1996; 41(4):674.
5. van Amerongen R, Rosen M, Winni KG, Horwitz J. Ventricular fibrillation following blunt chest trauma from a baseball. *Pediatr Emerg Care*. 1997; 13(2):107.
6. Darsee, JR. Pericardial disease. *Hosp Pract*. 1979; 14(2):138.
7. McSwain NE, Paturas J, Wertz EM, eds. *Pre-Hospital Trauma Life Support*. 3rd ed. St. Louis: Mosby; 1994.
8. Richardson JD, Miller FB. Injury to the lung and pleura. In: Feliciano DV, Moore EE, Mattox KL, eds. *Trauma*. 3rd ed. Stamford, Conn.: Appleton & Lange; 1996.
9. Wilson RF, Steiger Z. Thoracic trauma: chest wall and lung. In: Wilson RF, Walt AJ, eds. *Management of Trauma: Pitfalls and Practice*. Baltimore, Md.: Williams and Wilkins; 1996.
10. Wilson RF, Stephenson LW. Thoracic trauma: heart. In: Wilson RF, Walt AJ, eds. *Management of Trauma: Pitfalls and Practice*. Baltimore, Md.: Williams and Wilkins; 1996.
11. Britten S, Palmer SH. Chest wall thickness may limit adequate drainage of tension pneumothorax by needle thoracentesis. *J Accident Emer Med*. 1996; 13(6):426.
12. Jones KW. Thoracic trauma. *Surg Clin North Am*. 1980; 60:257.
13. Barrett J. Chest trauma. In: Kravis TC, Warner CG, eds. *Emergency Medicine: A Comprehensive Review*. Rockville, Md.: Aspen Publishers; 1987.
14. Hood RM. Trauma to the chest. In: Sabison DC, Spencer FC, eds. *Gobbon's Surgery of the Chest*. Philadelphia: WB Saunders; 1983.
15. LoCicero J, Mattox KL. Epidemiology of chest trauma. *Surg Clin North Am*. 1989; 69(1):15.
16. Kirsch M, Sloan H. *Blunt Chest Trauma: General Principles and Management*. Boston: Little, Brown; 1977.
17. Webb WR. Thoracic trauma. *Surg Clin North Am*. 1974; 54:1179.
18. Cohn R. Nonpenetrating wounds of the lungs and bronchi. *Surg Clin North Am*. 1972; 52:585.
19. Pate JW. Chest wall injuries. *Surg Clin North Am*. 1989; 69:59.
20. Beeson A, Saegesser F. *Color Atlas of Chest Trauma and Associated Injuries, 1*. Oradell, N.J.: Medical Economics Books; 1983.
21. Corso PJ. Chest trauma. *Primary Care*. 1978; 5:543.
22. Parham AM, Yarborough DR 3rd, Redding JS. Flail chest syndrome and pulmonary contusion. *Arch Surg*. 1978; 113:900.
23. Schaal, MA, Fischer RP, Perry JF Jr. The unchanged mortality of flail chest injuries. *J Trauma*. 1979; 19:492.
24. Blair E, Topuzlu C, Davis JH. Delayed or missed diagnosis in blunt chest trauma. *J Trauma*. 1971; 11:129.
25. Vukich DJ, Markovchick V. Thoracic trauma. In: Rosen P, et al, eds. *Emergency Medicine: Concepts and Clinical Practice*. 3rd ed. St. Louis: Mosby; 1992.
26. Symbas PN. Cardiac trauma. *Am Heart J*. 1976; 92:387.
27. Symbas PN. Traumatic heart disease. *Curr Probl Cardiol*. 1982; 7:3.
28. Shoemaker WC. Algorithm for early recognition and management of cardiac tamponade. *Crit Care Med*. 1975; 3:39.
29. Ramp JM, Hankins JR, Mason GR. Cardiac tamponade secondary to blunt trauma. *J Trauma*. 1974; 14:767.
30. Karrel R, Shaffer MA, Franaszek JB. Emergency diagnosis, resuscitation, and treatment of acute penetrating cardiac trauma. *Ann Emerg Med*. 1982; 11:504.

31. Ivatury RR, Rohman M. The injured heart. *Surg Clin North Am.* 1989; 69:93.

32. Symbas PN, Harlaftis N. Bullet emboli in the pulmonary systemic arteries. *Ann Surg.* 1977; 185:318.

33. Ivatury RR. Injury to the heart. In: Feliciano DV, Moore EE, Mattox KL, eds. *Trauma.* 3rd ed. Stamford, Conn.: Appleton & Lange; 1996.

34. Demetriades D, VanderVeen PW. Penetrating injuries of the heart: experience over two years in South America. *J Trauma.* 1983; 23:1034.

35. Hochstein E, Rubin AL. *Physical Diagnosis.* New York: McGraw-Hill; 1964.

36. Spodick DH. Electrical alternation of the heart: its relation to the kinetics of the heart during cardiac tamponade. *Am J Cardiol.* 1962; 10:155.

37. Steichen FM, Dargan EL, Efron G, Perlman DM, Weil PH. A graded approach to the management of penetrating wounds of the heart. *Arch Surg.* 1971; 103:574.

38. Feigenbaum H, Zaky A, Grabhom LL. Cardiac motion in patients with pericardial effusion. *Circulation.* 1966; 34:611.

39. Friedman HS, Gomes JA, Tardio AR, Haff JI. The electrocardiographic features of acute cardiac tamponade. *Circulation.* 1974; 50:260.

40. Alcan KE, Zabetakis PM, Marino ND, Franzone AJ, Michelis MF, Bruno MS. Management of acute cardiac tamponade by subxyphoid pericardiotomy. *JAMA.* 1982; 247:1143.

41. Markovchick VJ, Evans, GT, Rosen P, Haftel AJ. Traumatic acute pericardial tamponade. *Ann Emerg Med.* 1977; 6:562.

42. Griffith GL, Zook JV, Mattingly WT Jr., Todd EP. Right atrial rupture due to blunt chest trauma. *South Med J.* 1984; 77:715.

43. Calhoon JH, Hoffman TH, Trinkle JK, Harman PK, Grover FL. Management of blunt rupture of the heart. *J Trauma.* 1986; 26:495.

44. Mayfield W, Hurley EJ. Blunt cardiac trauma. *Am J Surg.* 1984; 148:62.

45. Pevec WC, Udekwu AO, Pietzman AB. Blunt rupture of the myocardium. *Ann Thorac Surg.* 1989; 48:139.

46. Martin TD, Flynn TC, Rowlands BT, Ward RE, Fischer RP. Blunt cardiac rupture. *J Trauma.* 1984; 24:287.

47. Shorr RM, Crittenden M, Indeck M, Hartunian SL, Rodriguez A. Blunt thoracic trauma: analysis of 515 patients. *Ann Surg.* 1987; 206:200.

48. Baldwin J, Edwards JE. Rupture of right ventricle complicating closed chest cardiac massage. *Circulation.* 1976; 53:562.

49. Pomerantz M. Traumatic wounds of the heart. *J Trauma.* 1969; 9:135.

50. Dimarco RF, Layton TR, Manzetti GW, Pellegrini RV. Blunt traumatic rupture of the right atrium and the right superior pulmonary vein. *J Trauma.* 1983; 23:353.

51. Markovchick V, Duffens KR. Cardiovascular trauma. In: Rosen P, et al, eds. *Emergency Medicine.* St. Louis: Mosby Yearbook; 1992.

52. Dow RW. Myocardial rupture caused by trauma. *Surgery.* 1982; 91:246.

53. Getz BS, Davies E, Steinberg SM, Beaver BL, Koenig FA. Blunt cardiac trauma resulting in right atrial rupture. *JAMA.* 1986; 255:761.

54. Leavitt BJ, Meyer JA, Morton JR, Clark DE, Herbert WE, Hiebert CA. Survival following non-penetrating traumatic rupture of the cardiac chambers. *Ann Thorac Surg.* 1987; 44:532.

55. Terry TR. Blunt injury of the heart. *Br Med J.* 1983; 286:805.

56. Weiss JP, Feld M, Sclafani SJ, Scalea T, Vieux E, Troaskin SZ. Traumatic rupture of the thoracic aorta. *Emerg Med Clin North Am.* 1991; 9:789.

57. Beel T, Harwood AC. Traumatic rupture of the thoracic aorta. *Ann Emerg Med.* 1980; 9:483.

58. Patterson RH, Willard BA, Frank JS. Rupture of the thoracic aorta: complication of resuscitation. *JAMA.* 1973; 226:197.

59. Merrill WH, Lee RB, Hammon JW, et al. Surgical treatment of acute traumatic tear of the thoracic aorta. *Ann Surg.* 1988; 206:699.

60. Lundell CJ, Quinn MF, Finck EJ. Traumatic laceration of the ascending aorta: angiographic assessment. *Am J Roentgenol.* 1985; 145:715.

61. Kirsh M, Orringer MB, Behrendt DM, Mills LJ, Tashian J, Sloan H. Management of unusual traumatic ruptures of the aorta. *Surg Gynecol Obstet.* 1978; 146:365.

62. Kirsh M, Behrendt DM, Orringer MB, et al. The treatment of acute traumatic rupture of the aorta: a 10-year experience. *Ann Surg.* 1976; 184:308.

63. Mattox KL. Injury to the thoracic great vessels. In: Moore EE, Mattox KL, Feliciano DV, eds. *Trauma.* 2nd ed. Norwalk, Conn.: Appleton and Lange; 1991.

64. Symbas PN, Tyras DH, Ware RE, Diorio DA. Traumatic rupture of the aorta. *Ann Surg.* 1973; 178:6.

65. Malm JR, Deterling RJ. Traumatic aneurysm of the thoracic aorta simulating coarctation. *J Thorac Cardiovasc Surg.* 1960; 40:271.

66. Mirvis SE, Pais SO, Jens DR. Thoracic aortic rupture: advantages of intra-arterial digital subtraction angiography. *Am J Roentgenol.* 1986; 146:987.

67. Dougall AM, Paul ME, Finley RJ, Holliday RL, Coles JC, Duff JH. Chest trauma: current morbidity and mortality. *J Trauma.* 1977; 17:547

68. Johnson JA, Cogbill T, Winga ER. Determinants of outcome after pulmonary contusion. *J Trauma*. 1986; 26:695.

69. Cowley RA, Conn A, Dunham CM, eds. *Trauma Care: Surgical Management*. Philadelphia: Lippincott; 1987.

70. Kuhlmann TP. Pulmonary injuries. *Emerg Care Q*. 1988; 4(1):29.

71. Trinkle JK, Richardson JD, Franz JL, Grover FL, Arom KV, Holstrom FM. Management of flail chest without mechanical ventilation. *Ann Thorac Surg*. 1975; 19:355.

72. Wiot JF. The radiologic manifestations of blunt chest trauma. *JAMA*. 1975; 231:500.

73. Barone JE, Pizzi W, Nealon T, Richman H. Indications for intubation in blunt chest trauma. *J Trauma*. 1986; 26:334.

74. Allen JE, Schwab CW. Blunt chest trauma in the elderly. *Am Surg*. 1985; 51:697.

75. Richardson JD, Adams L, Flint LM. Selective management of flail chest and pulmonary contusion. *Ann Surg*. 1982; 196:481.

76. Fabian TC, Mangiante EC, Patterson CR, Payne LW, Isaacson ML. Myocardial contusion in blunt trauma: clinical characteristics, means of diagnosis, and implications for patient management. *J Trauma*. 1988; 18:50.

77. Nirgiotis JG, Colon R, Sweeney MS. Blunt trauma to the heart: the pathophysiology of injury. *J Emerg Med*. 1990; 8:617.

78. Symbas PN. Traumatic heart disease. *Curr Probl Cardiol*. 1991; 16:543.

79. Doty DB, Anderson AE, Rose EF, Go RT, Chile CL, Ehrenhaft JL. Cardiac trauma: clinical and experimental correlations of myocardial contusions. *Ann Surg*. 1974; 180:452.

80. Lasky II, Nakum AM, Siegel AW. Cardiac injuries incurred by drivers in automobile accidents. *J Forensic Sci*. 1969; 14:13.

81. Saunders CR, Doty DB. Myocardial contusion. *Surg Gynecol Obstet*. 1977; 144:595.

82. Jackimczyk K. Blunt chest trauma. *Emerg Med Clin North Am*. 1993; 11(1):81.

83. Pearce W, Blair E. Significance of the electrocardiogram in heart contusion due to blunt trauma. *J Trauma*. 1976; 16:136.

84. Dubrow TJ, Mihalka J, Eisenhauer DM, et al. Myocardial contusion in the stable patient: what level of care is appropriate? *Surgery*. 1989; 106:267.

85. Illig KA, Swierzewski MJ, Feliciano DV, Morton JH. A rational screening and treatment strategy based on the electrocardiogram alone for suspected cardiac contusion. *Am J Surg*. 1991; 162:537.

86. Norton MJ, Stanford GG, Weigelt JA. Early detection of myocardial contusion and its complications in patients with blunt trauma. *Am J Surg*. 1990; 160:577.

87. Frazee RC, Mucha P Jr., Farnell MB, Miller FA Jr. Objective evaluation of blunt cardiac trauma. *J Trauma*. 1986; 26:510.

88. Baxter BT, Moore EE, Moore FA, McCroskey BL, Ammons LA. A plea for sensible management of myocardial contusion. *Am J Surg*. 1989; 158:557.

89. Bodin L, Rouby JJ, Viars P. Myocardial contusion in patients with blunt chest trauma as evaluated by thallium 201 myocardial scintigraphy. *Chest*. 1988; 94:72.

90. Moseley RV, Vernick JJ, Doty DB. Response to blunt chest injury: a new experimental model. *J Trauma*. 1970; 10:673.

91. Keller KD, Shatney CH. Creatinine phosphokinase-MB assays in patients with suspected myocardial contusion: diagnostic tests or tests of diagnosis? *J Trauma*. 1988; 28:58.

92. Parmely LF, Marion WC, Mattingly TW. Non-penetrating traumatic injury of the heart. *Circulation*. 1958; 18:371.

93. Cuadros CL, Hutchinson JE, Mogtader AH. Laceration of a mitral papillary muscle and the aortic route as a result of blunt trauma to the chest. *J Thorac Cardiovasc Surg*. 1984; 88:134.

94. Cline DM. Valvular emergencies and endocarditis. In: Tintinalli J, Ruiz E, Krome RL, eds. *Emergency Medicine: A Comprehensive Study Guide*. 4th ed. New York: McGraw-Hill; 1996.

95. Bryant LR, Dillon ML, Utley JR. Cardiac valve injury with major chest trauma. *Arch Surg*. 1973; 107:279.

96. Gelman R, Mirvis SE, Gens D. Diaphragmatic rupture due to blunt trauma: sensitivity of plain chest radiographs. *Am J Roentgenol*. 1991; 156:51.

97. Smithers BM, O'Loughlin B, Strong RW. Diagnosis of ruptured diaphragm following blunt trauma: results from 85 cases. *Aust N Z J Surg*. 1991; 61:737.

98. Ward RE, Flynn TC, Clark WP. Diaphragmatic disruption secondary to blunt abdominal trauma. *J Trauma*. 1981; 21:35.

99. Moore JB, Moore EE, Thompson JS. Abdominal injuries associated with penetrating trauma to the lower chest. *Am J Surg*. 1980; 140:724.

100. Kanowitz A, Markovchick V. Esophageal and diaphragmatic trauma. In: Rosen P, et al, eds. *Emergency Medicine: Concepts and Clinical Practice*. 3rd ed. St. Louis: Mosby; 1992.

101. Blumenthal DH, Raghu G, Rudd TG, Herman CM. Diagnosis of right hemidiaphragmatic rupture by liver scintigraphy. *J Trauma*. 1984; 24:536.

102. Heiberg E, Wolverson MK, Hurd RN, Jagonnodhara OB, Sundaram M. CT recognition of traumatic rupture of the diaphragm. *Am J Roentgenol*. 1980; 135:369.

103. Miller L, Bennett EV, Root HD, Trinkle JK, Grover FL. Management of penetrating and blunt diaphragmatic injury. *J Trauma*. 1984; 24:403.

104. Waldschmidt ML, Laws HL. Injuries of the diaphragm. *J Trauma*. 1980; 20:587.

105. Adamthwaite DN. Traumatic diaphragmatic hernia. *Surg Ann*. 1983; 15:73.

106. Van Vugt AB, Schoots FJ. Acute diaphragmatic rupture due to blunt trauma: a retrospective analysis. *J Trauma*. 1989; 29:683.

107. Sharma OP. Traumatic diaphragmatic rupture: not an uncommon entity. *J Trauma*. 1989; 29:678.

108. de la Rocha AG, Creel RJ, Mulligan GW, Burns CM. Diaphragmatic rupture due to blunt abdominal trauma. *Surg Gynecol Obstet*. 1982; 154:175.

109. Grimes OF. Traumatic injuries of the diaphragm. *Am J Surg*. 1974; 128:175.

110. Hood RM. Traumatic diaphragmatic hernia. *Ann Thorac Surg*. 1971; 12:311.

111. Lucido JL, Wall CA. Rupture of the diaphragm due to blunt trauma. *Arch Surg*. 1963; 86:989.

112. Waldhausen JA, Kilman JW, Helman CH, Battersby JS. The diagnosis and management of traumatic injuries of the diaphragm including the use of Marlex prostheses. *J Trauma*. 1966; 6:332.

113. Chen JC, Wilson SE. Diaphragmatic injuries: recognition and management in sixty-two patients. *Am Surg*. 1991; 57:810.

114. Olin C. Traumatic rupture of the diaphragm. *Chir Scand*. 1975; 141:282.

115. Hegarty MM, Bryer JV, Angorn IB, Baker LW. Delayed presentation of traumatic diaphragmatic hernia. *Ann Surg*. 1978; 187:229.

116. Kanowitz A, Marx JA. Delayed traumatic diaphragmatic hernia simulating acute tension pneumothorax. *J Emerg Med*. 1989; 7:619.

117. Feliciano D, Cruse PA, Mattox KL, et al. Delayed diagnosis of injuries to the diaphragm after penetrating injuries. *J Trauma*. 1988; 28:1135.

118. Ali J, Qi W. The cardiorespiratory effects of increased intra-abdominal pressure in diaphragmatic rupture. *J Trauma*. 1992; 33:233.

119. Symbas PN, Levin JM, Fernier FL, Sybers RG. A study on auto transfusion from hemothorax. *South Med J*. 1969; 62:671.

120. Eastridge CE, Hughes FA Jr., Pate JW, Cole F, Richardson R. Tracheobronchial injury caused by blunt trauma. *Am Rev Respir Dis*. 1970; 101:230.

121. Payne WS, DeRenue R. Injuries of the trachea and major bronchi. *Postgrad Med*. 1971; 49:152.

122. Relland J, Miller D, Carberry D. Traumatic rupture of the tracheobronchial tree. *NY State J Med*. 1973; 73:1291.

123. Urschel H, Razzuk M. Management of acute traumatic injuries of the tracheobronchial tree. *Surg Gynecol Obstet*. 1973; 136:113.

124. Baumgartner F, Sheppard B, deVirgilio C, et al. Tracheal and main bronchial disruptions after blunt chest trauma: presentation and management. *Ann Thorac Surg*. 1990; 50:569.

125. Mathisen DJ, Grillo H. Laryngotracheal trauma. *Ann Thorac Surg*. 1987; 43:254.

126. Shimazu T, Sugimoto H, Nishade K, et al. Tracheobronchial rupture caused by blunt chest trauma: acute respiratory management. *Am J Emerg Med*. 1988; 6:427.

127. Sealy WC. Rupture of the esophagus. *Am J Surg*. 1963; 105:505.

128. Bomback CT, Boyd DR, Nyhus LM. Esophageal trauma. *Surg Clin North Am*. 1972; 52:219.

129. Loop FD, Groves LK. Esophageal perforations: collective review. *Ann Thorac Surg*. 1970; 10:571.

130. Wichern WA. Perforation of the esophagus. *Am J Surg*. 1970; 119:534.

131. Glatterer MS Jr., Toon RS, Ellestad C, et al. Management of blunt and penetrating external esophageal trauma. *J Trauma*. 1985; 25:784.

132. Oparah RS, Maudal AK. Operative management of penetrating wounds of the chest in civilian practice. *J Thorac Cardiovasc Surg*. 1979; 77:162.

133. Pate JW. Tracheobronchial and esophageal injuries. *Surg Clin North Am*. 1989; 69:111.

134. Moore JD, Mayer JH, Gago O. Traumatic asphyxia. *Chest*. 1972; 62:634.

135. Jongewaard WR, Cogbill T, Landercasper J: Neurologic consequences of traumatic asphyxia. *J Trauma*. 1992; 32:28.

136. Brookes JG, Dunn RJ, Rogers, IR. Sternal fractures: a retrospective analysis of 272 cases. *J Trauma*. 1993; 35:46.

137. Wilson RF, Murray C, Antonenko DR. Nonpenetrating thoracic injuries. *Surg Clin North Am*. 1977; 57:17.

138. Richardson JD, McElvein RB, Trinkle JK. First rib fracture: a hallmark of severe trauma, *Ann Surg*. 1975; 181:251.

139. Antman E, Cargill V, Grossman W. Low-pressure cardiac tamponade. *Ann Intern Med*. 1979; 91:403.

140. Ramp J, Harkins J, Mason G. Cardiac tamponade secondary to blunt trauma. *J Trauma*. 1974; 14:767.

141. Zhang H, Spapen H, Vincent JL. Effects of dobutamine and norepinephrine on oxygen availability and tamponade-induced stagnant hypoxia: a prospective, randomized, controlled study. *Crit Care Med*. 1994; 22:299.

142. Harper RJ, Callaham ML. Pericardiocentesis and intracardiac injections. In: Roberts JR, Hedges JR, eds. *Clinical Procedures in Emergency Medicine*. Philadelphia: Saunders; 1998.

143. Kerber R, Ridges J, Harrison D. Electrocardiographic indications of atrial puncture during pericardiocentesis. *N Engl J Med*. 1979; 282:1142.

144. Kindig J, Goodman M. Clinical utility of pericardial fluid pH determination. *Am J Med*. 1983; 75:1077.

145. Permanyer-Miralda G, Sagrista-Sauleda J, Soler-Soler J. Primary acute pericardial disease: a prospective series of 231 consecutive patients. *Am J Cardiol*. 1985; 56:623.

146. Wong B, Murphy J, Chang CJ, Hassenein K, Dunn M. The risk of pericardiocentesis. *Am J Cardiol*. 1979; 44:1110.

147. Guberman B, Fowler N, Engel P. Cardiac tamponade in medical patients. *Circulation*. 1981; 64:633.

148. Krikorian J, Hancock E. Pericardiocentesis. *Am J Med*. 1978; 65:808.

149. Kwasnik E, Kostes J, Lazarus J. Conservative management of uremic pericardial effusions. *J Thorac Cardiovasc Surg*. 1978; 76:629.

150. Callahan J, Seward JB, Nishimura RA, et al. Two-dimensional echocardiographically guided pericardiocentesis: experience in 117 consecutive patients. *Am J Cardiol*. 1985; 55:476.

151. Bledsoe B, Porter R, Shade B. *Paramedic Emergency Care*. 2nd ed. Englewood Cliffs, N.J.: Prentice Hall; 1994.

152. Campbell, J. *Basic Trauma Life Support*. 3rd ed. Englwood Cliffs, N.J.: Prentice Hall; 1995.

153. Hatley T, Ma OJ, Weaver N, Strong G. Flight paramedic scope of practice: current level and breadth. *J Emerg Med*. 1998; 16.

154. Feliciano DV. Tube thoracostomy. In: Benumof JL, ed. *Clinical Procedures in Anesthesia and Intensive Care*. Philadelphia: JB Lippincott; 1992.

Chapter 14

Abdominal and Genitourinary Trauma

OBJECTIVES

Upon completion of this chapter, the reader should be able to:

- Describe the epidemiology of abdominal trauma.
- Describe the anatomy and physiology of each organ contained within the abdomen.
- Discuss the pathophysiology of injury to each of the abdominal organs.
- Delineate out-of-hospital assessment of patients with abdominal trauma and discuss emergency department assessment of such patients.
- Delineate out-of-hospital treatment of patients with abdominal trauma and discuss emergency department treatment of such patients.
- Describe the epidemiology of genitourinary trauma.
- Define the anatomy and physiology of each organ included within the genitourinary system.
- Discuss the pathophysiology of injury to each of these organ systems.
- Delineate out-of-hospital assessment of patients with genitourinary trauma and briefly discuss emergency department assessment of such patients.
- Delineate out-of-hospital treatment of patients with genitourinary trauma and briefly discuss emergency department treatment of such patients.

KEY TERMS

Body
Cardia
Cecum
Colon
Diagnostic peritoneal lavage (DPL)
Duodenum
Fundus
Gallbladder
Grey-Turner's sign
Ileum
Jejunum

Kidneys
Large intestine
Liver
Pancreas
Pylorus
Rectum
Small intestine
Spleen
Splenorrhaphy
Stomach

283

Abdominal trauma is often an occult entity and a source of unrecognized major hemorrhage in the unstable trauma patient. Like abdominal trauma, genitourinary trauma may be occult and a source of unrecognized hemorrhage. This chapter describes the epidemiology, anatomy and physiology, pathophysiology, assessment, and treatment of injuries to the gastrointestinal system and abdominal vascular structures as well as the urinary and genital systems.

ABDOMINAL TRAUMA

EPIDEMIOLOGY

Abdominal trauma accounts for between 7% and 15% of all trauma deaths.[1,2] A distinction is usually made between blunt and penetrating mechanisms. Mortality rates for blunt abdominal trauma range between 10% and 30% depending on access to sophisticated trauma care. Penetrating abdominal injury mortality rates have been reported to be less than 5%.[3]

Seventy-five percent of blunt abdominal trauma is due to high-speed motor vehicle crashes (MVCs).[4] Other etiologies include motorcycle collisions, vehicle ejection, falls, industrial injuries, and pedestrians struck by motor vehicles. The incidence of penetrating trauma, particularly in urban areas, has grown to such a proportion that some call it an epidemic.[5] The mix of blunt versus penetrating trauma varies greatly from area to area and depends on rural versus urban environment, drug traffic, and gun control laws.

ANATOMY AND PHYSIOLOGY

The organs of the abdominal cavity are contained within a large, continuous, serous sheath called the peritoneum. It is similar in structure to the pleura of the chest cavity. Organs within the torso but located behind the peritoneum are called retroperitoneal structures: kidneys, pancreas, and part of the small intestine (Figure 14-1). The omentum is a lacy, fatty portion of the peritoneum containing blood vessels and lies over the abdominal organs anteriorly. So, when opening the skin of the abdomen and entering the peritoneal cavity, the omentum is the first structure seen.

The **liver** is the largest organ within the abdomen. It lies in the upper right quadrant, is in direct contact with the diaphragm, and is partially protected by the most inferior ribs. Made up of two lobes (the large right and smaller left), the liver is a highly vascular structure with a massive blood supply (Figure 14-2). Between the two lobes of the liver lies the porta hepatis, the point of entry for the portal vein, hepatic arteries, nerves, lymph vessels, and the exit of the bile duct. The portal vein

drains the venous system of the entire digestive tract and dumps this nutrient-rich blood into the liver along with the oxygen-rich blood of the hepatic artery. The hepatic vein provides the conduit through which the blood, once processed by the liver, drains into the inferior vena cava to be recycled through the system.

The liver functions as a processing center for the nutrients absorbed by the digestive system. It is active in carbohydrate, fat, and protein metabolism. The liver also distributes the components of broken-down red blood cells and recycles the material to the bone marrow and other organs. Bile, partially composed of bilirubin from these broken-down red blood cells, is manufactured by the liver and is an essential component in the digestion of fats. Bile drains from the liver via the hepatic duct into the gallbladder for storage until needed by the digestive system.

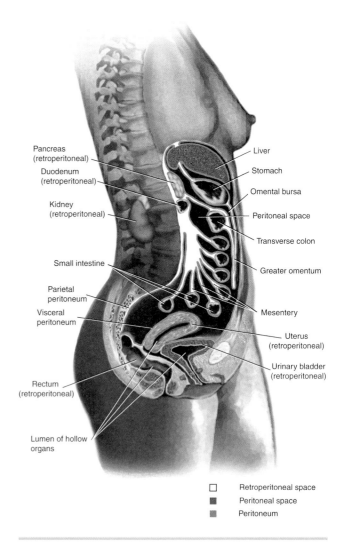

□ Retroperitoneal space
■ Peritoneal space
■ Peritoneum

FIGURE 14-1 Most of the abdominal organs lie anterior to the peritoneum. Those that do not (kidneys, pancreas, and portions of the small intestine) are called retroperitoneal organs.

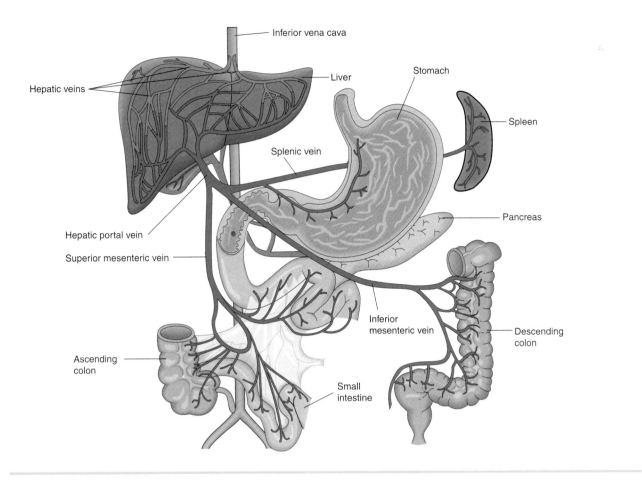

FIGURE 14-2 Hepatic portal circulation.

The **gallbladder**, a pear-shaped organ lying inferior to the liver, serves as a repository for collected bile until it is needed by the duodenum to process fatty material (Figure 14-3). It is attached to the common bile duct by a small, thin tube, the cystic duct. The confluence of the cystic and common hepatic ducts form the bile duct, through which bile is excreted into the duodenum. The liver is essential to life, but the gallbladder is removed with little consequence.

The **spleen** is a purplish, highly vascular organ situated in the left upper quadrant that is of variable size and shape depending on the person's age and underlying medical conditions. It lies against the diaphragm and is protected in part by the most inferior portion of the left rib cage. Because it is covered by a thick capsule, a small hemorrhage due to injury can easily be contained and perhaps tamponaded (Figure 14-3). The hilum of the spleen contains both the splenic artery and vein. The spleen serves as a filter, removing old or fragmented red blood cells, bacteria taken up by white blood cells, and particulate matter floating in the blood. Approximately 5% of the circulating blood volume is filtered through the spleen each minute.

The **pancreas** is an elongated organ lying in the mid-upper epigastric area of the abdomen at the level of the first lumbar vertebrae and is separated into several segments (Figure 14-3). The head of the pancreas extends to the right of the midline and lies within the curvature of the duodenum. The body of the pancreas lies in the midline and the tail extends to the left of the midline toward the hilum of the spleen. A ductal network carries the rich enzymatic juices of the pancreas to the pancreatic duct, which empties into the duodenum at the same location as the previously mentioned bile duct. The pancreas serves two major functions. First, it performs as an exocrine gland manufacturing and delivering enzymes to the gastrointestinal system to aid in digestion of food substances. Second, it executes an endocrine function by creating insulin within the islets of Langerhans cells, which regulates glucose within the body.

The **stomach** is a highly mobile organ that is fed by the esophagus from above and empties into the duodenum through the pyloric sphincter. It lies in the peritoneum, mostly in the left upper quadrant, although, when full, it can occupy a much larger area, extending into the midline. There are four portions of the stomach

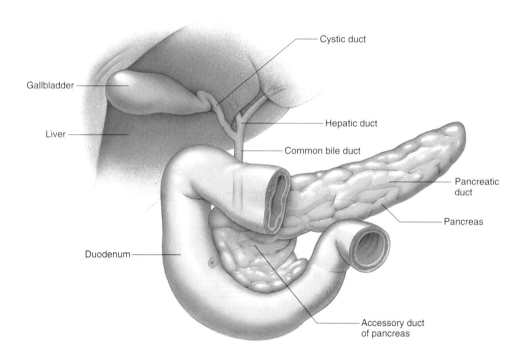

FIGURE 14-3 Gallbladder and bile ducts.

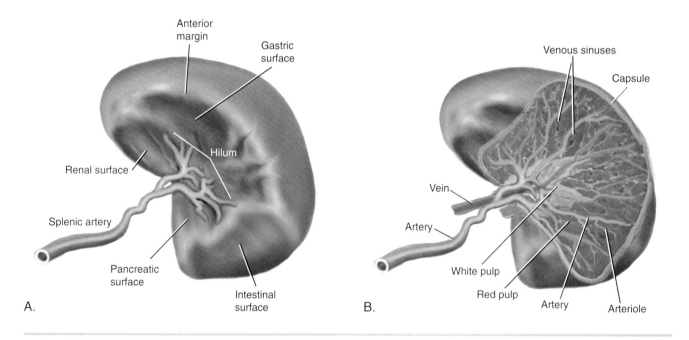

FIGURE 14-4 Surface anatomy (A) and sectional anatomy (B) of the spleen. The spleen is surrounded by a fibrous capsule that divides the organ into compartments. Small hemorrhages within the spleen may be contained and tamponaded by the capsule (subcapsular hematoma).

that bear note (Figure 14-5). The **cardia** is the portion of the stomach surrounding the gastroesophageal junction. The **fundus** is the superiormost portion and typically lies above the cardia. The **body** is the long curving portion in which the majority of food contents lie during

digestion. The **pylorus**, meaning gatekeeper in Greek, is the entryway for partially digested food to continue into the duodenum for additional breakdown. The stomach wall is comprised of four layers: three muscular layers and a mucous membrane that contain three distinct

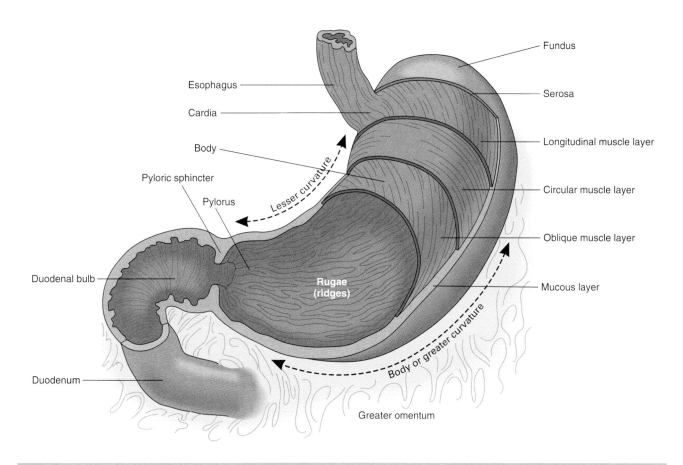

Esophagus

Cardia

Body

Pyloric sphincter

Pylorus

Duodenal bulb

Duodenum

Fundus

Serosa

Longitudinal muscle layer

Circular muscle layer

Oblique muscle layer

Mucous layer

Lesser curvature

Rugae (ridges)

Body or greater curvature

Greater omentum

FIGURE 14-5 External and internal anatomy of the stomach.

types of cells. Chief cells secrete digestive enzymes; mucous cells secrete mucous; and parietal cells secrete hydrochloric acid. Each of these play a role in the initial digestion or breakdown of food. Once the stomach's stretch receptors are activated with the ingestion of food or other substances, a peristaltic movement is initiated, leading to gastric emptying.

The **small intestine** extends approximately 21–23 feet in total length and is divided into three major sections: the duodenum, the jejunum, and the ileum. If the abdomen were opened and the omentum reflected upward, one would see the small intestine curled neatly in the central portion of the peritoneal cavity and the large intestine curving around the edges in a semicircle.

The **duodenum**, a retroperitoneal structure, is only a foot long. It is curved in the shape of a "C," with the pancreas residing in the middle of the curve. While the duodenum manufactures its own digestive enzymes, it also serves as a receptacle for bile from the bile duct and pancreatic enzymes from the pancreatic duct, both of which empty into the duodenum at the duodenal papilla. The **jejunum** is approximately 8 feet long and begins at the duodenojejunal junction (about the second lumbar vertebra). It fills the superior and

left portion of the abdominal cavity while the ileum fills the inferior and right portion of the cavity. The **ileum** is usually 12–13 feet in length. Both the jejunum and ileum are peritoneal structures and function as an absorption point for nutrients as they are broken down. They also shift fluid and electrolytes either into the lumen if there is an excess or out of the lumen if there is a deficit.

The **large intestine** surrounds the periphery of the small intestine in a long slow curve beginning at the ileocecal junction and terminating at the anus (Figure 14-6). It is composed of the cecum, colon, and rectum. All but the rectum are peritoneal structures. The **cecum** is a small sac approximately 2 inches long from which the appendix forms. It is continuous with the ascending portion of the **colon**. As the colon reaches the level of the liver, it turns to cross the abdomen and becomes the transverse colon. As it reaches the spleen, the colon turns downward toward the pelvis to become the descending colon. The sigmoid colon continues from the descending colon to the rectum. The **rectum** is usually about 5 inches long and lies just anterior to the sacrum and coccyx. It is a retroperitoneal structure. The anal canal is only 1–2 inches in length and is extremely muscular. The cecum and colon continue the

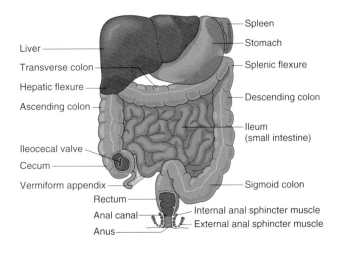

Spleen
Stomach
Liver
Splenic flexure
Transverse colon
Hepatic flexure
Descending colon
Ascending colon
Ileum
(small intestine)
Ileocecal valve
Cecum
Vermiform appendix
Sigmoid colon
Rectum
Anal canal
Internal anal sphincter muscle
Anus
External anal sphincter muscle

FIGURE 14-6 Anatomy of the large intestine.

process of shifting fluids and electrolytes either into or out of the lumen depending on the body's needs. The rectum is a conduit for fecal material; the anal canal and anus serve as the control point for expulsion of fecal material.

The aorta courses through the abdomen in the retroperitoneal space alongside the vertebral column. At the level of the fourth lumbar vertebrae, the aorta bifurcates into the internal and external iliac arteries. The external iliac artery then becomes the common femoral artery. The vena cava traverses the abdomen alongside the aorta and carries blood from the legs toward the heart. It begins at the confluence of the two common iliac veins at the level of the fifth lumbar vertebra and continues superiorly to the right atrium.[6,7]

INTERNET ACTIVITIES

Visit the University of North Carolina School of Medicine Web site at http://oisvideo2.med. unc.edu/ga/gaabcontent.ram and view the video on the anatomy of the abdominal cavity. This 25-minute video will play on your computer screen. You must have the RealPlayer media applicaton installed on your computer. If you do not have this program, it is available free of charge at http://www.real.com.

PATHOPHYSIOLOGY

Several factors play into the mortality rates reported in the literature. First, the length of time from injury to definitive trauma care certainly has a large impact on mortality and morbidity. The quality of delivered prehospital care has not been well studied, but the available data suggest that minimizing prehospital response,

scene, and transport times provide the patient with an optimal chance of surviving.[8–11] Second, it is important to deliver a patient to a trauma facility prepared and staffed to cope with the severity of the patient's injuries. Another factor in the morbidity of patients with abdominal trauma is that it rarely occurs as an injury to a single organ system.[12] These patients typically have multisystem or multiorgan injuries. The more systems or organs involved, the greater the mortality rate.

In blunt trauma, the spleen (20%–25%), liver (20%–29%), and intestines (large bowel 15% and small bowel 10%) are the most frequently injured abdominal organs.[12] All the other abdominal organs together account for the remaining 30%. Shoemaker reviewed 867 consecutive admissions to a level I trauma center and found massive hemorrhage with exsanguination in 11% of all patients admitted with blunt abdominal injury.[13] This 11% incidence of exsanguinating hemorrhage can be explained by the fact that the highly vascularized liver and spleen are the most frequently injured organs.

Penetrating trauma, with a mortality rate of less than 5%, typically affects the hollow abdominal organs as they take up the largest space within the abdominal cavity. In gunshot wounds, the small bowel, mesentery, liver, colon, and diaphragm are the most frequently injured organs. In stab wounds, the liver (being the largest organ), colon, small bowel, and stomach are most commonly injured. Feliciano studied 341 consecutive abdominal gunshot wound victims and found survival to range from 99% for those with single organ injury to 0% for those with eight or more injured organs.[14]

The liver is the largest solid organ in the abdomen and as such is highly vulnerable in both blunt and penetrating trauma. The vascular structure of the liver allows for profound hemorrhage when injured. Up to 60% of patients with liver injury are unstable at presentation to the emergency department and 45% have associated splenic injury.[15] The right lobe is injured more frequently and more severely than the left due to its relatively unprotected location.[15] In Kansas City, 16% of patients presenting to level I or II trauma centers with liver injury died, and approximately 25% of liver injury patients were in shock at the time of arrival to the hospital.[16] Overall, the reported mortality for liver injury is approximately 10%; but when considering blunt trauma as a distinct category, mortality from liver injury is 25%.[17] The mechanism of injury typically involves either direct compression of the liver itself with tearing or hematoma formation or avulsion injuries secondary to deceleration forces. Liver injuries are graded on a scale from I to VI.[18] Grade I and II injuries are subcapsular, nonexpanding hematomas involving less than 50% of the liver surface area or small lacerations. These are considered minor injuries and account for approximately 80%–90% of all liver injuries.[17] Grades III to VI are considered major life-threatening injuries and involve injuries ranging from large hematoma or laceration to complete avulsion of the liver from its vascular attachments.

The gallbladder and its associated ducts are injured in approximately 5% of all patients with abdominal trauma.[19,20] Of patients with biliary trauma, the gallbladder (80%) is much more frequently injured than the bile duct (30%). Injuries to the gallbladder and bile duct are almost never isolated injuries. In fact, in a study of blunt gallbladder injuries, all 22 cases studied occurred in the setting of other abdominal trauma.[21] Predisposing factors associated with gallbladder injury are (1) thin-walled normal gallbladder, (2) distended gallbladder, and (3) alcohol ingestion.[21] Although the association of alcohol ingestion and gallbladder injury is not immediately obvious, it is reported to be due to increased production and flow of bile with heightened ductal sphincter tone resulting in increased pressure in the biliary tract.[21] The nature of injury varies from simple contusion to complete avulsion. The most common injury is perforation or blow-out secondary to compressive forces.

The spleen is the most commonly injured abdominal organ in blunt trauma, with approximately 70% of all spleen injuries being due to a blunt mechanism.[22] Mortality from splenic injury is extremely low when the injury occurs as an isolated event. However, isolated splenic injury accounts for only 20% of all spleen injuries. As with other abdominal organs, splenic trauma is typically associated with other abdominal injuries, usually the kidney, liver, diaphragm, and major blood vessels. Mortality in the setting of associated injuries is reported to be as high as 8%–10%.[23] Injuries to the spleen are graded on the Organ Injury Scale accepted by the American Association for the Surgery of Trauma, or AAST (Table 14-1). Grade I and II injuries are small hematomas or simple lacerations. Grade III injuries involve large, expanding hematomas or deep lacerations. Grade IV injuries are lacerations involving the hilar blood vessels with resulting deprivation of blood to the spleen and major blood loss. A completely shattered spleen is a grade V injury, and a grade VI injury involves a hilar vascular disruption that completely devascularizes the spleen.[18]

Injury to the pancreas is uncommon, with a reported incidence between 2% and 12%.[24] Penetrating trauma is more frequently the cause of injury (60%). Because of its retroperitoneal location and close proximity to other abdominal organs, pancreatic injury is commonly associated (40%) with injuries to the liver, spleen, and major blood vessels.[25] The high rate of associated injuries combined with the isolated location of the pancreas in the retroperitoneum often leads to a missed or delayed diagnosis in pancreatic injury. Mortality rates for pancreatic trauma are high: up to 50% in blunt trauma, 25% for gunshot wounds, and 8% for stab wounds.[3] This includes those patients diagnosed at the time of injury as well as those presenting later after delayed diagnosis. Grades I and II injuries are those with minor hematomas or small lacerations. Grades III, IV, and V injuries are considered high-grade wounds and include injuries from major lacerations through complete disruption.

Isolated stomach injury is an exceedingly rare event, occurring in less than 2% of blunt injuries.[26] The typical mechanism of blunt injury is direct compression of a distended stomach (by food or air) with rupture of the contents into the abdominal cavity. The greater curvature of the stomach is the most common site of rupture.[27] Penetrating trauma is a far more common cause of gastric injury, accounting for 19% of all abdominal penetrating injuries.

The small intestine is most frequently injured in penetrating trauma (77%), probably because of its extensive surface area. In addition, it is not at all uncommon for the small intestine to be contused or ruptured in blunt trauma (particularly motor vehicle crashes) when it is pressed against the spinal column. In discussions of trauma to the small intestine, the duodenum is customarily discussed separately from the remainder of the small intestine as it is a retroperitoneal structure and the management varies slightly.

The duodenum is well protected, and injuries to this structure, by best estimates, occur in only 3.7%–5% of all patients with abdominal trauma.[28] Blunt injury mechanisms that lend themselves to duodenal injury are steering wheel or bike handlebar injuries, direct blows to the midabdomen, and deceleration injuries, as in falls from great height. Because of its close association with other organs, duodenal injuries rarely occur in isolation. The liver (17%), pancreas (12%), small intestine (12%), and colon (11%) are the organs most commonly associated with duodenal injury either by blunt or penetrating mechanism.[28] Grades I and II duodenal injuries encompass hematomas or lacerations involving less than 50% of the duodenal wall. Grade III injuries involve more than 50%–75% of the wall, and grade IV injuries encompass the entire wall, involve the pancreatic or bile ducts, or affect the blood supply to the duodenum. Grade V injuries involve either massive disruption of the duodenum or devascularization. These injuries usually require pancreaticoduodenectomy.[29]

The remainder of the small bowel (jejunum and ileum) is usually injured during penetrating trauma. The incidence of intestinal injury from penetrating trauma is 80%.[30] In blunt trauma, the most common sites of injury are the terminal ileum and proximal

Table 14-1
Grades of Splenic Injury

Grade*	Injury description	ICD-9	AIS 85	AIS 90
1. Hematoma	Subcapsular, nonexpanding, <10% surface area	865.11	2	2
Laceration	Capsular tear, nonbleeding, <1 cm parenchymal depth			
2. Hematoma	Subcapsular, nonexpanding, 10–50% surface area	865.11	2	2
	Intraparenchymal, nonexpanding, <2 cm in diameter			
Laceration	Capsular tear, active bleeding	865.12	2	2
3. Hematoma	Subcapsular, >50% surface area, or expanding	865.12	3	3
	Ruptured subcapsular hematoma, active bleeding			
	Intraparenchymal hematoma, >2 cm or expanding			
Laceration	>3 cm parenchymal depth or involving trabecular vessels	865.13	3	3
4. Hematoma	Ruptured intraparenchymal hematoma with active bleeding	865.13	3	4
Laceration	Laceration involving segmental or hilar vessels producing major devascularization (>25% of spleen)	865.13	3	4
5. Laceration	Completely shattered spleen	865.14	5	5
Vascular	Hilar vascular injury that devascularizes spleen	865.14	5	5

Abbreviations: ICD-9 = *International Classification of Diseases,* 9th edition; AIS 85 = Abbreviated Injury Scale, 1985; AIS 90 = Abbreviated Injury Scale, 1990.

*Advance one grade for multiple injuries to the same organ.

†Based on most accurate assessment at autopsy, laparotomy, or radiologic study.

jejunum. The same mechanisms of injury discussed above for the duodenum apply to the remainder of the small bowel as well. One additional injury that bears mentioning is bowel evisceration. This is a relatively rare event that is manifested by the extrusion of bowel content, typically the small bowel, through a laceration or tear in the abdominal wall to the exterior of the body.

The large intestine and rectum account for 5% of all abdominal injuries. There is a relatively high mortality, 2%–12%, and very high morbidity rate associated with large bowel injuries secondary to subsequent fecal contamination of the peritoneal cavity and resulting sepsis.[31] Almost 96% of all large bowel and rectal injuries are caused by penetrating trauma.[25] Other mechanisms of injury include impalement after falls, rectal perforation from placement of foreign objects in the rectal vault, and rectal laceration from bone shards in complex pelvic fractures. The transverse colon is the most commonly disrupted segment in both penetrating and blunt trauma. Colon and rectal injuries occur as an isolated event only 10%–25% of the time.

Abdominal vascular injuries are catastrophic events with a very high associated mortality rate, 30%–60%. Until recently, few of these patients actually arrived in the emergency department. As out-of-hospital care and access has improved, more of these patients are surviving to reach definitive care. The large majority of abdominal vascular injuries are from penetrating trauma. Approximately 15% of all patients with penetrating abdominal trauma admitted to a Houston hospital had an abdominal vascular injury.[14] Blunt trauma can cause various injuries, including simple contusion, intimal disruption, intramural hematoma, false aneurysm, dissection, or actual rupture.[32] The mortality associated with specific vasculature injury include: aorta, 50%–70%; iliac artery, 40%–53%; inferior vena cava, 30%–53%; portal and splenic veins, 40%–70%; and iliac vein, 38%.[25] Arterial injury may actually stop bleeding spontaneously as a result of the highly elastic nature of arterial vessels. The vessels curl inward and occlude the lumen of the artery, thereby obstructing continued hemorrhage. On the other hand, venous bleeding is frequently difficult to stop, particularly when the bleeding vessel is emptying directly into an open cavity such as the abdomen.

ASSESSMENT

The physical examination of blunt abdominal trauma patients is notoriously unreliable, with the examination accuracy reported to be as low as 65%.[33–35] Before the advent of the computerized tomography (CT) scanner and other diagnostic modalities currently in use, approximately 17% of persons with abdominal trauma died as a result of unrecognized hemorrhage.[36] It is, therefore, essential that the paramedic maintain a high index of suspicion when assessing high-risk individuals, such as those involved in high-speed motor vehicle collisions (MVCs), ejected from vehicles, or falling from heights greater than 15 feet or pedestrians struck by vehicles.[12,37] Persons with major chest trauma, pelvic fracture, or a history of hypotension in the field have an increased likelihood of intra-abdominal injury.[34]

Prehospital assessment of the trauma patient should include a rapid history and physical examination conducted in the most efficient and time-conscious

manner possible. It is important for the paramedic to investigate and factually report the details of the incident. In the event of an MVC, emergency department personnel need to know about ejection from the vehicle, use of restraint devices (seat belts, air bags), steering wheel or windshield damage, and patient position within the vehicle. Additionally, it is important to note the approximate speed of the vehicle(s) as well as direction and location of the impact. Patterns of injury can be suspected based on this information. For instance, lateral impact crashes are positively associated with abdominal injury. Drivers and front-seat passengers are more likely than other occupants to sustain abdominal injury.[38] Dashboard intrusion is associated with pelvic and femur fractures, closed head injuries, and intra-abdominal injuries.[39] While unrestrained occupants in an MVC are most likely to sustain liver and spleen laceration or rupture, occupants in either two- or, less commonly, three-point restraints are more likely to suffer hollow viscus injury (small or large bowel tears or perforations) or abdominal wall disruptions. In fact, the classic seat belt pattern of injury for two-point restraint devices is hollow viscus injury, flexion-distraction fractures of the lumbar spine, and abdominal wall disruptions.[40]

For penetrating trauma, it is important to note the caliber of the weapon, the estimated distance of the shooter from the victim, and the location of the wounds. Remember that penetrating trauma (gunshot or stabbings) to the lower chest is frequently associated with abdominal injury.[41] Eighty percent to 85% of gunshot wounds to the anterior abdomen violate the peritoneum and, of these, up to 98% require surgical intervention.[42,43] With stab wounds, it may be helpful to determine the size and length of the offending weapon. Stab wounds to the anterior abdomen violate the peritoneum 50%–70% of the time, and of these only half require surgical investigation.[42,43] Finally, falls from a height greater than 20 feet are associated with surgically significant abdominal injury about 3% of the time.[12] It is also important to note the position of the patient upon landing and the potential for spinal injury.

Once an adequate history has been established, including past medical history, current medications, and allergies, the paramedic can focus on the physical examination. Keep in mind that the entire history and physical examination should take less than 10 minutes in the setting of trauma and should occur concurrently with rapid movement of the patient to the ambulance. Attention should always first be directed to the airway, breathing, and circulation of the patient. Once these are taken care of, the abdomen should be fully exposed and inspected for visible wounds. The seat belt sign, which is positively correlated with abdominal injury, consists of skin abrasions and bruising of the abdomen, chest, or neck in the distribution of the restraint.[40] Wounds associated with penetrating trauma should be noted for exactly what they are: wounds. It is not possible in the prehospital setting to make an accurate determination of whether a wound was the entrance or exit site, and this information has no bearing on whether a patient needs to be treated or not. Sometimes, it is extremely difficult for a forensic pathologist to make this determination.

During the physical examination, it is relatively easy to inspect the anterior abdomen. The patient's back is frequently more difficult to inspect but is no less important. Many prehospital providers have missed a source of unrecognized hemorrhage, a bullet wound in the back.

After inspection, the abdomen should be auscultated quickly to assess whether bowel sounds are present. Each of the four quadrants of the abdomen should be gently palpated, looking for focal tenderness, guarding, or rebound. Focal tenderness in the left upper quadrant should raise suspicion about a splenic injury, just as right upper quadrant tenderness should peak concern about a liver injury. Lower rib border tenderness suggestive of rib fractures should also clue the provider into possible splenic or liver injury depending on which ribs are tender. In patients with left lower rib fractures, 20% will have splenic injury, and conversely, in patients with right lower rib fractures, 10% will have hepatic injury.[2,44] Guarding and rebound are subjective findings that, if present, should be conveyed to the trauma team, but these findings do not change field patient management. Other physical findings that may point to an abdominal injury are (1) loss of palpable pulses in the lower extremities indicating arterial disruption perhaps at the level of the descending abdominal aorta and (2) Kehr's sign, which is pain (not tenderness) in the left shoulder secondary to diaphragmatic irritation, usually due to blood from a splenic rupture.

Research has shown that the most common physical finding in blunt abdominal trauma is abdominal tenderness and guarding (75%).[35] Rebound and rigidity are present only 28% of the time. A large percentage may have no specific complaint or any evidence of an abnormal exam when first evaluated, and nearly 15% of these patients may reveal intra-abdominal injury upon later exploratory surgery. The initial physical examination is unreliable and merely serves as a baseline against which repeated examinations are compared.

In the emergency department, the trauma team reassesses the patient's airway, breathing, and circulation. They also repeat the abdominal examination. It is important for the paramedic to share the findings of the initial examination so that the team can compare the current findings to those from the prehospital arena. Beyond the prehospital evaluation, a rectal and perineal examination will be performed looking for evidence of injury or blood.

In addition to the physical examination, a set of routine blood work will be drawn. The hemoglobin and hematocrit are very helpful in determining ongoing blood loss and serve as a baseline against which to compare later measurements. It is extremely rare for a low hemoglobin or hematocrit to represent pretrauma anemia. Commonly, the white blood cell count will be elevated following trauma but is a nonspecific finding. Baseline measurements of the patient's renal and liver functions can be helpful. Abdominal radiographs are not helpful in blunt trauma and are used in penetrating trauma only to localize the projectile. Chest radiographs may demonstrate free air under the diaphragm suggesting bowel perforation, or rib fractures of the lower rib border suggestive of liver or spleen injury. The patient's blood will also be typed and crossmatched with available blood in the blood bank.

Patients with (1) a history not suggestive of abdominal trauma, (2) a negative abdominal physical examination, (3) normal vital signs, and (4) normal blood work usually do not undergo testing other than serial abdominal physical examinations. The notable exception to this pathway is patients who require prolonged anesthesia to repair other injuries. In this group, reliable serial abdominal examinations are not possible, and for that reason, most surgeons prefer further preoperative diagnostic testing rather than risk an intra-operative disaster.[45] Patients with obvious blunt abdominal trauma and unstable vitals signs, evisceration, or gunshot wounds to the anterior abdomen will go directly to the operating room for definitive management.

The large majority of abdominal trauma patients fall between the two extremes of no suspected injury and overtly obvious injury requiring emergent operative intervention. These patients cause the greatest anxiety in trauma surgeons. There are many available methods of searching for serious abdominal injury, and the challenge is to find the right test for the right patient. Patients with unstable vital signs from an undetected source cannot be taken safely to the radiology department for advanced imaging.

In 1965, Root developed the **diagnostic peritoneal lavage (DPL)**, a minimally invasive surgical technique for detecting abdominal trauma in the trauma bay.[46] After placement of a nasogastric tube and a Foley, the procedure involves making a small incision in the abdominal wall and penetrating the peritoneum with a small catheter (Figure 14-7). An attempt is made to withdraw fluid from the catheter. Removal of 10 mL of gross blood is considered a positive test. If there is no free blood, then 1 liter of warmed normal saline is infused into the peritoneal cavity, allowed to diffuse, and then removed by lowering the infusing bag to the floor and allowing the fluid to siphon off. The siphoned fluid is sent to the laboratory for analysis. A test is considered

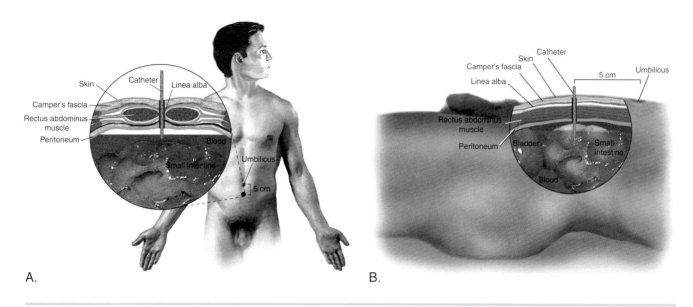

A.

B.

FIGURE 14-7 Diagnostic peritoneal lavage (DPL).

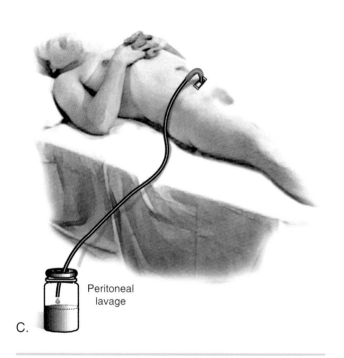

Peritoneal lavage

C.

FIGURE 14-7 Diagnostic peritoneal lavage (DPL).

positive if any of the following are present: (1) greater than 100,000/mm³ red blood cells (RBCs) for blunt trauma or 5,000/mm³ RBC for gunshot wounds, (2) greater than 500/mm³ white blood cells (WBCs), (3) greater than or equal to 20 IU/L amylase and 3 IU/L alkaline phosphatase, (4) any bile, or (5) gross contamination with fecal or digested food products.[42] The drainage of the infused fluid into the Foley, nasogastric tube, or a chest tube is also considered a positive test.

Diagnostic peritoneal lavage has a reported 93% accuracy rate and a complication rate of less than 1%.[4,47] In patients with unstable vital signs but no identified source of bleeding, surgeons are able to make a quick (5–10-minutes) determination of whether intra-abdominal bleeding is the cause. DPL is also useful in patients with an equivocal abdominal examination or no abdominal findings who will be undergoing prolonged anesthesia for other injuries. DPL is fast and relatively inexpensive and requires little training or expertise. The disadvantages of DPL are that it does not provide specific information about which organ system is injured, it is invasive with associated complications, it provides information about past bleeding but not about ongoing hemorrhage, and it is unable to detect hemorrhage in the retroperitoneal space.

Computed tomography has, in some situations, replaced DPL as the diagnostic test of choice for stable trauma patients with findings on abdominal physical examination or for those patients in whom a physical examination is confused by altered sensorium due to head injury or intoxicating substances. CT scans of the abdomen have an accuracy rate of 92% and a very low complication rate.[47] The abdominal CT has undergone recent advances that allow it to be completed in under 5 minutes in hospitals equipped with helical or spiral scanning techniques. There are many advantages to using CT scanning for the abdominal trauma patient, including (1) the ability to detect retroperitoneal injury or bleeding, (2) the ability to stage and nonoperatively manage some solid organ injuries, (3) the ability to examine other areas of the body during the same scanning session, (4) the ability to examine the vascular structures closely with intravenous contrast, and (5) its speed and repeatability. The disadvantages are that (1) the machinery is rarely located in the emergency department, which requires that the patient be transported and moved to the scanning table; (2) it is expensive; (3) a select number of patients are allergic to the intravenous contrast dye necessary for the scan; (4) small diaphragmatic, pancreatic, urinary bladder, or bowel injuries can be missed; and (5) a trained radiologist must be available to read the scan.[12,15]

Ultrasound may be the screening study of choice for abdominal trauma in the near future. It is commonly used in Europe for trauma victims to detect free peritoneal fluid or solid organ injury. It has an accuracy rate of 96% in detecting free fluid within the peritoneal cavity, which should prompt further investigation. The only disadvantages are that it is not helpful for hollow organ injury or for retroperitoneal hemorrhage. Advantages of ultrasonography are that it is (1) noninvasive, (2) very fast (less than 3 minutes), (3) done at the bedside, (4) without contraindications or complications, (5) repeatable, (6) inexpensive, and (7) suitable for both stable and unstable patients.[12,48] At present, it is used only in blunt trauma, as most penetrating trauma victims go quickly to the operating room without further imaging or testing.

The assessment of the abdominal trauma patient is grounded in ongoing and repeated examinations with multiple diagnostic modalities. Despite the best efforts of trauma surgeons, between 10% and 34% of trauma patients will have an injury that is missed in the initial evaluation phase.[49] This is typically due to more painful injuries masking less painful ones, substance abuse, head injury, or intubation. The importance of repeated physical examination cannot be emphasized enough.

INTERNET ACTIVITIES

Visit the University of North Carolina School of Medicine Web site at http://oisvideo2.med. unc.edu/mpac/allabdomen.ram and view the video on abdominal examination. This 16-minute video will play on your computer screen. You must have the RealPlayer media application installed on your computer. If you do not have this program, it is available free of charge at http://www.real.com.

MANAGEMENT

With the previously mentioned unreliability of the physical examination in abdominal trauma, coupled with the large number of highly vascular and vulnerable organs within the abdominal cavity, it is easy to see why abdominal trauma is such an occult source of

unrecognized hemorrhage. The task of the paramedic is to minimize the patient's time to definitive care, to provide the trauma service with the most complete physical assessment and scene description possible, and to provide state-of-the-art treatment during transport. There is no crime in failing to localize the source of hemorrhage; *the critical failure lies in failing to recognize and treat shock from occult bleeding.*

Rapid transport is the second most important intervention paramedics have to offer the trauma patient, the first being airway control. The prehospital trauma life support course emphasizes a maximum 10-minute scene time for nonentrapped victims of trauma.[50] Some systems are entertaining the idea of allowing nonmedical personnel, such as police officers, to rapidly transport trauma patients, particularly those with penetrating trauma, to the hospital. In a retrospective study from Philadelphia, assaulted patients transported via police did as well as those transported by EMS personnel.[51] Researchers in Los Angeles retrospectively reviewed trauma patients transported by private vehicle versus those transported by EMS. They found that patients brought to the emergency department by private vehicle arrived approximately 30 minutes sooner than patients brought by EMS and that those patients with severe trauma had a higher likelihood of survival if transported by private vehicle.[52] The reasons for this are fairly obvious. It takes time for the public to access the EMS system, for the EMS personnel to be dispatched and then to travel to the scene. The limited time most EMS personnel spend on the scene pales in comparison to the large amounts of time involved in actually getting to the scene. It is estimated that for every 10 minutes of delay in reaching definitive treatment, survival for critically injured trauma patients drops by 10%.[53] Several studies have demonstrated that extending prehospital time contributes to increased trauma mortality.[8,10,11,54–56]

In the past, military antishock trousers (MASTs) have been used indiscriminately to treat hypotension in trauma patients. More recently, some bold researchers have completed a series of well-conducted trials carefully examining the outcomes of trauma patients treated with and without MASTs.[57–59] They have demonstrated fairly conclusively that MASTs provide no improvement in survival, length of hospital stay, or hospital costs for trauma patients with blood pressures less than 90 mm Hg. There is a very small (0.02%) subset of hypotensive trauma patients with systolic blood pressures less than 50 mm Hg for whom MASTs may provide a small improvement in survival. It is thought that for this subset, rapid transport to a hospital for definitive surgical intervention provides the same level of improvement. Kenneth Mattox has said clearly that "these data support (in the urban setting) that a conscious patient with detectable hypotension should be transported with optimal oxygen provided and nothing to alter the blood pressure. In the patient in the urban scene with CNS (central nervous system) activity with no detectable blood pressure, we should optimize oxygen delivery and do something to elevate the blood pressure, but that something should not be MAST."[57]

Another prehospital management cornerstone undergoing reevaluation is the infusion of large amounts of intravenous fluids. Animal studies of uncontrolled hemorrhage have demonstrated increased mortality in those undergoing rapid intravenous resuscitation.[60,61] It is thought that rapid administration of intravenous fluids disrupts clot formation, increases bleeding, and, therefore, decreases survival. Additionally, there is evidence that infused intravenous fluid dilutes essential clotting factors and lowers blood viscosity, which then decreases the resistance to flow around a partially formed clot.[62]

In Houston, William Bickell performed a prospective trial of delayed fluid resuscitation for hypotensive victims of penetrating torso trauma (chest and abdomen) in an urban setting.[62] Patients were assigned to either the immediate fluid resuscitation or delayed resuscitation group on an alternating day basis. Immediate resuscitation meant that patients received a continuous infusion of intravenous fluid trying to keep systolic blood pressure in the 100 mm Hg range. Delayed resuscitation meant that patients had an intravenous catheter placed but received no fluid. Bickell found that those patients who received no fluid had a statistically better survival rate than did those receiving more traditional resuscitation. He concluded that "aggressive administration of intravenous fluids to hypotensive patients with penetrating injuries to the torso should be delayed until the time of operative intervention."[62] Other investigators have reached similar conclusions.[10,63,64] It is important to note that Bickell's study may not be generalizable to rural trauma, blunt trauma, or hypotension from injuries to body areas other than torso. More research is needed to determine the effect of intravenous fluid in these settings.

Evisceration is an uncommon injury but quite dramatic. The paramedic should cover the exposed bowel with a moistened, nonadherent, sterile dressing and minimize manipulation. Once in the emergency department, the patient will require operative repair of the abdominal wall defect and surgical repair of any torn or devascularized bowel. Impaled objects should be stabilized in the field but not removed. There are very rare occasions when the impaled object is firmly fixed to an external object or to the ground. These objects may need to be cut to free the victim. However,

it is best to seek the advice of medical control in those special cases as hospital personnel may need to respond to the scene to assist in advanced surgical interventions.

The hospital management of abdominal trauma has changed somewhat over the years as newer and more organ-specific diagnostic modalities have evolved. There are some situations where operative management is standard. Most patients with penetrating abdominal trauma will be explored in the operating room. The high incidence of multiorgan injury and the large number of bowel injuries usually preclude "watchful waiting" in this group of patients. Unstable trauma patients with positive DPL findings are also taken to the operating room without delay, as are patients with evisceration or impaled objects. Patients not falling into one of the above-mentioned categories, though, may not require urgent operative intervention.

Hemodynamically stable patients with blunt liver injury may, at the discretion of the surgeon, be managed nonoperatively. In a study of 184 patients with blunt hepatic injury from the Elvis Presley Regional Trauma Center in Memphis, 100 patients with liver injuries (inclusive of grades I–V) were assigned to the nonoperative group.[65] Only 12 of these patients went on to require operative management. There is a growing movement to manage as many hepatic injuries as possible in a nonoperative fashion. The criteria for nonoperative management, at present, is (1) hemodynamic stability, (2) absence of peritoneal signs, (3) neurological integrity, (4) CT scan delineation of injury, (5) absence of associated intra-abdominal injuries, (6) need for no more than two hepatic related blood transfusions, and (7) CT scan documented improvement or stabilization with time.[65] The overall success rate for nonoperative management is reported to be 94%.[66]

Approximately 10%–30% of patients with liver injury will have severe damage with ongoing hemorrhage and unstable vital signs. These injuries are very difficult to control in the operating room. The liver is an essential organ, one we cannot live without. Surgical techniques for dealing with severe injuries include omental packing, mesh wrapping, hepatic artery ligation, hepatic resection, atriocaval shunting, gauze packing, fibrin glue, or hepatic transplantation.[17,65] Patients with liver injuries of this magnitude require massive blood transfusions in the operative and immediate postoperative period. They are usually critically ill with poor outcomes. However, patients with successfully repaired liver injuries or those managed nonoperatively typically do very well once they survive the immediate posttrauma or surgery period. The liver regenerates itself and there is little long-term consequence to liver trauma.

Injuries to the gallbladder are commonly missed on initial examination. Good screening tests that specifically look for gallbladder injury do not exist. If the patient requires operative management for other injury, the gallbladder injury will probably be discovered. There is an average of 2.5–3.3 abdominal injuries in each patient with gallbladder injury, so operative management is likely.[21,67] If, however, gallbladder injury is not suspected and the patient is managed nonoperatively, there is a reported delay of 1–6 weeks before the injury is discovered. Normal, uninfected bile is not irritative enough to the peritoneum to produce findings on physical examination. Patients with a delayed or missed diagnosis present with fever, jaundice, nausea, vomiting, anorexia, light-colored stools and dark urine, or weight loss.[68,69]

The gallbladder is a nonessential organ and, in the event of injury, can simply be removed without consequence.[68] The more challenging injury is one to the bile duct, which is an essential element of the liver drainage system. If there is a partial tear of the duct, it may be repaired. Those injuries, though, that involve total disruption of the duct require a more creative approach. The surgeon may "patch" the disruption using portions of the gallbladder or may elect to perform a Roux-en-Y procedure, which rearranges the way the duct attaches to the duodenum to bypass the disrupted segment.[21,68,69] Occasionally, patients with repaired ductal systems experience duct stricture, duct leakage, or abscess formation postoperatively.

Over the last two decades, the management of traumatic splenic injury has evolved along with the evolution in radiological imaging techniques. In other words, we are now better able to keep an eye on what is happening with the spleen. As a result, surgeons have begun to consider a larger number of patients for nonoperative management of splenic injury. The generally accepted criteria for this approach is patients who are (1) hemodynamically stable, requiring fewer than three transfusions; (2) alert; (3) without peritoneal signs; and (4) with CT scan documentation of grades I–III splenic injury.[70] Approximately 30% of splenic injuries fall into this management strategy.[71] Reported failures of this strategy are in the range of 10%–20%.[71,72]

There is another group of patients with traumatic splenic injury (both blunt and penetrating) who are managed with surgical repair of the injured organ. This group comprises approximately 10%–66% of the spleen-injured population. The widely varying rate reflects surgeons' attempts to adjust to the changing management strategies for splenic injury. **Splenorrhaphy**, surgical repair of the spleen, has a complication rate, mostly rebleeding, of 1.7%–12%.[73,74] Techniques for surgical repair of the injured spleen include direct suturing of the splenic laceration, omental wrapping, splenic artery ligation, and partial

splenectomy.[70,71,75] Finally, in those patients who are hemodynamically unstable, have a large number of associated injuries, have extensive injuries involving the splenic hilum, or have massive splenic parenchymal destruction, the procedure of choice is splenectomy. Removal of the spleen is usually accomplished without untoward sequelae. There are a small number of patients (0.5%–2%) who will, after splenectomy, have overwhelming postsplenectomy infection (OPSI). OPSI carries a mortality rate as high as 50%–90%.[70,71,76] Because the spleen assists WBCs in fighting infection and ridding the body of invading organisms, its loss exposes the body to an infection risk. Most patients are able to continue the fight against infection despite the loss of the spleen, but there is a small group who succumb.

The pancreas is an essential organ and, fortunately, is well protected in the retroperitoneum. CT scanning detects most pancreatic injuries but not all. Some of these missed injuries are discovered during exploratory surgery for other injuries. Some are missed and present several days later with pain, nausea, vomiting, peritoneal signs, sepsis, or hypotension from bleeding. Once discovered, the current surgical dogma is to explore and repair pancreatic injuries. There is a small but growing body of literature proposing nonoperative management of low-grade pancreatic injuries, particularly in children.[77] Surgical repair of the injured pancreas can include simple drainage of the pancreas bed, simple resection, distal pancreatectomy, simple repair, or Roux-en-Y pancreaticojejunostomy. Complications of pancreatic injury are pancreatic pseudocyst (5%–10%), pancreatic fistula (12%–19%), abscess (10%–30%), pancreatitis (10%), and pancreatic necrosis (2%–5%).[77–79]

Gastric injuries are typically discovered upon recovery of blood following placement of a nasogastric tube or upon discovery of free air on either a chest or abdominal radiograph. These stomach wounds are repaired primarily in a two-layer closure during surgery. Because the stomach has an excellent blood supply, has relatively sterile contents, and lends itself to fairly easy detection of injury, there is little long-term consequence to gastric injury.[25] Complication of stomach rupture includes abdominal abscess, gastric fistula, sepsis, and wound infections.[27]

Though short, the duodenum causes the majority of the complicated small bowel injuries. It has several points of attachment that must be considered when planning a repair. The pylorus above and ileum below serve as the entrance and exit of material in the duodenum. In addition, the pancreatic and bile ducts link up with the second portion of the duodenum and can complicate a repair attempt. The most common injuries (60%–85%) are simple lacerations that can be repaired directly with two suture layers.[28,80] Intramural duodenal hematomas are associated with blunt trauma and are difficult to detect on initial presentation. A hematoma forms in the bowel wall that may be large enough to cause a narrowing of the lumen of the bowel. Patients present with epigastric or right upper quadrant pain, fever, nausea, and vomiting. These injuries are treated with bowel rest, nasogastric tube drainage, and watchful waiting for at least 2 weeks. The majority of duodenal hematomas resolve in this time period. For those that do not resolve, surgeons intervene and make a small incision in the bowel wall and drain the hematoma.

More complex injuries, such as devascularized tissue, tissue loss, or extensive destruction of tissue, require a creative repair approach. Keeping in mind the ductal system that needs to exit into the bowel, surgeons have repaired complex duodenal injury with the following techniques: (1) resection and primary anastomosis, (2) covering a large defect with a serosal patch using a loop of jejunum, (3) various diverting procedures (pyloric exclusion, tube duodenostomy, duodenal diverticulization, duodenojejunostomy), or (4) pacreaticoduodenectomy for a very small number of patients with extensive destruction and tissue loss.[79–81] Morbidity rates range from 38% to 125% (some patients had more than one complication) with average figures of 64%.[28] Complications associated with duodenal injury include duodenal fistula (2%–16%), duodenal obstruction (5%–8%), abscess (11%–18%), recurrent pancreatitis (2%–15%), and bile duct fistula (1%).[79–81] Duodenal fistula has a 2% mortality rate.[80]

Injuries to the jejunum and ileum are usually repaired with simple debridement and end-to-end anastomosis. Small lacerations or perforations are sutured. Rarely, a patient will require resection with diverting ileostomy. Complications associated with jejunal and ileal injury are breakdown of the surgical repair, abscess formation, and wound infection. There is a higher incidence of fecal contamination with colonic injury, thereby necessitating a diverting procedure more frequently.[82] With small perforations or lacerations, surgeons attempt to suture the defect. Other repair strategies include resection and end-to-end anastomosis and closure and proximal colostomy. Rectal perforation requires copious irrigation and debridement. Primary repair with a diverting procedure is the repair of choice for rectal perforation as the incidence of fecal contamination and the resulting infection rate is very high. Complications include wound infection, abscess formation, colonic obstruction, colocutaneous fistula, and bowel ischemia.[25]

The aorta is well protected and infrequently injured. However, when injury does occur, it has catastrophic implications. Surgical repair is undertaken as soon as the injury is identified. Surgical techniques include primary suturing, lateral repair, patch aortoplasty, end-to-end anastomosis, and insertion of an artificial conduit such as gortex grafting.[32,83] Careful attention must be paid to the numerous arterial branches exiting the aorta. Vena caval injuries are uncommon as well but can be equally catastrophic. These injuries must be promptly recognized and surgically repaired; techniques employed include direct sutured repair (most common), complete ligation for devastating infrarenal injuries, and atriocaval or ballooncaval shunts for devastating retrohepatic injuries.[84] Complications of vascular repairs include arteriovenous fistula, traumatic false aneurysm, graft failure, infection, thrombosis, and embolus.[32,83,84]

INTERNET ACTIVITIES

- Visit the e-medicine Web site at http://www.emedicine.com. Click on the Emergency Medicine on-line book and select Trauma and Orthopedics. Then click on Abdominal Trauma, Blunt. Review the chapter on the management of blunt abdominal trauma.
- Visit the e-medicine Web site at http://www.emedicine.com. Click on the Emergency Medicine on-line book and select Trauma and Orthopedics. Then click on Abdominal Trauma, Penetrating. Review the chapter on the management of penetrating abdominal trauma.

GENITOURINARY TRAUMA

EPIDEMIOLOGY

Of all patients with traumatic abdominal injuries, approximately 10%–15% have injuries to the genitourinary tract.[85] The organ most commonly injured in those with genitourinary trauma is the kidney (84%) followed by the bladder and urethra (8% each).[86] Other organs are rarely injured. Blunt trauma accounts for the majority of genitourinary injuries.

Genitourinary trauma rarely occurs as an isolated injury. It is most frequently found in association with pelvic fractures, lower rib fractures, gunshot wound (GSW) to the abdomen, and fractures of the lumbar transverse processes. In particular, injuries to the right kidney are associated with liver injury, and conversely, left kidney injuries are associated with splenic injuries, and both carry significant morbidity and mortality. Studies report from 6% to 12% mortality in renal trauma patients with associated abdominal injuries.[86,87]

Because of its occult nature and uncommon occurrence, genitourinary trauma is often overlooked. In the prehospital phase of the patient's care, there is little consequence to unrecognized genitourinary trauma. The uncompromising failure lies in not treating hypotension from an unrecognized source.

THE URINARY SYSTEM

ANATOMY AND PHYSIOLOGY

The **kidneys** are paired organs that lie in the retroperitoneal space on either side of the vertebral column between the twelfth thoracic and the third lumbar vertebrae (Figure 14-8). The typical size of an adult kidney is 11 cm long, 6 cm wide, and 3 cm thick. The left kidney is positioned slightly higher than the right. It is often extremely difficult, if not impossible, to palpate the kidneys during a physical examination.

Both kidneys are bounded by the psoas major muscle along the medial border and the transverse abdominus muscle along the lateral border. The upper half of the right kidney lies behind the liver, in contact with the diaphragm, and protected by the twelfth rib, while the lower half is covered by bowel. The upper portion of the left kidney, being slightly higher, is protected by the eleventh and twelfth ribs, is in contact with the diaphragm, and is covered by the stomach and spleen. The lower portion is covered by bowel. They

are each surrounded by a layer of fat and Gerota's fascia, which can contain and tamponade hemorrhage.

The kidneys are reddish brown, bean-shaped organs that have a long, smooth, convex lateral border and sharply indented medial border. The hilum is responsible for the deep indentation along the medial margin of the kidney and is composed of the renal vessels, lymphatics, and nerves that then enter the renal sinus. The renal pelvis, shaped like a funnel, also lies along the medial margin; it is comprised of the expanded upper end of the ureter. The renal parenchyma can be divided into the outer cortex and the inner medulla (Figure 14-9). The cortex consists of renal corpuscles and the convoluted portions of the renal tubules. The medulla contains the descending and ascending portions of the renal tubules and the collecting tubules.

The kidneys provide a complex system of waste product removal and electrolyte balance. The process includes filtration of blood, reabsorption of needed elements, and secretion of urine. The initial steps in urine formation occur in the cortex, where blood is filtered by the glomerular process. The final modification of urine occurs in the medulla, where the tubules complete the reabsorption process. Urine is secreted into the renal pelvis and from there into the ureters. Additionally, the kidneys secrete a variety of hormones, including angiotensin II, prostaglandins, and the kinins, which play a role in blood pressure control. Finally, the kidneys participate in the regulation of RBC synthesis through the formation of the hormone erythropoietin.

The ureters are also paired structures. As mentioned above, the renal pelvis, lying along the medial margin of the kidney, is comprised of the expanded upper end of the ureter. The ureter then courses out of the kidney and traverses the abdomen in a more or less vertical fashion to join the bladder. Each of the ureters functions as a conduit for urine from the kidney to the bladder.

The bladder is a hollow muscular reservoir for urine, lying behind the symphysis pubis. When empty, it is contained entirely within the bony pelvic ring. When full, however, it distends and rises into the abdominal cavity. In some persons, it may rise as high as the umbilicus.

The urethra is a hollow tube that passes urine from the bladder out of the body. It courses directly from the bladder to the urethral meatus and is shorter in women than men. As a result of this length difference, the urethra is more frequently injured in men than women. The female urethra is a simple tube running from the bladder neck to the meatus. It is tightly fused at its most external point to the anterior vaginal wall. It measures approximately 4 cm in length. The male urethra, on the other hand, is approximately 20

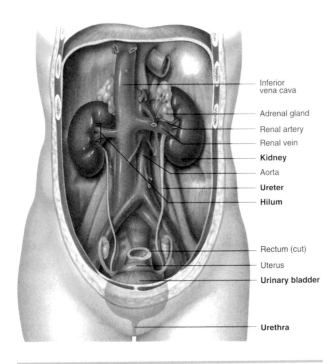

Inferior
vena cava

Adrenal gland

Renal artery

Renal vein

Kidney

Aorta

Ureter

Hilum

Rectum (cut)

Uterus

Urinary bladder

Urethra

FIGURE 14-8 Anatomy of the urinary system.

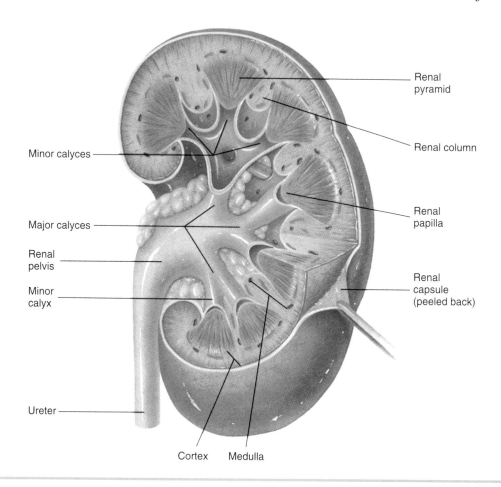

Minor calyces

Major calyces

Renal pelvis

Minor calyx

Ureter

Renal pyramid

Renal column

Renal papilla

Renal capsule (peeled back)

Cortex   Medulla

FIGURE 14-9 Coronal section of the right kidney.

cm in length and can be divided into several parts. The posterior urethra consists of the prostatic and membranous portions. The prostatic portion begins at the bladder neck and courses approximately 3 cm through the prostate itself. The membranous portion traverses the urogenital diaphragm and is approximately 2–2.5 cm in length. The anterior urethra consists of the bulbous and penile portions. The bulbous portion extends from the urogenital diaphragm to the base of the penis and the penile portion, as its name would suggest, courses the length of the penis.

PATHOPHYSIOLOGY

Renal injuries may be categorized based on the mechanism and degree of injury. The majority of renal injuries are caused by blunt trauma (80%–95%).[4,88] While the kidney is protected by the ribs for the most part, it is a very mobile organ, being attached only by the pedicle at the hilum. The pedicle consists of the renal artery, renal vein, and ureter. It is easy, therefore, to see how the kidney is frequently injured by acceleration-deceleration forces. The majority of renal injuries occur during

MVCs and motorcycle and pedestrian collisions, less commonly by falls and assaults.

Penetrating renal injuries are much less frequent than blunt injuries but result in a greater rate of renal loss following injury (39% vs. 5%).[89] Typically with penetrating injury, there are serious associated injuries that may cost the patient's life despite easy repair of the kidney itself. High-velocity wounds, such as those from hunting rifles, are nearly always associated with nephrectomy secondary to shattering of the kidney as the missile explodes through the organ. Low-velocity wounds cause damage to the affected kidney but usually result in salvage of the organ through operative repair. The larger the caliber of the bullet, the greater the destruction. Stab wounds are uncommonly associated with renal injury secondary to the protected location of the renal system. Deep stab wounds to the back or flank may penetrate the kidney but do not usually require operative intervention.

Renal injuries may be classified according to severity of injury. The classification of the Organ Injury Scaling Committee of the AAST is easy to use and correlates well with resulting patient condition (Figure 14-10).[90] Grade I includes simple contusions and subcapsular hematomas. Grade II is slightly larger hematomas that are nonexpanding and superficial lacerations through the capsule and into the parenchyma. These injuries affect the outer layers of the kidney and may result in the thrombosis of small veins and arteries. As a result, the cortex of the kidney may swell but bleeding is limited and there are usually no other associated abdominal injuries. Most renal injuries (85%–90%) fall into Grade I or II.[89,90]

Grade III injury indicates a laceration into the parenchyma of the kidney with collecting system disruption or urinary extravasation. Grade IV injury involves either a laceration extending through the cortex, medulla, and collecting systems or a major renal artery or vein injury with contained hemorrhage. These more serious injuries threaten the survival of the injured organ and may result in massive blood loss, thereby threatening the life of the patient. Con-

siderable force is required to cause this amount of damage, and thus there is frequently damage to other abdominal structures. Grade V injury results in a completely shattered kidney or avulsion of the renal hilum, causing devascularization. These patients sustain massive blood loss and are usually critically ill.[90]

Ureteral trauma is an uncommon entity. Most injuries to this structure occur as a result of penetrating injury, gunshot wounds more commonly than stab wounds. While gunshot wounds are estimated to cause 90% of all ureteral injuries, gunshot wounds to the abdomen cause ureteral injury only 2.2%–5% of the time.[91–93] The ureter is torn either partially or completely in the path of the projectile. It is usually a unilateral injury. Occasionally, the blast effect from a passing projectile will damage a ureter. While not torn or directly impacted by the missile, the ureter will necrose and perforate several days later, resulting in delayed diagnosis.[94] Obviously, there is a high rate (92%) of associated abdominal injury, most commonly to the bowel.[95] Rarely does blunt trauma result in ureter damage. When it does occur, the most common injury is disruption at the point of attachment to the bladder, the ureteropelvic junction.[96]

The bladder, when empty, is especially well protected from trauma by the bones of the pelvis. However, when the pelvis is fractured or the bladder is full, this organ can be easily ruptured. It is estimated that bladder injury is sustained in 5%–25% of pelvic fractures, while up to 70% of patients with bladder injury will have an associated pelvic fracture.[92] The injury to the bladder during pelvic fracture results either from (1) a tearing of the bladder away from its pelvic attachments or (2) penetration of the bladder by bone fragments or spicules. When blunt trauma is responsible for rupture of a full bladder without pelvic fracture, a blowout of the bladder dome is the most common injury seen.

Blunt trauma, typically MVCs, crush injuries, falls, or direct blows to the lower abdomen, is responsible for 75% of bladder injuries.[91,97] Less commonly, penetrating trauma causes bladder injury. Bladder injury should be suspected in patients with (1) pelvic fracture; (2) lower abdominal trauma, blunt or penetrating; (3) gross hematuria; or (4) inability to void.[98]

Female urethral trauma is uncommon and occurs almost exclusively as a result of direct trauma, e.g. a straddle injury or a severe pelvic fracture. There is usually concomitant injury to the vagina. Male urethral injuries are divided into anterior and posterior injuries. Anterior injuries are usually associated with a fall, straddle injury, or penetrating trauma. Posterior injuries are associated with pelvic fracture either from a shearing injury of the bony fragments or direct penetration by the fragments.[99] Five percent of male patients with pelvic fracture will have associated posterior urethral injury.[98]

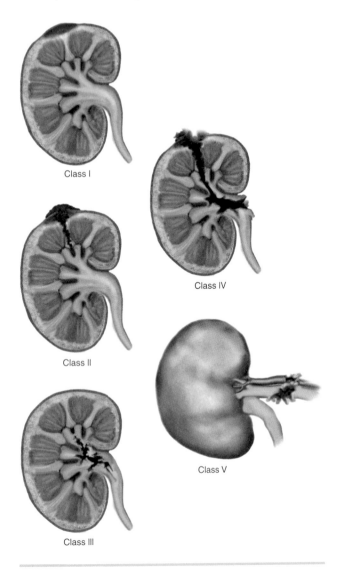

Class I

Class II

Class III

Class IV

Class V

FIGURE 14-10 Classification of renal injury.

Urethral trauma should be suspected in patients with (1) perineal trauma, (2) straddle injury, (3) pelvic fracture, (4) blood at the urethral meatus, (5) inability to void, (6) high-riding prostate on rectal examination, or (7) perineal, scrotal, or penile extravasation of blood or urine.[98]

ASSESSMENT

Out-of-hospital assessment should begin with a speedy but detailed history and physical examination. The challenge lies in expeditious assessment, treatment, and transport of the unstable trauma patient while still gathering enough background information to provide hospital personnel with an accurate snapshot of the incident. The mechanism of injury provides key clues in further assessment to detect genitourinary trauma in the emergency department. If time permits, obtain a brief focused history, including previous health history, allergies, medications, and last meal.

Field assessment of renal trauma is limited to inspection, auscultation, percussion, and palpation of the flank area. The flank area should be inspected for the presence of open wounds or impaled objects. **Grey-Turner's sign**, ecchymosis over the flank near the eleventh and twelfth ribs indicating retroperitoneal bleeding, may be present. Absence of this sign does not rule out renal trauma.[85] Auscultation of a renal artery bruit may indicate an intimal tear in the artery, but in the field, time should never be devoted to renal artery auscultation. Percussion of the flank may be dull if there is a large collection of fluid, such as blood or urine present. Finally, palpation of the kidneys is exceedingly difficult in even the thinnest, most cooperative patient and difficult, if not impossible, in the trauma patient. The presence of crepitus, mass, or pain in the flank area should raise the index of suspicion for renal trauma.

Emergency department assessment of renal trauma is delayed until life-threatening injuries of the cardiac, pulmonary, and neurological systems have been adequately addressed. Once these systems are secured, attention can be directed to the renal system. The trauma team will repeat the brief focused assessment already performed in the prehospital arena looking for changes since the initial examination. Then, diagnostic tests supplement the assessment.

Urine is assessed for the presence of blood. There is little or no correlation between the degree of hematuria and the extent of renal trauma. It has been suggested that only those patients presenting with (1) penetrating flank trauma or (2) blunt trauma with *either* (a) gross hematuria or (b) microscopic hematuria (greater than or equal to 3–5 RBCs/high-powered field) *and* shock [systolic blood pressure (SBP) less than or equal to 90 mm Hg] require evaluation beyond close observation and serial examinations.[100–103] Despite these suggestions, it is estimated that 10%–40% of blunt trauma patients with significant renal injury present without either gross or microscopic hematuria.[98]

Thus in blunt trauma patients, a high index of suspicion must be maintained. A decision about further diagnostic evaluation can be based on the following criteria: (1) sudden deceleration injury, (2) injury to flank soft tissue, (3) presence of microscopic or gross hematuria, (4) fractures of the lower ribs or upper lumbar vertebrae, (5) flank or abdominal mass, or (6) shock following blunt trauma.[98] If radiological evaluation is indicated, common methods for detecting renal trauma are intravenous pyelography, ultrasound, CT scan, and renal arteriography.

The field is not the appropriate place to diagnose ureter trauma. This diagnosis is difficult even with the sophisticated assessment tools available in the trauma center. The patient typically has no complaint specific to the ureter because there is usually no pain unless the ureter is obstructed. Transection produces no pain. Ureter injury should be suspected in the following situations: (1) penetrating injury in the vicinity of the ureter, (2) presence of gross or microhematuria, (3) deceleration injury with hyperextension of the spine, or (4) presence of a flank mass.[98] Microhematuria is present in approximately 90% of cases. Intravenous pyelography (IVP) is the most appropriate assessment tool. However, with a negative IVP and a continued high index of suspicion, a retrograde ureterogram may be performed.

In the field, the most prominent physical examination finding of bladder trauma will be suprapubic tenderness. There is a large association of bladder injury with trauma to other organs, especially the rectum, colon, and major vessels. In the emergency department, plain films of the pelvis may reveal a fracture or gross hematuria may be present; either of these should lead the clinician to pursue an investigation of bladder integrity. A retrograde cystogram can be performed in the trauma bay if the urethra is intact. Contrast is instilled through a Foley and serial X-rays are taken with the bladder fully distended and then fully evacuated, looking for extravasation of the contrast. If the urethra is not intact, then a Foley should not be placed and examination of the bladder can be performed during surgical repair of the urethra.[104] Computerized tomography can also demonstrate bladder disruption. Diagnostic peritoneal lavage is not a reliable test for bladder rupture. Bladder disruption in a female patient mandates careful gynecological examination in the emergency department for other injuries.

There are several types of bladder injury. Intraperitoneal rupture consists of a blowout of the bladder dome. This injury typically occurs in the patient with a full bladder who sustains a direct blow to the abdomen. Urine is extruded into the abdominal cavity. Extraperitoneal rupture involves a disruption or tear of the anteromedial segment near the bladder neck. Extraperitoneal injuries may occur as a result of (1) pelvic fracture fragments penetrating the bladder, (2) the ligamentous tearing of the bladder away from its attachments, or (3) severe compression of an empty bladder with resulting blowout similar to the mechanism described above for intraperitoneal injury.[105] Finally, the bladder wall may be severely contused or incompletely torn during trauma.

In the field, the paramedic may notice blood at the urethral meatus. This is a cardinal sign of urethral trauma, and its presence should be conveyed to the trauma team on hospital arrival. The patient may complain of pain at any point along the course of the urethra, or there may be a tender penile mass in male trauma patients. In the trauma bay, the urethra will be inspected for blood and, in male patients, the rectum will be palpated for the presence of a high-riding prostate. The scrotal or perineal area will also be inspected for hematoma. The presence of any of these abnormal findings precludes the placement of a Foley catheter.

Once urethral trauma is suspected, a retrograde urethrogram will be performed and serial X-rays taken. A Foley is placed at the urethral entrance and contrast material is slowly infused while radiographs are taken. Extravasation of contrast indicates a urethral disruption.[106] If the urethra is intact, then the Foley will be advanced into the bladder and a retrograde cystogram performed as described above for bladder trauma. The diagnosis of urethral injury is very difficult in women and requires a high index of suspicion. Urethrography is often not helpful in females, and the diagnosis is made either endoscopically or at the time of surgery.[106]

INTERNET ACTIVITIES

Visit the British Trauma Society Web site at http://www.trauma.org/abdo/renal/case.html and review the case presentation of a 32-year-old with renal trauma from a motor vehicle collision.

MANAGEMENT

In the field, the management of renal trauma should include (1) maintaining a high index of suspicion, (2)

aggressive treatment of hypotension in the absence of identified hemorrhage, and (3) rapid transport to a trauma center. Once renal trauma has been identified in the emergency department, a management decision about surgery must be contemplated. The vast majority of renal trauma can be managed nonsurgically. In general, only 8%–10% of blunt renal trauma requires immediate repair or exploration.[88] Specific indications for surgical management of blunt renal trauma include (1) an expanding, unconfined, or pulsatile hematoma; (2) extensive urinary extravasation; (3) large nonviable renal fragment; and (4) incomplete renal assessment secondary to other operative trauma. Penetrating trauma, which accounts for only a small percentage of overall renal trauma, usually mandates surgical exploration. Approximately 40% of stab wounds and 75% of gunshot wounds require surgical intervention.[107] Long-term complications of renal trauma include hypertension, arteriovenous fistula, and urinoma.[108]

Torn or disrupted ureters require surgical repair. Either the torn ends can be sewn together or, if the damage is extensive, the torn end of one ureter can be grafted onto its paired partner. The complications of ureter injury are stricture formation with resulting hydronephrosis, abscess formation, and urinoma formation if the diagnosis is delayed or missed.

Intraperitoneal rupture of the bladder and all penetrating injuries must be managed with surgical repair of the tear and drainage of the bladder through a suprapubic catheter.[109] Extraperitoneal rupture may be managed with Foley drainage and careful observation, provided that there is no coexisting injury.[97,110] Bladder contusion or partial tear of the bladder wall can also be managed with Foley drainage until the patient is able to void spontaneously and all bleeding has ceased. Complications of bladder injury include peritonitis, uroascites, and sepsis, particularly in those patients with delayed diagnosis. Rarely, patients will develop vesicocutaneous fistulas or prolonged healing with need for lengthy urinary Foley.[110,111]

Controversy exists as to the best method to manage blunt urethral trauma. Some advocate suprapubic drainage as a diverting procedure to allow the urethra to heal on its own. This approach is particularly applicable to anterior urethral injuries.[105,112] Others advocate prompt surgical repair.[104] Penetrating urethral trauma can be managed either conservatively with diverting drainage or with surgical repair depending on the extent of damage and associated injuries. Complications of urethral trauma include infection of the extravasated hematoma and urine, urethral stricture, urinary incontinence, and impotence in the male.

INTERNET ACTIVITIES

Visit the e-medicine Web site at http://www.emedicine.com. Click on the Emergency Medicine on-line book and select Trauma and Orthopedics. Then click on Trauma, Lower Genitourinary. Review the chapter on the management of genitourinary trauma.

THE GENITAL SYSTEM

The genital system consists of differing organs depending on the gender of the individual. In the female, the genital system is comprised of the paired ovaries and fallopian tubes, the uterus, and the vagina (Figure 14-11). In the male, the genital system is comprised of the prostate, the penis, and the testicles (Figure 14-12).

ANATOMY AND PHYSIOLOGY

The paired ovaries lie on either side of the female body in the ovarian fossa of the lateral pelvic wall. They are highly mobile organs attached to the uterus by the ovarian liga-

ment. The ovary contains, at birth, all the ova that will mature during the life of the woman. After the onset of puberty, ova begin to mature and develop. Each month during ovulation, an ovum traverses from the ovary through the fallopian tubes to the uterus for possible fertilization. The fallopian tubes are muscular tubes approximately 4 cm in length that extend laterally from each side of the uterus toward the ovaries. When an ovum is released from the ovary, it is swept into the end of the fallopian tube and heads toward the uterus. The nongravid uterus is a small pear-shaped organ situated between the bladder anteriorly and the rectum posteriorly.

The vagina is a muscular tube that extends from the exterior to the cervix or uterine entrance. It is bounded by the urethra and bladder anteriorly and the rectum posteriorly. It functions as the birth canal through which a fetus is expelled during labor, a conduit for menstrual flow, and as a passageway for the penis during intercourse. The vulva is the most external of the female genitalia. It consists of the paired labia majora and minora and the clitoris. Both the labia majora and minora are vascular skin folds that surround and protect the vaginal entrance. The clitoris is a highly sensitive organ located at the superior aspect of the joined pair of labia minora. The clitoris functions as a sexual arousal organ.

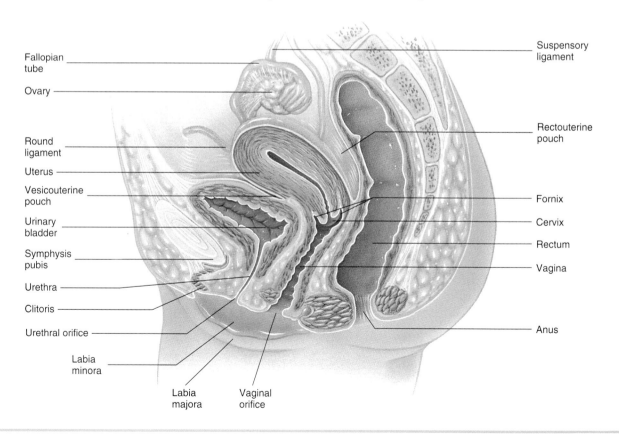

Fallopian tube
Ovary
Round ligament
Uterus
Vesicouterine pouch
Urinary bladder
Symphysis pubis
Urethra
Clitoris
Urethral orifice
Labia minora
Labia majora
Vaginal orifice

Suspensory ligament
Rectouterine pouch
Fornix
Cervix
Rectum
Vagina
Anus

FIGURE 14-11 Female urinary and reproductive structures.

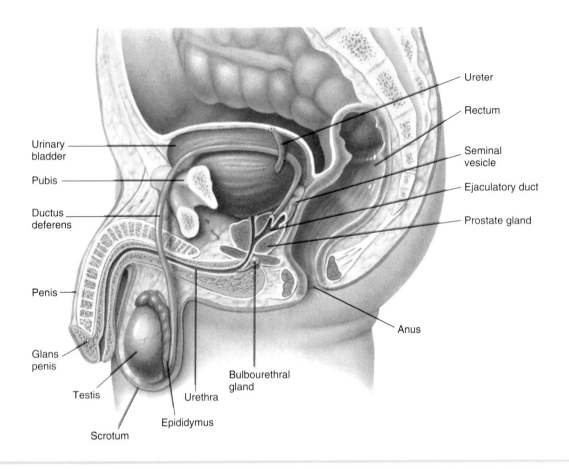

FIGURE 14-12 Male urinary and reproductive structures.

PATHOPHYSIOLOGY

The scrotum is a sac that hangs beneath the pubis in the male and behind the root of the penis. It is a complicated structure consisting of multiple fascial layers into which fluid can collect with inflammation or injury. The scrotal sac is divided into left and right halves, each of which contain one testicle. Each testicle measures approximately 4 by 3 by 2 cm and when palpated is a firm, ellipsoid organ. The testicle is the male gonad and, as such, functions to produce sperm and secrete the hormone testosterone. The epididymis, a compact collection of tubules through which sperm pass in their maturation process, is located at the superior pole of each testicle and pass superiorly to become the spermatic cord. The penis is comprised of two parts. The body of the penis hangs freely beneath the symphysis pubis just anterior to the scrotum. The root of the penis begins at the point the penis enters the pelvis. The penis functions as the male organ of copulation and as a conduit for urine and sperm.

Ovarian and fallopian tube injuries are exceedingly uncommon. Their size and mobility within the abdomen make them an unlikely target. Ovarian injuries range from simple contusion to complete avulsion or shattering. Fallopian tube injuries vary from simple hematoma to transection or devascularization. The nongravid uterus is injured rarely. Penetrating trauma is almost exclusively the etiology of injury, although blunt trauma may cause devascularization of the organ by disrupting its blood supply.[113] Grades I and II injuries involve contusions and superficial lacerations. Deep lacerations constitute grade III injury and lacerations involving the uterine artery define grade IV injuries. Avulsion or total devascularization are grade V injuries.[114] Injury to the gravid uterus is discussed in Chapter 25.

Vaginal injuries may occur with severe straddle injury, but most commonly, vaginal injury is a result of sexual assault or rape. Occasionally, vigorous consensual sexual activity will result in vaginal laceration. There are isolated case reports of vaginal injury after falling during water skiing, sliding down a water chute, and falling from a jet ski.[115–124] Injuries range from contusion and superficial laceration (grades I and II) to laceration into the cervix or peritoneum and injury involving other adjacent organs (grades IV and V).[114]

The vulva is typically injured during blunt trauma, either straddle injury or assault. Penetrating injuries from falls onto sharp objects, stabbing, gunshot wounds, or intentional impalement of objects by an assailant also occur. Injuries range from contusion or superficial laceration (grades I and II) to avulsion of tissue or injury to adjacent organs (grades IV and V).[114]

The scrotum and testicles can be injured in a variety of mechanisms: blunt trauma (most common), straddle injury, penetrating trauma, or entrapment in industrial/farm equipment.[125] Scrotal injury can result in large collections of fluid or blood within the sac or, if there is an entrapment or tearing injury, avulsion of large amounts of tissue. The testicles are rarely injured secondary to their mobility within the scrotal sac. They can, however, be ruptured due to blunt trauma or avulsed from the body by tearing or shear injury. On rare occasions, a testicle may be dislocated from the scrotum into the inguinal canal.[126]

Blunt trauma to the penis may result in extensive hematoma, avulsion of tissue, or penile fracture. Penile fracture, a rare entity, may also occur during sexual intercourse.[127–129] Penetrating trauma, ranging from pellet gun injury to shotgun blast, is also responsible for a large number of penile injuries.[130,131] There is, as would be expected, a high incidence of associated injuries with penetrating penile trauma. Concomitant trauma to the anterior urethra frequently occurs with penile injury. Amputation of the penis is an uncommon but devastating injury that may occur with either blunt or penetrating trauma.

ASSESSMENT

In the field there is no assessment tool or skill that leads to the diagnosis of ovarian or fallopian tube injury. There is no mechanism by which a trauma surgeon would identify ovarian or fallopian tube injury, unless it is incidentally noted on CT scan or during surgery for other injuries. Such an injury may be recognized much later in a woman undergoing an infertility work-up, although with an intact system on the other side, it might go unrecognized or explored.

In the field, uterine trauma is difficult to detect; time should not be devoted to searching for such an injury. The paramedic may notice vaginal bleeding if the injury is severe. In the emergency department, vaginal bleeding will be explored during a pelvic examination. Computerized tomography may demonstrate a substantial injury or hematoma. The injury may not be found until the time of exploratory surgery for penetrating trauma.

Patients with vaginal injury almost always present with bleeding and pain. The vagina is a highly vascular organ and can bleed quite profusely, even from a small laceration. Extensive injury can result in life-threatening bleeding. The paramedic should examine the vaginal area once bleeding is noted, taking great care to preserve the patient's privacy and dignity. Pay careful attention to clues to physical or sexual assault. Suspicions should be relayed to hospital personnel. In the emergency department, a speculum examination should be performed to delineate the extent of injury and decide the appropriate management.

In the field, the patient with vulvar injury will complain of pain and bleeding from the vaginal area. Again, assess for possible physical or sexual assault, and give a thorough report to hospital personnel. In the emergency department, a speculum examination will be performed to isolate the injury and any potential damage to adjacent organs. Penetrating injury requires further evaluation to determine the integrity of adjacent organs such as the bladder and rectum.

In the field, the patient with testicular or scrotal injury will complain of pain and bleeding. If there is avulsion of the testicles, these should be collected and preserved as with any other amputation. Inspection of the area may reveal massive edema or tissue loss depending on the injury mechanism. There should be two testicles within the scrotal sac. Absence of one or both testicles should be noted and relayed to the receiving trauma team. In the emergency department, the trauma team further evaluates the testicles with CT or ultrasonography.

In the field, those patients with penile injury will complain of pain and bleeding. The patient's pain may be severe and may mask other injuries that are more life threatening. Penile fracture will present as pain, swelling, discoloration, and deviation of the penis away from the site of fracture.[132,133] Penetrating penile trauma, especially if inflicted with a small-caliber weapon or in the setting of other penetrating injury, may easily be missed. Amputation of the penis can result in extensive hemorrhage and should be obvious to the examiner. Once in the emergency department, retrograde urethrography should be performed to assess urethral integrity. Other diagnostic modalities include CT, magnetic resonance imaging, or arteriogram.[134] In addition, a thorough assessment will be made of the rectum and bladder as there is a high association of other injuries with penile trauma, whether blunt or penetrating.[131]

MANAGEMENT

If ovarian or fallopian tube injury is recognized during exploratory surgery for other injury, the ovary or tube should be surgically repaired, if possible, or removed. The contralateral system should also be inspected for integrity at that time.

For patients with penetrating uterine injury, the defect should be oversewn, if possible, during exploratory surgery. Careful attention should be directed to preserving reproductive and hormonal function when possible. In the event of substantial injury or devascularization, removal of the uterus may be required.[113]

In the field, attempt to apply pressure dressings to a vaginal injury or, if adequate personnel are available to apply direct pressure to the vagina. If there is exsanguinating hemorrhage, fluid resuscitation should be initiated. There should be no delay in transport.

Simple vaginal lacerations in adult women can be repaired in the emergency department. Because children frequently require sedation or general anesthesia for even simple vaginal laceration repair, their injuries are often repaired in the operating room. In extensive injury, it may be very difficult to isolate the source of bleeding. Surgical management is focused on control of bleeding and restoration of normal anatomy and function.[113] On occasion, injury to the vaginal vascular supply can cause extensive hematomas that may bulge into the vagina. These hematomas should be evacuated and vascular repair undertaken in the operating room. Vaginal injuries tend to heal well without physical sequelae. On occasion, infections of large hematomas may occur. There may be emotional consequences as a result of injury whether caused by assault or not.

Vulvar lacerations can bleed profusely and attempts should be made to apply direct pressure. Impaled objects should not be removed; they should be stabilized as securely as possible to prevent further injury. Ice can be applied to vulvar hematomas to decrease the amount of swelling and to provide pain relief. In the hospital, large or expanding hematomas should be drained and bleeding vessels ligated. Large lacerations or avulsions are managed operatively to restore normal anatomy. Penetrating injury is usually explored and repaired in the operating room.

Scrotal and testicular trauma are rarely life threatening. These are, however, very dramatic and emotional injuries. All caregivers should thoroughly assess the patient, remembering that it is easy to focus on such an obvious injury while neglecting a more occult but life threatening injury. In the field, paramedics should control bleeding from the scrotum or testicles and collect/preserve any amputated tissue while maintaining the patient's dignity and privacy.

Scrotal and testicular injuries are repaired surgically. Salvage of scrotal tissue and cosmetic reconstruction frequently result in a good outcome. If there is extensive tissue loss and reconstruction is not possible, split-thickness skin grafts can be utilized to cover the testicles. When there is severe contamination of the wound, the testicles can be placed into subcutaneous pouches created in the medial aspect of the inner thigh, which approximates the temperature of the scrotum.[135] Dislocated testicles are recovered surgically and placed into the scrotal sac.[136]

Testicular rupture is managed with evacuation of scrotal hematoma and surgical repair of the injured testicle. While these testicles heal well after such a repair, they are typically useful only for hormone production but not spermatogenesis. On occasion, the testicle is so severely damaged that it cannot be repaired and an orchiectomy is necessary. Complications of testicular injury are impotence, infection, and a poor cosmetic appearance.

The paramedic should control penile bleeding as a first priority since open penile injuries can bleed quite freely. Direct pressure is the most appropriate method of hemorrhage control. If personnel are limited or there are other injuries requiring more immediate attention, a pressure dressing should be applied. Ice packs can be used for closed penile injuries to control swelling. Penetrating penile injury should be dressed as any other wound. Avulsed or amputated tissue should be recovered and preserved. Impaled objects should be stabilized and left in place.

In the hospital, penile rupture is usually repaired surgically by identifying torn tissue and restoring structural integrity.[129,133,137] This approach produces the fewest complications. Some practitioners advocate a conservative approach with urinary diversion, elevation, and pain control. This frequently results in permanent deformity, inadequate sexual function, and painful lumps.[138]

Penile reattachment after amputation requires a team of physicians, including urologists, plastic surgeons, and psychiatrists. If the ischemia time is less than 18 hours, the penis can usually be reattached providing there is not extensive functional tissue loss. Complications of penile amputation include inability to reattach the severed organ, permanent deformity, urethral stricture, sexual impotence, and emotional disability. Penetrating trauma should be surgically explored to achieve hemostasis, restore urethral integrity, and preserve penile function.[131,139,140]

► SUMMARY

Abdominal trauma is often an occult entity and a source of unrecognized major hemorrhage in the unstable trauma patient. The prehospital care provider must maintain a high index of suspicion in assessing the trauma patient, whether from blunt or penetrating mechanism. In blunt trauma, the spleen, liver, and intestines are the most frequently injured abdominal organs. In gunshot wounds, the small bowel, mesentery, liver, colon, and diaphragm are the most frequently injured organs. In stab wounds, the liver, colon, small bowel, and stomach are most commonly injured. The physical examination of abdominal trauma patients is notoriously unreliable, with the examination accuracy reported to be as low as 65%. Prehospital assessment of the trauma patient should include a detailed history and physical examination conducted in the most efficient and time-conscious manner possible. Prehospital treatment consists of rapid transport and judicious use of intravenous fluid. In-hospital treatment of injuries is organ specific. The task of the paramedic is to minimize the time to definitive care, to provide the trauma service with the most complete physical assessment and scene description possible, and to provide state-of-the-art treatment during transport. There is no crime in failing to localize the source of hemorrhage; the critical failure lies in failing to recognize and treat shock from occult bleeding.

Genitourinary trauma is often an occult entity and a source of unrecognized injury in the unstable trauma patient. The paramedic's focus should lie in rapid assessment and management of obvious injury, in treating unrecognized hemorrhage, and in rapid transport to a trauma center.

▶ REVIEW QUESTIONS

1. Abdominal trauma, as a whole, accounts for what percentage of total trauma fatalities?
   a. 1%–2%
   b. 7%–15%
   c. 25%–30%
   d. 85%

2. Which of the following is not a function of the liver?
   a. Manufacturing of bile
   b. Processing center for nutrients
   c. Production of insulin
   d. Recycling broken-down components of red blood cells

3. Name the two functions of the pancreas.

4. Which of the following is not commonly injured in blunt trauma?
   a. Gallbladder
   b. Intestines
   c. Liver
   d. Spleen

5. Which of the following is not a predisposing factor for gallbladder injury?
   a. Alcohol ingestion
   b. Distended gallbladder
   c. Pregnancy
   d. Thin-walled gallbladder

6. Missed injuries on initial examination can lead to increased morbidity and mortality. Which organ is *not* commonly missed on initial examination?
   a. Bowel
   b. Gallbladder
   c. Pancreas
   d. Spleen

7. Why is there a high infection rate with colon and rectal injuries?

8. Explain how arterial injuries may stop bleeding spontaneously.

9. How accurate is the examination of the blunt abdominal trauma patient?
   a. 15%
   b. 35%
   c. 65%
   d. 85%

10. Name three historical features of a motor vehicle collision that are important to emergency department personnel.

11. The classic seat belt pattern of injury is:
    a. Hollow viscus injury, flexion-distraction fractures of the cervical spine, abdominal wall disruption
    b. Hollow viscus injury, flexion-distraction fractures of the lumbar spine, abdominal wall disruption
    c. Hollow viscus injury, flexion-distraction fractures of the lumbar spine, diaphragmatic disruption
    d. Solid viscus injury, flexion-distraction fractures of the lumbar spine, abdominal wall disruption

12. Left lower rib border injuries should alert the prehospital care provider to what injury?
    a. Diaphragm rupture
    b. Pancreas injury
    c. Spleen injury
    d. Stomach injury

13. Which of the following patients would merit further evaluation and diagnostic tests before going to the operating room?
    a. Evisceration
    b. Gunshot wound to the anterior abdomen
    c. Obvious blunt trauma with unstable vital signs
    d. Stab wounds to the flank

14. A diagnostic peritoneal lavage is considered positive if which of the following is present?
    a. Gross blood (more than 10 mL)
    b. Greater than 8,000/mm^3 RBCs in blunt trauma
    c. Greater than 8 IU/L calcium
    d. Greater than 200/mm^3 WBCs

15. Which of the following is not a disadvantage of DPL?
    a. Does not provide organ-specific information
    b. Invasive with associated complications
    c. Requires a skilled radiologist

d. Unable to detect hemorrhage in the retroperitoneal space

16. For each 10 minutes of delay in reaching definitive treatment, survival for critically injured trauma patients drops by:
    a. 2%
    b. 10%
    c. 20%
    d. 50%

17. Infused intravenous fluid in the bleeding trauma patient is thought to do all of the following except:
    a. Decrease bleeding
    b. Dilute out essential clotting factors
    c. Disrupt clot formation
    d. Lower blood viscosity

18. The criteria for nonoperative management of liver injuries include all of the following except:
    a. Absence of peritoneal signs
    b. Absence of alcohol intoxication
    c. CT scan delineation of the injury
    d. Neurological integrity

19. Which of the following organs is not eligible for nonoperative management?
    a. Liver
    b. Pancreas
    c. Rectum
    d. Spleen

20. What is OPSI?

21. The organ most commonly injured in patients with genitourinary trauma is the:
    a. Bladder
    b. Kidney
    c. Ureter
    d. Urethra

22. Which of the following is not an injury associated with genitourinary trauma?
    a. Femur fractures
    b. Fractures of the transverse processes of lumbar vertebrae
    c. Gunshot wound to the abdomen
    d. Lower rib fractures

23. Of all patients with traumatic abdominal injuries, what percentage will have injuries to the genitourinary system?
    a. 2%–5%
    b. 10%–15%
    c. 25%–30%
    d. 70%–75%

24. The correct sequence of urinary organs from internal to external is:
    a. Kidney→ureter→meatus
    b. Kidney→ureter→urethra
    c. Kidney→urethra→ureter
    d. Urethra→bladder→ureter→kidney

25. Which of the following is *not* a function of the kidney?
    a. Blood pressure control
    b. Excretion of thyroxine
    c. Red blood cell production
    d. Urine formation

26. What anatomical characteristics of the kidneys make them particularly susceptible to injury in acceleration-deceleration accidents?

27. What is Grey-Turner's sign and what does its presence indicate?

28. Which of the following patients with suspected renal trauma do *not* require renal evaluation beyond close observation and serial examinations?
    a. 27-year-old male with penetrating flank trauma
    b. 34-year-old female with blunt trauma, microscopic hematuria, stable vital signs
    c. 41-year-old female with blunt trauma, microscopic hematuria, unstable vital signs
    d. 66-year-old female with blunt abdominal trauma and gross hematuria

29. Which of the following is *not* part of out-of-hospital management of renal trauma?
    a. Aggressive treatment of hypotension in the absence of identified trauma
    b. Auscultation for renal artery bruit
    c. High index of suspicion
    d. Rapid transport to a trauma center

30. Which one of these is *not* associated with bladder injury:
    a. Blunt trauma to a full bladder
    b. Pelvic fracture
    c. Tearing of the bladder from its pelvic attachment
    d. Transmitted trauma from the kidney

31. Bladder trauma should be suspected in patients who:
    a. Are over 65 years old
    b. Are unable to void
    c. Have associated splenic injury
    d. Have lumbar spine injuries

32. The urethra is much longer in the male than in the female. The correct order of the urethral segments in the male from bladder to meatus are:
    a. Bulbous→membranous→penile→prostatic
    b. Membranous→bulbous→prostatic→penile
    c. Prostatic→bulbous→membranous→penile
    d. Prostatic→membranous→bulbous→penile

33. Urethral trauma should be suspected in all of the following patients except:
    a. 15-year-old male with high-riding prostate on rectal examination
    b. 62-year-old male who cannot urinate spontaneously

c. 19-year-old male with renal injury

d. 22-year-old female with straddle injury

34. What is the cardinal sign of urethral trauma?

35. How is a retrograde urethrogram performed?

36. The mechanism of injury to the nongravid uterus is most commonly:
   a. Blunt trauma
   b. Electrical injury
   c. Penetrating trauma
   d. Acceleration-deceleration

37. The vagina may be injured in any of the following mechanisms except:
   a. Seat belt injury
   b. Sexual assault
   c. Straddle injury
   d. Water sports

38. Scrotal and testicular injuries are associated with each of the following mechanisms except:
   a. Blunt trauma
   b. Farm or industrial accidents
   c. Penetrating trauma
   d. Pelvic fractures

39. What is the appropriate treatment for testicular avulsion?

40. The presenting signs and symptoms for penile fracture include all of the following except:
   a. Brisk bleeding
   b. Deviation of the penis away from the site of fracture
   c. Pain
   d. Swelling

41. Which of the following is associated with penile trauma:
   a. Femur fracture
   b. Pelvic fracture
   c. Rectal injury
   d. Spleen laceration

▶ CRITICAL THINKING

● The mortality rate for blunt abdominal trauma ranges between 10% and 30%, whereas penetrating abdominal injury mortality rates are reported to be less than 5%. Why do you think there is such a disparity in mortality rates between these two injury mechanisms?

● Penetrating trauma is reported to be more prevalent in urban areas as opposed to rural and suburban areas. What may explain this phenomenon?

● You are dispatched to the scene of an MVC. Your patient is a 30-year-old male who struck a bridge abutment. Frontal damage to the vehicle is approx-

imately 20 inches. A lap restraint was worn, but the vehicle was not equipped with a shoulder harness or airbags. The patient is conscious and alert but confused. He denies pain. Breath sounds are clear and equal, neck veins flat, and heart sounds easily audible. The abdomen is diffusely tender to palpation. The abdomen also shows a seat belt abrasion and bluish discoloration around the umbilicus. The pelvis is stable and movement and sensation are present in all extremities. The skin is pale, cool, and clammy. Radial pulses are not palpable, but a rapid, weak carotid pulse is palpable. What is your impression of this patient? What are the possible injuries? What are your field treatment priorities?

▶ REFERENCES

1. Shackford SR, Mackersie RC, Holbrook TL, et al. The epidemiology of traumatic death: a population-based analysis. *Arch Surg.* 1993; 128:571.

2. Trunkey D, Hill A, Schecter W. Abdominal trauma and indications for celiotomy. In: Moore EE, Mattox K, Feliciano D, eds. *Trauma.* 2nd ed. Norwalk, Conn.: Appleton & Lange; 1991.

3. Anderson C, Ballinger W. Abdominal injuries. In: Zuidema G, Rutherford R, and Ballinger W, eds. *The Management of Trauma.* 2nd ed. Philadelphia: WB Saunders; 1973.

4. McAnena OJ, Moore EE, Marx JA. Initial evaluation of the patient with blunt abdominal trauma. *Surg Clin North Am.* 1990; 70:495.

5. Lacqua MJ, Sahdev P. The epidemic of penetrating trauma: a national dilemma. *J Emerg Med.* 1993; 11:747.

6. Crafts RC. *A Textbook of Human Anatomy.* 2nd ed. New York: John Wiley & Sons; 1979.

7. Berne RM, Levy MN. *Physiology.* St. Louis: CV Mosby Co; 1988.

8. Sampalis JS, Lavoie A, Williams JI, Mulder DS, Kalina M. Impact of on-site care, prehospital time, and level of in-hospital care on survival in severely injured patients. *J Trauma.* 1993; 34:252.

9. Cayten CG, Longmore W, Kuehl A, Gifford B. Basic life support vs. advanced life support for urban trauma. *J Trauma.* 1987; 27:651. Abstract.

10. Smith JP, Bodai BI, Hill AS, Frey CF. Prehospital stabilization of critically injured patients: a failed concept. *J Trauma.* 1985; 25:65.

11. Ferero S, Hedges JR, Simmons E, Irwin L. Does out-of-hospital EMS time affect trauma survival? *Am J Emerg Med.* 1995; 13:133.

12. Boulanger BR, McLellan BA. Blunt abdominal trauma. *Emerg Med Clin North Am.* 1996; 14:151.

13. Shoemaker WC, Corley RD, Liu M, et al. Development and testing of a decision tree for blunt trauma. *Crit Care Med.* 1988; 16:1141.

14. Feliciano DV, Burch JM, Spjut-Patrinely V, Mattox KL, Jordan GL. Abdominal gunshot wounds: an urban trauma center's experience with 300 consecutive patients. *Ann Surg.* 1988; 208:362.

15. Raptopoulos V. Abdominal trauma: emphasis on computed tomography. *Radiol Clin North Am.* 1994; 32:969.

16. Helling TS, Morse G, McNabney, WK. Treatment of liver injuries at level I and level II centers in a multi-institutional metropolitan trauma system. *J Trauma.* 1997; 42:1091.

17. Ochsner MG, Jaffin JH, Golocovsky M, Jones RC. Major hepatic trauma. *Surg Clin North Am.* 1993; 73:337.

18. Moore EE, Cogbill TH, Jurkovich GJ, Shackford SR, Malangoni MA, Champion HR. Organ injury scaling: spleen and liver (1994 revision). *J Trauma.* 1995; 38:323.

19. McNabney WK, Rudek R, Pemberton LB. The significance of gallbladder trauma. *J Emerg Med.* 1990; 8:277.

20. Posner MC, Moore EE. Extrahepatic biliary tract injury: operative management plan. *J Trauma.* 1985; 25:833.

21. Sharma O. Blunt gallbladder injuries: presentation of twenty-two cases with a review of the literature. *J Trauma.* 1995; 39:576.

22. Wilson RH, Moorehead RJ. Management of splenic trauma. *Injury.* 1992; 23:5.

23. Tjelmeland K. Abdominal and genitourinary trauma. In: Lee G, ed. *Flight Nursing.* St. Louis, Mo: Mosby Year Book; 1991.

24. Jurkovich GJ, Carrico CJ. Pancreatic trauma. *Surg Clin North Am.* 1994; 70:575.

25. Mason PJB. Abdominal injuries. In: Cardona VD, Hurn P, Mason P, Scanlon A, Veise-Berry S, eds. *Trauma Nursing.* 2nd ed. Philadelphia: WB Saunders Co; 1994.

26. Brunsting LA, Morton JH. Gastric rupture from blunt abdominal trauma. *J Trauma.* 1987; 27:887.

27. Fiorillo M, Ozuner G, Pomper S. Through-and-through isolated gastric perforation following blunt trauma. *Resident and Staff Physician.* 1996; 42:65.

28. Asensio JA, Feliciano D, Britt LD, Kerstein MD. Management of duodenal injuries. *Curr Probl Surg.* 1993; 1026.

29. Moore EE, Cogbill TH, Malangoni MA, et al. Organ injury scaling II: pancreas, duodenum, small bowel, colon, and rectum. *J Trauma.* 1990; 30:1427.

30. Nance FC, Wennar MH, Johnson LW, Ingram JC Jr., Cohn I Jr. Surgical judgment in the management of penetrating wounds of the abdomen: experience with 2212 patients. *Ann Surg.* 1974; 179:639.

31. Nance FC. Injuries to the colon and rectum. In: Moore EE, Mattox K, Feliciano D, eds. *Trauma.* 2nd ed. Norwalk, Conn.: Appleton & Lange; 1991.

32. Braithwaite CEM, Rodriguez A. Injuries of the abdominal aorta from blunt trauma. *Am Surg.* 1992; 58:350.

33. Powell DC, Bivens BA, Bell RM. Diagnostic peritoneal lavage. *Surg Gynecol Obstet.* 1982; 155:257.

34. Mackersie RC, Tiawary AD, Shackford SR, Hoyt DB. Intra-abdominal injury following blunt trauma. *Arch Surg.* 1989; 124:809.

35. Davis JJ, Cohn I, Nance FC. Diagnosis and management of blunt abdominal trauma. *Am Surg.* 1976; 183:672.

36. Perry JF. A five year survey of 152 acute abdominal injuries. *J Trauma.* 1965; 5:53.

37. Colucciello SA. Blunt abdominal trauma. *Emerg Med Clin North Am.* 1993; 11:107.

38. Orsay EM, Dunne M, Turnbull TL, Barrett JA, Langenberg P, Orsay CP. Prospective study of the effect of safety belts in motor vehicle crashes. *Ann Emerg Med.* 1990; 19:258.

39. Fox MA, Fabian TC, Croce MA, Mangiante EC, Carson JP, Kvosk VA. Anatomy of the accident scene: a prospective study of injury and mortality. *Am Surg.* 1991; 6:394.

40. Hayes CW, Conway WF, Walsh JW, Coppage L, Gervin AS. Seat belt injuries: radiologic findings and clinical correlation. *Radiographics.* 1991; 11:23.

41. Moore JB, Moore EE, Thompson JS. Abdominal injuries associated with penetrating trauma in the lower chest. *Am J Surg.* 1980; 140:724.

42. Marx JA. Penetrating abdominal trauma. *Emerg Med Clin North Am.* 1993; 11:125.

43. Lacqua MJ, Sahdev P. Effective management of penetrating abdominal trauma. *Hosp Pract.* 1993; 28:31.

44. Moore EE. Resuscitation and evaluation of the injured patient. In: Zuidema GG, Ballinger W, Rutherford R, eds. *The Management of Trauma.* 3rd ed. Philadelphia: WB Saunders Co; 1985.

45. Feliciano DV. Diagnostic modalities in abdominal trauma. *Surg Clin North Am.* 1991; 71:241.

46. Root HD, et al. Diagnostic peritoneal lavage. *Surgery.* 1965; 57:633.

47. Catre MC. Diagnostic peritoneal lavage versus abdominal computed tomography in blunt abdominal trauma: a review of prospective cases. *Can J Surg.* 1995; 38:117.

48. Pearl WS, Todd KH. Ultrasonography for the initial evaluation of blunt abdominal trauma: a review of prospective trials. *Ann Emerg Med.* 1996; 27:353.

49. Rizoli SB, Boulanger BR, McClellan BA, Sharkey PW. Injuries missed during initial assessment of blunt trauma patients. *Accid Anal Prev.* 1994; 26:681.

50. McSwain NE, Paturas JL, Wertz, E, eds. *PHTLS Basic and Advanced*. St. Louis, Mo.: Mosby-Year Book Inc; 1994.

51. Branas CC, Sing RF, Davidson SJ. Urban trauma transport of assaulted patients using nonmedical personnel. *Acad Emerg Med*. 1995; 2:486.

52. Demetriades D, Chan L, Cornwell E, et al. Paramedic vs private transportation of trauma patients. *Arch Surg*. 1996; 131:133.

53. Brill JC, Geiderman JM. A rationale for scoop and run: identifying a subset of time-critical patients. In: Brill JC, Geiderman JM, eds. *Topics in Emergency Medicine*. Rockville, Md.: Aspen Systems Corp; 1981.

54. Klauber MR, Marshall LF, Toole BM, Knowlton SL, Bowers SA. Cause of decline in head-injury mortality rate in San Diego County. *Calif J Neurosurg*. 1985; 62:528.

55. Shackford SR, Hollingworth-Fridlund P, Cooper GF, Eastman AB. The effect of regionalization upon the quality of trauma care as assessed by concurrent audit before and after institution of a trauma system: a preliminary report. *J Trauma*. 1986; 26:812.

56. Shackford SR, Mackensie RC, Hoyt DB, et al. Impact of a trauma system on outcome of severely injured patients. *Arch Surg*. 1987; 122:523.

57. Cayten CG, Berendt BM, Byrne DW, Murph JG, Moy FH. A study of pneumatic antishock garments in severely hypotensive trauma patients. *J Trauma*. 1993; 34:728.

58. Mattox KL, Bickell WH, Pepe PE, Mangelsdorff AD. Prospective randomized evaluation of antishock MAST in post-traumatic hypotension. *J Trauma*. 1986; 26:779.

59. Karch SB, Lewis T, Young S, Ho CH. Surgical delays and outcomes in patients treated with pneumatic antishock garments: a population-based study. *Am J Emerg Med*. 1995; 13:401.

60. Owens TM, Watson WC, Prough DS, Uchida T, Kramer CC. Limiting initial resuscitation of uncontrolled hemorrhage reduces internal bleeding and subsequent volume requirements. *J Trauma*. 1995; 39:200.

61. Bickell WH, Bruttig SP, Millnamon GA, O'Benar J, Wade CE. The detrimental effects of intravenous crystalloid after aortotomy in swine. *Surgery*. 1991; 110:529.

62. Bickell WH, Wall MJ Jr., Pepe PE, et al. Immediate versus delayed fluid resuscitation for hypotensive patients with penetrating torso injuries. *N Engl J Med*. 1994; 331:1105.

63. Kaweski SM, Sise MJ, Virgilio RW. The effect of prehospital fluids on survival in trauma patients. *J Trauma*. 1990; 30:215.

64. Pollack CV. Prehospital fluid resuscitation of the trauma patient: an update on the controversies. *Emerg Med Clin North Am*. 1993; 11:61.

65. Croce MA, Fabian TC, Menke PG, et al. Nonoperative management of blunt hepatic trauma is the treatment of choice for hemodynamically stable patients. *Am Surg*. 1995; 221:744.

66. Pachter HL, Hofstetter SR. The current status of nonoperative management of adult blunt hepatic injuries. *Am J Surg*. 1995; 169:442.

67. Soderstrom CA, Maekawa K, Dupriest RW Jr., Cowley RA. Gallbladder injuries resulting from blunt abdominal trauma. *Ann Surg*. 1981; 193:60.

68. Parks RW, Diamond T. Non-surgical trauma to the extrahepatic biliary tract. *Br J Surg*. 1995; 82:1303.

69. Feliciano DV. Biliary injuries as a result of blunt and penetrating trauma. *Surg Clin North Am*. 1994; 74:897.

70. Pachter HL, Spencer FC, Hofstetter SR, Liang HG, Hoballah J, Coppa GF. Experience with selective operative and nonoperative treatment of splenic injuries in 193 patients. *Ann Surg*. 1990; 211:583.

71. Hunt JP, Lentz CW, Cairns BA, et al. Management and outcome of splenic injury: the results of a five-year statewide population-based study. *Am Surg*. 1996; 62:911.

72. Malangoni MA, Cue JI, Fallot ME, Willing ST, Richardson JD. Evaluation of splenic injury by computed tomography and its impact on treatment. *Ann Surg*. 1990; 211:592.

73. Feliciano DV, Spjut-Patrinely V, Burgh JM. Splenorrhaphy: the alternative. *Ann Surg*. 1990; 211:569.

74. Beal SL, Spisso JM. The risk of splenorrhaphy. *Arch Surg*. 1988; 123:1158.

75. Shackford SR, Molin M. Management of splenic injuries. *Surg Clin North Am*. 1990; 70:595.

76. Krahenbuhl L, Berry AR. The management of splenic injuries in a district general hospital. *J R Coll Surg Edinb*. 1994; 39:249.

77. Keller MS, Stafford PW, Vane DW. Conservative management of pancreatic trauma in children. *J Trauma*. 1997; 42:1097.

78. Nwariaku FE, Terracina A, Mileski WJ, Mihel JP, Carrico CJ. Is octreotide beneficial following pancreatic injury. *Am J Surg*. 1995; 170:582.

79. Moncure M, Goins WA. Challenges in the management on pancreatic and duodenal injuries. *J Natl Med Assoc*. 1993; 85:767.

80. Carrillo EH, Richardson JD, Miller FB. Evolution in the management of duodenal injuries. *J Trauma*. 1996; 40:1037.

81. Davis K. The injured duodenum. *J Natl Med Assoc*. 1992; 84:177.

82. Wisner DH, Chun Y, Blaisdell FW. Blunt intestinal injury. *Arch Surg*. 1990; 125:1319.

83. Austin OM, Redmond HP, Burke PE, Grace PA, Bouchier-Hayes DB. Vascular trauma—a review. *J Am Coll Surg*. 1995; 181:91.

84. Cunningham PRG, Foil MB. The ripped cava. *J Natl Med Assoc*. 1995; 87:305.

85. Carroll PR, McAninch JW. Staging of renal trauma. *Urol Clin North Am*. 1989; 16:193.

86. Krieger JN, Algood CB, Mason JT, Copass MK, Ansell JS. Urological trauma in the Pacific Northwest: etiology, distribution, management, and outcome. *J Urol*. 1984; 132:70.

87. Sagalowsky AI, McConnell JD, Peters PC. Renal trauma requiring surgery: an analysis of 185 cases. *J Trauma*. 1983; 23:128.

88. Nguyen HT, Carroll PR. Blunt renal trauma: renal preservation through careful staging and selective surgery. *Semin Urol*. 1995; 13:83.

89. Guerriero WG. Etiology, classification, and management of renal trauma. *Surg Clin North Am*. 1988; 68:1071.

90. Moore EE, Shackford DR, Pachter HL, et al. Organ injury scaling—spleen, liver, & kidney. *J Trauma*. 1989; 29:1664.

91. Farrar J, Cottingham C, Rutter MM. Genitourinary injuries and renal management. In: Cardona VD, ed. *Trauma Nursing: From Resuscitation Through Rehabilitation*. Philadelphia: WB Saunders; 1995.

92. Peterson NE. Emergency management of urologic trauma. *Emerg Med Clin North Am*. 1988; 6:579.

93. Baniel J. The management of penetrating trauma to the urinary tract. *J Am Coll Surg*. 1994; 178:417.

94. O'Connell KJ, Clark M, Lewis RH, Christenson PJ. Comparison of low- and high-velocity ballistic trauma to genitourinary organs. *J Trauma*. 1988; 28(suppl):139.

95. Guerriero WG. Ureteral injury. *Urol Clin North Am*. 1989; 16:237.

96. Toporoff B, Scalea TM, Abramson D, Scalafani SJ. Ureteral laceration caused by a fall from a height: case report and review of the literature. *J Trauma*. 1993; 34:164.

97. Corriere JN, Sandler CM. Management of the ruptured bladder: seven years of experience with 111 cases. *J Trauma*. 1986; 26:830.

98. Hanno PM, Wein AJ. Urologic trauma. *Emerg Med Clin North Am*. 1984; 2:823.

99. Lowe, MA, Mason JT, Luna GK, Maier RV, Copass MK, Bencer RE. Risk factors for urethral injuries in men with traumatic pelvic fracture. *J Urol*. 1988; 140:506.

100. Guice K, Oldham K, Eide B, Johansen K. Hematuria after blunt trauma: when is pyelography useful? *J Trauma*. 1983; 23:305.

101. Mee SL, McAningh JW, Robinson AL, Auerbach PS, Carroll PR. Radiographic assessment of renal trauma: a 10-year prospective study of patient selection. *J Urol*. 1989; 141:1095.

102. Mee SL, McAninch JW. Indications for radiographic assessment in suspected renal trauma. *Urol Clin North Am*. 1989; 16:187.

103. Eastham JA, Wilson TG, Ahlering TE. Radiographic evaluation of adult patients with blunt renal trauma. *J Urol*. 1992; 148:266.

104. Cass AS. Diagnostic studies in bladder rupture: indications and techniques. *Urol Clin North Am*. 1989; 16:267.

105. Spirnak JP. Pelvic fracture and injury to the lower urinary tract. *Surg Clin North Am*. 1988; 68:1057.

106. Sandler CM, Corriere JN. Urethrography in the diagnosis of acute urethral injuries. *Urol Clin North Am*. 1989; 16:283.

107. McAninch JW, Carroll PR. Renal exploration after trauma: indications and reconstructive techniques. *Urol Clin North Am*. 1989; 16:203.

108. Peterson NE. Complications of renal trauma. *Urol Clin North Am*. 1989; 16:221.

109. Peters PC. Intraperitoneal rupture of the bladder. *Urol Clin North Am*. 1989; 16:279.

110. Corriere JN, Sandler CM. Management of extraperitoneal bladder rupture. *Urol Clin North Am*. 1989; 16:275.

111. Kotkin L, Koch MO. Morbidity associated with nonoperative management of extraperitoneal bladder injuries. *J Trauma*. 1995; 38:895.

112. Pierce JM. Disruptions of the anterior urethra. *Urol Clin North Am*. 1989; 16:329.

113. Sweet RL, Crombleholme WR. Gynecologic trauma in the nongravid and gravid patient. In: Trunkey DD, Lewis FR, eds. *Current Therapy of Trauma*. Philadelphia: BC Decker; 1991.

114. Moore EE, Jurkovich GJ, Knudson MM. Organ injury scaling VI: extrahepatic billiary, esophagus, stomach, vulva, vagina, uterus (nonpregnant), uterus (pregnant), fallopian tube and ovary. *J Trauma*. 1995; 39:1069.

115. McCarthy GF. Hazards of water-skiing. *Med J Austral*. 1969; 1:481.

116. Gray HH. A risk of water-skiing for women. *Western J Med*. 1982; 136:169.

117. Kalaichandran S. Vaginal laceration: a little known hazard for women water-skiers. *Can J Surg*. 1991; 34:107.

118. Edington RF. Vaginal injuries due to water-skiing. *Can Med Assoc J*. 1978; 119:310.

119. Morton DC. Gynaecological complications of water-skiing. *Med J Austral*. 1970; 1:1256.

120. Rudoff JC. Vulvovaginal water-skiing injury. *Ann Emerg Med*. 1993; 22:1072.

121. Niv J, Lessing JB, Hartuv J, Peyser MR. Vaginal injury resulting from sliding down a water chute. *Am J Obstet Gynecol*. 1992; 166:930.

122. Mushkat Y, Lessing JB, Jedwab GA, David MP. Vaginal trauma occurring while sliding down a water chute. *Br J Obstet Gynaecol.* 1995; 102:933.

123. Muller RJ. Jet-ski injury: a case history. *J Louisiana State Med Soc.* 1993; 145:27.

124. Wein P, Thompson DJ. Vaginal perforation due to jet-ski accident. *Austral NZ J Obstet Gynaecol.* 1990; 30:384.

125. Bowditch MG, Hamdy FC, Collins MC, Hastie KJ. Blast trauma and testicular rupture: an unusual civilian injury. *Br J Urol.* 1994; 74:805.

126. Lee JY, Cass A, Streitz JM. Traumatic dislocation of testes and bladder rupture. *Urology.* 1992; 40:506.

127. Cumming J, Jenkins JD. Fracture of the corpus cavernosa and urethral rupture during sexual intercourse. *Br J Urol.* 1991; 67:327.

128. Tsang T, Demby AM. Penile fracture with urethral injury. *J Urol.* 1992; 147:466.

129. Ruckle HC, Hadley HR, Lui PD. Fracture of penis: diagnosis and management. *Urology.* 1992; 40:33.

130. Bertini JE, Corriere JN. The etiology and management of genital injuries. *J Trauma.* 1988; 28:8.

131. Gomez RG, Castanheira ACC, McAninch JW. Gunshot wounds to the male external genitalia. *J Urol.* 1993; 150:1147.

132. Suzuki K, Shimizu N, Kurokawa K, Suzuki T, Yamanaka H. Fracture of the penis: magnetic resonance imaging of the rupture of the corpus carvernosum. *Br J Urol.* 1995; 76:800.

133. Kowalczyk J, Athens A, Grimaldi A. Penile fracture: an unusual presentation with lacerations of bilateral corpora cavernosa and partial disruption of the urethra. *Urology.* 1994; 44:599.

134. Brandes SB, Buckman RF, Chelsky MJ, Hanno PM. External genitalia gunshot wounds: a ten-year experience. *J Trauma.* 1995; 39:266.

135. McAninch, JW. Genitourinary trauma. In: Trunkey DD, Lewis FR, eds. *Current Therapy of Trauma.* Philadelphia: BC Decker; 1991.

136. Schwartz SL, Faerber GJ. Dislocation of the testis as a delayed presentation of scrotal trauma. *Urology.* 1994; 43:743.

137. Asgari MA, Hosseini SY, Safarinejad MR, Samadzadeh B, Bardideh AR. Penile fractures: evaluation, therapeutic approaches and long-term results. *J Urol.* 1996; 155:148.

138. Cass A. Genitourinary trauma. In: Kreis D, Gomez G, eds. *Trauma Management.* Boston: Little Brown; 1989.

139. Monga M, Moreno T, Hellstrom WJG. Gunshot wounds to the male genitalia. *J Trauma.* 1995; 38:855.

140. Hall SJ, Wagner JR, Edelstein RA, Carpinito GA. Management of gunshot wounds to the penis and anterior urethra. *J Trauma.* 1995; 38:439.

Chapter

15

Extremity Trauma

OBJECTIVES

Upon completion of this chapter, the reader should be able to:

- Describe the epidemiology and etiology of extremity trauma.
- Describe the normal anatomy and physiology of the extremities.
- Discuss the pathophysiology, assessment findings, and management of sprains, dislocations, fractures, and amputations.
- Explain the techniques for assessing extremity injuries.
- Describe the general principles of splinting.
- List the complications of extremity injury.
- List the associated blood loss of various fracture sites.
- Explain the healing process of fractures.
- List and describe the various types of fractures.

KEY TERMS

Colles' fracture
Compartment syndrome
Coxae
Fracture
Galeazzi's fracture
Local crush injury

Menisci
Olecranon process
Open fracture
Smith fracture
Systemic crush syndrome
Two-point discrimination

Extremity trauma is commonly encountered by paramedics in the field. Although rarely life threatening, injured extremities produce major disability and loss of earning capacity. Proper treatment and rehabilitation of musculoskeletal injuries (MSIs) can return the majority of patients to or close to their previous level of function.

Although extremity injuries, fractures in particular, have been diagnosed and treated since the beginning of time, treatment methods have changed slowly. Many of the extremity injury management principles and techniques used outside the hospital today remain exactly as they have been for centuries. In the third century B.C., Hippocrates used two men to apply traction and countertraction to reduce and stabilize fractures.[1] Similarly, trained physicians of those times recognized that the outcome of extremity trauma was

315

influenced by fracture stability and the amount of neurovascular damage incurred.[2]

In the late 1800s, Sir Hugh Owen Thomas invented the full-leg traction splint for which he is remembered. It was invented not as an emergency treatment device but as an adjunct for alignment and reduction of the fractured femur. His nephew, Sir Robert Jones, and other British and American surgeons during World War I modified the full-ring to a half-ring traction splint and began using it as an immediate treatment aid for injured soldiers. A study of injured soldiers of that time showed that the resultant reduction of continuing hemorrhage in the thigh after traction application reduced mortality from 80% to approximately 15%.[3]

In addition, other improvements in MSI management in the last two centuries include advances in surgical technique, antibiotic development, and fluid resuscitation. While military conflict has stimulated the greatest number of changes, advances in civilian prehospital care have overshadowed previous military advances for first-hour care post injury.

An evolution in prehospital assessment and treatment is occurring even as this is being written. Previously, extremity injuries received minor attention when compared to the more life-threatening trauma of the head, chest, and abdomen. Paramedics rightfully concentrated their attentions on that which was most likely to result in the demise of their patients. As shoulder and lap seatbelt restraining systems are now more frequently combined with vehicle air bag systems, both injury severity and mortality rates from motor vehicle collisions (MVCs) are decreasing. When used together, it is expected that a 45% decrease in mortality will ultimately occur.[4] This decrease in upper body trauma allows caregivers to focus comparatively more attention on extremity injuries. Logically, this could lead to a further decrease in mortality and morbidity.

EPIDEMIOLOGY AND ETIOLOGY

Musculoskeletal injuries are predominately injuries to the extremities; however, most epidemiological studies also include data concerning bone and muscle injuries of the trunk and neck. Musculoskeletal injuries are the most common type of trauma seen in hospitals in the United States. The National Center for Health Statistics (NCHS) reported that in the 1991 National Hospital Discharge Survey, the most common injury and diagnosis at time of inpatient hospital discharge was fracture, representing 37% of all patients.[5] A staggering 53% of all reported injuries in the National Health Interview Survey (NHIS) from 1985 to 1988 involved the musculoskeletal system with an incidence of 13.8 per 100 persons.[6,7] Of these injuries, sprains and dislocations

accounted for 44.7%, followed by open wounds (28.9%), fractures (18.8%), and crushing injuries (0.9%).[6,7] Injuries are more common in males and reach a peak incidence of 20.7 per 100 persons in the 18–44 age group.[6,7] Overall, the incidence of fractures is 2.6 per 100 persons.[6,7] Fractures are more common in males than females under 44 years of age, but there is a dramatic reversal in the trend after that point. In the elderly aged 85 and over, fractures are four times more common in females, with an incidence of 6.4 per 100 persons.[6,7] Like all injuries, the most common place of occurrence for musculoskeletal trauma is at home, followed by industrial sites. For multiple trauma patients, 83% will have MSI, with over half of these patients sustaining two or more musculoskeletal injuries.[8] For patients admitted to trauma centers for skeletal injuries, the most common cause is (MVCs).[9]

ANATOMY AND PHYSIOLOGY

The musculoskeletal system is comprised of bones (206) and their joints, skeletal muscles, nerves, tendons, ligaments, and blood vessels. The bones work with the body's tissues to allow movement, while forming a supportive and protective framework for the body. In addition, bone marrow produces red blood cells (erythropoiesis) and some white blood cells, and stores/releases calcium and phosphorus.

The bones of the upper extremity include the clavicle (collarbone), scapula (shoulder blade), humerus (arm), radius and ulna (forearm), carpals (wrist), metacarpals (hand), and phalanges (fingers). The head of the humerus articulates with the scapula at its proximal end and the radius and ulna at its distal end (Figure 15-1).

The **olecranon process** is the prominent bony projection of the ulna that may be felt medially at the elbow. The distal end of the ulna articulates with the bones of the wrist and the radius. Associated neurovascular structures of the upper extremities include the subclavian, axillary, brachial, radial, median, and ulnar arteries (Figures 15-2A and B). The nerves are the axillary, radial, median, and ulnar. These nerves branch from the brachial plexus and include both sensory and motor function (Figure 15-2C).

The lower extremities are divided into the pelvis, upper leg, lower leg, and foot. The bones of the pelvis are the ilium, ischium, and pubis (Figure 15-3). The superior portion of the ilium is known as the iliac crest. This crest begins anteriorly as the anterior-superior iliac spine and ends posteriorly as the posterior-superior iliac spine. On each side of the pelvis during development, these three bones fuse together to form the **coxae** (or hip bones). The coxae are joined to the body anteriorly by the pubic bones at the symphysis pubis, and the iliac

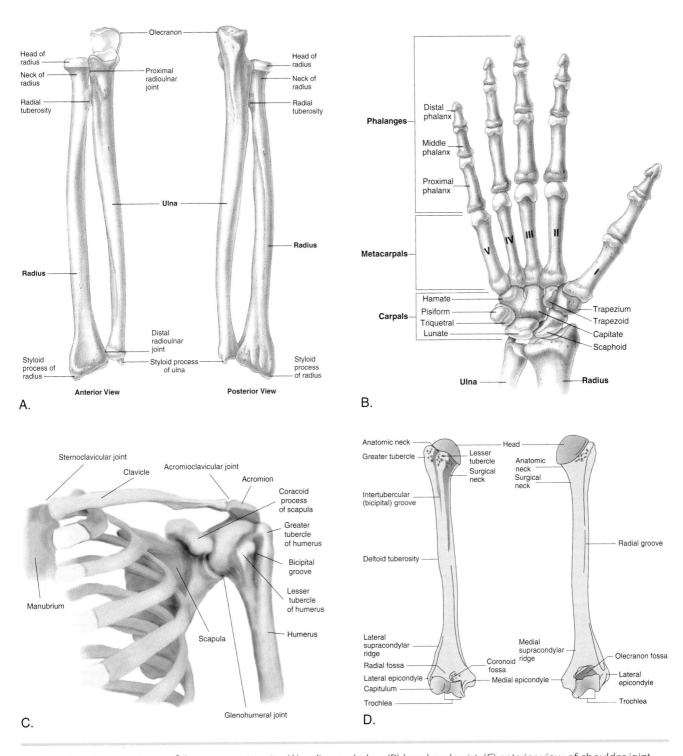

FIGURE 15-1 Bony anatomy of the upper extremity: (A) radius and ulna; (B) hand and wrist; (C) anterior view of shoulder joint; (D) humerus.

bones attach to the sacrum of the vertebral column posteriorly. A projection on the ischium known as the ischial tuberosity anchors the posterior thigh muscles and is used by field providers as the anchoring point for most types of traction splints. Each coxa has a fossa on the lateral surface known as the acetabulum. This is the loca-

tion at which the head of the femur articulates with the pelvis. The obturator foramen is a hole in the anterior portion of each coxa through which the neurovascular and muscular components of the lower extremity pass through the pelvis. The gluteal muscles (buttocks) are posterior to the pelvis, attaching to the femur. The pelvic

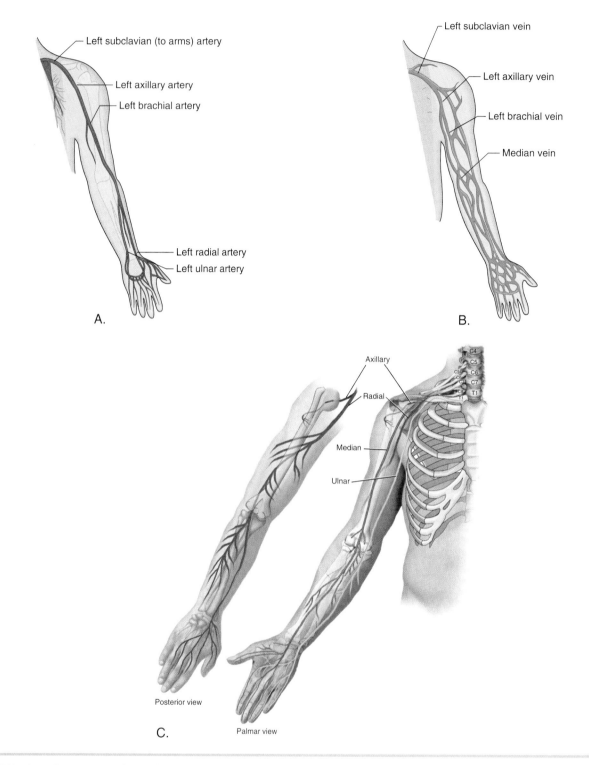

FIGURE 15-2 Nerves and vasculature of the upper extremity: (A) arteries; (B) veins; (C) nerves.

structure is designed to protect the intestine and large vessels that pass through it. Damage to the pelvic ring and its associated structures may provoke blood loss in excess of 3 liters.[10]

The bones of the upper leg include the femur and patella. Of all bones in the body, the femur is the longest. Its proximal portion has a prominent head that articulates with the pelvic acetabulum (Figure 15-4). The greater and lesser trochanters are tuberosities on the femoral shaft that serve as attachment sites for muscles that connect the hip to the thigh. The distal femur has the lateral and medial condyles that articulate with the patella and their tibial counterparts. The upper leg has some of the longest muscles in the body.

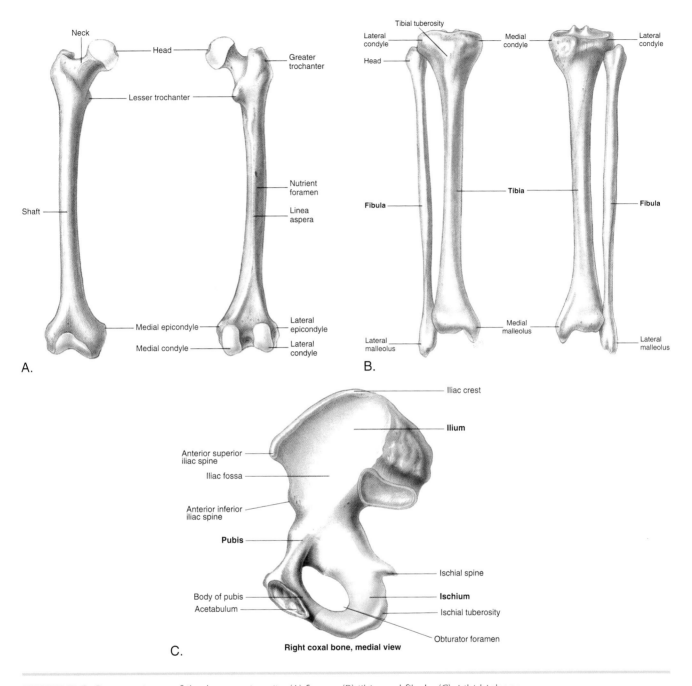

FIGURE 15-3 Bony anatomy of the lower extremity: (A) femur; (B) tibia and fibula; (C) right hipbone.

Femur fracture and damage to this musculature can lead to blood loss in excess of 1 liter.[11]

The tibia and fibula are the bones of the lower leg. The tibia is the larger and supports most of the weight. The distal end of the tibia ends in the medial malleolus, which forms the medial side of the ankle. The fibula, while not articulating with the femur, does articulate with the tibia, via its small proximal head. Distally, the fibula forms the lateral malleolus, giving shape to the lateral portion of the ankle.

The foot is formed of the tarsal bones (talus, calcaneus, navicular, cuboid, and three cuneiform bones), the metatarsals, and the phalanges (Figure 15-5). The talus is the articulation surface for the tibia and fibula. The calcaneus (heel) is inferior to the talus and serves as the attachment for the muscles of the calf. The remainder of the bones are supporting structures for the foot in much the same composition as those of the hand.

Associated neurovascular structures of the lower extremities include the abdominal aorta and femoral, popliteal, and anterior/posterior tibial arteries. The nerves include the sciatic, tibial, and peroneal (Figure 15-6).

Joints are of several types:

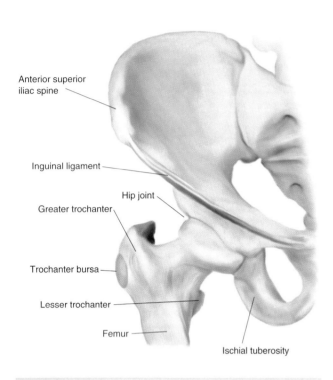

control) with light and dark colorings known as striations and are enclosed in a layer of connective tissue known as fascia. While tendons connect muscle to bone, another connective tissue, ligament, connects bone to bone.

While the skeletal muscles comprise the bulk of musculoskeletal soft tissue, nerves, tendons, ligaments, and blood vessels add to both this mass and the complications that can ensue in musculoskeletal trauma.

INTERNET ACTIVITIES

Visit the University of North Carolina School of Medicine Web site and view the videos on gross anatomy of the extremities. The site addresses are http://oisvideo2.med.unc.edu/ga/gathigh.ram (a 27-minute anatomy review of the thigh), http://oisvideo2.med.unc.edu/ga/galegreview.ram (a 14-minute anatomy review of the leg), and http://oisvideo2.med.unc.edu/ga/gabrachplex.ram (a 36-minute review of the arm and brachial plexus).

FIGURE 15-4 Anatomy of the hip joint.

- Ball and socket joint — shoulder, acetabulum (hip)
- Hinge — elbow, knee
- Gliding (plane) — vertebrae
- Saddle — carpal, metacarpal
- Minimal rotation (or ellipsoid) — sacroiliac
- Pivot — atlas, axis

Skeletal muscles attach to bones by tendons. These muscles form the largest mass of muscle tissue in the body. These are voluntary muscles (conscious

ASSESSMENT

In the multiple trauma patient, extremity and orthopedic injuries are not evaluated or treated until the initial

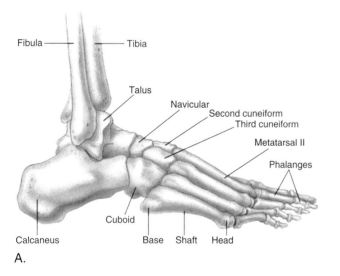

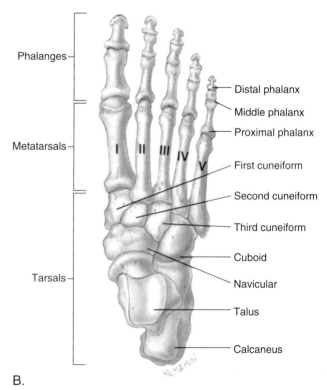

FIGURE 15-5 Anatomy of the foot: (A) lateral view; (B) superior view.

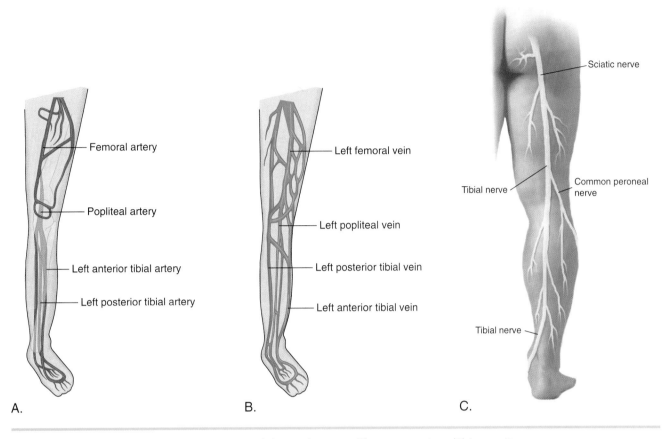

A. B. C.

FIGURE 15-6 Neurovascular structure of the leg: (A) arterial system; (B) venous system; (C) innervation.

assessment has been completed and all life-threatening injuries stabilized.

HISTORY

The chief complaint and mechanism of injury are sufficient to predict most extremity injuries. When these are combined with a careful history and physical examination, including degree of pain and neurovascular changes, the radiographic findings for orthopedic injuries can be predicted with a high degree of accuracy.[12] Specific historical information obtained should include patient position on arrival; details about the mechanism of injury, such as the amount of force applied and the mechanism of forces involved, including the amount and/or speed, weight, and distance of fall; whether the mechanism of force was direct, indirect, or rotational; the age of the patient; and the history of current symptoms and preexisting medical conditions.

PHYSICAL EXAMINATION

Evaluation of the extremities in the field is dependent on both patient symptomatology and physical examination of their circulation, sensory/motor function, and skeletal/joint function. The basic physical examination elements of inspection, palpation, and auscultation are used to assess extremity injuries. Most importantly for field evaluation, the patient must be assessed for neurological and vascular function distal to the injury.

The patient should have all clothing surrounding potential injuries removed. The safest method to gain visual access without aggravating potential injuries is to cut the clothing from the extremity. This will allow an adequate visual inspection for deformities, angulations, swelling, edema, and discoloration. The extremity should then be palpated for defects, deformities, tightness, crepitus, and point tenderness. The distal pulses, capillary refill, and skin temperature should be assessed and recorded. Neurological status for distal sensory and motor function should be assessed. In the emergency department, range of motion and joint stability will be assessed by a physician. While these last two elements are important parts of the physical examination, it is best to defer these assessments for a more controlled environment.

Circulation

Injury to the major blood vessels supplying the limbs can occur with penetrating or blunt trauma. Fractures can produce injury to the vessels by direct laceration or by stretching, which causes the vessel lining (intima) to sag. This can immediately occlude distal flow or can expose critical intimal cells leading to platelet aggregation and delayed occlusion. Because of this potential delay in occlusion, repeated examination of the circulatory function of the limb is mandatory until the patient is delivered to definitive care. Nail color and warmth of the skin of the distal extremity must be assessed and compared to the uninjured extremity. Distal pallor and asymmetric regional hypothermia could mean a vascular injury. Brachial, radial, and ulnar pulses should be evaluated when the upper extremities are involved. The lower extremities require assessment of the femoral, popliteal, posterior tibial, and dorsalis pulse sites. Blood loss and hypothermia tend to make pulses difficult to assess. In the field the pulse of obese individuals can also be difficult to evaluate; therefore temperature and color become key indicators. If available, auscultation of blood flow by Doppler is helpful. Auscultation for bruits is performed over major vessels and injury sites. Any suspected major arterial injury should be treated as a surgical emergency.

Sensory and Motor Function

Nerve function may be impossible to assess in an unconscious or uncooperative patient. Whenever possible, however, it is important to establish the status of nerve function in the distal extremity. Initial findings can then be periodically compared with additional examinations during transportation. Deteriorating neurological status of an extremity has important implications for definitive care of the patient.

Motor and sensory examinations should be carefully documented. It is important that the neuromuscular examination be performed prior to any manipulation or intervention.[13] For the upper extremity, all sensory and motor components of the brachial plexus should be evaluated. This is accomplished by examination of the six muscles and corresponding sensory areas listed in Table 15-1. Sensory function is assessed with regard to light touch and **two-point discrimination**, which is performed by placing the ends of two paper clips or other sharp instruments against the skin approximately 1 cm apart. The objects are then moved closer together until reaching a distance at which the patient can no longer differentiate between one and two points. Inability to discriminate between the two points down to a minimal distance is considered abnormal. Minimal distances are listed in Table 15-2. Muscle function should be assessed by observing active function and evaluating muscle strength against resistance. It is not necessary for the patient to fully abduct or adduct the extremity; rather the examiner palpates the muscle groups as the patient

pushes against resistance.[13] This is much more comfortable for the patient.

Sensory testing of the hand can be done using light touch and two-point discrimination (described above). However, it is important to test radial, ulnar, and median nerves as all three provide sensory innervation of the hand (Figure 15-7). Similarly, motor testing should evaluate all three nerves. To test the ulnar nerve, the patient is asked to forcefully spread the fingers against resistance while palpating the first dorsal interosseus muscle on the radial side of the index finger (Figure 15-8). Motor function of the radial nerve is assessed by asking the patient to extend the wrist against resistance (Figure 15-9). Various testing methods are possible for evaluating the median nerve, including opposing the thumb to the small finger,

Table 15-1
Sensory and Motor Components of the Brachial Plexus

Nerve	Muscle	Sensory Area
Axillary	Deltoid	Lateral arm
Suprascapular	Shoulder external rotation	Lateral forearm (variable)
Musculocutaneous	Biceps	
Radial	Thumb interphalangeal extensor	
Median	Index finger flexor	Index fingertip
Ulnar	Interossei	Little fingertip

Source: Szalay EA, Rockwood CA. Injuries of the shoulder and arm. *Emerg Med Clinics North Am.* 1984; 2:279.

Table 15-2
Minimal Distances of Two-Point Discrimination

Location	Minimal Distance (MM)
Fingertips	2–8
Toes	3–8
Palm of hand	8–12
Chest	40
Forearms	40
Back	40–70
Upper arms	75
Thigh	75

Source: Malasanos L. *Health Assessment,* 4th ed. St. Louis, MO: CV Mosby Co.; 1989.

Radial nerve
Median nerve
Ulnar nerve

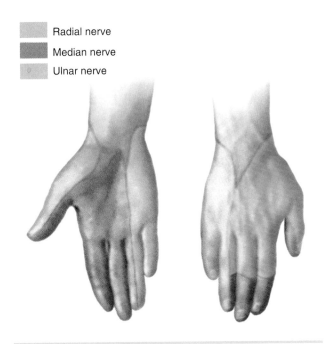

FIGURE 15-7 Sensory innervation of the hand.

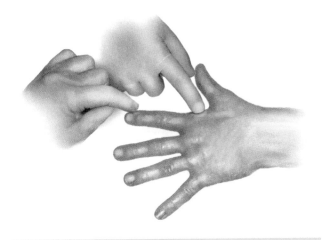

FIGURE 15-8 Ulnar nerve test. Abduction of fingers against resistance.

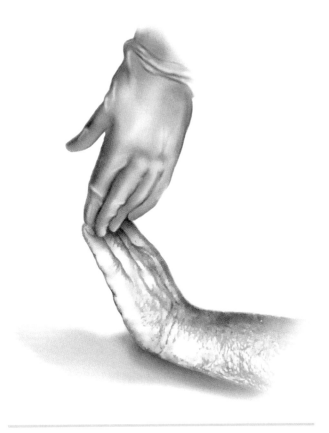

FIGURE 15-9 Radial nerve test. Extension of wrist and fingers against resistance.

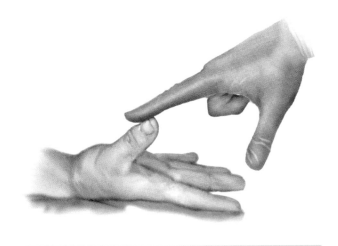

FIGURE 15-10 Median nerve test. Abduction of thumb against resistance.

forming a circle with the thumb and index finger, and laying the dorsum of the hand on a flat surface and asking the patient to palmar abduct the thumb against resistance (Figure 15-10).

Nerve testing of the lower extremity should include the femoral nerve and the sciatic nerve and its major branches (peroneal, saphenous, and tibial nerves). Injury to the femoral nerve will result in marked weakness of knee extension, though some extension of the knee against gravity is possible.[14] Sensory testing of this nerve is performed slightly superior and medial to the patella. Sciatic nerve injury results in varying degrees of paresis or paralysis of the hamstring muscles and the muscles distal to the knee and sensory loss of the posterior thigh and most of the leg distal to the knee. If spinal cord injury is a potential complication, the presence or absence of the Babinski reflex (dorsiflexion of the great toe) should be noted.

SKELETAL FUNCTION

The long bones of the lower extremity serve as the two structural supports for locomotion. Those of the upper extremity stabilize the soft tissues, which allow positioning of the hand in space. An angulated deformity should alert the examiner to the existence of a fracture; appropriate splinting should be performed after the limb is aligned with axial traction. Palpable crepitus confirms the diagnosis. Other than noting the degree and orientation of the limb's position when the victim is found, there is no reason to delay aligning and splinting fractures. Making the distinction between joint injuries and intra-articular or very proximal or distal fractures is difficult for even the experienced practitioner and must wait until the patient arrives at a definitive care facility. Similarly, distinguishing a ligamentous injury from a fracture of the wrist or ankle is difficult. Since the field care of these classes of injuries is identical, knowledge of the exact injury is not required for treatment in the field.

JOINT FUNCTION

Muscle forces act across the joints to improve the position of the lower limbs for ambulation and of the hand for manipulating objects. Each joint has a certain minimum function that allows stability and normal range of motion. Making the diagnosis of a joint injury in the field allows appropriate splinting and prevents further damage during transport.

Palpation of the long bones should begin distally and proceed across all joints. Palpable crepitus at the joint level requires that the joint be splinted. If the situation allows and the patient is able, the examiner should request that the patient move every joint through an active range of motion. This will focus the examination on the location of the injury. When this is not possible, passive motion at each joint can be evaluated after palpation of the joint for crepitus and swelling. Crepitus, swelling, deformity, or decreased range of motion necessitates the application of a splint. If the joint is dislocated, depending on local protocol, it should be promptly reduced following completion of the neurocirculatory examination. Reduction of the joint will relieve the patient's discomfort considerably. Remember that joints with associated fractures are frequently unstable after reduction. Particularly in these circumstances or if reduction cannot be accomplished, consideration should be given to splinting the involved joint to prevent additional swelling or repeated dislocation. Details of the reduction maneuver, including orientation of the pull, amount of force involved, degree of patient sedation, and residual instability of the joint, should be reported to the emergency department physician and clearly documented by the paramedic.

EMERGENCY DEPARTMENT

Additional evaluations in the emergency department will include radiographic examinations, special imaging studies, and possible joint aspiration. Radiographic evaluations will typically involve at least two views for evaluating fractures, dislocations, and foreign bodies. Special imaging studies may include computerized tomography (CT), which is particularly good for assessing fracture displacement and articular surfaces, and magnetic resonance imaging (MRI), which can assess ligaments and other soft tissue structures. Vascular imaging studies are employed when major vascular injury is suspected. Although rarely indicated when a patient presents with a clear history of trauma, joint fluid can be aspirated for examination.

INTERNET ACTIVITIES

Visit the University of North Carolina School of Medicine Web site at http://oisvideo2.med.unc.edu/mpac/muscneuroex.ram and view the video on physical examination of the extremities. This 22-minute video will play on your computer screen. You must have the RealPlayer media applicaton installed on your computer. If you do not have this program, it is available free of charge at http://www.real.com.

PATHOPHYSIOLOGY

AMPUTATIONS

Extremity amputations are infrequently seen but do have the potential to be life-threatening injuries. Usually the mechanism causing an amputation has enough force to cause multisystem trauma and/or serious hemorrhage. While direct pressure over the bleeding stump may be required, tourniquet application is a rare necessity. The torn/sheared blood vessels usually spasm and retract into the stump, tamponading the blood flow. The amputated part is usually viable for reimplantation from 14–18 hours postinjury. The best out-of-hospital method of preserving viable body parts is to surround the amputated tissue in a damp (not wet) saline gauze and place it in a plastic bag and then place that bag on ice.[15] However, the amputated tissue must not be allowed to freeze or suffer frostbite. The amputated part should accompany the victim to the hospital when possible, but transport of severely injured patients should not be delayed while making an exhaustive search for an amputated part. Instead, the patient should be promptly transported while other rescuers locate and transport the amputated tissue.

INTERNET ACTIVITIES

Visit the e-medicine Web site at http://www.emedicine.com. Click on the Emergency Medicine on-line book and select Trauma and Orthopedics. Then click on Replantation. Review the chapter on the replantation of amputated extremities.

COMPARTMENT SYNDROMES

A **compartment syndrome** exists when locally increased tissue pressure compromises local circulation and neuromuscular function. Compartment syndromes most frequently occur in association with crush injuries, fractures, electrical burns, snake bites, tight casts, and hematoma within a compartment.[15, 16] This syndrome can also occur when the victim has been lying for some time across a limb with the body weight occluding arterial blood supply. The prolonged use of the pneumatic/military antishock garment/trouser (PASG or MAST) has been associated with compartment syndrome by prolonging muscle ischemia.[17]

The lower leg and forearm are the most common sites for a compartment syndrome because tight fascia encase the muscle compartments in these regions and because these areas frequently suffer fractures or severe contusions. Compartment syndromes have also been described in the thigh, hand, foot, and gluteal regions.

The conscious patient complains of severe limb pain that seems out of proportion to the injury. The muscle compartment feels extremely tight and applied pressure, passive stretch, and active contraction increase the pain. The cooperative patient notes decreased sensation to light touch and pinprick stimuli in the areas supplied by the nerve(s) traversing the compartment. Most commonly this is noted on the dorsum of the foot in the first web space, caused by pressure affecting the deep peroneal nerve in the anterior compartment of the leg. Paresthesia and loss of distal pulses are late signs and portend a poor outcome.[15,16] These signs and symptoms are often capsulized as the "six P's of compartment syndrome" — pain, paresis, paralysis, puffiness, pallor, and pulselessness.

For optimum results, a compartment syndrome must be definitively treated in the first 6–8 hours after onset of this condition. Emergency fasciotomy, the treatment of choice, is performed to relieve the pressure, which can produce muscle and nerve cell death within 12 hours. Compartment syndrome is discussed in detail in Chapter 16.

CRUSH INJURY

Entrapment by a heavy object for several hours causes two crush injuries: local crush injury and systemic crush syndrome. **Local crush injury** occurs when weight is allowed to push on tissue for hours, crushing the musculoskeletal structure. Removing the weight off the patient is the goal, but often the local damage has already occurred.

Systemic crush syndrome occurs when muscle tissue disintegrates and myoglobin, potassium, and phosphorus leak into the circulation. It seems to develop once reperfusion of the area occurs. Crush syndrome then provokes hypovolemic shock, hyperkalemia, and eventual renal failure. Prehospital treatment centers around forcing diuresis by infusing 500 mL of intravenous fluid per hour and administration of sodium bicarbonate[18] (see Chapter 16).

DISLOCATIONS AND SPRAINS

A dislocation is derangement of the normal articulation of bones at the joint space. Sprains, or ligament injuries, are categorized into three grades. A first-degree sprain involves partial disruption of some of the ligament fibers with mild interior hemorrhage, but the joint remains stable and range of motion is normal. Second-degree injury involves complete disruption of some portion of the ligament fibers with moderate hemorrhage, but the joint remains stable. Third-degree sprain consists of complete disruption of the ligament fibers, marked disability, and usually an unstable joint. The various dislocations of the extremities are discussed below and summarized in Table 15-3.

Sternoclavicular Joint

The sternoclavicular joint is one of the least frequently injured joints in the body, accounting for only 1% of all dislocations.[19] The usual mechanism of injury is MVCs or sports injuries involving significant force. Anterior dislocations result from anterolateral forces applied to the shoulder while posterior dislocations result either from a direct blow to the medial clavicle or from a posteriolateral blow to the shoulder.[19] Although posterior dislocations account for only 10% of sternoclavicular dislocations, when present, they are frequently associated with life-threatening chest injuries.[20]

Patients present with the injured extremity supported tightly against the body and complaining of pain with movement or palpation of the joint. Anterior dislocations present with palpable deformity of the dislocated medial end of the clavicle, while the clavicular notch of the sternum may be palpated in posterior

Table 15-3
Common Dislocations

Body Area	Mechanism of Injury	Clinical Findings	Treatment
Shoulder Anterior	Fall on outstretched arm or direct impact on shoulder	Arm abducted; cannot bring elbow down to chest or touch opposite ear with hand	Splint in position of comfort; reduce as soon as possible
Posterior	Rare; strong blow in front of shoulder; result of violent seizures	Arm held at side, unable to externally rotate	As above
Elbow (radius and ulna)	Fall on outstretched hand with elbow in extension	Loss of arm length, painful motion, and rapid swelling; nerve lesions may occur	As above. Surgical repair if dislocation is associated with fracture to radial head or olecranon.
Radius head (children)	Pulled or nursemaid's elbow due to sudden pull, jerk, or lift on child's wrist or hand	Pain, refusal to use arm; limited supination; can flex and extend at elbow; may not be accompanied by deformity	Reduce, place in sling; advise parents that this may recur until age 5 years
Hip (usually posterior)	Blow to knee while hip is flexed and adducted (sitting with crossed knees); common in passengers seated in front seat	Hip flexed, adducted, internally rotated, and shortened; may have associated fracture of femur; sciatic nerve injury (lies posterior)	Splint in position of comfort; reduce as soon as possible
Patella	May be spontaneous	Knee flexed, can palpate patella lateral to femoral condyle	Reduce (may occur spontaneously); immobilize with cast or splint
	Associated with other trauma	Excessive swelling, tenderness, and palpable soft tissue defect	Surgical repair of soft tissue injury or fractures
Knee (rare)	Direct severe blow to upper leg or forced hyperextension of knee	Ligamentous instability (requires disruption of structures to occur); inability to straighten leg; peroneal nerve and popliteal artery injury common—must assess distal neurovascular function	Immediate neurovascular assessment; reduce
Ankle	Ankle is complex joint, with multiple ligaments providing stability; dislocation is usually associated with other injury such as fracture and soft tissue trauma	Swelling, tenderness, and loss of alignment and function	Splint; usually necessitates open reduction, as this joint has complex motion and must have accurate alignment

Source: Adapted from Emergency Nurses Association (ENA). *Emergency Nursing Core Curriculum.* 4th ed. ENA: 1994.

dislocations. Treatment of these injuries is best accomplished with a figure-eight splint (Figure 15-11).

Acromioclavicular Joint

Most acromioclavicular (AC) joint injuries or shoulder separations are the result of contact sports such as football and wrestling but may also result from MVCs and falls.[21] The mechanism typically involves a direct blow to the point of the shoulder or a fall on an outstretched hand. The force displaces the scapula downward and medial to produce the dislocation.[22] The presentation of AC joint dislocation varies considerably and is dependent upon the severity of damage to the AC and coracoclavicular ligaments.[21] Minor injuries present with mild tenderness and swelling, full range of motion, and no deformity. Severe injuries present with severe pain, deformity of the distal end of the clavicle, adduction of the arm close to the body, and a slumping shoulder.[22] Deformity of the joint can best be appreciated with the patient in a seated or standing position (Figure 15-12).[22] The AC joint separation should be immobilized with a sling and swathe.

Glenohumeral Joint

The glenohumeral joint (shoulder) is the most frequently dislocated major joint in the body, accounting for over 50% of major joint dislocations.[23] The glenohumeral joint can dislocate anteriorly, posteriorly, inferiorly, or superiorly (Figure 15-13). Anterior dislocations account for up to 97% of all glenohumeral dislocations, with posterior dislocations accounting for the bulk of the remainder; inferior and superior dislocations are extremely rare.[13,20] Glenohumeral separations, regardless of type, should be initially immobilized using a sling and swathe.

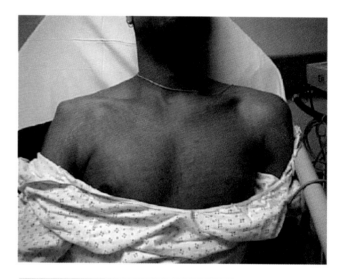

FIGURE 15-12 Acromioclavicular dislocation.

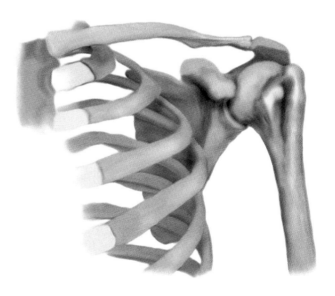

A.   **Normal Glenohumeral Anatomy**

FIGURE 15-13 Types of glenohumeral dislocation: (A) normal anterior, (1) subcoracoid, (2) subglenoid, (3) subclavicular, (4) intrathoracic; (B) posterior; (C) inferior. *(continues)*

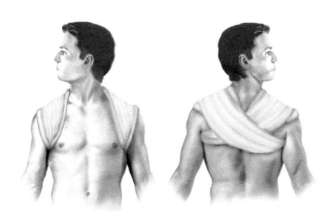

FIGURE 15-11 Figure-eight splint.

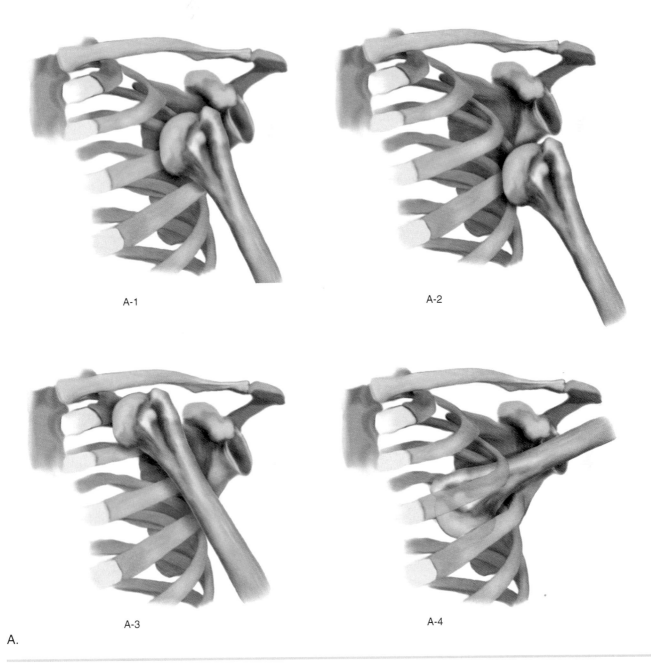

A-1   A-2

A-3   A-4

A.

FIGURE 15-13 (continued) Types of glenohumeral dislocation: (A) anterior, (1) subcoracoid, (2) subglenoid, (3) subclavicular, (4) intrathoracic.

Anterior dislocations may result from indirect or direct forces, typically those sustained by young individuals participating in athletics or older patients who fall on an outstretched arm.[24] The patient presents with severe pain with the arm abducted and externally rotated. The victim will generally have an absence of normal shoulder contour and an inability to move the shoulder joint. The acromion process is prominent and the anterior shoulder appears full. Neurovascular assessment is paramount as brachial plexus, axillary nerve, axillary artery, or radial nerve damage occurs in

up to 12% of anterior dislocations. Anterior shoulder instability recurs in 30%–50% of individuals.[25]

Posterior dislocations typically result from a fall onto an outstretched arm held in flexion, adduction and internal rotation, or occasionally a direct blow.[20,26] Nearly all posterior dislocations result in the humeral head assuming a subacromial position, but subglenoid and subspinous positions are also possible.[27] The patient presents with severe pain, adduction and internal rotation of the affected limb, prominent acromion and coracoid processes, and an abnormal shoulder contour.[20] The

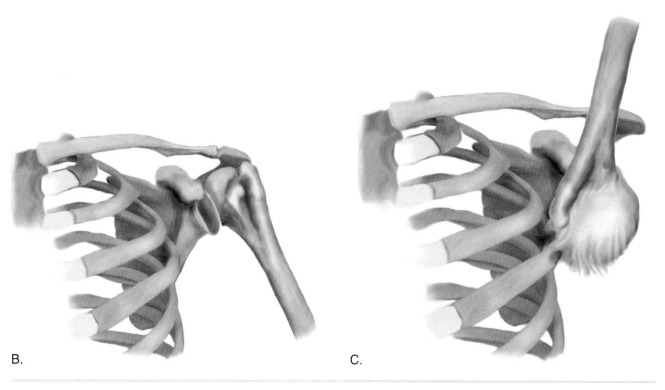

B.

C.

FIGURE 15-13 (continued) Types of glenohumeral dislocation: (B) posterior; (C) inferior.

patient will not allow external rotation or abduction because of pain.[28] The humeral head may also be palpable below the acromion process posteriorly.[20] Neurovascular injuries are less frequent with posterior dislocations than with other glenohumeral dislocations.

Inferior glenohumeral dislocations are rare, accounting for less than 0.5% of all shoulder dislocations.[29] The usual mechanism is an indirect force that thrusts the humeral head below the inferior rim of the glenoid fossa. The patient presents with the arm locked overhead, typically with elbow flexed and the hand either on or behind the head.[28] This injury is frequently accompanied by neurovascular and soft tissue damage.

Elbow

Dislocations of the elbow occur from a fall on an outstretched hand with the arm abducted or extended. The vast majority of these dislocations are posterior, although anterior, medial, or lateral dislocations are possible (Figure 15-14). Up to 40% of elbow dislocations are associated with fractures of adjacent bony structures.[30] The examination will show an elbow locked in moderate flexion (45°) with shortening of the forearm and marked prominence of the olecranon.[31] Perform a careful examination of the distal sensory, motor, and circulatory status as injury to the brachial artery, ulnar nerve, or median nerve occurs in up to

21% of patients.[31] A padded board or wire ladder splint should be applied to the arm in the position found, if distal sensation/circulation is intact.

Radiocarpal Joint

Radiocarpal (wrist) dislocations may be accompanied by carpal fractures. This injury typically occurs as a result of falling on a dorsiflexed wrist, although falls onto a palmar flexed wrist are also possible. Virtually every bone in the wrist is palpable, and tenderness and swelling suggest fracture, dislocation, or soft tissue injury in that region.[32] Neurovascular assessment is crucial because the radial and ulnar arteries and median, ulnar, and radial nerves all lie superficial and can easily be injured. A padded board splint, wire ladder splint, or pillow splint should be applied. Follow up with a sling and swathe.

Hip

Hip dislocations account for 10%–15% of all dislocations.[33] In the normal, adult hip, tremendous force is required to dislocate the femoral head from the acetabulum. The majority of these are sustained in MVCs. Other mechanisms include displacement of hip prostheses and athletic injuries where dislocations can occur with even minimal force.

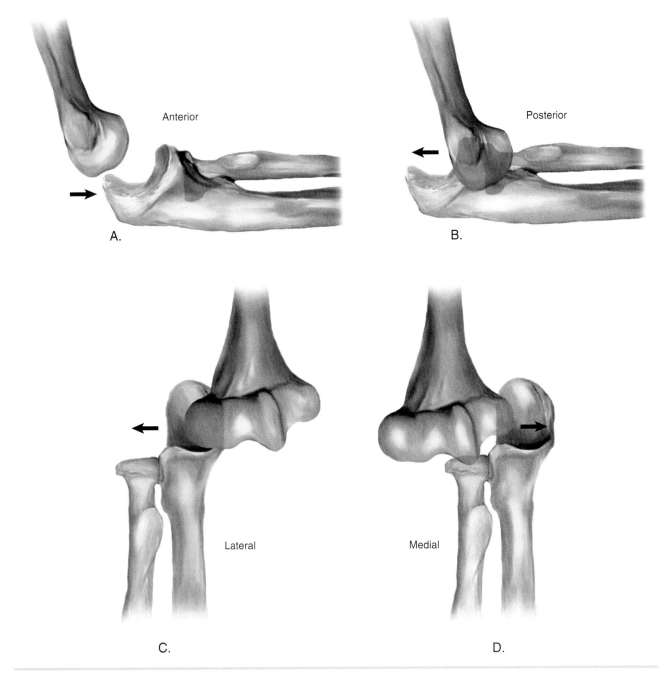

FIGURE 15-14 Types of elbow dislocations: (A) anterior; (B) posterior; (C) lateral; (D) medial.

Posterior dislocations account for 80%–90% of hip dislocations.[33] The most common mechanism is MVCs, where the knees of the unrestrained occupant strike the dashboard pushing the head of the femur posteriorly through the joint capsule (Figure 15-15). The classic presentation is a shortened, flexed, adducted, and internally rotated extremity. Up to 50% of these injuries are accompanied by fractures and 15% result in sciatic nerve injury.[33] Depending upon which nerve fibers are involved, the patient may be unable to flex the knee or may exhibit decreased sensation on the posterolateral leg and sole of the foot.[34]

Anterior dislocations are classified as superior iliac, superior pubic, and inferior obturator, depending on the final position of the femoral head (Figure 15-16).[34] In both superior iliac and superior pubic dislocations, the femoral head rests anterolaterally and superiorly, resulting in external rotation and abduction of the extremity with slight flexion.[33,34] The femoral head is palpable in the area of the anterosuperior iliac

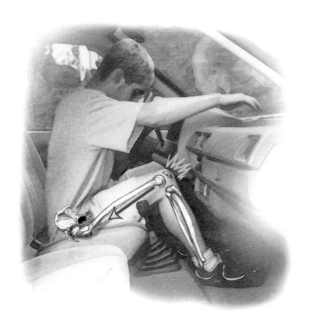

FIGURE 15-15 Posterior hip dislocation resulting from dashboard impact.

spine in the iliac type or below the femoral artery in the pubic type of dislocation.[34] Involvement of the femoral artery or nerve may result in decreased quadriceps function, knee-jerk reflex, sensation of the anteromedial thigh, and peripheral pulses.[34]

Treatment of hip dislocations includes placing the patient supine to perform a complete assessment of the body, remembering that substantial forces are required to dislocate the hip and other, more serious injuries

may be present. In the absence of life-threatening injuries, the distal limb should be carefully examined for appropriate neurovascular condition and associated fractures. Splinting should immobilize the victim in the position found. This splinting may utilize blankets or pillows between the legs so as to secure them together as comfortably as possible. Another alternative splinting technique is to use a Kendrick Extrication Device (KED).™ This extrication vest is placed on the abdomen with the head/neck portion placed on the upper thigh of the affected extremity. The buckles normally secured around the chest are secured around the abdomen. The portion of the splint normally used for head and neck immobilization is then secured around the thigh of the hip that has been dislocated.[35] As always, recheck neurovascular status after splinting to assure intact function.

Knee

The knee is a hinge joint with a range of motion of 0° in full extension to 130° of full flexion.[33] Because the joint is positioned between the upper and lower legs, which act as levers, the knee is prone to injury when subjected to even moderate amounts of energy. In addition, the knee is inherently unstable; all stability is provided by the ligaments surrounding the joint, making the knee even more susceptible to injury. Anterior and posterior stability is provided by the anterior and posterior cruciate ligaments while lateral stability is provided by the lateral and medial collateral ligaments (Figure 15-17).

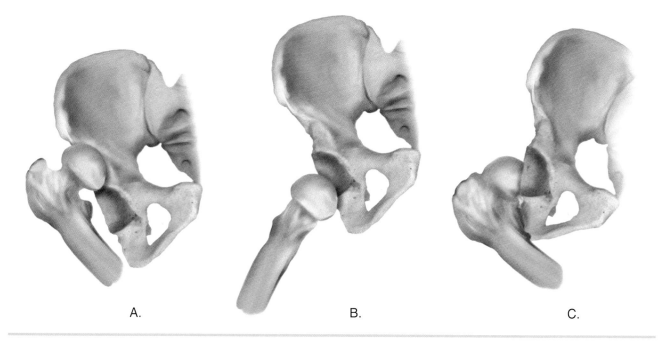

A.   B.   C.

FIGURE 15-16 Types of anterior hip dislocations: (A) superior iliac; (B) superior pubic; (C) inferior obturator.

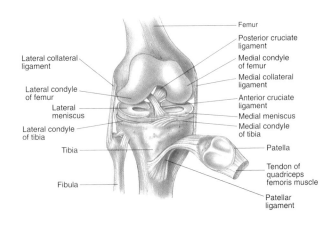

FIGURE 15-17 Ligaments of the knee.

Dislocation of the knee is one of the few true orthopedic emergencies owing to the high rate of associated vascular and nerve damage. Dislocations of the knee are described by the position of the tibia with respect to the femur, of which there are five types: anterior, posterior, medial, lateral, and rotatory (Figure 15-18). Of these, anterior and posterior dislocations account for 50%–60% of all knee dislocations.[36] Vascular damage occurs in approximately 40% of knee dislocations, and of these, one-half will eventually result in amputation.[36] The amputation rate associated with injury to the popliteal artery is higher than with injuries to any other artery, including the brachial artery.[36] This is because viability of the lower leg is vitally dependent upon the popliteal artery, even more so than the arm is dependent upon the brachial artery.[36]

Anterior dislocations are the most common, resulting from a hyperextension injury. Anterior dislocations result in tears to the posterior capsule and the posterior cruciate ligament. Posterior dislocations require much greater force than anterior dislocations and often result from a direct blow to the anterosuperior tibia with the knee in a flexed position, such as the knee striking the dashboard in an MVC.[36] Medial, lateral, and rotary dislocations require forces with varus (toward the midline), valgus (away from the midline), or rotary forces. Medial and lateral dislocations require severe direct forces applied to the distal femur or upper tibia. Medial dislocation is associated with varus forces that tear the cruciates and lateral ligaments while lateral dislocation occurs with valgus forces that tear the cruciates and medial ligaments.[37]

Patellar dislocations are more common in females than males because of the increased femorotibial angle in females. Dislocation of the patella may result from a twisting injury or asymmetric quadriceps contraction during a fall. These mechanisms routinely occur with energetic sports like running, hiking, and football. Neurovascular compromise is rare with this injury.

Treatment of knee dislocations should begin with a thorough history, including the type of activity immediately prior to the injury and the severity and direction of applied forces. Inspection of the knee should be accomplished while the patient is supine. This position relaxes the leg muscles, making findings more noticeable.[38] The knee should then be inspected for swelling, deformity, and ecchymosis. It should be noted that the lack of deformity does not rule out a dislocation due to

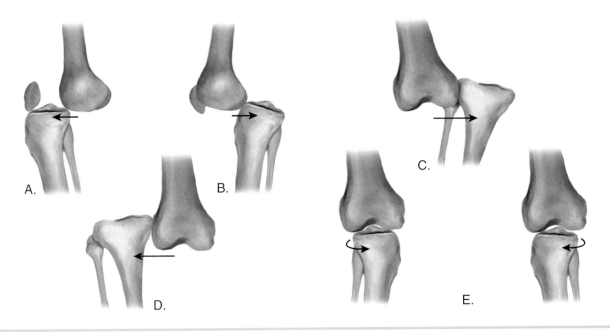

FIGURE 15-18 Types of knee dislocations: (A) anterior; (B) posterior; (C) medial; (D) lateral; (E) rotatory.

the high rate of spontaneous reduction in knee injuries. Inspection should be followed with a thorough palpation of the joint capsule and associated ligaments. A thorough evaluation of distal neurovascular function is essential, given the high incidence of concomitant neurovascular injuries. In general, knee dislocations should be splinted in the position found, unless distal circulation is absent, in which case the leg may be repositioned once in an effort to improve circulation. If transport times are long, field reduction should be attempted. This is accomplished with sedation followed by longitudinal traction of the lower leg with countertraction of the femur.[33,36] Following reduction, distal pulses and nerve function are reassessed and a splint applied with the leg at 15°–20° of flexion.

Medial Collateral Ligament Sprain

Medial collateral ligament (MCL) injuries usually result from a blow to the outer part of the knee such as sustained in contact sports. The valgus stress placed on the knee causes stretching or tearing of the MCL. The patient will complain of medial knee pain and joint instability. Physical examination may reveal tenderness, swelling, and pain and/or instability with valgus stress. To test the MCL for instability, firmly grasp the ankle and the knee and apply opposing forces (medial against the knee and lateral against the ankle) while palpating and visualizing the medial joint space (Figure 15-19). A gap in the joint space or a "clunk" heard when the opposing forces are relieved indicates an MCL injury. The clunk is the sound of the tibia and femur coming together due to a lack of MCL support as they close.[39]

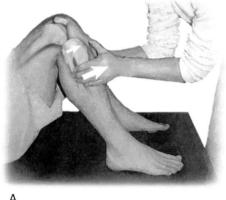

A.

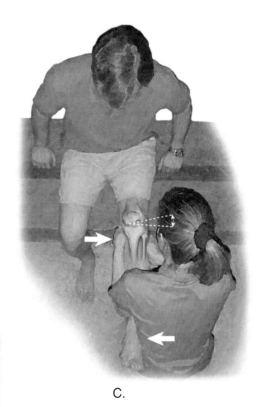

C.

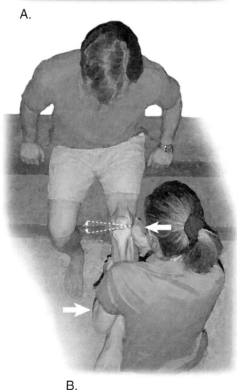

B.

FIGURE 15-19 Testing of (A) ACL, (B) MCL, and (C) LCL.

Lateral Collateral Ligament Sprain

The lateral collateral ligament (LCL) is rarely injured, but when injured, often results from varus stress. The patient will complain of tenderness over the head of the fibula with lateral instability. To test the LCL, reverse the hand position used for the MCL test to open the knee joint on the lateral side (Figure 15-19). Palpate the lateral joint line for gaps and observe for clunking of the femur and tibia as varus stress is released and the joint space closes.[39]

Posterior Cruciate Ligament Sprain

Posterior cruciate ligament (PCL) trauma is usually the result of sports-related injuries or MVCs and is usually accompanied by injury to other ligaments of the knee. Isolated injury to the PCL may occur, however, during a fall onto a flexed knee or a dashboard injury to a flexed knee.[40] Hyperextension of the knee may tear the PCL, but only after the ACL has been disrupted.[33] The patient will complain of posterior knee pain and may walk with the knee flexed slightly to avoid terminal extension of the joint. Ecchymosis and swelling may be observed in the posterior popliteal space. To test the PCL, place the leg in a flexed position with an assistant holding the foot flat against the ground. Firmly grasp the knee below the patella and push the tibia backwards. If the tibia slides backward on the femur, the PCL is probably damaged.[41]

Anterior Cruciate Ligament Sprain

The anterior cruciate ligament (ACL) is the most commonly injured ligament of the knee, occurring predominantly as a result of noncontact sports where an athlete is running, plants his or her foot, and then cuts in the opposite direction or where a ski binding fails to release during a fall while skiing. The patient may note a "pop" at the time of injury followed by severe instability of the joint. The injury is accompanied by varying degrees of pain as there are few pain fibers in the area. When present, pain will be located in the posterolateral area accompanied by immediate swelling. Testing of the ACL is similar to testing the PCL, except the direction of the force is reversed (Figure 15-19).

Treatment of ligament injuries of the knee is the same regardless of the specific ligament injured. The joint should be immobilized in the position found provided that distal neurocirculatory function is intact. Early ice application reduces swelling and provides some pain relief.

Meniscus Injury

The **menisci** are two semilunar cartilages in the capsule of the knee joint that act as shock absorbers, lubricate the joint, and more evenly distribute weight to the femoral condyles and the tibial plateau.[33] The medial meniscus is more frequently injured than the lateral meniscus. The typical injury mechanism is a twisting motion. Because of their limited vascular supply, an injured meniscus does not always heal well, even when repaired. If the meniscus must be removed or becomes avascular and degenerates, the articular surface contact forces will rise substantially, leading to degenerative changes in the joint.

The patient will complain of medial or lateral joint line tenderness with exacerbation of pain at the extremes of normal knee motion. Often, swelling is delayed and the joint remains stable, prompting many athletes to continue to play following the injury.[39] If the meniscus is severely torn and becomes incarcerated within the joint space, the knee is locked in position with severe limitation of flexion and extension.

Ankle

Ankle dislocations are almost always accompanied by fractures of both malleoli. These dislocations generally occur with falls on uneven surfaces or during twisting injuries. Dislocations are of four types: posterior, anterior, upward, and lateral (Figure 15-20). The area about the ankle should be carefully observed for open injuries. A baseline neurocirculatory examination should be conducted in conjunction with the detailed assessment. The ankle joint should then be splinted with a posterior splinting device such as a Velcro, pillow, or vacuum splint. During transport the limb should be elevated above the level of the heart.

Ankle sprain is one of the most common musculoskeletal injuries. The medial ligament complex consists of the deltoid ligament, which runs from the medial mallets to the talus (Figure 15-21). The ligament complex on the lateral side consists of three separate ligaments: the calcaneofibular ligament, the anterior talofibular ligament, and the posterior talofibular ligament. The lateral ligament complex is the most frequent site of an inversion injury. The examination of the site should include palpation of each ligament for tenderness and the anterior drawer test [Stabilize the tibia with one hand and grasp the posterior heel, pulling the foot forward with the other hand (Figure 15-22). If the talus slides forward, the injury may be presumed to be a grade 3 disruption.] Splint the foot and ankle with an air, pillow, vacuum, or Velcro splint. If there is no instability, the joint may be properly immobilized with an elastic bandage or taping.

Hindfoot

The subtalar joint may infrequently be dislocated in a significant fall or jump when an individual lands off balance or on an uneven surface. The calcaneus may be

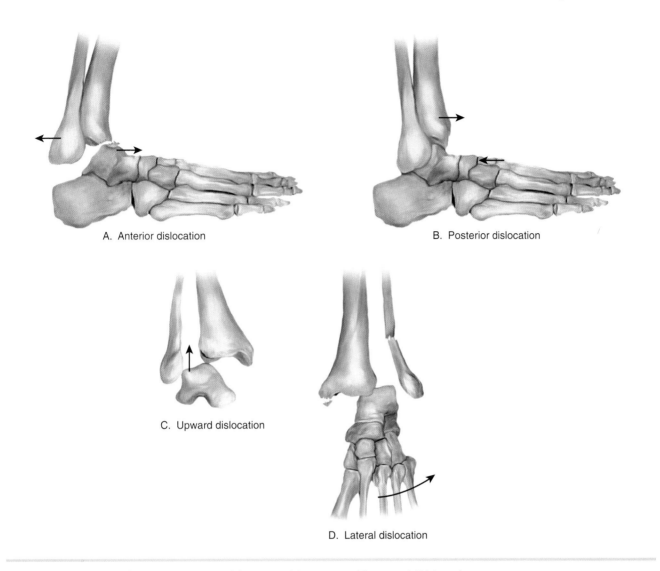

A. Anterior dislocation

B. Posterior dislocation

C. Upward dislocation

D. Lateral dislocation

FIGURE 15-20 Types of ankle dislocations: (A) anterior; (B) posterior; (C) upward; (D) lateral.

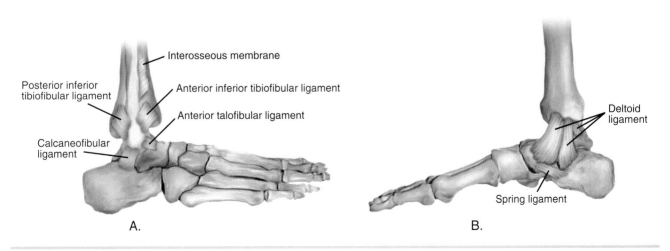

Interosseous membrane

Posterior inferior tibiofibular ligament

Anterior inferior tibiofibular ligament

Anterior talofibular ligament

Calcaneofibular ligament

Deltoid ligament

Spring ligament

A.

B.

FIGURE 15-21 Ankle ligaments: (A) lateral view; (B) medial view.

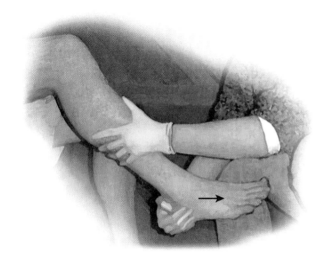

FIGURE 15-22 Anterior drawer test.

dislocated medially or laterally relative to the talus, the latter being slightly more common. The position of the heel relative to the ankle should be assessed. A posterior splint is applied and the leg elevated above the level of the heart.

Midfoot

Midfoot dislocations are generally associated with one or more fractures at the base of the metatarsals, most commonly the second and fifth metatarsals. Midfoot dislocations occur with axial loading of the foot in maximum plantar flexion. The forefoot is generally displaced laterally relative to the midfoot when the injury is initially unstable. More commonly the foot is normally aligned. There is significant swelling and tenderness at the base of the first, second, third, and fifth metatarsals. With dorsal-plantar-oriented force, instability and crepitus are frequently noted. If the forefoot is unstable and associated with significant swelling, pain, or crepitus, a midfoot dislocation is considered to be present. Short-leg-type splints are appropriate here, and the injured extremity should be elevated above the heart during transportation.

Toe

Metatarsophalangeal joint dislocations of the toes are uncommon but can occur in the large toe with moderate force. Crush injuries can produce this injury. Injuries of this type may be associated with fractures of the metatarsal or phalanx, but the dislocation is usually distal. The lesser metatarsophalangeal joints are generally dislocated laterally or medially. The most common mechanism for this injury is striking bare toes against immovable objects.

INTERNET ACTIVITIES

Visit the e-medicine Web site at http://www.emedicine.com. Click on the Emergency Medicine on-line book and select Trauma and Orthopedics. Then Click on Dislocation. Review the chapters on the management of various joint dislocations.

FRACTURES

In orthopedics, **fracture** is a nonspecific term used to describe a break involving bone or cartilage. Bone is a highly vascular tissue and all fractures will almost universally bleed, some to a greater extent than others. In conscious patients, fractures are almost always painful. Truly "occult" fractures are extremely rare. Physical signs and symptoms are almost always present, though they may be subtle even for the most astute clinician.[42] Sometimes deformity is obvious, particularly in bones that lie near the surface, such as the clavicle, wrist, and ankle.

A fracture may be closed or open. An **open fracture** is one that has a break in the skin that communicates with the fracture site. Although usually caused by the sharp edge of the fractured bone penetrating the overlying skin, a mechanism of injury causing external trauma (e.g., gunshot) may also be a causative factor. These types of injuries are generally treated as closed fractures, except that they are not usually realigned into a position of function. Splinting them as they lie is generally the best method to minimize additional wound contamination. Controlling active hemorrhage is an occasional necessity, as is covering the wound itself. There is detailed language specific to orthopedics to precisely describe these injuries. Table 15-4 lists the commonly used fracture terminology.

Fracture healing begins with a hematoma that bridges the bone ends, progresses to an inflammatory phase, and ends with remodeling. The rate of healing is affected by the type of bone (cancellous heals faster than cortical), degree of fracture, and systemic states such as hyperthyroidism and hypoxia. In addition to the damage to the bone itself, fractures have several associated complications. Because of the rich blood supply to the skeleton, fractures may result in significant hemorrhage, particularly fractures of the pelvis and femur (Table 15-5). Nerve injuries are also a frequent complication of fractures. In addition to these serious complications, other complications of fracture and immobility following fracture are possible (Table 15-6). Each type of fracture is discussed below and summarized in Table 15-7.

Scapula

The scapula is well protected by muscle and soft tissue and requires a great deal of force to fracture.

Table 15-4
Fracture Terms and Descriptions

Term	Description
Angulated	Loss of normal alignment along the long axis of the bone.
Avulsion	Fracture with fragment pulled away by ligament or muscle contraction.
Closed	Skin overlying the fracture is closed; no communication to outside environment. Also known as simple.
Comminuted	Fracture with more than two fragments.
Complete	Fracture line involves both cortices.
Displaced	Fracture with fragment moved from its normal anatomical position.
Greenstick	Incomplete fracture resulting from bending the bone.
Impacted	Fracture with forceful compression of bone fragments. Specific types include compressed, as seen in the vertebrae, and depressed, as seen in the skull.
Incomplete	Fracture line involves only one cortex.
Oblique	Fracture line occurs at oblique angle to long axis of bone.
Open	Fracture site communicates to outside environment by any manner. Also known as compound.
Pathological	Fracture involving diseased bone. Can occur with a relatively minor mechanism of injury.
Spiral	Fracture line spirals the shaft of the bone. Results from rotational injury.
Stress	Fracture that results from repeated, low-intensity trauma, such as marching.
Transverse	Fracture line occurs at right angle to long axis of bone.

Source: Geiderman J. Fractures. In: Hardwood-Nuss A, ed. *The Clinical Practice of Emergency Medicine.* Philadelphia: JB Lippincott; 1991.

Consequently, scapular injuries are relatively uncommon injuries, accounting for less than 1% of all fractures and usually occurring in young men.[43,44] The usual mechanisms of injury are falls, MVCs, or crush injuries.[45] One should be alert to other injuries, including injury to the chest wall, shoulder girdle, vertebrae, clavicle, and humerus, as well as pneumothorax, hemothorax, pulmonary contusion, and neurovascular injury. The mortality associated with scapular injury is 4%–10%.[44,45]

Table 15-5
Blood Loss by Fracture Site

Fracture	Associated Blood Loss (L)
Humerus	1.0–2.0
Elbow	0.5–1.5
Radius	0.25–0.5
Radius/ulna	0.5–1.0
Pelvis	1.5–4.0
Hip	1.5–2.5
Femur	1.0–2.0
Knee	1.0–1.5
Tibia and fibula	0.5–1.5
Ankle	0.5–1.5

Source: Chipman C, et al. Basic principles of emergency orthopedics. In: Chipman C, ed. *Emergency Department Orthopedics.* Rockville, Md: Aspen Publications; 1982.

Table 15-6
Complications of Fractures

Complications of Fractures
- Hemorrhage
- Nerve injuries
- Compartment syndrome
- Volkmann's ischemic contracture
- Avascular necrosis
- Reflex dystrophy
- Fat embolism

Complications of Immobility
- Pneumonia
- Deep venous thrombophlebitis
- Pulmonary embolism
- Urinary tract infection
- Wound infection
- Decubitus ulcers
- Muscle atrophy
- Stress ulcers
- Gastrointestinal bleeding
- Psychiatric disorders

Source: Geiderman J. Orthopedic injuries: management principles. In: Rosen P, et al, eds. *Emergency Medicine: Concepts and Clinical Practice,* 3rd ed. St Louis, Mo: Mosby; 1992.

Table 15-7
Common Fractures

Bone	Mechanism of Injury	Clinical Findings	Treatment
Humerus Neck	Fall on outstretched arm (may occur with dislocated shoulder)	Ecchymosis of shoulder, upper arm, and chest wall	Immobilize with sling; may splint or internally reduce if severe
Shaft	Direct trauma, twisting of arm	Radial nerve injury often occurs with fracture of lower third of bone	Immobilize with sling; use hanging arm cast if able to be mobile
Supracondylar	Fall on extended, outstretched arm (usually occurs in children)	Rapid swelling of elbow; pain	Admit to hospital for close neurovascular observation and definitive care
Radius Head	Fall on outstretched arm	Swelling; pain on lateral side of elbow; decreased range of motion in elbow; may have associated wrist injury	Immobilize; treatment varies according to range of motion and association with dislocated elbow
Shaft	Usually occurs with falls, altercations, and motor vehicle crashes	Pain along bone (bones are mostly subcutaneous, therefore easy to palpate)	Splint for comfort (tight muscular compartments and interosseous membrane provide stabilization against movement)
Distal	Colles' fracture (angulated dorsally)—fall on outstretched hand Smith's fracture (angulated toward volar surface)—fall on dorsum of hand	Distal fragment is deviated dorsally ("silver fork") Reverse of Colles' fracture	Immobilize with splint; reduce if displaced, cast
Radius—Galeazzi's fracture	Oblique fracture at junction of middle and distal thirds of radius with disruption of distal radio-ulnar joint—fall or blow on dorsal and lateral side of wrist and distal radius (commonly occurs in adults)	Wrist and radial shaft tenderness and shortening	Usually unstable; needs open reduction
Ulnar Monteggia's fracture	Fracture of proximal third of ulna with anterior dislocation of radial head	Pain and swelling around elbow, pain worse with attempts at rotation; radial dislocation may be missed if elbow not included in radiograph	Immobilize for comfort; closed reduction for children, open for adults
Nightstick fracture	Isolated fracture of midshaft of ulna as result of sharp blow	If ulna is angulated, injury to radius is also present	Immobilize; these fractures require 8–16 weeks to heal
Wrist—carpus (navicular)	Usually occurs with falls on outstretched hand or direct blow; common in young men whose strong muscles prevent injury to lower radius (navicular is longest of carpal bones)	Pain in wrist, most severe in anatomical snuff-box; swelling; radiographs should include oblique view	Immobilize; cast for at least 3 months to be sure fracture has reunited

(continues)

Table 15-7 (continued)

Bone	Mechanism of Injury	Clinical Findings	Treatment
Pelvis	Low velocity—elderly; high velocity—all age groups (MVC, falls, and crushing forces)	Hypovolemia—retroperitoneal space can hold 4 liters of blood; associated with multi-system trauma, especially genitourinary; tenderness with ilial wing compression or palpation of symphysis; ecchymosis (late sign) in flank and peritoneal area	Splint to immobilize; begin fluid resuscitation; evaluate for sacral spine injury and genitourinary injury
Femur			
Head or neck (intracapsular)	Due to fall or spontaneous break (osteoporosis)	Pain in hip or referred to knee; leg shortened and externally rotated	Splint for comfort; avoid traction splint; surgical care
Trochanter (extracapsular)	As above	Has greater blood supply, therefore blood loss is heavier	As above
Shaft	Associated with high force	Powerful muscle groups cause angulation and overriding to produce deformity; severe pain; major blood loss into tissue	Traction splint; admit for definitive care
Tibia			
Plateau (extends into knee joint)	Fall on extended leg, direct blow; rotation stress on extended leg (in pedestrians)	If radiographs are questionable or normal, may aspirate joint; usually associated with soft tissue injuries	Splint for comfort, compressive dressing; refer to orthopedist for definitive care
Shaft	Direct trauma—its position at distal end of leg exposes it to more trauma (e.g., car bumper); or rotation and leverage strain (as with stepping into deep hole while running); open fractures more common because bone is subcutaneous on its anterior and medial surfaces	Associated with fractures in rest of body (ipsilateral extremity or elsewhere); must determine if fibula is also fractured, as it acts as splint if intact. Prone to complications: (1) Increased incidence of compartment syndrome (tibia borders three of four myofascial compartments of lower leg) (2) Arterial injuries common with fractures of upper third	Splint for comfort
Fibula			
Proximal	Direct blow to side of leg	May have concomitant peroneal nerve injury	Splint
Shaft	As above	Considered minor	Symptomatic care
Distal	As above	Associated with ankle injuries	Splint
Ankle	Varies	Sprained ankles in children are uncommon	Splint; usually requires open reduction

Source: Adapted from Emergency Nurses Association (ENA). *Emergency Nursing Core Curriculum,* 4th ed. ENA: 1994.

Obvious deformity is usually lacking in scapular injuries due to the masking effect of the overlying soft tissue. Other than local signs of injury, such as ecchymosis, swelling, and tenderness, the patient will have difficulty raising the arm and some respiratory difficulty. Pain similar to that of pleurisy may also be present on the side of injury. The scapula can be splinted with a sling and swathe. Because spinal injury may also be a possibility with this injury, spinal immobilization may be indicated.

Clavicle

The clavicle is the most frequently fractured bone, accounting for 5% of all fractures. Fractures of the middle third of the clavicle are most common, accounting for 80% of all clavicular fractures,[46] and are usually the result of forces applied to the lateral aspect of the shoulder. Fractures of the lateral third result from a direct blow to the top of the shoulder and account for an additional 15% of clavicular fractures.[20] Fracture to the proximal third of the bone are relatively rare, accounting for only 5% of all clavicular fractures, and are typically associated with direct blows to the anterior chest.[20]

The patient presents with the affected extremity held close to the body with complaints of pain over the fracture site.[20] The pain will be increased with motion of the arm or shoulder. Gentle palpation should identify the location of tenderness and thus the fracture site. Crepitus at the clavicle strengthens the diagnosis. A thorough neurocirculatory examination of the affected extremity should be performed as brachial plexus or vascular injury may accompany the fracture. In addition, breath sounds should be evaluated for equality since clavicular fractures are associated with pneumothorax. Field treatment may utilize a sling and swathe combination, but a figure-eight bandage will often provide more pain relief once applied.

Humerus

Proximal humeral fractures account for 4%–5% of all fractures, occur primarily in older populations, and are the result of direct forces against the upper arm, axial loads transmitted through the elbow, or a high-velocity fall onto an outstretched and abducted arm.[19,47] These fractures are often difficult to differentiate from a shoulder dislocation. The patient typically presents with the arm held closely to the body. Pain with associated deformity and crepitus are the usual symptoms that confirm humeral fracture. The extremity should be splinted with a padded board splint on the posterolateral aspect of the upper arm. A sling and swath will

further immobilize the site while providing increased comfort. Complications of proximal humeral fractures include adhesive capsulitis ("frozen shoulder"), axillary artery injury, and injury to the axillary nerve or brachial plexus.[19,20]

Midshaft humeral fractures most often result from direct trauma from falls and motor vehicle collisions. Midshaft fractures usually have a greater degree of deformity than proximal fractures, with the deformity influenced by the location of the fracture. Fractures above the pectoralis major muscle cause the proximal fragment of the humerus to abduct and rotate. If the fracture occurs between the pectoralis major and the deltoid, the proximal fragments will adduct.[30] Other signs and symptoms include pain, diminished range of motion, and shortening or rotation of the arm depending on the displacement of the fracture fragments.[30] Midshaft humeral fractures have several immobilization options available: padded board or wire ladder splint applied with the elbow at 45° or 90° of flexion may be used as well as the Velcro or vacuum-type splints. If the board/wire ladder splint is used, a sling and swathe are necessary for adequate immobilization. Complications of this fracture include radial nerve injury, occurring in 15%–20% of humerus fractures, and vascular injury.[30]

Distal humeral fractures are usually the result of a fall on an outstretched hand or direct blow to the elbow. Depending on the location of the fracture, clinical presentation may include localized tenderness and swelling, exaggeration or absence of the normal olecranon prominence, abnormal positioning of the elbow, crepitus, pain, and diminished range of motion. As with other humeral injuries, neurovascular assessment is paramount. Immobilization is the same as for other humeral injuries.

Radius

Although MVCs and falls are the usual mechanisms of injury for these fractures, they are also seen in the setting of twisting injuries at industrial accidents. The typical etiology of injury is a direct blow to the forearm. Fractures of the radial shaft are usually located at the junction of the middle and distal thirds where the bone is relatively unprotected by surrounding musculature.[32] Fracture of the proximal two-thirds is relatively uncommon due to the protection afforded by the ulna and the surrounding musculature.[28] Fracture of the distal third of the radius is usually the result of a fall on an outstretched hand or a direct blow and is frequently associated with a radioulnar joint dislocation (**Galeazzi's fracture**).[28] Galeazzi's fracture requires open reduction and fixation.

A fracture involving the distal radius with dorsal displacement of the distal radius is referred to as **Colles' fracture** and is the most common fracture of the wrist. The injury mechanism is usually a fall on an outstretched hand that results in dorsiflexion of the wrist. The resulting deformity provides the "silver fork" deformity at the wrist that is pathognomonic of Colles' fracture.

The **Smith fracture**, sometimes referred to as a "reversed Colles' fracture," typically results from a direct blow to the dorsal surface of the hand while the hand is in a flexed position. The injury results in volar and proximal displacement of the distal fracture fragment.[32]

A radial head fracture generally is the result of a fall on an outstretched hand. Displacement of the radial head fragment suggests substantial forces were involved and increases the likelihood of injury to the surrounding soft tissues.[48] A fracture of the radial head will cause elbow pain with loss of full extension. Pain may be reproduced on the lateral side of the elbow with gentle pressure and rotation of the forearm.

Fractures of the radius are usually immobilized from the wrist to the elbow using a rigid splint followed by application of a sling and swathe. When necessary, a wire ladder splint may be substituted.

Ulna

Fractures of the proximal ulna (olecranon) occur as a result of a fall onto the posterior elbow. Pain, edema, and ecchymosis will usually be prominent on exam. The olecranon may have a palpable gap and an open fracture may be present. After the distal neurocirculatory examination is complete and examination of the shoulder and wrist has been performed, a splint similar to that for the radial fracture should be applied with the hand in a position of function.

An isolated ulnar shaft fracture's most frequent mechanism of injury is direct force applied to the shaft itself. Ulnar shaft fractures are most often associated with fractures of the radius at the same level. Pain, localized swelling, and crepitus are present. Any splint suitable for other forearm fractures will work well here. Again, splint with the hand in a position of function.

Carpal

Wrist (carpal) fractures occur because of significant rotational force or with falls onto the hand. Pain followed by swelling of the wrist with limited mobility will be the patient's chief complaint. Any use of the hand or rotation of the forearm will produce significant pain. A combination radial/ulnar fracture may also produce a fractured wrist with the classic silver fork deformity (Colles' fracture). Many fractures of the carpal bones are associated with wrist dislocations. A sling and swathe may be used along with a padded board/wire ladder splint or a pillow splint. Immobilize in the position found with a bulky hand dressing, such as a roll of gauze bandage.

Metacarpal

Fractures of the base or shaft of one or more metacarpals occur with crushing injuries or with direct blows when immovable objects are struck. Tenderness, crepitus, and occasionally deformity are present. These should be managed by taping to an adjacent uninjured finger and securing to a tongue blade or aluminum splint. If more than one digit is compromised, it may be more efficient to immobilize the entire hand on a padded board splint with a bulky dressing.

Phalanges

Fractures of the phalanges occur as a result of crush injuries or when the digits are caught in equipment. Deformity and crepitus make these fractures obvious. They should be immobilized by taping the injured digit to the neighboring uninjured digit or by taping the digit to a hand splint. Nailbed fractures or crushes should be cleaned and a dressing applied.

Injuries to the Pelvis

Fractures of the pelvis are generally associated with falls (30%) and vehicular trauma (60%).[49] Mortality from pelvic fracture ranges from 6% up to 19%, but may be as high as 50% when pelvic fractures are associated with hypotension.[50–53] Thus, hemorrhage should be suspected with any major pelvic fracture.[54]

Pelvic fractures have been described by a number of classification schemes over the years, but the Key and Conwell scheme is a widely used model that orders fracture types with respect to increasing complexity (Figure 15-23).[55,56] Type I fractures comprise nearly one-third of all pelvic fractures and are divided into (1) avulsion fractures, (2) fracture of the pubis or ischium, (3) fracture of the iliac wing, (4) fracture of the sacrum, and (5) fractures of the coccyx. In general, these injuries are stable, have the lowest incidence of associated injuries, lack disruption of the pelvic ring, and, with bed rest, are prone to fairly rapid healing.[57]

Type II fractures involve a single fracture of the pelvic ring and include unilateral fractures of both pubic rami, subluxation of the symphysis pubis, and fractures near or subluxation of the sacroiliac (SI) joint.

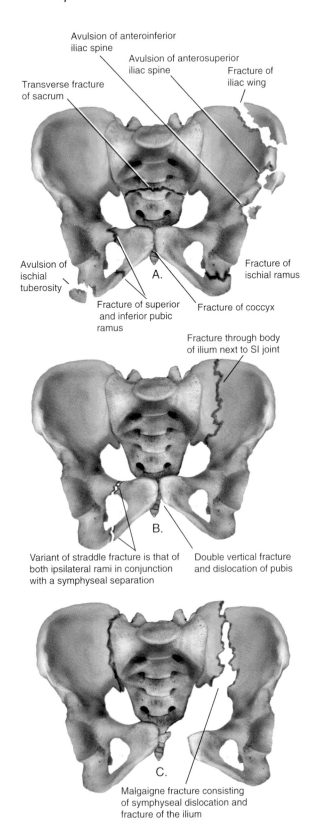

Avulsion of anteroinferior iliac spine

Avulsion of anterosuperior iliac spine

Fracture of iliac wing

Transverse fracture of sacrum

Avulsion of ischial tuberosity

Fracture of ischial ramus

Fracture of superior and inferior pubic ramus

Fracture of coccyx

A.

Fracture through body of ilium next to SI joint

B.

Variant of straddle fracture is that of both ipsilateral rami in conjunction with a symphyseal separation

Double vertical fracture and dislocation of pubis

C.

Malgaigne fracture consisting of symphyseal dislocation and fracture of the ilium

FIGURE 15-23 Types of pelvic fractures. (A) Type I fractures. Fracture of individual bones without disruption of pelvic ring. (B) Type II fractures. Single break in the pelvic ring. (C) Type III fractures. Double break in pelvic ring.

If the pelvis were truly rigid, it would be impossible to have a single break in the ring. However, the pelvis is not completely rigid due to mobility at the symphysis pubis and sacroiliac joints. This allows a single fracture to occur. However, it is necessary to thoroughly examine the pelvic ring to ensure that a second break does not exist. In addition, should there be displacement of the fracture fragments, a thorough search needs to take place for the second disruption, which is usually the ipsilateral SI joint.[56] Overall, type II fractures are stable and treated conservatively with bed rest, and they have the lowest incidence of associated injuries.[33]

Type III fractures, with an incidence of roughly 33%, involve two or more sites and include straddle fractures, Malgaigne fracture, pelvic dislocation, and "open book" injury.[55] Because type III fractures involve multiple breaks of the pelvic ring, they are all unstable, but the degree of instability will vary with the configuration of the fracture. Because it takes considerable trauma to cause a double break in the pelvic ring, these fractures carry a higher association of retroperitoneal hemorrhage, intraperitoneal injuries, and injury to the urinary bladder and urethra.[34,58] The mortality rate has been reported to be between 11% and 50%.[52,59,60]

Type IV fractures involve the acetabulum and occur in approximately 20% of all pelvic fractures in adults, are associated with hip dislocations or fractures, and are frequently the result of major trauma, such as MVCs, falls, and pedestrian–motor vehicle collisions.[33,61]

Associated Injuries Injuries to the lower pelvis may be associated with hemorrhage, abdominal trauma, injuries to the bladder or urethra, colon, nerves, and components of the reproductive system. Hemorrhage is a major cause of death in pelvic injuries; up to 65% of patients who die as a result of pelvic fractures exsanguinate from related hemorrhage.[50,62,63] Hemorrhage from pelvic fractures occurs most frequently in patients with type III fractures and results from lacerations to the rich vascular network of the pelvis.[33] The major arterial supply to the pelvis originates from the internal iliac arteries, which course at the level of the SI joints and run in close proximity to the posterior pelvic arch. The venous system also has many branches within the pelvis. Because the venous system of the pelvis is thin walled, it lacks the ability to constrict and slow blood loss when injured.[34] In addition, the innominate bones are major hematopoietic sources with a rich blood supply that provide an additional source of hemorrhage when fractured. Overall, estimates of hemorrhage associated with pelvic fracture range between 1 and 2 liters, but the retroperitoneal space may accommodate up to 6 liters of occult hemorrhage when bleeding extends into this area.[64]

The urinary bladder may or may not be injured depending upon the magnitude of blunt force applied, volume of urine within the bladder, and whether a pelvic fracture exists. An empty bladder will likely not be injured unless there is a pelvic fracture, whereas a full bladder is more susceptible to injury regardless of the presence of pelvic fracture.[34,57] Urethral injury is also commonly associated with pelvic fracture. Because of its anatomical structure, the urethra is more commonly injured in men. Signs of urological injury include blood at the urethral meatus, inability to void, scrotal swelling, and inability to pass a urinary catheter. In addition, male impotence is associated with urethral rupture.[34] In women, gynecological injuries are rare, but when present, laceration of the vagina is most common.[64] The short female urethra is unlikely to be injured.

The bowel and rectum may also be injured by pelvic fracture. Transmitted forces that fracture the pelvis may also injure portions of the bowel. In addition, bony fragments of the fractured pelvis may penetrate the bowel or rectum, resulting in an open fracture. These fractures have a very high rate of sepsis and abscess and must be aggressively treated with a diverting colostomy, washout of the distal colon, and antibiotics.

The signs and symptoms of pelvic fracture may include pain, pelvic ring instability and crepitus, deformity, swelling, ecchymosis, and shortening of the leg on the affected side. Evaluation of the pelvic injury should include careful palpation of the pelvic ring. First compress the pelvis lateral to medial through the iliac crests, then palpate anterior to posterior through the iliac crests, followed by anterior to posterior through the symphysis pubis, feeling for instability and crepitus. Because pelvic fractures may also injure the cauda equina, sacral nerves, lumbosacral plexus, and peripheral nerves, the lower extremities should be evaluated for abnormal sensation and motor weakness.[65] In addition, these nerve injuries may result in disruption of the autonomic innervation of the bowel, bladder, and sex organs. It is therefore important to inspect for priapism and incontinence, indicating nerve injury, as well as blood around the urethral meatus and rectal bleeding, which may indicate urological or bowel injury.

The key factor in initial management of pelvic fractures is identifying posterior injury to the pelvic ring. Posterior fractures or dislocations are associated with more significant hemorrhage, nerve injury, and mortality than other pelvic fractures. The diagnosis of a posterior ring fracture is based on instability of the pelvis associated with posterior pain, swelling, and ecchymosis. Some EMS systems advocate placing and inflating the PASG for both splinting of fractures and hemorrhage control.[66,67] Because the mechanism of injury for pelvic fractures is similar to that for spinal injury, immobilizing these patients on a split (or scoop)

stretcher or backboard should be done, with care taken to minimize leg and torso movement. Remember that a backboard, while allowing ease of transfer of the patient from ground to board, is a sliding device as well as a splint. As such, it will not allow the comfort or positive immobilization that can be achieved with the scoop. Movement of the patient during foot or vehicular transport can be minimized by use of a blanket folded in thirds, rolled from both ends toward the middle, and placed upside down over the patient's hips. Secure this roll to the device with a strap.

In general, lateral compression injuries are stable injuries with impaction of the posterior structures. These fractures usually have anterior instability along with ramus fractures that cause gapping of the pubic symphyses. These fractures may cause bladder, prostatic, or urethral injury. Prehospital care is immobilization as above with an eye toward prevention of hypovolemic shock.

Femur and Patella

In general, young individuals fracture the proximal femur in falls from great height, high-speed collisions, and gunshot wounds. As patients age, they tend to have more fractures with less mechanism due to changes in bone density. These fractures occur in the neck of the femur and are the most common musculoskeletal injury requiring hospitalization in the United States.[68] The patient will complain of pain in the area of the proximal thigh. There is usually little swelling or deformity around the hip. Movement of the affected leg can produce significant pain. There is often noticeable shortening and external rotation of the extremity. After exposing the area and completing the necessary sensory, motor, and circulatory examination, the leg should be realigned and a traction splint applied. If none is available, the alternative is to create a traction splint with a scoop stretcher (see General Management and Splinting Techniques) or immobilize on a backboard, with the legs tied, strapped, or taped together. If a traction splint is contraindicated (fractured pelvis, displaced hip injury, major knee injury, avulsion/amputation to knee, open fracture, fractured tibia or fibula, ankle injury, or sciatic nerve injury), the MAST may be an alternative splinting device. Remember that episodes of compartment syndrome have been associated with prolonged MAST application.[15,17]

Fractures of the femoral shaft have the same mechanisms of injury as do proximal fractures. Crepitus and serious deformity will be noted at the midthigh. The treatment is the same as with proximal femur fractures. Open fractures often result in significant hemorrhage. Direct pressure and pressure dressings are usually effective for these wounds. Application of traction via a traction splint in cases of open femur fracture is controversial. Some authors do not recommend traction that will retract exposed bone ends because of the risk of infection.[14]

Fractures of the distal end of the femur are frequently intra-articular and occur with high-velocity loading when the knee is flexed. With axial loading of the femur, the patella becomes the driving wedge and the femoral condyles are impacted. A patellar fracture may result or the condyles of the distal femur may be split. With a fractured patella, the injury may be obvious on deep palpation. These injuries are often open, since there is very little soft tissue overlying this bone. The initial exam of nerve and vessel function should be performed after exposing the site; then the limb should be realigned. Crepitus may be noted as well as significant instability in the case of a distal femur fracture, which will not be seen with a patellar fracture. A posterior splint (traction splint without applied traction works well) should be applied to the realigned limb for transportation.

Tibia and Fibula

The tibial plateau is the broad surface of the proximal tibia that articulates with the distal femur. Vehicle collisions and falls and jumps from heights are the most common mechanisms for injury. Pain, swelling, and deformity are obvious on initial examination. These fractures bleed fairly profusely, causing rapid onset of joint edema. Because the popliteal artery is tethered by the soleus fascia, arterial injuries may be seen with these fractures when associated with knee dislocation. Distal pulses and capillary refill should be closely watched, along with the requisite neurocirculatory examination. The possibility of a compartment syndrome must be kept in mind. After initial examination, the limb should be carefully realigned and a padded board/wire ladder splint, vacuum splint, or Velcro splint applied. The toes should be visible after splinting to allow for ease of determining neurocirculatory status.

Tibial shaft fractures are accompanied by fibular shaft fractures in most cases. These fractures result from high-impact torsional trauma, usually due to the body rotating around a fixed foot. When this injury is suspected, a careful inspection of the affected limb's circulation and neurological function is necessary, as this is the most common location for compartment syndrome. Splint with a device providing the same posterior support as for proximal tibial fractures.

Ankle

The distal tibia, medial malleolus, distal fibula, or any combination of these may be involved in an ankle fracture, generally produced by large amounts of torsion around a fixed foot. With the distal tibia, axial loading from a fall or jump may also be involved. The patient generally experiences significant pain and swelling. Palpation along the medial and lateral malleoli will confirm the injury.

If there is a rotational deformity, the ankle should be realigned with gentle traction before application of a splint. While a pillow splint works well here, any splint that provides posterior support for the ankle will provide adequate immobilization. Transport with the injured extremity elevated.

Tarsal

The calcaneus and talus are most often fractured during jumps or falls when the victim lands on the feet. With a calcaneus fracture, significant heel pain, deformity, and crepitus are immediately evident when the shoe is removed. A talus fracture causes tenderness and swelling distal to the malleoli. If tenderness and deformity are at the level of the malleoli, the injury is probably due to a fractured ankle. Treatment is similar to that for other foot injuries.

Metatarsal

Fractures at the bases of the metatarsals often occur in combination with midfoot dislocation. These injuries usually occur with axial loading of the foot while it is in maximum plantar flexion. This mechanism is seen in vehicular trauma. The victim complains of midfoot pain and swelling; once the shoe is removed, crepitus and tenderness are noted at the base of the metatarsals. The foot should be placed in a well-padded splint. Commercial splints that function well at providing support include pneumatic or vacuum splint or a pillow splint. Elevate whenever possible. Under no circumstances should a victim with a suspected midfoot fracture-dislocation be allowed to ambulate, since swelling would worsen and further injury may result.

Metatarsal shaft fractures occur with crush injuries and with falls or jumps from moderate heights. Midshaft metatarsal fractures also occur as stress fractures. These injuries are often the result of prolonged hiking or running with poor preconditioning. These fractures are splinted as for other foot injuries.

Phalanx

Toe phalanges are fractured by crush injuries or when heavy objects are dropped on the foot. These injuries can be prevented by the use of hard-toed boots. Prehospital treatment of phalanx fractures are managed by taping the toe to an adjacent uninjured toe, padding between them.

GENERAL MANAGEMENT AND SPLINTING TECHNIQUES

All patients with fractures should first have airway, breathing, and circulation stabilized. Control all bleeding and cover all wounds. Then evaluate distal circulatory and neurological function before and after splinting. Evaluate the injured extremity, comparing it with the uninjured one. Also evaluate the joints above and below the fracture site prior to splinting. Immobilize those same joints above and below the fracture site when splinting. Provide proper padding to prevent soft tissue injury. Always avoid unnecessary movement. When in doubt, treat any questionable fracture as though it is fractured.

Straighten angulated fractures prior to splinting unless resistance is met. When splinting fractures in the position found is compared to reduction prior to splinting, improved results are seen with reduction, then splinting with longitudinal traction or an air splint.[69,70] However, do not reduce open fractures out of hospital. Cover wounds with sterile pressure dressings and then splint. Splint joint injuries in the position found when distal neurovascular function is intact.

When splinting limbs, particularly the upper extremities, the primary goal is to immobilize the limb securely in the functional position until definitive care can be reached. For fractures or dislocations around the shoulder, a commercially available sling or improvised triangular bandage will suffice and will provide considerable relief by taking the weight of the arm off the injured structure(s).

Hand splints should be applied with the metacarpophalangeal joints flexed 90° and the interphalangeal joints extended. This position (position of function) places the hand at rest in its most comfortable position while keeping the collateral ligaments at maximum length. This will prevent later joint contracture if the hand is immobilized for excessive periods of time or becomes paralyzed.

Any patient with suspected pelvic injury should be transported on a board or scoop stretcher with the addition of the previously described blanket roll to stabilize the pelvis during transport. Restraint of the lower extremities will also prevent lower body motion.

The lower extremity should be positioned for transport with the hip and knee extended and the ankle in neutral. In cases of hip or femur fractures or dislocations, traction should be applied whenever possible, improvising when necessary. Most commonly a commercial Thomas-type splint with a Spanish windlass is available. The ring of the splint rests against the patient's ischium and pubis, and traction is applied via the windlass. This supposedly stabilizes the joint or

fracture fragments. However, in the author's experience, this is not necessarily true. Those generic and commercial bipolar traction splints that resemble the Thomas design have a flaw that is frequently overlooked. The proximity of the ischial pad (in its posterior position) to the proximal segment of a femur fracture usually seems to cause proximal third displacement of the fractured femur. Modifying its position by placing the pad on the lateral portion of the fractured extremity seems to alleviate this condition somewhat, but it does not prevent it. While there is currently very little literature to support alternatives, the unipolar-style traction splint seems to have some promise. Always placed on the medial or lateral aspect of the injured extremity with the traction originating from a single strut prevents proximal femur segment displacement. While there is again little literature to support this contention, these results have been demonstrated by radiography. In addition, this style splint lends itself well to splinting of bilateral femur fractures.

Splinting an angulated femur fracture is a difficult venture, particularly if it is open. A commercial bipolar splint (REEL™) is available that will provide an alternative method of immobilization with or without traction applied. It may also be used preextrication and for some upper extremity fractures.[71]

If commercial splints are impractical or unavailable, adapting available material to suit the situation is one of the hallmarks of a classic field provider of emergency care. An injured extremity can be splinted against the body or, in the case of the lower extremities, against the opposite leg. Both the backboard and the split frame (scoop) stretcher also serve admirably as splinting devices. It is even possible to create traction via the split-frame stretcher.[72]

For the lower leg, commercial splinting devices include metal splints, Velcro splints, cardboard splints, vacuum splints, and wood splints. Pneumatic (air) splints, while still available, have lost favor with professional emergency medical providers because of their tendency to develop leaks and provide less than optimum splinting stability. Pillows make excellent splinting devices for the hand and ankle. They are generally secured with roller gauze or elastic-type bandages.

Another treatment that is dramatic in its implications but rarely performed is the field amputation. This procedure has been performed most frequently in urban areas following motor vehicle accidents. In one five-year study of 143 surveys completed, 18 respondents reported 26 out-of-hospital amputations (13%) performed. Trauma surgeons and emergency physicians performed 89.6% of these amputations. Only two EMS systems had a protocol regarding in-field amputations. Of the 143 surveys, 96% reported no training available through their agencies related to performing an out-of-hospital amputation.[73] The study concluded that there exists a need for established protocols and training regarding this topic.

INTERNET ACTIVITIES

Visit the e-medicine Web site at http://www.emedicine.com. Click on the Emergency Medicine on-line book and select Trauma and Orthopedics. Then click on Fractures. Review the chapter on the management of the various extremity fractures.

SUMMARY

Extremity injuries, while rarely life threatening, occur with alarming frequency and, when treated improperly, may result in permanent disability. In addition, some extremity injuries, such as femur fractures and pelvic fractures, are associated with significant hemorrhage. Furthermore, improper management of extremity trauma may result in complications that limit the patient's lifestyle, such as delayed union or nonunion of bone ends, osteomyelitis, contractures, and paralysis. Consequently, it is incumbent upon the paramedic to be able to properly assess and manage extremity trauma.

REVIEW QUESTIONS

1. Fractures are more common in males under the age of 44 and females above age 44.
   a. True
   b. False

2. The functions of bone include:
   a. Movement, support, protection
   b. Erythropoiesis
   c. Storage and release of calcium and phosphorus
   d. All of the above

3. Arteries of the upper extremities include:
   a. Subclavian
   b. Axillary
   c. Radial
   d. All of the above

4. Nerves of the upper extremities include:
   a. Axillary
   b. Radial
   c. Median
   d. All of the above

5. Fractures of the pelvis are associated with blood loss of up to:
   a. 1/2 liter
   b. 1 liter
   c. 2 liters
   d. 3 liters

6. What do tendons connect?
   a. Muscle to muscle
   b. Bone to bone
   c. Muscle to bone
   d. None of the above

7. Delayed occlusion following fractures may result due to intimal sagging and platelet aggregation.
   a. True
   b. False

8. To test the ulnar nerve, the patient is instructed to:
   a. Abduct the thumb
   b. Spread the fingers against resistance
   c. Extend the wrist against resistance
   d. Oppose the thumb and small finger

9. When properly managed, amputated parts are viable for reimplantation for up to how many hours?
   a. 4
   b. 8
   c. 18
   d. 24

10. What are the two most common sites of compartment syndrome?
    a. Thigh, lower leg
    b. Lower leg, forearm
    c. Upper arm, forearm
    d. Upper arm, thigh

11. List the six "P's" of ischemia.

12. Which of the following are complications of crush syndrome?
    a. Hyperkalemia
    b. Renal failure
    c. Hypovolemic shock
    d. All of the above

13. A dislocation with complete disruption of some portion of the ligament fibers with moderate hemorrhage is a _____-degree dislocation.
    a. First
    b. Second
    c. Third
    d. Fourth

14. Posterior sternoclavicular dislocations are frequently associated with life-threatening chest injuries.
    a. True
    b. False

15. Most glenohumeral dislocations are inferior dislocations.
   a. True
   b. False

16. Assuming distal neurocirculatory function is intact, elbow dislocations should be splinted in the position found.
   a. True
   b. False

17. The most common mechanism of posterior hip dislocation is:
   a. MVCs
   b. Falls
   c. Osteoporosis
   d. None of the above

18. Knee dislocation is a true orthopedic emergency.
   a. True
   b. False

19. A widened medial joint space when applying medial pressure to the thigh and lateral pressure to the medial ankle indicates an injury to the:
   a. ACL
   b. LCL
   c. MCL
   d. PCL

20. The most commonly injured ligament of the knee is the:
   a. ACL
   b. LCL
   c. MCL
   d. PCL

21. Pain along the medial joint line of the knee is most likely due to injury of the:
   a. ACL
   b. LCL
   c. Meniscus
   d. PCL

22. The most frequently fractured bone is the scapula.
   a. True
   b. False

23. Radial fractures with dorsal displacement of the distal fragment are commonly referred to as:
   a. Galeazzi's fracture
   b. Smith's fracture
   c. Colles' fracture
   d. None of the above

24. Which of the following injuries may accompany a pelvic fracture?
   a. Bladder rupture
   b. Bowel laceration
   c. Lacerated internal iliac artery
   d. All of the above

25. Which of the following devices should be used to splint an open femur fracture?
   a. PASG
   b. Padded board splints
   c. Traction splint
   d. Sager splint

▶ CRITICAL THINKING

1. You are dispatched to the scene of an MVC. Upon arrival, you are escorted by a police officer to a 1971 Chevrolet pickup truck. Seated in the driver's seat is a 52-year-old male who is conscious, alert, and oriented ×3. He states that he swerved to miss a car that pulled into the roadway from a side street, ran off the road, and struck a utility pole. There is minimal damage to the vehicle. Being an older model vehicle, the truck was not equipped with restraints other than a lap belt, which was not worn. He denies any loss of consciousness and complains only of right knee pain and an inability to move the joint. Physical examination reveals a small laceration under the right patella with minimal bleeding. Distal neurocirculatory function is intact. There are no other complaints and the remainder of the physical exam is unremarkable. The patient is immobilized on a spine board and prepared for transport. Just prior to leaving the scene, the police officer appears at the back doors of the ambulance and asks the patient for the key to the vehicle, stating the vehicle did not require towing and would be moved off the roadway and could be retrieved later. The patient stated the key was in the ignition switch. The police officer leaves only to return moments later, stating the key was not in the ignition.

   • What knee injuries may present with the joint in a locked position? What are the consequences of injury to the popliteal artery from a knee injury? Where is the key to the truck?

2. What is the significance of a posterior sternoclavicular dislocation? What are the treatment priorities?

3. A patient with an obvious pelvic fracture presents with signs and symptoms of hemorrhagic shock. In addition, the physical exam reveals priapism, incontinence, blood around the urethral meatus, and varying sensory and motor dysfunction to the lower extremities. Are these findings associated with the pelvic fracture or do they represent other injuries? What is their significance? What are your treatment priorities?

REFERENCES

1. Hippocrates, 350 BC.
2. Peltier L. *Fractures: A History and Iconography of Their Treatment.* San Francisco: Norman Publishing; 1990.
3. Gray H. *The Early Treatment of War Wounds.* 1919.
4. Blackskin MF. Patterns of fractures after air bag deployment. *J Trauma.* 1993; 35:840.
5. *Hospitalizations for Injury and Poisoning in the United States.* National Center for Health Statistics;1991.
6. Praemer A, Furner S, Rice DP. *Musculoskeletal Conditions in the United States.* Park Ridge, Ill: American Academy of Orthopedic Surgeons; 1992.
7. *National Health Interview Survey.* Data tapes. National Center for Health Statistics; 1985–1988.
8. Burgess A, Poka A. Musculoskeletal trauma. *Emerg Med Clin North Am.* 1984; 2:871.
9. Child SA. Musculoskeletal trauma. *Crit Care Nurs Clin North Am.* 1994; 6:483.
10. Trufton, PG. Orthopedic emergencies. In: Mills J, et al, eds. *Current Emergency Diagnosis and Treatment,* 2nd ed. Stamford, Conn: Appleton & Lange; 1985.
11. Caroline NL, *Emergency Care in the Streets.* 2nd ed. Boston: Little, Brown and Company: 1991.
12. Geiderman J. Orthopedic injuries. In: Rosen P, et al, eds. *Emergency Medicine: Concepts and Clinical Practice,* 2nd ed. St Louis, Mo: CV Mosby; 1988.
13. Szalay EA, Rockwood CA. Injuries of the shoulder and arm. *Emerg Med Clin North Am.* 1984; 2:279.
14. Gruber J. Proximal femur and femoral shaft. In: Rosen P, et al, eds. *Emergency Medicine: Concepts and Clinical Practice,* 3rd ed. St Louis, Mo: Mosby; 1992.
15. Graber MA. Extremity Trauma, Internet—The Virtual Hospital: University of Iowa Family Practice Handbook. Retrieved Feb 1997.
16. Mabee, JR. Compartment syndrome: a complication of acute extremity trauma. *J Emerg Med.* 1994; 12:651.
17. Aprahamian C, Gessert G, Bandyk DF, Sell L, Stiehl J, Olson BW. Mast-associated compartment syndrome (MACS): a review. *J Trauma.* 1989; 29: 549.
18. Odeh M. The role of reperfusion-induced injury in the pathogenesis of the crush syndrome. *N Engl J Med.* 1991; 324:1417.
19. Neer CS, Rockwood CA. Fracture and dislocations of the shoulder. In: Rockwood CA, Green DP, eds. *Fractures in Adults,* 2nd ed. Philadelphia: JB Lippincott; 1984.
20. Daya M. Shoulder. In: Rosen P, et al, eds. *Emergency Medicine: Concepts and Clinical Practice,* 3rd ed. St. Louis, Mo: Mosby; 1992.
21. Allman F. Fractures and ligamentous injuries of the clavicle and its articulation. *J Bone Joint Surg.* 1967; 49(A):774.
22. Wickiewicz T. Acromioclavicular and sternoclavicular joint injuries. *Clin Sports Med.* 1983; 2:429.
23. Simon R, Koenigsknecht S, Stevens C. *Emergency Orthopedics: The Extremities,* 2nd ed. Norwalk, Conn.: Appleton and Lange; 1987.
24. Kroner K, Lind T, Jensen J. The epidemiology of shoulder dislocations. *Arch Orthop Trauma Surg.* 1989; 108:288.
25. Hovelius L, Eriksson K, Fredin H, et al; Recurrences after initial dislocation of the shoulder: results of a prospective study of treatment. *J Bone Joint Surg.* 1983; 65A:343.
26. May V. Posterior dislocation of the shoulder: habitual, traumatic and obstetrical. *Orthop Clin North Am.* 1980; 11:271.
27. Orban D. Shoulder. In: Rosen P, et al, eds. *Emergency Medicine: Concepts and Clinical Practice,* 2nd ed. St. Louis, Mo: Mosby; 1988.
28. Uehara D, Rudzinski J. Injuries to the shoulder complex and humerus. In: Tintinalli J, Ruiz E, Krome R, eds. *Emergency Medicine: A Comprehensive Study Guide,* 4th ed. New York: McGraw-Hill; 1996.
29. Saxena K, Stavas J. Inferior glenohumeral dislocation. *Ann Emerg Med.* 1983; 12:718.
30. Magnusson R. Humerus and elbow. In: Rosen P, et al, eds. *Emergency Medicine: Concepts and Clinical Practice,* 3rd ed. St. Louis, Mo: Mosby; 1992.
31. Ueheara D, Chin H. Injuries to the elbow, forearm, and wrist. In: Tintinalli J, Ruiz E, Krome R, eds. *Emergency Medicine: A Comprehensive Study Guide,* 4th ed. New York: McGraw-Hill; 1996.
32. Chin H, Propp D, Orban D. Forearm and wrist. In: Rosen P, et al, eds. *Emergency Medicine: Concepts and Clinical Practice,* 3rd ed. St. Louis, Mo: Mosby; 1992.
33. Stewart C. Extremity trauma: Part I. *Emerg Med Services.* 1999; 28:43.
34. Cwinn A. Pelvis and hip. In: Rosen P, et al, eds. *Emergency Medicine: Concepts and Clinical Practice,* 3rd ed. St. Louis, Mo: Mosby; 1992.
35. Dick T. Personal communication. 1984.
36. Mayeda D. Knee and lower leg. In: Rosen P, et al, eds. *Emergency Medicine: Concepts and Clinical Practice,* 3rd ed. St. Louis, Mo: Mosby; 1992.
37. Roman P, Hopson C, Zenni E. Traumatic dislocation of the knee: a report of 30 cases and literature review. *Orthop Rev.* 1987; 16:917.

38. Lombardo JA. The athlete's knee: an orderly examination. *Emerg Med.* 1984; 16:34.

39. Ward B, Godbout B. Foul play: field evaluation of athletic knee injuries. *JEMS.* 1999; 24:67.

40. Covey D, Sapega A. Current concepts review: injuries of the posterior cruciate ligament. *J Bone Joint Surg.* 1993; 75A:1376.

41. Hoppenfeld S. *Physical Examination of the Spine and Extremities.* East Norwalk, Conn: Appleton, Century and Croft; 1976.

42. Rosenthal RE. Emergency department evaluation of musculoskeletal injuries. *Emerg Med Clin North Am.* 1984; 2:219.

43. McGinnis M, Denton R. Fractures of the scapula: a retrospective study of 40 fractured scapula. *J Trauma.* 1989; 29:1488.

44. Rowe C. Fractures of the scapula. *Surg Clin North Am.* 1963; 43:1565.

45. Armstrong C, Van der Spuy J. The fractured scapula: importance and management based on a series of 62 patients. *Injury.* 1984; 15:324.

46. Eiff MP. Management of clavicle fractures. *Am Fam Phys.* 1997; 55:121.

47. Hawkins R, Angelo R. Displaced proximal humeral fractures. *Orthop Clin North Am.* 1987; 18:421.

48. Lombardo J. Around the elbow. *Emerg Med.* 1983; 15:14.

49. Kinzl L, Burri C, Coldewey J. Fractures of the pelvis and associated intrapelvic injuries. *Injury.* 1982; 14:63.

50. Rothenberger D, Fischer RP, Strate RG, Velasco R, Perry JF. The mortality associated with pelvic fractures. *Surgery.* 1978; 84:356.

51. Mucha P, Farnell M. Analysis of pelvic fracture management. *J Trauma.* 1984; 24:379.

52. McMurtry R, Walton D, Dickinson D, Kellam J, Tile M. Pelvic disruption in the polytraumatized patient: a management protocol. *Clin Orthop.* 1980; 151:22.

53. Gordon R, Fast A, Aner H, Shifrin E, Siew F, Floman Y. Control of massive retroperitoneal bleeding associated with pelvic fractures by angiographic embolization. *Isr J Med Sci.* 1983; 19:185.

54. Mucha P, Welch TJ. Hemorrhage in major pelvic fractures. *Surg Clin North Am.* 1988; 68:747.

55. Rockwood C, Green D. *Fractures in Adults.* Philadelphia: JB Lippincott; 1984.

56. Jerrard D. Pelvic fractures. *Emerg Med Clin North Am.* 1993; 11:147.

57. Kane W. Fractures of the pelvis. In: Rockwood C, Green D, eds. *Fractures in Adults.* 2nd ed. Philadelphia: JB Lippincott; 1984.

58. Calapinto V. Trauma to the pelvis: urethral injury. *Clin Orthop.* 1980; 151:46.

59. Trunkey D, Chapman MW, Lim RC, Dunphy JE. Management of pelvic fractures in blunt trauma injury. *J Trauma.* 1974; 14:912.

60. Ward R, Clark D. Management of pelvic fractures. *Radiol Clin North Am.* 1981; 19:167.

61. Rogers L. *Radiology of Skeletal Trauma.* New York: Churchill Livingstone; 1982.

62. Brown J, Greene F, McMillin R. Vascular injuries associated with pelvic fractures. *Am Surg.* 1984; 50:150.

63. Cryer H, Miller F, Ever, B. Pelvic fracture classification: correlation with hemorrhage. *J Trauma.* 1988; 28:973.

64. Waeckerle J, Steele M. Trauma to the pelvis, hip and femur. In: Tintinalli J, Ruiz E, Krome R, eds. *Emergency Medicine: A Comprehensive Study Guide,* 4th ed. New York: McGraw-Hill; 1996.

65. Huittinen V. Lumbosacral nerve injury in fracture of the pelvis: a postmortem radiographic and patho-anatomical study. *Acta Chir Scand Suppl.* 1972; 429:1.

66. Pons P, Cason D (eds). Paramedic field care. *Am Coll Emerg Phys.* Dallas, 1997.

67. County of San Diego, Division of Emergency Medical Services. *Paramedic Policy/Procedure/ Protocol Manual.* San Diego: County of San Diego; 1991.

68. *National Hospital Discharge Survey* Data tapes. National Center for Health Statistics; 1985–1988.

69. Tscherne H. The management of open fractures. In: Tscherne H, ed. *Fractures with Soft Tissue Injuries.* Berlin: Springer-Verlag; 1984.

70. Bone LB. Emergency treatment of the injured patient. In: Browner BD, et al, eds. *Skeletal Trauma.* Philadelphia: WB Saunders; 1992.

71. Auerbach PS, Geehr EC, Ryv RK. The reel splint: experience with a new traction splint apparatus in the prehospital setting. *Ann Emerg Med.* 1984; 13:419.

72. Dick T. Personal communication. 1986.

73. Kampen KE, Krohmer JR, Jones JS, Dougherty JM, Bonness RK. In-field extremity amputation: prevalence and protocols in Emergency Medical Services. *Prehosp Disaster Med.* 1996; 11:63.

Chapter 16
Compartment Syndrome and Crush Injuries

OBJECTIVES

Upon completion of this chapter, the reader should be able to:

- Describe the epidemiology and etiology of crush injury and compartment syndrome.
- Define compartment syndrome and crush syndrome.
- List the injuries most commonly associated with compartment syndrome.
- Describe the anatomical features common to the locations that develop compartment syndrome.
- Discuss the role of reperfusion as a contributing factor in compartment syndrome.
- Describe the basic surgical procedure used for pressure release in compartment syndrome.
- Describe the clinical presentation of compartment syndrome.
- Describe what actions should be taken when compartment syndrome is suspected in the field.
- Discuss the complications of crush injury.
- Describe the mechanisms of injury in crush injury.
- List the signs and symptoms of crush injury.

KEY TERMS

Compartment syndrome
Crush injury
Crush syndrome
Disseminated Intravascular Coagulation (DIC)
Fascia
Hydrostatic forces

Mangled Extremity Severity Score (MESS)
Oncotic forces
Osteofascial compartments
Rhabdomyolysis
Starling equation

The ischemic complications of extremity fractures were described by Volkmann over 100 years ago, laying the foundation for what we now call compartment syndrome.[1,2] **Compartment syndrome** is defined as necrosis of muscle and nerve within a contained area secondary to increased tissue pressure. It is now known that compartment syndrome and crush injuries are not limited to the extremities but can lead to the life-threatening systemic complication of crush syndrome. This chapter will provide an overview of compartment syndrome, crush injuries, and crush syndrome.

EPIDEMIOLOGY AND ETIOLOGY

Acute compartment syndrome (CS) is most often seen as a complication of trauma. Extremity fracture accounts for 45% of all CS.[3,4] The most common cause of CS is a closed tibia fracture, with an incidence of 3%–17%.[5] Other common fracture sites include the fibula, distal radius (Colles' fracture), and distal humerus (supracondylar fracture). Compartment syndrome is also seen in open fractures, with an incidence of 6%–9%.[4–6] Other causes of acute CS include minor crush injuries without fracture, vascular injuries, snake bites, electrical injuries, infiltration of intravenous fluids, intraosseous fluid administration, compression from immobility, position during surgery, fracture casting, anticoagulation therapy, and extreme exercise.[7–18]

ANATOMY AND PHYSIOLOGY

Acute compartment syndrome almost exclusively occurs in the **osteofascial compartments**. In many locations of the body, these discrete compartments are formed when **fascia**, a tough and inelastic membranous connective tissue, connects with bone (Figure 16-1). These chambers, or osteofascial compartments, typically contain skeletal muscle, nervous system tissue, and vascular structures. Of the body's 46 fascial compartments, the ones commonly involved with CS are in the extremities.

In the upper extremity, the arm has two fascial compartments: anterior and posterior. The anterior fascial compartment of the arm contains the flexor muscles and the major nerves for the upper extremity. The posterior fascial compartment of the arm contains the extensor muscles.

In the forearm there are three main fascial compartments: anterior, lateral, and posterior. The anterior fascial compartment of the forearm contains the flexor muscles for the distal extremity. The lateral fascial compartment of the forearm contains a major flexor muscle for the forearm at the elbow. The posterior fascial compartment of the forearm contains mainly extensor muscles for the distal extremity. Each fascial compartment in the forearm contains the associated nerves for their muscle groups.

In the lower extremity, the thigh has three fascial compartments: anterior, medial, and posterior. The anterior fascial compartment of the thigh contains the large flexor muscles for the thigh and extensor muscles for the leg. This compartment also contains the femoral artery. The medial fascial compartment of the thigh

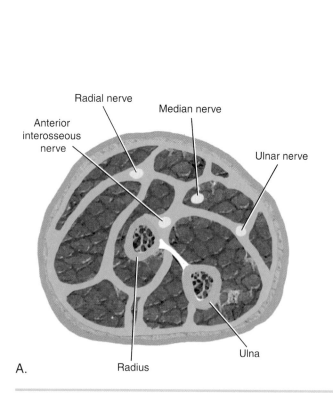

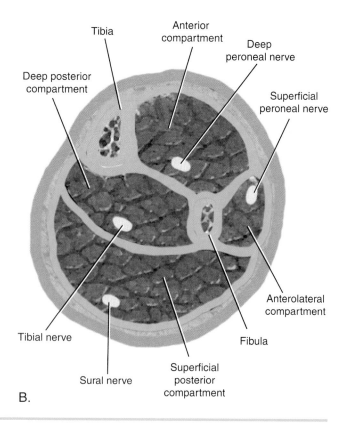

FIGURE 16-1 (A) Compartments of the forearm. (B) Compartments of the lower leg.

contains the adductors for the thigh. The posterior fascial compartment of the thigh contains mainly flexors for the leg and also contains the sciatic nerve.

In the lower leg there are four fascial compartments: anterior, lateral, superficial posterior, and deep posterior. The anterior fascial compartment of the leg contains the extensors for the foot (dorsiflexion) and toes. The anterior tibial artery and deep peroneal nerve are located in the compartment. This is the most common location for CS. The lateral fascial compartment for the leg contains flexors for the foot (plantar flexion.) This is a common location for CS. The superficial posterior fascial compartment of the leg contains the main flexors for the foot (plantar flexion). The deep posterior fascial compartment of the leg contains the main flexors for the toes. This compartment also contains the tibial artery and nerve.

In addition to the main fascial compartments of the extremities listed above, a few others deserve mention. The gluteal region in the buttocks contains three fascial compartments. The outermost gluteal compartment contains the gluteus maximus muscle for extending the thigh at the hip joint. The sciatic nerve is in close proximity and deep to this compartment. A tensor muscle is located in the most anterior fascial compartment. The gluteus medius and minimus are located under a layer of fascia between these two compartments. A second consideration is that the hand and foot each contain multiple small compartments, all of which are subject to CS.

MICROCIRCULATION AND PERFUSION

In the microvasculature, fluid flows through the capillary lumen and across the capillary wall. The fluid exchange across the capillary wall is described by the **Starling equation**. This equation determines direction and rate of flow based on three factors: (1) the permeability of the capillary wall, (2) hydrostatic forces, and (3) oncotic forces. **Hydrostatic forces** refer to the physical pressure of the fluid. When the hydrostatic pressure inside the capillary exceeds the hydrostatic pressure on the outside, fluid will be filtered out of the capillary. **Oncotic forces** can be thought of as chemical pressure to attract fluid. The principal oncotic force in the microvasculature is protein in the blood. When the oncotic pressure inside the capillary exceeds the oncotic pressure on the outside, fluid will be absorbed into the capillary. Oncotic or hydrostatic forces can cause both filtration and absorption. The net flow from all of these forces in the normal microvasculature is for fluid filtration at the arterial side of the capillary and fluid absorption at the venous side of the capillary. In CS, this balance is disrupted.

PATHOPHYSIOLOGY

COMPARTMENT SYNDROMES

In its simplest definition, CS requires (1) tissue confined within a fixed compartment with minimal capacity to expand and (2) an increase in pressure within the compartment.[1] The pathology of CS results from compromised perfusion, ultimately leading to tissue ischemia and necrosis. Most commonly, this condition is seen in osteofascial compartments as a complication of a fracture. However, any condition that causes increased tissue pressure within a fixed compartment can lead to CS.

Tissue pressure can be elevated by several mechanisms. Because the capacity of the compartment is limited and fixed, any increase in volume will result in an increase in pressure. In trauma, compartmental bleeding and edema are common causes of increased tissue volume. A second mechanism for increasing tissue pressure is to reduce the size of the compartment while keeping the tissue volume constant. This can be accomplished by applying external compression forces to the compartment. MAST garments, extremity entrapments, and circumferential burns are examples of potential mechanisms for this type of compression.

When the pressure in the compartment rises above a critical point, the microcirculation fails and tissue perfusion decreases. While intuitively this seems reasonable, the physics and physiology involved are quite complex and there are numerous theories to explain this phenomenon.[19–22] Normal intramuscular capillary pressure is about 25 mm Hg, and when the interstitial and tissue pressures become greater than the capillary pressure, the net flow of blood through the microcirculation decreases and the tissue becomes ischemic. One popular theory is that microcirculation fails secondary to compression of the venous end of the capillary, resulting in decreased capillary blood flow.[1,21,23] However, failure of the microcirculation does not necessarily imply complete impedance of blood flow through the extremity.

An important anatomical consideration is that the metarterioles that supply the capillaries also have the ability to shunt blood around the capillary bed and empty directly into the venous system. Because these vessels operate at higher pressures than the capillaries, they can preserve blood flow through the extremity when the tissue pressures in CS exceed the capillary pressure by a small margin. Therefore, in CS arterial pulses and capillary refill may be intact, but the tissue at the cellular level can be unperfused and ischemic secondary to microcirculation failure.

Compartment syndrome results in local tissue changes that exacerbate the underlying pathology of increased compartment pressure. Tissue ischemia alters the permeability of cell membranes, resulting in increased cellular fluid volume. In the capillaries, ischemia in the vessel walls allows proteins to leak out of the vascular space. The resulting decreased capillary oncotic pressure leads to increased filtration and interstitial fluid volume. In addition, occlusion of the venous end of the capillary would result in increased capillary hydrostatic pressure, again favoring fluid filtration into the interstitial space. The intercellular and interstitial edema worsens the elevated compartment pressure. This promotes a cycle of swelling-ischemia-swelling that can only be halted with release of the tissue pressure (Figure 16-2).

The critical points for the development of CS are tissue pressures of 30–40 mm Hg for more than 4–6 hours. Irreversible tissue changes occur with tissue pressure above 50 mm Hg. Full recovery is generally possible if pressure is released within 4 hours. Exposure to pressure for longer than 8 hours carries a poor prognosis. However, the amount of tissue damage is a function of both duration of exposure and pressure level. Higher pressures result in earlier injury, and damaged tissue appears to be more vulnerable to the ischemic effects. The nervous system tissue within the compartment is particularly vulnerable to the effects of CS, leading to sensory deficits, motor dysfunction, and pain. In addition to local tissue necrosis, CS can lead to systemic complications. Commonly, the injured muscle cells will leak myoglobin and electrolytes, resulting in electrolyte disturbances and potential renal complications.

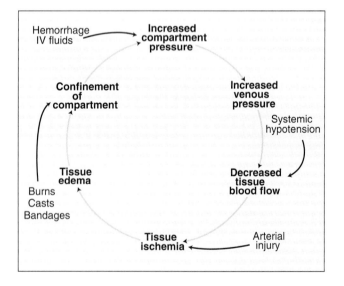

FIGURE 16-2 Pathophysiology of compartment syndrome. (From McGee DL, Dalsey WC. The mangled extremity: compartment syndrome and amputations. *Emerg Med Clin North Am.* 1992; 10(4)784. Reprinted with permission.)

INTERNET ACTIVITIES

Visit the Wheeless' Textbook of Ortho-paedics Web site at http://www.medmedia.com/oa2/72.htm and review the section on compartment syndrome.

UNUSUAL COMPARTMENT SYNDROMES

Although most CS will involve the extremities, other unusual locations include the orbital globe and kidney.[24] Two other unusual locations deserve mention: the gluteal compartment and the abdominal compartment. Gluteal CS is rare, but it is occasionally seen and has a high potential for delayed diagnosis.[25] In addition to trauma, other reported causes include prolonged immobility secondary to substance abuse and unconsciousness.[14,25,26] In these situations, the external pressure placed on the compartment from patient position is the etiology of the CS. Because of the large muscle mass involved, these patients may also develop a crush syndrome.[26]

The abdominal compartment syndrome is caused by an acute increase in intra-abdominal pressure. The condition is usually caused by an intra-abdominal hemorrhage and is most commonly seen in postoperative abdominal trauma patients.[27] Like the other CS discussed, the underlying pathology is related to elevated compartment pressure and the treatment is surgical decompression. In this syndrome, potentially catastrophic cardiovascular, pulmonary, and renal compromise are the main concerns, not muscle ischemia. The multisystem dysfunction is directly related to the mechanical compression of vital organs. The elevated intra-abdominal pressure decreases cardiac output by impairing venous return and increasing peripheral resistance. Pulmonary function is compromised by displacing the diaphragm and hindering ventilation. Renal output is decreased by directly compressing the kidney. These patients present with a multisystem failure despite aggressive treatment. The diagnosis is largely clinical, but intra-abdominal compartment pressure or bladder pressures can be measured.

CRUSH INJURIES

In clinical practice, the term *crush injury* is used liberally and applied to a wide range of injuries. Crush injury has been described in the chest, abdomen, and pelvis.[28–31] In these locations, the term *crush* is most frequently used to describe a mechanism of injury involving a specific type of blunt-force trauma. Most commonly, **crush injury** refers to a type of extremity trauma that can lead to the well-defined systemic complication of crush syndrome.

Used in this manner, the term *crush injury* implies more than a mechanism of injury.

Crush injury is often described as a specific type of extremity trauma resulting from continuous and prolonged pressures on the limb.[32,33] This type of injury results from entrapment of the extremities with objects exerting great force for hours prior to release. This mechanism can be seen in patients trapped under debris of collapsed buildings after earthquakes, bombings, or other disasters. The presentation after extrication for this type of trauma is a patient with minimal pain, severe sensory deficit, flaccid paralysis, intact pulses, and no edema.[32] Later, striking edema in the injured extremity dominates the clinical picture. Although difficult to palpate through the edema, pulses remain intact and the extremity remains perfused. The patient later develops hypovolemic shock and systemic changes consistent with crush syndrome. The pathophysiology is not well known for this injury but is related to massive muscle damage and is distinct from CS. Unlike CS, compartment pressures are initially normal and muscle damage precedes any elevation of compartment pressure. Treatment of crush injury is aimed at preventing crush syndrome. Surgical management is controversial, but fasciotomy is typically not indicated.[32,34]

Less rigidly defined discussions of extremity crush injury are also found in the literature.[35] This broadly defined type of crush injury often refers to severe extremity trauma, or "mangled limbs," and is commonly considered in conjunction with degloving injuries. These can be devastating injuries and the surgeon determines if the limb is salvageable.[36] Restoration of useful limb function is unlikely when combinations of the following are present: major avulsions, multiple fractures, near-complete traumatic amputations, major neurological injury, and severe crush with prolonged ischemia. Other important factors in determining if a limb is salvageable are (1) the patient's general condition, such as age and coexisting medical problems; (2) preexisting condition of the extremity; and (3) other injuries and treatment priorities.[37] The **Mangled Extremity Severity Score (MESS)** has been developed as a guideline for assessing the viability of severely injured limbs (see Table 16-1). Limbs with MESS scores of 6 or less are likely to be salvageable while limbs with scores of 7 or more typically require amputation.[37]

INTERNET ACTIVITIES

Visit the Marcus Healthcare, Inc. Web site at http://www.024u.com/Crush.htm and review the indications for the use of hyperbaric oxygen therapy for crush injury and compartment syndrome.

Table 16-1
MESS Variables

Skeletal/soft tissue injury	
Low energy [stab, simple fracture, GSW (low-powered weapon)]	1
Medium energy (open or multiple fractures, dislocation)	2
High energy [close-range shotgun or GSW (high-powered weapon) crush injury]	3
Very high energy (as above with gross contamination, soft tissue avulsion)	4
Limb ischemia	
Pulse reduced or absent but perfusion normal	1*
Pulseless, parasthesias, diminished capillary refill	2*
Cool, paralyzed, insensate, numb	3*
Shock	
Systolic blood pressure always >90 mm Hg	0
Hypotensive transiently	1
Persistent hypotension	2
Age (yr)	
<30	0
30–50	1
>50	2

Source: Adapted from Johansen K, et al. Objective criteria accurately predict amputation following lower extremity trauma. *J Trauma*. 1990; 30:568.

*Score doubled for ischemia >6 hr.

CRUSH SYNDROME

The multiple systemic complications of soft tissue injury and the disruption of muscle integrity following a crush injury or CS are recognized as **crush syndrome**. These complications include rhabdomyolysis, electrolyte disturbances, hypovolemia, renal failure, acidosis, and disseminated intravascular coagulation.[38] Crush syndrome can also be a cause of CS.[38]

At the cellular level, damage and ischemia of skeletal muscle and soft tissue lead to multiple electrolyte and fluid imbalances.[32,33,38,39] The compromised cellular membrane releases intracellular contents into the serum, resulting in elevated serum potassium, creatinine, creatine phosphokinase (CPK), phosphate, and lactic acid. In addition, extracellular electrolytes such as sodium, chloride, and calcium move into the cell. The electrolyte imbalances cause fluid to shift into the interstitial space ("third spacing") and intracellular compartment. The depletion of intravascular fluid can cause hypotension, shock, and decreased renal output. The electrolyte disturbances also have other potentially devastating effects. Hypocalcemia can cause decreased cardiac function. Hyperkalemia may lead to potentially lethal cardiac conduction abnormalities. Hyperphosphatemia may result in mental status changes. Most of the electrolyte imbalances lead to neuromuscular dysfunction and irritability. Acidosis results from the release of lactic acid and the products of anaerobic metabolism into the circulation. The compromised renal function secondary to intravascular hypovolemia exacerbates the electrolyte disturbances and acidosis.

Rhabdomyolysis is the destruction of skeletal muscle cell membranes.[32,33,38,40] One major complication of rhabdomyolysis is caused by the release of myoglobin into the serum. Myoglobin is a compound found in skeletal muscle that is similar to hemoglobin. Once in the serum it is filtered by the kidney, causing a redbrown color in the urine. Although not fully understood, myoglobin in the kidney results in tubular necrosis and renal failure. The toxic effects of myoglobin are accentuated by the intravascular hypovolemia and decreased renal function.

Disseminated intravascular coagulation (DIC) can also be seen in crush syndrome.[38] This is a complex disorder of bleeding in the face of massive activation of the coagulation system. Clinically this condition presents as generalized oozing, bleeding, and abnormal clotting parameters. In crush syndrome the release of thromboplastin from damaged cells is the likely trigger to activate the coagulation cascade.[38]

Reperfusion of a previously ischemic compartment plays a complex role in the development of crush syndrome. It is thought that much of the rhabdomyolysis occurs during reperfusion and that compressive forces of entrapment may provide some protection from the systemic consequences of muscle injury.[38,40,41] The reperfusion of previously ischemic tissue allows the release of multiple mediators of injury, such as oxygen free radicals and inflammatory agents, from damaged cells that accelerate tissue injury.

A pseudo–crush injury syndrome has been reported in victims of torture.[42] In these patients, repeated beatings were the cause of muscle injury. In the setting of forced dehydration, the patients developed myoglobinuria and renal failure.

ASSESSMENT

The history is the key to identifying CS in the field. Delays in diagnosis can lead to irreversible neurological injury or loss of limb. Unfortunately, the diagnosis is occasionally missed and treatment is delayed. Compartment syndrome accounts for about 2% of all malpractice claims in the United States; most cases of CS arise while the patient is under direct medical care.[43]

HISTORY

The patient history coupled with a high index of suspicion is important to the identification of CS. High-energy mechanisms of injury, such as motor vehicle collisions, are more commonly associated with CS.[5] The greater the degree of soft tissue injury, the higher the risk of CS. Fractures with surrounding soft tissue contusion and crush are more likely to have CS.[44]

PHYSICAL EXAMINATION

The variability in clinical presentations and physical findings can make the identification of CS difficult.[45] The classic criteria are (1) pain out of proportion to the existing injury, (2) pain on passive stretch of the muscle in the involved compartment, and (3) decreased sensation and loss of motor function. Pain is typically an early symptom and tends to become progressively worse as pressure rises in the compartment. The most reliable physical finding is sensory deficit, which is often associated with muscle weakness.[1] The presence of distal pulses and capillary refill does not rule out CS. The extremity may feel tight to palpation. The six P's of ischemia (pain, pallor, paresthesia, pulselessness, puffiness, and paralysis) are late findings.

The physical examination should include serial assessments of distal pulses, capillary refill, skin temperature and color, sensory function, motor function, and sensation to passive range of motion. The mechanism of injury and the nature of the underlying pathology will dictate which of these assessment parameters are appropriate for field evaluation. The assessment must not aggravate or exacerbate existing injuries. A patient with an obvious fracture should have the extremity appropriately immobilized, which limits the field assessment for range of motion and motor function. Vital signs and hemodynamic status monitoring are also important.

EMERGENCY DEPARTMENT EVALUATION

In the hospital, invasive needle manometer devices can be used to obtain measurements of compartment pressure. The procedure involves inserting a needle (16 gauge) into the compartment, attaching a fluid-filled line, then measuring the pressure in the column of fluid with a manometer or arterial pressure transducer (Figure 16-3). The normal compartment pressure is 0–8 mm Hg.[1] The threshold pressure for surgical intervention varies, with most recommending 30–45 mm Hg or within 30 mm Hg of the patient's diastolic blood pressure.[1,5,21,46] In addition to compartment pressure measurements, factors such as physical examination findings, duration of exposure to the pressure, amount of underlying tissue damage, and the overall hemodynamic status are used to determine if surgery is indicated. If CS is diagnosed, it is a surgical emergency.

Other studies, such as arteriograms and venograms, are sometimes employed depending on the underlying injury. Laboratory tests include CPK, blood urea nitrogen (BUN), and urine myoglobin to monitor for renal failure. Elevated CPK of 100–5,000 units/mL (normal <130 units/mL) and myoglobinuria are suggestive of CS but are not specific.[1,47]

MANAGEMENT

Supportive care is the primary initial field treatment of suspected CS. Ensure that the patient is adequately oxygenated and hemodynamically stable. Bleeding should be controlled with direct pressure, but massive hemorrhage is not typically associated with crush injury, even when the extremity is mangled.[35] Systolic hypotension and shock are associated with increased incidence of acute CS.[23] Aggressive treatment with intravenous hydration is almost universally indicated. If possible, fluid hydration should begin while extrication is in progress. Early hydration may help protect against the renal complications associated with rhabdomyolysis.[38,48] For an isolated crush limb injury, isotonic crystalloid, such as normal saline or lactated Ringer's, at a rate of 1.5 liters/h for several hours is recommended.[39]

Specific measures include the immobilization of the extremity. In suspected CS, remove any constricting casts, splints, or dressings. The extremity should be kept level. Avoid elevation of the affected extremity because it will further decrease arterial flow and exacerbate the ischemia.[49] Lowering the extremity should also be avoided because it will decrease venous return and increase intracompartmental pressure.[46]

Although controversial, efforts to correct hyperkalemia are recommended. High levels of circulating potassium are associated with cardiac dysrhythmias. Fifty to 100 mEq of sodium bicarbonate may be administered intravenously to drive potassium intracellularly. To be effective, the sodium bicarbonate should be administered prior to the release of pressure on the extremities.

Finally, the paramedic must weigh the risk of prolonged extrication of patients with life-threatening injuries. In some circumstances, field amputation of mangled extremities may be indicated and a surgeon should be summoned to the scene.

At the hospital, surgical decompression of the compartment with fasciotomies can be a limb-saving procedure. This decompression is often indicated in the setting of major vascular or severe soft tissue injury

to an extremity. The skin is widely incised and the fascia is divided to decompress the compartment (Figure 16-4). Underlying fractures are repaired and damaged

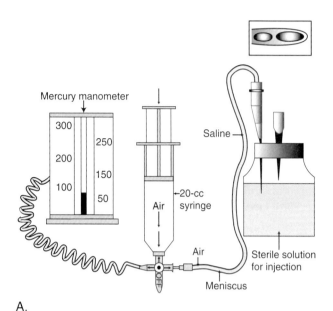

A.

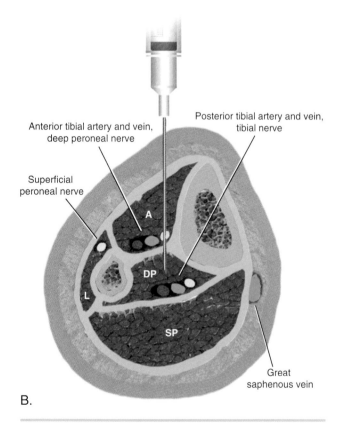

B.

FIGURE 16-3 (A) Assembly of equipment used for compartment tissue pressure measurements. (B) Placement of the needle into the fascial compartment for tissue pressure measurements.

tissue is debrided during the surgery. Typically, the incision is packed and left open for several days. The extremity is splinted and given daily physical therapy with passive range of motion to prevent contracture. Patients may require multiple trips to the operating room and skin grafts for final closure. While associated with some complications, this limb-saving procedure seems to contribute little to long-term morbidity.[50]

In addition to specific surgical procedures that may be employed to salvage the limb, treatments will focus on preventing and reducing the systemic complications of CS and crush injuries. Patients will receive aggressive intravenous hydration and correction of electrolyte abnormalities. After stabilization of systemic hemodynamics, patients may be given diuretics, like mannitol, and alkalizing agents, like sodium bicarbonate, until myoglobin clears from the urine.

INTERNET ACTIVITIES

Visit the Royal Infirmary of Edinburgh Web site at http://www.orthopaedic.ed.ac.uk/compartment/sld001.htm and review the lecture on compartment syndrome of the hand and forearm.

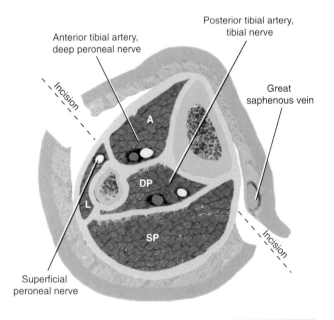

Anterior tibial artery, deep peroneal nerve

Posterior tibial artery, tibial nerve

Great saphenous vein

Incision

Incision

A

DP

L

SP

Superficial peroneal nerve

FIGURE 16-4 Double-incision fasciotomy. The medial incision allows access into the deep posterior (DP) and superficial posterior (SP) compartments of the lower leg. The lateral incision allows access into the anterior (A) and lateral (L) compartments.

EXPERIMENTAL TREATMENTS AND CURRENT RESEARCH

HYPERBARIC OXYGEN

Hyperbaric oxygen (HBO) has been used in the treatment of severe crush injuries and CS. In a small but well-controlled study, HBO improved wound healing and outcome in patients with crush injury.[51] In this study, a subgroup of patients older than 40 with severe soft tissue injuries showed the most benefit from HBO. This subgroup showed a reduced need for repetitive and new surgical procedures, such as skin flaps, skin grafts, vascular surgery, and amputation.

REDUCTION OF CELL INJURY

Oxygen free radicals are highly reactive particles that have been implicated as one of the most important mediators of cell membrane injury during ischemia. These substances react with the cell membrane through the process of lipoperoxydation, resulting in increased membrane permeability and cellular edema. Reperfusion of ischemic tissue results in elevated levels of oxygen free radicals. Multiple pharmacological agents have been investigated for their potential to reduce oxygen free-radical injury. Mannitol, mainly known as an osmotic diuretic, also has oxygen free-radical scavenging properties and has demonstrated protective effects in acute ischemia-reperfusion injuries.[52–55] Mannitol, especially when combined with aggressive fluid therapy and sodium bicarbonate, may reduce acute renal failure secondary to rhabdomyolysis in CS, decrease compartmental pressure without fasciotomy in CS, and improve postoperative outcome of ischemic extremities.[39,52,53] Other free-radical scavenging agents such as allopurinol have been investigated with varied degrees of success.[56–58]

SUMMARY

Crush injury typically is the result of blunt trauma and/or compressive forces to the extremities. Treatment for crush injury is generally supportive. Similar to crush injury, compartment syndrome may be the result of blunt trauma to the extremities; it can also be caused by other etiologies, such as electrical injury, snakebite, MAST application, and fractures. The mechanism of injury behind compartment syndrome is swelling-ischemia-swelling with an increased risk to the limb until the sequence is halted. Treatment of compartment syndrome includes relief of pressure, hydration, and maintenance of circulation.

The multiple systemic complications of soft tissue injury and the disruption of muscle integrity following a crush injury or CS are recognized as crush syndrome. These systemic manifestations include rhabdomyolysis, electrolyte disturbances, hypovolemia, renal failure, acidosis, and disseminated intravascular coagulation. Crush syndrome can also be a cause of CS.

In addition to surgical procedures that may be employed to salvage the limb, treatment focuses on preventing and reducing the systemic complications of CS and crush injuries. Patients receive aggressive intravenous hydration and correction of electrolyte abnormalities. After stabilization of systemic hemodynamics, patients may be given diuretics, like mannitol, and alkalizing agents, like sodium bicarbonate, until myoglobin clears from the urine.

► REVIEW QUESTIONS

1. The most common cause of compartment syndrome is:
   a. Tibial fracture
   b. Ulnar fracture
   c. Snakebite
   d. Fracture cast

2. The "compartments" prone to compartment syndrome are formed by:
   a. Ligaments
   b. Tendons
   c. Fascia
   d. Skin

3. The compartments most likely to develop compartment syndrome are located in the:
   a. Arms
   b. Legs
   c. Gluteal region
   d. All of the above

4. Fluid exchange across the capillary wall is dependent upon which of the following?
   a. Capillary wall permeability
   b. Hydrostatic forces
   c. Oncotic forces
   d. All of the above

5. The principal oncotic force in the microvasculature is:
   a. Sodium
   b. Protein
   c. Potassium
   d. Calcium

6. The primary mechanism of compartment syndrome is:
   a. Hypotension
   b. Hypovolemia secondary to dehydration

   c. Ischemia secondary to hypoxia
   d. Increased pressure within an osteofascial compartment

7. Which of the following are involved in the cyclical mechanisms of compartment syndrome?
   a. Increased compartment pressure
   b. Decreased blood flow
   c. Ischemia and increased capillary permeability
   d. Edema
   e. All of the above

8. Compartment pressures are initially _____ in crush injury.
   a. Elevated
   b. Decreased
   c. Normal

9. The systemic complications of compartment syndrome and crush injury are known as:
   a. Crush toxidrome
   b. Rhabdomyolysis
   c. Crush syndrome
   d. Mangled extremity syndrome

10. Complications that may arise from the crush syndrome include:
    a. Electrolyte imbalance
    b. Renal failure
    c. DIC
    d. All of the above

11. The primary signs and symptoms of compartment syndrome are:
    a. Pain out of proportion to the injury
    b. Pain on passive stretch of the muscle in the involved compartment
    c. Decreased sensation and loss of motor function
    d. All of the above

12. The primary field intervention for treating compartment syndrome is:
    a. Aggressive fluid administration
    b. Administration of vasodilators
    c. Administration of vasoconstrictors
    d. Fasciotomy

13. Drugs that may be used in the management of compartment syndrome include:
    a. Calcium chloride
    b. Sodium bicarbonate
    c. Potassium
    d. Vasoconstrictors

14. Which of the following treatments are contraindicated in the management of compartment syndrome?
    a. PASG
    b. Tourniquets
    c. Tightly applied bandages
    d. All of the above

► CRITICAL THINKING

● You are dispatched to a private residence for a fall with injuries. Upon your arrival you find a 63-year-old female who has fallen down a flight of stairs. She states she fell at approximately 10 PM last evening, about 12 hours ago. She is positioned on her right side with her right leg beneath her. She states that she was unable to move due to pain in her hip and legs and has remained in this position since the fall. Upon physical examination, you note a mass in the inguinal area of the right leg, with shortening and external rotation of the extremity. Distal pulses are palpable and the leg is insensate. There is no pedal edema. No other injuries are noted and the remainder of the physical examination is unremarkable. In addition to the obvious anterior hip dislocation, what other pathologies may be present? In addition to immobilization, how will you treat this patient?

● As part of a mutual aid response, you are dispatched to the scene of an earthquake in a neighboring city. You are directed to an apartment complex where you are met by rescuers who have been on the scene for the past 36 hours. You are led into a collapsed building where you find a 27-year-old female who is trapped from the waist down by debris. Fire department personnel indicate they are preparing to lift the debris with a pneumatic jack and wanted you to be present in the event the patient needed treatment. The patient is conscious and alert and is quite relieved that she will finally be freed from her would-be tomb. Her only complaint is that her legs are numb. A cursory physical examination of the exposed portion of her body does not reveal any injury. As a matter of protocol, you establish an IV of normal saline and place her on oxygen. She reluctantly accepts the treatment stating, "I'm fine, I just want out of here and to get the feeling back in my legs." Just as the fire department removes the heavy debris, the patient experiences sudden cardiac arrest.

1. What do you think precipitated cardiac arrest in this patient? Could it have been prevented? What additional treatments were needed for this patient prior to removing the debris from her legs?

2. Treating hyperkalemia is a high priority in managing patients with crush syndrome. In addition to sodium bicarbonate, what other drugs can be used to manage hyperkalemia?

► REFERENCES

1. Moore RE 3rd, Friedman RJ. Current concepts in pathophysiology and diagnosis of compartment syndromes. *J Emerg Med*. 1989; 7(6):657.
2. Volkmann R. Die Ischaemischen Muskallahmangen und Kontnakturen. *Zentralbl Chir*. 1881; 8:801.
3. Christenson JT, Wulff K. Compartment pressure following leg injury: the effect of diuretic treatment. *Injury*. 1985; 16:591.
4. Mabee JR. Compartment syndrome: a complication of acute extremity trauma. *J Emerg Med*. 1994; 12(5):651.
5. Gulli B, Templeman D. Comparment syndrome of the lower extremity. *Orthop Clin North Am*. 1994; 25(4):677.
6. DeLee JL, Stiehl JB. Open tibia fracture with compartment syndrome. *Clin Orthop*. 1981; 160:175.
7. Aerts P, De Boeck HD, Casteleyn PP, Opdecam P. Deep volar compartment syndrome of the forearm following minor crush injury. *J Pediatr Orthop*. 1989; 9(1):69.
8. Martin RR, Mattox KL, Burch JM, Richardson RJ. Advances in treatment of vascular injuries from blunt and penetrating limb trauma. *World J Surg*. 1992; 16(5):930.
9. Vigasio A, Battison B, De Filippo G, Branelli G, Calabrese S. Compartment syndrome due to viper bite. *Arch Orthop Trauma Surg*. 1991; 110(3):175.
10. Schepsis AA, Lynch G: Exertional compartment syndromes of the lower extremity. *Curr Opin Rheumatol*. 1996; 8(2):143.
11. Mann R, Gibran N, Engrav L, Heimboch D. Is immediate decompression of high voltage electrical injuries to the upper extremity always necessary? *J Trauma*. 1996; 40(4):584.
12. d'Amato TA, Kaplan IB, Britt LD. High-voltage electrical injury: a role for mandatory exploration of deep muscle compartments. *J Natl Med Assoc*. 1994; 86(7):535.
13. Vidal R, Kissoon N, Gayle M. Compartment syndrome following intraosseous infusion. *Pediatrics*. 1993; 91(6):1201.
14. Prynn WL, Kates DE, Pollak CV Jr. Gluteal compartment syndrome. *Ann Emerg Med*. 1994; 24(6):1180.
15. Goldsmith AL, McCallum MI. Compartment syndrome as a complication of the prolonged use of the Lloyd-Davies position. *Anaesthesia*. 1996; 51(11): 1048.
16. Hawkins BJ, Bays PN. Catastrophic complication of simple cast treatment: case report. *J Trauma*. 1993; 34(5):760.

17. Griffiths D, Jones DH. Spontaneous compartment syndrome in a patient on long-term anticoagulation. *J Hand Surg Br*. 1993; 18(1):41.

18. Ouellette EA, Kelly R. Compartment syndromes of the hand. *J Bone Joint Surg Am*. 1996; 78(10):1515.

19. Shrier I, Magder S. Presssure-flow relationships in vitro model compartment syndrome. *J Appl Physiol*. 1995; 79(1):214.

20. Seebodee D, Scheidt H, Schmid-Schonbein H. A pressure chamber to simulate the microcirculation of compartment syndromes. *Microvasc Res*. 1994; 47(3):338.

21. Mabee JR, Bostwick TL. Pathophysiology and mechanisms of compartment syndrome. *Orthop Rev*. 1993; 22(2):175.

22. Har-Shai Y, Silbermann M, Reis ND, et al. Muscle microcirculatory impairment following acute compartment syndrome in the dog. *Plast Reconstr Surg*. 1992; 89(2):283.

23. Ross D. Acute compartment syndrome. *Orthop Nurs*. 1991; 10(2):33.

24. Schein M, Wittman DH, Aprahamian CC, Condon RE. The abdominal compartment syndrome: the pathophysiology and clinical consequences of elevated intra-abdominal pressure. *J Am Coll Surg*. 1995; 180:745.

25. Bleicher RJ, Sherman HF, Latenser BA. Bilateral gluteal compartment syndrome. *J Trauma*. 1997; 42(1):118.

26. Schmalzried TP, Neal WC, Eckardt JJ. Gluteal compartment and crush syndromes. Report of three cases and review of the literature. *Clin Orthop Related Res*. APR 1992; (277):161.

27. Burch JM, Moore EE, Moore FA, Francoise R. The abdominal compartment syndrome. *Surg Clin North Am*. 1996; 76(4):833.

28. Brathwaite CE, Rodriguez A, Turney SZ, Dunham CM, Cowley R. Blunt traumatic cardiac rupture. A 5-year experience. *Ann Surg*. 1990; 212(6):701.

29. Brathwaite CE, Rodriguez A. Injuries of the abdominal aorta from blunt trauma. *Am Surg*. 1992; 58(6):350.

30. Reisman JD, Morgan AS. Analysis of 46 intra-abdominal aortic injuries from blunt trauma: case reports and literature review. *J Trauma*. 1990; 30(10):1294.

31. Smejkal R, Izant T, Born C, DeLong W, Schwab W, Ross SE. Pelvic crush injuries with occlusion of the iliac artery. *J Trauma*. 1988; 28(10):1479.

32. Michaelson M. Crush injury and crush syndrome. *World J Surg*. 1992; 16:899.

33. Reis ND, Michaelson M. Crush injury to lower limb. *J Bone Joint Surg*. 1986; 68A(3):414.

34. Michaelson M, Taitelman U, Bshouty Z, Bar-Joseph G, Bursztein S. Crush syndrome: experience from the Lebanon War. *Isr J Med*. 1982; 20:305.

35. Carter PR. Crush injury of the upper limb. *Orthop Clin North Am*. 1984; 14(4):719.

36. Mattox K, ed. *Complications of Trauma*. New York: Churchill Livingstone; 1994.

37. Johansen K, Daines M, Howley T, Helfet D, Hansen ST Jr. Objective criteria accurately predict amputation following lower extremity trauma. *J Trauma*. 1990; 30:568.

38. Cheney P. Early management and physiologic changes in crush syndrome. *Crit Care Nurs Q*. 1994; 17(2):62.

39. Better OS. The crush syndrome revisited (1940–1990). *Nephronology*. 1990; 55:97.

40. Better OS, Stein JH. Early management of shock and prophylaxis of acute renal failure in traumatic rhabdomyolysis. *N Engl J Med*. 1990; 322:825.

41. Peck SA. Crush syndrome: pathophysiology and management. *Orthop Nurs*. 1990; 9:33.

42. Bloom AI, Zarnir G, Muggia M, Friedlander M, Gimmon Z, Rivkind A. Torture rhabdomyorhexis—a pseudo-crush syndrome. *J Trauma*. 1995; 38(2):252.

43. Shirreffs TG Jr. Compartment syndrome: an extremity at risk. *Emerg Med*. 1990; 22(6):102.

44. Tscherne H, Gotzen L, eds. *Fractures with Soft Tissue Injuries*. New York: Springer-Verlag; 1984.

45. Matsen FA III, Winquist RA, Krugmire RB Jr. Diagnosis and management of compartment syndromes. *J Bone Joint Surg*. 1980; 62A:286.

46. Cook T, Brown D, Roe J. Hypokalemia, hypophosphatemia, and compartment syndrome of the leg after downhill skiing on moguls. *J Emerg Med*. 1993; 11:709.

47. Clayton JM, Hayes AC, Barnes RW. Tissue pressure and perfusion in the compartment syndrome. *J Surg Res*. 1977; 22:333.

48. Better OS, Rubinstein I, Winaver J. Recent insight into the pathogenesis and early management of the crush syndrome. *Semin Nephrol*. 1992; 12:217.

49. Matsen FA. *Compartment Syndromes*. New York: Grune and Stratton; 1980.

50. Vitale GC, Richardson JD, George SM Jr, Miller FB. Fasciotomies for severe, blunt and penetrating trauma of the extremity. *Surg Gynecol Obstet*. 1988; 166(5):397.

51. Bouachour G, Cronier P, Gouello JP, Toulemonde JL, Talha A, Alquier P. Hyperbaric oxygen therapy in the management of crush injuries: a randomized double-blind placebo-controlled clinical trial. *J Trauma*. 1996; 41(2):333.

52. Shah DM, Bock DE, Darling RC 3rd, Chang BB, Kupinski AM, Leather RP. Beneficial effects of hypertonic mannitol in acute ischemia-reperfusion injuries in humans. *Cardiovasc Surg.* 1996; 4(1):97.

53. Ferreira TA, Pensado A, Dominguez L, Aymench H, Molins N. Compartment syndrome with severe rhabdomyolysis in the postoperative period following major vascular surgery. *Anaesthesia.* 1996; 51(7):692.

54. Better OS, Zinman C, Reid DN, Har-Shai Y, Rubenstein I, Abassi Z. Hypertonic mannitol ameliorates intracompartmental tamponade in model compartment syndrome in the dog. *Nephron.* 1991; 58(3):344.

55. Buchbinder D, Karmody AM, Leather RP, Shah DM. Hypertonic mannitol: its use in the prevention of revascularization syndrome after acute arterial ischemia. *Arch Surg.* 1981; 116:414.

56. Hakaim AG, Corsetti R, Cho SI. The pentafraction of hydroxyethyl starch inhibits ischemia-induced compartment syndrome. *J Trauma.* 1994; 37(1):18.

57. Ricci MA, Graham AM, Corbisiero R, Baffour R, Mohamed F, Symes JF. Are free radical scavengers benefical in the treatment of compartment syndrome after acute arterial ischemia? *J Vasc Surg.* 1989; 9(2):244.

58. Ferrari RP, Battison B, Brunelli G, Casella A, Caimi L. The role of allopurinol in preventing oxygen free radical injury to skeletal muscle and endothelial cells after ischemia-reperfusion. *J Reconstr Microsurg.* 1996; 12(7):447.

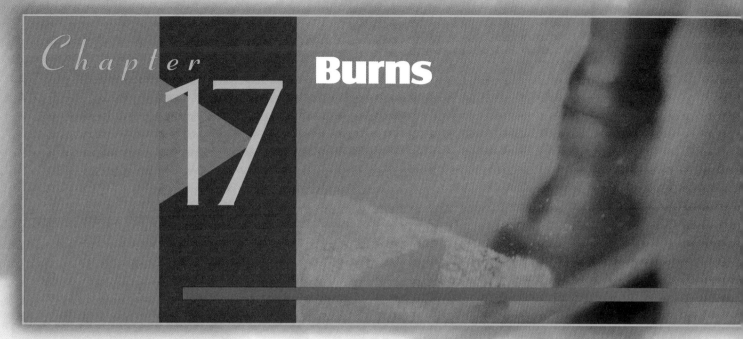

Chapter 17 Burns

OBJECTIVES

Upon completion of this chapter, the reader should be able to:

- Describe the epidemiology of burn injury.
- Describe the anatomy and physiology of the skin.
- List the four basic functions the human skin performs as a vital organ.
- Outline and define the American Burn Association classification of burns.
- Describe the appearance of the following:
  1. First-degree (superficial partial-thickness) burns
  2. Second-degree (deep partial-thickness) burns
  3. Third-degree (full-thickness) burns
- Identify methods utilized to calculate the total body surface area (TBSA) burned.
- Outline principles and methods of emergency assessment, stabilization, and transfer of the burn-injured person from the scene of injury to admission to the burn care facility.
- Outline the major pathophysiological processes following thermal injury.
- Outline the pathophysiology, assessment, and management of an inhalation injury.
- Outline techniques of assessing and monitoring the cardiovascular, pulmonary, renal, gastrointestinal, and neurological system in the emergent and acute phases of burn injury.
- Identify potential complications of these systems secondary to burn injuries.
- Describe the principles of fluid resuscitation, including the Parkland formula, for the burn-injured patient.
- Describe the prehospital management of pain for the burn-injured patient.
- Discuss the epidemiology, pathophysiology, assessment, and treatment of the patient with an electrical injury.
- Discuss the epidemiology, pathophysiology, assessment, and treatment of the patient with a chemical injury.
- Discuss the unique factors of the pediatric burn patient.

KEY TERMS

Burn shock

Circumferential burn

Corium

Dermis

Epidermis

First-degree burn

Full-thickness burn

Joule's law

Lund and Browder chart

Moderate-deep partial-
thickness burn

Ohm's law

Parkland formula

Partial-thickness burn

Rule of nines

Second-degree burn

Stratum corneum

Subcutaneous tissue

Third-degree burn

Zone of coagulation

Zone of hyperemia

Zone of stasis

Shortly after man discovered fire, he discovered burn injuries. Records of burn care can be traced to the early writings of ancient Egypt, Greece, and Europe. Documentation carefully describes the removal of foreign bodies, suturing, and wound protection with clean materials.[1] Burn care has progressed through the years from the documented use of herbs by the early Romans to the application of onions, leeks, and animal dung in the seventh century. In the 1800s, Lister and Semmelweis recognized the influence of bacteria on wound sepsis and the infectious process; thus, the use of vegetables and animal dung was greatly lessened.[2]

Modern-day burn care has progressed to include a highly specialized team of health care professionals. In 1947, the first official burn unit was established at Brooke Army Medical Center, Fort Sam Houston, in San Antonio, Texas. Today, there are approximately 138 burn care facilities (about 1,700 beds) designated specifically for the care of the burn patient.[3] The paramedic, in order to effectively treat the burn patient and his or her family, must have a full comprehension of the burn injury, its etiology, and the confidence to provide critical care needed in the first moments following a burn injury.

EPIDEMIOLOGY

It is estimated that 1.2 million Americans are burned each year. Approximately 51,000 individuals will require hospitalization for the care of their burn wounds. Burns account for approximately 5,500 deaths per year.[4] Fire and burn injuries are the second leading cause of unintentional deaths in children 1–4 years of age and the third leading cause of injury and death for ages 1–18.[5] According to the National Committee for Injury Prevention and Control, fire and burns in older adults are the third leading cause of unintentional deaths, preceded by falls and motor vehicle collisions.[6] A burn involves the destruction of skin cells and sometimes the underlying structures of muscle, subcutaneous tissue, and bone. A burn occurs when these structures absorb more heat than their capacity to dissipate it.

BURN-PRONE PATIENTS

The very young (children less than 4 years of age) and the elderly (individuals over the age of 65) are the most vulnerable to burn injury. These injuries occur for several reasons: their inability to care for themselves, curiosity, sensory changes associated with the aging process, and the inability to thoroughly comprehend "cause and effect." Burn-prone patients also include those who are physically and mentally challenged and persons with psychiatric disorders.

ANATOMY AND PHYSIOLOGY

The skin is the largest organ of the body. It serves as the first line of defense against infection and trauma. The skin also aids in the regulation of temperature, production of vitamin D, and retention of body fluids. The sense of pressure, pain, touch, and temperature, which allow individuals to interact with their environment and respond to danger, are found in the skin. Psychosocially, the skin may be used to identify or describe individuals by race, distinguishing marks, or fingerprints. Because the skin is a visible organ, there are also cosmetic factors; many people are concerned about the texture, condition, and appearance of their skin. The skin consists of two layers: the epidermis and the dermis (corium). The subcutaneous tissue is under the dermis but is not considered a layer of skin. Muscle and bone lie underneath the subcutaneous tissue. Figure 17-1 illustrates the various layers of the skin.

EPIDERMIS

The **epidermis** is the outer layer of skin and is composed of five cellular layers: stratum corneum, stratum lucidum, stratum granulosum, stratum sponsor, and

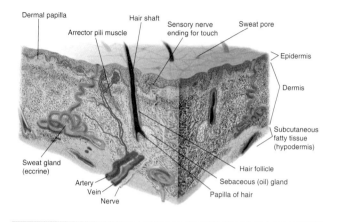

Dermal papilla
Hair shaft
Arrector pili muscle
Sensory nerve ending for touch
Sweat pore
Epidermis
Dermis
Subcutaneous fatty tissue (hypodermis)
Sweat gland (eccrine)
Artery
Vein
Nerve
Hair follicle
Sebaceous (oil) gland
Papilla of hair

FIGURE 17-1 Various layers of skin.

stratum germinativum. The two layers most significant in burn injuries are the stratum corneum, or surface layer, and the deepest layer, the stratum germinativum. The **stratum corneum** acts as a vapor barrier to the body and protects the body from microorganisms and chemicals. The stratum corneum is composed mostly of dead keratinized cells surrounded by a lipid mono-layer. When the stratum corneum becomes damaged by burns, body fluids (water, electrolytes, and albumin) escape. New epithelial covering of the stratum corneum are provided by cellular regeneration of the stratum germinativum. The epidermis contains no blood vessels but receives nourishment from capillaries in the upper part of the dermis. Layers of the epidermis vary in thickness and according to age. It is thickest (0.24 in./0.61 cm) on the upper back and thinnest (0.02 in./0.05 cm) on the eyelids.[7] Individuals exposed to the same temperature for the same length of time may have varying degrees of burn injury on different parts of the body due to the age factor. The skin of the very young and the very old is thin and translucent, making an accurate assessment of burn depth difficult. By virtue of the fact that their skin is thinner, these two age groups may sustain more severe burns at lower temperatures and in less time than an average adult. For example, children under the age of 2 have dispro-portionately thin skin that may result in full-thickness, third-degree burns that initially may appear to be partial-thickness burns. Persons in the age group from birth to preteen have greater stamina and endurance, generally better health, and fewer incidences of past medical problems. Because of the increased metabolic rate, tissue regeneration is usually faster in this age group than in other populations. After a burn injury, the vulnerability of an older adult is demonstrated by impaired tissue regeneration, decreased functional

reserves, poorer immunological function, and pro-longed tissue regeneration. These contribute to a reduced ability to cope with the constant and pro-longed stress of a burn injury.

DERMIS

The **dermis** is the second layer of skin and is com-posed primarily of collagen and fibrous tissue. It is also known as the **corium**, or true skin, since it is continu-ously being shed and replaced, as is the epidermis. The surface of the dermis is uneven because of papillae that attach it to the epidermis. Arterioles and capillaries receive blood from arteries beneath the dermis. The corium is interlaced with sensory nerve endings that identify the sensations of touch, pressure, pain, and temperature. This is a protective mechanism that allows an individual to adapt to changes in the physical environment. The dermis also contains the lymphatic system of the skin.

SUBCUTANEOUS TISSUE

Subcutaneous tissue (also known as superficial fas-cia) lies below the dermis and is firmly attached to the dermal layer of skin by collagen fibers. It is composed of areolar, adipose, and loose connective tissue. This layer of tissue varies in thickness because of the varying amounts of adipose tissue in each individual. The deep fascia layer lies underneath the superficial fascia and surrounds muscles and blood vessels. This layer is con-nected to the periosteum of bones.

BURN WOUND DEPTH

A burn involves the destruction of skin cells and some-times the underlying structures of muscle, fascia, and bone. A burn occurs when the heat that is absorbed surpasses the capacity to dissipate it. The depth of the burn wound depends upon the exposure time (duration of contact) and the causative energy source, such as heat, caustic chemicals, or electricity. Another factor affecting burn wound depth is related to the individual who has been burned. Children and older adults, by virtue of the fact that their skin is thinner, may sustain more severe burns at lower temperatures and in less time than a younger adult. Exposure for just 3 seconds to water that is 140°F, (44°C) (the temperature of the average home's hot water as it comes from the tap) can result in a full-thickness or third-degree burn that may require hospitalization and skin grafts.[8] The severity of the burn injury depends upon the burn agent and burn circumstances, location, age, concomitant injuries, and preexisting conditions of the individual.

There are three dimensions of a burn wound. The superficial outer zone is referred to as the **zone of hyperemia** and is similar to a sunburn. The middle layer is known as the **zone of stasis**. Because of the damage done to microcirculation, capillary permeability allows fluid to leak into the extravascular spaces. The formation of edema and potential burn shock may be associated with this phenomenon. The innermost layer is known as the **zone of coagulation** or necrosis. At this level of destruction, there is obstruction of the microcirculation, which prevents the humoral defenses of the immune response from reaching the burned tissue.[9] The depth of the burn wound determines the type of wound care required and the time required for healing. Figure 17-2 reveals the depths of burn wounds.

SUPERFICIAL PARTIAL-THICKNESS BURNS

Burns in which only the epidermis has been injured may be classified as **partial-thickness burns** or **first-degree burns**. These burns may have a pink or light red appearance and are considered minor burns. The burned tissue may be dry and painful and with or without small blister formation. This injury is often compared to a mild-moderate sunburn. Individuals, such as construction workers, agricultural workers, and gardeners, who work predominately out of doors are highly susceptible to this type of injury. The patient may experience mild hypersensitivity (pain) as a result of this injury. This burn usually heals in 5–10 days.[10] Figure 17-3 is an example of a first-degree (superficial partial-thickness) burn injury.

INTERNET ACTIVITIES

Visit the e-medicine Web site at http://www.emedicine.com. Click on the Emergency Medicine on-line book and select Environmental Emergencies. Then click on Sun Burn. Review the chapter on the management of sunburn.

DEEP PARTIAL-THICKNESS BURNS

Second-degree or **moderate-deep partial-thickness burns** involve the epidermal and varying degrees of the dermal layers of skin. The second-degree burn injury is further divided into superficial and deep dermal injuries. Superficial injuries are the result of brief contact with hot liquids, flashes of flames, or brief exposure to flames. Typically, this injury has a bright red or mottled (dull) red appearance and a moist surface and exhibits extreme sensitivity to stimuli (even a

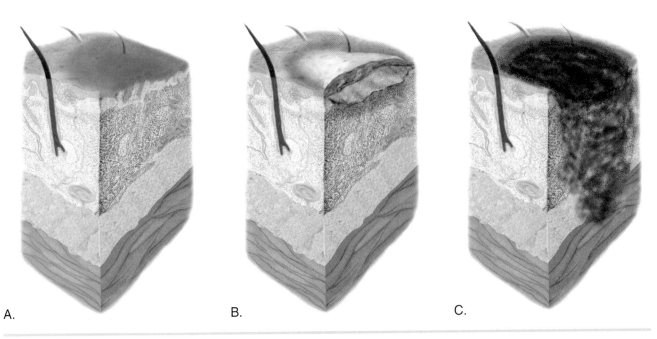

A. B. C.

FIGURE 17-2 Depth of burn wounds. (A) Superficial partial-thickness burn, (B) moderate–deep partial-thickness burn, (C) full-thickness burn.

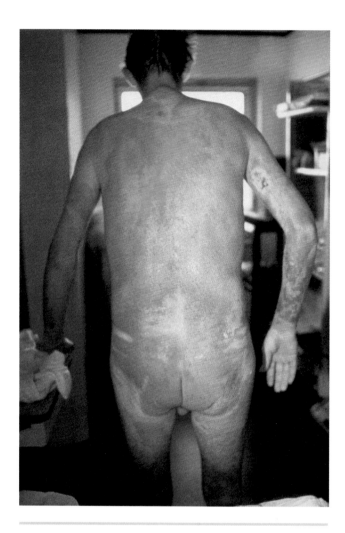

FIGURE 17-3 A first-degree burn received by an elderly patient who was unable to turn off the hot water from the shower in time to prevent him from being burned.

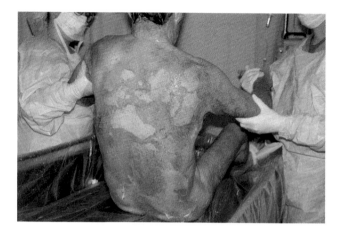

FIGURE 17-4 A partial-thickness burn injury received by a patient who unintentionally spilled boiling hot water on himself. Note the blisters and loose skin.

current of air). The skin remains soft and pliable, but some edema may be present. Formation of blisters is very common for this degree of injury. Blisters should be kept as intact as possible as breakage may increase the chance for infection. This injury should heal in approximately 1–2 weeks.[10,11] An example of a second-degree burn is noted in Figure 17-4.

Deeper second-degree injury (deep partial-thickness burns) involves the entire epidermal and dermal layers of the skin. Sweat glands and hair follicles remain intact. These burns are very painful because sensory nerve endings are partially destroyed. Deep partial-thickness burns are dark red or yellow-white in color, have a slightly moist surface, and exhibit decreased pin-prick sensation but intact deep pressure sensation. These burns require more than 3 weeks for natural healing but may also require skin grafting procedures to help speed the healing process.[10,11] An example of a deep partial-thickness burn injury is noted in Figure 17-5.

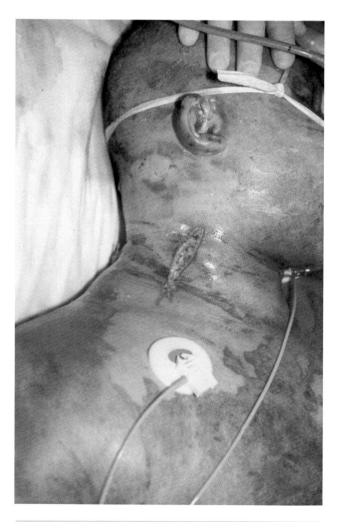

FIGURE 17-5 A deep partial-thickness burn received from a house fire. Note the cherry red appearance of the skin.

FULL-THICKNESS BURNS

Third-degree, or **full-thickness burns**, extend into the subcutaneous tissue and may involve muscle and bone. This injury may be caused by exposure to concentrated chemicals, high-voltage electricity, flame, and prolonged contact with hot objects. Full-thickness burns have a white, waxy appearance, charred/parchment tan appearance, or black appearance. The skin texture typically is hard, dry, and leathery. Edema is prevalent because fluid is absorbed from underlying tissues by the leaking wound. The diagnostic finding of full-thickness burns is a lack of sensation and pain because of the destruction of nerve endings, unless the burn is surrounded by areas of partial-thickness burns. Thrombosed superficial veins, a lack of capillary refill,

and the leathery skin texture are also characteristics of a full-thickness injury. All epithelial elements are destroyed, rendering the burn incapable of self-regeneration. Grafting is required for wound closure. Figure 17-6 is an example of a full-thickness burn injury. Table 17-1 reflects clinical characteristics of partial-thickness and full-thickness burn wounds.

EXTENT OF INJURY

The depth of a burn wound is not the only factor that affects the magnitude of these injuries. Illness and death may be related to surface area involved, depth of the burn, age of the patient, prior state of health of the patient, location of the burn wound, and severity of any

Table 17-1
Clinical Characteristics of Partial-Thickness and Full-Thickness Burn Wounds

	Partial -Thickness Burns		Full-Thickness or Third-Degree Burns
	Second-Degree Burns		
First-Degree Burns	**Superficial**	**Deep Dermal**	

Cause*
Sun
Minor flash
	Hot liquids
	Flashes of flame
	Brief exposure to
	    dilute chemicals
		Hot liquids
		Flashes of flame
		Brief exposure to
		    dilute chemicals
			Flame
			High-voltage electricity
			Exposure to concentrated
			    chemicals
			Contact with hot metal

Color* Pink or light red	Bright red or mottled red	Dark red or yellow-white	Pearly white or charred Translucent and parchment- like
Surface* Dry or small blisters	Variably sized bullae Moist and weeping	Large bullae often ruptured Slightly moist	Dry with shreds of nonviable epidermis Thrombosed vessels visible

Texture*
Soft with minimal edema
    and later superficial
    exfoliation
	Thickened by edema
	    but pliable
		Moderate edema with
		    decreased pliability
			Inelastic and leathery

Sensation*
Hypersensitive
	Hypersensitive	Decreased pinprick
		    sensation
		Intact deep pressure
		    sensation
			Hypalgesic

Healing* 3–6 days	10–21 days	>21 days	Grafting required

*These criteria apply to all categories of burns.

Source: Pruitt BA, Goodwin CW. *Textbook of Clinical Surgery.* St Louis: Mosby Yearbook; 1995.

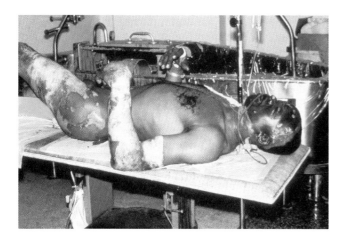

FIGURE 17-6 A full-thickness burn injury received from a house fire. Note the tan/khaki-colored, leathery texture of the skin.

and does not allow for differences in proportion in infants, children, and adults.

The use of the rule of nines designed for the adult is not accurate when assessing burns in children associated injuries. An estimation of the extent of the burn injury should be ascertained by the paramedic. Two of the most common methods used for calculation of the percent total body surface area burned are the rule of nines and the Lund and Browder chart. The **rule of nines** (Figure 17-7) is the most common universal guide used to determine the extent of a burn injury. This method divides the body into segments whose areas are either 9% or multiples of 9% of the total body surface area (TBSA); the perineum is counted as 1%. This formula is easy and quick to use for an initial assessment; however, it is often inaccurate

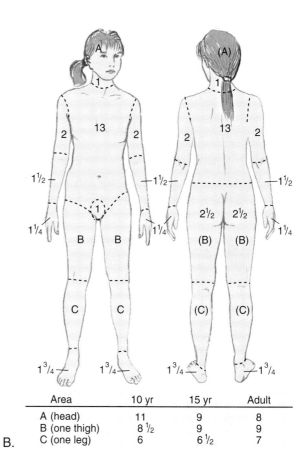

Area	10 yr	15 yr	Adult
A (head)	11	9	8
B (one thigh)	8 ½	9	9
C (one leg)	6	6 ½	7

B.

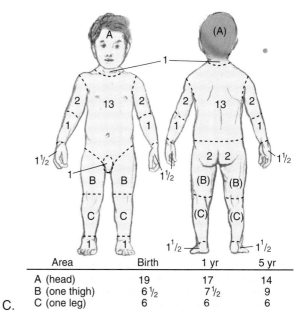

Area	Birth	1 yr	5 yr
A (head)	19	17	14
B (one thigh)	6 ½	7 ½	9
C (one leg)	6	6	6

C.

A.

FIGURE 17-7 Rule of nines for an adult and estimation of child burn percentages. (A) Adult, (B) Ages 10 years to dault, (C) Ages birth to 5 years.

or burns that may be scattered over the body. The distribution of surface area by body parts is quite different in infants and children, in whom the head and neck represent a considerably greater percentage of the total body surface area than in the adult. Hence the pediatric rule of nines (sometimes referred to as the rule of nineteen) should be used when assessing burns in this population. In children, during the first year of life, the head and neck are 19% of the body surface and each lower extremity is $12\frac{1}{2}$%. With each year of age, subtract 1% from the head and neck and add it to the lower extremity. By age 10, the surface area distribution approximates that of the adult (see Figure 17-7).[12]

The use of the **Lund and Browder chart** provides a more accurate and precise estimation of burn injuries. The Lund and Browder chart is an age-related anatomic scale or diagram in which the percentage of anatomical body parts such as hands, feet, upper arm, and lower arm allows for more accurate estimation of the extent of the burn.

An adaptation of both methods utilizes the palm of the patient's closed hand. This is commonly referred to as the rule of palm. This method refers to the palmar side of the patient's hand (minus the fingers) as 1% of the body surface area and allows for the estimation of irregularly disposed burns. However, for children, the Lund and Browder chart is recommended (See Figure 17-8).[12,13]

INTERNET ACTIVITIES

Visit the Wake Forest University Web site at www.wfubmc.edu/burnunit/index.html and examine and explore the SAGE II computerized burn diagramming tool used to determine percentages and to note depths of burns.

BURN CLASSIFICATION

The American Burn Association categorizes burns as minor, moderate, or major, based on depth of tissue destruction, TBSA affected, age, cause of the injury, body part affected, preexisting disease, and trauma, as follows:

● Minor burns are first- and second-degree burns in the adult that are less than 15% TBSA or less than

Lund and Browder's Burn Estimate Diagram

AREA	Inf.	1-4	5-9	10-14	15	Adult
HEAD	19	17	13	11	9	7
NECK	2	2	2	2	2	2
ANT. TRUNK	13	13	13	13	13	13
POST. TRUNK	13	13	13	13	13	13
R. BUTTOCK	2.5	2.5	2.5	2.5	2.5	2.5
L. BUTTOCK	2.5	2.5	2.5	2.5	2.5	2.5
GENITALIA	1	1	1	1	1	1
R.U. ARM	4	4	4	4	4	4
L.U. ARM	4	4	4	4	4	4
R.L. ARM	3	3	3	3	3	3
L.L. ARM	3	3	3	3	3	3
R. HAND	2.5	2.5	2.5	2.5	2.5	2.5
L. HAND	2.5	2.5	2.5	2.5	2.5	2.5
R. THIGH	5.5	6.5	8	8.5	9	9.5
L. THIGH	5.5	6.5	8	8.5	9	9.5
R. LEG	5	5	5.5	6	6.5	7
L. LEG	5	5	5.5	6	6.5	7
R. FOOT	3.5	3.5	3.5	3.5	3.5	3.5
L. FOOT	3.5	3.5	3.5	3.5	3.5	3.5

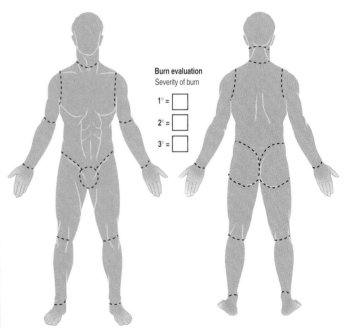

Burn evaluation
Severity of burn

1° = □
2° = □
3° = □

FIGURE 17-8 Lund and Browder chart.

10% TBSA in children, and third-degree burns less than 2% full thickness. Minor burns do not involve special care areas such as the face, eyes, ears, hands, feet, or perineum.

- Moderate burns are mixed partial- and full-thickness burns of 15%–25% TBSA in adolescents and young adults, 10%–20% partial thickness in children under the age of 10 and adults over age 40, and full-thickness burns of less than 10% TBSA not involving special care areas.

- Major burns are all burn injuries totaling more than 25% TBSA in adolescents and young adults; burns involving more than 20% TBSA in children under 10 and adults over 40; full-thickness burns of 10% TBSA or more; all burns involving the hands, feet, face, eyes, ears, or perineum that are likely to result in either functional or cosmetic impairment; all inhalation, chemical, high-voltage electrical injuries, or burns complicated by fractures or other major trauma; and burns that occur in high-risk patients, such as infants, the elderly, and patients with diabetes, heart disease, renal disorders, or other health problems such as cerebral vascular accidents, head injury, psychiatric disabilities, or closed-space injuries.[14]

EMERGENCY BURN CARE

The paramedic must be aware that the burn injury should be treated the same as any other trauma injury. First, evaluate the scene for safety. Carefully remove the patient from the burning source, such as heat, chemical, or electrical contact. Instruct the patient to stop, drop, and roll if still aflame or use a coat, blanket, or heavy rug to extinguish the fire. After the flame has been smothered, pour cool water from a faucet, garden hose, or any other available source over the burned skin. Normal saline should be used if a ready source of tap water is not available. Covering the burn with a moist sterile dressing will assist in pain relief and help stop the burning process. Cooling should be done just to the temperature of unburned skin and should be performed within 10–15 minutes of the injury. If more time has elapsed, radiative loss of heat and heat transfer by the circulation at the periphery of the burn will have returned tissue temperature to essentially normal levels. Any attempts to wipe the burned area may result in further skin damage. Do not apply ice; it accelerates the loss of body heat through the broken skin, causing further tissue damage, and increases the risk of hypothermia and shock. All clothing, jewelry, and other objects on the body should be immediately removed because they trap heat and may constrict circulation as edema begins to form. Care should be used when removing

these objects to prevent further skin damage. Any clothing still attached can trap heat (in the case of thermal burns) next to the body and should be removed. Use scissors to trim away the clothing as broken bones and hidden objects piercing the body may go undetected. No attempts should be made to debride the burned tissue. Most importantly the paramedic should remember the 3 Cs when assessing the burn patient: *cool, cover, and carry.* The patient should be covered with a clean sheet and then a blanket to conserve body heat and minimize the risk of hypothermia.

INITIAL ASSESSMENT

The initial assessment is a thorough assessment of the airway, breathing, circulation, and cervical spine stabilization, especially if the burn involved an explosion, car collision, or electrical injury. The initial assessment sets into motion the proper care that is needed to decrease the morbidity and mortality of the burn patient.

Airway

Assessment of the patient's airway for patency must be very thorough. The paramedic should observe the chest to evaluate the patient's breathing. Listening to breath sounds will help determine the presence of a pneumothorax or other complications. The decision to administer oxygen, intubate, and ventilate the patient is dependent on the extent of TBSA burn or the presence of facial burns. Burns to the chest may further complicate respiratory efforts as they may produce a tourniquet-like effect, making chest expansion and breathing difficult to impossible. Remember to assess other signs of inadequate oxygenation of the body such as nasal flaring, stridor, or hoarseness and signs of cyanosis in the nail beds, gums of the mouth, and sclera of the eyes. The level of consciousness (impaired sensorium) of the patient will also assist with this assessment. Pulse oximetry should be employed as a helpful tool but should not be heavily depended upon because a false reading can occur; hemoglobin combined with carbon monoxide (and other end products of combustion inhaled by the patient) is not detected. The percentage saturation of oxyhemoglobin may appear normal. Endotracheal intubation is indicated if the patient is semiconscious or unresponsive, has deep burns to the face and neck, or is otherwise critically injured. Intubation should be done early in all doubtful cases since delayed intubation will be difficult to achieve in cases associated with upper airway edema and/or injury. An emergency cricothyrotomy or tracheostomy may be necessary under difficult circumstances. Particular attention should be given to the airway while en route to the hospital and should be assessed repeatedly. With the exception of minor burns, patients should receive high-flow humidified oxygen during transport.

Circulation

Circulation should be assessed as well. Baseline vital signs, including pulse, blood pressure, and respiratory rate, should be obtained at the scene and during transport. Pay close attention to extremities, which may have suffered a **circumferential burn** (a burn in which the injury completely surrounds a body part). Circulatory demise to extremities due to edema formation may occlude venous blood flow. If this is not corrected, arterial blood flow will be reduced to a low level, resulting in ischemia, necrosis, and eventually development of gangrene. Prolonged circulatory compromise could result in muscle or nerve damage and lead to compartment syndrome. A thorough examination of the pulse should include the ability to palpate a pulse, observation of the nail beds for cyanosis, and complaints of numbness, pain, or tingling sensation by the patient. Prior to and during transport the paramedic should elevate burned extremities above the level of the heart to slow the process of edema formation.

HISTORY AND PHYSICAL EXAMINATION

Conduct a thorough history and physical examination of the burned patient. This is a head-to-toe examination to rule out further injuries. The burn is often the most obvious injury, but other serious, even life-threatening injuries may be present. The paramedic should focus on a systematic approach when performing the physical examination, making certain to examine each of the body's systems. During this examination, it is important to obtain a thorough history of the incident. This may require asking questions of the patient, family, coworkers, or bystanders for more details. Find out if the incident happened within an enclosed space, if there was an explosion, or if chemicals were involved. A medical history of the patient is extremely important. The paramedic collects a history of allergies, medications, and tetanus immunization. Preexisting illnesses or diseases should also be considered, such as diabetes, hypertension, and cardiac or renal disease. The use of alcohol and drugs should be documented and reported to emergency department staff. If the patient is a child or elder and the burn wound looks suspicious, check for cigarette, scalding, or immersion burns as well as other signs of possible abuse and trauma, such as broken bones and bruises. Any reasons to suspect attempted self-immolation should also be documented. This should be considered when a reasonable explanation of the mechanism of the burn is lacking.

BURN SHOCK

Burn shock describes a specific type of hypovolemic shock in which smaller components of blood are lost from the vascular space. Burn shock is due to the loss of fluid from the vascular compartment into the area of injury. The bigger the burn, the greater the degree of shock. The greatest loss of fluid occurs within the first 8–12 hours. Fluid loss occurs as a result of the altered capillary permeability, severe hypoproteinemia, and the shift of sodium into the cells. Burn shock at the cellular level is caused by a decrease in cell membrane potential from a normal of –90 mV to levels of –80 to –70 mV. Cell death occurs at –60 mV.[2] At these lowered potentials, sodium and water shift into the cell, causing intracellular swelling. The cause of the decreased cell membrane potential is believed to be a failure of the energy-dependent enzyme systems [adenosine triphosphatase (ATPase)] that maintain the normal sodium-potassium gradient.[15] The sodium pump slows down due to hypoxia, leading to an increase of sodium chloride inside the cell and potassium outside the cell. Initially, the patient has hyperkalemia from the release of potassium from the cells and fluid shifts from the intravascular space. Perfusion to this area is diminished, not only because of the hypovolemia associated with capillary permeability changes, but also because of the formation of microvascular thrombi caused by direct heat injury and venous stasis.

Insensible water loss, such as from normal respiration, also contributes to burn shock. Fluid loss from burned skin is 5–10 times greater than that from undamaged skin. If a patient has burns on 50% of his or her body, water loss can amount to 4,000–5,000 mL/day. Heat loss may also result in hypothermia. Approximately 2,000–4,000 calories may be expended in the evaporation process, resulting in hypothermia. Both water and heat loss may contribute to a hypermetabolic state. The systemic response to burn shock is noted in several body tissues. In a very real sense, the burn patient is truly the universal trauma model. The systemic response to burn injury involves all organ systems.[15]

CARDIOVASCULAR INVOLVEMENT

Cardiovascular instability may be related to microvascular changes and hypovolemia. Cardiac output is decreased initially because of hypovolemia. Without treatment, hypovolemia, caused by the progressive loss of fluid through the burn wound, reduces cardiac filling and further decreases cardiac output. This results in diminished blood flow to the kidneys and other organs. The combination of hypovolemia and decreased cardiac output generates a vasoconstrictive response as the body attempts to compensate for the loss of blood volume. Also noted is a dramatic increase in the heart rate and blood pressure. Keep in mind that children have a very labile cardiovascular system; pulse, rather than blood pressure, is a better indicator of change.

PULMONARY INVOLVEMENT

The pulmonary system is reasonably well protected from the early edema process. There are no significant alterations in pulmonary function unless the patient is suffering from an inhalation injury. The patient may hyperventilate early postburn, but this will not persist unless pulmonary complications set in. Pulmonary edema is uncommon during the resuscitation period unless there is a superimposed inhalation injury. Some researchers report a release of pulmonary vasoconstrictors, such as catecholamines, thromboxane, and serotonin. These substances can cause transient pulmonary artery hypertension, resulting in hyperventilation.[16] Pulmonary complications are discussed in the section on inhalation injury.

RENAL INVOLVEMENT

The response of the kidney to burn injury is directly related to the hemodynamic changes. Early postburn reduction of renal blood flow and glomerular filtration rate results in oliguria because of a decrease of free water and endogenous creatine clearance. If resuscitation measures are inordinately delayed and the hypovolemia progresses, acute renal failure may occur. Other causes of renal damage include occlusion of the nephron and tubules due to buildup of hemoglobin released from destroyed red blood cells (RBCs) in the early stages of the burn and/or the accumulation of myoglobin from the destruction of muscle mass in electrical burns.

GASTROINTESTINAL (GI) INVOLVEMENT

Cessation of normal peristaltic activity is the initial response of the GI tract to a significant burn injury. The resulting ileus that occurs is the net effect of the hypovolemic process and the neurological and endocrine response to the injury. Circulatory supply will be altered as a compensatory mechanism in response to shock. The body shunts blood from the GI periphery to the major organs. The insertion of a nasogastric tube to prevent aspiration in patients with extensive burns is indicated.

HEMATOLOGICAL INVOLVEMENT

The elements of the blood are affected in direct proportion to the extent of the burn. Destruction of RBCs

occurs in the burned area with reduced red cell half-life secondary to increased fragility. Anemia results from red cell damage and reduced half-life. Red blood cells usually remain inside the blood vessels during the fluid shift, which often results in an increase in the hematocrit and hemoglobin in the immediate postburn period. As fluid leaks into the extravascular space, the cellular components of the blood become more concentrated, resulting in an increased hematocrit and sluggish blood flow. This causes ischemia in the underlying tissue to a depth of perhaps 3–7 times the thickness of the directly damaged tissue. Thrombi may develop in the blood vessels, which also may contribute to ischemia.[17] White blood cells and macrophages migrate to the burn area by chemotaxis (response to the release of chemical mediators by neutrophils, monocytes, and injured tissue). This migration is aided by the increased capillary permeability. The process of phagocytosis prepares the injured area for healing.

Fibrinogen (essential for clot formation) normally occurs in the injured area to decrease bleeding. Two elements, albumin and globulin, which normally do not pass through the capillary walls, escape into the interstitial area. The albumin molecules are smaller than globulin; therefore, more albumin molecules leak out. The fluid loss into the interstitial spaces is no longer available for circulation. Instead, the albumin and globulin increase the concentration of protein in the interstitial fluid and pull more fluid from the vascular space by osmosis. This results in edema formation. This edema resolves when the walls of the capillaries regain their normal integrity and osmotic pressure is reestablished. Fluid is reabsorbed into the bloodstream and excreted via the kidneys, causing the patient to have profound diuresis 48–72 hours after the burn injury.[15] Figure 17-9 provides an example of burn wound edema formation.

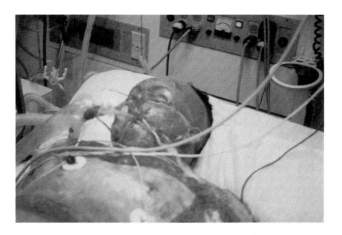

FIGURE 17-9 Burn wound edema. Note the facial swelling.

ENDOCRINE INVOLVEMENT

As a result of the burn injury, all body systems of the burn patient are stressed. The body moves from an anabolic (energy storage) mode to a catabolic (energy-utilizing) mode. Much of this is due to the hypermetabolic state caused by the burn injury and much is also due to the hormonal changes after the burn injury. The body increases the secretion of catecholamines, cortisol, glucagon, renin-angiotensin, antidiuretic hormone (ADH), and aldosterone. The consequence is a tendency toward retention of sodium and water and excretion of potassium by the kidneys. Catecholamines (epinephrine and norepinephrine) are released by the adrenal glands immediately after the injury. Epinephrine stimulates glycogenolysis and promotes hyperglycemia. Norepinephrine causes an initial vasoconstriction after the burn injury. Cortisol stimulated by the adrenal cortex is formed by the adrenocorticotropic hormone (ACTH) immediately after the burn injury. Cortisol is a factor in the early phase of the catabolic response because of its regulatory action in the metabolism of fats, carbohydrates, sodium, potassium, and proteins. Aldosterone secretion is increased in response to the decrease in intravascular sodium and hypovolemia.[17]

FLUID RESUSCITATION

Patients who are intubated and those with serious burns of 20% or more of the body surface area need fluid replacement to counteract the hypovolemic process. This is indicated by a change in the blood pressure, increase in heart rate, and in late stages, loss of consciousness. A large-bore intravenous line (IV), 14–16 gauge or larger, should be established, preferably through nonburned intact peripheral tissue. The antecubital vein should be used if cannulation through burned tissue is necessary. Two large-bore IVs should be established in the event of burns larger than 25% TBSA. Correction therapy for burn shock is mostly concerned with the restoration of fluid, electrolyte, and protein deficiencies. Optimal fluid volume replacement during this period is essential to cardiac output, renal perfusion, and tissue perfusion. This may be accomplished via several recognized fluid replacement formulas; however, the most commonly used formula in the United States is the Parkland formula.[18]

THE PARKLAND FORMULA

The **Parkland formula** provides for fluid replacement based on the patient's weight in kilograms and the percent of the TBSA burned. Because the greatest loss of plasma occurs in the first 24 hours postburn, the greatest replacement also needs to occur during this period. It is important to remember that any formula used is only a guideline for fluid replacement and that continuous monitoring of the patient's status (vital signs, urinary output, electrolyte balance, and hemodynamic pressures) is essential to successful resuscitation.

The consensus fluid resuscitation formulas for the first few hours postburn are as follows:

- Adults: 2–4 mL lactated Ringer's × body weight in kilograms (kg) × percent TBSA burn
- Children: 3–4 mL lactated Ringer's × body weight in kilograms (kg) × percent TBSA burn
  The formula is given as follows:
- One-half in the first 8 hours (the first 8 hours refers to the 8 hours after the burn occurred, not the time of the arrival of EMS or of the patient in the emergency department)
- Second half in the following 16 hours

The patient's response to the formula should be monitored.

Following an estimation (or actual accounting) of the patient's weight and the calculation of fluid requirement, the rate of fluid infusion is regulated so that one-half of the estimated volume will be infused during the first 8 hours postburn. During the subsequent 16 hours of the first postburn day, the remaining half of the estimated resuscitation should be administered. For example, a 70-kg adult patient with a 60% burn would require 4 mL × 70 kg × 60% burn = 17 liters for the first 24 hours with half of that volume (8.5 liters) delivered in the first 8 hours. The volume of fluid actually infused is guided by physiological monitoring of the patient's response to the burn injury and treatment. In the field, a general guideline for paramedics to use is lactated Ringer's solution at the rate of 2 L/hr in adults and 500 mL/hr in children (150 mL/hr under age 4).[11] Lactated Ringer's solution is used because it mimics intravascular fluid.

The following criteria should be used by the paramedic to monitor the effectiveness of fluid resuscitation. Signs of adequate fluid resuscitiation are

1. Urine output of 2–50 mL/hr (or 1 mL/kg body weight) per hour in children and 30–70 mL/hr in adults
2. Pulse rate of 100–120 in children and 80–100 in adults
3. Clear sensorium
4. Absence of ileus or nausea
5. Balanced acid-base

Signs of inadequate fluid resuscitation are

1. Hypotension/tachycardia
2. Tissue hypoxia/changes in levels of consciousness (restlessness, disorientation)

3. Acute organ failure (particularly renal failure)

4. Pulmonary edema

5. Cerebral edema

6. Myoglobinuria

Although the replacement of fluid loss with colloids has been examined, this has proven to be nonbeneficial.[19] This is because the cell wall permeability does not usually return to normal until after the first 24 hours. The use of colloids (albumin, plasma, or other volume expanders) exerts little influence on intravascular retention of fluid and would not minimize the amount of fluid needed during this time period. Colloids are best used after the return of capillary wall integrity, during the second 24-hour period postburn. Intravenous therapy during the second 24 hours consists of glucose and water; a hypotonic salt solution to replace evaporative losses and the addition of plasma protein to maintain adequate circulating volume may also be considered.[19]

ALTERATION IN FLUID RESUSCITATION NEEDS

Although the standard formula for fluid therapy replacement benefits most burn patients, the effectiveness of such therapy may be altered under certain conditions. Each patient reacts differently to the burn injury and the resuscitation process. Patients who may require more fluids than predicted by formula include the following: (1) patients with electrical injury; (2) patients with an inhalation injury; (3) patients in whom the resuscitation process has been delayed; (4) patients who sustain a burn injury while intoxicated; and (5) patients who may have prolonged hypothermia.

Patients who may be considered "volume sensitive" (requiring less fluid resuscitation therapy) would include the following: (1) patients with preexisting cardiopulmonary disease, renal disease, or head trauma and (2) patients at either end of the age spectrum (less than 2 years of age or greater than 50 years of age).[20]

It is important that the paramedic remember the need for frequent assessment and monitoring of the burn patient's general condition. In assessing patients who continue to have oliguria (diminished urinary output), the infusion of dopamine or another inotropic agent may be used to improve myocardial function and renal perfusion.

ELECTROLYTE AND HORMONAL RESPONSES

Mild **hyponatremia** commonly observed during the resuscitation process may be manifested by a serum sodium concentration similar to that of lactated Ringer's solution (130 mEq/L). Such low levels infrequently cause symptoms and are corrected by reducing the fluid infusion rate. Symptomatic hyponatremia occurs most commonly in burn patients in whom the administration of electrolyte-free fluid has depressed the serum sodium concentration to 120 mEq/L or less. A possible side effect of hyponatremia is seizures, especially in children. Other causes of hyponatremia in burn patients include the inappropriate secretion of ADH.[21]

Hypernatremia is the most common electrolyte abnormality following the reabsorption of excessive fluid. Causes of this condition may include inadequate replacement of water loss, elevated urinary glucose concentration caused by preexisting diabetes mellitus, or excessive glucose administration. Large evaporative water loss secondary to increased ventilatory rate and increased body temperatures may also contribute to mild to severe cases of hypernatremia.[21]

In hyperkalemia potassium should not be added to initial resuscitation fluids. Modest hyperkalemia is commonly produced by the destruction of RBCs and other tissue injured by the burn and the subsequent release of intracellular potassium. The paramedic should observe the patient for changes in cardiac dysfunction if the serum potassium levels become too elevated. These changes may be manifested by prolonged PR interval, wide QRS, a tall, tented T wave, or ST depression on electrocardiogram. Hyperkalemia from inadequate resuscitation may also result from impaired tissue perfusion in which acidosis has developed.[21]

Hypokalemia may occur during the diuretic phase after resuscitation. Additional hypokalemia may result if the patient suffers from diarrhea because potassium is lost in the stool.

In patients with burns of 30% or more TBSA, a mild hypocalcemia is common. However, such decreased levels are nondetrimental and are consistent with the decrease observed in calcium-binding proteins.[21]

PAIN CONTROL

Pain control presents a major problem in the care of the burn patient. Interpreting behavior and assessing pain are often among the most difficult aspects of emergency burn care. The degree of pain experienced depends largely on the depths of injury, the individual's perception of pain, and the level of anxiety experienced. The need for analgesia in the burn patient is inversely proportional to the depth of the burn. Full-thickness burns, in which the cutaneous nerve endings have been destroyed, are generally insensate to pain, whereas partial-thickness burns (particularly superficial partial-thickness burns) can be extremely painful. Pain is best controlled with the use of intravenous rather than intramuscular narcotics. Changes in fluid volume and circulation make absorption of any drug given intramuscularly or subcutaneously irregular.

Morphine is the narcotic of choice for the control of burn pain. Narcotics should be given in the smallest doses sufficient to control pain and only after signs of adequate burn shock resuscitation have been observed. This is necessary because the administration of narcotics may cause peripheral vasodilatation and narcotics administered before fluid resuscitation can potentiate the profound effects of shock. Other methods the paramedic could consider may include the use of meperidine IV, which has also been proven successful at relieving burn pain, and/or the elevation of the burned extremity. Naloxone hydrochloride should be readily available to reverse the actions of narcotics administered if respiratory depression is noted. The administration of sedatives and/or tranquilizers to decrease anxiety may also be considered. Anxiety may exaggerate the pain experience. It is important for the paramedic to remember that any environmental stimuli can trigger intense pain.

MANAGEMENT

The immediate management of the burn wound generally requires that it be protected from further harm and the environment. The wound usually requires the application of a clean dressing or sheet to the involved body parts. The treatment modality may vary as to the application of dry or moist dressings. The paramedic should be familiar with local EMS and receiving facility protocols that address treatment modalities. The application of moist dressings may minimize pain but may also rapidly induce hypothermia.

ESCHAROTOMY

Further assessment of the burn wound may be required if the wound is found to be circumferential. Circumferential burns to body parts such as the chest, arms, legs, and neck could greatly impede blood flow. To reduce edema and pain, burned extremities should be elevated at all times. The application of wound dressings should be applied from the distal to the proximal limbs, taking care not to further constrict blood flow. Pulse checks of involved extremities should be performed every 15 minutes. Hallmark signs of impending vascular compromise include the following: progressive decrease or absence of pulses distal to the burn, numbness, complaints by the patient of deep aching pain or throbbing, loss of capillary refill,

cyanosis, and cool/cold extremities. Frequently assess pulse intensity and strength of the burned patient. Use of a Doppler flowmeter assists with this process when palpation of pulses becomes difficult. An immediate escharotomy may be indicated when increased pressure symptoms occlude blood flow or restrict chest wall expansion. This procedure is rarely necessary in the field. A preanesthetic agent is usually not required for the performance of an escharotomy because the incisions made will pass through necrotic tissue. Incisions should be made on both the lateral and medial aspects of the limb. With the exception of the digits, the entire length of the burn should be incised. Bleeding is usually minimal and may be controlled with direct pressure. If circumferential chest wall burns are restricting adequate chest excursion, escharotomies of the chest may be required. The chest escharotomy should be performed by making two parallel incisions along the anterior axillary line to the waist. A third incision may be made to create an inverted "V" near the xiphoid process. This will allow for both lateral and anterior-posterior excursion as well as adequate diaphragmatic movement. Figure 17-10 shows preferred escharotomy sites. Figure 17-11 is an example of an escharotomy being performed, and Figure 17-12 is an example of a completed escharatomy of the chest and arms.

BURN INJURIES

Based on the source of injury, there are essentially four types of burns: thermal, electrical, chemical, and radiation. Regardless of the severity of the injury, expertise in emergency burn care is essential. The paramedic must possess the skills and knowledge of up-to-date treatment techniques to stabilize the burn patient, provide comfort, and prevent further complications.

THERMAL BURNS

The majority of thermal burns are caused by flames, hot liquids, heated metals, and steam. Flame burns most often are third degree (full thickness), particularly if the clothing has caught fire. Liquid burns are most often second degree in nature. The full depth of a liquid burn may not be readily apparent in the very young or in older adults. Both boiling water and hot grease can produce a full-thickness burn with little contact time. Metals and melted synthetics may also cause full-thickness burns. Both substances will adhere to the skin surface, resulting in the absorption of most of the heat. A good example of this is a tar burn to the hand. Prolonged exposure will result in a deeper than anticipated injury, as the outer layer of tar is cooled but the tar in contact with the skin is still molten hot. Hot liquids

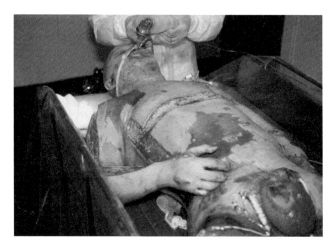

FIGURE 17-12 Complete escharotomy of chest and arms.

such as coffee or tea, at low temperatures (130°F–150°F), may also cause full-thickness injuries from prolonged contact. The elderly, the very young, and individuals who may be physically or mentally challenged are most affected by injuries of this type. Steam, which has the heat-carrying capacity 4,000 times that of hot air, is usually the only kind of injury that causes direct airway injury to the lung, but this is very rare.[22] Steam used in the industrial setting may produce partial- to full-thickness burns depending upon the length of exposure.

Inhalation Injury

Inhalation injuries account for 20%–30% of the patients admitted to burn centers and 60%–70% of the patients who die in the burn center.[23] Inhalation injury is caused by three basic mechanisms, alone or in combination: carbon monoxide poisoning, direct heat injury, and chemical damage. For clarification, carbon monoxide poisoning is not an injury, but an intoxication, and is the major cause of fire-related deaths in urban environments.[23] Direct heat injury is rare and primarily affects the upper airway. The heat-carrying capacity of air is quite low, and hot vapors are rapidly cooled to body temperature as they pass through the pharyngeal area and upper airway. Cyanide, acroleins, aldehydes, anhydrides, carbon, and sulfur dioxides are the most common chemicals inhaled in a house fire. These products of incomplete combustion produce a chemical tracheobronchitis on contact with mucosal surfaces. Unlike hot air, these toxic products can be inhaled deeply into the lungs and commonly cause severe damage to the respiratory tree. Burns to the upper airway should be anticipated in all patients with burns of the neck and face. Signs of inhalation injury vary, depending upon the kind of damage sustained.

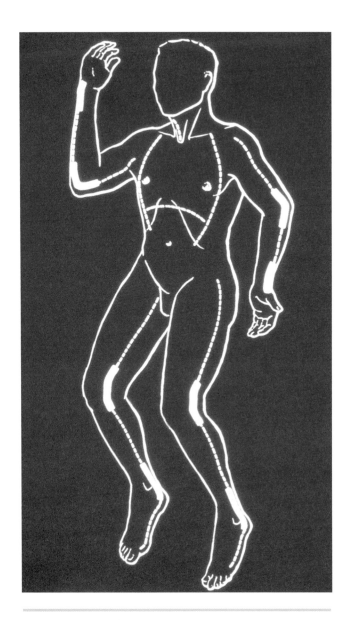

FIGURE 17-10 Preferred escharotomy sites.

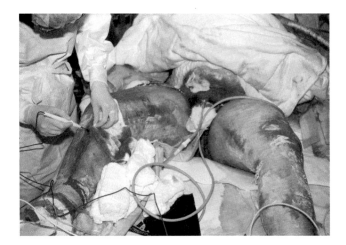

FIGURE 17-11 Escharotomy being performed.

Redness or blistering around the mouth, singed nasal hairs, sore throat, or visible burns indicate upper airway injury. Symptoms include changes in respiration or pulse, stridor or hoarseness, cyanosis, and impaired sensorium. The patient's airway may become occluded by laryngeal edema. Inhalation injuries require the administration of 100% oxygen and intubation.

Carbon Monoxide Poisoning   Carbon monoxide (CO) poisoning must be considered with every patient suspected of having an inhalation injury, especially if there is a history of closed space confinement. Carbon monoxide is a colorless, odorless gas resulting from incomplete burning of organic substances, such as gasoline, coal products, tobacco, and building materials. Any physical evidence of inhalation should warrant close observation by the paramedic. A late sign of a high concentration of CO is cherry red skin and lips. The use of pulse oximetry (which cannot distinguish between carboxyhemoglobin and oxyhemoglobin) for oxygen saturation content may be misleading and should not be relied upon as the only assessment tool to confirm potential CO intoxication. Arterial blood gases and carboxyhemoglobin levels must be obtained upon arrival to the emergency department. Levels of carboxyhemoglobin above 5% in nonsmokers and above 10% in smokers could indicate CO poisoning. Carbon monoxide has an affinity for hemoglobin that is 200–250 times greater than that of oxygen. The CO displaces oxygen and produces a leftward shift in the oxyhemoglobin dissociation curve. In other words, the half-life at which the hemoglobin molecule is saturated is lowered. Carboxyhemoglobin formation also prevents release of oxygen from unaltered hemoglobin to the tissues. In addition, CO binds with the myoglobin in muscle cells and interferes with cellular respiration. The result is a patient who is both hypoxic and in a state of metabolic acidosis.[22] Without the rapid administration of oxygen therapy, CO poisoning is fatal. Most persons found dead at the scene of a fire have little or no burn of the skin but have died of CO poisoning.

Table 17-2 summarizes symptoms commonly associated with CO poisoning. Initial symptoms of mild CO poisoning (less than 20% carboxyhemoglobin) are manifested by headache, slight dyspnea, mild confusion, and diminished visual acuity. Moderate poisoning (20%–40% carboxyhemoglobin) leads to irritability, impairment of judgment, dim vision, nausea, and fatigability. Severe poisoning (40%–60% carboxyhemoglobin) produces hallucinations, confusion, ataxia, collapse, and coma. Levels of 60% or more are usually fatal. Initial treatment for suspicion of CO poisoning includes the insertion of the largest oral endotracheal tube feasible for a patient. Oxygen therapy should include 100% humidified oxygen to slow pharyngeal

Table 17-2
Carbon Monoxide Poisoning

Carboxyhemoglobin Level	Severity	Symptoms
<20%	Mild	Headache, mild dyspnea, visual changes, confusion
20%–40%	Moderate	Irritability, diminished judgment, diminished vision, nausea, easy fatigability
40%–60%	Severe	Hallucinations, confusion, ataxia, collapse, coma
>60%	Fatal	

Source: Way LW. *Current Surgical Diagnosis and Treatment,* 10th ed. East Norwalk, Conn.: Appleton & Lange; 1994:248. With permission.

edema and loosen secretions. Oxygen administration should be initiated at the scene, as this intervention is the single most effective therapy for CO toxicity.

Hyperbaric oxygen (HBO) therapy not only enhances CO elimination but also appears to decrease the incidence of neurological complications. Hyperbaric oxygen therapy improves the neurological status by maintaining the viability of neurons in the ischemic brain until circulation is restored by reducing cerebral edema, which occurs secondary to diffuse anoxia and CO poisoning. Controversy exists concerning if and when HBO is needed for the treatment of CO poisoning. Some clinicians suggest that any patient with a carboxyhemoglobin level greater than 20%, a history of loss of consciousness, persistent neurological deficits, and cardiac abnormalities should be referred to hyperbaric therapy. Others would suggest that patients with carboxyhemoglobin levels greater than 40% need HBO because this level represents a significant exposure and the risk of secondary complications is increased. Certainly any patient who receives 100% oxygen therapy for several hours with minimal neurological improvements, even if carboxyhemoglobin levels return to normal, should be referred.[22]

Upper Airway Injury

Burns of the upper respiratory tract include those involving the nasal cavity, pharynx, supraglottis, trachea, and larger bronchi. Injuries of the upper airway are manifested by hoarseness, stridor, audible air-flow turbulence, the production of carbonaceous sputum, or bronchorrhea. Airway edema and eventual obstruction of the airway may result in as little as 30 minutes to 48 hours after injury. In patients with potential obstruction, immediate intubation in the field and the administration of 100% oxygen is necessary to protect occlusion of the airway. Upon arrival to the hospital, a bronchoscopic procedure may be performed.

Lower Airway Injury

Injury to the lower airway primarily involves the terminal bronchioles and alveoli. Because the specific heat of air is very low and the heat-exchanging mechanism of the upper respiratory tract is so efficient, even superheated air is cooled considerably by the time it reaches the tracheobronchial tree. Usually, the cause of most lower airway injuries is extreme, prolonged exposure to chemicals as by-products of combustion. The primary complications of lower airway injury include impaired ciliary activity, bronchospasm, airway edema, pneumonia, and pulmonary edema. Initial emergency care is the same as that of the patient with upper airway injuries.[22,23]

INTERNET ACTIVITIES

Visit the e-medicine Web site at http://www. emedicine.com. Click on the Emergency Medicine on-line book and select Environmental Emergencies. Then click on Thermal Burns. Review the chapter on the management of thermal burn injuries.

ELECTRICAL INJURY

Electrical injuries account for approximately 6% of admissions to burn centers across the United States.[24] Electrical burns result from contact with an electrical power source or from the arcing of current near the body. The electrical injury occurs most often to men between the ages of 20 and 34 and is usually job related. The groups at highest risk for injury are electrical and construction workers, golfers who fail to seek shelter during electrical storms, and teenage thrill seekers. Toddlers are another high-risk group who may sustain an electrical injury because of their curiosity and/or fascination with electric supply cords and outlets.[25,26] To understand the damage from an electrical current, it is necessary to have a knowledge of Ohm's and Joule's laws. **Ohm's law** states that electrical current is directly proportional to voltage and inversely proportional to resistance:

$$I = \frac{E}{R}$$

where E is voltage, I is current in amperes, and R is resistance in ohms.

Voltage is an electrical potential, resistance is the opposition offered by an object to the passage of a steady flow of electricity, and current is the flow of the electric charge. If a high voltage meets with high resistance, the current will be small, but if the voltage is high and meets with little resistance, the resulting current also will be high.

Joule's law depicts the relationship between heat production, current, and resistance:

$$J = I^2RT$$

where J is heat in joules, I is current in amperes, R is resistance in ohms, and T is time in seconds. From Joule's law it can be seen that heat is produced when electric current meets resistance over time. The amount of heat produced is directly related to current, resistance, and time (duration of contact). If any of these factors increases, the amount of heat produced will also be increased. Each type of body tissue offers its own resistance to current flow. Certain areas of the skin, such as the palms of the hands and soles of the feet, have higher resistance due to the thickness (callous formation) of the skin. Resistance of the skin can vary due to the presence or absence of water.[26] Bone offers the greatest resistance of the body to electrical current. Electrical current travels through the body following the path of least resistance—through tissue fluid, blood vessels, and nerves. Table 17-3 lists the body tissues in order from greatest to least resistance. As illustrated in Table 17-3, it may be presumed that bone generates more heat than other tissues. Severity of an electrical injury is also determined by other factors. These factors are outlined in Table 17-4.

Table 17-3
Tissue Resistance to Electricity (Greatest to Least)

Bone
Fat
Tendon
Skin
Muscle
Blood vessels
Nerves

Electrical current can be high or low voltage, and either direct (DC) or alternating (AC) current. Low-voltage direct current is less dangerous than low-voltage alternating current due to the tetanic muscle contractions produced by alternating current. Alternating current is capable of producing ventricular fibrillation, respiratory failure, and convulsions at a very low voltage, because it has a repetitive fibrillatory stimulus that occurs 60 times a second. Current that passes through muscles may cause spasms severe enough to produce long-bone fractures or dislocations. Conversely, high-voltage direct current is more frequently fatal than high-voltage alternating current. Lightning is an example of high-voltage, high-amperage direct current.

Pathophysiology

In general, there are three types of electrical injury and three types of injury caused by lightning. First, thermal injuries may be caused by the ignition of clothing from heat or flames produced by an electrical spark or arcing. Second, an arc-type or flash injury may be produced by the leaping of electrical current to the skin producing severe, deep muscle damage. This arcing is produced by the resistance of the air between the patient and the current source being so small that the current flows through the air to the patient. As the current arcs, it produces skin temperatures high enough to cause charring and burning. Third, a true electrical injury is caused by direct contact of the body with an electrical source. As the current travels through the body, it heats up, causing deep tissue and muscle necrosis and also producing an entrance and exit wound. An entrance wound may be described as having an indentation as the current entered the body producing a depressed gray or yellow area of full-thickness destruction surrounded by a sharply defined zone of hyperemia (Figure 17-13). The vast majority of entrance and exit

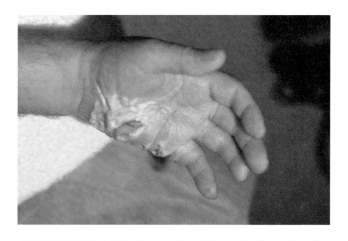

FIGURE 17-13 The zones of hyperemia.

sites are in the upper and lower extremities.[23] Because these areas have relatively small cross-sectional diameters and a large bone-to-tissue ratio, they are quite susceptible to thermal injury. The exit wound may be described as having a flared appearance (Figure 17-14).

Lightning has been described as occurring in three forms as well. First, ground current can produce damaging effects by creating a circuit between the ground and the legs of the patient. Flash or discharge injury is another form of lightning injury that occurs when lightning "splashes" to a victim from a nearby struck object such as a tree. This is also known as a side flash. A direct strike occurs when the patient is struck directly because of a metal object such as an umbrella, which attracts electrical energy. In this case, the current travels through the patient's body. Wounds are frequently superficial, with "feathering" or "spidery" patterns that disappear after several days.[27]

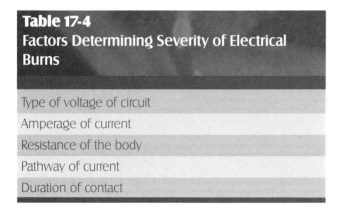

Table 17-4
Factors Determining Severity of Electrical Burns

Type of voltage of circuit
Amperage of current
Resistance of the body
Pathway of current
Duration of contact

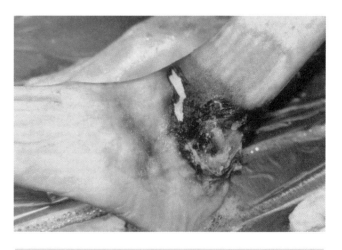

FIGURE 17-14 An exit wound.

Emergency Care

When examining the patient with an electrical injury, the paramedic should take care not to touch an individual who may still be in contact with the electrical source. Immediate concern at the scene focuses on turning off the power supply. This may be accomplished by turning off a nearby main power switch or by notifying the utility company to turn off the power source. The use of non-conductive objects such as a wooden pole or ax handle is not recommended as these objects may still conduct alternating current. The paramedic should remember that electrically injured patients are trauma patients with a crush injury until proven otherwise. If possible, cervical spine immobilization should be performed before extricating the patient. Next, assess the need for the initiation of cardiopulmonary resuscitation and defibrillation; current passing through the body can cause ventricular fibrillation or cardiac standstill. Patients sustaining a cardiac arrest should undergo continuous ECG monitoring for at least 24–48 hours.[28] Assess the patient's airway, breathing, and circulation, and initiate life-saving treatment as required.

Because blunt trauma and skeletal injury may both coexist with an electrical injury, a thorough physical examination is essential. Occult hemorrhage secondary to associated trauma may be present, resulting in hypotension and hypovolemia. The insertion of a large-bore IV line and the infusion of lactated Ringer's or normal saline will help maintain blood pressure and intravascular volume and will reduce the risk of renal failure from the formation of myoglobin.[26] The risk of renal complication is relatively high in patients with electrical injury.[29] There is a higher incidence of hemoglobinuria and hematuria from damaged tissue. Damaged muscle releases myoglobin in the urine, which can lead to acute tubular necrosis and renal failure (see Figure 17-15). Renal failure may also occur as a result of the flow of electrical current through the renal arteries or kidney or both. Initial fluid therapy should be crystalloid infusion sufficient enough to maintain a urinary output of 75–100 mL/hr to maintain myoglobin clearance and maintain adequate urinary output. Additional therapy may include the administration of one ampule (50 mL) of sodium bicarbonate or 12.5 grams of mannitol to each liter of IV fluid to clear the pigmentation of the urine and to maintain an alkaline urinary output.[30] Care should be taken to maintain a high urinary output as underestimation of deep tissue damage may result in inadequate resuscitation and the development of oliguria.

Electrical energy may cause damage to muscle tissue (Figure 17-16). This is initially due to edema formation and later to a progressive loss of sufficient blood supply. The patient may complain of numbness,

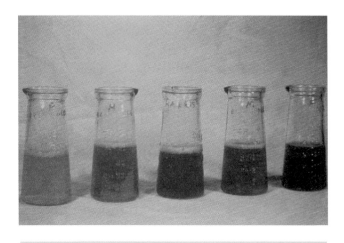

FIGURE 17-15 Pigmented urine.

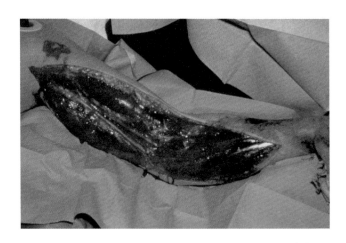

FIGURE 17-16 Muscle damage after an electrical injury.

tingling, or pain at the site. Further examination should assess for pulses, capillary bed refill, temperature, and cyanosis of involved body parts. If a critical decrease in perfusion is evident (e.g., diminished pulses, cyanosis), the patient should be prepared for a fasciotomy.

Assess all electrically injured patients for deficits involving peripheral nerves, the spinal cord, and cerebral functioning. This may occur as a result of minor compression fractures of the vertebrae or the disruption of the blood supply to the spinal cord. This compression may lead to transient paresthesia or permanent quadriplegia. The patient should be assessed frequently for neurological deficits. Such deficits may present as confusion, convulsions, decreased levels of consciousness, and respiratory depression or failure. Care should also be taken to assure that the cervical spine is immobilized when attempting to move the patient. The use of the log roll technique may be beneficial at this point.[30,31]

INTERNET ACTIVITIES

Visit the e-medicine Web site at http://www. emedicine.com. Click on the Emergency Medicine on-line book and select Environmental Emergencies. Then click on Electrical Injury. Review the chapter on the management of electrical injuries.

CHEMICAL INJURY

The potential for chemical injury exists in our work, home, and recreational environments. Burns caused by chemical exposure may come from several sources, such as the industrial setting, agricultural products, and the home environment. Chemicals coming into contact with the body may be classified as alkali, acid, or organic compounds.[30]

Males are the most likely to be injured by chemical exposure in the work environment. Chemical burns are rarely seen in children, although esophageal strictures in children are caused by the ingestion of caustic chemicals from household items. Chemical burns usually occur most frequently on upper and lower extremities, followed by injury to the trunk. Inhaled chemicals can damage the respiratory system and may be more difficult to neutralize and treat.[30] Specific chemicals, their uses, and exposure effects are identified in Table 17-5.

Table 17-5
Chemicals: Uses and Exposure Effects

Chemicals	Uses	External Effects	Internal Effects
Oxidizing agent Chromic acid	Metal cleaning	Ulcerates and coagulates tissue	Violent gastroenteritis, peripheral vascular collapse, vertigo, muscle cramps, coma, toxic nephritis with glycosuria
Potassium permanganate	Disinfectants, bleach, medicine for skin disorders	Concentrated solutions and dry crystals create a thick brown-purple eschar of coagulated protein	Edema of the glottis after swallowing; no systemic effects
Sodium hypochlorite	Disinfectants, bleaches, deodorants	Released chlorine coagulates cutaneous protein as well as mucous membrane proteins	Esophageal stricture (late complication); vomiting; circulatory collapse; edema of larynx, glottis, and pharynx
Reducing agents Hydrochloric acid	Industrial laboratories	Converts protein to respective chloride or nitrate salt; causes erythema with blister formation	Ingestion can cause an esophagitis with stricture; inhalation of the fumes can result in pulmonary injury
Gasoline	Fuel	Causes erythema and blister formation	Produces CNS, pulmonary, cardiovascular, renal, and hepatic injuries; absorption is rapid once skin is broken
Corrosives Phenols	Deodorants, sanitizers disinfectants	Extensive protein denaturation forms a white or dull grey stain with soft eschar and shallow ulcer formation; causes demyelination of nerve fiber; thus, there is absence of pain or discomfort	Absorbed rapidly percutaneously leading to pulmonary edema, hemolysis, and cardiovascular collapse; can also lead to nephrotoxicity and hepatic failure

(continues)

Table 17-5 (continued)

Chemicals	Uses	External Effects	Internal Effects

Lyes
  Potassium
    hydroxide
  Sodium hydroxide
  Ammonium
    hydroxide
  Lithium hydroxide
  Barium hydroxide
  Calcium hydroxide
  Sodium metal
	Industrial cleaning
	Washing powders
	Drain cleaners
	Urine-sugar reagent
	  tablets
	Cement
	Agriculture
		Causes liquifaction necrosis—
		  a gelatinous, friable, often
		  brown eschar forms;
		  saponifies tissue cells
			Ingestion causes severe pain,
			  spasms, leading to circulatory
			  collapse, asphyxia from
			  glottal or laryngeal edema,
			  pulmonary and gastrointest-
			  inal problems

White phosphorus	Incendiaries, insecticides,
	  fertilizers
		Painful second- and third-
		  degree burns occur due to
		  thermal activity when exposed
		  to air; cellular dehydration
		  due to chemical activity
			Absorbed and causes
			  systemic toxicity, as
			  evidenced by hepatic and
			  renal failure and hematemesis

Protoplasmic poisons
  Acids
    Tungstic
    Sulfosalicylic, Tannic
    Trichloroacetic,
    Cresylic, Acetic
    Formic
	Industrial use	Forms thin to hard, thick eschars	Hepatic necrosis or
			  nephrotoxicity may result
			  after ingestion or systemic
			  absorption
			Rapidly penetrates causing
			  metabolic acidosis, hemolysis,
			  and renal failure

Oxalic acid	Industrial use	Chalky, white, indolent ulcers form	Causes hypocalcemia

Hydrofluoric acid	Glass etching, plastics
	  production, component
	  of rust removers
		Painful, deep ulcerations form
		  under coagulated eschar;
		  bone decalcifies
			Fluoride ion penetrates tissue,
			  causing continued injury over
			  a period of time; chemical
			  pneumonitis can result from
			  inhalation of fumes; corneal
			  loss due to eye exposure;
			  severe hypocalcemia
			  produces refractory cardiac
			  dysrhythmias

Desiccants
  Sulfuric acid
 	
  Muriatic acid
	Toilet bowl cleaner,
	  industrial use
	
	Sheet-metal work,
	  plumbing
		Forms coagulation necrotic
		  eschar with deep indolent
		  ulcers; extremely painful due
		  to the exothermic reaction
		Coagulation necrosis is slow
		  and deep; more severe ulcers
		  are produced
			Ingestion causes oral burns,
			  injury to the hypopharynx and
			  epiglottis; esophageal injury is
			  a frequent complication
			(Same as sulfuric acid)

Vessicants
  Cantharides
  Dimethyl sulfoxide
    (DMSO)
  Mustard gas
	Veterinary aphrodisiac
	Linement carrier
	
	Military use
		Produces blisters and edema;
		  liberates histamine and
		  serotonin at the site; may also
		  cause local tissue anoxia	

Alkalis

Strong alkali exposure usually produces a tissue necrotic phenomenon known as "liquifaction necrosis." This involves the breakdown of protein and collagen, saponification of fats, dehydration of tissues, thrombosis of blood vessels, deep penetrating injury, and little pain. The amount of tissue damaged will depend upon the concentration of the agent, quantity of the agent, length of exposure, mechanism of action, and depth of penetration.[30] Examples of common alkali products include oven cleaners, drain cleaners, fertilizers, and heavy-duty industrial cleaners. Figure 17-17 is an example of an alkali burn.

Acids

Acids differ from alkalis in their destruction of tissue. Acids cause coagulation necrosis and immediate pain. The formation of coagulation necrosis involves eschar formation, which tends to shield the deeper tissues from injury. Acids are found in everyday household products such as bathroom cleaners, rust removers, and industrial-strength drain cleaners. The amount of tissue damaged depends upon the concentration of the agent, quantity of the agent, length of exposure, mechanism of action, and depth of penetration.[30] Figure 17-18 is an example of an acid burn.

Organic Compounds

Organic compounds such as phenols, creosotes, and petroleum products produce systemic toxicity with prolonged contact to the body. Hydrocarbon molecules of these products absorbed by the body can cause damage

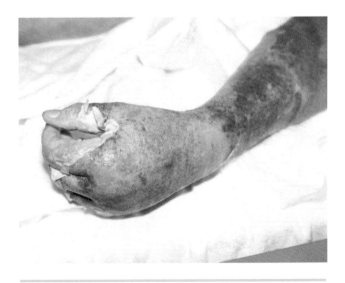

FIGURE 17-17 An alkali burn.

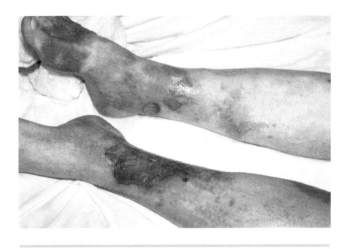

FIGURE 17-18 An acid burn.

to the hepatic, renal, and pulmonary systems, in addition to skin surface damage. The amount of tissue and organ damage depends upon the quantity and concentration of the agent, length of exposure, mechanism of action, and depth of penetration.[30]

Emergency Treatment

Tissue injury can be minimized if the chemical agent is removed from contact with exposed body surfaces. The paramedic should don protective clothing, goggles, and gloves to avoid contact with the chemical agent. A consultation with the local hazardous materials team for level of suits may be required before primary care is initiated. When rendering care to the patient, all clothing, including shoes, socks, and underwear (especially if the injury is above the waist), should be removed rapidly and copiously irrigated with water. While acids may be removed in as short as an hour, alkalis may require several hours of irrigation and lavage. Neutralizing agents should be avoided, since an intense exothermic reaction may be produced by contact with the chemical and cause further thermal damage.[32,33]

Chemical Burns to the Eyes

Chemical burns of the eyes are ocular emergencies. Chemical burns to the eyes should be treated with copious lavage of water or saline. This is essential to retain vision and minimize damage to the globe and surrounding structures. Extended irrigation is necessary in patients with injuries caused by strong alkalis. Usually the patient will present with swelling and/or spasms of the eyelid. The initial irrigation is most easily done by everting the eyelids and using a continuous drip of normal saline through intravenous tubing, with the stream directed into the conjunctival sacs. Care must be taken to avoid further eye damage. Check for contact lenses, which should be removed before irrigation.

RADIATION INJURY

Exposure to ionizing radiation can follow one of three patterns. First, it can be the result of a small-scale accident (e.g., in a laboratory and where resources will be available to cope); second, it can be due to a large industrial accident (e.g., the nuclear reactor explosion in Chernobyl, USSR, in 1986), where resources may be stretched in coping; and third, exposure may follow the detonation of a nuclear device in a military conflict, where resources are totally overwhelmed or unavailable and associated multiple and combined injuries also exist. A significant radiation accident is one in which an individual exceeds at least one of the following criteria:

- Whole-body dose equal to or exceeding 25 rem (0.25 Sv)

- Skin dose equal to or exceeding 600 rem (6 Sv)

- Absorbed dose equal to or greater than 75 rem (0.75 Sv) to other organs or tissues other than skin from an external source

- Internal contamination equal to or exceeding one-half the maximum permissible body burden (MPBB) as defined by the International Commission on Radiological Protection (this number is different for each radionuclide)

- Medical misadministrations, provided they result in a dose or burden equal to or greater than the criteria already listed above

Radiation accidents should be reported to the Radiation Assistance Center/Training Site at Oak Ridge Associated Universities in Oak Ridge, Tennessee 37831-0117 (Tel. 615-576-3130).[34]

The paramedic must remember that time spent in any potentially contaminated area should be kept to a minimum. When it is known or highly suspected that a high-level radiation exposure has occurred, it may be necessary to delay rescue efforts until properly trained and equipped personnel are on the scene. Part of the rescue efforts may require the wearing of positive-pressure SCBA and other protective equipment specified by references such as the *DOT Emergency Response Guidebook* or the *CANUTEC Initial Emergency Response Guide.*[35]

Once clearance has been given, take reasonable precautions to avoid contact with radioactive material. The patient should be removed from the contaminated area as soon as possible. The patient's clothing, jewelry, and shoes should be removed and quickly isolated. Immediate assessment of the airway should be performed and patency assured. Normal resuscitation procedures must be followed (e.g., airway, breathing, circulation). If the patient is having trouble breathing or is unconscious, nasotracheal intubation for airway control is warranted. Perform cardiopulmonary resuscitation (CPR) if necessary. Start an IV of lactated Ringer's solution to support vital signs. The patient should be monitored for shock, seizures, or convulsion and treated accordingly. Routine emergency care should be performed for any associated injuries. If possible, decontamination of the skin at the scene may be performed by rinsing with water and soap or detergent. Package the patient using reverse isolation procedures such as transportation bags, plastic, or blanket. This helps prevent the spread of contamination during transport. The emergency department should be notified that a potentially contaminated patient is en route and supplied with all available information concerning the identity and nature of the contaminant.[35]

BURNS SPECIFIC TO PEDIATRICS

Thermal injury is the second leading cause of unintentional death in children between the ages of 1 and 15 in the United States. Thirty thousand children are admitted to hospitals and burn facilities each year for treatment of significant burns.[36] Scalds from hot liquids are the most common cause of nonfatal burns in children under age 3. Curious toddlers exploring their environment often pull pots or cups of hot liquids onto their faces, neck, arms, and chest (Figure 17-19). Preschoolers often sustain burns when playing with lighters or matches.[37] Emergency management of the pediatric burn patient requires the use of specialized assessment skills by the paramedic. A thorough knowledge of normal physiology and its changes with age are important when implementing care for the pediatric burn patient.

EMERGENCY TREATMENT

Emergency treatment for the pediatric burn patient should follow the established guidelines as listed for

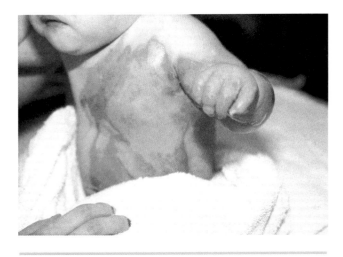

FIGURE 17-19 Scald injury of a toddler.

thermal burns. Appropriate prehospital management can decrease the mortality and morbidity of the pediatric burn patient. Burns in infants and small children pose a special problem because the TBSA in children is much larger in proportion to the total body mass than in adults. Refer to the pediatric rule of nines discussed earlier in this chapter (Figure 17-7). There are important considerations that the paramedic must remember when providing care to the pediatric burn patient. Factors to remember are:

- The child has a greater evaporative water loss relative to weight than an adult.
- Temperature regulation in infants and toddlers is influenced by the body surface area involved, which may compromise conservation of body heat. It is essential that a warm environment be maintained.
- The extent of the injury will be dependent upon the age, body surface area involved, and depth of the burn injury.
- Thin skin may make the initial determination of the severity of the burn difficult.
- Hypoglycemia may occur in infants because of limited glycogen storage.

When venous cannulation cannot be accomplished, the pediatric patient can be administered fluid volumes in excess of 100 mL/hr directly into the bone marrow. The low fat content of the marrow in children may account for the rare incidence of embolic complications with this procedure. A 16–18-gauge bone marrow aspiration needle can be used to cannulate the bone marrow compartment, although spinal needles or butterfly needles can be pushed through the porous bone of a child. The anterior tibial plateau, medial malleolus, anterior iliac crest, and distal femur are preferred sites for intraosseous infusion. The needle should be introduced into the bone, taking care to avoid the epiphysis,

either perpendicular to the bone or at a 60° angle with the bevel facing the greater length of the bone.[34]

The events leading to the thermal injury and the past medical history are extremely important when evaluating the infant and child. The potential for child abuse must always be considered, particularly in children under the age of 4.

Child Abuse

Most frequently associated with child abuse are contact burns or scald injuries. Each member of the health care team must be alert to the thermal components of child abuse. Alerting factors include the history of injury, the compatibility of the history with the injury, and the physical aspect of the injury. Burns that are symmetrical may strongly suggest child abuse in the patient under 4 years of age. This pattern of injury is reflective of the developmental ability of children at this age. The index of suspicion may also be heightened by physical examination of the child. Evidence of multiple injuries (e.g., previous history of broken bones, bruises, cigarette burns, radiator burns, immersion/symmetrical burns to legs or buttocks, burns with specific patterns such as an iron or coil pattern from a stove isle), the reaction of the child to the physical exam, and an incomplete or inconsistent history can provide further evidence of abuse. The goal in the management of child abuse is the protection of the child from further injury. Whenever abuse is suspected, appropriate authorities (social services, police) must be notified. A federal law, the Child Abuse Prevention and Treatment Act, requires professionals who work with children to report suspected abuse or neglect. The law further protects the individuals from liability should the suspicions prove false.[38] Figure 17-20 is an example of child abuse.

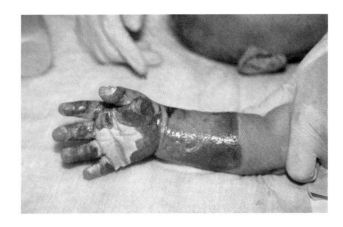

FIGURE 17-20 Intentional child abuse. Note the circumferential burn to the arm.

INTERNET ACTIVITIES

Visit the National Library of Medicine Web site at http://www.ncbi.nlm.nih.gov/PubMed. Conduct a literature search on burn injuries. Review the abstracts of the search results. Ask your librarian to assist you in obtaining the journals with the five most relevant articles. Review these articles and summarize their findings.

SUMMARY

Burn injury of any magnitude can be a serious injury. A major burn is one of the most traumatic events that an individual and his and her family can experience. It is imperative that the paramedic understand the physiological and psychological effects the burn injury can have on the body system. Due to the time period between the initial injury and the initiation of treatment, the paramedic must be prepared to meet the challenge this injury may present.

REVIEW QUESTIONS

Mr. James Dodson's wife calls 911 to report that her husband has sustained burns of his entire anterior chest and abdomen, entire right arm, and entire right leg. The incident occurred when gasoline ignited while he was cleaning the engine of his motorcycle. You are dispatched to the home to render assistance.

1. In relation to emergency care at the time of the incident, it is generally agreed that it would have been best to care for Mr. Dodson's burn areas by:
   a. Pouring cool water over the areas
   b. Applying clean, dry dressings to the area
   c. Rinsing the areas with a warm, mild soap solution
   d. Applying a mild antiseptic ointment over the area

2. Using the rule of nines, the burned areas indicated by the description above on Mr. Dodson's body would be calculated as:
   a. 18%
   b. 27%
   c. 45%
   d. 64%

3. Mr. Dodson's burns are called into the local emergency department as deep partial and full thickness. The paramedic should recognize that deep partial-thickness burns are defined as burns that involve:

   a. The epidermis and subcutaneous tissue
   b. The epidermis only
   c. The epidermis and varying degrees of the dermis

4. A full-thickness burn is characterized by:
   a. No sensation of pain
   b. Tan, brown, or black color
   c. Surface that is dry and leathery
   d. All of the above
   e. None of the above

5. Which of the following descriptions best defines the term eschar?
   a. Scar tissue in a developmental stage
   b. Crust formation without a blood supply
   c. Burned tissue that has become infected
   d. Viable living tissue with a rich blood supply

6. The paramedics obtained intravenous access through the left antecubital vein. What intravenous fluid must be started?
   a. 5% dextrose in 0.45% saline
   b. 0.9% normal saline
   c. 0.45% saline
   d. Ringer's lactate solution
   e. Hyperalimentation solution

7. In a major burn patient, which is the most important indicator of adequate fluid therapy?
   a. Initial estimate by a burn fluid formula
   b. Serum osmolarity
   c. Hemoglobin, hematocrit, and serum sodium
   d. Pulse, blood pressure, and urine output

8. During transport, the patient begins to complain of pain in his right hand. The paramedic's initial action at this time should be to:
   a. Obtain a blood pressure in the unburned arm
   b. Compare radial pulses and capillary refill bilaterally
   c. Elevate the involved extremity
   d. Continue to cool the right arm

9. All of the following are appropriate interventions for a person with thermal burns except:
   a. Removing clothing and jewelry as soon as possible
   b. Applying ice water to extensive burns to help arrest the burning process
   c. Covering burns with a clean sheet
   d. Cutting around clothing that sticks to the skin
   e. Withholding pain medication until the shock state is under control

10. Upon arrival to the emergency department, the physician inserts a subclavian line and orders several laboratory tests. Mr. Dodson had begun to complain of shortness of breath. What laboratory test may be obtained to prevent life-threatening complications?

a. Urinalysis
b. Complete blood count
c. Arterial blood gas with co-oximetry
d. Blood-urea-nitrogen and creatine
e. Electrolytes

11. Mr. Dodson has an indwelling Foley catheter placed. The generally accepted minimum safe range for the hourly output of urine during the first few hours after a burn such as Mr. Dodson's is:
a. 10–21 mL
b. 30–70 mL
c. 70–100 mL
d. 10–150 mL

12. The paramedic can anticipate that the most commonly ordered route for administering Mr. Dodson's pain medication is:
a. Oral
b. Rectal
c. Intravenous
d. Intramuscular

13. The paramedic should be aware that fluid shifts in Mr. Dodson result from an increase in:
a. Permeability of capillary walls
b. Total volume of intravascular plasma
c. Total volume of circulating whole blood
d. Permeability of the tubules in the kidneys

14. Which of the following complications is sometimes observed in patients with burns and appears to be the result of prolonged stress?
a. Paralytic ileus
b. Gastric dilatation
c. Nitrogen imbalance
d. Gastrointestinal ulceration

15. Mr. Dodson is ordered to receive morphine sulfate via the intravenous route. In addition to respiratory depression, which one of the following problems is most likely to occur if Mr. Dodson is given narcotics in large doses for the control of pain?
a. Suppression of urine
b. Camouflage of other symptoms
c. Depression of peripheral nerve endings
d. Stimulation of the central nervous system

16. The paramedic is assisting the nursing staff with the application of bandages to Mr. Dodson's wounds. Which one of the following techniques should be used when applying bandages to his hands to maintain functional alignment?
a. Wrapping the thumb and each finger separately
b. Wrapping the closed fist with recurrent bandages
c. Curving the fingers and thumb over a roll of gauze

d. Securing the fingers to a flat, well-padded handboard

17. The paramedic is assisting with the transport of Mr. Dodson to the burn center located 3 hours away. While in transport, the following laboratories drawn 1 hour before are transmitted to the ambulance: hemoglobin 17%g; hematocrit 50%. The paramedic also obtained vital signs at this time: blood pressure 90/70; pulse 120. Other data are: central venous pressure 2 mm Hg; urine output 8 cc/hr. What is the next step to be taken?
a. Irrigate the Foley catheter.
b. Administer furosemide (Lasix) or mannitol.
c. Begin dopamine infusion.
d. Administer whole blood.
e. Increase crystalloid infusion.

18. Most electrical burns are considered third-degree burns. Which of the following is also of primary consideration?
a. Where the incident occurred
b. Appearance of the wound
c. Heart rhythm
d. Age of the patient
e. None of the above

19. What is the most common complication of an electrical burn injury?
a. Retrograde amnesia
b. Sepsis
c. Hypotension
d. Ventricular fibrillation
e. None of the above

20. The appropriate field management for a chemical burn is:
a. Do not waste time; rush the patient to the emergency department for definitive care.
b. Irrigate for 30 minutes with a neutralizing acid.
c. Irrigate with water for 5 minutes and take the patient to the emergency department for administration of a neutralizing solution specific to the chemical.
d. Irrigate 10–15 minutes immediately with large volumes of water.
e. None of the above.

Mrs. Olivia Newsome's clothing ignited as she started a charcoal fire with gasoline. She was planning a party with guests due to arrive in 15 minutes. Prehospital care was rendered and she was rushed to the hospital by the paramedics.

21. Her third-degree burns involved the entire anterior trunk, excluding genitalia, and the entire anterior surface of both legs. What is the percentage of body surface burned?
a. 18%

b. 27%

c. 36%

d. 54%

22. The primary cause of a rising hematocrit in the first few hours postburn is:

a. Plasma loss

b. Erythrocyte loss

c. Gastric hemorrhage

d. Dehydration

23. You are monitoring the patient for shock. The result that indicates a serious problem is:

a. Central venous pressure of 11 mm Hg

b. Pulse of 100 beats per minute

c. Red blood cells 5.0 × 10.6

d. Urine output of 10 cc/hr

24. Four hours after admission, Mrs. Newsome begins to moan in pain, and the doctor orders morphine 5 mg IV. The paramedic should realize that the reason for this route of administration is:

a. It provides relief more quickly.

b. The circulation is impaired.

c. It avoids damage to potential donor site.

d. She is prone to hypotension with larger doses.

25. In assessing the burn patient, which of the following would alert the paramedic to suspect pulmonary/inhalation injury?

1. Burns to the face

2. Burns that occurred within a closed space

3. Carbonaceous sputum

4. Burns caused by electric shock

  a. 1 only

  b. 1 and 3

  c. 1, 2, 3

  d. All of the above

26. Burns are classified as first, second, or third degree according to:

a. Extent of body surface burned

b. Depth of skin damage

c. Cause of burn

d. Degree of sensory and motor loss

The paramedics are called to a local manufacturing plant in which an employee was burned while attempting to light a cigarette in the chemical storage area. The explosion and fire that occurred due to the chemical fumes in the air caused the patient to be thrown 30 feet against a wall and the patient to receive burns covering his entire left arm, the front of his left leg, and the entire front of the trunk. When asked why he was smoking in the chemical area, the patient replied that it was too cold to go outside to smoke.

27. Which of the following would be the best first-aid measures for this patient after assuring scene safety?

  a. Application of warm/moist dressings to keep him from freezing

b. Application of cool/moist dressings

c. Application of ointments

d. Application of local anesthetic to reduce the pain/discomfort

28. If the patient had received burns of the neck and face, which of the following would pose the greatest concern during the paramedic's initial assessment?

a. Respiratory damage

b. Brain damage due to a lack of oxygen

c. C-spine stabilization

d. Psychological problems due to disfigurement

▶ CRITICAL THINKING

- You are dispatched to the scene of a "sick call." Upon your arrival, you are met by a distraught mother who says her child has been complaining of headache, fatigue, nausea, and vomiting for the past 24 hours. She thought he was suffering from some form of viral infection because the rest of the family has been complaining of the same symptoms. This morning she went to awaken him and found him very difficult to arouse and called 911. Upon entering the home, you note the smell of exhaust fumes. Upon questioning the mother, you find that her husband operates an automotive shop part time in the adjoining garage. Upon further questioning, you discover that he has been behind in his repairs and, to appease his customers, has worked almost continuously for the past 36 hours. Your patient, a 12-year-old male, is found responsive only to pain. His bedroom is adjacent to the garage. What do you suspect as the cause of this patient's symptoms? What are your immediate actions? How will you treat this patient? Is treatment necessary for the other members of the household?

- You are dispatched to the scene of an industrial accident. Upon your arrival, you are escorted by the site foreman to the back of a building that is under construction. You find a 25-year-old male sitting in a chair talking with his coworkers. He indicates that he was testing some electrical circuits when he accidentally touched a bare wire with a screwdriver. A quick survey of the electrical panel indicates that the line was 220 volt alternating current. He further states that it "kicked like a mule" and knocked the screwdriver from his hand. He denies syncope and states "I feel OK now." Upon physical examination you notice a small, blackened entry wound about the size of a pinhead. The vital signs are normal and the ECG shows sinus rhythm at 90 beats per minute. The patient refuses transport to the hospital. Is emergency treatment necessary for this patient? Why or why not? What treatments will be required at the hospital if he is transported? What further assessment should be performed while en route to the hospital? Describe the pathophysiology of this injury. Why is this injury serious despite the apparent lack of physical findings?

● Upon arrival at the scene of an apartment fire, you are led to a 23-year-old female who has suffered burns over 30% of her body, including the face, neck, and scalp. The burns appear to be partial thickness. She is complaining of pain to the burned areas. You note that her eyebrows are singed as well as her nasal hairs and her voice is raspy. She has no previous medical history. How will you manage this patient?

▶ REFERENCES

1. Bryan CP. *Ancient Egyptian Medicine: The Papyrus Ebers*. London: Ares; 1930.
2. Haynes BW. The history of burn care. In: Boswick JA, ed. *The Art and Science of Burn Care*. Rockville, Md.: Aspen Publishers; 1987.
3. Macmillan BG. The development of burn care facilities. In: Boswick JA, ed. *The Art and Science of Burn Care*. Rockville, Md.: Aspen Publishers; 1987.
4. Brigham PA, McLoughlin E. Burn incidence and medical care use in the United States: estimated, trends, and data sources. *J Burn Care Rehab*. 1996; 17:95.
5. National Fire Protection Association (NFPA). Uniform fire incident reporting system data. Boston: NFPA; 1990.
6. National Committee for Injury Prevention and Control. *Injury Prevention: Meeting the Challenge*. Oxford: Oxford University Press; 1989.
7. Bayley EW, Smith GA. The three degrees of burn care. *Nursing*. 1987; 17(3):34.
8. Burn Awareness Coalition (BAW). Burn Awareness Kit. Encino, Calif.: BAW; 1993.
9. Zimmerman TJ, Krizek TJ. Thermally induced injury: a review of pathophysiological events and therapeutic interventions. *J Burn Care Rehab*. 1984; 5(33):193.
10. Achauer BM, Martinez SE. Burn wound pathophysiology and care. *Crit Care Clin*. 1985; 1(1):47.
11. American College of Emergency Physicians. *Minor Burns: Evaluation and Treatment*. Kansas City, Mo.: Marion Laboratories, Scientificom; 1979.
12. Burgess MC. Initial management of a patient with extensive burn injury. *Crit Care Nurs Clin North Am*. 1991; 3:65.

13. Trofino RB. *Nursing Care of the Burn Injured Patient*. Philadelphia: FA Davis; 1991.
14. American Burn Association. Guidelines for service standards and severity classifications in the treatment of burn injury. *Am Coll Surg Bull*. 1984; 69:24.
15. Robins EV. Burn shock. *Crit Care Nurs Clin North Am*. 1990; 2:229.
16. Kramer GC, Herndon DN, Linares HA. Effects of inhalation injury on airway blood flow and edema formation. *J Burn Care Rehab*. 1989; 10:45.
17. Trofino RB, Braun AE. Pathophysiology of burns. In: Trofino RB, ed. *Nursing Care of the Burn Injured Patient*. Philadelphia: FA Davis; 1991.
18. Berkowitz RL. Burns. In: Krupp MA, Schroeder SA, Tierney LM, eds. *Current Medical Diagnosis and Treatment*. Norwalk, Conn.: Appleton & Lange; 1987.
19. Baxter CR. Fluid volume and electrolyte changes in the early postburn period. *Clin Plast Surg*. 1974; 1:693.
20. Nebraska Burn Institute (NBI). *Advanced Burn Life Support Course Manual*. 2nd ed. Lincoln, Neb.: NBI; 1990.
21. Loven L, Norstrom H, Lennquist S. Changes in calcium and phosphate and their regulating hormones in patients with severe burn injuries. *Scand J Plast Reconstr Surg*. 1984; 1:18.
22. Bayley EW. Care of the burn patient with an inhalation injury. In: Trofino RB, ed. *Nursing Care of the Burn Injured Patient*. Philadelphia: FA Davis; 1991.
23. Pruitt BA, Goodwin CW. Thermal injuries. In: Davis JH, et al, eds. *Clinical Surgery*. St. Louis, Mo.: Mosby; 1987.
24. Wittman MI. Electrical and chemical burns. In: Richard RL, Staley MJ, eds. *Burn Care and Rehabilitation: Principles and Practice*. Philadelphia: FA Davis Company; 1993.
25. Seward PN. Electrical injuries: trauma with a difference. *J Emerg Med*. 1992; 6:157.
26. Boswick JA. *The Art and Science of Burn Care*. Rockville, Md.: Aspen Publishers; 1987.
27. Trofino RB, Orr PA. Types of burns. In: Trofino RB, ed. *Nursing Care of the Burn Injured Patient*. Philadelphia: FA Davis; 1991.
28. Solem L, Fischer RP, Strate RG. The natural history of electrical injury. *J Trauma*. 1977; 17:487.
29. Divincenti FC, Moncrief JA, Pruitt BA Jr. Electrical injuries: a review of 65 cases. *J Trauma*. 1969; 9:497.
30. Trofino RB, Orr PA. Types of burns. In: Trofino RB, ed. *Nursing Care of the Burn Injured Patient*. Philadelphia: FA Davis; 1991.
31. Pruitt BA Jr. The burn patient: initial care. *Current Prob Surg*. 1979; 16:43.
32. Nebraska Burn Institute (NBI). *Advanced Burn Life Support Course Manual*, 2nd ed. Lincoln, Neb.: NBI; 1990.

33. Saydjari R, Abston S, Desai MH, Hemdon DN. Chemical burns. *J Burn Care Rehab*. 1986; 5:397.

34. Milner SM, Thuan TN, Herndon DN, Rylah LT. Radiation injuries and mass casualties. In: Herndon DN, ed. *Total Burn Care*. Philadelphia: WB Saunders; 1996.

35. Bronstein AC, Currance PL. *Emergency Care for Hazardous Material Exposure*, 2nd ed. St. Louis, Mo.: Mosby Year-Book; 1994.

36. Clark JR. Managing burns in children. *J Emerg Med Serv*. 1990; 4:90.

37. Carajal HF. Burns. In: Behrman RE, Vaughn VC, eds. *Nelson Textbook of Pediatrics*, 13th ed. Philadelphia: WB Saunders; 1987.

38. Myers JEB. *Legal Issues in Child Abuse and Neglect*. Newbury Park, Calif.: Sage; 1992.

Airway and Ventilatory Management

OBJECTIVES

Upon completion of this chapter, the reader should be able to:

- Describe the anatomy and physiology of the respiratory system.
- Describe the five major types of airway and respiratory pathologies.
- Discuss methods for maintaining airway patency in the patient with cervical spine injuries.
- Explain the basic interventions in airway and ventilatory management.
- Describe the advanced methods of airway control and list the indications, advantages, and disadvantages for each.
- Discuss the indications, contraindications, and procedures for surgical airway control.
- Explain the indications, contraindications, and procedures for rapid-sequence intubation.
- Describe in detail the dosage, mechanisms of action, and side effects of the neuromuscular blocking agents most commonly employed in the prehospital setting.
- Discuss the setup and operation of chest drainage systems.
- List and describe the ventilator modes most commonly used in the management of trauma patients.
- Determine the initial settings for mechanical ventilation.
- Describe the techniques used to assess patient response to mechanical ventilation.
- Explain the physiological responses to intubation and mechanical ventilation.
- Explain the procedure for obtaining arterial blood gas samples.
- Discuss the interpretation of arterial blood gas values.
- Discuss the interpretation of end-tidal carbon dioxide monitoring.

KEY TERMS

Assist control ventilation (ACV)
Capnography
Cellular respiration
Combitube
Controlled mandatory ventilation (CMV)

Cricothyrotomy
Esophageal gastric tube airway (EGTA)
Esophageal obturator airway (EOA)
Expiratory center
Hering-Breuer reflex

(continues)

(continued)

Inspiratory center
Intermittent mandatory ventilation (IMV)
Laryngeal mask airway (LMA)
Laryngospasm
Nasopharyngeal airway (NPA)
Oropharyngeal airway (OPA)
Pharyngeotracheal lumen airway (PTLA)
Pneumotaxic center

Pulmonary respiration
Retrograde tracheal intubation (RTI)
Synchronized intermittent mandatory
    ventilation (SIMV)
Transillumination intubation
Translaryngeal jet insufflation (TJI)
Ventilation

Of all the skills used in caring for the trauma patient, none is more important than airway control and ventilatory management. Total airway obstruction leads to permanent CNS damage after 4 minutes and may result in cardiac arrest within 4–10 minutes.[1,2] Because of the serious sequelae of airway compromise, paramedics must be capable of quickly and effectively establishing a patent airway and ensuring adequate ventilation and oxygenation. Consequently, a thorough knowledge of airway anatomy and physiology, as well as skill in various airway and ventilatory techniques, are essential in the management of the trauma patient.

ANATOMY OF THE RESPIRATORY SYSTEM

The nose is the anatomically superior part of the airway containing the paired nasal cavities, which continue posteriorly and perpendicular to the face to open into the nasopharynx. The common medial wall of the nares is the septum, which, when deviated, may create nasal obstruction. Projecting medially from the lateral wall are three horizontal turbinates, each over a corresponding meatus. The anterior aspect of the nasal cavity receives its blood supply from the internal carotid artery and the posterior aspect is supplied by the external carotid artery. The trigeminal nerve, cranial nerve five (CN V), supplies sensation to the nasal cavities, and olfactory receptors provide the sense of smell via the olfactory nerve (CN I).

The nose serves several functions, including humidifier, heat exchanger, voice resonator, filter for inhaled particulate matter, and a conduit for air.[3,4] Endotracheal intubation bypasses these functions, delivering cool, dry, unfiltered air to the lower respiratory system.[4]

The mouth serves as a conduit for air flow and alimentation. The oral cavity is bounded by the dental arches, tongue, and hard and soft palates, opening posteriorly into the oropharynx (Figure 18-1). The tongue is innervated by the hypoglossal nerve (CN XII) and protects the airway from obstruction by foreign matter. If this nerve is injured or impaired, such as with uncon-scious or intoxicated patients, the tongue falls into the posterior oropharynx, causing obstruction.[4] Snoring is the clinical sign indicative of acute airway obstruction by the tongue. Basic airway maneuvers, such as the trauma jaw thrust, move the tongue anteriorly, thereby eliminating the obstruction.

The larynx forms the boundary between the upper and lower airway (Figure 18-1). The larynx functions as an open valve during respiration, a partially closed valve for speech, and a closed valve for protecting the airway against aspiration during swallowing.[5] It extends from the tip of the epiglottis to the lower border of the cricoid cartilage. In the adult, the larynx is at the C-3 to C-5 level of the spinal column. The epiglottic, thyroid, and cricoid cartilages form the basic structure of the larynx and provide major internal (epiglottis) and external (cricoid and thyroid cartilage) anatomical landmarks.[4]

The thyroid cartilage is the largest laryngeal cartilage and is attached superiorly to the hyoid bone by the thyrohyoid ligament. Inferiorly, the thyroid cartilage articulates with the cricoid cartilage via the cricothyroid membrane and ligament. The cricothyroid membrane measures 1 by 3 cm in the adult, is relatively avascular, superficial, and distant to other major structures in the neck, and is easily identified, making it a suitable site for surgical airway access. Similar in shape to a signet ring, the cricoid cartilage forms the only complete cartilaginous ring of the airway.[6] Because it forms a complete skeletal ring, pressure applied to the anterior surface of the cricoid cartilage will be transmitted to the esophagus. Cricoid pressure will also displace the vocal cords posteriorly.[7] Consequently, cricoid pressure, also called the Sellick maneuver, serves two purposes: (1) it promotes visualization of the vocal cords during laryngoscopy and (2) it closes the esophagus, thus preventing regurgitation into the airway.[8]

The larynx is one of the most powerful sphincters in the body. **Laryngospasm** is a reflexive, forceful contraction of all the laryngeal muscles and occurs when a foreign body enters the larynx. Although laryngospasm is a defensive mechanism designed to protect the airway, it may exacerbate airway obstruction, prevent positive-pressure ventilation, and hinder the

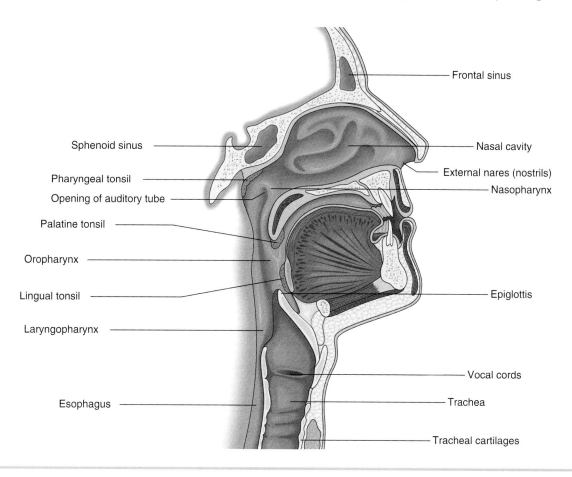

Frontal sinus

Sphenoid sinus

Nasal cavity

External nares (nostrils)

Pharyngeal tonsil

Nasopharynx

Opening of auditory tube

Palatine tonsil

Oropharynx

Lingual tonsil

Epiglottis

Laryngopharynx

Vocal cords

Esophagus

Trachea

Tracheal cartilages

FIGURE 18-1 Anatomy of the upper airway.

passage of an endotracheal tube.[3] Forcing an endotracheal tube through the vocal cords may dislocate an arytenoid cartilage, resulting in permanent hoarseness.[9]

The adult trachea is 9–16 mm in diameter and extends about 10–15 cm from the lower border of the cricoid cartilage to the carina. Formed by 16–22 C-shaped cartilaginous rings, the trachea is bordered posteriorly by the esophagus and cervical spine. The carina is formed by the division of the trachea into the left and right mainstem bronchi at the sternomanubrial joint (angle of Louis), or the level of T-5 posteriorly (Figure 18-2). The right bronchus is less angulated (25° angle from the trachea) than the left (45° angle) and is more readily entered by an endotracheal tube advanced too far.[10] The average distance from the incisors to the carina is 27 cm in the adult male and 23 cm in the female.[10] A properly positioned endotracheal tube should rest at the 18–22-cm level at the incisors.[4] The distance from the nares to the carina is about 4 cm longer.[10] An endotracheal tube passed nasally should exit the nare at the 22–26-cm level.

Like the trachea, the primary bronchi are supported by C-shaped cartilaginous rings. As the bronchi divide into smaller and smaller divisions, the bronchi become increasingly muscular until no cartilage is found. The primary bronchi divide into secondary bronchi, providing two lobar bronchi for the left lung and three for the right. The right upper lobe bronchus originates from the right bronchus approximately 2 cm from the carina, whereas the left arises about 5 cm from the carina. As a result, foreign bodies tend to gravitate into the right upper and lower lobes.[3] The secondary bronchi continue to divide until they reach a diameter of approximately 1 mm, at which point they become bronchioles. Although the size of the individual airways decreases with each successive branching, the total area available for gas exchange increases from the mainstem bronchi to the terminal bronchioles and alveoli.

The lungs extend from the diaphragm to slightly above the clavicles. They lie against the ribs both anteriorly and posteriorly. The medial surface is concave, allowing room for the heart and major structures of the mediastinum. The primary bronchi and pulmonary blood vessels form the root of the lung and enter each lung through an opening on the medial surface called the hilum. The left lung consists of two lobes while the right has three. Each lung consists of innumerable tubes of decreasing diameter that form the bronchial

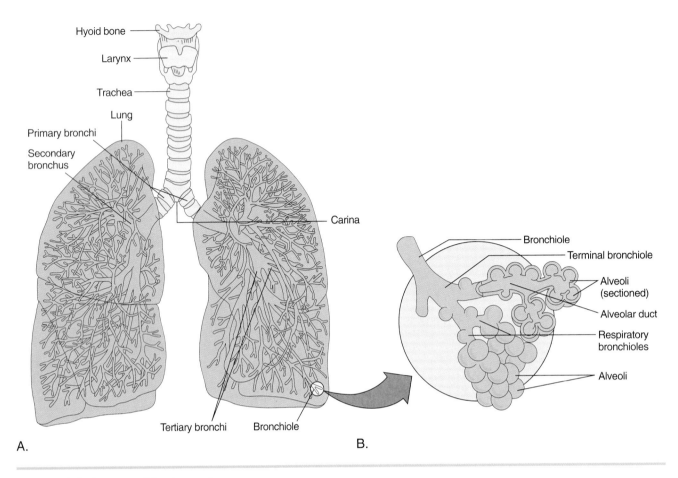

FIGURE 18-2 Anatomy of the lower airway.

tree. The smallest tubes terminate at the alveoli, where gas exchange occurs. The lungs contain approximately 300 million alveoli with a surface area of 70 m², forming an effective mechanism for gas exchange.

The lungs are covered by the pleura. The parietal layer of the pleura lines the entire thoracic cavity, adhering to the internal surface of the ribs and the superior surface of the diaphragm. The outer surface of the lungs are covered by the visceral pleura. The parietal and visceral pleura are separated only by the small amount of pleural fluid within the pleural space. As the intercostal muscles contract, the ribs pull the parietal pleura outward. The cohesion between the pleural layers cause the visceral pleura to also be pulled outward, allowing the lung to inflate.

PHYSIOLOGY OF RESPIRATION

Respiration is the exchange of gases between the human body and the environment and is comprised of three components: (1) ventilation, (2) pulmonary respiration, and (3) cellular respiration. **Ventilation** is the mechanical process of moving atmospheric gases into and out of the lungs. **Pulmonary respiration** occurs

in the lungs and involves the transfer of gases between the alveoli and the red blood cells. **Cellular respiration** is the transfer of gases between the red blood cells and the various tissues in the body. Each respiratory component is discussed below.

VENTILATION

The difference in gas pressures between two different areas is known as the pressure gradient. When a pressure gradient exists, gas will flow freely from the area of higher pressure to the area of lower pressure. Ventilation is dependent upon a pressure gradient between atmospheric pressure and intrapulmonary pressure.

Atmospheric pressure is the combined pressures exerted by all gases in atmospheric air. At sea level, atmospheric pressure is 760 mm Hg, but declines as altitude increases. Intrapulmonary pressure is the pressure of gas within the alveoli and varies throughout the respiratory cycle. During inspiration, the diaphragm and intercostal muscles contract, increasing the volume of the thorax and decreasing intrapulmonary pressure by 1 mm Hg below atmospheric pressure.[11] The result is a negative intrapulmonary pressure gradient, and atmospheric air rushes into the lungs. At the end of inspiration, the thorax stops expanding and air ceases to flow into the lungs as soon as equilibrium is reached between intrapulmonary and atmospheric pressures (i.e., the pressure gradient no longer exists). As the diaphragm and intercostal muscles relax, the elasticity of the chest wall, lungs, and diaphragm reduces intrathoracic volume and increases intrathoracic pressure by 1 mm Hg, creating a positive-pressure gradient. Air rushes out of the lungs until equilibrium is once again reached between intrapulmonary and atmospheric pressure. This represents one respiratory cycle and the movement of approximately 500 mL of air into and out of the lungs, known as the tidal volume. Minute ventilation is the product of tidal volume and respiratory rate. Normally, the respiratory rate in an adult is 12 breaths per minute (bpm), yielding a normal tidal volume of 6 L/min (500 mL × 12 bpm).

The airways of the respiratory system consist of 23 generations (or branchings) from the trachea to the alveoli. Of these, the first 16 generations comprise the conducting airways and do not take part in gas exchange but merely function as a conduit for air flow.[12] These airways hold roughly 150 mL of air and are called the anatomic dead space. Therefore, 30% of the tidal volume does not reach the alveoli to participate in gas exchange. In addition, not all alveoli are functional due to atelectasis or because they lack blood flow. Because these alveoli do not function in gas exchange, they are considered to be pathological dead space. When combined, the anatomical dead space and pathological dead space are called the physiological dead space. In the normal individual, where nearly all alveoli are functional, anatomical dead space and physiological dead space are nearly equal. However, in patients with poorly perfused alveoli, physiological dead space may be greater than 60% of the tidal volume.[13]

In managing the trauma patient's ventilations, the goal is to ensure adequate delivery of oxygen to the alveoli for gas exchange. This is accomplished by aggressive management of injuries that interfere with ventilation, such as pneumothorax, hemothorax, flail chest, and airway obstruction, and by providing positive-pressure ventilation when indicated. Once ventilation is provided, the next step is to ensure adequate oxygenation, which is the focus of the next section.

PULMONARY AND CELLULAR RESPIRATION

Along with adequate ventilation, the other items necessary for adequate oxygenation of tissues are adequate blood flow through the lung (pulmonary perfusion), normal gas diffusion, and delivery of the oxygen-bound hemoglobin to the tissues.

Gas Exchange

The combination of the pressures exerted by all gases in a gas mixture is the total pressure of the mixture. Atmospheric air has a total pressure of 760 mm Hg at sea level. If atmospheric air were divided into its subcomponents, each gas would have a contribution to the total pressure. The pressure exerted by each individual gas is known as the partial pressure. The partial pressure of each gas in atmospheric air can be determined by multiplying the concentration of each gas by atmospheric pressure. For example, atmospheric air contains roughly 21% oxygen, yielding a partial pressure in atmospheric air of roughly 160 mm Hg (21% × 760 mm Hg).

Oxygen and carbon dioxide transfer between the alveoli and capillary through diffusion. The transfer across the alveolar-capillary (A-C) membrane is dependent upon the difference in the partial pressure of the gas on each side of the membrane (pressure gradient) as well as the thickness of the membrane. The alveolar-arterial pressure gradient in room air is normally 2–10 mm Hg. As the fraction of inspired oxygen (FiO_2) is increased, the pressure gradient increases, as does the uptake of oxygen. By a similar mechanism, carbon dioxide is transferred from the area of higher concentration (capillaries) to the areas of lower concentration (alveoli).

Once oxygen is transferred across the A-C membrane, it is dissolved in plasma. Once dissolved, the oxygen continues to exert its partial pressure. The partial pressure of dissolved oxygen is measured as arterial blood gases. Normally, the partial pressure of oxygen in arterial blood (PaO_2) is 80–100 mm Hg at sea level. Normal PaO_2 is lower at higher altitudes and declines with age, falling 3–4 mm Hg per decade after the second or third decade of life.

Despite the relatively efficient mechanism for dissolving oxygen in blood, very little of this oxygen is made available to the tissues. Instead, oxygen delivery is dependent upon hemoglobin. Each gram of hemoglobin, when fully saturated, can carry 1.34 mL of oxygen. Thus, a patient with a normal hemoglobin of 15 g/dL can transport 20 mL of oxygen per 100 mL of blood when O_2 saturation is 100%. In comparison, each mm Hg of PaO_2 represents only 0.0031 mL of dissolved oxygen in 100 mL of blood. Thus, a patient with a PaO_2 of 100 mm Hg has only 0.31 mL of oxygen dissolved in the plasma.

The amount of oxygen carried on hemoglobin combined with the oxygen dissolved in plasma is known as the oxygen content of arterial blood (CaO_2) and is calculated as:

$$CaO_2 = [Hb](1.34)(SaO_2/100) + (PaO_2)(0.003)$$

The oxygen content equation illustrates several essential components that must be present for oxygenation of the trauma patient. They include an adequate amount of hemoglobin, a high ratio of saturated hemoglobin, and an adequate PaO_2.

Ensuring an adequate oxygen content in itself does not preclude hypoxia. The oxygen must also be delivered to the tissues. Oxygen delivery (DO_2) is determined by both oxygen content and cardiac output (CO). Oxygen delivery is calculated as:

$$DO_2 = (10 \times CaO_2)(CO)$$

Consider the patient with the following values:

Hemoglobin	15 g/dL
PaO_2	100 mm Hg
Cardiac output	5 L/min
O_2 saturation	98%

The oxygen delivery would be $[(10)(15)(1.34)(98/100) + (100)(0.003)](5)$ or roughly 1,000 mL/min. If hemoglobin were to drop to 10 g/dL as the result of hemorrhage, oxygen delivery would fall to 672 mL/min. Reductions in any of the other components in the equation, such as cardiac output or O_2 saturation, would also result in lower oxygen delivery to the tissues.

The arterial oxygen content and oxygen delivery equations illustrate the importance of proper ventilation, sufficient hemoglobin, and adequate cardiac output for tissue oxygenation. When applying these concepts to the trauma patient, it is easy to identify the principles that guide the paramedic in treatment. They include providing a patent airway, ensuring ventilation, administering high FiO_2, controlling the loss of hemoglobin, and normalizing cardiac output.

REGULATION OF RESPIRATIONS

The nerve impulses that control breathing originate in the brain. The respiratory control center consists of two divisions: the inspiratory center and the expiratory center. The **inspiratory center** intermittently fires, causing contraction of the diaphragm and intercostal muscles. Normally, exhalation is passive and does not require intervention by the expiratory center, unless breathing becomes labored. In this case, the **expiratory center** synchronizes impulses with the inspiratory center to produce forceful inhalation followed by forceful exhalation.

The normal rhythm and depth of respirations are regulated by the **Hering-Breuer reflex**. As the lungs inflate, baroreceptors within the lungs are stimulated, which send inhibitory impulses to the inspiratory center in the medulla via the vagus nerve. These inhibitory signals cause inspiration to cease, the diaphragm and intercostal muscles relax, and exhalation ensues. Then, when the lungs are sufficiently deflated to inhibit the lung baroreceptors, inhalation resumes. This reflex functions as a protective mechanism and prevents overinflation and pulmonary barotrauma.

The **pneumotaxic center** in the upper part of the pons is thought to control respiratory rhythm. Whenever the inspiratory center is stimulated, impulses are sent to the pneumotaxic center as well as the diaphragm and intercostal muscles. After a brief delay, the pneumotaxic center stimulates the expiratory center, which in turn sends inhibitory impulses to the inspiratory center and exhalation begins. It is believed that the primary control of rhythm is the Hering-Breuer reflex and the pneumotaxic center is active only during labored breathing.

In the lower portion of the pons lies the apneustic center. The apneustic center also stimulates the inspiratory center but is overridden by the superimposed pneumotaxic center.

The complex arrangement of respiratory control centers in the brain ensures adequate respiratory rate, depth, and rhythm. In addition to recognizing altered breathing patterns and the need for airway intervention, knowledge of the functions of these centers will assist the paramedic in localizing lesions in brain-injured patients.

Chemoreceptors

The partial pressures of arterial oxygen and carbon dioxide, along with the pH of arterial blood, influence respirations. The $PaCO_2$ acts on the chemoreceptors in the medulla that are sensitive to carbon dioxide and hydrogen ion concentration. Increases in $PaCO_2$ stimulate the medulla to increase the rate and depth of respiration. Mild decreases in $PaCO_2$ have the opposite effect.

A decrease in arterial blood pH and PaO_2 has a stimulating effect on the chemoreceptors in the carotid and aortic bodies. Once stimulated, the carotid and aortic bodies send signals to the medulla and respirations increase. Compared to $PaCO_2$ and pH, PaO_2 has a much less significant role in the regulation of respirations.

MEASURING RESPIRATORY FUNCTION

A number of diagnostic tools are available to the paramedic for evaluating the adequacy of ventilation and oxygenation, beginning with a good history and physical assessment. The physical examination provides signs and symptoms of inadequate ventilation and oxygenation (Table 18-1). In addition to these clinical signs and symptoms, arterial blood gas (ABG) analysis provides useful

Table 18-1
Signs and Symptoms of Inadequate Ventilation and Oxygenation

Inadequate Ventilation	Inadequate Oxygenation
Tachypnea	Pallor
Hyperpnea	Cyanosis
Hypopnea	Decreased mentation
Bradypnea	Decreased PaO_2
Altered respiratory patterns	Decreased SpO_2
Rhonchi	
Rales	
Wheezing	
Snoring	
Diminished or absent breath sounds	
Asymmetrical chest wall movement	
Chest injury	
Tracheal deviation	
Elevated $PaCO_2$	
Decreased $PetCO_2$	
Decreased pH	

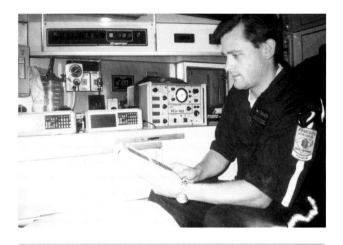

FIGURE 18-3 Field ABG analysis is possible with a hand-held analyzer.

information on the patient's ventilatory, oxygenation, and acid-base status and should become a routine field procedure in the care of the critical trauma patient.

Obtaining an ABG Sample

Hand-held ABG analyzers are now available for field use and provide a fast and convenient method for blood gas analysis (Figure 18-3). Once the patient is en route to the hospital, and if time permits, an arterial sample is drawn and inserted into the analyzer cartridge (Figure 18-4). Within 2 minutes, measurements are available for the partial pressures of oxygen and carbon dioxide, HCO_3, and pH. These machines are also capable of analyzing hemoglobin, hematocrit, and electrolyte levels from venous blood samples.

Interpreting PaO_2 and $PaCO_2$

Direct measurement of arterial carbon dioxide tension $(PaCO_2)$ is the most accurate method of assessing a patient's ventilatory status.[14] A decrease in pH accompanied by an increase in $PaCO_2$ reflects hypoventilation and respiratory acidosis. This condition may be corrected by increasing the rate and/or tidal volume of

ventilations. While a seemingly simple solution, increasing the respiratory rate or tidal volume may involve invasive procedures such as intubation, needle thoracotomy, and positive-pressure ventilation.

Oxygenation is easily assessed by measuring arterial oxygen tension (PaO_2). A decreased PaO_2 reflects tissue hypoxia. Table 18-2 provides a guideline for interpretation of oxygenation status. In general, a decreased PaO_2 accompanied by an increase in alveolar-arterial oxygen tension gradient $[P(A-a)O_2]$ reflects a diffusion defect, ventilation/perfusion (V/Q) mismatch, or shunt. A decrease in PaO_2 without an increase in $P(A-a)O_2$ is likely due to hypoventilation and will be accompanied by an elevated $PaCO_2$.[15]

The alveolar-arterial oxygen gradient is the difference between alveolar oxygen tension (PAO_2) and arterial oxygen tension and can be calculated by

$$P(A-a)O_2 = PAO_2 - PaO_2$$

The PaO_2 is obtained from the ABG, while PAO_2 is calculated by

$$PAO_2 = (Pb - PH_2O) \times FiO_2 - (PaCO_2/R)$$

where Pb is the barometric pressure (760 mm Hg at sea level), PH_2O is water vapor pressure (generally 47 mm Hg), R is the respiratory quotient (generally a constant value of 0.8, but may be eliminated when $FiO_2 > 0.60$), and FiO_2 is the fraction of inspired oxygen.

A quick evaluation of PaO_2, PCO_2, and $P(A-a)O_2$ will indicate the underlying pathology. An elevated $PaCO_2$ and decreased PaO_2 reflect hypoventilation. Treatment is aimed at improving ventilation and increasing oxygenation. Increasing FiO_2 alone will not improve oxygenation.

When the PaO_2 is decreased with little or no change in $PaCO_2$, a V/Q mismatch or intrapulmonary shunting is suspected. Hypoxemia caused by V/Q

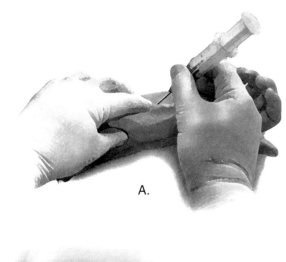

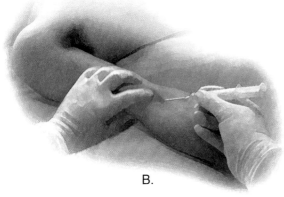

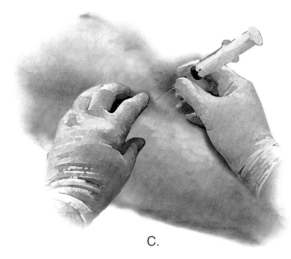

FIGURE 18-4 Obtaining the arterial blood sample from (A) radial artery; (B) brachial artery; (C) femoral artery.

mismatch, such as pulmonary embolism or circulatory shock, responds to oxygen therapy. However, hypoxemia resulting from intrapulmonary shunt does not respond well to oxygen therapy because the shunted blood does not come into contact with the ventilated alveoli. Conditions such as atelectasis lead to intrapulmonary shunting. Correction of hypoxemia due to

Table 18-2
Interpretation of Oxygenation Status

Parameter	Criteria	Interpretation
PaO_2	80–100 mm Hg 60–79 mm Hg 40–59 mm Hg < 40 mm Hg	Normal Mild hypoxemia Moderate hypoxemia Severe hypoxemia
$P(A-a)O_2$	Room air 1.0 FiO_2	Should be less than 4 mm Hg for every 10 years of age, otherwise hypoxemia Every 50 mm/Hg difference approximates 2% shunt

Source: Adapted from Chang DW. *Clinical Application of Mechanical Ventilation.* Albany, NY: Delmar Thomson Learning; 1997.

intrapulmonary shunts usually requires positive end-expiratory pressure (PEEP) in addition to oxygenation. If an elevated $PaCO_2$ is also present, ventilatory assistance will also be necessary.

Diffusion abnormalities cause hypoxemia by three mechanisms: (1) low oxygen pressure gradient, (2) increased alveolar-capillary thickness, and (3) decreased alveolar surface area.[14] Low alveolar-arterial oxygen tension gradient is usually due to a reduction in alveolar oxygen (PAO_2). The paramedic may encounter this mechanism of hypoxia when treating patients found in environments with low oxygen concentrations such as confined spaces, high altitudes, or house fires. Treatment is aimed at increasing the $P(A-a)O_2$ gradient by providing high FiO_2. With the exception of carbon monoxide poisoning, these patients respond well to oxygen therapy.

Increased alveolar-capillary thickness is seen in conditions such as pulmonary and interstitial edema from toxic inhalations, near drowning, and aspiration. In mild cases, this type of hypoxemia responds to oxygen therapy.[14]

The last type of diffusion abnormality, decreased alveolar surface area, is usually the result of underlying disease processes such as emphysema and pulmonary fibrosis. Although not trauma induced, injured patients may present with these concomitant disease processes. The diffusion problem may be partially corrected by oxygen therapy.

Limitations of Blood Gases

Arterial blood gas analysis provides useful information to the paramedic in managing the acutely injured patient. However, as with any diagnostic procedure, there are limitations to ABGs and the paramedic must be cognizant of these limitations.

First, ABGs are a "snapshot" of the patient's ventilatory and oxygenation status. They reflect only the patient's condition at the time the arterial sample was drawn. Because the trend of the patient's condition is important, ABGs need to be repeated often and supplemented by other means of monitoring such as pulse oximetry and end-tidal CO_2 monitoring.

Second, ABGs reflect only the partial pressures of gases dissolved in the plasma. As stated earlier, oxygen dissolved in plasma contributes very little to tissue oxygenation. The majority of the oxygen delivered to the tissues is provided by hemoglobin. Therefore, without adequate levels of hemoglobin, tissues will be hypoxic even if the PaO_2 is normal.

Third, oxygen delivery and oxygen use by the tissues are impaired in the presence of certain chemicals such as carbon monoxide and cyanide. In these cases, the patient may have normal arterial oxygen tensions and hemoglobin levels but will nevertheless be hypoxic.

Finally, the ability of hemoglobin to release oxygen to the tissues is affected by temperature, pH, and $PaCO_2$. Again, even when PaO_2 is normal, tissues may be hypoxic.

AIRWAY AND RESPIRATORY PATHOLOGIES

A wide variety of airway and respiratory pathologies exist, each of which warrants some type of emergency intervention. These pathologies can be pedagogically divided into five broad categories: airway obstruction, central nervous system (CNS) dysfunction, mechanical dysfunction, toxic inhalations, and V/Q mismatch. Regardless of the etiology of airway and respiratory compromise, its rapid identification and management are top priorities in trauma care.

AIRWAY OBSTRUCTION

Tongue

The most obvious and urgent indication for airway management is obstruction. Many obstructive causes of airway compromise are possible. The most common type of obstruction, however, is mechanical obstruction caused by the tongue (Figure 18-5). Normally, the submandibular muscles keep the tongue retracted away from the posterior pharynx. In the absence of adequate muscle tone, however, the tongue relaxes and forms an occlusion against the posterior oropharynx. While this mechanism of airway obstruction is most often associated with unconscious patients in the supine position, it

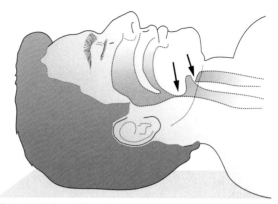

Obstructed airway (tongue against pharynx)

FIGURE 18-5 The tongue is the most common airway obstruction encountered in the field.

can occur irrespective of the patient's position. Fortunately, this type of obstruction is readily corrected by basic airway maneuvers such as the trauma jaw thrust (TJT) and trauma chin lift (TCL).

Foreign Body

Any patient who develops sudden respiratory distress should be suspected of foreign body airway obstruction (FBAO). Most FBAOs are the result of pieces of food becoming lodged in the airway during a meal. However, such possibilities should not be overlooked in the trauma patient given today's "eat-on-the-run" lifestyle where meals may be eaten while driving. Other possible causes of FBAO in the trauma patient include dislodged teeth and dentures, blood, vomitus, chewing gum, and tobacco products, resulting in either partial or complete obstruction. In the partially obstructed airway, the voluntary cough generates the greatest air flow (2,700 mL/sec).[16,17] In these instances, the patient should be encouraged to persist with spontaneous coughing, with due regard for potential spinal injuries. Basic maneuvers, such as the Heimlich maneuver and finger sweeps, are currently recommended by the American Heart Association for complete obstruction.[18] However, when possible, such as in an unconscious patient, direct visualization by laryngoscopy and extraction of the foreign body using Magill forceps should take priority over these indirect methods.

Trauma

Direct laryngeal trauma, especially when associated with fractures of the cricoid cartilage, can result in a loss of support of the vocal cords, causing them to collapse into the laryngeal lumen and obstruct the airway. Such injuries are recognized by subcutaneous emphysema, dysphagia, and throat discomfort that increases with swallowing. This life-threatening injury may exist with or without any evidence of external injury. These injuries are usually the result of the patient's neck striking the steering wheel in motor vehicle collisions.

Blunt or penetrating trauma to the neck may also produce obstruction from expanding hematomas. The neck is rich in vascular structures, yet lacks a surrounding skeletal structure for protection. Structures at risk include the carotids, aortic arch, subclavian, vertebral, and innominate arteries, jugular veins, innominate vein, and subclavian veins. The expanding hematomas that may result from injuries to these vessels can cause airway obstruction from deviation of the larynx and from mechanical compression of the trachea.[20]

Blunt transection of the airway is an uncommon injury, typically the result of steering wheel strikes, that usually occurs at the cricotracheal junction.[20] The trachea retracts into the lower neck, but the surrounding soft tissues provide a "pseudoairway."[20] External compression of the anterior neck or intubation attempts may result in loss of the pseudoairway, creating a difficult-to-manage airway obstruction. Open neck injuries may also produce discontinuity of the airway and obstruction due to tracheal collapse, clotted blood, or laryngeal edema.[20]

Facial fractures may also lead to airway obstruction. Maxillary fractures such as the Le Fort II and III fractures may compromise the airway, either through direct obstruction or through bleeding and soft tissue edema. Bilateral mandibular fractures may also result in obstruction through the loss of support for the tongue, allowing it to fall into the posterior oropharynx.

Laryngeal Spasm and Edema

Because the glottis is the narrowest portion of the adult airway, it is of particular concern in airway control. Edema may form as a result of blunt injury, thermal injury, near drowning, strangulation, toxic inhalations, and other inflammatory processes. Even moderate laryngeal edema may create a potentially lethal airway obstruction. Once present, laryngeal edema resolves slowly, requiring aggressive airway interventions to prevent asphyxiation.

Laryngeal spasm may be precipitated by foreign body aspiration, toxic inhalations, blunt trauma, near drowning, or intubation attempts. The result is a forceful closure of the glottis. Once spasm has ensued, forceful intubation attempts are discouraged as soft tissue trauma may result. Instead, topical anesthesia may be applied to relax the spasm.

CNS DYSFUNCTION

Head and Spinal Cord Injury

Head injuries can result in an airway and ventilatory problem through two different mechanisms: obstruction and impaired respiratory drive. Head-injured patients frequently lose consciousness through disruption of the reticular activating system (RAS). During this time, the patient lacks the usual protective mechanisms of gag and cough reflexes, as well as the ability to prevent airway occlusion by the tongue. In addition, head-injured patients are prone to vomiting, particularly when ethanol intoxication is superimposed. Without proper airway management, any of these mechanisms may lead to obstructive airway compromise.

The control centers that regulate respirations are dispersed throughout the cerebral hemispheres and brain stem, each responsible for a unique respiratory pattern. The pattern is associated with the level of intracranial injury and the degree to which rising intracranial pressure affects the brain stem. Most of these altered respiratory patterns result in a loss of respiratory drive, hypoventilation, hypoxia, and hypercapnia and require advanced airway procedures.

Even with an adequate respiratory drive and a clear airway, damage to the spinal cord may result in inadequate respiratory function. The muscles of inspiration (intercostal muscles and diaphragm) are composed of skeletal muscle and must be stimulated to contract. Stimulating impulses arrive from the brain via the spinal cord. Two phrenic nerves responsible for stimulating the diaphragm originate from the third, fourth, and fifth cervical spine nerves. The 11 pairs of intercostal nerves originate from the first through eleventh thoracic spinal nerves. Disruption of the spinal cord prevents delivery of impulses to the intercostal muscles that are innervated below the level of the cord injury, resulting in hypoventialtion. High cervical cord injuries risk not only total loss of control of the intercostal muscles but also loss of innervation of the diaphragm. In this case, the patient suffers apnea even in the presence of a clear airway, adequate respiratory drive, and pulmonary function. Without aggressive management these injuries are rapidly fatal.

Toxins

The respiratory drive can also be depressed by circulating toxins. Such toxins include narcotics, sedatives, asphyxiants, and especially, ethanol. In addition to providing airway and ventilatory interventions, the paramedic must also address the underlying toxins themselves, which are often superimposed on other traumatic injuries.

MECHANICAL DYSFUNCTION

The lungs lack any intrinsic mechanism to expand or contract. Ventilation, therefore, relies upon changes in pressure within the chest to effect respiration. The pressure changes are accomplished by contraction of the diaphragm and intercostal muscles. Contraction of the diaphragm increases the size of the thoracic cavity and, thus, thoracic volume. In addition, contraction of the intercostal muscles expands the chest wall, to which the parietal pleura is attached. Between the visceral and parietal pleura is a negative pressure and a small amount of fluid that maintains a "seal" between them. As the intercostal muscles contract, the chest wall expands and the lungs assume the contour of the thoracic cavity. The result is a further increase in thoracic volume. This increase in thoracic volume creates a decrease in intrathoracic pressure and air rushes in to fill the lungs. As the intercostal muscles and diaphragm relax, pressure within the lungs increases and air rushes out. Injuries to the diaphragm, pleura, intercostal muscles, ribs, or lungs interfere with the normal mechanical process of breathing.

Pneumothorax

A simple pneumothorax is caused by the presence of air within the pleural space. The air may originate from a defect in the chest wall (open pneumothorax) or from a lesion within the respiratory tract. The air decreases the adhesion of the visceral and parietal pleura. As the size of the pneumothorax increases, the lung begins to collapse. The large reserve capacity of the ventilatory and circulatory systems usually prevents serious consequences from a simple pneumothorax in young, healthy patients.[21] Older patients and those with preexisting disease or concomitant injuries are less likely to tolerate such injuries. However, as the pneumothorax expands, decompensation will occur even in young and previously healthy patients.

In some cases, air continues to enter the thoracic cavity through defects in the respiratory tract and/or chest wall and pressure begins to rise in the pleural space. Eventually, the lung collapses on the affected side. If the pneumothorax goes untreated, pressure continues to rise, resulting in a tension pneumothorax and a mediastinal shift to the opposite side. The mediastinal shift results in compression of the heart and great vessels and limits inflation of the opposite lung. Left untreated, these injuries are rapidly fatal.

Diaphragmatic Rupture

Trauma to the anterior chest and abdomen may produce large increases in intra-abdominal pressure and herniation of abdominal contents into the thoracic cavity. Typically occurring on the left, perforations are created in the diaphragm, allowing loops of bowel to enter the chest cavity. The bowel contents limit inflation of the lung and may lead to respiratory decompensation. Endotracheal intubation or assisted positive-pressure ventilation improves oxygenation.

Hemothorax

The presence of blood in the lungs affects ventilation and oxygenation in two ways: mechanical interference and loss of circulating hemoglobin. Bleeding within the chest may originate from several different sources, such as intercostal vessels, pulmonary vessels, or the lung itself. As bleeding continues, blood collects in the pleural space, limiting inflation of the lung. Each hemithorax can accommodate up to 3,000 mL of blood and may result in tension hemothorax.

In addition to the mechanical disruption of air flow due to hemothorax, the blood lost from the circulatory system is no longer available to transport oxygen to the tissues. Thus, management is directed at both airway control as well as management of hemorrhagic shock.

Rib Fractures

As described above, the intercostal muscles and ribs play an important role in normal respiration. When fractured, ribs are no longer able to provide the elastic recoil of the chest wall necessary for adequate respiration. In addition, jagged and displaced bone ends may damage surrounding tissue, particularly the pleura and lung parenchyma.

Hypoventilation often accompanies rib fractures. Pain associated with rib fractures is often intense, and patients are reluctant to take deep, full ventilations. The resulting shallow ventilations lead to hypoventilation, poor pulmonary toilet, atelectasis, and pneumonia.

Flail Segments

Flail segments result when two or more adjacent ribs are fractured in two or more places. The fractured area loses its bony support and floats freely. During inspiration, the flail segment moves inward, and during exhalation, the segment moves outward. This paradoxical movement leads to hypoventilation, hypoxia, and hypercarbia.

Chest Wall Compression

Even when uninjured, the chest wall must be unencumbered and free to expand. Prolonged circumferential pressure prevents chest excursion and normal ventilation. Chest wall compression typically occurs with structural collapse, cave-ins, and falls into grain elevators. The resulting external pressure on the chest caused by grain, dirt, or debris inhibits movement of the chest wall and inspiration.

Burns are also another mechanism of chest wall compression. Deep burns of the chest, especially when circumferential, lead to inelastic eschar formation. As tissue edema forms following the burn injury, the inelastic eschar functions as a vise, limiting chest excursion. The result is inadequate tidal volume, hypoventilation, hypoxia, and hypercarbia.

ASPIRATION AND TOXIC INHALATIONS

Aspiration

Aside from providing ventilation and supporting respiration, active airway management is aimed at protecting the airway against aspiration of gastric contents. Even patients without any evidence of respiratory compromise may require advanced airway procedures. Such patients include those with diminished mentation where there exists the risk of aspiration. Gastric aspirate has been found in the respiratory tract following intubation in 8% of anesthetized patients and in up to 50% of patients undergoing emergency intubation.[22,23]

Aspiration occurs as a result of the loss of the laryngeal reflex coupled with the loss of tone in the lower esophageal sphincter. Normally, the gastroesophageal sphincter is contracted and exerts a pressure of 10 cm H_2O, higher than intragastric pressure, thus preventing regurgitation. Increased intragastric pressure, such as with bag-valve mask (BVM) ventilations, exceeds the limits of the sphincter, permitting regurgitation. Other conditions such as pregnancy, hiatal hernia, obesity, nasogastric tubes, and paralytic agents predispose patients to regurgitation and aspiration.

Aspiration of gastric contents sets the stage for three separate syndromes: (1) chemical pneumonitis due to the direct damage caused by gastric contents, (2) obstruction of smaller airways by food particles, and (3) infection.[24] Within seconds of aspiration, the gastric fluid can reach the aveolar space and may cause any of the following: (1) destruction of aveolar cells, (2) loss of surfactant, and (3) edema and bleeding within the alveoli. The clinical picture is one of bronchospasm, tachypnea, rales, wheezing, hypoxemia, hypotension, and shock.

The mortality rate associated with aspiration is related to the volume (0.4 mL/kg to be clinically significant), distribution, and acidity of the aspirate. The mortality rate of aspiration correlates inversely in an almost linear fashion with pH.[25] Aspirate with a pH of less than 2.5 carries a 40% mortality rate, which increases to nearly 100% as the pH approaches 1.8.[26,27] The mortality rate is higher with infected aspirate than with the normally sterile aspirate.

Management of aspiration is aimed initially at prevention. Intubation attempts should be limited as multiple intubation attempts increase the risk of aspiration. Proper ventilation with the BVM prevents gastric insufflation and increased intragastric pressures. The use of the Sellick maneuver and a cuffed endotracheal tube also decreases the likelihood of aspiration.

Once aspiration has occurred, the airway should be secured with an endotracheal tube and endotracheal suctioning immediately performed. Bronchial lavage has been performed with alkaline solution but with minimal effectiveness, owing to the rapid progression of the aspirate into the aveoli. Corticosteroids and antibiotics have shown no practical benefit.[28]

Chemical

Inhalation of toxic substances may be the result of transportation mishaps, structure fires, industrial accidents, faulty heating units, and improperly functioning ventilation systems. Pathologies arising from toxic inhalations include airway edema, laryngospasm, pulmonary edema, disruption of alveolar/capillary membranes, and interference with oxygen absorption.

In addition to the risks associated with thermal injury, structure fires produce toxic byproducts of combustion, along with smoke, that contain many toxic substances. The increased use of plastics and synthetic materials in the home exposes fire victims to many toxic products, including carbon monoxide, hydrochloric acid, potassium cyanide, and hydrogen sulfide. Once inhaled, these substances are capable of producing chemical burns or systemic poisoning.

Aside from carbon monoxide and chlorine, no single gas causes a significant number of chemical inhalation injuries, but many gases are capable of producing bronchopulmonary injury.[29] Each gas may lead to pulmonary edema, local pulmonary injury, or interfere with oxygenation.

Regardless of the injury mechanism of these chemical agents, all warrant airway and ventilatory intervention. In some cases, laryngeal edema may require a surgical airway and pulmonary edema may be so severe as to require intubation, mechanical ventilation, PEEP, and tracheal suctioning.

VENTILATION AND PERFUSION MISMATCH

Ventilation distributes oxygen into the alveoli and blood flow brings CO_2 to the alveoli. Exchange of oxygen and carbon dioxide across the alveoli requires a balance between ventilation and blood flow. Adequate ventilation does not result in adequate tissue oxygenation in the absence of adequate blood flow and vice versa. Several mechanisms of V/Q mismatching may be encountered in the prehospital trauma patient.

Any mechanism that produces fluid in the lung interferes with ventilation of alveoli. Such mechanisms include hemothorax, pulmonary edema secondary to toxic inhalation, and water-filled lungs of a near-drowning victim. Such V/Q mismatches are termed right-to-left shunts because blood is flowing to alveoli that are not being ventilated. A similar mechanism is responsible for a V/Q mismatch in patients with atelectasis resulting from hypoventilation, rib fractures, flail segments, and prolonged compression of the chest.

The opposite syndrome occurs when sufficient amounts of blood do not pass adequately ventilated alveoli. Such conditions occur during shock or injuries to the pulmonary vasculature. The final product is the same, inadequate gas exchange leading to hypoxemia and hypercapnia.

AIRWAY MANAGEMENT

Given the myriad of airway and ventilatory pathologies, it is incumbent on the paramedic to become competent in airway management. Because paramedics often encounter unique patient presentations, it is important to develop skill in a variety of airway procedures. With a large arsenal of airway techniques, it becomes easier for the paramedic to find a technique suitable for any situation. The following sections describe the indications, advantages, and disadvantages of various airway techniques as well as airway challenges posed by the trauma patient.

CERVICAL SPINE INJURY AND AIRWAY MANAGEMENT

The incidence of cervical spine (C-spine) fracture or injury in the setting of blunt trauma patients has been estimated at 1%–12%, and one series of traffic fatalities recognized that 21.1% of victims sustained C-spine injuries.[30–36] In addition, victims of passenger cars sustaining enough damage to require towing from the scene have a 1:300 chance of sustaining severe neck injuries.[37] Given the potential for C-spine injury in blunt trauma, the concern for producing iatrogenic injury during airway procedures is well justified.

There is great controversy concerning the possibility of injury to the spinal cord during airway maintenance, particularly orotracheal intubation. A few studies have suggested that C-spine injuries can be predicted in the field using a set of exclusionary criteria, such as patients who are awake and alert, without a history of syncope, and that exhibit no signs of spinal injury.[38,39] However, these low-risk patients are unlikely to require emergency airway management, and these criteria have little utility in managing multisystem trauma patients in need of agressive airway interventions. Therefore, it must be assumed that in any patient who has sustained blunt injury of a magnitude sufficient to warrant emergency airway management, a significant risk of concomitant C-spine injury exists.[40]

For the trauma patient whose C-spine status has not been established, the airway management options must be restricted to those that can be performed without manipulation of the C-spine. The accepted basic airway maneuvers are the chin lift and trauma jaw thrust (discussed below).[41] However, neither of these techniques is devoid of C-spine movement. In a cadaver model in which C5–C6 instability was surgically created, Aprahamian et al. found that both techniques increased the disc space in excess of 5 mm.[42] Notwithstanding Aprahamian's findings, these basic maneuvers are considered the standard of care in the setting of trauma. However, the advanced airway procedures are more controversial.

The incidence of C-spine injury in multisystem trauma patients mandates that all patients be immobilized on a long spine board, cervical collar, head immobilization device, and straps. The suggested approaches to advanced airway management of these patients are blind nasotracheal intubation, oral intubation with manual immobilization, and surgical airway. The following paragraphs will discuss these techniques in the context of C-spine injury. The procedure for each technique is described in a later section.

Blind nasotracheal intubation is widely advocated in managing the airway in the immobilized blunt trauma patient.[43] The technique does not require laryngoscopy and, therefore, does not require manipulation of the head and C-spine. In the investigation by Aprahamian et al., 2 mm of posterior subluxation was noted with this procedure.[42]

The application of distracting force to the unstable C-spine is the primary disadvantage of orotracheal intubation. In the nontraumatized patient, the head and neck are repositioned in the "sniffing position" to facilitate visualization of the glottis. This positioning is contraindicated in the trauma patient. However, the use of "manual stabilization" has been suggested as an adjunct that will permit orotracheal intubation without C-spine manipulation.[44] Several studies have shown manual stabilization during orotracheal intubation to be a safe and effective technique.[45–47] In addition, Majernick et al. found no difference in C-spine movement between intubations using straight or curved blades.[47] The key element among these studies is that the C-spine must be meticulously immobilized during intubation by someone other than the intubator. In addition, it is important to discriminate between manual in-line stabilization and "traction." The former does not involve distracting forces as does the latter. The American College of Surgeons considers both nasal and oral intubations to be acceptable and recommends that the intubator use the technique in which he or she is most skillful.[41]

The surgical airway is the last of the widely accepted airway control techniques for the trauma patient. There have been no investigations of C-spine movement during cricothyrotomy.[43] However, the only force applied during the procedure is to the airway itself and should not aggravate an unstable spine.[43] However, while there is little movement of the C-spine, the technique is not routinely practiced, most likely due to its invasive nature and the need for considerable skill by the clinician.

These techniques are the most widely accepted methods of advanced airway management in the trauma patient. The choice of technique should ultimately be based on the clinical presentation, urgency, local protocol, and skill of the intubator.

BASIC AIRWAY MANAGEMENT

In unresponsive patients, the tongue becomes flaccid and, by the force of gravity, falls into the posterior pharynx. This is the most common form of airway obstruction. Fortunately, because the tongue is attached to and moves with the mandible, this form of airway obstruction is easily remedied by basic maneuvers such as the trauma jaw thrust and trauma chin lift. Both techniques relieve the obstruction without undue manipulation of the C-spine.

Trauma Jaw Thrust

The trauma jaw thrust is performed by grasping the patient's head by placing the thumbs on the zygoma. While the head and C-spine are stabilized, the index and long fingers grasp the mandible at the angle and push forward without moving the head or C-spine (Figure 18-6). As the mandible is displaced forward, the tongue is removed from the posterior oropharynx.

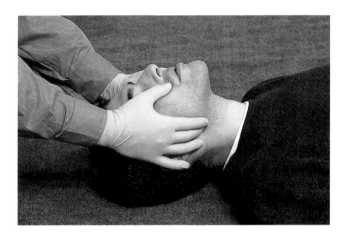

FIGURE 18-6 Trauma jaw thrust.

Trauma Chin Lift

The trauma chin lift is another means of opening the airway of an unconscious trauma patient with suspected C-spine injury. With this technique, the mandible is pulled forward by grasping the chin and the lower incisors and lifting (Figure 18-7). Again, as the mandible is displaced anteriorly, the tongue is lifted from the posterior oropharynx. However, this technique carries a risk of biting injuries to the paramedic and should be reserved for deeply unconscious patients.

AIRWAY ADJUNCTS

Following basic maneuvers to open the airway, adjuncts may be used to maintain airway patency. During initial assessment and treatment of the trauma patient, the most readily available and rapidly inserted devices that provide an adequate airway should be used. These devices can be replaced later when time

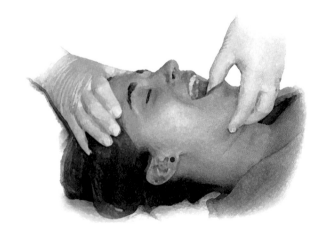

FIGURE 18-7 Trauma chin lift.

permits or additional personnel are available to perform the more invasive procedures. However, if at any time a basic adjunct fails to provide a proper airway, it should immediately be replaced by an advanced airway.

Oropharyngeal Airway

The most basic and simplest to use airway device is the **oropharyngeal airway (OPA)**. The OPA is a semi-circular device constructed of rigid plastic. It is designed to overcome soft tissue obstruction and may also serve as a bite block. There are two basic designs: the Guedel, which is a tubular design, and the Berman, which possesses channels on each side of the device (Figure 18-8). The Guedel airway is preferred for children because it is easier to insert and less traumatic. When inserted, either device holds the tongue away from the posterior wall of the pharynx.

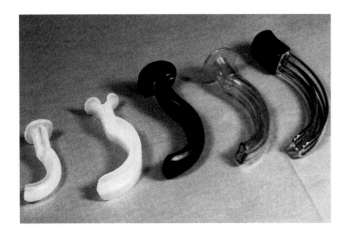

FIGURE 18-8 Oropharyngeal airways.

The OPA is available in an assortment of sizes (Table 18-3). To measure the device, the flange is placed against the patient's incisors with the body of the device parallel to the palate. The tip of the properly sized OPA rests at the angle of the jaw. Alternatively, the device should reach from the corner of the mouth to the earlobe. Once properly sized, the OPA is inserted by inverting the device 180° and inserting the tip into the mouth. After advancing the tip past the crest of the tongue, the OPA is rotated 180° into anatomical position. The airway is further inserted following the curvature of the oropharynx until the flange rests against the lips. Inserting the OPA in a rotated position limits the risk of inadvertently pushing the tongue into the back of the oropharynx. Alternatively, the tongue can be displaced inferiorly and anteriorly with a tongue blade and the OPA inserted following the natural curvature of the oropharynx. With this method it is unnecessary to invert the OPA prior to insertion. This alternative method of inserting the OPA is preferred in children.

When properly inserted, the OPA prevents soft tissue obstruction, provides access for oral suctioning, and serves as a bite block. However, the device does not protect against aspiration, stimulates the gag reflex and laryngospasms, and does not provide direct access to the lungs. In addition, the trauma jaw thrust is still necessary when this device is used. Therefore, the OPA is a temporizing airway and should be used only in unconscious patients, and then only until a more definitive airway can be provided.

Nasopharyngeal Airway

The **nasopharyngeal airway (NPA)** is an excellent airway adjunct for the trauma patient. It is a tube made from soft latex rubber with a beveled tip and a proximal

Table 18-3
Approximate Oropharyngeal and Nasopharyngeal Airway Sizes

Patient Size	OPA		NPA
	Berman	**Guedel**	**NPA**
Extra large adult	110 mm		9.0 mm i.d. (36 French)
Large adult	100 mm	Guedel #4	8.0 mm i.d. (32 French)
Medium adult	90 mm	Guedel #3	7.0 mm i.d. (29 French)
Small adult	80 mm	Guedel #2	6.0 mm i.d. (26 French)
Adolescent	70 mm	Guedel #1	5.0 mm i.d. (23 French)
Child	60 mm	Guedel #0	4.0 mm i.d. (20 French)
Infant	50 mm	Guedel #00	
Neonate	40 mm		

flange (Figure 18-9). The advantage of the NPA over the OPA is that it is well tolerated in conscious patients and does not invoke laryngospasms or stimulate the gag reflex, especially when the tip is lubricated with an anesthetic jelly. In addition, preparation of the tip with an alpha sympathomimetic will constrict the mucosal vasculature and facilitate passage of the airway.

The NPA secures an airway by providing a conduit past the tongue for air flow. As with the OPA, several sizes of NPA are available (Table 18-3). Sizes range from 17 to 36 French. Each French unit measures the inside diameter of the device and equals approximately $\frac{1}{3}$ mm. To insert the NPA, the device is measured by selecting the device that approximates the distance from the nares to the earlobe. An NPA of appropriate length has an external diameter that is slightly smaller than the internal diameter of the nares. The beveled side is passed along the medial aspect of the nose, which is devoid of the rich blood supply of the lateral mucosa, thus limiting the risk of trauma and bleeding. The NPA is constructed such that it is designed for the right nare (bevel to the septal side). However, the device may be inserted on the left side by rotating the device 180° and rotating it back to its original position once the tip has passed the nasopharynx. Therefore, the paramedic should select the nare that provides the largest and most direct access to the nasopharynx and adjust the insertion procedure accordingly.

Once the tip of the NPA has been prepared, it is inserted into the nare with the bevel toward the septum. The device is gently passed along the floor of the nare, which is parallel to the palate. The most common insertion error is to insert the device in an upward direction. If resistance is met, twisting the device gently may facilitate passage. After insertion, the airway rests in the posterior pharynx behind the tongue. If the patient begins to gag, the tip of the tube may be stimulating the posterior pharynx and should be withdrawn slightly. As with the OPA, it is important that the mandible be displaced using the trauma jaw thrust in the unconscious patient.

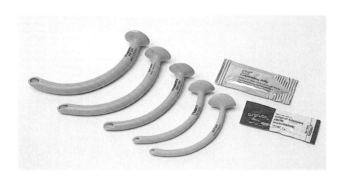

FIGURE 18-9 Nasopharyngeal airways.

Disadvantages of this airway include trauma to the nasal mucosa with bleeding, inability to protect against aspiration, pressure necrosis if left in place for extended periods, and stimulation of laryngospasm and gag reflex when improperly positioned. There is also a potential to pass the NPA into the cranial vault in the presence of a basilar skull fracture. In addition, because of the small internal diameter of the device, the NPA can easily become occluded by mucus, blood, vomitus, soft tissues, and foreign bodies. The NPA is an effective and well-tolerated device that should be used only temporarily and replaced as soon as possible with a more advanced device.

Bag-Valve Unit

The bag-valve unit is a descendant of the anesthesia bag and consists of a self-inflating bag and a nonrebreathing valve. The device delivers positive-pressure ventilation to patients with inadequate respirations or apnea. The bag-valve unit may be used with a mask, endotracheal (ET) tube, or other invasive airway device. The ideal unit consists of a self-refilling bag, a port for supplemental oxygen, reservoir attachments for delivering high-concentration oxygen, a nonrebreathing valve, standard 15- and 22-mm connectors, and bag units and face masks of assorted sizes.

The BVM unit is the first means of ventilating the trauma patient. When used properly, usually in conjunction with a nasopharyngeal or oropharyngeal airway, the BVM is capable of delivering 10–15 mL/kg of pure oxygen as recommended by the American Heart Association.[18] However, the device requires considerable practice to acquire proficiency. Several investigations have reported limited ability of prehospital personnel to adequately ventilate with the BVM.[48–50] Inadequate ventilations have been attributed to size of the operator's hand, inadequate seal with the face mask, dead space under the mask, and inadequate compression of the bag.[11,51] As a result, it is recommended that the device be used by two operators when possible. If extra personnel are not available, an alternative is to add extension tubing between the mask and the bag, allowing the operator to squeeze the bag against his or her thigh to increase delivered tidal volumes; however, this method is less effective than two-person ventilation (Figure 18-10).[21,52] The use of low-dead-space face masks will also increase delivered tidal volumes.[51]

To use the BVM, the operator stands at the patient's head. He or she may use his or her knees to maintain cervical immobilization or this may be done by an assistant.[21,52] The airway should be free of blood, vomitus, or other obstructions before ventilating. Once the airway is cleared, the mask is placed on the patient's

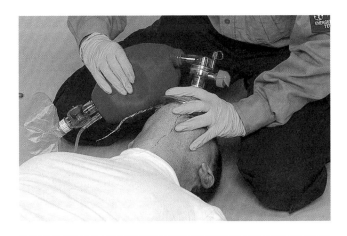

FIGURE 18-10 When forced, the paramedic may have to use the BVM alone. Adequate tidal volumes are best achieved by squeezing the bag against the operator's thigh.

face, ensuring a proper seal. The bag is then compressed against the operator's knee (one-person technique) or by the assistant. The bag should be compressed quickly and smoothly, delivering 500–800 mL of oxygen to the average-sized adult patient. Proper tidal volumes can be ensured by observing the rise and fall of the chest with each ventilation. Supplemental oxygen and a reservoir device should be added to the BVM.

When properly used, the BVM offers several advantages: (1) rapid means of providing initial ventilations, (2) does not require intubation, (3) ability to provide a wide range of ventilatory pressures and tidal volumes, (4) can be used to assist patients with shallow or ineffective respiratory efforts, (5) ability to provide varying degrees of oxygen concentration (21% to nearly 100%), (6) allows operator to gauge lung compliance and detect conditions such as pneumothorax, and (7) can be used in conjunction with advanced airways.

INTERNET ACTIVITIES

Visit the e-medicine Web site at http:// www.emedicine.com. Click on the Emergency Medicine on-line book and select Emergency Medical Services. Then click on Prehospital Airway Devices. Review the chapter on airway control techniques.

Esophageal Obturator Airway and Esophageal Gastric Tube Airway

Efforts to overcome the unpleasantries and gastric distention associated with mouth-to-mouth ventilation led to the development of the precursor to the esophageal airway in 1968.[51] Later refined by Gordon, the device became known as the **esophageal obturator airway (EOA)**.[53] The EOA resembles an elongated (34-cm) cuffed ET tube 13 mm in diameter with sixteen 3-mm perforations in the proximal one-third of the tube (Figure 18-11). The proximal end of the tube has an adaptor that attaches to a face mask. The distal end of the tube is closed, with a 35-mL inflatable balloon located just proximal to the closed end. When properly positioned, the balloon rests below the tracheal bifurcation and occludes the esophagus when inflated. When gas is introduced via the face mask, it exits the perforations, which are now at the level of the pharynx. With proper sealing of the face mask and inflation of the balloon, air is forced into the trachea.

The **esophageal gastric tube airway (EGTA)** was introduced to overcome some of the criticisms of the EOA. Instead of the distal end being sealed, the EGTA has an open end to allow a nasogastric tube to be passed for gastric decompression. The EGTA also lacks perforations for air flow in the proximal portion of the tube. Instead, air is introduced via a second hole in the face mask that does not communicate with the tube (Figure 18-12). Air is forced into the trachea similar to the BVM, with the added advantage of the esophagus being sealed by the EGTA.

With laryngoscopy and intubation being commonly practiced in the prehospital setting, the EOA

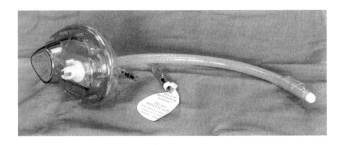

FIGURE 18-11 Esophageal obturator airway.

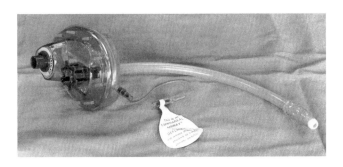

FIGURE 18-12 Esophageal gastric tube airway.

and EGTA have experienced declining use. Despite the widespread use of ET, the EOA or EGTA may still be appropriate when intubation is not possible or is unsuccessful. Contraindications include children under 16 years of age, presence of a gag reflex, conscious or semiconscious patient, caustic ingestion, known esophageal disease or injury, and massive facial injuries that would preclude an adequate seal with the face mask. The age restriction is related more to the size of the patient than to age per se. The balloon will not rest in the proper position in patients under 5 feet or over 7 feet in height. The tube will be too long for the short patient, and the balloon will be improperly positioned above the carina in the tall patient. Because the cartilaginous rings of the trachea are "C" shaped with the open portion on the posterior surface, they lack rigid structure on the posterior surface. In tall patients where the EOA balloon lies above the carina, the trachea can be occluded when the balloon is inflated.

Despite the ease of insertion, the EOA and EGTA suffer from a relatively high complication rate. Investigations comparing arterial blood gases, ventilation, and oxygenation between the EOA and ET intubation in prehospital cardiac arrest patients have produced variable results.[54–57] In addition, Bryson et al. noted substantially lower mean tidal volumes using the EOA as compared with using a mask and oral airway.[58] They also noted the difficulty in obtaining an adequate mask-to-face seal. Similarly, Harrison et al. noted a lower tidal volume with the EOA compared to the ET tube.[59] The overall effectiveness of the EOA and EGTA is best summarized by Pepe et al.: "Our conclusions from reviewing the available studies are that, with some operators, the EOA/EGTA occasionally can be as effective as the endotracheal tube. However, it is never more effective, and, in some cases, the EOA/EGTA is significantly inferior to the endotracheal tube in providing adequate oxygenation and ventilation."[60]

Other reported complications with the EOA and EGTA include esophageal perforation (up to 2% of cases), inadvertent tracheal intubation (1%–10% of cases), inability to intubate the esophagus (5%–12% of cases), and esophageal mucosal damage (10% of cases).[54,61–63] Table 18-4 summarizes the indications, contraindications, advantages, and disadvantages of the EOA and EGTA.

Insertion of the EOA or EGTA begins with hyperventilation using 100% O_2 and lubricating the tube with surgical lubricant. The patient's neck is placed in the neutral position with manual stabilization of cervical alignment. Grasping the tongue and lower jaw with the thumb and index finger, the mouth is fully opened. The tube with attached mask is inserted blindly into the esophagus following the curvature of the pharynx. The mask is sealed against the patient's face and the patient ventilated. The paramedic should

Table 18-4
Indications, Advantages, Disadvantages, and Contraindications of the EOA and EGTA

Indications	Advantages	Disadvantages	Contraindications
Failure of other techniques of airway control	Blind procedure	Less effective means of ventilation compared to ETI	Less than 16 years of age
Inability to visualize anatomical landmarks during laryngoscopy due to vomitus or blood	Requires less technical skill than endotracheal intubation (ETI)	Requires proper seal between face and mask	Greater than 7 feet in height
Inability to visualize anatomical landmarks due to traumatic disruption	Requires less time to perform than ETI	Does not protect lungs from aspirating blood and foreign bodies from upper airway	Less than 5 feet in height
	Does not require manipulation of the head for insertion	Esophageal injury and perforation	Esophageal injury
	Provides access for gastric decompression (EGTA only)	Restrictions on patient size	Preexisting esophageal disease
	Once inserted, serves as an esophageal marker and lessens the likelihood of esophageal intubation during ETI		Ingestion of caustic substances
			Presence of a gag reflex
			Massive facial trauma that would preclude adequate interface between face and mask

auscultate over the lungs and stomach to ensure proper tube position. If the tube is in the esophagus, the balloon should be inflated with 30–35 mL of air. If ET is necessary, the mask is removed and the patient intubated around the EOA or EGTA tube. If removal of the EOA or EGTA is necessary, the balloon is deflated and the tube withdrawn following the curvature of the pharynx. Suction should be available because patients frequently regurgitate during removal.

Pharyngeotracheal Lumen Airway

The **pharyngeotracheal lumen airway (PTLA)** was developed to overcome the limitations of the EOA and EGTA, principally those of inadvertent tracheal intubation and the reported problems of obtaining a proper face-to-mask seal.[60] The PTLA is a double-lumen tube with a twin-balloon system (Figure 18-13). The lumens are of unequal length and run parallel, each with a proximal adaptor for ventilation. The first tube is 31 cm in length with an internal diameter of 8 mm and contains a semirigid stylet for maintaining the curvature of the tube. A small, low-volume balloon is attached to the end of this tube, giving it the appearance of an ET tube. The second tube is 21 cm in length and is attached to the larger of the two balloons at its distal end.

The PTLA is inserted blindly, much like the EOA and EGTA. The balloons are inflated simultaneously through the 15-mm adaptor using a BVM. The upper balloon seals off the oropharynx while the lower balloon seals either the trachea or the esophagus, depending upon the placement of the tube. The shorter tube is ventilated first and the patient observed for chest rise. If the chest rises and breath sounds are heard, the longer tube is positioned in the esophagus and ventilation continues through the short tube (Figure 18-14A). When the PTLA is in this esophageal position, it functions similar to an EGTA. If the chest does not rise, the PTLA is in a tracheal position (Figure 18-14B). The paramedic should remove the stylet from the longer

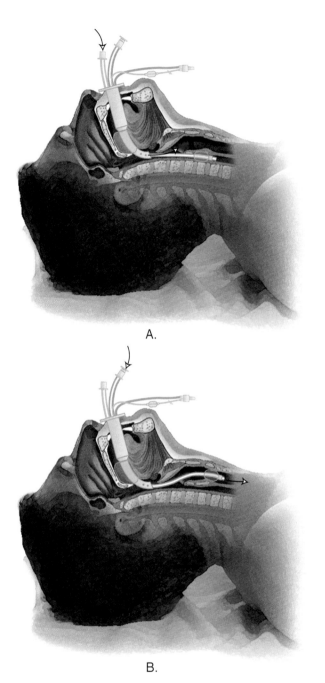

FIGURE 18-14 (A) PTLA in esophageal position. (B) PTLA in tracheal position.

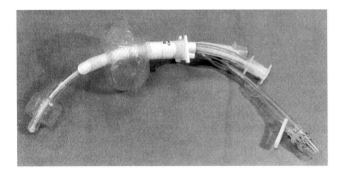

FIGURE 18-13 Pharyngeotracheal lumen airway.

tube and ventilate through this tube. In this position, the PTLA functions similar to an ET tube.

The indications, contraindications, and complications of the PTLA and the Combitube (discussed below) are similar to those of the EOA/EGTA and are summarized in Table 18-5. The primary advantage of the PTLA over the EOA/EGTA is that it cannot be improperly positioned. Regardless of whether the airway assumes a tracheal or esophageal position, it will provide a means of ventilation. Sufficient data from clinical trials to fully evaluate the effectiveness of the PTLA are lacking.[64] However, after reviewing the available data, Pepe et al. concluded that the PTLA appears to offer oxygenation and ventilation similar to that achieved with an ET tube.[60] Complications associated with the PTLA include an inadequate seal of the pharyngeal balloon, difficulty intubating around the device, esophageal rupture, and undetected bleeding below the pharyngeal balloon.[60,65] Inflation of the pharyngeal balloon has also been noted to push the tube out of position.[66] The overall complication rate of the PTLA is less than 1%.[65]

Combitube Airway

The **Combitube** is a double-lumen, double-balloon system similar in structure and function to the PTLA (Figure 18-15). The distal balloon is inflated through a proximal pilot balloon with a one-way valve and is designed to hold 15–20 mL of air. The proximal balloon, designed to seal off the mouth and nasopharynx, holds 100–140 mL of air and is also inflated through a proximal pilot balloon-valve system.[64] One lumen of the device is perforated near its midpoint and has a sealed distal end. The other lumen is nonperforated and is open at its distal tip.

Similar to the PTLA, the Combitube is inserted blindly and the proximal balloon is first inflated with 100 mL of air, followed by the distal balloon with 15 mL of air. The patient is then ventilated through the

Table 18-5
Indications, Advantages, Disadvantages, and Contraindications of the PTLA and Combitube

Indications	Advantages	Disadvantages	Contraindications
Same as EOA/EGTA	Blind procedure	Inadequate seal of pharyngeal balloon has been reported with PTLA	Less than 14 years of age
	Requires less skill to perform than ETI	Difficult to pass endotracheal tube around these devices	Esophageal injury
	Requires less time to perform than ETI	Esophageal rupture possible	Preexisting esophageal disease
	Does not require manipulation of the head for insertion	Lethal complications with misdiagnosed placement	Ingestion of caustic substances
	Provides access for gastric suctioning	Infrapharyngeal bleeding may be obscured by balloon and go undetected	Presence of gag reflex
	Functional airway regardless of whether it is placed in trachea or esophagus		
	Possibility of spontaneous respirations through unused lumen in case of undiagnosed misplacement (Combitube only)		
	Less likely to produce esophageal rupture than EOA/EGTA		
	Improved ventilation over EOA/EGTA		
	Does not require the use of a face mask negating the problem of mask seal associated with BVM, EOA, and EGTA		

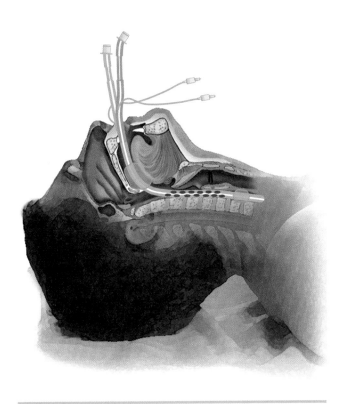

FIGURE 18-15 Combitube airway in esophageal position.

longer lumen and the patient observed for chest rise. If the patient's chest rises and breath sounds can be heard, the tube is in an esophageal position and ventilation continues through this lumen. If not, the patient is ventilated through the shorter lumen, indicating a tracheal position. Success rates of insertion range between 69% and 100%.[67,68]

The indications, contraindications, and complications of the Combitube are similar to those of the PTLA and are summarized in Table 18-5. An advantage of the Combitube over the PTLA is that, in the event of misdiagnosed tracheal placement, a spontaneously breathing patient may breathe through the perforations in the unused lumen.[60] In addition, the pharyngeal balloon can be deflated independently of the distal balloon, allowing for pharyngeal suctioning.

The complication rate of the Combitube is very low, and in one study involving 470 prehospital cardiac arrest patients, the Combitube had the fewest complications with ventilation when compared with the PTLA, laryngeal mask airway, and OPA.[69] There were no significant differences in blood gases or spirometry among the devices.[69] Other studies have used crossover techniques to evaluate the effectiveness of the Combitube when compared to ETI.[68,70–73] The results of these clinical trials indicate that the Combitube can ventilate as well as and occasionally better than the ET tube. However, the occasional marginal improvement

in ventilation with the Combitube, while statistically significant, is not of clinical importance.[60] The improvement is thought to be related to a PEEP effect created by the higher resistance to air flow observed with the Combitube than with the ET tube.[60]

Endotracheal Intubation

Endotracheal intubation is the "gold standard" of airway management in patients who cannot protect their own airway or who require assisted ventilation. Several challenges face the clinician who must intubate a trauma patient in the field, such as poor lighting, awkward positions of both rescuer and patient, and the omnipresent need to maintain neutral alignment of the C-spine. Although direct orotracheal intubation should be considered the primary technique of intubation, the procedure is not always easily accomplished. Fortunately, there are several methods of intubation from which the paramedic can choose to determine the one best suited for each situation. Consequently, the paramedic must be proficient in the use of many intubation techniques. The following section describes several intubation methods suitable for field use.

Orotracheal Technique. The standard technique of orotracheal intubation is largely preserved in the setting of trauma. The only major deviation from the standard technique in the setting of trauma is the need to maintain manual in-line cervical immobilization and avoid the "sniffing position." In general, an assistant maintains cervical immobilization during the procedure. This can be accomplished from the patient's side or, alternatively, the assistant can be positioned astraddle the patient. Regardless of position, it is important that the assistant not allow the neck to be manipulated during intubation. Application of a cervical collar may offer further protection of the C-spine during intubation. Although a single paramedic can simultaneously maintain cervical immobilization during BVM ventilation, it is not recommended that the intubator also provide cervical immobilization using his or her knees during intubation attempts.

Despite the inability to place the patient in the sniffing position prior to intubation, several steps can be taken to increase the likelihood of successful orotracheal intubation. For patients who are electively intubated but do not require immediate intubation, such as patients with burn injuries or head trauma with patent airway and respirations, it may be possible to examine the airway and predict the likelihood of successful orotracheal intubation. Mallampati proposed a system for identifying patients at risk for difficult intubation.[74] This system classifies intubation difficulty into four categories based on the visibility of intraoral structures (Figure 18-16A).

Patients in classes III and IV are at high risk for difficult intubation and the paramedic may abandon orotracheal intubation in favor of other airway techniques. Obviously, predicting difficult intubations with this system requires a cooperative patient, which minimizes its utility in many cases. In these circumstances, intubation difficulty is predicted during laryngoscopy (Figure 18-16B). In patients with difficulty grades of 3 or 4, orotracheal intubation is unlikely and the paramedic should abandon repeated attempts at intubation in favor of other airway techniques.

Altering the position of the intubator can also increase the likelihood of successful intubation. Because trauma patients often present in awkward positions, it is advantageous for the paramedic to become comfortable intubating while prone and

seated. In addition, these positions will sometimes offer better visualization over the standard position.

Because neutral alignment of the C-spine limits visualization during laryngoscopy, often cricoid pressure will bring the glottis into view. Cricoid pressure can be applied by the assistant maintaining cervical alignment as long as it does not interfere with his or her ability to protect spinal integrity. Furthermore, the use of neuromuscular blocking agents may facilitate visualization during difficult intubations by reducing resistance to displacement of the mandible.

Finally, it may be possible that orotracheal intubation is not the appropriate technique for airway control. As previously described, Mallampati classes III and IV and intubation difficulty grades 3 and 4 should probably be intubated using methods other than

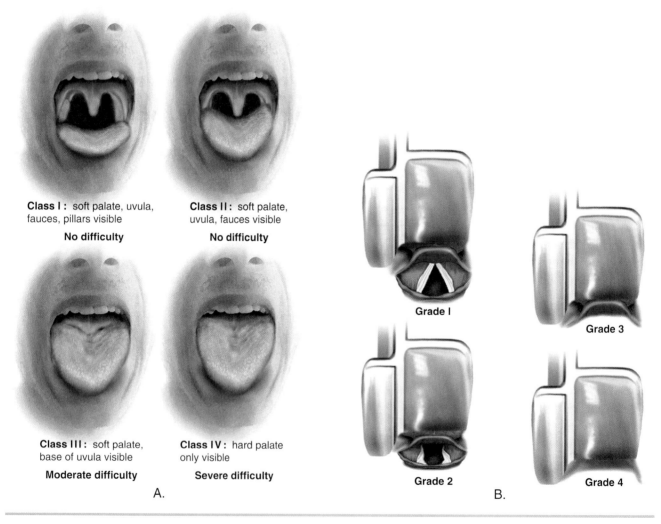

Class I: soft palate, uvula, fauces, pillars visible

No difficulty

Class II: soft palate, uvula, fauces visible

No difficulty

Class III: soft palate, base of uvula visible

Moderate difficulty

Class IV: hard palate only visible

Severe difficulty

A.

Grade I

Grade 2

Grade 3

Grade 4

B.

FIGURE 18-16 (A) Mallampati classifications for predicting difficulty of orotracheal intubation. (B) The grades of difficulty of endotracheal intubation based on the best view obtained during laryngoscopy. Grade 1: All or most of glottis visible; no difficulty anticipated. Grade 2: Only posterior aspect of glottis visible; slight difficulty anticipated. Grade 3: Only epiglottis, no part of glottis, visible; fairly severe difficulty anticipated. Grade 4: Not even epiglottis visible; intubation impossible except by special techniques.

orotracheal intubation. The paramedic should decide, based upon clinical judgment, whether orotracheal intubation is appropriate. Table 18-6 summarizes the indications, contraindications, advantages, and disadvantages of orotracheal intubation and Table 18-7 summarizes the procedure.

Seated Orotracheal Intubation. Despite the importance of aggressive airway mangement, occassionally patients present in awkward positions. One such presentation is that of the patient pinned by automobile wreckage in a seated position . The paramedic must be able to adapt to the situation and effectively manage the airway, particularly if extrication time will be lengthy. Despite the unique position of the patient, standard orotracheal intubation techniques can be adapted to effect airway control.[75]

Intubation of the seated patient begins with C-spine control, hyperventilation, and preparation of equipment. There are two variations of the technique: the superior approach and the frontal approach. The superior approach is technically similar to intubating the supine patient. The paramedic is positioned behind the patient, typically in the back seat of the auto. Intubation proceeds in the usual manner except that the intubator is required to lean over the patient (Figure 18-17). Care must be taken to ensure that the laryngoscope is manipulated in the proper direction (i.e., 45° anterocaudal direction relative to the patient).

Table 18-7
Procedure for Orotracheal Intubation

1. Assistant maintains cervical spine alignment.
2. Patient is hyperventilated with 1.0 FiO_2.
3. Laryngoscope is inserted into the right side of the patient's mouth, sweeping the tongue to the left.
4. When a curved blade is used, the blade is inserted into the vallecula. If a straight blade is used, the blade tip is inserted under the epiglottis.
5. The blade is lifted forward at a 45° angle and cricoid pressure is applied to bring the glottis into view.
6. The tube is advanced along the right side of the oropharynx.
7. After the glottis is visualized, the tube is passed through the vocal cords to the proper depth. If a stylet was used, it should now be removed.
8. The cuff is inflated with 5–10 cc of air.
9. Tube placement is confirmed.
10. An oropharyngeal airway is inserted and the position of the tube at the incisors (22 cm in average-sized adult) is noted.
11. The tube is secured to the head with tape or a commercially available device designed for this purpose.

Table 18-6
Indications, Advantages, Disadvantages, and Contraindications of Orotracheal Intubation

Indications	Advantages	Disadvantages	Contraindications
First choice of airway control when basic maneuvers fail	Most familiar technique among paramedics	Produces some movement of cervical spine	Predicted difficult orotracheal intubation (Mallampati III/IV)
Unable to ventilate with BVM	Rapidly performed	Visualization more difficult due to need for neutral alignment	Major maxillofacial trauma
Loss of pharyngeal (gag) reflexes	Can be performed in a variety of patient positions	Requires two clinicians	Inability to control cervical spine during procedure
Head injury with Glasgow Coma Scale of <8	High success rate	Requires laryngoscopy	Laryngeal trauma*
Prevention of aspiration	Requires minimal equipment	Potential for trauma to teeth and oropharynx	
Correct hypoxia and hypercarbia		Increased intracranial pressure	
Obstructed airway		Vagal stimulation and bradycardia	
Pulmonary toilet in near drowning and toxic inhalations		Laryngospasm	

*Relative contraindication.

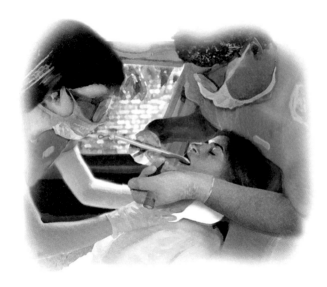

FIGURE 18-17 Seated orotracheal intubation using the superior approach.

It may be necessary to maintain spinal alignment from the front seat in order to provide enough room to perform the procedure. Removal of the vehicle's roof prior to intubation may also be necessary .

The frontal approach requires greater modification of technique. Facing the patient, the intubator places the laryngoscope in the right hand and in an inverted position (Figure 18-18). The intubator is posi-

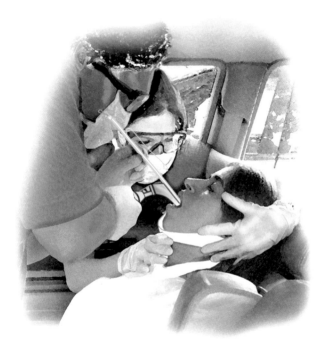

FIGURE 18-18 Seated orotracheal intubation using the frontal approach.

tioned in front of or to either side of the patient. While alignment of the C-spine is maintained, the laryngoscope blade is inserted and the tongue moved to the patient's left. The mandible is then displaced by pulling the laryngoscope anteriorly and caudally relative to the patient. Cricoid pressure and a stylet improve visualization and passage of the tube. In addition, a curved blade is better suited for this technique.

Intubation of Laterally Positioned Patients. Occasionally, patients may present in a lateral position and cannot be immediately repositioned for intubation. Alternatively, the presence of excessive oral hemorrhage may necessitate the patient being placed in a lateral position to facilitate drainage and suctioning. In either case, it is possible to intubate the patient in this position.

Barring anatomical distortion from trauma or edema, the patient's anatomy does not change when the patient's position changes. If the patient is turned to the side to facilitate drainage, placement on the left side facilitates ventilation and intubation. One assistant must control spinal alignment, allowing a second to ventilate. Positioning the patient on the left permits the ventilator to secure a seal of the mask with the left hand and ventilate with the right. Furthermore, because the laryngoscope is a left-handed device, positioning the patient on the left permits intubation in the usual manner. If the patient is positioned on the right side (whether by circumstance or by choice), the equipment must be reversed.

The procedure for intubation proceeds as usual. The blade is inserted on the right side (the "up" side for a patient positioned on the left side) and the tongue pushed to the left. Once in position, the laryngoscope blade is "lifted" at the usual angle relative to the patient. There will be less resistance to the blade because the weight of the head will be noticeably absent. Therefore, care must be taken not to compromise spinal alignment. The remainder of the procedure is similar to the standard orotracheal intubation technique.

Digital Intubation.   First described in 1796, digital, or tactile, orotracheal intubation was the original technique for securing an airway.[76] The technique remained widely practiced even after the introduction of the laryngoscope.[77] The technique then fell into disuse until its revival by Stewart as an emergency airway procedure.[78] Despite the obvious hazards of placing the fingers into the mouth of an unconscious patient, the procedure is well suited for certain patient groups, particularly those in whom C-spine trauma is suspected. The indications, contraindications, advantages, and disadvantages of digital intubation are summarized in Table 18-8.

Table 18-8
Indications, Advantages, Disadvantages, and Contraindications of Digital Intubation

Indications	Advantages	Disadvantages	Contraindications
Comatose patients with head and neck trauma	Does not require laryngoscopy	Blind procedure requires diligence in confirming correct placement	Patients with small mouths
Obese or short-necked patients	Minimal manipulation of C-spine	Risk of trauma to intubator's hand	Intubators with oversized or undersized hands
As a back-up procedure during rapid sequence intubation (RSI)	Can be performed under less than ideal circumstances such as poor lighting, cramped space, and awkward position		Patients with intact gag reflexes
Facial trauma where anatomical disruption prevents visualization			
When suctioning is unable to adequately remove blood or vomitus			
When other methods have failed			

As with any intubation attempt, the patient must first be prepared for the procedure, including preoxygenation, and the equipment assembled. The same size of tube that would be used for standard orotracheal intubation should be selected and a stylet inserted to within ½ inch of the distal end. The tube/stylet combination should be formed into an open "J" configuration with a prominent bend at the distal end. Facing the patient, the intubator places the middle and index fingers of the left hand into the right side of the patient's mouth (Figure 18-19A). While pressing downward and pulling forward on the tongue, the intubator "walks" down the tongue until the epiglottis is palpated (Figure 18-19B). The ET tube is then slid alongside the side of the middle finger, which remains in contact with the epiglottis. The tube is advanced distally and the middle finger lifted to press the tube tip against the epiglottis (Figure 18-19C). Cricoid pressure is then applied as the fingers "walk" the tube into the glottic opening. Once the tube is in the intratracheal lumen, it is held

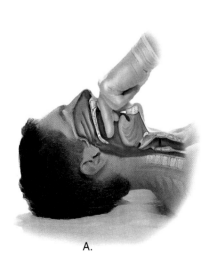
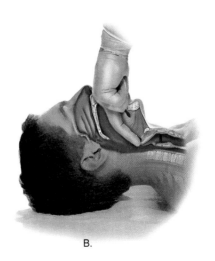
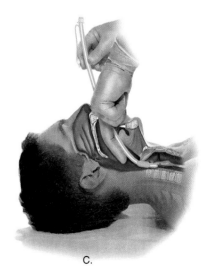

A.   B.   C.

FIGURE 18-19 Digital intubation technique. (A) Fingers are introduced into the right side of the patient's mouth. (B) "Walking" down the patient's tongue. (C) The middle finger presses the tube against the epiglottis and guides it into the glottic opening.

securely while the stylet is removed. The tube can then be advanced to an appropriate depth, its position confirmed, and secured.

Nasotracheal Intubation. Blind nasotracheal intubation (BNI) was first reported by Kuhn in 1902.[79] However, the technique was not commonly practiced until World War I.[80] Rowbotham and Magill popularized the technique for use by anesthetists prior to the introduction of muscle relaxants.[81] Following the introduction of muscle relaxants and rapid induction methods, the technique fell into disuse until its revival as a method for emergency airway control.[4]

Blind nasotracheal intubation involves the blind insertion of an ET tube into the trachea via the nasopharynx. The procedure is considered technically more difficult and requires more time to perform than orotracheal intubation. One series revealed that the time required for BNI averaged 62 seconds, approximately 2.5 times longer than for intubations via the oral route.[82] Investigations of BNI success rates indicate failure to intubate in 8%–9% of cases compared with a 4% rate for the orotracheal route.[83–85] Despite the added technical difficulty of BNI, there are several occasions where BNI is advantageous or even preferred. Table 18-9 summarizes the indications, contraindications, advantages, and disadvantages of BNI.

Portions of Table 18-9 deserve further discussion, particularly the contraindications of apnea and head injury. A survey of the literature reveals nine published reports of cranial vault penetration by introduction of an adjunct into the nasopharynx, of which only three were nasotracheal tubes.[86] Of these only two were the result of passing a nasotracheal tube through a fracture in the roof of the nasopharynx, the most commonly cited concern for nasotracheal intubation in the setting of trauma.[87,88] The other often-cited reports of penetration of the cranial vaults actually involve nasogastric (NG) tubes.[89–92] Because of its smaller diameter and lack of rigidity, it would appear to be easier to inadvertently pass an NG tube into the cranial vault than an ET tube. Given that only two documented cases of intracranial penetration by BNI appear in the English language medical literature, this complication is likely overstated.

Apnea is judged by many authorities to be a contraindication to BNI.[11,93] The reason cited is that spontaneous respirations are usually required to assist the intubator in guiding the ET tube into the trachea. However, apnea is a contraindication only for the standard blind technique and nasotracheal intubation can still be accomplished using a lighted stylet or any of the other techniques, such as tactile, inflated cuff, or stylet-assisted techniques discussed below.

The standard technique of nasotracheal intubation is a blind procedure in which the tube is inserted without the benefit of directly visualizing the cords. The appropriate size tube for nasotracheal intubation is

Table 18-9
Indications, Advantages, Disadvantages, and Contraindications of BNI

Indications	Advantages	Disadvantages	Contraindications
Inaccessible oral cavity (trismus, seizures, wired jaws, trauma)	Patient unable to bite tube	Prone to nasopharyngeal trauma and epistaxis	Apnea*
Sniffing position contraindicated	Better tolerated in conscious patient	Necrosis of nares	Severe maxiollofacial trauma*
Difficult direct laryngoscopy	Requires minimal equipment	Potential for retropharyngeal perforation	Obstruction of the nasopharynx
Need for long-term ventilation	Does not require laryngoscopy	Potential for esophageal intubation due to blind procedure	Upper airway foreign body
Paralytics contraindicated	No cervical spine manipulation		
Patients in awkward positions	Reduced oropharyngeal secretions		
Conscious or semiconscious patients requiring intubation (e.g., burns, overdose)			

*Relative contraindication.

a cuffed ET tube approximately 1 mm smaller in inside diameter than would be used for oral intubation. While the intubator prepares and checks the equipment, the patient should be prepared for the procedure. The patient should be hyperventilated with 100% O_2 using a BVM for at least 2 minutes prior to intubation. This provides a pulmonary reservoir of oxygen, decreases pulmonary carbon dioxide and nitrogen, and reduces intracranial pressure.[93] The nares are then examined for patency. To evaluate the nares, a nasopharyngeal airway is lubricated with 2%–4% lidocaine jelly and used to explore each nare. The nare with the largest diameter and most direct passageway should be used for BNI. Once a nare is selected, a second application of lidocaine jelly can be applied to the NPA, along with a vasoconstrictor such as phenylephrine, and the NPA reinserted and left in place while equipment is prepared. This will lubricate, anesthetize, and dilate the nare in preparation for the procedure.

The ET tube should then be lubricated with water-soluble or lidocaine jelly. The tube is introduced into the nare with the beveled edge facing the septum. This placement prevents mucosal abrasion and trauma to the turbinates. If the right nare is used, the curvature of the tube will be inferiorly. When introduced into the left nare, the curvature will be superiorly. In this case, the tube will need to be rotated 180° once it has entered the posterior pharynx so that the curvature of the tube corresponds with the anatomical curvature of the nasopharynx. Once positioned in the external nare, the tube should be gently advanced perpendicular to the frontal plane. The temptation to advance the tube superiorly should be avoided. If resistance is met, gently twisting the tube may facilitate passage. The tube should be advanced until there is a loss of resistance, indicating that the tube has entered the posterior pharynx. The tube is gently advanced, listening for air flow through the tube. The tube should be directed toward the air flow during inspiration. Inspiration opens the vocal cords to their widest, increasing the likelihood of proper placement. Cricoid pressure also facilitates proper position of the tube. When performing BNI in noisy environments, the head of a stethoscope may be removed and the tubing inserted into the proximal end of the ET tube. Air flow can then be more easily appreciated through the stethoscope. The normal position of a nasotracheal tube at the nares is 26 cm in the average-sized adult male and 22 cm in the average-sized female.[94] Once in place, tube position should be confirmed and secured.

Occasionally, difficulty is encountered while attempting to advance the ET tube. The tendency is for the tube to enter the esophagus because it will not curve after entering the oropharynx. Several options are available to increase success in these cases. The first is to simply coil the tube prior to insertion so that the distal end nearly touches the proximal end. The "memory" of this curvature will tend to guide the tube into proper position. The second option is to use a type of ET tube known as the Endotrol tube. This tube has a pull ring near the proximal end of the tube. Pulling the ring causes the distal end of the tube to curve anteriorly, allowing the intubator to manipulate the tip of the tube into position. The third option is to insert the fingers into the oropharynx and manipulate the tube manually, as discussed earlier. The fourth option is to use the Magill forceps to direct the tip of the tube anteriorly (Figure 18-20). This is probably a better alternative than digital manipulation because it removes the risk of the patient biting the hand of the intubator.

The fifth technique of nasotracheal intubation is somewhat more involved than the previous methods. This technique involves the use of a malleable stylet and considerable finesse on the part of the intubator. The stylet is inserted into the tube in the standard manner and the tube/stylet combination is straightened (Figure 18-21A). A 90° bend is then formed at the distal end of the tube, approximately four finger-breadths from the tip for the average-size adult (assuming the

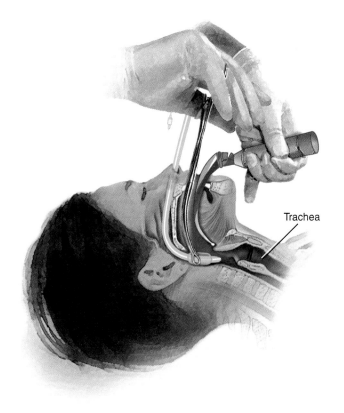

Trachea

FIGURE 18-20 Magill forceps may be used to facilitate passage of the tube during nasotracheal intubation.

intubator's hand is also of average size) (Figure 18-21B). The tube is then lubricated and introduced into the nare at a 90° angle to the frontal plane and a 90° angle to the sagittal plane (Figure 18-21C) and inserted up to the level of the bend in the tube (Figure 18-21D). The tube is then rotated 90° until it is congruent with the midsagittal line (Figure 18-21E). Next, the tube is rotated superiorly until it is perpendicular with the frontal plane (Figure 18-21F). In this position, the tube should be directed slightly anteriorly in the hypopharynx in the direction of the laryngeal opening (Figure 18-21G). Holding the stylet in place, the intubator should slide the tube from the stylet, much in the same manner as one would slide the Teflon catheter from an over-the-needle IV catheter (Figure 18-24H). The stylet can then be removed by reversing the insertion procedure. The tube should then be checked for position.

The hazards of this technique should be apparent. By introducing a stylet into the nasopharynx, there is the potential to traumatize soft tissue. Therefore, considerable care should be taken not to force the tube should it encounter resistance.

A better technique to direct the tip of the tube into the trachea is the inflated cuff technique. This technique involves inserting the tube in the usual manner. However, once the tube has reached the oropharynx, the cuff is inflated with the standard amount of air, usually 5–10 cc (Figure 18-22A and B). The tube is then advanced until it meets resistance. The resistance is the result of the cuff contacting the epiglottis (Figure 18-22C). However, the distal 1 cm of the tube should be positioned in the tracheal lumen. The cuff is deflated and the tube advanced to the proper depth and the cuff reinflated. The tube should then be in proper position (Figure 18-22D).

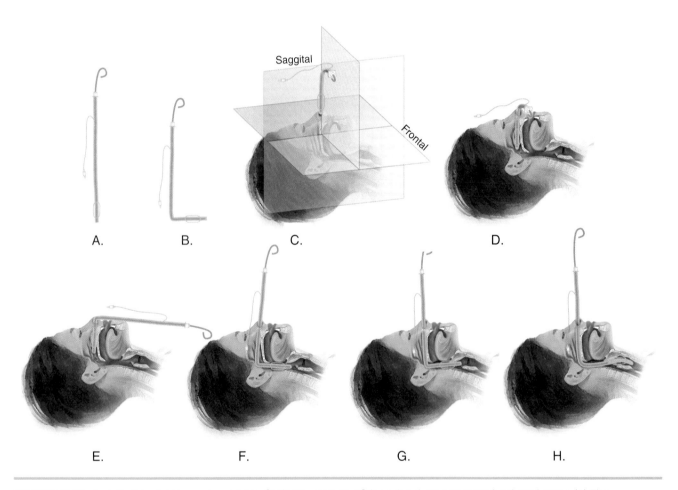

A.   B.   C.   D.

E.   F.   G.   H.

FIGURE 18-21 A malleable stylet may be used to facilitate passage of the tube during nasotracheal intubation. (A) The tube/stylet combination is straightened. (B) A 90° bend is formed four finger-breadths from the distal end of the tube. (C) The tube/stylet is inserted into the nare at a 90° angle to the midsagittal and frontal planes. (D) The tube/stylet is inserted up to the level of the 90° bend. (E) The tube/stylet is then rotated 90° to where it rests perpendicular to the midsagittal plane. (F) The tube/stylet is rotated 90° to the frontal plane. (G) With the tube in this position, the distal end of the tube is directed toward the glottic opening. (H) With the stylet held in place, the tube is advanced over the stylet.

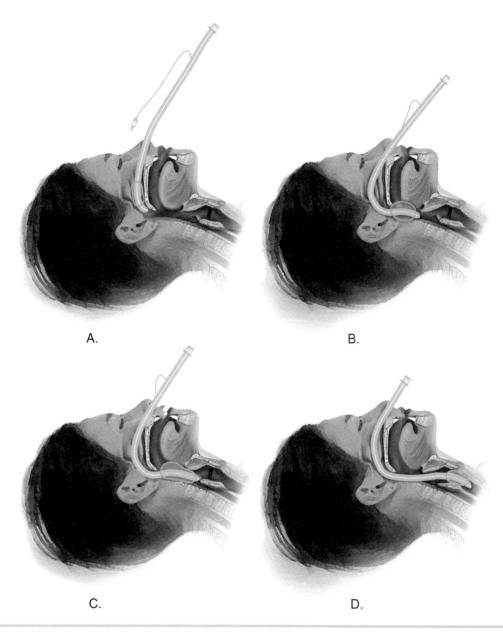

FIGURE 18-22 Inflation of the cuff may be used to facilitate passage of the tube during nasotracheal intubation. (A) The tube is advanced into the oropharynx in the usual manner. (B) The cuff of the tube is then inflated with 5–10 cc of air. (C) The tube is then advanced until resistance is met, indicating contact of the cuff with the epiglottis. (D) The cuff is then deflated and the tube advanced through the glottic opening.

Transillumination Intubation. **Transillumination intubation**, or lighted stylet orotracheal intubation, is another method of intubation that may prove useful in managing the airway of the traumatized patient. Transillumination intubation uses a lighted malleable stylet to illuminate the structures of the neck and guide the intubator to the glottic opening. Similar to digital intubation, transillumination is not a replacement for direct laryngoscopy, but rather an alternative when direct visualization is impossible or impractical. First described by MacIntosh and Richards, transillu-

mination was not initially used as a method of intubation, but rather as an adjunct to illuminate the airway during laryngoscopy.[95] The possibility of using transillumination as an intubation technique was not suggested until some time later.[96,97]

As with digital intubation, the advantage of transillumination intubation is that it can be accomplished without extending the patient's neck. The technique is, therefore, particularly suited for the trauma patient where movement of the C-spine is contraindicated. In addition, it is possible to perform the technique from various positions, making it a versatile procedure for the prehospital setting where patients often present in awkward positions. In one study, the technique had an 88% field success rate when used by resident physicians in an urban EMS system, with a mean intubation time of 20 seconds.[98] The indications, contraindications, advantages, and disadvantages of transillumination intubation are listed in Table 18-10.

The intubation procedure begins with preoxygenation of the patient and preparation of equipment. The lighted stylet is lubricated and inserted into a standard orotracheal tube of appropriate size. The tube/stylet combination is lubricated and the distal tip is formed into a slightly greater than 90° angle (Figure 18-23A). The tube is then inserted at the labial angle and slid down the tongue toward the epiglottis (Figure 18-23B). The location of the tube can be seen through the soft tissues of the neck. If the tip is in either pyriform fossa, a dim glow is recognized lateral to the midline.[99] Esophageal position is indicated by a dim, diffuse glow in the midline. Intratracheal positioning is recognized by a bright, sharply circumscribed glow in the midline below the laryngeal prominence. Once intratracheal positioning is observed, the tube is gently advanced to ensure the tip extends beyond the vocal cords. The intubator then withdraws the stylet while firmly holding the ET tube. The tube is then secured in the usual fashion.

The lighted stylet can also be used in conjunction with nasotracheal intubation and digital intubation. Using the insertion procedure standard with these two techniques, the lighted stylet can assist the intubator by providing visual clues to the position of the ET tube. The lighted stylet can also be used to confirm proper tube position in patients intubated by other procedures.

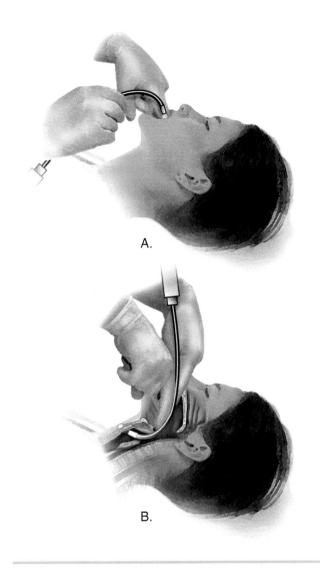

A.

B.

FIGURE 18-23 Transillumination intubation. (A) A bend is formed in the distal end of the tube/stylet combination. (B) The tube/stylet combination is inserted at the labial angle.

Table 18-10
Indications, Advantages, Disadvantages, and Contraindications of Transillumination Intubation

Indications	Advantages	Disadvantages	Contraindications
Suspected cervical spine injury	Rapidly performed	Difficult to visualize glow from stylet in environments with high-intensity ambient light	Similar to oral intubation
Facial trauma	Can be performed in a variety of patient positions		
Difficult direct laryngoscopy	High success rate	Potential for esophageal intubation due to blind procedure	
Patients in awkward positions	No manipulation of cervical spine		
Patients immobilized on spine boards	Does not require laryngoscopy		
Confirmation of tube placement in intubated patients			

Laryngeal Mask Airway. The **laryngeal mask airway (LMA)** has been used as an alternative to ET intubation for many years in Europe and Australia, and is gaining popularity in the United States.[83] Several experimental investigations suggest that paramedics and other allied health professionals can be easily trained in the insertion procedure.[100–102] In certain circumstances the LMA provides an alternative to surgical airways in difficult-to-intubate patients encountered in the prehospital setting.[100–105] Indications, advantages, disadvantages, and contraindications of the LMA are summarized in Table 18-11.

Developed in London by anesthesiologist Archie Brain, the LMA is made of silicon rubber and looks like a short ETI tube with an oval-shaped mask on the distal end (Figure 18-24). It was designed to form a seal around the laryngeal perimeter with the tip of the mask resting against the upper esophageal sphincter,

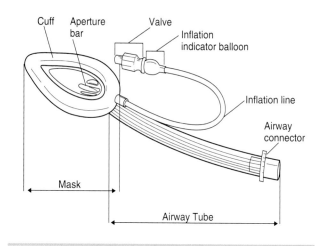

FIGURE 18-24 Laryngeal mask airway.

Table 18-11
Indications, Advantages, Disadvantages, and Contraindications of the LMA

Indications	Advantages	Disadvantages	Contraindications
Inability to intubate using standard techniques Suspected C-spine injury	Requires minimal training Ease of insertion Rapidly inserted (<15 sec) Blind insertion technique avoids the need for special equipment Endotracheal intubation can be achieved through the LMA Manipulation of the head and neck is not necessary for insertion Less negative cardiovascular response as compared with ETI insertion[†] Less soft tissue trauma as compared with endotracheal intubation No danger of inadvertent passage of the LMA into a mainstem bronchus Can be inserted with the patient in a variety of positions, including lateral recumbent	Does not protect against aspiration or regurgitation Potential for malpositioning	Gross obesity Inability to open the mouth wider than 1.5 cm Pregnancy Recent ingestion of opiates Decreased pulmonary compliance Subglottic obstruction

[†] Data from Fujii Y, Tanaka H, Toyooka H. Circulatory responses to laryngeal mask airway insertion or tracheal intubation in normotensive and hypertensive patients. *Can J Anaesth.* 1995; 42:32.

the sides facing the pyriform fossae, and the upper edge positioned below the base of the tongue.[106] This ideal positioning occurs in approximately 50%–60% of cases. Although the actual position of the LMA often deviates from the intended position, ventilation is rarely impaired, occurring in only 1%–5% of cases.[83]

To insert the LMA, the appropriate size mask must be selected. The LMA is available in six sizes and the appropriate size mask is selected based upon the size of the patient (Table 18-12). The mask is inflated, checking for abnormal bulging of the cushion or air leaks. Next, the cushion is deflated and a lubricant is applied to the posterior surface of the LMA. It is important that the anterior surface not be lubricated nor should lubricant be allowed to trickle into the bowl of the mask. Lubrication in these areas may be aspirated or result in blockage of the mask's aperture.

The patient's mouth is opened and the LMA inserted under direct vision. The mask tip is pressed upward against the hard palate, continuously pressing upward as the mask advances into the pharynx until resistance is felt (Figure 18-25A and B). It should be possible to insert the mask in one fluid movement. Without holding the tube, the mask is inflated with the appropriate amount of air (Table 18-12). Typically, the tube will move outward 1–2 cm as the cushion seats itself in position. Once inflated, the tube is held until its position is confirmed and the tube secured.

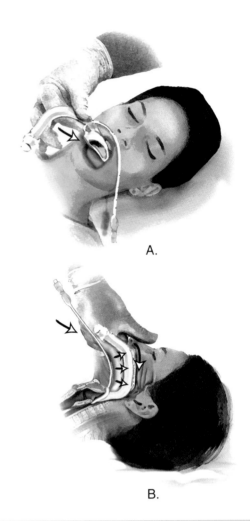

A.

B.

FIGURE 18-25 Insertion of the laryngeal mask airway. (A) Under direct vision, mask tip is pressed upward against the hard palate. The index finger continues pressing upward to advance the mask into the pharynx to ensure the tip remains flattened and avoids the tongue. (B) Pushing continues with the ball of the index finger, guiding the mask downward into position. By withdrawing the other fingers and slight pronation of the forearm, it is usually possible to push the mask fully into position in one fluid movement.

INTERNET ACTIVITIES

- Visit the British Trauma Society Web site at http://www.trauma.org/anaesthesia/airway.html. Review the material on airway management of the trauma patient.
- Visit the British Trauma Society Web site at http://www.trauma.org/eates/ectc/ectc-airway.html. Review the material on airway management.

Table 18-12
LMA Sizes, Inflation Volumes, and Endotracheal Tube Accommodations

Size	Patient Size	Inflation Volume (mL)	Size of ET That Can Pass Through LMA
1	Neonates/infants up to 6.5 kg	2–4	3.5 mm uncuffed
2	Infants and children up to 20 kg	5–10	4.5 mm uncuffed
2.5	Children 20–30 kg	10–15	5.0 mm uncuffed
3	Children and small adults over 30 kg	15–20	6.0 mm cuffed
4	Normal and large adults	20–30	6.5 mm cuffed

Once inserted, the LMA may initially allow backflow around the device. This typically occurs when ventilation pressures reach 15–20 cm H_2O. The leak is transient, however, and will disappear as the soft tissue molds itself around the cushion.[83] If a leak exists when ventilatory pressures are less than 15 cm H_2O, the most likely cause is an undersized mask. The LMA should be removed and a larger mask inserted. It is important that the mask not be overinflated to compensate for an undersized mask. Overinflation dislodges the mask from around the larynx.

While simple to insert, the LMA should be used with caution. Because the LMA does not seal the trachea, and because the LMA may be malpositioned with the esophageal opening within the cushion in 10%–15% of insertions, there is a risk of aspiration. Therefore, the LMA should be reserved for cases in which ET intubation is impossible. Additionally, once inserted, the LMA can be used as a guide for blind and fiberoptically directed ET intubation. Up to a size 6.5-mm cuffed ET tube can be passed down the lumen of a size 4 LMA and into the trachea. The ET tube must be rotated 15°–90° to pass the bevel of the ET tube through the aperture of the LMA. Once the ET tube has passed through the aperture (at about the 20-cm level), the tube is rotated back into anatomical position. Blind intubation through the LMA is possible in about 90% of cases and, with experience, can be accomplished within 30 seconds.[106] Alternatively, an ET tube changer can be used to remove the LMA and pass a properly sized ET tube.

SURGICAL AIRWAYS

On rare occasions it is impossible to establish airway patency using the more common approaches such as orotracheal intubation and BNI. These instances require more invasive airway techniques, such as translaryngeal jet insufflation, cricothyrotomy, and retrograde intubation.

Translaryngeal Jet Insufflation

Translaryngeal jet insufflation (TJI) involves the insertion of a cannula through the cricothyroid membrane that is connected to an intermittent high-pressure oxygen source. This technique was introduced by Hooke over 300 years ago.[107] The modern technique arose at the turn of the century but was not evaluated further until 1954, when Reed provided the basis for the presently accepted procedure.[108] Translaryngeal jet insufflation is indicated when other methods have failed or when anatomic disruptions of the face or supralaryngeal areas prevent the use of more traditional approaches. Table 18-13 summarizes the indications, advantages, disadvantages, and contraindications of TJI.

Table 18-13
Indications, Advantages, Disadvantages, and Contraindications of Translaryngeal Jet Insufflation

Indications	Advantages	Disadvantages	Contraindications
Inaccessible oral cavity (trismus, seizures, trauma, wired jaws)	Less invasive than surgical cricothyrotomy	Potential for subcutaneous emphysema and pneumothorax with misdirected cannula	Inability to locate cricothyroid membrane
Difficult direct laryngoscopy	Paramedics more comfortable with IV catheter than scalpel	Relatively poor air exchange	Total airway obstruction at or above the level of the cords (complete expiratory obstruction)
Severe facial trauma	Provides a temporary airway while other methods are attempted	Temporizing procedure	
Supralaryngeal obstruction		Barotrauma	Infralaryngeal obstruction
Anatomical disruption of upper airway		Potential esophageal perforation	Primary laryngeal injury
Failure of standard techniques		Requires specialized equipment	Children less than 5 years of age
		Does not protect against aspiration	
		Permits accumulation of CO_2	

The procedure begins by locating the cricothyroid membrane. The most reliable landmark is the thyroid notch, which is easily palpated at the superior aspect of the thyroid cartilage (Figure 18-26). Proceeding inferiorly from the thyroid notch, the cricothyroid membrane lies within a few centimeters and above the cricoid cartilage (the next palpable structure proceeding inferiorly).

Once identified, the cricothyroid membrane is prepared with antiseptic solution. The membrane is then punctured with a 12- or 14-gauge IV catheter with attached syringe directed inferiorly at a 45° angle (Figure 18-27). Air is then aspirated to ensure proper position of the catheter. The stylet is removed and the catheter secured in place and connected to the O_2 source.

The oxygen source must be capable of delivering 1,200 mL/sec at 50 psi of pressure. Three devices are commonly employed for O_2 delivery: BVM, demand valve, and commercial transtracheal jet insufflators. For the BVM and demand valve, a 15-mm adaptor from a 3-mm ET tube can be used as a connector for the IV catheter. While this procedure is widely described in paramedic texts, the delivered tidal volumes are suboptimal (Figure 18-28).[109] Therefore, the recommended delivery device is the translaryngeal jet insufflator, which is designed to deliver the proper flow rate and pressure.

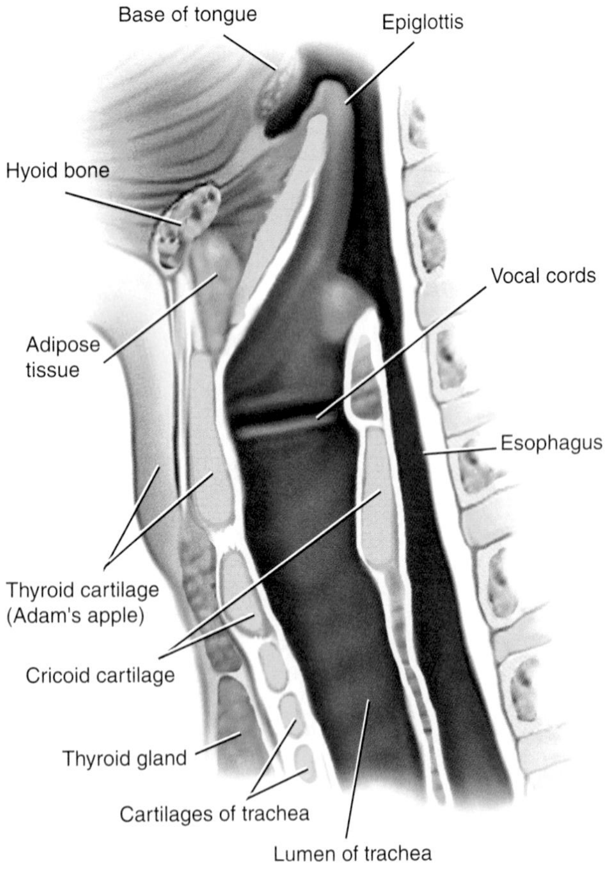

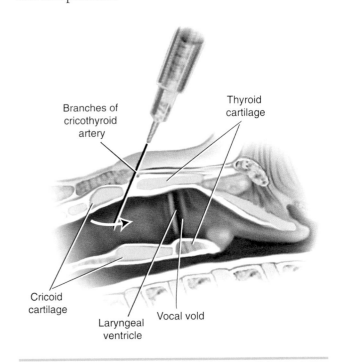

FIGURE 18-27 During translaryngeal jet insufflation, the catheter/syringe combination is inserted inferiorly at a 45° angle into the cricothyroid membrane.

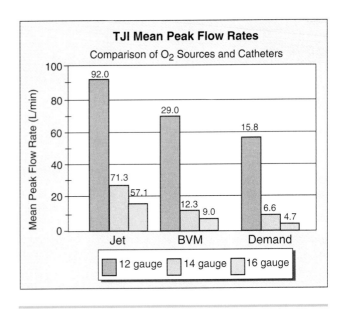

FIGURE 18-28 Tidal volumes generated during translaryngeal jet insufflation. (*Source:* Yealy et al. Myths and pitfalls in emergency translaryngeal ventilation: correcting misimpressions, *Ann Emerg Med.* 1988; 17(7):690-692.

FIGURE 18-26 Location of the cricothyroid membrane.

The ventilatory rate should be 12–20 breaths per minute, with insufflation time being about 1 second (or until rise of the chest is observed). Because insufflation is done under pressure and exhalation is a passive process, more time is required for exhalation. Therefore, an inspiratory-expiratory ratio of 1:4 is recommended.[21] It is also good practice to hold the cannula during insufflation as displacement of the cannula during ventilation has been reported.[110]

Surgical Cricothyrotomy

Cricothyrotomy is an opening established in the trachea at the level of the cricothyroid membrane. The technique has been performed for over 200 years. The first published report of the modern technique was by Jackson in 1909, who outlined the principles that reduced the high mortality rate (50%) associated with early use of the procedure.[111] Following the work of Jackson, mortality associated with cricothyrotomy was reduced to 3%, which compares favorably with modern-day complication rates of 6%.[111,112] In the prehospital setting, cricothyrotomy has been shown to be safe and effective in managing the difficult airway. Jacobsen et al. reported a 94% success rate and a 4% complication rate for the procedure in a series of 50 patients treated in an urban EMS system.[113] The complications most commonly reported with the procedure are bleeding, subglottic stenosis, tracheoesophageal fistula, infection, and extratracheal tube placement.[114]

The indications for surgical cricothyrotomy are similar to those for TJI. Cricothyrotomy, however, is preferred in cases of complete inspiratory and expiratory obstruction.[109] Table 18-14 summarizes the indications, contraindications, advantages, and disadvantages of cricothyrotomy.

The procedure for cricothyrotomy begins with identification of the cricothyroid membrane and, if time permits, cleansing the neck with alcohol or other antiseptic agent. Using a number 11 scalpel, a 2-cm horizontal incision is made over the cricothyroid membrane (Figure 18-29A). The incision is opened by inserting the blunt handle of the scalpel into the incision and rotating 90° or by inserting and spreading a clamp (Figure 18-29B and C). With the opening dilated by the scalpel or clamp, a 6.0 or 7.0 ET tube is inserted for the average-sized adult (Figure 18-29D). Tube placement should be confirmed and then secured in place. The excess tube can be trimmed for convenience.

As an alternative to the surgical approach to cricothyrotomy, several commercial kits have been developed. Common among these kits is a device for percutaneous puncture of the cricothyroid membrane through which a tracheostomy tube, metal airway tube, or other form of airway lumen is inserted. In practice, however, these devices offer few, if any, advantages over the standard surgical approach. In one investigation, the standard surgical approach was compared with the Nu-Trake airway device (International Medical Devices Inc., Northridge, Calif.).[115] Paramedic students established cricothyrotomies in cadavers using the Nu-Trake device and the standard surgical approach. The investigators report a higher success rate with the surgical approach than with the Nu-Trake

Table 18-14
Indications, Advantages, Disadvantages, and Contraindications of Cricothyrotomy

Indications	Advantages	Disadvantages	Contraindications
Poor visualization of oral cavity (trismus, trauma, wired jaws)	Improved ventilation over TJI	Potential for subcutaneous emphysema and pneumothorax with misdirected ET tube	Inability to locate cricothyroid membrane
Supralaryngeal obstruction	Prevents aspiration		Infralaryngeal obstruction
Difficult direct laryngoscopy	Longer term airway when compared with TJI	Potential esophageal perforation	Supralaryngeal obstruction
Severe facial trauma	Access to lungs for drug administration or pulmonary toilet	Requires specialized equipment	Primary laryngeal injury
Anatomical disruption of upper airway		Paramedics less comfortable using scalpel	Children less than 10 years of age
Failure of standard techniques	Does not require laryngoscopy		Preexisting subglottic stenosis
Back-up procedure during RSI	High success rate	Invasive procedure	Coagulopathy
	Does not require manipulation of the neck	Potential for bleeding, infection, and subglottic stenosis	Expanding hematoma of the neck

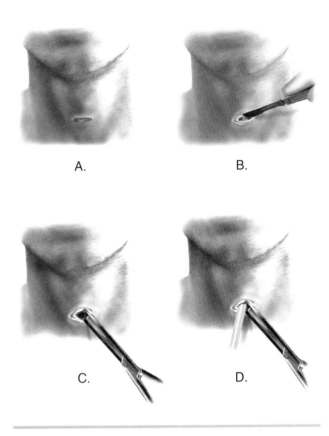

A.   B.

C.   D.

FIGURE 18-29 Surgical cricothyroidotomy. (A) A horizontal incision is made in the cricothyroid membrane with a scalpel. (B) The incision is opened by rotating the scalpel handle. (C) Alternatively, the incision may be opened with forceps. (D) Once the incision is opened, the endotracheal tube is passed through the incision.

(86% vs. 73%). In addition, the surgical approach was significantly faster (mean time to airway of 46 seconds vs. 103 seconds). The authors conclude that the standard surgical approach may be faster and less difficult to perform.

Retrograde Tracheal Intubation

Retrograde tracheal intubation (RTI) was first described in 1960 and consisted of passing a catheter through a tracheostomy into the pharynx and the subsequent use of the catheter as a guide for passing an ET tube.[116] The technique has undergone subsequent modifications, and the technique used today abandons the use of tracheostomy in favor of passing a guide wire via cricothyroid membrane puncture.[117,118] The indications for the procedure are similar to TJI and cricothyrotomy and, in general, RTI can be considered an alternative to either of these procedures.[118] The complications associated with the procedure are mainly those related to cricothyroid membrane puncture.[117–120] In the only known investigation of the technique in the prehospital setting, Barriot and Riou reported 100% success rate with no serious complications in a series of 19 trauma patients treated by EMS units staffed by nurses and physicians.[121] While no investigation exists of the procedure performed by nonphysician personnel, the technique is easily taught and may be a useful field technique for paramedics.[122] Table 18-15 summarizes the indications, contraindications, advantages, and disadvantages of RTI.

The RTI procedure is technically similar to TJI. The cricothyroid membrane is identified and prepared similar to TJI. The difference with RTI is that the

Table 18-15
Indications, Advantages, Disadvantages, and Contraindications of Retrograde Tracheal Intubation

Indications	Advantages	Disadvantages	Contraindications
Same as for cricothyrotomy	Same as for cricothyrotomy Less invasive than cricothyrotomy	Requires specialized equipment Potential for bleeding, infection, and subglottic stenosis Requires more time to perform than cricothyrotomy More steps in procedure than cricothyrotomy Potential esophageal perforation	Inability to locate cricothyroid membrane Infralaryngeal obstruction Inability to open mouth for catheter removal Coagulopathy Expanding hematoma of the neck Preexisting subglottic stenosis

needle enters the cricothyroid membrane at a 90° angle to the frontal plane and, once intratracheal positioning is confirmed by aspirating free air, the needle is rotated cephalad into a 30°–45° angle (Figure 18-30A). Repeat aspiration of air confirms intratracheal placement.

Holding the needle in place, the syringe is removed and the guide wire is passed through the needle and retrieved from the mouth using Magill forceps (Figure 18-30B and C). The needle is then removed and a clamp placed on the distal end of the guide to prevent its passage through the puncture site (Figure 18-30D). The proximal end of the guide is passed through the side hole of the ET tube (Murphy's eye) (Figure 18-30E). With tension pulled on the proximal end of the guide wire, the ET tube is passed down the guide and through the trachea until it will pass no farther. The tube now rests against the wire at the level of the cricothyroid membrane (Figure 18-30F). With the tube held firmly in place, the clamp is released on the distal end of the guide wire and the guide is removed through the mouth. Withdrawing the guide through the mouth prevents contamination of the soft tissues of the puncture site with oral flora.

While the procedure enjoys a high success rate and is considered an alternative to cricothyrotomy, the procedure is more involved than cricothyrotomy, is more labor intensive, and requires specialized equipment to perform. Prepackaged kits are available that conveniently contain all necessary equipment.

The preceding has illustrated the variety of advanced airway procedures available to the paramedic. In general, the ET tube is considered the "gold standard" of airway management. However, ETI is not always easily accomplished. In these instances, the paramedic must evaluate the effectiveness, advantages, and disadvantages of each of the alternative devices and select the most appropriate one for the situation. The preceding provided an overview of the effectiveness of each device, and these findings are summarized in Table 18-16.

CONFIRMING TUBE PLACEMENT

Following intubation from any technique, it is important to confirm that the tube is properly positioned in the trachea. Occasionally a tube is improperly placed in the esophagus or a mainstem bronchus. This does not pose a problem as long as it is immediately recognized and corrected. There are several methods of confirming tube placement that can be used to ensure that the ET tube is properly positioned. These methods are summarized in Table 18-17.

Table 18-17
Methods for Confirming Correct Placement of the Endotracheal Tube

1. Visualizing the tube passing between the vocal cords during direct laryngoscopy
2. Breath sounds over all lung fields during ventilation
3. Absence of gurgling sounds over epigastrium during ventilation
4. Chest excursion during ventilation
5. Condensation within the tube during ventilation
6. Appropriate color change of end-tidal CO_2 monitor
7. Appropriate waveform of capnogram
8. Normal pulse oximetry values
9. Intratracheal verification by lighted stylet

Table 18-16
Comparison of Endotracheal Intubation, Esophageal Devices, LMA, TJI, and Cricothyrotomy

Device	Placement Success (%)	Overcoming Obstruction	Prevention of Aspiration	Oxygenation	Ventilation	Complications
ETI	88%–97%	0 to +1	+2	+2	+2	Up to 50%
EOA	88%–95%	0 to –1	+1	0 to +1	0	Up to 18%
EGTA	88%–95%	0 to –1	+1	0 to +1	0	Up to 18%
PTLA	82%–83%	0 to –1	+2	+1 to +2	+1	Less than 1%
Combitube	69%–100%	0 to –1	+1	+1 to +2	+1 to +2	None reported
LMA	50%–100%	0 to –1	–2	+1 to +2	+1 to +2	Up to 6%
TJI		+1	0	0 to -2	0 to -2	Unknown
Cricothyrotomy	88%	+1 to +2	+2	+2	+2	28%–32%

Source: Adapted from ref. 64, p 70.

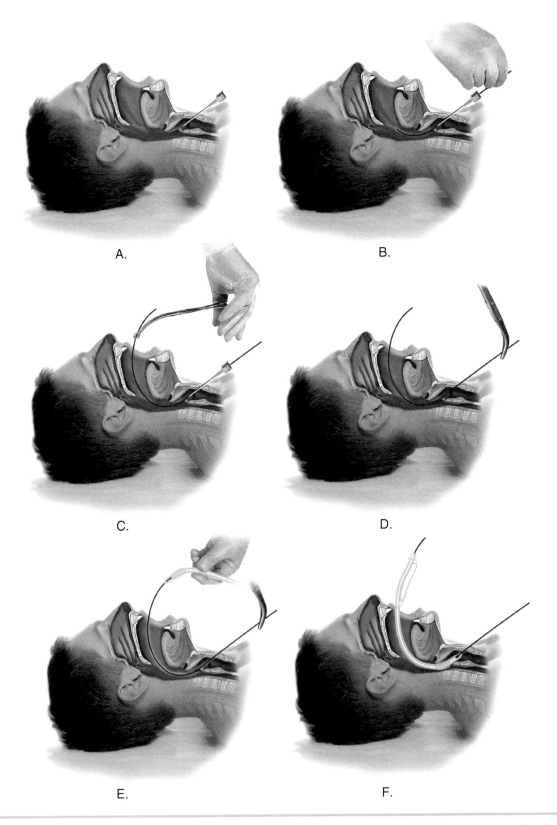

A.

B.

C.

D.

E.

F.

FIGURE 18-30 Retrograde intubation. (A) Once the syringe is inserted into the cricothyroid membrane, it is directed cephalad at a 45° angle. (B) The guide wire is inserted through the needle. (C) The wire is retrieved from the mouth with Magill forceps. (D) The needle is removed from the neck and the distal end of the guide wire clamped with a Kelly clamp. (E) The guide wire is passed through the Murphy eye of the tube. (F) The tube is advanced until resistance is met. The tube now rests at the level of the cricothyroid membrane.

One definitive method of confirming tube placement is capnography. **Capnography** is a waveform measurement of the partial pressure of carbon dioxide in a gas sample (Figure 18-31A). In intubated patients, capnography analyzes the end-tidal partial pressure of carbon dioxide ($PetCO_2$) with each exhalation. The exhaled carbon dioxide ($PeCO_2$) is measured by a sensor attached to the proximal end of the ET tube. During inspiration $PeCO_2$ is zero (point *A* of Figure 18-31A). At the beginning of expiration, the $PeCO_2$ remains at zero as dead-space volume exits the airway. The $PeCO_2$ then rises rapidly as alveolar gas begins mixing with the dead-space gas (point *B* of Figure 18-31). The waveform then plateaus for a period of time as pure alveolar gas exits the airways (point *C* of Figure 18-31A). The end of the alveolar plateau is the $PetCO_2$. A capnogram of 35–45 mm Hg is considered normal indicating tracheal positioning of the ET tube and adequate ventilation. Capnography can be used to detect esophageal intubation, ET tube cuff leaks, and airway obstructions and provide real-time evaluation of ventilation, but will not detect a main bronchus intubation (Figures 18-31B and C).

RAPID-SEQUENCE INTUBATION

Most patients requiring aggressive airway control can be intubated without difficulty. Occasionally, however, patients may be combative or retain reflexes that make intubation problematic. These patients are candidates for rapid-sequence intubation (RSI), a technique that relies on neuromuscular blocking agents to induce total muscle relaxation. Neuromuscular blocking agents have a long history of use by anesthesiologists in the operating room. More recently, RSI has been extended into field care with success rates similar to that attained in the emergency department setting.[123] When used correctly, RSI offers a safe, effective means of achieving airway control. Used incorrectly, however, RSI can lead to hypoxia and death. Therefore, it is imperative that the paramedic fully understand the indications and technique.

Mechanisms of Action of Neuromuscular Blocking Agents

The drugs used in RSI interfere with the normal events of muscle contraction at the neuromuscular junction. The neuromuscular junction is where the terminal axon (presynaptic membrane) and the muscle cell membrane (postsynaptic membrane) meet. The two membranes are separated by a small cleft known as the synapse. As a nerve impulse travels down the axon, it causes a release of acetylcholine into the synaptic cleft. Acetylcholine then crosses the synapse and connects with receptor sites on the postsynaptic membrane,

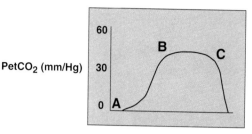

A. Normal capnogram

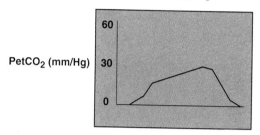

B. Capnogram indicating airway obstruction

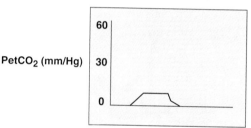

C. Capnogram indicating esophageal intubation

FIGURE 18-31 End-tidal capnography: (A) normal capnogram; (B) capnogram indicating airway obstruction; (C) capnogram indicating esophageal intubation.

resulting in muscular contraction (Figure 18-32A). After the muscle contraction begins, acetylcholine is rapidly hydrolyzed by acetylcholinesterase, resulting in termination of the contraction.

There are two major categories of neuromuscular blocking agents, depolarizing and nondepolarizing, so named because of the way they interfere with the normal muscle contraction sequence. The depolarizing neuromuscular blockers, such as succinylcholine, mimic the action of acetylcholine, except that depolarization of the synapse persists (Figure 18-32B). This results in a brief contraction called a fasciculation. The fasciculation is followed by relaxation because the membrane remains depolarized and cannot be further stimulated.

The nondepolarizing neuromuscular blockers, such as pancuronium, directly compete with acetylcholine for receptor sites on the postsynaptic membrane. Once they have occupied the receptor sites, these drugs block the effects of acetylcholine and prevent muscular contraction (Figure 18-32B). Table 18-18 summarizes the neuromuscular blockers used in airway management.

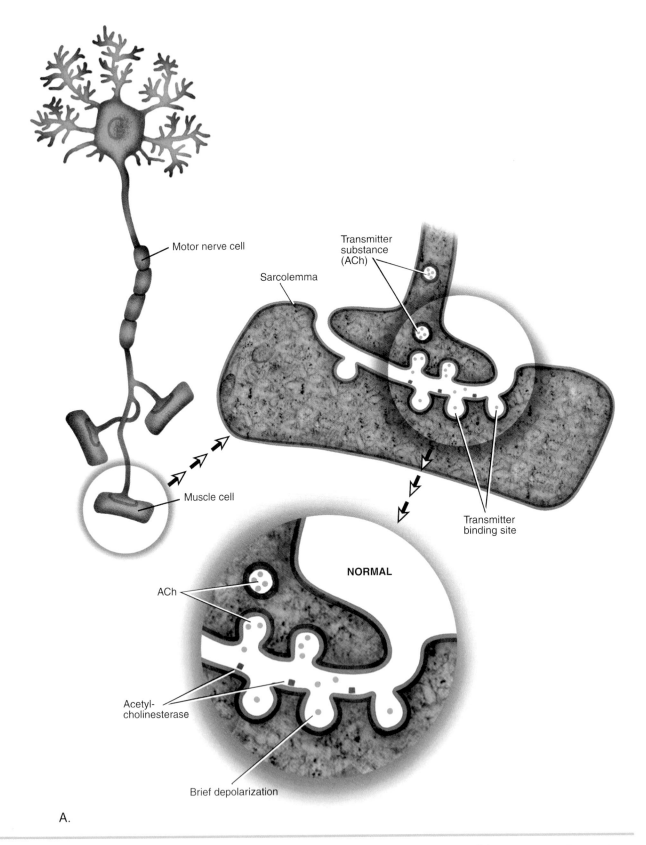

FIGURE 18-32 Mechanism of action of neuromuscular blocking agents. (A) Normal physiology of the neuromuscular junction. There is uninhibited access for acetylcholine at the postjunctional receptors. *(continues)*

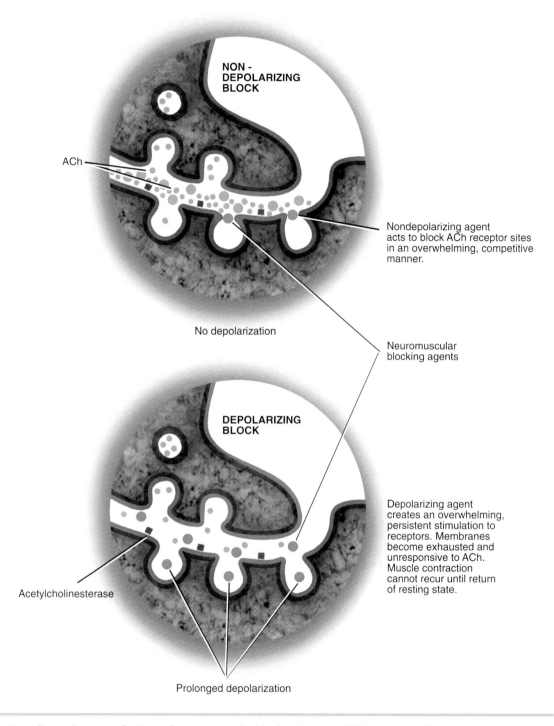

NON-DEPOLARIZING BLOCK

ACh

Nondepolarizing agent acts to block ACh receptor sites in an overwhelming, competitive manner.

No depolarization

Neuromuscular blocking agents

DEPOLARIZING BLOCK

Depolarizing agent creates an overwhelming, persistent stimulation to receptors. Membranes become exhausted and unresponsive to ACh. Muscle contraction cannot recur until return of resting state.

Acetylcholinesterase

B.

Prolonged depolarization

FIGURE 18-32 (continued) Mechanism of action of neuromuscular blocking agents. (B) Illustrations of the proposed mechanisms of action for the two major classes of neuromuscular blocking drugs.

Side Effects of Neuromuscular Blockers

The fasciculations caused by succinylcholine can increase intraocular pressure. Although the pressure rise is usually small (less than 10 mm Hg), there is the potential for intraocular contents to extrude through traumatic defects in the globe. The fasciculations may also be of concern in the setting of unstable fractures, particularly those involving cervical vertebrae.

Succinylcholine also causes transient increases in intracranial pressure (ICP). The increases average 5 mm Hg though the clinical significance of this rise is unknown.[124] Lidocaine, when administered prior to

Table 18-18
Summary of Commonly Used Neuromuscular Blocking Agents

Drug	Class	Dose (mg/kg IVP)	Onset	Duration (min)	Side Effects
Succinylcholine (Anectine)	Depolarizing	1.5	30–60 sec	4–6	Fasciculations Dysrhythmias Hyperkalemia Increased intracranial pressure Increased intraocular pressure Increased intragastric pressure Rhabdomyolysis Histamine release
Pancuronium (Pavulon)	Nondepolarizing	0.1	2–5 min	60–90	Tachycardia Increased peripheral vascular resistance (PVR) Prolonged recovery time in patients with hepatorenal dysfunction
Vecuronium	Nondepolarizing	0.1	2–3 min	25–40	Prolonged recovery time in patients with hepatorenal dysfunction

induction, has been shown to decrease this rise in ICP.[125]

The effects of succinylcholine on vagal ganglia, compounded by the vagal effect of laryngoscopy, may lead to bradycardia or asystole in children.[124] For this reason, children should be premedicated with atropine prior to RSI with succinylcholine.

The side effects of nondepolarizing agents are limited to tachycardia and increased peripheral vascular resistance. These side effects are associated to a greater extent with pancuronium than with vecuronium.

Reversal of Neuromuscular Blockade

Occasionally, it is necessary to reverse the effects of neuromuscular blockade, such as when paralysis complicates the physical assessment or when efforts at intubation have been unsuccessful and spontaneous respirations must be restored. While several agents exist to reverse the neuromuscular blockade of nondepolarizing drugs, pharmacological reversal of succinylcholine is not possible. The only means of reversing succinylcholine-induced paralysis is to allow the drug to "wear off," which is a function of drug clearance. Fortunately, the half-life of succinylcholine is much shorter than the half-life of the nondepolarizing drugs.

Because nondepolarizing neuromuscular blockers compete directly with acetylcholine for receptor sites, their effects can be reversed by increasing the concentration of acetylcholine at the synapse. Reversal agents inhibit the action of cholinesterase, the enzyme that breaks down acetylcholine. The result is an accumulation of acetylcholine at the synapse that competes with the nondepolarizing agent for receptor sites and restores normal muscular contraction. The reversal agents are summarized in Table 18-19.

Procedure for Rapid-Sequence Induction

1. Assemble all equipment, including BVM, laryngoscope and blades, ET tubes, stylet, syringe, and tape.
2. Hyperventilate the patient with 100% O_2 via BVM.

Table 18-19
Summary of Neuromuscular Blockade Reversal Agents

Neostigmine 0.05 mg/kg and atropine 15 μg/kg
Pyridostigmine 0.2 mg/kg and atropine 10 μg/kg
Edrophonium 0.2 mg/kg and atropine 10 μg/kg

3. Attach the patient to a cardiac monitor.

4. Premedicate the conscious patient with a sedative/hypnotic or narcotic agent.

5. Premedicate children with atropine 0.01 mg/kg to prevent bradycardia.

6. Premedicate head-injured patients with 1.0–1.5 mg/kg lidocaine to prevent further increases in ICP.

7. Administer the muscle relaxant.

8. Monitor for adequate relaxation, demonstrated by decreased resistance to BVM ventilations and relaxation of the jaw.

9. Perform ET intubation in the usual manner, securing the tube once proper placement has been confirmed.

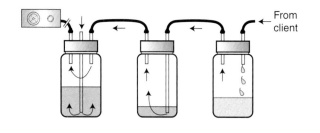

FIGURE 18-33 Traditional three-bottle chest drainage system.

ADVANCED TOPICS

CHEST DRAINAGE SYSTEMS

Air moves in and out of the thorax based on changes in intrathoracic pressure. Normally, there is always negative pressure in the pleural cavity (-4 cm H_2O during exhalation). This negative pressure between the visceral and parietal pleura helps to maintain lung expansion. During inspiration, the diaphragm moves downward and the intercostal muscles contract, expanding the rib cage and further increasing the negative pressure within the thorax to -8 cm H_2O and air rushes in to inflate the lungs. Whenever there is a disruption in negative pressure within the pleural cavity, such as with pneumothorax or hemothorax, the normal mechanics of respiration are lost resulting in pulmonary compromise. The treatment is to drain the air or blood through a chest tube. The procedure for inserting a chest tube was discussed in Chapter 13. The following section focuses on the techniques of incorporating the chest tube into a chest drainage system.

Overview of the Chest Drainage Systems

Traditionally, chest drainage was accomplished with a three-bottle system. In this system, each glass bottle has a separate function (Figure 18-33). Single-unit, disposable systems such as the Pleur-evac have replaced the traditional system, but their function is similar (Figures 18-34A and B). The first chamber of the chest drainage system corresponds with the first bottle in the traditional system and functions as the collection chamber. This chamber is nearest the patient and connects to the chest tube. Fluid and/or air from the patient's pleural cavity drains into this chamber. The chamber is also graduated to allow rapid measurement of blood or effusate.

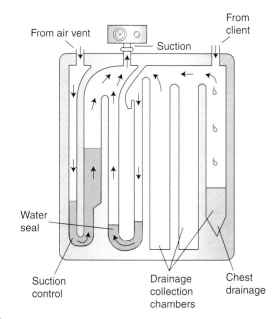

A.

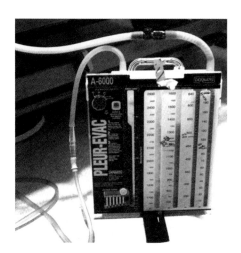

B.

FIGURE 18-34 Self-contained chest drainage system.

The second chamber correlates with "Bottle 2" of the traditional system and functions as a water seal. The purpose of the water seal is to serve as a one-way valve allowing air to escape from the pleural cavity but preventing its return. The water seal thus preserves the negative pressure within the pleural cavity. In addition to functioning as a water seal, the second chamber is calibrated to measure the amount of negative pressure in the pleural cavity. The water level rises in the chamber as intrapleural pressure becomes more negative.

The third chamber limits the amount of suction that can be applied to the pleural cavity and correlates with "Bottle 3" of the traditional system. The suction control chamber is essentially a safety mechanism that limits the amount of suction applied to the pleural cavity, regardless of the amount of suction applied to the drainage system. The height of the water in the column regulates the amount of suction applied to the pleural cavity. A suction pressure of –20 cm H_2O is recommended, but lower levels may be indicated for infants or adults with lung disease.

Clinical Application of Chest Drainage

To assemble the equipment needed, use the following steps:

1. Attach a funnel to the suction tubing connector, crimp the tubing, and fill the funnel with approximately 70 mL of sterile water. Release the crimp to fill the chamber. The water-seal chamber should be filled to the 2-cm water level. If necessary, additional water may be added through the injection port with a needle and syringe.

2. Remove the cover from the suction control chamber and fill the chamber with water to the dotted line or the desired level of suction.

3. Using sterile technique, connect the tubing from the collection chamber to the chest tube.

4. Attach the tubing from the suction control chamber to a suction source. Adjust the suction until gentle, continuous bubbling occurs.

Monitoring the Chest Drainage System

Once connected, the chest drainage unit must remain upright. Dependent loops in the patient tubing should be avoided because this causes resistance to drainage. Air leaks can be detected by monitoring the water seal. Normally, a small amount of bubbling may occur with exhalation. If it occurs with inhalation, look for a leak in the system. If there is no bubbling, the water level should rise and fall with the patient's respirations. This is normal and reflects the normal intrapleural pressure

changes associated with breathing. If the patient is breathing spontaneously, the water level should rise during inhalation and fall during exhalation. If the patient is receiving positive-pressure ventilation via BVM or ventilator, the water level should fall during inspiration. If the patient is receiving PEEP, the oscillations will be dampened. They may also be absent if the lung is fully expanded and the lung is occluding the holes in the chest tube.

The complication of most concern when using chest drainage systems is tension pneumothorax. If the paramedic suspects a tension pneumothorax in a patient with a chest drainage system, the most likely cause is an obstruction in the patient tubing. The system should be thoroughly inspected and any obstruction removed. The other likely cause of tension pneumothorax is clamping the patient tubing for transport or manipulation of the drainage system. If air is still escaping from the pleural cavity via the patient tubing, clamping the tubing will allow air to accumulate in the pleural space. Therefore, the tubing should never be clamped. If the drainage system is not functioning or has been knocked over, it is preferable to temporarily submerge the tubing in a bottle of sterile water or leave the tubing open to air while system patency is reestablished. The small amount of air that could enter the pleural space is not as dangerous as the potential for a tension pneumothorax if the tubing is clamped.[126]

MECHANICAL VENTILATION

Mechanical ventilation permits patients to survive illness and injuries that were routinely fatal only a few decades ago.[127] Mechanical ventilation is used to improve arterial oxygenation, supplant inadequate ventilation, improve carbon dioxide elimination, relieve the patient from the work of breathing, and free the paramedic from the task of manually ventilating the intubated patient with a BVM during transport. The paramedic may use a mechanical ventilator to ventilate patients during transport from the scene, but more often ventilators are used for interfacility transport of trauma patients. In either case, it is important for the paramedic to understand the basic operations of mechanical ventilators and how to assess the patient's response to mechanical ventilation.

Modes of Ventilation

There are many parameters that control how a ventilator functions. A set of these parameters is called the ventilator mode and describes how the ventilator is triggered into inspiration and cycled into exhalation and whether ventilations are spontaneous, mandatory, or both.[14] The result is a plethora of ventilator modes and settings that results in confusion for clinicians who do not use them regularly.[127] Fortunately, the settings are already determined for trauma patients being transferred to other facilities; the paramedic merely adjusts the settings on the transport ventilator to match those on the hospital ventilator. Additionally, only a few settings are truly necessary for the acute management of patients between the scene and the emergency department.

Controlled Mandatory Ventilation.

With the **controlled mandatory ventilation (CMV)** mode, the ventilator delivers a preset tidal volume at a time-triggered respiratory rate. Because the ventilator controls both tidal volume and rate, the patient's minute volume is entirely controlled by the ventilator. The patient cannot spontaneously increase the rate or volume of respirations by breathing spontaneously. Because this mode would be psychologically troubling to the conscious patient, it should only be used in unconscious patients or those properly medicated with a combination of sedatives and neuromuscular blockers. The CMV mode is indicated in patients with tetanus or seizure activity that interrupts the delivery of mechanical ventilation, with chest wall injury in which inspiratory efforts produce paradoxical movement, or in patients who are apneic and unconscious.[128,129]

Assist Control Ventilation.

The **assist control ventilation (ACV)** mode provides the patient with a set respiratory rate and ensures that a set tidal volume is delivered with each spontaneous breath. The patient may increase the ventilator rate (assist) in addition to the preset mechanical respiratory rate (control). The mandatory mechanical breaths may be triggered either by the patient's spontaneous breaths or time triggered by a preset mechanical rate. If the patient's spontaneous ventilatory rate drops below the preset mechanical rate, the ventilator delivers the mechanical rate. This mode supports the respiratory effort of patients who cannot consistently maintain adequate respiratory rate, tidal volume, ventilation, or oxygenation.[130]

The ACV mode is most often used to provide full ventilatory support to patients when initially placed on mechanical ventilation.[14] The ACV mode is used for patients who have an adequate respiratory drive and can trigger the ventilator into inspiration. The time-triggering (control) mechanism is essentially a failsafe mechanism to be used only in the event that the patient stops triggering the ventilator at an acceptable rate. An advantage of the ACV mode is that it allows the patient to adjust his or her spontaneous respiratory

rate in order to normalize the pH to compensate for any changes in $PaCO_2$ levels.

Intermittent Mandatory Ventilation.

Intermittent mandatory ventilation (IMV) is a mode that delivers breaths at a set rate and volume. Between mechanical breaths, a fresh gas supply is available for the patient's spontaneous breaths. However, the ventilator does not assist the spontaneous breaths but merely offers supplemental oxygen at the preset FiO_2.

The primary complication associated with IMV is the chance for delivering a mechanical breath on top of a spontaneous breath. This occurs when the patient is at the end of a spontaneous breath and the ventilator is time triggered into delivering a mechanical breath at the same time. The risk of the IMV mode is high lung volume and airway pressures that may result in barotrauma, a dangerous complication in the trauma patient where a pneumothorax may already exist.

Synchronized Intermittent Mandatory Ventilation.

Because of the risk of delivering stacked breaths, the IMV mode has been largely replaced with the **synchronized intermittent mandatory ventilation (SIMV)** mode. This mode delivers mechanical breaths at or near the beginning of a spontaneous breath. By synchronizing mandatory breaths with the patient's spontaneous efforts, breath stacking is avoided. If the patient makes no effort, the preset breaths are delivered. If the patient's intrinsic rate is faster than the preset mechanical rate, breaths are not assisted (in comparison to the ACV mode where all breaths, spontaneous and mechanical, are assisted).

The primary use of SIMV is to provide partial ventilatory support. Typically, when a patient is placed on mechanical ventilation, full ventilatory support is used to relieve the patient from the work of breathing, at least for the first 24 hours.[14] Following the initial period of full support, the patient is placed on partial support with SIMV. By doing so, the patient is transitioned back into spontaneous control of respirations and the work of breathing. The benefits of transitioning with SIMV is that it avoids atrophy of respiratory muscles, decreases mean airway pressure, and facilitates weaning. Ventilatory modes are summarized in Table 18-20.

Initial Ventilator Settings

Although there are many other modes of mechanical ventilation, CMV, ACV, and SIMV are the ones most likely to be encountered by the paramedic. In the field setting where the paramedic will be initiating mechanical ventilation, the ACV and SIMV modes are the best

Table 18-20
Comparison of Ventilator Modes

Mode	Response to Apnea	Response to Spontaneous Breaths	
		Rate	Volume
CMV	Set rate and volume delivered	None	None
ACV	Set rate and volume delivered	Set by patient	Delivered at set volume (assisted)
IMV	Set rate and volume delivered	Set by patient	Set by patient (not assisted)
SIMV	Set rate and volume delivered	Set by patient	Set by patient

modes for initial ventilation. During this acute phase of management, there is no important clinical difference between ACV and SIMV. The clinician should choose one and use it consistently unless there is a compelling reason to favor another mode.[127]

The initial tidal volume is usually set between 10 and 15 mL/kg of ideal body weight (IBW). The patient's actual weight can be used for determining tidal volume unless the patient is significantly underweight or overweight.[14] In these cases, the following formulas should be used:

Male:
IBW (kg) = {106 + [6 × (height in inches - 60)]} / 2.2

Female:
IBW (kg) = {105 + [5 × (height in inches - 60)]} / 2.2

The respiratory rate is usually set at 10–12 breaths per minute for adults. When coupled with a tidal volume of 10–15 mL/kg, this rate usually provides a minute volume sufficient to normalize the patient's $PaCO_2$. Mechanical rates greater than 20 breaths/minute are associated with auto-PEEP and should be avoided.[131]

An alternative method of selecting the initial respiratory rate is to first estimate the patient's minute volume requirement using the following formulas:

Male: minute volume = 4 × body surface area

Female: minute volume = 3.5 × body surface area

The body surface area is estimated from a nomogram such as the Dubois body surface area chart (Figure 18-35). Once the minute volume is determined, the initial respiratory rate can be calculated as follows:

Respiratory rate = estimated minute volume/tidal volume

For nearly all trauma patients, the initial FiO_2 should be set at 100%. Once the patient is stabilized, the FiO_2 may be lowered based upon arterial blood gas analysis. If possible, the FiO_2 is best kept below 50% to avoid oxygen-induced lung injury.[131]

Rarely will PEEP be required in the prehospital setting. Usually, PEEP is used to treat refractory hypoxia such as that encountered in posttrauma patients who develop adult repiratory distress syndrome (ARDS). Therefore, PEEP is encountered almost exclusively during interfacility transports where the paramedic sets the PEEP level to match the settings used in the hospital. If the paramedic is ordered to initiate PEEP, the usual

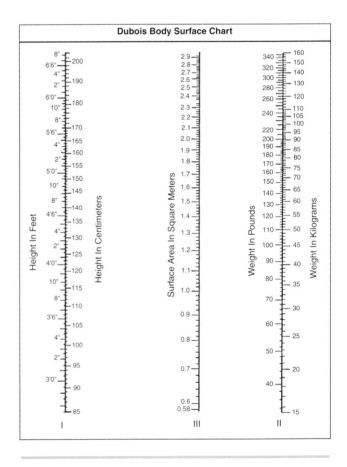

FIGURE 18-35 Dubois body surface area chart. *Source:* Dubois EF. *Basal Metabolism in Health and Disease.* Philadelphia: Lea & Febiger; 1924. Reprinted with permission.)

starting level is 5 cm H_2O. Subsequent changes in PEEP should be based on ABGs, tolerance of PEEP, and effects on the cardiovascular system.

Depending upon the model of the ventilator, there are a number of alarms that must be set. Of these, the inspiratory pressure alarm is of major importance when using mechanical ventilation in the trauma patient. In the presence of a tension pneumothorax, higher pressures are required to expand the lungs. This is usually detected by increasing resistance to ventilations with the BVM. However, in patients being ventilated mechanically, this early sign of tension pneumothorax is lost. To avoid developing a potentially life-threatening tension, most ventilators are equipped with an inspiratory pressure alarm. The inspiratory pressure alarm monitors the amount of pressure required to deliver the set tidal volume during each ventilation. It is initially set at 10–15 cm H_2O above the observed peak inspiratory pressure. When the alarm activates, the ventilator goes into the expiratory cycle, thus avoiding dangerously high inspiratory pressures. When the alarm activates, the cause of the alarm must be determined. In addition to tension pneumothorax, causes include bronchospasm, water in the ventilator circuit, kinking or biting of the ET tube, and secretions in the airway.[14] Because of the potential for an undetected tension pneumothorax, ventilators without an inspiratory pressure alarm must not be used in the trauma patient. Additionally, patients with a pneumothorax should not be placed on mechanical ventilation until a chest tube is in place.

Assessment of Mechanical Ventilation

Once mechanical ventilation has been instituted, it is important to continually reassess the patient's ventilatory and oxygenation status. The paramedic cannot simply attach the patient to a ventilator and assume that airway and breathing are controlled. In addition to monitoring the ventilator alarms, the patient's pulse oximetry and end-tidal CO_2 readings, ABGs, lung sounds, and other clinical signs must be frequently reevaluated.

The best measure of a patient's ventilatory status is the $PaCO_2$. A $PaCO_2$ of greater than 45 mm Hg indicates hypoventilation. The most common approach to improving ventilation is to increase the respiratory rate. It is generally not desirable to increase the ventilator tidal volume beyond that which is appropriate for the patient's ideal body weight. Doing so increases the risk of barotrauma as well as having undesired effects on the cardiovascular system.

The following equation estimates the respiratory rate required to normalize the $PaCO_2$:

$$\text{New respiratory rate} = \frac{(\text{original rate} \times \text{present } PaCO_2)}{(\text{desired } PaCO_2)}$$

Other means of improving ventilation include using the largest ET tube possible and cutting off any excess tube to reduce airway resistance, using a low-compliance ventilator circuit, and, lastly, increasing mechanical tidal volume.

Oxygenation is dependent upon adequate ventilation, diffusion, and perfusion. In addition to the usual clinical signs to evaluate oxygenation, the PaO_2 provides a general and quantifiable measure of oxygenation. The normal PaO_2 is 80–100 mm Hg. Correcting a low PaO_2 begins with ensuring adequate ventilation. If ventilation is normal, increasing FiO_2 is the next corrective measure. As previously stated, an FiO_2 of 1.0 is appropriate in the field setting. When it is necessary to more finely adjust the FiO_2, the following formulas are used:

- Step 1: Determine the PAO_2 needed:

  $$PAO_2 \text{ needed} = PaO_2 \text{ desired}/(\text{a/A ratio})$$

  where the PAO_2 needed is the alveolar oxygen tension needed for a desired PaO_2 and the a/A ratio is the arterial/alveolar oxygen tension ratio (PaO_2/PAO_2 before changes) and PaO_2 is obtained from ABGs and PAO_2 is obtained from the alveolar oxygen tension equation described earlier.

- Step 2: Determine the FiO_2 needed:

  $$FiO_2 \text{ needed} = (PAO_2 \text{ needed} + 50)/713$$

Oxygen therapy alone may not be sufficient to correct hypoxia. If the hypoxia is caused by intrapulmonary shunting, PEEP may be required. If the cause of hypoxia is poor perfusion, cardiac output must also be restored to normal. In addition, while restoring circulating volume with crystalloid IV fluid may improve cardiac output, it will not in itself correct hypoxia. Adequate levels of hemoglobin are also required. Once the hemoglobin level is corrected, normal oxygen-carrying capacity and oxygen content will be restored.

PHYSIOLOGICAL RESPONSE TO INTUBATION AND MECHANICAL VENTILATION

The act of ET intubation and mechanical ventilation can have profound effects on patients, particularly on the cardiovascular system. The cardiovascular response to intubation is mediated by the autonomic nervous system.[132] Transient increases in heart rate and blood pressure are common and have been reported in the range of 15–30 bpm and 25–37 mm Hg, respectively.[133,134] Bradycardia has also been reported as a consequence of intubation.[132]

Under certain circumstances, atropine and lidocaine have been used to counteract the cardiovascular effects of intubation. Lidocaine, given topically to the larynx and trachea or intravenously, has been shown to reduce the increases in heart rate and blood pressure associated with ET intubation.[135–138] Four milliliters of 4% topical lidocaine may be administered by the laryngotracheal anesthesia set, producing complete anesthesia of the oropharynx within 60 seconds.[137] Alternatively, lidocaine 1.5 mg/kg may be administered intravenously 1 minute prior to intubation. Studies suggest that while both routes of administration provide anesthesia, intravenous lidocaine is more effective in blunting increases in heart rate and intracranial pressure.[137] Reflex bradycardia in children from intubation attempts can be managed with intravenous atropine. Atropine 0.01 mg/kg may be administered intravenously prior to intubation attempts.[124] However, atropine administration may aggravate the associated tachycardic, hypertensive, and dysrhythmic responses to intubation in adults.[139]

Positive-pressure ventilation has beneficial and negative physiological effects on the pulmonary, cardiovascular, and other major organ systems. When positive pressure is used for ventilation, the pressures in the airways and lungs are increased during inspiration, opposite of the normal decrease in airway pressure observed during spontaneous respirations. Positive-pressure ventilation increases the mean airway pressure (MAWP), which compresses pulmonary blood vessels, reducing stroke volume and cardiac output.[14] The reduced cardiac output causes a V/Q mismatch leading to reduced oxygen delivery to the tissues. In addition, the lower cardiac output reduces blood flow to major organs such as the kidneys, liver, and brain. However, this decrease in cardiac output due to positive-pressure ventilation can usually be managed with intravascular volume expansion and positive inotropic drugs.[14]

INTERNET ACTIVITIES

Visit the e-medicine Web site at http://www.emedicine.com. Click on the Emergency Medicine on-line book and select Special Aspects of Emergency Medicine. Then click on Ventilator Management. Review the chapter on the management of ventilators and ventilator-dependent patients.

SUMMARY

As with any patient, managing the trauma patient begins with airway patency, ventilation, and oxygenation. Further patient evaluation and treatment cannot proceed until the airway is secure and respirations restored. In addition, in the setting of trauma, consideration must be given to C-spine manipulation. The risk of aggravating spinal injuries, coupled with the sometimes awkward patient presentations encountered in the field, restricts the paramedic's options for airway control. Fortunately, there are several techniques at the paramedic's disposal for effectively managing the airway and ventilations of the trauma patient. It is imperative that the paramedic be knowledgeable of these procedures and technically proficient in their implementation.

REVIEW QUESTIONS

1. A common cause of airway obstruction is occlusion of the oropharynx by the tongue. When functioning properly and unimpeded by trauma, drugs, or alcohol intoxication, which cranial nerve is responsible for controlling the tongue and protecting the airway?
   a. Vagus, CN X
   b. Hypoglossal, CN XII
   c. Trigeminal, CN V
   d. Olfactory, CN I

2. Which functions of the nasopharynx are bypassed in the intubated patient?
   a. Humidification
   b. Humidification, filtration, alimentation
   c. Humidification, filtration, alimentation, heat exchange
   d. Humidification, filtration, heat exchange, voice resonation

3. Because it is the only complete cartilaginous ring of the airway, which of the following structures is used to perform the Sellick maneuver?
   a. Cricoid cartilage
   b. Thyroid cartilage
   c. Tracheal ring
   d. Arytenoid cartilage

4. Which of the following corresponds with the level of the carina?
   1. Fourth intercostal space
   2. Sternomanubrial joint
   3. Fifth thoracic vertebrae
   4. Sternoclavicular joint
      a. 1 only
      b. 2 only
      c. 2 and 3
      d. 1 and 4

5. The average distance from the incisors to the carina is 27 cm in the adult male and 23 cm in the adult female. Therefore, at what level should a

properly positioned endotracheal tube rest at the incisors?
a. 18–22 cm
b. 23–27 cm
c. 29–32 cm
d. 22–26 cm

6. At what level should a properly positioned naso-tracheal tube in the adult male exit the nare?
a. 18 cm
b. 32 cm
c. 23 cm
d. 29 cm

7. Aspirated foreign bodies tend to gravitate to which areas of the lungs?
a. Left middle lobe
b. Left upper lobe and right upper lobe
c. Right upper lobe and right lower lobe
d. Right lower lobe and left lower lobe

8. Which of the following occurs during inspiration?
1. Contraction of diaphragm and intercostal muscles
2. Expansion of the thoracic cavity
3. Relaxation of diaphragm and intercostal muscles
4. Decrease in intrapulmonary pressure
5. Increase in intrapulmonary pressure
   a. 1, 2, 4
   b. 1, 2, 5
   c. 3, 5
   d. 3, 4

9. Normal minute volume in the resting, adult male is:
a. 500 cc
b. 1 liter
c. 3 liters
d. 6 liters

10. Which of the following conditions hold true in the healthy individual?
a. Anatomic dead space > physiological dead space
b. Anatomic dead space < physiological dead space
c. Anatomic dead space = physiological dead space
d. Anatomic dead space = physiological dead space/2

11. Which of the following relationships hold true at the alveolar-capillary membrane?
1. $\uparrow$ FiO_2 $\rightarrow\downarrow$ oxygen uptake
2. $\uparrow$ FiO_2 $\rightarrow\uparrow$ oxygen uptake
3. $\uparrow$ FiO_2 $\rightarrow\uparrow$ oxygen pressure gradient
4. $\uparrow$ FiO_2 $\rightarrow\downarrow$ carbon dioxide uptake
   a. 1, 4
   b. 2, 3

c. 1, 3
d. 2, 4

12. PaO_2 represents the amount of oxygen dissolved in plasma and, thus, the amount available to tissues.
a. True, when hemoglobin is 15 g/dL
b. True, regardless of hemoglobin levels
c. True, when hemoglobin, carboxyhemoglobin, and pH are normal
d. False, regardless of hemoglobin, carboxyhemo-globin, and pH levels

13. Which of the following is a protective mechanism that prevents barotrauma to the lungs?
a. Hering-Breuer reflex
b. Pneumotaxic reflex
c. Apneustic reflex
d. Chemoreceptive reflex

14. Which of the following may result in loss of air-way patency?
1. Laryngeal fracture
2. Penetrating neck trauma
3. Expanding hematoma of the neck
4. Le Forte III fracture
   a. 2
   b. 2, 3, 4
   c. 1, 3, 4
   d. 1, 2, 3, 4

15. In the setting of aspiration, when do gastric con-tents reach the alveoli?
a. Within seconds
b. Within 1–2 min
c. Within 10 min
d. During the second day postaspiration

16. The mortality rate associated with aspiration:
a. Is related to the volume, distribution, and acid-ity of the aspirate
b. Is decreased by intubation and bronchial lavage
c. Correlates directly with the pH of the aspirate
d. Is lowered by the early administration of antibiotics

17. Under ideal circumstances, the BVM is capable of delivering _____ of oxygen-enriched air.
a. 500 mL
b. 600 mL
c. 700 mL
d. 800 mL

18. The first line of airway control in the apneic trauma patient should be:
a. Endotracheal intubation
b. Trauma jaw thrust, OPA, and BVM
c. Trauma jaw thrust and intubation
d. Demand valve

19. Which of the following are true of the EOA and EGTA?
  1. Can be inserted without manipulation of the cervical spine
  2. Can be used for gastric evacuation (EGTA) only
  3. Are as effective as intubation
  4. Are safer means of airway control in children less than 15 years of age when compared to endotracheal intubation
  5. Relieve the paramedic from the need to maintain a seal with the face mask
    a. 1 only
    b. 1, 2, 4
    c. 1, 2
    d. 1, 2, 3, 4, 5

20. The advantages of the PTLA over the EOA and EGTA include:
  1. The PTLA does not require C-spine control during insertion.
  2. The PTLA offers ventilation and oxygenation comparable to intubation.
  3. The PTLA provides an airway regardless of whether it is inserted into the esophagus or trachea.
  4. The face mask of the PTLA is easier to seal than that of the EOA and EGTA.
  5. The complication rate of the PTLA is lower than that of the EOA and EGTA.
    a. 1, 2, 3
    b. 1, 2, 3, 5
    c. 2, 3, 4
    d. 2, 3, 5

21. The primary advantage of the Combitube over the PTLA is that:
  a. There is less manipulation of the C-spine associated with insertion of the Combitube.
  b. The Combitube provides better oxygenation and ventilation.
  c. In the event of misdiagnosed placement, a spontaneously breathing patient may breathe through the perforations of the unused lumen.
  d. The complication rate is significantly lower with the Combitube than with the PTLA.

22. Which of the following Mallampati classifications suggest that the paramedic abandon orotracheal intubation in favor of other techniques?
  1. Mallampati I
  2. Mallampati II
  3. Mallampati III
  4. Mallampati IV
    a. 1 only
    b. 4 only
    c. 1 and 2
    d. 3 and 4

23. When intubating the seated patient using the frontal approach, the intubator holds the laryngoscope:
  a. In the right hand in an inverted position
  b. In the right hand in the standard position
  c. In the left hand in an inverted position
  d. In the left hand in the standard position

24. When intubating the seated patient using the frontal approach, the laryngoscope is lifted relative to the patient:
  a. Anteriorly and caudally
  b. Superiorly and caudally
  c. Anteriorly and cephalad
  d. Superiorly and cephalad

25. If a backboarded patient must be turned to facilitate drainage of blood and vomitus, yet requires BVM ventilation, the patient is best turned:
  a. To the right side
  b. To the left side
  c. To either side
  d. Only briefly for suctioning, then returned to the supine position

26. Which of the following are considered contraindications to the use of digital intubation?
  1. Cervical spine injury
  2. Oversized hands of the intubator
  3. Undersized hands of the intubator
  4. Patients without gag reflexes
  5. Patients with small mouths
    a. 1, 3, 5
    b. 2, 4, 5
    c. 2, 3, 5
    d. 2, 3, 4

27. Which of the following are true of blind nasotracheal intubation (BNI)?
  1. The technique has been commonly practiced since World War I.
  2. The procedure takes 2–3 times longer to perform than orotracheal intubation.
  3. In the presence of basilar skull fracture, the procedure frequently results in inadvertent passage of the tube into the cranial vault.
  4. Apnea is an absolute contraindication.
  5. Exploration of the nares for patency using a nasopharyngeal airway coated with 2% lidocaine is recommended.
    a. 1, 2, 3
    b. 2, 4, 5
    c. 1, 4, 5
    d. 1, 2, 5

28. Which of the following may facilitate passage of the nasotracheal tube?
  1. Use of a malleable stylet

2. Inflation of the balloon in the oropharynx, advancement until resistance is met, then deflation and passage of the tube
3. Gentle twisting when resistance is met
4. Preforming the tube by coiling the tube prior to insertion
5. Lubrication of the tube with surgical or lidocaine jelly
   a. 2, 3, 4
   b. 3, 4, 5
   c. 2, 3, 4, 5
   d. 1, 2, 3, 4, 5

29. Transillumination intubation may be used in which of the following circumstances?
1. Failure of orotracheal intubation
2. As the first-line technique for airway control in the setting of cervical spine injury
3. In the setting of upper airway obstruction
4. In the setting of trismus
5. To confirm tube placement in intubated patients
   a. 1, 3
   b. 1, 2, 3
   c. 1, 2, 5
   d. 2, 4, 5

30. Which of the following are advantages of the laryngeal mask airway?
1. High placement success rates among paramedics in U.S. EMS systems
2. Endotracheal intubation can be performed through a properly positioned LMA
3. Does not require manipulation of the cervical spine
4. Can be inserted with the patient in a variety of positions
5. Protects the airway from aspiration
   a. 1, 2, 5
   b. 2, 3, 4
   c. 1, 3, 4
   d. 1, 3, 5

31. Which of the following are disadvantages of translaryngeal jet insufflation?
1. Cannot be performed in a timely fashion
2. Requires special equipment
3. Less invasive than cricothyrotomy
4. Permits accumulation of CO_2
5. Provides poor air exchange
   a. 1, 2, 4, 5
   b. 2, 3, 4, 5
   c. 1, 2, 3, 4
   d. 1, 3, 4, 5

32. The proper ventilatory pressure and ventilation/exhalation ratio for translaryngeal jet insufflation are:

   a. 50 psi and 1:2
   b. 100 psi and 1:4
   c. 50 psi and 1:2
   d. 50 psi and 1:4

33. The most commonly reported complications of cricothyrotomy include:
1. Bleeding
2. Subglottic stenosis
3. Tracheoesophageal fistula
4. Infection
5. Extratracheal tube placement
   a. 1, 4, 5
   b. 1, 2, 3
   c. 1, 2, 3, 4, 5
   d. 1, 2, 4, 5

34. Cricothyrotomy is preferred over translaryngeal jet insufflation in which of the following circumstances?
1. Complete inspiratory and expiratory obstruction
2. Primary laryngeal injury
3. Coagulopathy
4. Backup procedure during rapid-sequence intubation
5. Endotracheal drug administration
   a. 2, 3, 4
   b. 1, 4, 5
   c. 3, 4, 5
   d. 1, 2, 4

35. Which of the following statements are true of depolarizing neuromuscular blocking agents?
1. They mimic the action of acetylcholine.
2. They do not result in fasciculations.
3. They work by blocking acetylcholine receptor sites at the postsynaptic membrane.
4. They can be easily reversed with neostygmine.
5. They can increase intracranial pressure.
   a. 2, 3
   b. 1, 5
   c. 4, 5
   d. 1, 2

36. When administering succinylcholine, which of the following should be available?
1. Equipment for cricothyrotomy
2. Lidocaine
3. Atropine
4. Edrophonium
5. Valium
   a. 1, 2, 3, 5
   b. 1, 3, 4, 5
   c. 1, 2, 3, 4
   d. 2, 3, 5

37. Which of the following are complications of rapid-sequence intubation?

1. Hypoxia
2. Increased intracranial pressure
3. Increased intraocular pressure
4. Bradycardia
5. Fasciculations
   a. 1, 2
   b. 1, 2, 4
   c. 1, 2, 3, 4, 5
   d. 1, 2, 4, 5

38. The amount of suction exerted by a chest drainage system is controlled by:
   a. Amount of suction applied to the drainage system
   b. Water level in "Bottle 3" of the system
   c. Length of the chest drainage tubing
   d. Height of the collection chamber

39. The recommended suction level for the adult patient is:
   a. –20 cm H_2O
   b. –30 cm H_2O
   c. –40 cm H_2O
   d. –50 cm H_2O

40. Bubbling with exhalation in the water seal chamber indicates that:
   a. The system is functioning properly.
   b. There is a leak in the system.
   c. The lung has reinflated.
   d. The wall suction level is set too high.

41. The ventilatory mode that delivers a preset rate and volume of breaths and provides supplemental oxygen supply for spontaneous breaths is:
   a. Assist control mode
   b. Intermittent mandatory ventilation mode
   c. Synchronized intermittent mandatory ventilation mode
   d. Controlled mode

42. The best modes for initial ventilatory management by the paramedic are:
   a. Assist control and control
   b. Intermittent mandatory ventilation and control
   c. Synchronized intermittent mandatory ventilation and control
   d. Synchronized intermittent mandatory ventilation and assist control

43. The initial tidal volume for ventilation is:
   a. 8–10 mL/kg
   b. 10–12 mL/kg
   c. 8–12 mL/kg
   d. 10–15 mL/kg

44. Because of the risk of unrecognized tension pneumothorax, which alarm must be available on the ventilator used for initial management of the trauma patient?
   a. Low inspiratory pressure
   b. Low volume
   c. High inspiratory pressure
   d. High volume

45. Which of the following are side effects of mechanical ventilation?
   1. Increased mean airway pressure during inspiration
   2. Decreased stroke volume
   3. Decreased cardiac output
   4. Increased blood pressure
   5. Decreased mean airway pressure during inspiration
   a. 1, 2, 3
   b. 2, 3, 5
   c. 1, 3, 4
   d. 1, 4, 5

▶ CRITICAL THINKING

● The laryngeal mask airway (LMA) is a relatively new device in emergency medicine. Under what circumstances would you choose to use this device in the field? What other options exist for airway control? What are their limitations? What are the limitations of the LMA?

● You have just begun transport of a 17-year-old male involved in a high-speed MVC. He is unconscious and suffering from a head injury and fractured ribs on the right. His blood pressure is 132/86, heart rate 110, respirations 3 and agonal. Your transport time is 35 minutes. What settings will you use for mechanical ventilation for this patient?

● While en route with the patient described above, the high-pressure alarm on the ventilator sounds. What are the possible causes for the alarm? What assessments will you perform? What actions will you take?

● You are dispatched to the scene of a shooting. Upon arrival, you are escorted by police to a 21-year-old male who has sustained a shotgun blast to the face. While the nose and eyes are recognizable, all facial features below the nose are obliterated. The patient shows signs of respiratory effort but no signs of actual air exchange. What options exist for establishing an airway in this patient? What are the advantages and disadvantages of each? Which would you choose? Why?

▶ REFERENCES

1. Kastendieck J. Airway management. In: Rosen P, Barkin R, Braen C, eds. *Emergency Medicine: Concepts and Clinical Practices*. 2nd ed. St. Louis: Mosby; 1988.

2. Safar P. Sequential steps of emergency airway control. In: Safar P, ed. *Advances in Cardiopulmonary Resuscitation*. New York: Springer Verla; 1977.

3. Young GP. Clinical airway anatomy. In: Dailey RH, Simon B, Young GP, Stewart RD, eds. *The Airway. Emergency Management*. St Louis: Mosby Yearbook; 1992.

4. Morris I. Airway management. In: Rosen P, Barken R, Braen C, (eds). *Emergency Medicine: Concepts and Clinical Practices*. St. Louis: Mosby Yearbook; 1992.

5. Ellis H. *Clinical Anatomy. A Revision and Applied Anatomy for Clinical Students*. 6th ed. Oxford: *Blackwell Scientific Publications*; 1977.

6. Graney DO. Basic science: anatomy. In: Cummings CW, et al., eds. *Otolaryngology: Head and Neck Surgery*. St Louis: CV Mosby Company; 1986.

7. Dripps RD, Eckenhoff JE, Vandam LD, eds. In: *Introduction to Anesthesia. The Principles of Safe Practice*. 5th ed. Philadelpia: W.B. Saunders Company; 1982.

8. Scott J. Oral endotracheal intubation. In: Dailey RH, Simon B, Young GP, Stewart RD, eds. *The Airway. Emergency Management*. St Louis: Mosby Yearbook; 1992.

9. Holley HS, Gildea JE. Vocal cord paralysis after tracheal intubation. JAMA. 215:281; 1971.

10. Atkinson RS, Rushman GB, Lee JA. *A Synopsis of Anesthesia*. 8th ed. Bristol, UK: John Wright and Sons; 1977.

11. Sanders MJ. *Mosby's Paramedic Textbook*. St Louis: Mosby Lifeline; 1994.

12. Mezzanotte WS, Rodman DM. Ventilation and oxygenation. In: Dailey RH, Simon B, Young GP, Stewart RD, eds. *The Airway. Emergency Management*. St Louis: Mosby Yearbook; 1992.

13. Wilson RF, Barton C. Blood gases. pathophysiology and interpretation. In: Tintinalli JE, Ruiz E, Krome RL eds. *Emergency Medicine: A Comprehensive Study Guide*. 4th ed. New York: McGraw-Hill; 1996.

14. Chang DW. *Clinical Application of Mechanical Ventilation*. Albany, NY: Delmar Publishers; 1997.

15. Tobin MJ. Respiratory monitoring during mechanical ventilation. *Crit Care Clin*.1990; 6:679.

16. Gordon AS, Belton MK, Ridolpho PF. Emergency management of foreign body airway obstruction. In: Safar P, ed. *Advances in Cardiopulmonary Resuscitation*. New York: Springer-Verlag; 1977.

17. Baker FJ, Strauss R, Walter JJ. Cardiac arrest. In: Rosen P, et al, eds. *Emergency Medicine: Concepts and Clinical Practice*. 2nd ed. St Louis: C. Mosby; 1988.

18. *Advanced Cardiac Life Support*. Dallas, TX: American Heart Association; 1997.

19. Safar P. Sequential steps of emergency airway control. In: Safar P, ed. *Advances in Cardiopulmonary Resuscitation*. New York: Springer-Verlag; 1977.

20. Mulder DS. Airway management. In: Feliciano DV, Moore EE, Mattox KL, eds. *Trauma*. 3rd ed. Stanford, CT: Appleton and Lange;1996.

21. McSwain NE, Paturas JL, Wertz E, eds. PHTLS. *Basic and Advanced Pre-hospital Trauma Life Support*. 3rd ed. National Association of Emergency Medical Technicians; 1994.

22. Chokshi SK, Asper RF, Khandheria BK. Aspiration pneumonia: a review. *Am Fam Phys*. 1986; 33:195.

23. Kinni ME, Stout MM. Aspiration pneumonitis predisposing conditions and prevention. *J Oral Maxillofac Surg*. 1986; 44:378.

24. Wolfe R. Aspiration. In: Dailey RH, Simon B, Young GP, Stewart RD, eds. *The Airway. Emergency Management*. St Louis: Mosby Yearbook; 1992.

25. Dines DE, Baker WG, Sweantland WA. Aspiration pneumonitis. *Mayo Clin Proc*. 1970; 45:347.

26. Cameron JL, Zuidema GD. Aspiration pneumonia. magnitude and frequency of problem. *JAMA* 1972; 219:119.

27. Cameron JL, Mitchell WH, Zuidema GD. Aspiration pneumonia. Clinical outcome following documented aspiration. *Arch Surg*. 1973;106:49.

28. Chapman RL, Downs JB, Modell JH. The Ineffectiveness of steroid therapy in treating aspiration of hydrochloric acid. *Arch Surg*. 1974;108:858.

29. Bailery TD, Brenner BE, Simon RR. Miscellaneous Respiratory Emergencies. In: Kravis TC & Warner CG, eds. *Emergency Medicine. A Comprehensive Review*. 2nd ed. Rockville, MD: Aspen Publishers; 1987.

30. Cadoux CG, White JD, Hedberg MC. High-yield roentgenographic criteria for cervical spine injury. *Ann Emerg Med*. 1987; 16:738.

31. Gbaanador GBM, Fruin AH, Taylon C. Role of routine emergency cervical radiography in head trauma. *Am J Surg*. 1986; 152:643.

32. MacDonald RL, Shwartz ML, Mirich D, Sharkey PW, Nelson WR. Diagnosis of cervical spine injury in motor vehicle crash victims how many x-rays are enough? *J Trauma*. 1990; 30:392.

33. McNamara RM, O'Brien MC, Davidheiser S. Posttraumatic neck pain. A prospective and follow-up study. *Ann Emerg Med*. 1988; 17:906.

34. Neifeld GL, Keene JG, Hevesy G, Leikin J, Proust A, Thisted RA. Cervical injury in head trauma. *J Emerg Med*. 1988; 6:20.

35. Roberge RJ, Wears RC, Kelly M, et al. Selective application of cervical spine radiography in alert victims of blunt trauma: a prospective study. *J Trauma*. 1988; 28:784.

36. Alker GJ, Oh YS, Leslie EV, Lehotay J, Panarova, Eschner EG. Postmortem radiology of head and neck injuries in fatal traffic accidents. *Radiology*. 1975; 114:611.

37. Huelke DF, O'Day J, Mendelsohn RA. Cervical injuries suffered in automobile crashes. *J Neurosurg*. 1981; 54:316.

38. Shani R, Menegazzi J, Mossesso V. Paramedic evaluation of clinical indicators of cervical spine injury. *Prehosp Emerg Care*. 1997; 1(1):16.

39. Domeier RM, Evans RW, Swor RA, Rivera-Rivera EJ, Frederikesen SM. Multicenter prospective validation of out-of-hospital clinical spinal clearance crieteria. *Acad Emerg Med*. 1997; 4(6):643.

40. Walls RM. The multiple trauma patient. In: Dailey RH, Simon B, Young GP, Stewart RD, eds. *The Airway. Emergency Management*. St Louis: Mosby Yearbook; 1992.

41. American College of Surgeons: *Advanced Trauma Life Support Student Manual*. 5th ed. Chicago, IL:. American College of Surgeons; 1993.

42. Aprahamian C, Thompson BM, Finger WA, Darin JC. Experimental cervical spine injury model: evaluation of airway management and splinting techniques. *Ann Emerg Med*. 1984; 13:584.

43. Menn SJ, Roth R. Airway management. In: Kravis TC, Warner CG, et al, eds. *Emergency Medicine: A Comprehensive Review*. 2nd ed. Rockville, MD: Aspen Publishers; 1987.

44. Campbell WH, Cantrill SV. Neck trauma. In: Dailey RH, Simon B Young, GP, Stewart RD, eds. *The Airway. Emergency Management*. St Louis: Mosby Yearbook; 1992.

45. Rhee KJ, Green W, Holcroft JW, Mangili JA. Oral intubation in the multiply injured patient: the risk of exacerbating spinal cord damage. *Ann Emerg Med*. 1990; 19:511.

46. Dula DJ. Trauma to the cervical spine. *JACEP*. 1979; 8:13.

47. Majernick TG, Bieniek R, Houston JB, Hughes HG. Cervical spine movement durin g orotracheal intubation. *Ann Emer Med*. 1986; 15:417.

48. Cummins RO, Austin D, Graves JR, Litwin PE, Pierce J. Ventilation skills of emergency medical technicians: a teaching challenge for emergency medicine. *Ann Emerg Med*. 1986; 15:1187.

49. Rhee KJ, O'Malley RJ, Turner JE , Ward RE. Field airway management of the trauma patient: the efficacy of bag mask ventilation. *Am J Emerg Med*. 1988; 6:333.

50. Augustine JA, Seidel DR, McCabe JB. Ventilation performance usng a self-inflating aneshtesia bag: effect of operator characterisitcs. *Am J Emerg Med*. 1987; 5:267.

51. Don Michael TA, Lambert EH, Mehran A. Mouth-to-lung airway for cardiac resuscitation. *Lancet*. 1968; 2:1329.

52. Campbell JE. *Basic Trauma Life Support for Paramedics and Advanced EMS Providers*. 3rd ed. Englewood Cliffs, NJ: Brady Publishing;1995.

53. Don Michael TA, Gordon AS. The esophageal obturator airway: a new device in emergency cardiopulmonary resuscitation. *Br Med J*. 1980; 281:1531.

54. Smith JP, Bodai BI, Seifkin A, Palder S, Thomas V. The esophageal obturator airway: a review *JAMA*. 1983; 259:1081.

55. Hammargren Y, Clinton JE, Ruiz E. A standard comparison of esophageal obturator airway and endotracheal tube ventilation in cardiac arrest. *Ann Emerg Med*. 1985; 14:953.

56. Auerbach PS, Geehr EC. inadequate oxygenation and ventilation using the esophageal gastric tube airway in the prehospital setting. *JAMA*. 1983; 250:3067.

57. Meislin HW. The esophageal obturator airway: a study of respiratory effectiveness. *Ann Emerg Med*. 1980; 9:54.

58. Bryson TK, Benumof JL, Ward CF. The esophageal obturator airway: a clinical comparison to ventilation with mask and oropharyngeal airway. *Chest*. 1978; 74:537.

59. Harrison RR, Maull KI, Keenan RL, Boyan CP. Mouth-to-mask ventilation: a superior method of rescue breathing. *Ann Emerg Med*. 1982; 15:1187.

60. Pepe PE, Zachariah BS, Chandra NC. Invasive airway techniques in resuscitation. *Ann Emerg Med*. 1993; 22:2 Part 2:393.

61. Shea SR, MacDonald JR, Gruzinski G. Prehospital endotracheal tube airway or esophageal gastric tube airway: a critical comparison. *Ann Emerg Med*. 1985; 14:102.

62. Don Michael TA. The role of the esophageal obturator airway in cardipulmonary resuscitation. *Circulation*. 1986; 74(suppl IV):134.

63. Donen N, Tweed WA, Dashfsky S, Guttormson B. The esophageal obturator airway: an appraisal. *Can Anaesth Soc J*. 1983; 30:194.

64. Birnbaumer DM, Niemann JT. Esophageal airways. In: Dailey RH, Simon B, Youn GP, Stewart RD eds. *The Airway. Emergency Management*. St Louis: Mosby Yearbook; 1992.

65. McMahan S, Ornato JP, Ract EM, Cameron J. Multi-agency prehospital evaluation of the pharyngeo-tracheal lume (PTL) airway. *Prehosp Disaster Med*. 1992; 7:13.

66. Merrifield AJ, Waldemann C, Blundell MD. Ventilation through a new emergenc airway in an anesthetized man (abstract). *Proc Anaes Res Soc*. 1983; 55:1155.

67. Atherton GL , Johnson JC. Ability of paramedics to use the combitube in prehospital cardiac arrest. *Ann Emerg Med*. 1963; 22:1263.

68. Frass M, Frenzer R, Rauscha F, Weber H, Pacher R, Leithner C. Evaluation of the esophageal tracheal combitube in cardiopulmonary resuscitation. *Crit Care Med*. 1986; 15:609.

69. Rumball CJ, MacDonald D. The PTL Combitube laryngeal mask and oral airway: a randomized preshospital comparative study of ventilatory device effectiveness and cost-effectiveness in 470 cases of cardiorespiratory arrest. *Prehosp Emerg Care*. 1997; 1:1.

70. Frass M, Rodler S, Frenzer R, Ilias W, Leithner C, Lackner F. Esophageal tracheal combitube endotracheal airway and mask: comparison of ventilatory pressure curves. *J Trauma*. 1989; 29:1476.

71. Frass M, Frenzer R, Rauscha F, Schuster E, Glogar D. Ventilation with the esophageal tracheal combitube in cardiopulmonary resuscitation: promptness and effectiveness. *Chest*. 1988; 93:781.

72. Frass M, Frenzer R, Mayer G, Popovic R, Leithner C. Mechanical ventilation with the esophageal tracheal combitube (ETC) in the intensive care unit. *Arch Emerg Med*. 1987; 4:219.

73. Frass M, Frenzer K, Zdrahal F, Hoflehner G, Porges P, Lackner F. The esophageal tracheal combitube: preliminary results with a new airway for CPR. *Ann Emerg Med*. 1987; 16:768.

74. Mallampati SR, Gatt SP, Gugino LD, et al. A clinical sign to predict difficult tracheal intubation: a prospective study. *Can Anaesth Soc J*. 1985; 32:429.

75. Hubble MW. Seated orotracheal Intubation. *Emergency* . 1996; 28:18.

76. Herholdt JD, Rafn CG. Life-saving measures for drowning persons. *Copenhagen H Tikiob*. 52:1796.

77. Sykes WS. Oral endotracheal intubation without laryngoscopy: a plea for simplicity. *Curr Res Anaesth Analg*. 1937; 16:133.

78. Stewart RD. Tactile orotracheal intubation. *Ann Emerg Med*. 1984; 13:175.

79. Kuhn F. Die pernasale Tubage. *Muenchen Med Wochenschr*. 1902; 49:1456.

80. Tintinalli JE, Claffey J. Complications of nasotracheal intubation. *Ann Emerg Med*. 1981; 10:142.

81. Magill IW. Technique in endotracheal anaesthesia. *Br Med J*. 1930; 2:817.

82. Depoit JP, Depoix JP, Malbezin S, Videcoq M, et al. Oral Intubation v. nasal Intubation in adult cardiac surgery. *Br J Anaest*. 1987; 59:167.

83. Whitten CE. *Anyone Can Intubate. A Practical Step-by-Step Guide for Health Professionals*. 4th ed. San Diego, Calif: K-W Publications; 1997.

84. Iserson KV. Blind nasotracheal Intubation. *Ann Emerg Med*. 1981; 10:468.

85. Danzyl DF, Thomas DM. Nasotracheal intubation in the emergency department. *Crit Care Med*. 1980; 8:677.

86. Wingfield WE. Blind nasal intubation. *Emergency*. 1997; 29(4):14.

87. Horellou M, Mathe D, Feiss P. A hazard of nasotracheal intubation. *Anesthesia*. 1978; 33:73.

88. Taylor T , Major E. *Hazards and Complications of Anaesthesia*. 2nd ed. Naperville, Ill: Churchill Livingstone ;1993.

89. Seebacher J, Nozik D, Mathieu A. Inadvertent intracranial introduction of nasogastric tube: a complication of severe maxillofacial trauma. *Anesthesiology*. 1975; 42:100.

90. Wyler A, Reynolds A. An intracranial complication of nasogastric intubation. *J Neurosurg*. 1977; 47:297.

91. Bouzarth W. Intracranial nasogastric tube insertion. *J Trauma*. 1978; 18:818.

92. Fremstad J, Martin S. Lethal complication from insertion of nasogastric tube after severe basilar skull fracture. *J Trauma*. 1978; 18:820.

93. Pointer JE. Nasotracheal intubation. In: Dailey RH, Simon B, Young GP, Stewart RD, eds. *The Airway: Emergency Management*. St Louis: Mosby Yearbook; 1992.

94. Danzl DF. Advanced airway support. In: Tintinalli JE, Ruiz E, Krome RL, eds. *Emergency Medicine: A Comprehensive Study Guide*. 4th ed. New York: American College of Emergency Physicians; 1996.

95. Macintosh R, Richards H. Illuminated introducer for endotracheal tubes. *Anaesthesia*. 1957; 12:223.

96. Raj P, Forestner J, Watson TD, Forris RE, Jenkins MT. Techniques for fiberoptic laryngoscopy in anesthesia. *Anaesth Analg*. 1974; 53:708.

97. Ducrow M. Throwing light on blind intubation (letter). *Anaesthesia*. 1979; 34:677.

98. Vollmer TP, Stewart RD, Paris PM, Ellis D, Berkebile PE. Use of a lighted stylet for guided orotracheal intubation in the prehospital setting. *Ann Emerg Med*. 1985; 14:324.

99. Verdile VP. Digital and transillumination intubation. *Emerg Care Q*. 1987; 3:77.

100. Reinhart DJ, Simmons G. Comparison of placement of the laryngeal mask airway with endotracheal tube by paramedics and respiratory therapists. *Ann Emerg Med*. 1994; 24:260.

101. Deakin CD. Prehospital management of the traumatized airway. *Eur J Emerg Med*. 1996; 3:233.

102. Roberts I, Allsop P, Dickinson M, Curry P, Eastwick-Field P, Eyre G. Airway management training using the laryngeal mask airway: a comparison of two different training programs. *Resuscitation*. 1997; 33:211.

103. Sasada MP, Gabbott DA. The role of the laryngeal mask airway in prehospital care. *Resuscitation*. 1994; 28:97.

104. Martin SE, Ochsner MG, Jarman RH, Agudelo WE. Laryngeal mask airway in air transport when intubation fails: case report. *J Trauma*. 1997; 42:333.

105. Brimacombe J, Berry A. Laryngeal mask airway insertion: a comparison of the standard versus neutral

position in normal patients with a view to its use in cervical spine instability. *Anaesthesia*. 1993; 48:670.

106. Brain A. *The Intavent Laryngeal Mask: Instruction Manual*. Berkshire, UK:Brain Medical Limited; 1992.

107. Hooke R. Account of an experiment made by R. Hooke of preserving animals alive by blowing through their lungs with bellows. *Philos Trans R Soc Lond*. 1667; 2:539.

108. Reed JP, Kemph JP, Hamelberg W, et al. Studies with transtracheal artificial respiration. *Anesthesiology*. 1954; 15:28.

109. Yealy DM. Surgical methods of emergency airway control. *Emerg Care Q*. 1987; 3:11.

110. Ravussn P, Freeman J. A neck transtracheal catheter for ventilation and resuscitation. *Can J Anaesth*. 1985; 32:60.

111. Jackson C. Tracheostomy. *Laryngoscope*. 1909; 19:285.

112. Brantigan CO, Grow JB. Cricothyroidotomy: elective use in respiratory problem requiring tracheotomy. *J Thorac Cardiovasc Surg*. 1976; 71:71.

113. Jacobson LE, Gomez GA, Sobieray, RJ, Rodman GH, Solotkin KC, Misinski ME. Surgical cricothyroidotomy in trauma patients: analysis of its use by paramedics in the field. *J Trauma*. 1996; 41:15.

114. Esses BA, Jafek BW. Cricothyroidotomy: a decade of experience in Denver. *Ann Otol Rhinol Laryngol*. 1987; 96:519.

115. Johnson DR, Dunlap A, McFeeley P, Gaffney J, Busick B. Cricothyrotomy performed by prehospital personnel: a comparison of two techniques in a human cadaver model. *Am J Emerg Med*. 1993; 11:207.

116. Butler FS, Cirillo AA. Retrograde tracheal intubation. *Anesth Analg*. 1960; 39:333.

117. Yealy D, Paris P. Recent advances in airway management. *Emerg Med Clin North Am*. 1989; 7:8.

118. McNamara RM. Retrograde intubation of the trachea. *Ann Emerg Med*. 1987; 13:175.

119. Purcell T. Retrograde tracheal intubation. In: Dailey RH, Simon B, Young GP, Stewart RD, eds. *The Airway. Emergency Management*. St Louis:Mosby Yearbook ;1992.

120. Lyons GD, Garrett ME, Fourier DG. Complications of percutaneous transtracheal procedures. *Am J Otolayngol*.1977; 86:633.

121. Barriot P, Riou B. Retrograde technique for tracheal intubation in trauma patients. *Crit Care Med*. 1988; 16:712.

122. King HK, Wang LF, Wooten DJ. Endotracheal intubation using translaryngeal guide intubation vs. percutaneous retrograde guidewire insertion (letter*)*. *Crit Care Med*. 1987; 15:183.

123. Hedges JR, Dronen SC, Feero S, Hawkins S, Syverud SA, Schultz B. Succinylcholine-assisted intubations in prehospital care. *Ann Emerg Med*. 1988; 17:469.

124. Storer DL. The pharmacology of airway control. *Emerg Care Q*. 1991; 7:64.

125. White PE, Schlobehm RM Pitts LH, Lindauer JM. A randomized study of drugs for preventing increases in intracranial pressure during endotracheal suctioning. *Anesthesiology*. 1982; 57:212.

126. Deknatel DSP. *Understanding Chest Drainage*. Tucker, Ga: Deknatel; 1995.

127. English DK. Ventilators. In: Dailey RH, Simon B, Young GP, Stewart RD, eds. *The Airway: Emergency Management*. St Louis: Mosby Yearbook; 1992.

128. Burton GB, Gee GN, Hodgkin JE. *Respiratory Care: A Guide to Clinical Practice*, 3rd ed. Philadelphia; J.B. Lippincott; 1991.

129. Linton DM, Wells Y, Potgieter PD. Metabolic requirements in tetanus. *Crit Care Med*. 1992; 20:950.

130. Bolton PJ, Kline KA. Understanding modes of mechanical ventilation. *Am J Nurs*. 1994; June .

131. Shapiro BA. A historical perspective on ventilator management. *New Horiz*. 1994; 2:8.

132. Gibbs JM. The effects of endotracheal intubation on cardiac rate and rhythm. *NZ Med J*. 1967; 66:465.

133. Stoelting RK. Endotracheal intubation. In: Miller RD, ed. *Anesthesia*. 2nd ed. New York: Churchill-Livingstone; 1986.

134. Takashimi K, Nodak, Higaki M. Cardiovascular response to rapid anesthesia induction and endotracheal intubation *Anesth Analg*. 1964; 43:201.

135. Denlinger JK, Ellison N, Ominsky AJ. Effects of intratracheal lidocaine on circulator responses to tracheal intubation. *Anesthesiology*. 1974; 41:409.

136. Abou-Madi MN, Keszler H, Yacoub JM. Cardiovascular reactions to laryngoscope and tracheal intubation following small and large intravenous doses of lidocaine. *Ca Anaesth Soc*. 1977; J 24:12.

137. Hamill JF, Bedford RF, Weaver DC, Colohan AR. Lidocaine before endotracheal intubation: intravenous or laryngotracheal? *Anesthesiology*. 1981; 55:578.

138. Youngberg JA, Graybar G, Hutchings D. Comparison of intravenous and topical lidocaine in attenuating the cardiovascular respones to endotracheal intubation. *South Med*. 1983; 76:1122.

139. Fassoulaki A, Kaniaris P. Does atropine premedication affect the cardiovascular response to laryngoscopy and intubation? *Br J Anaesth*. 1982; 54:1065.

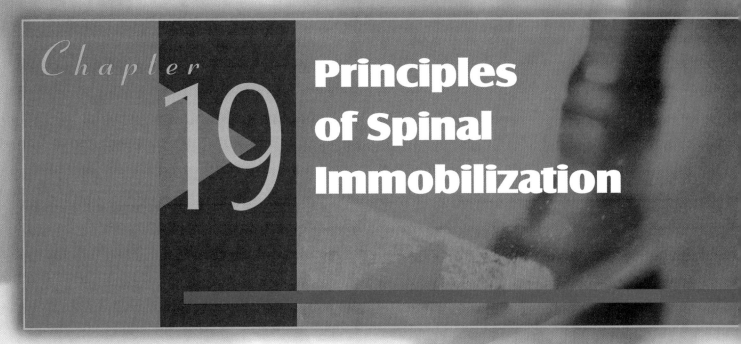

Chapter 19

Principles of Spinal Immobilization

OBJECTIVES

Upon completion of this chapter, the reader should be able to:

● Describe the importance of proper and timely management of patients with possible spinal injuries.

● Explain the difference between spinal stabilization and spinal immobilization.

● Describe the proper method to stabilize the head and neck in a neutral position of a seated or standing patient.

● Describe the proper method to stabilize the head and neck in a neutral position of a patient in a supine position.

● Explain the proper method of applying a cervical collar.

● Identify other ways to stabilize the neck when a cervical collar cannot be used.

● Explain the purpose of immobilizing a patient in a seated position before placement on a backboard.

● Describe the general principles of applying a short spine device.

● Understand the objectives of immobilizing a patient on a long backboard or similar device.

● Describe various types of straps that are available and the objectives of proper strapping techniques.

● Explain the proper technique for securing the head onto a long board.

● Describe when a standing takedown should be used.

● Explain the steps in performing a standing takedown.

● Describe the risks associated with the use of a rapid extrication.

● Explain the steps for carrying out a rapid extrication.

● List some considerations that should be taken when managing infants and children.

● Describe general principles of managing spinal injuries related to sports injuries.

● Explain the criteria and steps for removing a helmet from a patient with a possible spinal injury.

● Describe special considerations for managing a spinal injury in the water.

● Understand the criteria used to clear the spine in the field.

KEY TERMS

Immobilization
Stabilization

In Chapters 10 and 11 various types of injuries that may result from trauma to the spine and head were discussed. This chapter will review the principles of properly managing patients with head and spinal injuries. While the focus of this chapter is on spinal immobilization, remember that any patient with a possible head injury should be treated as if a spinal injury were also present.

When dealing with a spinal injury, mishandling or improper care may result in serious injury and permanent disability. Studies show that proper and rapid stabilization and immobilization in the field are correlated with fewer medical complications resulting in shorter hospital stays.[1] In order to successfully manage spinal injuries, paramedics need to know the objective of providing care, to do no "further harm." This is accomplished by preventing any further movement of the head or spine that may aggravate any preexisting or acute injuries.

When dealing with spinal trauma you are likely to be dealing with multisystem trauma in which the paramedic needs to manage the potential spinal injury while assuring that the patient has a secure airway, is receiving proper oxygenation, and maintains proper circulation. For example, a patient with serious trauma may have an unstable airway or possible spinal injury and may be going into hemorrhagic shock. This requires the paramedic to secure the airway by performing a trauma intubation, the application of PASG without manipulating the spine, and finally immobilizing the patient to protect the head and spine, all within a short time span.

This chapter will not provide the answers to every possible situation; however, it will present the principles of immobilization that will provide the paramedic with the knowledge and skills necessary to manage a patient with a spinal injury.

STABILIZATION VERSUS IMMOBILIZATION

Paramedics need to understand the concept of and difference between stabilization and immobilization. **Stabilization** is defined as the process of making firm or steady.[2] In other words, keeping the injured part from moving. This concept is typically emphasized when splinting extremities. When it comes to stabilizing the head and back, the need to prevent or minimize any further movement to the head, neck, and back is critical. This is primarily accomplished by maintaining the head in a neutral, in-line position.

Immobilization of the spine is defined as a procedure that involves placing the body in an immobile position to protect the spinal cord when injury is suspected.[3] More specifically, this includes securing the

patient's head, torso, and extremities to a backboard or similar device to keep the spine from moving. A good way to remember the difference between the two is that stabilization is temporary and immobilization is more permanent. This is why manual in-line stabilization is performed when first arriving on the scene, not immobilization, which is accomplished after the patient is fully secured to a backboard device.

STABILIZATION

The first principle when dealing with a spinal injury is the concept of stabilization. Positioning the head in a neutral in-line position provides the best alignment of the spinal canal and allows the maximum opening for the spinal cord if it begins to swell from an injury. When stabilizing the head and neck of a patient, especially of a seated or standing patient, consider the following:

- The average weight of the adult human head is 15–17 pounds.
- The head is connected and supported to the spinal column by the first two small vertebrate, the atlas and axis, and skeletal support muscles
- When there is severe injury to the neck, these support muscles are weakened, and the weight of the head is supported only by the two vertebrate. This may result in compression of the spinal cord.

These points are important to remember when trying to stabilize the head and neck. When stabilizing the head and neck, it is important to support the back or occipital region of the head and the front part of the head (Figure 19-1). This is easily accomplished by supporting the back of the patient's head with the thumbs while supporting the mandible and face with the middle and index fingers. The other two fingers help support the cervical spine. This position also keeps the ears exposed so the patient can hear. Holding the head solely from the sides does not help alleviate the weight bearing down on the vertebrate.

If the patient is in a supine position, compression is not much of a concern; however, lateral rotation is. To accomplish stabilization on a supine patient, the paramedic should spread his or her hands and place them evenly on either side of the patient's head. The paramedic's elbows should rest on the ground stabilizing his or her arms to prevent accidental movement of the patient's head, should the paramedic shift body position (Figure 19-2). This position also allows easy monitoring of the airway and permits the paramedic to open the airway using the jaw-thrust technique if needed.

There are some situations in which the paramedic should not attempt to place the patient's head in a neutral position. These include:

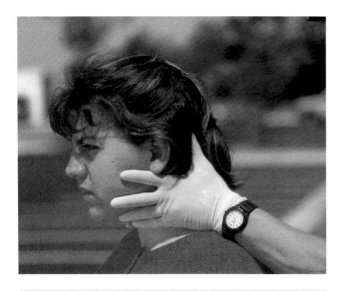

FIGURE 19-1 Manual in-line stabilization. (Rick Brady, photographer.)

- Patient complaint of severe pain, pressure, or numbness when attempting to move the head.
- Resistance felt when trying to move the head.
- The patient's head is severely angulated and movement is painful.

In these situations, the paramedic should hold the head in place and immobilize the patient in the position found.

Stabilization of the head is one of the most important skills in immobilization. All paramedics should be proficient in properly stabilizing the patient's head.

The Use of Cervical Collars

There are many devices on the market to assist the paramedic in accomplishing in-line stabilization. The use of rigid cervical or extrication collars has been a standard in prehospital care since the early 1970s.

A cervical collar is designed to help the paramedic maintain the patient's head in a neutral in-line position. Cervical collars serve two roles: to help alleviate the pressure placed on the cervical spine by the head as a result of weakened muscles from overstretching, such as in a hyperextension or flexion injury, and to limit movement of the neck. A cervical collar alone does not provide adequate stabilization or immobilization of the head and neck. A cervical collar should always be accompanied by in-line stabilization.

A wide variety of collars have been marketed and several studies have evaluated their effectiveness.[4] The early collars used in prehospital care were made of soft foam. In the 1970s, collars made of stronger materials, originally designed to be used in the hospital, such as the Philadelphia collar, proved to be better than the soft foam collars.[5] However, these collars were not made specifically for prehospital care. Later, one-piece polyethylene collars were developed, such as California Medical's Stifneck Extrication collar. Studies showed that one-piece hard collars were more effective in minimizing cervical spine movement.[6] Since then many other manufacturers such as Jobst, Ambu, and Jerome Medical have developed extrication collars (Figure 19-3). In 1991, Philadelphia introduced its Red EM Philadelphia Cervical Collar. This red collar was designed to be used in the field.[7] A study done by Ducker in 1990 showed that two-piece collars such as the NecLoc collar were better than one-piece collars.[8] These plastic collars come in various sizes, requiring the

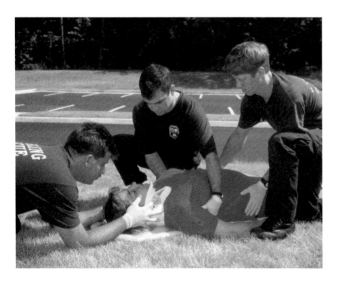

FIGURE 19-2 In-line stabilization of the supine patient. (Rick Brady, photographer.)

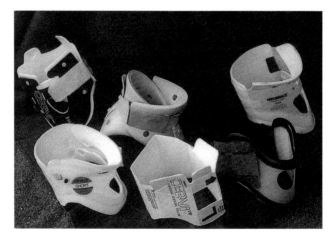

FIGURE 19-3 Over time various types and styles of collars have been developed for prehospital care.

paramedic to know how to measure the patient for the proper size collar. While there are no recent studies on the effectiveness of different types of collars, Table 19-1 presents results of a study done in the mid-1980s showing that polyethylene (rigid plastic) collars were more effective for prehospital care.[6] The study showed that the polyethylene-1 collar was most effective. Although the polyethylene-2 collar scored better in measuring extension and lateral bending, these scores were not statistically significant.

Recently, manufacturers have developed single adjustable collars to replace the various sized collars. These include Laerdal's Stifneck SELECT collar and Ambu's Perfit ACE adjustable collar. However, to date there have been no clinical investigations of their effectiveness. One concern is that the collars adjust for neck height in the front but are not adjustable in the back. A new collar on the market, the WIZ LOC by the Kohlbrat+Bunz Corporation, may address this concern. This collar provides an occipital adjustment. Studies have shown that prolonged use of collars may cause irritation to the occipital lobe and the chin area since these are the two support points for collars.[9] Completely adjustable collars may help ease these complications. The overwhelming number of collar designs requires the paramedic to be proficient and familiar with the collars that are used. Regardless of the type of collar chosen, there are certain points to remember:

- The collar must be for prehospital use. Soft foam collars and collars used for rehabilitation should not be used.
- The paramedic must be familiar with the proper way to size the collar(s) being used.
- The paramedic must know the proper steps in applying a cervical collar.

- The paramedic should understand the purpose of a cervical collar and appreciate the importance of proper collar application.

The use of rigid cervical collars has been demonstrated to be effective for stabilizing the spine. However, if not properly used, cervical collars can also create complications. A study done by Houghton and Curley showed that if a collar is too small or too tightly placed it may restrict laryngeal movement during swallowing, which can be misinterpreted as a neuromuscular function disorder.[10] A collar that is too small applies pressure on the throat and can result in a decrease of venous return or may cause the patient to experience hypotension from vagal nerve stimulation. These concerns are even greater with collars that do not have an opening in the middle allowing access to monitor the trachea and jugular veins.

Proper Application of Cervical Collars

The effectiveness of a cervical collar is based on the proper application of the device. A collar that is improperly measured or applied can result in harm to the patient. Applying a collar that is too large can result in hyperextension, whereas applying a collar that is too small may lead to hyperflexion. In addition, as studies have shown, a collar that is applied improperly can result in airway compromise.

The first step in applying a collar is selecting the proper size. Many collars on the market today come in four sizes: extra small (no neck), small, medium, and large. Since there are many more sizes of necks than there are collars, there will not always be an exact fit. However, in determining the proper size, the most reliable indicator is whether the collar is accomplishing its goals. Is the head maintained in a neutral in-line position? Is the collar providing proper support to the head? Is the collar applied snugly without compromising the airway? Answering these questions will help in determining if the selected collar has been properly sized.

While there are many ways to measure for a collar, it is important to follow the manufacturer's recommendations. A popular method for measuring collars is the finger-width technique. This method was originally designed to measure the Stifneck collar,[11] but it has been adopted for use with other collars.

To use the finger-width technique on a standing or sitting patient, a paramedic places the fingers of one hand next to the patient's neck, while another paramedic is maintaining in-line stabilization. An imaginary line is drawn across the top of the patient's shoulders, the trapezius muscle, and across the chin (Figure 19-4). The space between these two imaginary lines is measured using the fingers. After determining how many finger-widths there are between these two "key dimensions,"

Table 19-1
Effectiveness of Cervical Immobilization Collars: Average Rank Scores (±SD)

Collar	Flexion	Extension	Lateral Bending
Polyethylene-1[a]	1.29±.49	2.79±.81	2.14±.85
Polyethylene-2[b]	2.57±1.13	2.50±1.19	1.71±.70
Philadelphia[c]	3.07±.45	2.00±1.15	3.00±.76
Extrication[d]	2.07±1.24	3.14±1.21	3.14±1.46

[a]Stifneck type.

[b]Nec-Loc type.

[c]Tan collar.

[d]Foam collar.

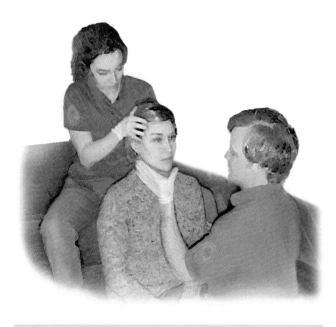

FIGURE 19-4 Sizing for a collar involves measuring the area between the top of the patient's shoulder and an imaginary line across the level of the chin.

the space between the edge of the hard plastic and the black peg on the Stifneck collar is measured and a determination is made as to which collar has the same finger-width as the patient's key dimensions. Other collars have a similar notch or measurement line that matches the finger-width measurement. Often, paramedics measure the angle of the jaw or the bottom of the ear; however, the correct landmark is an imaginary line across the chin. Other collars such as the Philadelphia or the Necloc require only that the paramedic visualize the proper size and assure that the patient is in a neutral position when the collar is in place.

Once the proper size has been determined, the paramedic is ready to apply the collar. Follow these steps:

- If you are using a collar that has been lying flat or was just assembled, preform the collar to give it a round shape.
- Grasp the collar from the front and place the collar against the patient's chest.
- Slide the collar up into position, under the neck, and begin to wrap the collar around the patient's neck.
- Reach behind the patient and grab the loose end of the collar, bring it around the patient, and secure the Velcro. When tightening the collar, support the front of the collar by grabbing the tracheal opening hole. This keeps the collar steady and keeps it from moving as the collar is tightened around the patient's neck.

- The collar should be under the chin, supporting the mandible without digging into the soft part of the neck. The collar should be wrapped around the patient's head and secured.
- Once the collar has been applied, make sure that the collar is positioned properly. The patient should be in a neutral position with the eyes straight ahead. If the patient's eyes are positioned toward the ceiling or to the floor, the collar is not the correct size.
- Despite proper measurement, there may be occasions when the collar does not fit properly. If this occurs, remove the collar and place another collar without releasing manual stabilization at any point.

One of the biggest challenges to providers is applying the collar around the person maintaining in-line stabilization. The manual in-line stabilization method described earlier allows for easy application of a cervical collar. The back of the head is supported by the thumbs while the front and sides are supported by the middle and index fingers, leaving the ring and small fingers free. From this position the paramedic stabilizing the head can spread his or her fingers apart while still maintaining in-line stabilization. This technique is called "spreading your wings" (Figure 19-5).

Special Situations

If the patient is lying supine, the application of a collar is more challenging. Remember that the application of a collar in a supine position is primarily to minimize movement. The finger-width method can be used to measure for a collar in the same manner as it is done

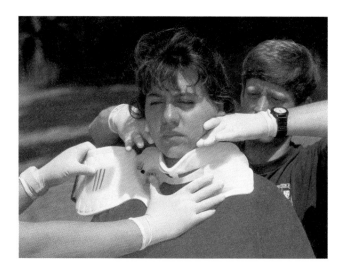

FIGURE 19-5 Using the "spreading your wings" technique while stabilizing the head and neck allows for easy collar placement. (Rick Brady, photographer.)

for a sitting patient. Unfortunately, the measurement on a supine patient may be more difficult depending on the patient's position and whether the shoulders are relaxed or in a shrugged position.

To apply the collar simply slide the front of the collar under the chin into position. While holding the collar in place, feed the end of the collar under the patient's head. While maintaining the front piece of the collar in place, wrap the end of the collar around the patient and secure it in place making sure that the head is in a neutral position.

There may be some instances when no collar fits properly or a collar cannot be placed because of the patient's position, such as a severe angulation of the head and spine. In these cases the paramedic must improvise. A rolled-up towel or sheet may be placed around the patient's neck for support (Figure 19-6). If a collar cannot be applied and local protocols require the use of a collar, it is important to document the reasons why a collar could not be applied.

IMMOBILIZATION OF THE SEATED PATIENT

A common situation the paramedic encounters is immobilizing a patient with a possible spinal injury in a seated position, typically after a car crash. In this situation, the patient's head and neck are the most vulnerable for injury. Therefore, the head and cervical spine need to be secured before the patient is removed from the car.

There are several devices on the market for seated spinal immobilization. The simplest device is the short backboard or half spine board that has been used in pre-hospital care since the early 1970s. This device, although very useful, lost its popularity with the introduction of the

vestlike devices, the most common being the Ferno Kendrick Extrication Device, known as the KED, introduced in 1978 (Figure 19-7). Changes in vehicle construction such as bucket seats also made the standard short-board device more difficult to use. Continuous evolution in car manufacturing and spinal management have led to the development of other vestlike devices. These devices wrap around the patient and provide a snug fit around the patient. Other devices, such as the Kansas board, the Oregon Splint II, and the XP-One, are also on the market. Some EMS systems also use a narrower version of the traditional short board

All stable or potentially unstable patients should be immobilized in a seated position before being moved onto a long board. Many times paramedics believe that the time taken to do this delays patient care and prolongs on-scene time. Others may fail to see the benefit of seated immobilization. Regardless, the standard of care is that any patient with a suspected spinal injury but without an immediately life threatening injury should be fully immobilized. Paramedics need to be comfortable and proficient in immobilizing a patient on a short-board device.

It is important to ascertain neurological status before and after any intervention. The paramedic

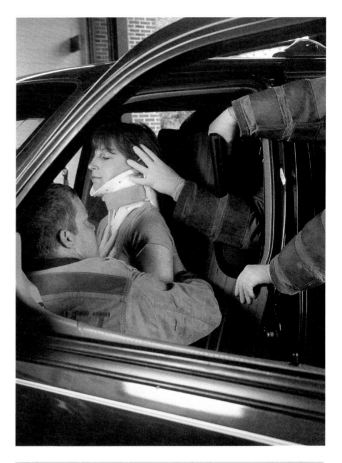

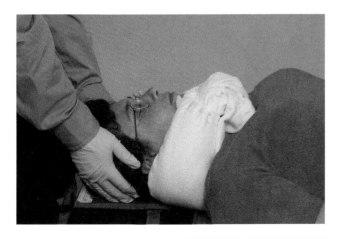

FIGURE 19-6 In some situations the paramedic can use a rolled towel as a cervical collar.

FIGURE 19-7 The Ferno Kendrick Extrication Device.

should assess the extremities for pulses, movement, and sensation (Table 19-2). Once the neurological assessment has been completed, a short spine device can be applied.

Short-Board Devices

A common type of short spine device is the short backboard. The short backboard was the standard of care for many years before the evolution of new devices in the late 1970s. The biggest drawback of the short board is its poor adaptation to bucket or contour seats.

There are various strapping techniques used for the short board. The best technique is the one that works best for the patient. To apply a short-board device:

1. Stabilize the patient's head, assess distal pulses and motor and sensory function in all extremities, and apply a cervical collar.

2. Move the patient forward as a unit and place the board behind the patient.

3. Move the patient back into position. Make sure the top of the short board is even with the top of the patient's head.

4. Secure the patient's torso. A common way is using the crisscross technique. Rest the buckle of the strap on the patient's shoulder. Feed the end of the strap through the top hole of the short board. Feed the strap through the hole at the bottom from behind the board. Pull the strap through the hole across the patient to the top of the opposite shoulder and feed it through the top hole of the board. Feed the strap behind the board and

through the bottom hole back across the patient and attach it to the buckle. A second strap can be attached around the bottom as a seat belt to secure the bottom of the board.

5. Secure the patient's head to the short board using cravats, tape, or roller gauze. Make sure the patient's head remains in a neutral position.

6. Assess distal pulses and motor and sensory function in all extremities and prepare the patient to be moved to the long board.

Once application of the short board is completed, the patient's head and upper torso should be immobile. Some strapping techniques call for the inclusion of the legs when securing the patient to the short board. This depends on local protocol and preferred strapping techniques.

Vest-Type Devices

When applying the KED or any vest-type device, it is important that manual stabilization is maintained throughout the process and that a cervical collar is in place. To place the device behind the patient, the patient may need to be moved forward as a unit. To do this, one paramedic maintains stabilization of the head while a second paramedic supports the patient's upper torso. One hand is placed behind the patient to support the neck and back, while the other hand is placed on the chest with the forearm parallel to the sternum for support. On the count of the paramedic at the head, the patient is moved forward. The second paramedic now takes the device and places it behind the patient. Once the device is in position, the second paramedic supports the patient's body, as the patient is placed back in a neutral position. The paramedic at the head once again counts to initiate the move.

Once the patient is in place, the paramedic should make sure the device is properly positioned. This entails having the device centered and the flaps of the device right under the armpits. The next step is to secure the torso. This includes securing the torso straps in the proper order. For the KED device the recommendation is the middle and bottom torso straps followed by the leg straps, which must be released when the patient is placed supine, securing the head and finally the top torso strap. The order of application of the torso straps is not too critical; it is important to remember that the top chest strap should be tightened last since it may affect breathing. When securing the top strap, the paramedic should tell the patient to exhale and then take a deep breath. The strap is tightened in this position since the chest will be fully expanded. If the top strap is tightened while the victim is exhaling, breathing will be hindered by limiting chest excursion.

Table 19-2
Circulatory/Neurological Assessment

Upper extremities

    Check for the presence of radial pulses.

    Ask patients if they can feel you touch their hands.

    Ask patients to wiggle their fingers.

    Ask patients to squeeze your finger.

Lower extremities

    Check for presence of pedal pulses.

    Ask patients if they feel you touching their feet.

    Ask patients to wiggle their toes.

    Ask patients to push down with their feet.

    Ask patients to pull up with their feet.

This assessment should be done before and after immobilizing a patient.

In 1989, another vestlike device, the Oregon Spine Splint II by Skedco, Inc., was introduced. This device, although similar to the KED, offers some additional features. It is secured in position by the use of shoulder straps, which prevents the device from moving up and down. The flaps on this device do not reach around the front of the victim which allows for complete access to the anterior chest. The torso straps are used to hold the device to the patient. The leg straps are actually groin straps that are pulled up between the legs and on either side of the patient. However, they will not interfere with circulation when the legs are lowered on a backboard. Similar to the KED, the head is secured to the device using Velcro straps (Figure 19-8).

The key steps to applying a vest-type device are:

1. Maintain manual stabilization, check pulses and motor and sensory function, and apply a cervical collar.
2. Move the patient forward as a unit and place the device behind the patient.
3. Move the patient back into a neutral position and make sure the device is aligned properly.
4. Secure the torso straps.
5. Secure the leg straps.
6. Secure the head straps.

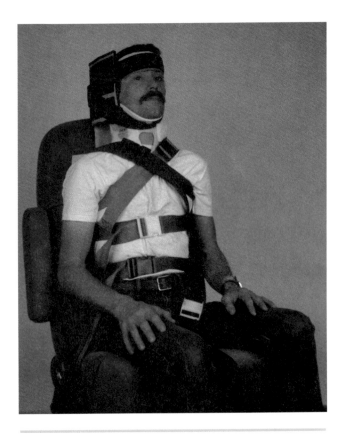

FIGURE 19-8 The Oregon Spine Splint II.

Note: When securing the head, fill any necessary voids between the head and the device. Remember that too much padding causes the head to hyperflex when the patient is in a supine position. If possible, the person maintaining stabilization should try to bring the device to the patient, minimizing the void between the device and the patient.

7. Check pulses and motor and sensory functions and prepare to move the patient.

IMMOBILIZATION OF THE SUPINE PATIENT

Any patient with a suspected spinal injury should be secured to a spine board to fully immobilize the spine. This has been the standard in the industry for over 30 years. The original boards were made out of wood. However, recently they are more commonly made of fiberglass or plastic.

Use of Long-Board Devices

Recently, there have been studies questioning the effectiveness of immobilizing patients on rigid boards. In a study of healthy individuals placed on a board for 30 minutes, the subjects all developed pain from lying on rigid boards. Some individuals developed additional symptoms such as headache, back and neck stiffness, nausea, and sciatica 48 hours after being on a board.[12] This raises concern about the consequences of keeping patients on these devices.

New devices on the market attempt to minimize these problems while still immobilizing the patient. One such device is Hartwell's Vacuum Splint. This device looks like an air mattress and is placed under then shaped around the patient. Air is then withdrawn from the device using a pump. As air is removed, the device hardens and molds to the patient. This allows the patient to be immobilized without the discomfort of lying on a rigid board. Goldberg et al., comparing symptoms developed after standard backboard immobilization and immobilization with a vacuum mattress splint, discovered that subjects were three times more likely to have symptoms from being immobilized on a backboard.[13] The study also showed that subjects were seven times more likely to complain of occipital pain and four times more likely to complain of pain to the lumbar sacral region when immobilized on a rigid board versus a vacuum mattress. In a similar study by Johnson et al., the vacuum splint was judged to be more comfortable.[14] It also provided better immobilization of the torso and less slippage when the device was tilted. The vacuum splint is applied in a similar time frame as the long board with comparable, if not better, immobilization. While more studies are showing the positive effects of vacuum-type devices, the cost and tracking of these devices within an EMS system make widespread adoption unlikely.

One of the challenges faced by paramedics when caring for a patient with a possible spinal injury is placing the patient on the board. For many years the log roll has been the standard method of placing a patient on a backboard. However, studies have shown that the log roll may not be as effective as once believed. This is partly because when a patient is rolled on the side, he or she is not in an in-line position. As the person is rolled on the side, the pelvis is the widest point. The body then tapers down the legs. In order to properly roll a patient on the side, the legs need to be kept in line with the rest of the body. This requires that the paramedic supporting the lower legs hold the legs in-line as the person is turned. This also means that the lower legs are kept off the ground when the person is rolled, keeping the body in an in-line position. Failure to do so allows the weight of the legs to bend the spine laterally toward the ground (Figure 19-9). Since the log roll is not effective in maintaining in-line position, other techniques should be considered, such as using a straight lift or a scoop stretcher to place the person on a backboard.

Another challenge when placing a patient on a backboard is how to center the patient on the board. Many times, after being placed on the board, the patient is not centered properly and paramedics are faced with having to move the patient, jeopardizing the integrity of the spine. Two techniques can be used to center the patient while minimizing the movement on the spine.

The first technique requires the paramedic to place the top third of the backboard higher than the patient. Once the patient is rolled onto the board, the patient can be slid up on the board as a unit in an up-

and-over motion. This centers the patient on the board. Moving the patient along the axis minimizes movement to the spine. An approach that can be used when there is no room to place the board higher than the patient is to roll the patient on the board, then slide the patient down and then up again into position. This technique also minimizes movement of the spine. This technique is sometimes referred to as the "Z" slide.

While using either technique, it is important that the patient is properly moved. Ideally, this should be done with three paramedics. One paramedic stabilizes the patient's head while the second paramedic supports the patient under the armpits and the third paramedic supports the patient from the pelvis. In this manner, the patient's largest and strongest body parts are secured.

Straps and Strapping Techniques

One area of controversy is the use of straps. There are many types and styles of straps (Figure 19-10). While paramedics are sometimes limited to whichever straps are available, it is important to remember that the best straps and the best strapping technique is the one that meets the objectives of immobilizing the spine. When immobilizing the spine, it is important that the patient's head, thorax, pelvis, and upper legs be secured. How many straps are used or how they are applied is not important as long as the patient can not move (Figure 19-11).

Several types of straps, such as speed clips, allow quick application of straps across the body. However, they have been scrutinized for their limitations since they can only be applied where there are pins on the board. These pins also make it harder to grab the board while wearing leather gloves.

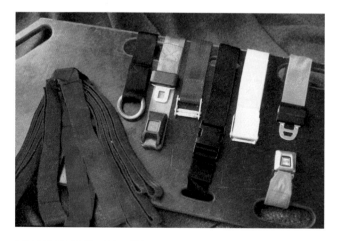

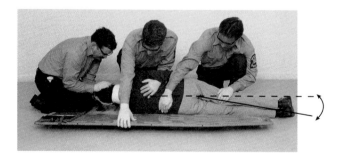

FIGURE 19-9 When performing a log roll paramedics must keep the patient in an in-line position. This requires elevating the legs.

FIGURE 19-10 Various types and styles of buckles and straps are available on the market today. (Courtesy of Jose Salazar & Associates, Sterling, VA.)

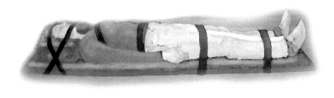

FIGURE 19-11 A patient fully immobilized is secured at the head, chest, pelvis, upper legs, and lower legs.

Another popular type of strap is the Spider or quick strap. The Spider strap is one strap with several straps attached to it. While this strap can have some advantages, there are also certain limitations. To properly apply the strap, two paramedics are needed to secure the strap simultaneously on both sides. This is necessary to maintain equal pressure on both sides while adjusting the strap. To properly align this type of strap, it should be applied beginning at the shoulders and then tightened as the strap is applied down the body. When applying the strap, it should be aligned over the bony structures of the body. These include the chest, pelvis, and upper legs. A strap over the lower legs restricts their movement.

Individual straps provide more flexibility and can be adapted to meet virtually all strapping needs. While some paramedics believe that using individual straps is more time consuming and difficult to accomplish, it is really a matter of practice.

When using individual straps, single-buckle straps are recommended. This type of strap allows the buckle to be left in place while the other, buckleless end can be fed through the holes of the backboard. These straps should also be at least 10 feet in length. Some experts recommend using a crisscross pattern over the chest and straps over the lower half of the body. Regardless of the strapping technique used, remember the following:

- Always secure the torso before the head.
- Make sure that straps are placed over the thorax, pelvis, and upper legs.
- Pad any areas where straps will come in direct contact with skin and any voids between the patient and the board.
- When tightening straps, do not simply pull the strap through the buckle, but feed the strap through the buckle as you tighten the strap.
- When strapping small patients and children, pad the board with blankets to ensure there are no voids between the patient and the straps.
- Always use the best technique for the patient's needs, not your needs.
- When immobilizing a pregnant patient, make sure to tilt the board about 15° to the left to relieve any

pressure the gravid uterus may place on the mother's blood vessels when she is lying completely supine. This position avoids supine hypotension syndrome. (See Chapter 25.)

IMMOBILIZATION OF THE HEAD

Once the body has been secured, the last step is to secure the head to the backboard. This is an important step and should not be overlooked. Transporting a patient to the hospital with the head improperly secured defeats the purpose of immobilizing the patient in the first place.

Before securing the head, make sure that the head is in a neutral position and not tilted back. In some patients this may necessitate placing a pad under the head. Several studies have investigated the use of padding under the head. DeLorenzo et al. showed that the optimal position of the head for neutral alignment is a slight hyperflexion that can be achieved by raising the head about 2 cm.[15] This positioning provides the greatest opening between the spinal canal and the spinal cord. Because spinal cord swelling may result from an injury to the spine, providing a greater canal opening reduces the chance of additional injury. Depending on the device being used to secure the head, this padding may already be in place.

Devices for securing the head have also evolved. Years ago, a blanket rolled up and shaped like a horseshoe was wrapped around the head and secured with cravats and/or tape. Since then devices such as the Ferno Head Immobilizer, the Bashaw CID, the Laerdal Headbed, the Auto Cradle, and many other similar devices ranging from foam blocks to cardboard head immobilizers are in use today. Again, many devices are available to meet the various needs and budgets of providers. Sandbags should never be used because they can cause injury when patients need to be turned if they begin to vomit.

Paramedics need to be familiar with local head immobilization equipment. For example, the Laerdal Headbed utilizes a two-strap system. One strap fits around the patient's head and keeps the flaps in place, while the top strap secures the head firmly to the board. If either strap is used improperly, the device may not work. The Ferno Head Immobilizer uses two head blocks attached with Velcro to a base and then strapped in place. However, if the base is not positioned on the board before the patient is placed on the board, the head blocks cannot be used. Many providers still rely on the use of simple blocks with tape to secure the head. Unfortunately, the head is not always secured properly with tape.

Many EMT students were told to turn the tape over or to place a piece of gauze on the forehead of the patient to avoid catching the eyebrows. While this may be acceptable in the classroom, it is not acceptable in the field. The presence of gauze or upside-down tape over the eyebrows means that the patient's head is not immobilized. The patient's head can slide under the tape. In order to properly secure the patient's head, the tape must go directly over the patient's forehead. When properly placed, the head will not be able to move from side to side.

A chin or collar strap is also used to help secure the head; however, the use of a chin strap is contraindicated. Some providers now use a collar strap, but again, airway management is a concern. A collar strap should only be used when there is constant monitoring of the patient's airway. The collar strap should be removed if the patient begins to vomit.

INTERNET ACTIVITIES

● Visit the British Trauma Society Web site at http://www.trauma.org/eates/ectc/ectc-spine.html and review the material on spinal injury assessment and management.
● Visit the British Trauma Society Web site at http://www.trauma.org/anaesthesia/cspine anaes.html and review the material on spinal injury assessment, management, presentation, and complications.

SPECIAL SITUATIONS

This chapter has addressed the principles of spinal management for most patients. There may be some situations in which the paramedic will have to approach spinal immobilization in a different manner. Two common situations paramedics face are patients that are standing or walking and complaining of neck pain, and unstable or critical patients that need to be rapidly removed from a vehicle. Techniques have been developed to assist providers with management of these situations.

STANDING TAKEDOWN

Upon arrival at the scene of a motor vehicle crash, paramedics may encounter a patient standing outside his or her vehicle complaining of neck pain. Having the patient lie down on the stretcher can cause excessive spine movement. In this situation, the use of a standing or rapid takedown should be used.[16] This technique ensures in-line stabilization while the patient is still standing by lowering the patient to the ground with a backboard already in place.

To complete a standing takedown, follow these steps:

1. One paramedic instructs the patient to stop moving and stabilizes the head. Initially this can be done from the front until another provider arrives to assist. Approaching a patient from behind and grabbing the head can startle the patient and cause him or her to jerk. Once in-line stabilization is achieved, a quick neurological assessment is performed and a cervical collar applied.

2. While maintaining in-line stabilization, a second paramedic places the backboard behind the patient by sliding the board between the arms of the paramedic who is maintaining in-line stabilization (Figure 19-12).

3. A third paramedic helps place the board directly behind the patient. The patient's head should rest against the board (Figure 19-13).

4. Each paramedic at the side grasps the handhold that is slightly above the patient's armpit with the hand closest to the patient while facing the paramedic who is holding in-line stabilization (Figure 19-14).

5. On the count of the paramedic at the head, the two paramedics on the side begin to lower the board by walking forward. These paramedics will end up kneeling on one knee. The paramedic supporting the head carefully rotates his or her hands while maintaining stabilization as the

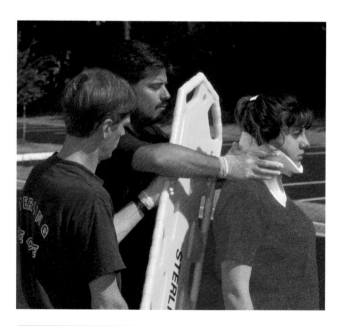
FIGURE 19-12 While maintaining stabilization, paramedics place the backboard behind the patient. (Rick Brady, photographer.)

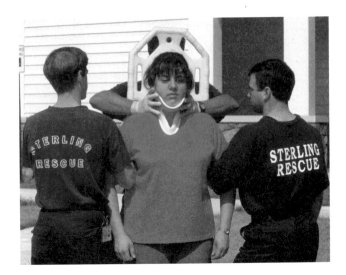

FIGURE 19-13 One paramedic on each side of the patient grabs the backboard. (Rick Brady, photographer.)

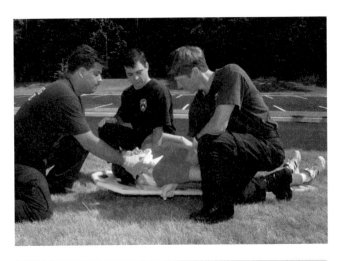

FIGURE 19-15 Proper bending techniques should be used while lowering the patient to the ground. (Rick Brady, photographer.)

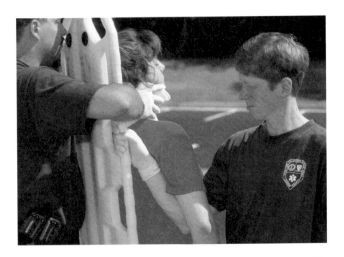

FIGURE 19-14 Hands are placed in handholds above the patient's armpit. (Rick Brady, photographer.)

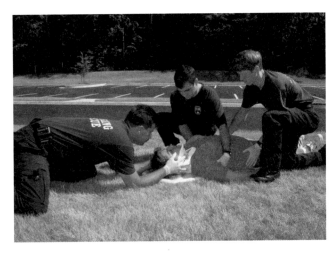

FIGURE 19-16 While maintaining in-line stabilization, the paramedics properly align the patient on the board. (Rick Brady, photographer.)

patient is lowered. The patient's head should remain in contact with the board at all times (Figure 19-15).

6. Once the patient is lowered onto the backboard, the patient is centered and raised on the board as necessary. The paramedic at the head calls for the move while one paramedic supports the patient under the arms and the other paramedic supports the patient from the pelvis (Figure 19-16).

After the patient is positioned on the backboard, the patient can be fully immobilized. This technique is based not on strength but rather on technique and coordination. Through practice this technique can be done quickly and efficiently. It is important that para-medics bend from the knees and not the waist to avoid back injury. One of the paramedics should continuously explain the procedure to the patient.

RAPID EXTRICATION

There may be some situations in which a patient in critical condition needs to be removed from a vehicle quickly and paramedics lack the time to apply a vest-type immobilization device, but some type of spinal integrity needs to be maintained. The rapid extrication technique should only be used on patients who are crit-ical these patients cannot afford the time required to be fully immobilized in a short spine device and then onto a long board. These are the same situations in which there is not time to remove doors or the roof. In these cases, the paramedic's objective is to rapidly remove the patient onto a backboard with only a cervical collar in place. This technique requires at least three trained paramedics and a bystander and should be practiced before it is done in the field. To perform a rapid extrication, follow these steps:

1. One paramedic performs an initial assessment while another paramedic stabilizes the C-spine. Once it has been determined that the patient requires a rapid extrication, a collar is placed on the patient.

2. One paramedic is positioned at the head, another paramedic outside the vehicle, and the third paramedic inside the vehicle on the other side of the patient. While the paramedic on either side of the victim lifts the patient about 1 inch off the seat, a fourth paramedic or bystander places the backboard under the patient (Figure 19-17).

3. On the count of the paramedic at the head, the patient is turned a quarter turn toward the door. The paramedic outside supports the patient under the arms, while the third paramedic begins to free the patient's legs. At this point the paramedic at the head will not be able to continue to support the head since the car's "B" post will be in the way (Figure 19-18).

4. The paramedic on the outside takes over in-line stabilization, and the paramedic at the head comes out of the back seat and supports the patient under the arms. The patient is turned and

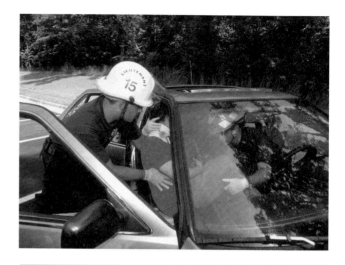

FIGURE 19-18 On the count from the paramedic at the head, the patient is turned a quarter turn. (Rick Brady, photographer.)

lowered to the board. If available, the ambulance cot should be placed under the board for additional support (Figure 19-19).

5. Once the patient is lowered, the patient is pulled onto the board. The board is then secured to the cot (Figure 19-20).

While every attempt is made to minimize movement of the spine, this technique greatly jeopardizes the spine. Therefore, it should only be used in situations where the patient is in critical condition or unstable. It should not be used as a shortcut for quickly removing stable patients from vehicles.

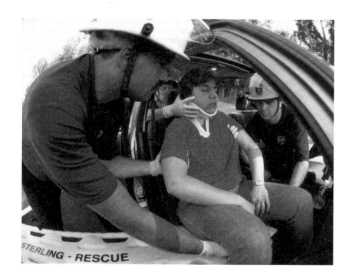

FIGURE 19-17 As two paramedics lift the patient the backboard is positioned under the patient. (Rick Brady, photographer.)

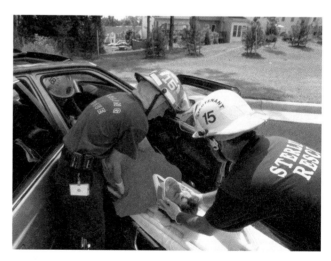

FIGURE 19-19 The rescuer outside takes over in-line stabilization as the other two rescuers turn and lower the patient to the board. (Rick Brady, photographer.)

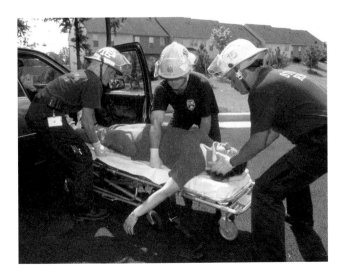

FIGURE 19-20 Once the patient is supine on the board, the patient is removed from the vehicle. (Rick Brady, photographer.)

PEDIATRIC IMMOBILIZATION

When dealing with an infant or child with a possible spinal injury, it is important to remember that there are certain differences between caring for these patients versus an adult patient. There are significant anatomical differences between children and adults.

The head of a child (8 years of age or younger) is larger in proportion to the rest of the body. As a result, when a child is placed in a supine position, the head flexes forward. In order to place a child in a neutral position, padding, such as a towel, is placed under the shoulders to maintain a neutral position and prevent the head from flexing. Since a child has a larger head, most of the injuries to a pediatric patient are in the cervical region and result from falls.[17]

It is often easier to immobilize infants or small children in their car seats. Using towels and blankets to pad the sides of the car seat, the child can be immobilized. If the car seat has been damaged, it should not be used. If needed, lay the child down and rapidly extricate out of the car seat.

Pediatric immobilizers such as the Ferno Pedi-Pac and the LSP Pediatric Immobilization Board are specially designed for children. If a child is being secured to an adult-size backboard, padding may be added around the sides of the board to fill any voids that may exist. A short backboard may work well as a long board for small children and infants.

The pediatric patient may be very agitated and scared and begin to thrash about and resist being immobilized. In this situation, it may be best to stop any intervention and allow the child to calm down, thus minimizing movement.

HELMET AND EQUIPMENT REMOVAL

In most situations, when dealing with a patient who may have a spinal injury and is wearing a helmet such as a motorcycle or sports helmet, it does not have to be removed. Helmets should only be removed if there is an airway problem (Figure 19-21 A–E). Most biker and sport helmets are custom fitted and provide support for the head.

When dealing with football and hockey helmets, the face piece can usually be cut off, allowing access to the airway. If a patient is wearing shoulder pads and the helmet has been removed, the shoulder pads also need to be removed; otherwise, hyperextension of the head will result. Alternatively, padding can be placed behind the patient's head. Individuals such as athletic trainers are familiar with this equipment and can be very helpful at the scene.

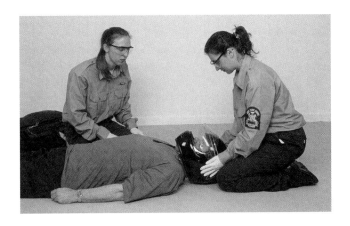

FIGURE 19-21 Helmet removal procedure. (A) Initial stabilization is provided by grasping the sides of the helmet.

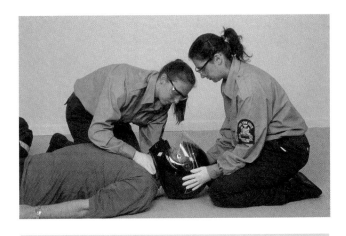

FIGURE 19-21 (B) The first paramedic loosens the chin strap and grasps the mandible with one hand. The other hand is placed under the occiput. The second paramedic takes over in-line stabilization of the head.

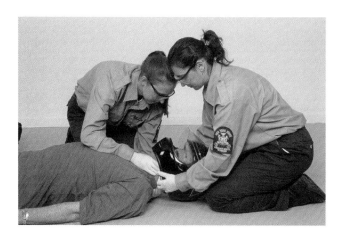

FIGURE 19-21 (C) The first paramedic now releases the sides of the helmet and grasps the lower rim of the helmet on both sides. The helmet is spread apart and rotated gently so that it clears the nose. The second paramedic continues to support the head.

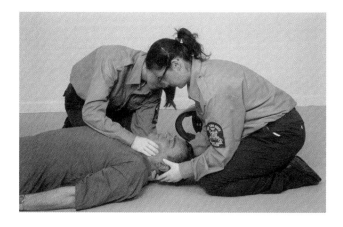

FIGURE 19-21 (D) The helmet is gently rotated until it is completely removed. The first paramedic then assumes manual stabilization of the head.

SPINAL INJURIES IN WATER

A paramedic may be called to an aquatic facility for a spinal injury. One study showed that the most common sport resulting in spinal injury is swimming. Typically, these injuries result from people misjudging water depth and diving into shallow water.[18]

If the incident occurs at a guarded facility, the paramedic should assist the lifeguards with immobilization. Lifeguards are usually trained for water immobilization. Their techniques may vary slightly due to the different environment. For example, some agencies do not train lifeguards in the use of collars. This is acceptable for the aquatic environment. If the paramedic feels that a collar is needed, it can be placed on the

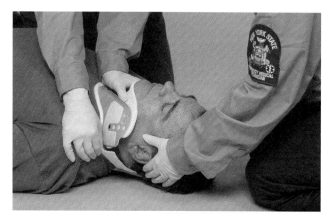

FIGURE 19-21 (E) Once the helmet is removed, padding may need to be placed under the head to maintain cervical alignment. A cervical collar is then applied.

patient once the patient is on land. Paramedics without specialized aquatic training should not attempt immobilization in deep water.

There may be many other unique situations the paramedic may face in which a patient may have a possible spinal injury. While not all situations can be addressed in this chapter, it is important that the paramedic understand the objectives of spinal management. The integrity of the spine needs to be maintained. The spine needs to be kept in-line. Care should focus on immobilizing the spine, according to the presenting situation.

CLEARING THE SPINE IN THE FIELD

One emerging trend, and a subject of much controversy, is clearing the cervical spine in the field. Currently, most patients involved in motor vehicle crashes are immobilized based on mechanism of injury. While immobilization is a very important aspect of patient care for trauma patients, certain experts believe that patients are being immobilized more than necessary.

The most important question raised is whether paramedics in the field can obtain enough diagnostic information to clear the spine without the aid of radiographic imaging. In some EMS systems, protocols exist for ruling out cervical spine injuries in the field.[19] In order to rule out the need for immobilization, the following criteria are used. The patient must not have:

- An altered level of consciousness
- Pain or tenderness along the vertebrae
- Neurological deficit
- Evidence of intoxication or drug use
- Presence of a distracting injury such as fractures, severe lacerations, or amputations

If a patient meets the criteria, then he or she is not immobilized. If all the criteria cannot be met with certainty, the patient is immobilized. This type of protocol has been found to be effective in systems where there are many minor vehicle crashes.[20] Several clinical investigations have validated these criteria, showing that paramedics can accurately identify patients for whom spinal immobilization is unnecessary.[21-23] While protocols of this nature seem promising, it by no means should diminish the value and need for proper spinal immobilization of patients with suspected spinal injury.

INTERNET ACTIVITIES

Visit the British Trauma Society Web site at http://www.trauma.org/resus/moulagefour/moulagefour.html and review the material on spinal clearing. What are the similarities and differences when compared with the field spine clearing protocols published by the National Association of EMS Physicians?

SUMMARY

This chapter provides an overview of the principles of caring for spinal injuries in the field. Proper initial in-line stabilization followed by placement of a cervical collar, application of short spine devices, and full immobilization is essential in the management of spinal injuries. Paramedics need to be familiar with various types of equipment and techniques used for spinal immobilization. Proficiency with skills such as rapid takedown and rapid extrication can be beneficial when applied properly. Just as a paramedic needs to think and react to various medical emergencies, the same holds true for managing spinal injuries. While protocols for clearing the spine in the field may become a useful tool, the need for constant training and proficiency in caring for spinal injuries must always remain a priority for the paramedic.

REVIEW QUESTIONS

1. Compare and contrast stabilization and immobilization.
2. The patient's head should not be placed in the neutral position when:
   a. The patient complains of severe pain, pressure, or numbness upon moving the head.
   b. Resistance is felt when moving the head.
   c. The patient's head is severely angulated and movement is painful.
   d. All of the above.
3. Neutral in-line stabilization is no longer required once a cervical collar is applied.
   a. True
   b. False
4. List the two functions of the cervical collar.
5. Which of the following is the most effective means for immobilizing the cervical spine?
   a. Rigid plastic, two-piece cervical collar
   b. Philadelphia-style cervical collar
   c. Foam cervical collar
   d. Towel roll
6. Which of the following are complications of a tightly fitting cervical collar?
   a. Restriction of laryngeal movement
   b. Decreased venous return from the head
   c. Vagus nerve stimulation
   d. All of the above
7. A cervical collar that is too large will likely result in:
   a. Hyperextension
   b. Hyperflexion
   c. Lateral flexion
   d. Cervical distraction
8. Vest-type immobilization devices should be used on all patients found in a seated position.
   a. True
   b. False
9. When should pulses, motor function, and sensation be assessed in the extremities?
   a. Prior to spinal immobilization
   b. After spinal immobilization
   c. Upon arrival at the hospital
   d. All of the above
10. Complications from immobilization on a long spine board include:
    a. Pain
    b. Neck stiffness
    c. Both b and c
    d. No complications have been attributed to immobilization
11. The vacuum mattress provides superior immobilization when compared to the long spine board.
    a. True
    b. False
12. To maintain in-line positioning, the legs must be elevated off the ground when performing a log roll.
    a. True
    b. False
13. The head should always be secured to the long spine board before the torso.
    a. True
    b. False

14. Rapid extrication techniques should be used on all patients found seated in a motor vehicle following a collision.
a. True
b. False

15. It is not always necessary to remove a motorcycle helmet.
a. True
b. False

16. List the criteria for clearing the spine in the field.

▶ CRITICAL THINKING

- You are dispatched to the scene of an MVC. Upon arrival you find a single vehicle that left the roadway, traveled down a steep embankment, and overturned. Inside the vehicle, you find an unconscious elderly female seated in the driver's seat. She is wearing a lap and shoulder restraint and hanging upside down in the vehicle. How will you protect this patient's spinal column and extricate her from the vehicle? What assessments and treatments will you perform prior to extrication?

- Upon arrival at the scene of an industrial accident, you are led to the loading dock where you find an 18-year-old male pinned between the back doors of a large truck and the loading dock. The bystanders state that the patient attempted to open the trailer doors before the truck came to a stop. He then fell from the loading dock and was pinned against the loading dock by the back of the trailer before he could move out of the path of the truck. The patient is conscious and alert and pinned in a standing position. He is complaining of pain in his pelvis and abdomen. How will you immobilize this patient? What actions will you take prior to moving the truck?

- You are dispatched to the scene of a fall. You arrive to find an elderly female lying at the bottom of a flight of stairs. She is conscious and alert and states that she became faint while climbing the stairs and fell backward, falling nearly the entire length of the stairs. She is lying supine and complains of pain in her left thigh. Upon physical examination you discover a fractured left femur, an unstable pelvis, and diminished sensory and motor function of both legs. What injuries do you suspect? How will you immobilize her pelvis, femur, and spine? How will you move her to the backboard?

▶ REFERENCES

1. Campagnolo DI, Esquieres RE, Kopacz KJ. Effect of timing of stabilization on length of stay and medical complications following spinal cord injury. *J Spinal Cord Med.* 1997; 20:331.

2. Garcia B. *Mosby's Emergency Dictionary*, 2nd ed. St. Louis: Mosby-Yearbook; 1998:316.

3. Garcia B. *Mosby's Emergency Dictionary*, 2nd ed. Mosby-Yearbook, St. Louis, 1998:176.

4. Podolsky S, Baraff LJ, Simon RR, Hoffman JR, Larmon B, Ablon W. Efficacy of cervical spine immobilization methods. *Trauma.* 1983; 23:461.

5. Johnson RM, Hart DL, Simmon EF, Ramsby GR, Southwick WO. Cervical orthoses: a study comparing their effectiveness in restricting cervical motion in normal subjects. *J Bone Joint Surg.* 1977; 59:332.

6. McCabe JB, Nolan DJ. Comparison of the effectiveness of different cervical immobilization collars. *Ann Emerg Med.* 1986; 15:93.

7. Philadelphia Corp. *New RED E.M. Cervical Collar Training.* [video]. 1991.

8. Ducker TB. *Restriction of Cervical Spine Motion by Cervical Collars.* Poster presentation at Annual Meeting of American Association of Neurological Surgeons; 1990; Nashville, Tenn.

9. Blaylock B. Solving the problem of pressure ulcers resulting from cervical collars. *Ostomy Wound Manage.* 1996; 42:26.

10. Houghton DJ, Curley JW. Dysphagia caused by a hard cervical collar. *Br J Neurosurg.* 1996; 10:501.

11. Laerdal Corporation. *Issues in Spinal Care: Proper Use of the Stifneck Extrication Collar Instructor's Manual.* Laerdal Corp; 1990:4.

12. Chan D, Goldberg R, Tascone A, Harmon S, Chan L. The effect of spinal immobilization on healthy volunteers. *Ann Emerg Med.* 1994; 23:48.

13. Goldberg R, Chan D, Mason J, Chan L. Standard spinal immobilization versus a vacuum mattress splint: a comparison of symptoms generated. *J Emerg Med Services.* 1996; 14:3.

14. Johnson DR, Hauswald M, Stockhoff C. Comparison of a vacuum splint device to a rigid backboard for spinal immobilization. *Am J Emerg Med.* 1996; 14.369.

15. DeLorenzo, RA, Olson JE, Boska M, et al. Optimal positioning for cervical immobilization. *Ann Emerg Med.* 1996; 28:301.

16. Elling R, Pollitis J. Backboarding the standing patient. *J Emerg Med Services.* 1987; 9:64.

17. Turgut M, Akpinar G, Akalan N, Ozcah OE. Spinal injuries in the pediatric age group: a review of 82 cases of spinal cord and vertebral column injuries. *Eur Spine J.* 1996; 5:148.

18. Noguchi T. A survey of spinal cord injuries resulting from sports. *Paraplegia.* 1994; 32:170.

19. Monk MD. Maine taps medics spinal skills. *J Emerg Med Services.* 1997; 3:77.

20. Myers R. Personal communication; March 1997.

21. Brown LH, Gough JE, Simonds WB. Can EMS providers adequetely assess trauma patients for cervical spine injury? *Prehosp Emerg Care.* 1998; 2:33–6

22. Domeier RM, Swor RA, Evans RW, Hancock JB, Fales W, Krohmer J, et al. The reliability of prehospital clinical evaluation for potential spinal injury is not affected by the mechanism of injury. *Prehosp Emerg Care.* 1999; 3(4):332–7.

23. Muhr M, Seabrook D, Wittwer L. Paramedic use of a spinal injury clearance algorithm reduces spinal immobilization in the out-of-hospital setting. *Prehosp Emerg Care.* 1999; 3(1):1–6.

Chapter 20

Fluid Resuscitation

OBJECTIVES

Upon completion of this chapter, the reader should be able to:

- Name the different blood groups and types in humans and their approximate percentages in the U.S. population.
- Describe the basic blood components that may be utilized in emergency medicine and the indications for the use of each product.
- Explain how the decision to use blood resuscitation is made.
- Describe the term autotransfusion and the role it plays in transfusion medicine.
- Describe the selection of blood in an emergency situation.
- Define the advantages and disadvantages of blood substitutes.
- List the rationale in the choice of needle size, filter type, and concurrent fluids utilized in a transfusion.
- Describe the more common transfusion reactions and the treatment for each.
- Compare and contrast crystalloid and colloid solutions.
- Discuss the existing controversy over fluid resuscitation in the hemorrhaging patient.
- Explain the various techniques that can be used to insert large-bore catheters.
- List the most common sites used for venous access.
- Explain the technique for adult intraosseous infusions.
- Explain the procedure for intravenous access using the Seldinger technique.
- Explain the technique for external jugular cannulation.
- Explain the technique for saphenous vein cutdown.
- Explain the technique for femoral vein cannulation.

KEY TERMS

Albumin
Autotransfusion
Colloid solutions
Crystalloid solutions
Dextran

Hydroxyethyl starch (hetastarch)
Immunohematology
Perfluorocarbons
Seldinger technique
Stroma-free hemoglobin

The body maintains homeostasis, or balance, through the functioning of a seemingly effortless system of automatic processes designed to turn on and off without conscious thought or aid. Maintenance of blood pressure, circulation, and oxygen delivery each occur exactly as programmed by the body until an incident or disease interferes with this function. Even when there is interference with homeostasis, the body systems respond by altering innate safety procedures that are designed to return the perfect level of function. These systems, however, have limits beyond which even the miraculous workings of the body cannot recover unassisted.

The use of crystalloid and colloid therapy to aid the body in making repairs in areas grossly affected by trauma or disease has been one of the most relied upon means of field treatment in the injured and distressed. Loss of oxygen transport due to cardiac pump failure or hemorrhage can have devastating effects on the body tissues, creating a wasteland of dead and dying cells. Replacement fluids assist in maintaining circulating volume allowing delivery of limited oxygen supplies to those vital areas of the heart, kidneys, and brain that are the absolute minimum for survival. The body's homeostatic mechanisms perform this function until the blood volume deficit is so low that multisystem failure is irreversible.

The body maintains vascular volume and blood pressure by manipulating the colloid osmotic pressure (COP) in such a way that it draws fluid into the vascular space from the intracellular space and vice versa. In other words, fluid shifts from areas of low, or hypotonic, concentration to areas of higher, or hypertonic, concentration to create a balance between the two. Normally, when the fluid volume is low, the brain sends a signal in the form of thirst; by drinking, the "tank" is topped off. If fluid is not replaced by drinking, the body responds by constricting capillaries, forcing the remaining blood volume to pass through a smaller space, which in turn maintains blood pressure. Additionally, organs such as the digestive tract and kidneys decrease function to conserve both oxygen and energy use. This is why renal output is a measure of hydration and why people who have been traumatized or dehydrated often suffer impaired bowel motility. In trauma and other states of severe disease, brain signals are lost or the outside fluid shifts are so sudden that the body is unable to compensate rapidly enough to prevent the decompensation that follows. At this point intervention with isotonic fluids is necessary.

ucts. Advantages include the lack of allergic or anaphylactic response, low cost of the product in relation to colloids, long shelf life, and minimal storage restrictions. Perhaps the greatest disadvantages are its inability to transport oxygen, the amount of fluid that must be infused to replace the lost volume of blood, and the subsequent effects of that fluid volume on the cardiorespiratory system. Current standards of practice use isotonic 0.9% normal saline (osmolarity of 310 mosm) and lactated Ringer's solution (osmolarity of 275 mosm) interchangeably.

Hypertonic crystalloid solutions are used in situations that require rapid shifts from interstitial and intracellular areas into the intravascular space, such as occurs in burn patients.[1,2] There are two products currently being studied against conventional saline treatment. The first is hypertonic saline/dextran (HSD), composed of 7.5% sodium chloride in 6% dextran. Groups under study had fewer complications [adult respiratory distress syndrome (ARDS), renal failure, and coagulopathy] in clinical trials than the normal saline controls; also, swine models demonstrated improved cardiovascular function.[1–5]

A second product, known as hypertonic saline (HTS), is a solution of 7.5% saline which trials have shown increase cardiac output and mean arterial pressure, shift fluids into the intravascular compartment rapidly, and increase the duration of intravascular volume expansion.[1,3,6] Both HDS and HTS decrease the amount of fluid required to expand the depleted vascular system, decreasing the likelihood of pulmonary edema or cardiovascular overload.

The major drawback of these solutions remains the risk of causing a hyperosmolar state, which can trigger seizure activity.[6] Infiltration of hypertonic saline solutions can lead to tissue damage and necrosis.[7] In addition to hypernatremia and hypokalemia, the most important potential complication is the increased risk of hemorrhage demonstrated in numerous studies.[8–11] Furthermore, neither of these products supplies additional oxygen for cellular use.

Research into the use of hypertonic saline solutions is ongoing, and results thus far have produced varied findings in terms of survival rates and increasing the rate of hemorrhage. To date no definitive answer is available. Current protocols reflect the lack of scientific evidence in support of these solutions and continue to recommend lactated Ringer's or normal saline for fluid resuscitation.

CRYSTALLOIDS

Crystalloid solutions are a balanced salt product currently used for volume resuscitation, both with and without the concomitant use of blood and blood prod-

COLLOIDS

Colloid solutions are composed of large-molecule compounds that act primarily in the intravascular space by drawing fluid from both the intracellular and interstitial spaces into the bloodstream. Colloids are useful in resuscitation because small-volume infusions can produce significant elevations in blood pressure secondary to rapid osmotic shifts. Colloids have been shown to expand plasma volume three to one compared to crystalloids.[1,12,13] Several types of colloids are currently in use and others are being investigated.

SERUM ALBUMIN

A biological protein derived from human blood, **albumin** remains in the intravascular space for approximately 16 hours. Although it rarely causes side effects and is processed to remove the threat of blood-borne disease, albumin may impair the immune system, rendering the recipient susceptible to infections following administration.[14] Additionally, albumin is expensive, is dependent on human donors, may exacerbate interstitial edema, may precipitate pulmonary edema or ARDS if infused too rapidly, and does not have the capacity to carry oxygen. Recommended infusion rates are 2–4 mL/min of 5% albumin or 1 mL/min of the 25% product.[3]

DEXTRAN

Dextran is a large, synthetic glucose polymer used to expand intravascular blood volume in patients by shifting fluid from the interstitial and intracellular spaces into the vascular space using its high osmolarity. Advantages include biodegradability, long dwell time (12–24 hours), and extended shelf life. Dwell time is important because the length of time the molecule remains in the vascular space is directly proportional to how much fluid has to be infused. Here small amounts of fluid provide big gains in vascular volume. While it is less expensive than albumin and disease free, dextran can cause platelet dysfunction and coagulation abnormalities and impair immune system function.[3] Glucose readings may be falsely elevated, and dextran may interfere with cross-matching. Dextran will induce diuresis and may obviate the use of urine output as an indicator of renal perfusion. It is available in two molecular weights: dextran 40 comes in D_5W, or 10% normal saline, and dextran 70 comes in D_5W, or 6% normal saline. Dextran will increase intravascular volume up to two times the volume of the infusion but does not have the capacity to carry oxygen.[3] Administration is limited to 2 mg/kg of body weight.

HYDROXYETHYL STARCH

Also known as hetastarch, **hydroxyethyl starch (hetastarch)** is another synthetic macromolecule used to expand plasma volume. Other than coagulation problems, few side effects have been noted with the use of this product. Like dextran, hetastarch comes in a 6% normal saline solution that has been demonstrated to remain in the circulation for up to 24 hours. Infusion of hydroxyethyl starch is recommended at 1,500 mL per 24 hours or 20 cc/kg.[3] Expansion of blood volume approximates the volume infused, limiting its usefulness in patients who have lost more than a liter of blood. Hydroxyethyl starch does not have the capacity to carry oxygen.

BLOOD SUBSTITUTES

STROMA-FREE HEMOGLOBIN

Stroma-free hemoglobin, still under development, is designed to carry large amounts of oxygen to the cells of patients who have lost significant amounts of blood. The product is made by hemolyzing outdated red blood cells and removing all of the stroma (cell membrane). While the hemoglobin molecule does exhibit a tremendous affinity for oxygen, research has yet to develop a way to encourage the molecule to release the oxygen to the cells. Rather, the oxygen remains attached to the hemoglobin and is carried out of the body via the renal system approximately 3 hours following infusion. A further difficulty is the stability of the hemoglobin, which degrades outside of the red cell wall and raises the level of free hemoglobin in circulation, precipitating toxic effects on some organs. Other nonbiological substances that carry oxygen are also being developed.

PERFLUOROCARBONS

Perfluorocarbons are new and promising man-made products not currently available on the market. While remaining chemically and biologically inert, perfluorocarbons display high gas solubility, are stable at room temperature, and are able to dissolve large amounts of oxygen, nitrogen, and carbon dioxide.[1,15,16] Because perfluorocarbons do not produce or contain antibodies, there is no need for crossmatching. Unlike colloids, perfluorocarbons carry oxygen to the cells and remove carbon dioxide waste. The greatest disadvantages are the conditions that limit its application for prehospital use. Due to the rapid excretion rate of the product, infusion must be constant. Current preparations must be stored frozen and then thawed and reconstituted prior to use. Research suggests that "small amounts administered in the prehospital setting may be beneficial in restoring metabolic function and may result in a more stable patient."[15]

Both perfluorocarbons and stroma-free hemoglobin require further research and development prior to widespread use. They offer unique and exciting benefits not previously realized by any other products on the market, namely that of oxygen delivery. Additionally, neither product contains antigens, which makes crossmatching unnecessary. Use of these non-biological products would virtually eliminate the concern of disease transmission.

INTERNET ACTIVITIES

Review the lecture on blood substitutes at http://www.sciencefriday.com/pages/1999/Jan/hour1_011599.html. You must have the Real Player media application installed on your computer. If you do not have this program, it is available free of charge from http://www.real.com.

CRYSTALLOID AND COLLOID RESUSCITATION VERSUS THE USE OF BLOOD

A debate rages over the use of crystalloids versus colloids. While most experts can agree that some combination of these products should be used in traumatic hemorrhagic shock, the timing of administration, amount of fluid, and type of fluid remain hotly contested. Any number of clinical trials have demonstrated improved outcomes using one type over the other, but to date, none are conclusive. Experts agree that timely,

definitive surgical intervention to control hemorrhage is essential to the success of any fluid resuscitation. But are fluids best given before surgery or withheld until bleeding is controlled? Is a moderate amount of hypotension actually beneficial? Should fluid be aggressively administered in the prehospital setting or cautiously given to maintain minimum circulation? These questions continue to occupy researchers who are conducting clinical trials in large cities and teaching hospitals around the world.

Another debated issue, the timing of blood transfusion, has vague guidelines at best. Most practitioners use estimated blood loss as their guide for initiation of blood and other fluids. Table 20-1 displays guidelines from the American College of Surgeons on estimating blood loss; however, in practice it is up to the physician to decide when and if blood or blood products are used.[17] This decision is often driven by physician preference. Current standards advise the use of crystalloid fluid with or without the concomitant use of colloids, reserving blood use for those patients who have lost more than 20% of their total blood volume.[18,19] Increased cardiac output and blood pressure are achieved by both the crystalloid and nonblood colloid solutions. Table 20-2 compares the advantages and disadvantages of crystalloid and colloid solutions.

Hemodilution, often the end result of prolonged fluid resuscitation with crystalloids, produces anemia in the hemorrhaging patient. While the increase in volume generated by the crystalloid improves cardiac output and facilitates oxygen delivery, the oxygen content of the blood is significantly decreased. While this is

Table 20-1
Estimated Fluid and Blood Losses

	Class I	Class II	Class III	Class IV
Blood loss (mL)	Up to 750	750–1,500	1,500–2,000	2,000 or more
Blood loss (% BV±)	Up to 15%	15%–30%	30%–40%	40% or more
Pulse rate	<100	>100	>120	140 or higher
Blood pressure	Normal	Normal	Decreased	Decreased
Pulse pressure	Normal or increased	Decreased	Decreased	Decreased
Capillary refill test	Normal	Positive	Positive	Positive
Respiratory rate	14–20	20–30	30–40	>35
Urine output (mL/hr)	30 or more	20–30	5–15	Negligible
Mental status	Slightly anxious	Mildly anxious	Anxious; confused	Confused; lethargic
Fluid replacement (3:1 ratio)	Crystalloid	Crystalloid	Crystalloid + blood	Crystalloid + blood

Amounts are based on the patient's initial presentation. BV = blood volume. Values based on 70-kg male.

Source: American College of Surgeons (ACS) Committee on Trauma. *The Advanced Trauma Life Support Student Manual.* Chicago: American College of Surgeons; 1993: 86. Used with permission.

Table 20-2
Comparison of Crystalloid and Colloid Fluids

	Crystalloid	Colloid
Action	Intracellular, extracellular; short-acting volume increase, usually less than 1 hour	Intravascular only; long intravascular dwell time, from 12 hours to several days
Cost	Inexpensive	Expensive
Blood pressure support	Gradual increase	Rapid increase
Anaphylaxis	No risk for anaphylaxis	Higher risk with some products
Volume expansion	3:1 ratio	1:1 ratio
Risk of disease transmission	No risk	Potential risk of blood-borne disease
Colloid osmotic pressure	Decreased	Increased
Metabolic	Dilutional acidosis	Hyperkalemia, decreased ability to metabolize lactate
Cardiac output	Increased	Increased
Oxygen	Improves delivery but does not transport oxygen	Only blood will supply oxygen, other colloids do not

used in some surgical and medical situations, hemodilution is never recommended for trauma patients.[20] Do not forget that poor response to fluids may be due to occult hemorrhage, cardiac pump failure, or other injuries. Indeed, controversy exists over the need to administer any intravenous fluid (IVF) until such time as the hemorrhaging is surgically controlled. One study using sheep models demonstrated that giving IVF caused a twofold increase in the rate and volume of hemorrhage.[21] The same study found oxygen delivery capacity greater in the group that received no IVF.[21] Another study, this one using rat models, postulated that IVF administration increases the risk of blood loss because not only did hemodilution cause a decrease in tissue perfusion, but by lowering the oxygen level in the blood it also prevented the formation of clots necessary for hemostasis. Additionally, the authors found the clots, if formed, were often washed away by the increases in blood pressure generated by IVF therapy.[22] These findings have led some to question the benefits of IVF therapy.

If too much fluid is given to a patient with uncontrolled hemorrhage, are we risking exsanguination when the blood pressure increases due to IVF administration? Several scientists have theorized that a moderate level of hypotension may actually exert a protective effect on the patient, allowing clots to form and controlling hemorrhage spontaneously. Other researchers contend that the damaging effects of "sludging" in the

microcirculation support the need for aggressive IVF intervention. In another study, a computer model was used to run simulations of various rates of both blood loss and fluid replacement. It demonstrated that the increase in preload and afterload as a result of fluid resuscitation actually increased myocardial oxygen consumption. Additionally, although coronary circulation improved, the falling hematocrit and decreased oxygen-carrying capacity ultimately resulted in an overall oxygen deficit. The model also suggested that slowing the infusion rate to less than 50 mL/min extended the rate of decline.[3]

There is no question that further studies must be done before a definitive change in current IVF therapy can occur. One author judiciously suggests that fluids should be administered over the same time frame as that in which the loss occurred. This is intuitively a good suggestion; however, until such time as there is a product able to replace lost blood with a fluid capable of replacing not only the volume of blood lost but also the oxygen required by the body for proper functioning, only warmed lactated Ringer's or normal saline is available.

In making a choice to administer fluids, observation of the patient's condition and the response to intervention is the best guide to resuscitation. Is the patient improved by the intervention, unchanged, or worsened? Actions in response to these observations must be cautious and based on a sound understanding of physiology and standards of emergency care.

ADMINISTRATION OF CRYSTALLOIDS AND COLLOIDS

Hemorrhage necessitates rapid control of bleeding and administration of volume support via intravenous lines. Advances in catheter style, preassembled kits, the use of trauma tubing (Figure 20-1), and advanced training allow EMS personnel to access standard anatomical sites with greater ease. There are three ways of inserting catheters: catheter over the needle, catheter through the needle, and catheter inserted over a guidewire.

1. Catheter over the needle (Figure 20-2) is the standard access method in both field and hospital settings. Figure 20-3 shows a variety of catheters currently available on the market. Although the lumen are the same size, the shorter catheters will deliver a more rapid infusion because infusion rate is inversely proportional to the length of the catheter. This type of catheter allows for patient movement and removes the needle from the site after the vein is accessed. The twin catheter (Figure 20-4) is often used to allow IVF administration to occur simultaneously with IV push drugs or administration of antibiotics. Drugs should be placed in the distal port to avoid interaction with hanging fluid.

2. Inserting a catheter through the needle (Figure 20-5) carries the risk of shearing off part of the catheter. After the catheter is threaded through the needle, the needle is pulled out of the site but

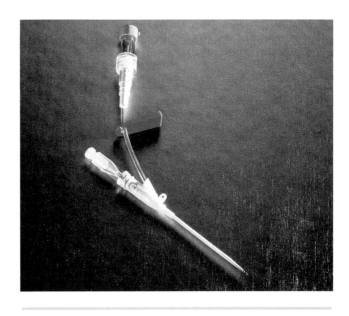

FIGURE 20-2 Catheter over the needle. (Courtesy of Arrow International.)

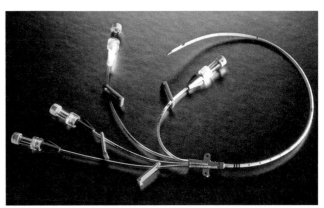

A.

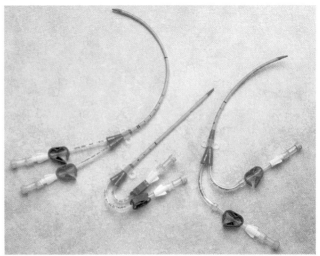

B.

FIGURE 20-3 (A) Multilumen catheter; (B) Twin-Cath catheters. (Courtesy of Arrow International.)

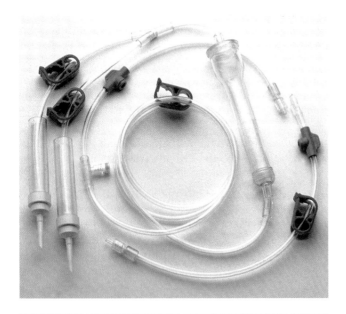

FIGURE 20-1 Trauma tubing. (Courtesy of Arrow International.)

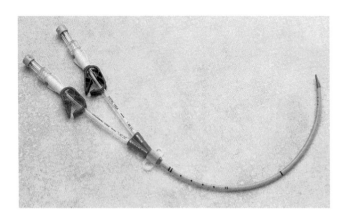

FIGURE 20-4 Twin catheter. (Courtesy of Arrow International.)

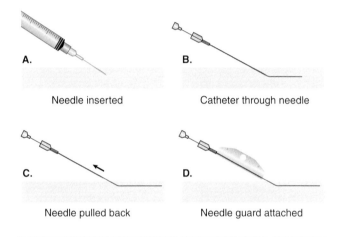

A. Needle inserted

B. Catheter through needle

C. Needle pulled back

D. Needle guard attached

FIGURE 20-5 Catheter through the needle.

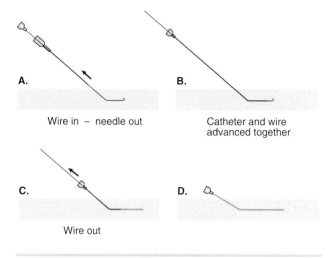

A. Wire in – needle out

B. Catheter and wire advanced together

C. Wire out

D.

FIGURE 20-6 Seldinger technique.

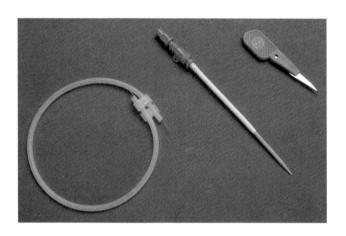

FIGURE 20-7 Knife, J wire, and introducer used to perform Seldinger technique. (Courtesy of Arrow International.)

remains attached to the catheter. Great care must be taken not to shear off the catheter while manipulating the attached needle. This technique has been gradually replaced by the other two catheter styles.

3. The **Seldinger technique**, shown in Figure 20-6, uses a guidewire to thread the catheter into the vein, allowing the user to insert a standard IV catheter into a peripheral vein and convert the site to a much larger bore in a matter of seconds; this technique has long been used in emergency departments. Several commercially prepared kits are available on the market for use in the field or hospital setting (Figure 20-7). The beauty of this technique is the ease with which a 20-gauge catheter can be transformed into a line with as large a lumen as an 8.5 French, facilitating the life-saving administration of blood and other fluids.

It should be understood that while access to the venous circulation is vital, on-scene delay for the pur-

pose of initiating IV lines is not acceptable. One study suggests that on-site IVF replacement may not be beneficial and when coupled with long scene times may actually increase morbidity.[3] If it takes more than 90 seconds to access a peripheral site, the patient should be loaded and further attempts at IV access made en route to the emergency department. Standard IV initiation sites are displayed in Figures 20-8A,B and 20-9A,B.

The external jugular vein is an alternate site when the antecubital fossa is not accessible in patients with burns, trauma, or other injury that prevents its use (Figure 20-10). To locate the external jugular vein, turn the patient's head away from you (assuming there is no spinal injury) and place the patient in a Trendelenburg position. Trace a line from below and slightly behind the ear downward and back toward the middle of the clavicle crossing the sternomastoid muscle. After preparing the site as usual, begin insertion midway between the angle of the jaw and the clavicle, at a 45°

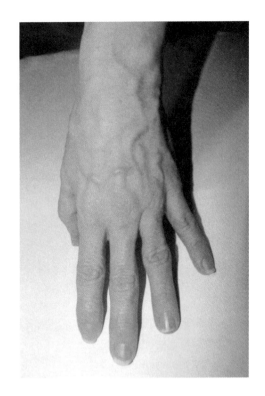

A.

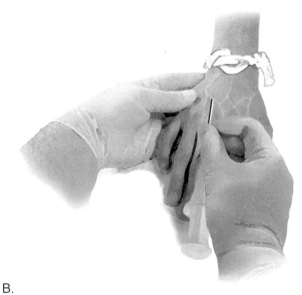

B.

FIGURE 20-8 (A) Typical venous pattern. (Courtesy of Mark Zeringue.) (B) Venipuncture sites of the hand.

angle down toward the shoulder. The vein should be held firmly between thumb and forefinger for stabilization. Secure the catheter, but *do not* tape or wrap gauze all the way around the neck as this could create an airway obstruction.

Chest trauma, cardiopulmonary resuscitation (CPR), and rigid cervical collar or intubation may interfere with cannulation of the jugular veins. A femoral line

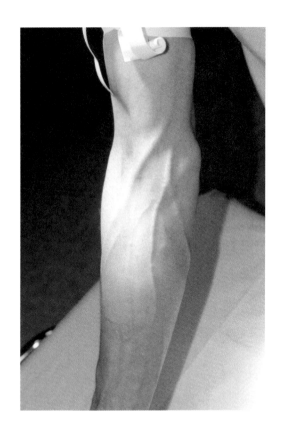

A.

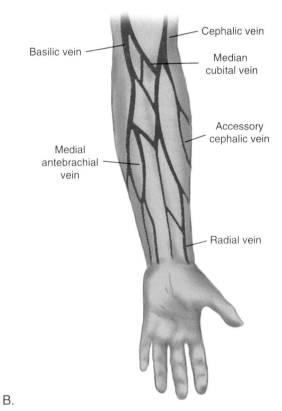

B.

FIGURE 20-9 (A) Venous configuration in the forearm. (Courtesy of Mark Zeringue.) (B) Anatomy of veins of upper extremity. *(continues)*

is a good choice for a large-bore IV line and is often away from the "action" at the top half of the body. Locate the femoral vein by placing your middle finger on the symphysis pubis, your thumb on the anterior superior iliac spine. The femoral artery should cross the middle of the line with the femoral vein located just medial to the artery (Figure 20-11). If a pulse is present, insert the catheter medial to the pulse; however, remember that CPR can make finding the vein difficult because the pulse may be a venous pulse. Attach the catheter to a 5- or 10-cc syringe (Figure 20-12) and draw back on the plunger, gently aspirating blood to identify placement. Be sure to use a needle and catheter of sufficient length to thread into the vein (Figure 20-13). Secure the catheter in place with a suture, if possible.

Do not forget the availability of the intraosseous route when faced with trauma in children 6 years and under. In addition to crystalloid fluids, both drugs and blood can be administered via the intraosseous route, which is accessed by placing an intraosseous needle 2 fingers breadth beneath the tibial tuberosity and pressing gently but firmly in a downward motion, rotating the needle slightly. Too much pressure applied to the needle can cause it to pass through the bone and out the other side. For this reason, never place your free hand beneath the patient's leg; rather grip the leg distal to the insertion site for balance and stability. The catheter is then secured with tape and the IV line attached (Figure 20-14).

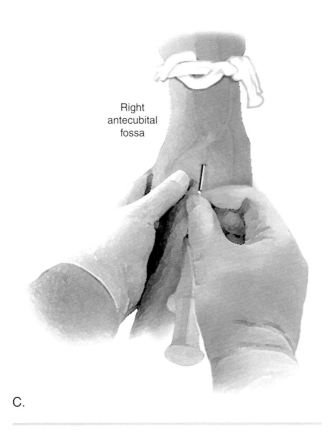

Right antecubital fossa

C.

FIGURE 20-9 (continued) (C) Antecubital venipuncture.

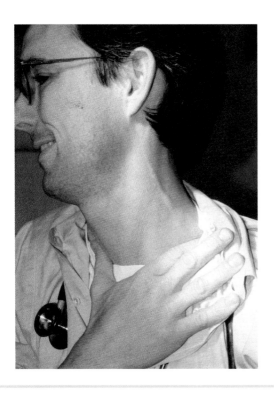

A.

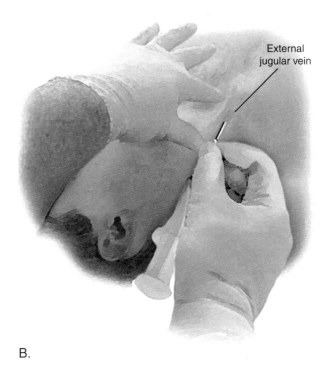

External jugular vein

B.

FIGURE 20-10 (A) Configuration of the external jugular vein. (Courtesy of Mark Zeringue) (B) Cannulation of the external jugular vein.

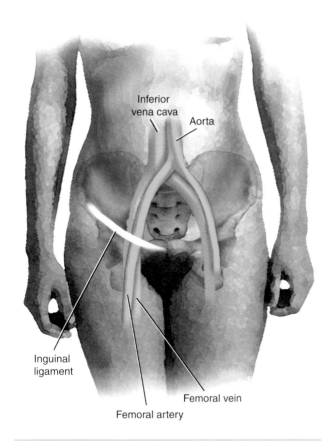

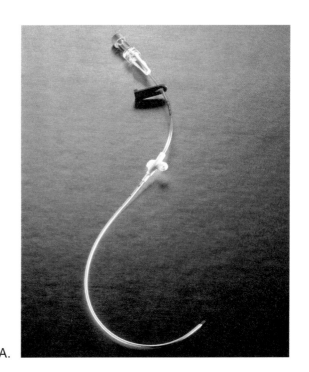

A.

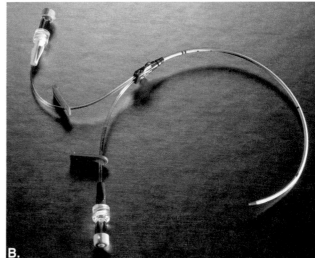

B.

FIGURE 20-11 Femoral vein.

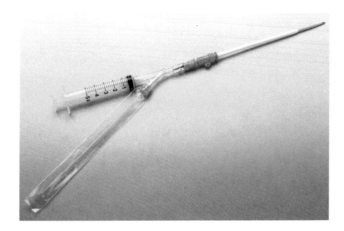

FIGURE 20-12 Needle with 5-cc syringe used for cannulating the femoral vein. (Courtesy of Arrow International.)

While pediatric intraosseous (IO) infusion has been a routine procedure for many years, it has only recently been introduced as an alternative access route for adult patients. Two new spring-actuated devices have entered the market for quickly obtaining intraosseous access in adults: the bone injection gun (BIG) and the F.A.S.T.-1 IO system. There are few

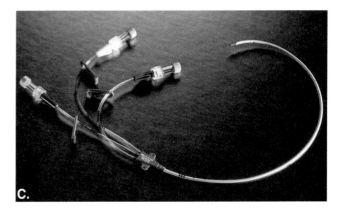

C.

FIGURE 20-13 Femoral catheters: (A) single, (B) double, and (C) multilumen. (Courtesy of Arrow International.)

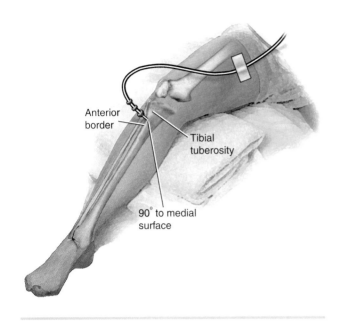

Anterior
border

Tibial
tuberosity

90° to medial
surface

FIGURE 20-14 Intraosseous cannulation.

reports of intraosseous infusion in adults, and even fewer evaluations of adult IO techniques performed by paramedics.[31–34] One study reported the successful use of the BIG among paramedic students using a cadaver model.[35] In this randomized, cross-over study comparing the ability of paramedic students to use the BIG versus saphenous vein cutdown, the BIG proved superior. Success rates for establishing venous access were higher for the intraosseous route (92.3%) than for the cutdown technique (69.2%), but these differences did not achieve statistical significance. The time required to initiate fluid flow was 3.91 minutes by the intraosseous route and 7.57 minutes by venous cutdown. In a report of prehospital IO infusions that included adult patients, Glaeser et al. reported a 50% success rate among 14 patients using an 18-gauge iliac Jamshidi sternal bone marrow needle.[32] More recently, Macnab and colleagues reported their investigation of the F.A.S.T.-1 IO system.[36] In their series of 50 patients, the device was successfully placed in the sternum of 42 patients (84%); 29 attempts were made by paramedics in the field and 21 by physicians in the hospital. Flow rates of up to 80 mL/min were reported with this device when coupled with a pressure infuser. The mean time to infusion, measured as the interval from opening the package to commencement of fluid flow, was 77 seconds. While still a relatively new technique, adult IO infusion appears to be a promising route for adult patients in whom access is problematic.

If peripheral percutaneous and intraosseous cannulation cannot be performed, a venous cutdown is an alternative means of vascular access. However, the technique is associated with a higher rate of complica-

tions and may take as long as 10 minutes to perform. Nevertheless, venous cutdown of the saphenous vein offers EMS personnel an alternative of last resort for intravenous access in the severely injured trauma patient. The technique is summarized in Figure 20-15.

Choosing the appropriate venous access technique is a matter of training and experience. Proficiency and familiarity with all types of setup and infusion systems are necessary. It is often left up to the EMS provider to decide which approach will be used at what site. Intravenous access limitations due to location of injury, CPR, or the inexperience of the paramedic are expected and should be part of the training in any program. The first catheter placed should be the largest bore catheter that the paramedic is confident of placing because he or she may not get access to a second site.

HISTORY OF BLOOD THERAPY

The science of blood transfusions began with William Harvey's discovery and exploration of blood circulation in 1628.[23] The first human-to-human transfusion occurred in London in 1818.[18] Prior to this time there had been experiments with animal-to-human transfusions resulting in many recorded reactions and deaths. It was not understood why some transfusions were successful while others failed. Additionally, there were problems storing blood. Until the development of anticoagulants, a major obstacle in blood therapy was clotting of stored blood. A mixture of sodium citrate and glucose, the first anticoagulant that did not damage red blood cells or produce harmful toxins, was developed in 1914.[24]

Reactions following transfusions continued to occur, and it was not until 1901, when Karl Landsteiner discovered the ABO blood groups, that science began to understand why this was happening.[24] Four separate blood groups were recognized, each genetically determined. The four blood groups are O, A, B, and AB; all groups are not compatible with each other.

BASICS OF BLOOD THERAPY

Many separate products or components may be obtained from a single unit of donated blood. The greatest advantage of using blood components is that several people may benefit from the donation of a single unit of blood. Components help to increase the inventory available to hospitals and medical centers. The use of component therapy versus whole-blood therapy became widely accepted in the 1970s.[23]

Today the emphasis is on appropriateness of care for the patient. Physicians are held accountable for their ordering practices and must have sound reasons

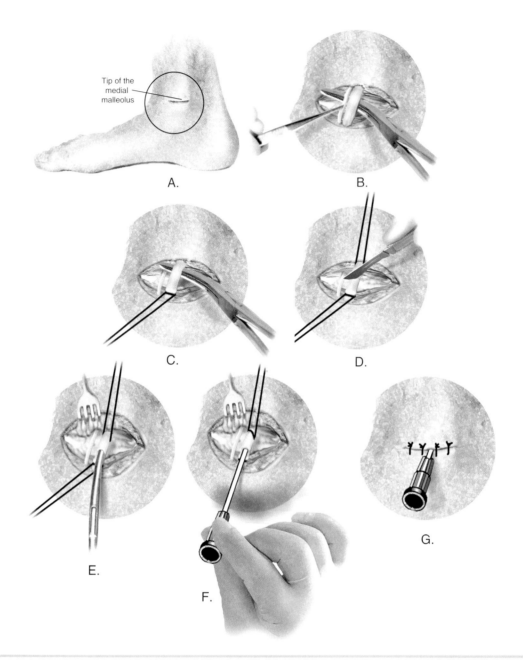

A.

B.

C.

D.

E.

F.

G.

FIGURE 20-15 Venous cutdown procedure. 1. The primary site of cutdown is the saphenous vein at the ankle. 2. To prevent damage to the cannula of vein by ankle movements, infants and children need restraining during the procedure. This can be done by strapping the foot and lower leg to a padded armboard or Papoose Board. 3. Apply a rubber tourniquet to the upper half of the calf. 4. Prep the skin of the ankle with povidone-iodine and drape. 5. Infiltrate the skin overlying the saphenous vein with 0.5% lidocaine. 6. Make a transverse incision through the area of anesthesia. A 2 to 2.5 cm incision should suffice (Fig. 20-15A). 7.Once teh skin is incised full thickness, spread the subcutaneous fat gently with a curved hemostat. 8. Identify the saphenous vein traversing the incision in a slightly oblique direction. 9. Free up the vein from the surrounding tissue by gentle spreading movements. The saphenous nerve runs parallel to the saphenous vein (Fig. 20-15B). 10. Elevate the vein from its bed for a distance of 1.5 to 2 cm and separate the saphenous nerve from the vein. 11. Place a suture tie at the lower end of the mobilized vein & leave it in place for traction (Fig. 20-15C). 12.Pass a catgut tie behind the vein above the lower tie. 13. Make a small transverse incision in the anterior wall of the vein. A brisk flow of blood will occur because of the tourniquet applied above. Control the bleeding by slight traction on the upper loose tie (Fig. 20-15D). 14. Introduce a plastic cannula into the vein through the venotomy and hold it in place by tying the upper tie about the vein. The cannula should be inserted almost to its hub (Fig. 20-15E and F). 15. Then close site with simple interupted sutures (Fig. 20-15G). 16. Apply a topical antibiotic ointment followed by a sterile dressing.

for ordering a transfusion of blood products. Although there are many blood components that may be transfused, only a few are routinely encountered in the trauma situation: packed red blood cells (PRBCs), whole blood, fresh frozen plasma (FFP), and platelets.

PACKED RED BLOOD CELLS

Packed red blood cells are probably the most common blood component encountered in the emergency situation. They are made by expressing most of the plasma from the unit of whole blood at the time of processing. This renders an enriched product of red blood cells without the excess volume. An average unit of PRBCs has an approximate volume of 250 mL (Figure 20-16B). Red blood cells are stored at 1°C–6°C. The normal life span of a red blood cell is 120 days. The type of anticoagulant used in collecting the unit of blood determines the expiration date of the product. Acid-citrate-dextrose (ACD) and citrate-phosphate-dextrose (CPD) are the most popular anticoagulants for storing red blood cells. The viability of the red blood cells after storage and their ability to survive normally after transfusion are the deciding factors when determining the expiration date. The shelf life for both ACD and CPD is 21 days. Longer expiration dates may be achieved when certain preservatives are added, such as adenine to CPD. This can increase the expiration date to 42 days by preserving red cell blood viability.[25]

Packed red blood cells are used to increase the oxygen-carrying capacity in patients with acute or chronic blood loss. Packed red blood cells are the primary source of red blood cells stocked in most hospital blood banks. They are the component of choice when fluid overload is a clinical concern; however, this is not usually an initial issue in the trauma situation.

WHOLE BLOOD

Whole blood is the entire unit of blood as collected from the blood donor (Figure 20-16A). There is no extraction of plasma, platelets, or other products during the processing phase. Whole blood is stored at 1°C–6°C. The same anticoagulants and preservatives used in red blood cells are also utilized in whole blood. Expiration dates depend upon the anticoagulant and preservative used in the collection process.

Whole blood restores oxygen-carrying capacity while increasing the blood volume or mass. Fresh whole blood is the best choice to use in an acute hemorrhage. Fresh whole blood contains viable platelets and coagulation factors necessary to aid in clotting. Whole blood is considered the resuscitation fluid of choice in the trauma situation.[23] It should be noted that this component is not routinely stocked in many hospital blood banks, though it may be found in some military situations.[23] While whole blood is necessarily utilized in exchange transfusions and is often used to prime the blood pump in cardiac bypass surgery, it is more efficiently utilized after processing into specific components for therapy.

FRESH FROZEN PLASMA

Fresh frozen plasma contains all coagulation factors present in the bloodstream. These coagulation factors are destroyed upon storage of blood. The plasma is expressed from a fresh unit of blood within 8 hours of collection and quickly frozen to preserve these factors. Fresh frozen plasma is stored at –18°C or lower for a maximum of 1 year.[18]

The primary use of FFP is to treat coagulation deficiencies. It should not be used as a plasma expander. Crystalloids and other colloids are more effective for this purpose. Severe burns may require the addition of plasma after several hours of fluid treatment to aid in the repair of damaged capillaries and to restore coagulation factors (Figure 20-17).

PLATELETS

Platelets play an essential role in hemostasis and maintenance of capillary integrity. Platelets are produced in the bone marrow and remain in the bloodstream for up to 12 days. The platelet component is prepared by one

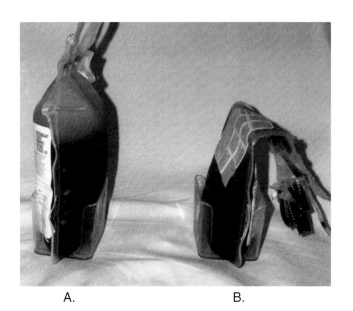

A.   B.

FIGURE 20-16 (A) Whole-blood unit, volume 500 cc; (B) packed red blood cell unit, volume 250 cc. (Courtesy of M. Elaine Frye.)

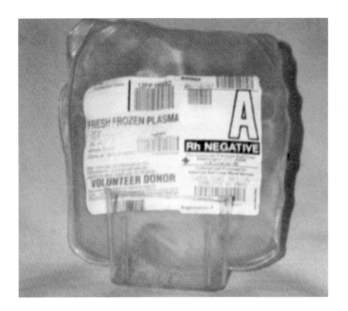

FIGURE 20-17 Fresh frozen plasma (FFP). (Courtesy of M. Elaine Frye.)

of two methods. Platelets may be prepared by centrifugation of the freshly donated unit of whole blood for separation and used as random donor platelets or through platelet pheresis. A platelet concentrate is collected from a single donor using some type of hemapheresis equipment. Each pack of pheresis platelets, shown in Figure 20-18, is equivalent to approximately six units of random donor platelets.[26] The optimal storage temperature of platelets is 20°C–24°C. Cold storage reduces the survival rate of the stored platelets as well as decreases the survival rate of transfused platelets. Currently, the expiration date of platelets stored at room temperature and receiving gentle, continuous agitation is 5 days. The agitation aids in maintaining the pH of the component.

Platelet units are transfused to patients suffering from thrombocytopenia. Normal platelet count ranges from 150,000 to 350,000 depending upon the method utilized in measuring the platelets. Platelet transfusions are considered when the total count is lower than 20,000, in preoperative patients with counts lower than 50,000, and in those patients with impaired production as well as impaired function of platelets.[18] Platelet infusions are commonly given to patients with acute leukemia and other neoplastic conditions.

BLOOD SELECTION FOR TRAUMA SITUATIONS

The patient's blood is routinely grouped and typed when a blood transfusion is ordered by the attending physician. Blood of the same group and type is selected

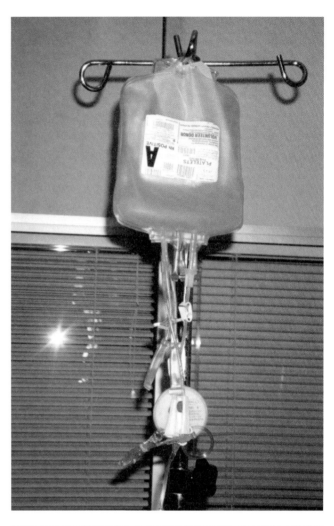

FIGURE 20-18 A bag of platelets. (Courtesy of M. Elaine Frye.)

for transfusion; however, compatibility of the selected blood is determined by combining the donor's blood with the possible recipient's blood. A series of tests are performed on the combined blood. Body conditions are simulated serologically to predict compatibility. This series of tests are performed in vitro and are referred to as a crossmatch. After completion of the crossmatch, the unit is declared compatible if no adverse reactions are encountered. This is the best method for determining compatibility. The procedure requires at least 1 hour for completion. An antibody screen on the patient's blood is also essential for determining possible adverse reactions. The antibody screen procedure searches for the presence of antibodies that could cause significant transfusion problems. These antibodies could react with like antigens present on the donor's red blood cells. When like antigens and antibodies are combined, agglutination of the red blood cells occurs. The antibody screen procedure requires at least 1 hour for completion.

A procedure known as the type and screen is utilized in some situations. This test includes a group and type along with antibody screen for significant antibodies. It is of significant use in potential transfusion candidates, such as, surgical patients. The antibody screen requires at least 1 hour to perform. Decreased costs, smaller blood inventory requirements, and better ordering practices by the physicians make this an attractive test. The type and screen should be used when there is a low likelihood of the patient needing the blood. The trauma patient may be a good candidate for this test since other fluids should be used when possible. The type and screen may be utilized for trauma patients that may be transported to another facility and can give the attending physician useful information if the need for an emergency transfusion arises. The probability of an incompatible transfusion is low when un-crossmatched blood is transfused to a patient with a negative antibody screen.

INTERNET ACTIVITIES

Visit the National Library of Medicine Web site at http://www.ncbi.nlm.nih.gov/PubMed/. Conduct a literature search on the use of prehospital fluid resuscitation in the setting of hemorrhagic shock. Review the abstracts of the search results. Ask your librarian to assist you in obtaining the journals with the five most relevant articles. Review these articles and summarize their findings.

EMERGENCY RELEASE OF BLOOD

Time is one of the most critical factors in treating the trauma patient. The physician must determine which poses the greatest risk, giving un-crossmatched blood or waiting 60 minutes until compatible blood is obtained. Prompt intervention in the trauma situation often requires giving un-crossmatched blood. Many institutions have a legal document stating that the risk of giving un-crossmatched blood outweighs the risk of waiting for compatible blood to be obtained and which must be signed by the physician. The physician must be aware that serologic testing has not been performed on the donor's or the recipient's blood and that compatibility has not been determined. However, while the un-crossmatched blood is being administered to the patient, compatibility testing and antibody screening is performed, which is helpful in predicting delayed reactions.

O-NEGATIVE PACKED CELLS: THE UNIVERSAL DONOR

In many traumas, time is such a critical factor that no time can be spared for grouping and typing of the patient. In these cases O-negative packed red blood cells is the fluid of choice. A unit of O-negative red blood cells does not contain the A, B, or D antigen and is the universal donor. During the Vietnam era O-negative whole blood was used without adverse consequences.[27]

Unfortunately, the person whose blood group and type is O negative cannot receive any blood other than O negative. O negative blood is a precious commodity worldwide and in short supply all the time. Note that only 6%–8% of the population is O negative.

Some medical air transport teams carry one or two units of O-negative packed red blood cells on board to trauma scenes where it is likely to be needed. Strict adherence to proper storage, handling, and usage protocols is necessary to ensure the safety of the patient.[28]

GROUP AND TYPE SPECIFIC EMERGENCY TRANSFUSIONS

Some emergencies allow enough time for the laboratory personnel to group and type the patient. This procedure requires only 10–15 minutes. This practice enables the patient to receive group and type specific blood, preserving the O-negative supply. However, the difficult decision to give blood as an emergency transfusion is most commonly made by a physician.

AUTOTRANSFUSION

The term **autotransfusion** refers to the reinfusion of one's own blood. Autologous blood is blood that has been donated and stored in the blood bank by a patient prior to surgery. If blood is needed, the patient will receive his or her own blood. The use of autologous blood is a form of autotransfusion that has become very popular. Autotransfusion may also refer to intraoperative blood and postoperative salvage. The blood is filtered, washed, and then reinfused.

Autotransfusions and autologous transfusions have a distinct advantage over the use of banked blood due to the reduction in complications that could occur in stored blood. Perhaps the complication of the greatest significance is disease transmission. The risk of disease transmission has led many patients to choose autologous donation for pending surgery, thus avoiding transfusion reactions. The trauma patient, theoretically, is an ideal candidate for autotransfusion due to the massive blood loss of some victims as well as the unavailability of stored blood in the field. However, the need for a machine to process the collected blood before reinfusion becomes an inherent problem in prehospital and emergency department environments.

Bacterial contamination, which often leads to sepsis, is an inherent risk in autotransfusion. Consequently, abdominal blood is unsuitable for reinfusion because of the chance of contamination by enteric bacteria. However, thoracic blood is suitable blood for reinfusion.

In addition to bacterial contamination, other complications include the development of renal failure following the release of large quantities of free hemoglobin by damaged red blood cells; coagulation problems in response to the presence of coagulation factors activated following trauma; and the possibility of an air embolism. For these reasons prehospital use of autotransfusion devices is not advisable. It should be utilized only in those life-threatening situations where banked blood is not available.[20]

BLOOD ADMINISTRATION

Only isotonic saline should be used concommitantly when administering blood products. Many commonly used crystalloids will damage red blood cells causing hemolysis or clot formation. The use of D_5W will cause hemolysis. Ringer's lactate may initiate coagulation within the infusion set itself. Also, many drugs will affect the integrity of the final product. Therefore, nothing should be infused in the same intravenous line with blood except 0.9% normal saline. The fluid of choice in hemorrhage is blood with or without crystalloid IVF, but it is in short supply compared to crystalloids.

Prior to the administration of any blood products a secure IV line must be initiated. Blood and blood products must be filtered during administration to remove small clots and cellular debris that form during storage. Some blood sets may contain this filter; others require that the filter be added to the line. Filter type and size may vary depending upon the product being infused. Standard in-line intravenous filters are not acceptable. For administration of blood products, nothing smaller than an 18-gauge catheter should be used. Smaller lumens damage the cells, resulting in hemolysis and clot formation, negating the benefits of the transfusion.

PATIENT IDENTIFICATION

Proper identification of the patient and the blood component is essential for patient safety. The principal cause of most transfusion-related deaths is clerical error.[29] Therefore, identification procedures are developed for all medical personnel involved in the transfusion. Patients receiving blood or blood prod-

ucts are usually identified with a unique identification bracelet containing the name of the patient as well as a unique blood bank identification number. The bracelet is placed on the patient when blood is drawn for crossmatching purposes. EMS personnel administering blood must follow stringent identification procedures before hanging the product. The purpose of this rigorous identification process is to prevent clerical errors from occurring. Laboratory personnel insist upon proper labeling of blood drawn for testing and will not use tubes that are not completely labeled. Proper identification procedures provide a way to ensure that transfusion-related deaths do not occur due to clerical errors.

INITIATING AND MONITORING THE TRANSFUSION

After the decision is made to administer blood or blood products whether emergently or routinely, certain procedures must be followed to assure safe and timely administration. Table 20-3 outlines a standard procedure for transfusion therapy. Before performing a blood transfusion procedure, become familiar with current policy. Some states require written consents or other documentation signed by the patient or a legal representative prior to administering blood. Even in emergency situations legal documentation may be required and failure to obtain it may lead to disciplinary or legal action.

Table 20-3
Procedures for Initiation and Monitoring of Blood Products

- Identify the patient and verify a match of the blood bank identification numbers on both the blood and the patient.
- Visually inspect the blood product for impurities.
- Obtain a full set of baseline vital signs, including temperature.
- Ascertain that normal saline is hanging with the Y set to avoid occlusion of tubing.
- Hang blood unit and observe the patient closely during the first 15 minutes of transfusion. This is the most likely time for reactions to occur and the most dangerous time for the patient.
- Change blood filters every 2 units.
- Observe and inspect the IV site frequently for signs of infiltration and phlebitis.

Along with proper consents, documentation of the transfusion is of paramount importance. Table 20-4 suggests minimum parameters that should be covered in the documentation. Monitoring the patient for complications, including infiltration, phlebitis, embolism, or transfusion reactions, is essential and should be noted.

Prior to hanging a bag of blood or blood product, always examine it carefully for sediment, clots, bubbles, cloudiness, or areas of dark color, which could indicate bacterial contamination. It is essential that the numbers on the blood bag match the identification bracelet worn by the patient. Even with emergency release units, a blood bank ID number is assigned and a bracelet placed on the patient. Always administer blood via a Y set IV tubing with 0.9% normal saline (Figure 20-19). Do not substitute any other crystalloid fluid for the normal saline. The IV lines are primed with normal saline prior to spiking the blood bag. Filters used with blood tubing should be changed every 2 units. Because they are collecting particles, microclots, and cellular debris, filters can become clogged, slowing the transfusion. Further, the blood particles in the filter are at room temperature and bacteria can multiply rapidly in this environment. A standard unit of blood is 250 cc and should be infused within 4 hours of obtaining the blood from the refrigerated source. Most trauma patients will receive multiple units in that time frame, but patients transported with blood infusing may not be receiving a rapid infusion and require that close attention be paid to hanging time.

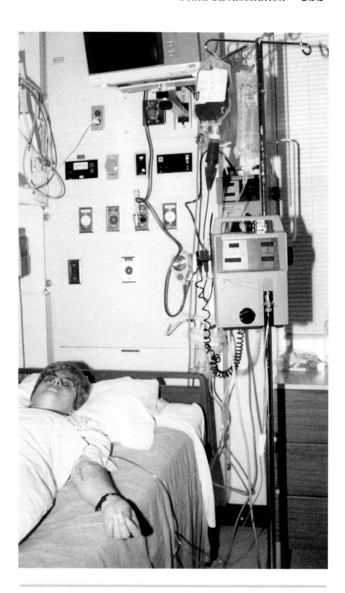

FIGURE 20-19 Patient attached to Y tubing of blood setup. (Courtesy of Mark Zeringue.)

Table 20-4
Documentation Parameters

Baseline vital signs	Febrile reactions are defined by a rise in temperature.
Type of blood product infused	Emergency release, O negative, type specific, crossmatched, PRBC, FFP, whole blood, etc.
Time infusion began and ended	Blood must be used within 4 hours of removal from the refrigerator.
Patient response after each unit	Improved, unchanged, worsening, possible reaction.
Vital signs	Depending on patient's condition, but not less than every 15 minutes.
Amount of blood and saline infused	Total amounts of all fluids received during the resuscitation effort must be documented.

INTERNET ACTIVITIES

Visit the Web site of the British Trauma Society at http://www.trauma.org/resus/massive. html and review the material on massive blood loss and replacement transfusion.

RATE OF INFUSION

The physician will use the patient's clinical condition to determine the rate of blood infusion, bearing in mind that a "rapid" rate of fluid administration is somewhat subjective and is often influenced by the type of tubing in use, catheter size and placement, filters, and overall condition of the patient. Using a Y set, the blood is piggybacked with normal saline to decrease its viscosity and enable the blood to run into the patient more readily. The primary goal of fluid/blood administration is restoration of tissue perfusion. Patients with certain underlying medical conditions should receive blood at a slower rate to decrease the chance of cardiac overload. However, cardiac overload is an infrequent occurrence during exsanguinating hemorrhage. Under normal circumstances most patients tolerate transfusion rates of 1 unit over $1\frac{1}{2}$–2 hours. In trauma situations expect blood to be administered in minutes rather than hours, keeping in mind that each unit transfused increases the risk of adverse reactions.

The American Association of Blood Banks (AABB) stipulates that blood should be infused within 4 hours after the start of the transfusion because bacterial growth within the blood product is accelerated at room temperature.[29] For this reason blood should be initiated immediately upon arrival of the product and not left lying about while other procedures are performed. Paramedics who anticipate long transport times should clearly mark the unit with an expiration time, discontinue the unit when it expires, and initiate a fresh, refrigerated one.

Whole blood and packed red blood cells are stored at 1°C–6°C in the blood bank refrigerator until needed. Refrigerators and freezers used in blood storage are monitored constantly for temperature and equipped with alarms. Strict guidelines are in place to ensure that the blood supply is free from bacterial contamination.

GENERAL PRINCIPLES OF BLOOD TYPES

The study of antigens and antibodies and their relationship to blood is called **immunohematology**. Antigens are located on the red blood cell surface, while antibodies are found in the plasma. Awareness of the existence of both antigens and antibodies and the reactions that can occur with the combination of like antigens and antibodies is important for the EMS provider.

A person's blood group is inherited genetically from their parents. A gene from each parent combines to form the ABO blood group antigen(s). The blood group antigens are A, B, and O, and the presence or absence of each plays a role in determining the blood group. The A and B antigens are codominant over the O antigen. Therefore, if a person is group O, an O antigen must be inherited from each parent. If an A antigen is inherited from one parent and an O antigen from the other, the blood group will be A (Table 20-5).

The patient's blood type is determined by the presence or absence of the D antigen: Rh positive or Rh negative (Table 20-6). The D antigen is the most important antigen in the Rh blood system, discovered

Table 20-5
Genetic Combinations and Their Interpretations

Genetic Code Combinations	Blood Group Interpretations
AA	A
AO	A
BB	B
BO	B
AB	AB
OO	O

Table 20-6
Blood Type Interpretation

Blood Type	D Antigen
Rh Positive	Present
Rh Negative	Absent

in the 1930s.[27] Rh antigens are also located on red blood cells. The Rh system is important because of the potential for antibody formation and future reactions. Antigens to many other blood groups also exist on the red blood cell and are inherited genetically.

Antibodies are proteinlike substances that are formed in response to antigenic stimuli. The primary mode for blood group antibody production is through transfusion or pregnancy. An antibody screen is performed on all potential blood recipients to ensure that no clinically significant antibodies are present. Examples of such antibodies are anti-Kell, anti-Lewis, and anti-Duffy. The ABO blood group system, however, has "naturally occurring" antibodies to the dominant antigen lacking on the red blood cells. A person with group A blood would have the A antigen on the red blood cells and the B antibody in his or her plasma (Table 20-7).

Table 20-7
ABO Blood Type Antigens and Antibodies

ABO Group	Antigens on Red Cells	Antibodies In Plasma
A	A	B
B	B	A
AB	A and B	None
O	None	A and B

COMPLICATIONS OF TRANSFUSIONS

EMS personnel should remember that blood transfusions are not without risks. As with medications, life-threatening reactions can and do occur. The act of transfusing blood can be compared with an organ transplant. When blood is infused, living cells are transplanted into the patient. The threat of rejection can be greatly reduced by following guidelines set forth for blood banking practices. Reactions vary from minor to severe and, on occasion, death. Until proven otherwise, all reactions are assumed to be hemolytic.

The paramedic cannot become complacent about the act of transfusing blood. Education about the products being used, the symptoms associated with reactions, and common modes of treatment is necessary. Quick intervention when a severe reaction occurs can mean the difference between life and death. The reactions listed below are the most commonly occurring reactions; however, other reactions do exist. The reader should be aware of this fact and inform the physician of any adverse symptom(s) noted.

FEBRILE

The febrile reaction is the most common reaction encountered. Most symptoms of a febrile reaction are mild. These reactions occur much more often in patients who have had previous blood transfusion reactions. Febrile reactions are reactions formed in response to the antigens on the transfused white blood cells. If these transfused white blood cells are reduced, the incidence of a febrile reaction is greatly decreased. Signs and symptoms of febrile reaction include fever with or without chills, hypotension (rare), tachycardia (rare), and dyspnea (rare). When these symptoms are recognized, the paramedic should stop the transfusion, keep the IV line open with normal saline, notify the attending physician of the possible reaction, and be prepared to administer antipyretics such as aspirin or acetaminophen.

Patients requiring blood who have a history of repeated febrile reactions may require the use of blood with reduced white blood cells or leukocytes. This can be done by using components such as leukocyte-depleted blood. Leukocytes are depleted in these units shortly after collection. In-line filters are used during the component preparation process to accomplish this reduction. Washed red blood cells, another product with reduced leukocytes, are prepared by washing the unit of cells with saline prior to infusion. In order to wash red blood cells, the blood unit must be unsealed. This reduces the shelf life to 24 hours. Leukocyte-depleted cells and/or washed red blood cells are not readily available in some hospitals. A leukocyte filter may be utilized at the bedside in lieu of such products as washed red blood cells. This filter eliminates the majority of white blood cells, accomplishing an effect similar to washing the cells. If white blood cell filtration is performed at the patient's bedside, the shelf life of the blood is unaffected. Infusion rates should not be appreciably slowed with the use of this filter. These filters are not routinely used because of the added costs. They are often reserved for those patients with documented, recurrent febrile reactions. Premedication with antipyretics is sometimes used in the patient with a history of febrile reactions; however, antipyretics are not used in all transfusions since masking of symptoms may occur.[25]

ALLERGIC (URTICARIAL)

Allergic reactions are the second most common transfusion reaction. The definitive cause of this type of reaction is not clearly known. Production of histamines appears to be responsible. Allergic reactions are not usually dangerous but can cause profound discomfort to the patient. Signs and symptoms of allergic reaction include redness, itching, hives, and possibly fever. Once an allergic reaction is recognized, the paramedic should stop the transfusion, keep the IV line open with normal saline, and notify the attending physician of the possible reaction. Antihistamines such as diphenhydramine are used in the treatment of the allergic reaction. Severe reactions may warrant the use of theophylline, epinephrine, or steroids. Premedication with antihistamines is not uncommon in a transfusion.

ANAPHYLACTIC

Anaphylactic reactions are similar to allergic reactions but are more severe. The most probable cause is histamine release. Symptoms develop quickly, within minutes of receiving the first few milliliters of blood. Anaphylactic reactions can cause severe respiratory distress and are potentially fatal. This reaction usually involves anti-immunoglobulin A (anti-IgA) in high titers found in the recipient. The IgA is the predominant immunoglobulin found in body secretions. Its principal role is the removal of antigenic substances without an inflammatory response. When the antibody to IgA is found in large quantities in the recipient, a complement is activated. The complement's main function is to promote the inflammatory response. Signs and symptoms of an anaphylactic reaction include flushing, bronchial spasms, urticaria, shock, hypotension, unconsciousness, dyspnea, angioedema, and nausea. Fever is not observed. Treatment of the anaphylactic reaction includes stopping the transfusion, keeping the IV line open with normal saline, notifying the attending physician of the reaction, administering epinephrine, maintaining blood pressure with crystalloids, administering oxygen, and stabilizing vital signs.

CIRCULATORY OVERLOAD

Although not initially a concern in the trauma patient, circulatory overload occurs when a patient receives too much volume within too short a period of time. This may lead to congestive heart failure and possibly pulmonary edema. High-risk groups of patients include pediatrics, geriatrics, and people with chronic anemia. Blood should be administered at a slower rate for these high-risk individuals, but care should be taken not to exceed 4 hours per unit as previously stipulated. Control of infusion rate and volume is key in alleviating these reactions.

Units of blood containing smaller volumes than routinely encountered are available for use with pediatric patients. Donation of a single unit of whole blood may yield up to four pediatric units. Dosing varies greatly in the pediatric patient depending upon the clinical condition of the child as well as the age. Dosing is based upon the weight of the child. The transfusion of 10 mL/kg of weight increases the hemoglobin approximately 3 g/dL.[30] Signs and symptoms of circulatory overload include chest pain, coughing, cyanosis, tachycardia, dyspnea, and hypertension. To treat circulatory overload, the paramedic should stop the transfusion, keep the IV line open with normal saline, notify the attending physician of the possible reaction, monitor vital signs, and administer oxygen and IV diuretics per protocol or order.

SEPSIS

Sepsis is a rare transfusion reaction but can occur quickly and lead to death. Symptoms usually occur within the first 30 minutes of the transfusion. Bacterial contamination of the transfused blood product is the cause of this reaction. EMS providers should be alert for contaminated units, examining all units closely before hanging the product. Contaminated units may be hemolyzed, turbid, or discolored or contain "fuzz balls" or "cottonlike balls" not routinely seen in the component. Blood bank personnel should be consulted if a unit is in question. Blood should be left refrigerated or kept on ice until ready for infusion to decrease the chance of bacterial contamination. Signs and symptoms of sepsis include fever, shaking chills, abdominal cramps, dryness and flushing of skin, vomiting, and

possibly shock, renal failure, and disseminated intravascular coagulation (DIC). Treatment includes stopping the transfusion, keeping the IV line open with normal saline, notifying the attending physician of the possible reaction, supporting vital signs with dopamine, and administering broad-spectrum antibiotics.

HEMOLYTIC REACTIONS

A hemolytic reaction is the destruction of red blood cells by one of two methods: intravascular hemolysis or red blood cell lysis. Intravascular hemolysis releases hemoglobin along with other red blood cell parts leading to hemoglobinuria. Red blood cell lysis does not occur intravascularly and no hemoglobin is released into the circulating blood. Reactions to intravascular hemolysis are swift, with effects that can be life threatening. Extravascular hemolytic reactions (red blood cell lysis) are milder reactions. When symptoms of a reaction are first displayed, its classification is not always obvious. Many reactions display similar symptoms. Therefore, all transfusion reactions should be investigated. Patients must be monitored throughout and immediately following a transfusion for any signs and symptoms of a reaction. The severity of a hemolytic reaction is dose related. The more blood that is received by the patient, the more severe the reaction. When possible, transfusions should be started at a slow rate and the patient monitored closely in the initial 15 minutes of the transfusion.

Acute Hemolytic Reaction

Acute hemolytic reactions are almost always due to an ABO incompatibility between the transfused blood and the patient. Clerical error is the major reason for the administration of incompatible blood. Signs and symptoms of an acute hemolytic reaction include fever, chills, DIC, nausea, chest pain, dyspnea, flank pain, hypotension, abdominal pain, flushing, hemoglobinuria, and acute renal failure. Treatment includes stopping the transfusion, keeping the IV line open with normal saline, notifying the attending physician of the possible reaction, increasing renal cortical perfusion using IV saline or Ringer's lactate in large doses, and maintaining volume and blood pressure using crystalloids and possibly dopamine. Dopamine supports the blood pressure, increases cardiac output and renal cortical perfusion, and combats shock and renal failure.

Delayed Hemolytic Reaction

The delayed hemolytic reaction is due to an amnestic response in the patient who has been previously sensitized by pregnancy or previous transfusions. Sensitization is achieved by the building up of antibodies via exposure to foreign antigens. When exposed to these antigens, antibodies react by destroying the transfused red blood cells containing this antigen. These antibodies may not be detectable when performing the antibody screen on the patient during the pretransfusion testing if the antibodies exist in low titers. The signs and symptoms of the delayed hemolytic reaction are somewhat milder than the acute reaction. Timing of the delayed hemolytic reaction may occur 1–14 days following a transfusion. Excess antibody production causes lysing of the transfused cells and anemia. Essentially, the transfused red blood cells containing the appropriate antigen are destroyed. Signs and symptoms of delayed hemolytic reaction include fever with or without chills, anemia, and mild jaundice. Usually no treatment is required. If severe reactions do occur, treatment is the same as for acute hemolytic reactions.

▶ SUMMARY

Fluid resuscitation using crystalloid solutions remains the standard of treatment for EMS providers. Crystalloid fluids, while composed of naturally occurring components, can cause serious complications, even death. Judicious use of the proper intravenous fluid or blood product is essential to the resuscitation effort. It is critical that all personnel involved with the care of the patient receiving blood be familiar with the use of blood or blood products and be alert for adverse reactions. Continuous monitoring during transport is essential.

Although long the purview of hospital nurses and physicians, the life-saving administration of blood in the hemorrhaging patient is likely to be used at the scene of traumas with increasing frequency. However, field administration of blood products by EMS personnel is limited due to product storage requirements, limited space on emergency vehicles, and the need for specialized training.

▶ REVIEW QUESTIONS

1. The blood group and type considered to be the universal donor is:
   a. A positive
   b. O positive
   c. AB negative
   d. O negative
2. The primary reason for utilizing a large-bore needle in a blood transfusion is:
   a. To allow the blood to be given quickly
   b. To prevent damage to the red blood cell

   c. To be able to give other fluids with the blood
   d. To prevent an occlusion of the vein
3. A rise in temperature with no other symptoms of a reaction noted is mostly which of the following?
   a. Urticarial
   b. Delayed hemolytic
   c. Circulatory overload
   d. Febrile
4. Until proven otherwise, all transfusion reactions are treated as if they are:
   a. Febrile
   b. Circulatory overload
   c. Hemolytic
   d. Sepsis
5. Symptoms of sepsis would include all of the following except:
   a. Fever
   b. Chills
   c. Urticaria
   d. Flushing of skin
6. Packed red blood cells or whole blood may hang for a maximum of 4 hours.
   a. True
   b. False
7. Filter size is of no importance when transfusing blood.
   a. True
   b. False
8. Abdominal blood is a good source for autotransfusion.
   a. True
   b. False
9. What is the most common cause of a fatal transfusion reaction?
10. What single advantage does the infusion of red blood cells have over crystalloid or nonblood colloidal resuscitation?
11. A catheter lumen that is less than _____ gauge will _____ red cells.
12. Compare and contrast crystalloid and colloid fluids.
13. Discuss the controversies surrounding the administration of intravenous fluids.
14. Identify three sites most frequently used for intravenous access.
15. The three types of catheter insertion techniques are:
   a. Subclavian, peripheral, and over the needle
   b. Through the needle, over the needle, and under the needle
   c. Over a guide wire, through the needle, and over the needle

d. Seldinger technique, over a guide wire, and over the needle

16. The Y set IV tubing is always primed with:
  a. Blood or blood product
  b. Normal saline
  c. Lactated Ringer's solution
  d. Any crystalloid solution

17. Discuss the differences between isotonic, hypotonic, and hypertonic solutions.

▶ CRITICAL THINKING

● What are the disadvantages of aggressively resuscitating a patient with crystalloid fluids during active internal hemorrhage?

● Some researchers believe that hemorrhaging patients should be resuscitated with only enough crystalloid fluid to maintain moderate hypotension (≈90 mm Hg systolic). What are your thoughts on this proposed treatment regimen?

● Under what circumstances would you elect to perform the following procedures: (1) external jugular cannulation, (2) femoral vein cannulation, (3) large-bore catheter insertion using the Seldinger technique, (4) saphenous vein cutdown, and (5) intraosseous infusion? What are the advantages and disadvantages of each venous access technique?

▶ REFERENCES

1. Pollack CV. Prehospital fluid resuscitation of the trauma patient. *Emerg Med Clin North Am.* 1993; 11:1.
2. Kreimeier U, Messmer IK. Future trends in emergency fluid resuscitation: small volume resuscitation by means of hypertonic saline dextran. *Intens Care World.* 1992; 9:3.
3. Crisp CB. Fluid resuscitation in the traumatized patient: a review of crystalloid and colloid therapy. *Emerg Care Q.* 1988; 3:4.
4. Vassar MJ, Holcroft JW. Use of hypertonic-hyperoncotic fluids for resuscitation of trauma patients. *J Intens Care Med.* 1992; 7.
5. Wade CE, Hannon JP, Bassone CA, Hunt MM. Superiority of hypertonic saline/dextran over hypertonic saline during the first 30 min of resuscitation following hemorrhagic hypotension in conscious swine. *Resuscitation.* 1990; 49:1:20.
6. Mattox KL, Maningas PA, Moore EE, et al. Prehospital hypertonic saline/dextran infusion for post-traumatic hypotension. *Ann Surg.* 1991; 213:5.
7. Cox DM. Trauma fluid resuscitation. *Emergency.* 1994; 26(4):22–6.
8. Gross D, Landau EH, Klin B, Krausz MM. Quantitative measurement of bleeding following hypertonic saline therapy in 'uncontrolled' hemorrhagic shock. *J Trauma.* 1989; 29.
9. Reed RL 2nd, Johnston TD, Chen Y, Fischer RP. Hypertonic saline alters plasma clotting times and platelet aggregation. *J Trauma.* 1991; 31:1.
10. Krausz MM, Bar-Ziv M, Rabinovici R, Gross D. "Scoop and run" or stabilize hemorrhagic shock with normal saline or small volume hypertonic saline. *J Trauma.* 1992; 33:1:6.
11. Bickell WH, Bruttig SP, Millnamow GA, O'Behar J, Wade CE. Use of hypertonic saline/dextran versus lactated Ringer's solution as a resuscitation fluid after uncontrolled aortic hemorrhage in anesthetized swine. *Ann Emerg Med.* 1992; 9:21.
12. Imm A, Carlson RW. Fluid resuscitation in circulatory shock. *Crit Care Clin.* 1993; 9:2.
13. Wyngaarden JB, Bennett JC, Smith LH. Shock. *Cecil's Textbook of Medicine.* 19th ed. Philadelphia: WB Saunders. 1992.
14. Barker WJ. Vascular techniques and volume support. In: Rosen P, Barkin R, eds. *Emergency Medicine.* 3rd ed. St Louis: Mosby Year Book. 1992.
15. Goodin TH, Grossbard EB, Kaufman RJ, et al. A perfluorochemical emulsion for prehospital resuscitation of experimental hemorrhagic shock: a prospective, randomized, controlled study. *Crit Care Med.* 1994; 22:4.
16. Greenberg AG, Kim HW. Use of donor blood in the surgical setting: potentials for application of blood substitutes. *Art Cells Blood Subs Immob Biotech.* 1997; 25:1.
17. Kennedy M, Carmen J. Transfusion therapy. In: Harmening D, ed. *Modern Blood Banking and Transfusion Practices.* 3rd ed. Philadelphia: FA Davis; 1994:320.
18. Labidie LL. Transfusion therapy in the emergency department. *Emerg Med Clin North Am.* 1993; 11:384.
19. Pisciotto P, eds. *Blood Transfusion Therapy; a Physician's Handbook.* 4th ed. Bethesda, Md: American Association of Blood Banks; 1993:24.
20. Kennedy M, Carmen J. Transfusion therapy. In: Harmening D, ed. *Modern Blood Banking and Transfusion Practices.* 3rd ed. Philadelphia: FA Davis; 1994; 330.
21. Sakles JC, Sena MJ, Knight DA, Davis JM. Effect of immediate fluid resuscitation on the rate, volume, and duration of pulmonary vascular hemorrhage in a sheep model of penetrating thoracic trauma. *J Surg Res.* 1996; 63:2.

22. Leppaniemi A, Sottero R, Burris D, et al. Fluid resuscitation in a model of uncontrolled hemorrhage: too much too early, or too little too late? *J Surg Res*. 1996; 63:2.

23. Fisher A. *The Healthy Heart*. Alexandria, Va: Time-Life Books; 1981; 8.

24. Harmening DM, Harrison CR, Dawson RB. Blood preservation: historic perspectives, review of metabolism, and current trends. In: Harmening DM, ed. *Modern Blood Banking and Transfusion Practices*. 3rd ed. Philadelphia: FA Davis; 1994; 2.

25. Moore GP, Jordan R, eds. Hematologic/oncologic emergency. *Emerg Med Clin North Am*. 1993; 11:2.

26. Pisciotto P, et al, eds. *Blood Transfusion Therapy, A Physician's Handbook*. 4th ed. Bethesda, Md: American Association of Blood Banks; 1993; 9.

27. Harmening DM, Firestone D. The ABO blood group system. In: Harmening DM, ed. *Modern Blood Banking and Transfusion Practices*. 3rd ed. Philadelphia: FA Davis; 1994; 87.

28. Kennedy M, Carmen J. Transfusion therapy. In: Harmening D, ed. *Modern Blood Banking and Transfusion Practices*. 3rd ed. Philadelphia: FA Davis; 1994; 325.

29. Thurer RL, Hauer JM. *Autotransfusions and Blood Conservation: Current Problems in Surgery*. Chicago, Ill: Year Book Medical Publishers; 1982; 97.

30. Krugh D. Emergency transfusion during medical air transport. *Lab Med*. 1994; 25:5: 318.

31. Waisman M, Waisman D. Bone marrow infusion in adults. *J Trauma*. 1997; 42:288–293.

32. Glaeser P, Hellmich T, Szewczuga D, Losek J, Smith D. Five-year experience in prehospital intraosseous infusions in children and adults. *Ann Emerg Med*. 1993; 22:1119–1124.

33. Iserson K. Intraosseous infusions in adults. *J Emerg Med*. 1989;7:587–591.

34. Waisman M, Roffman M, Bursztein S, Heifetz M. Intraosseous regional anesthesia as an alternative to intravenous regional anesthesia. *J Trauma*. 1995; 39:1153–1156.

35. Hubble M, Trigg D. Training prehospital personnel in saphenous vein cutdown and adult intraosseous Access Techniques. *Prehosp Emerg Care*. 2001; 5(2):181–189.

36. Macnab A, Christenson J, Findlay J, Horwood B, Johnson D, Jones L, et al. A new system for sternal intraosseous infusion in adults. *Prehosp Emerg Care*. 2000; 4:173–177.

BIBLIOGRAPHY

American College of Surgeons (ACS). *Shock: Advanced Trauma Life Support*. 5th ed. Chicago, Ill: ACS; 1995; 75.

Anderson KC, Ness PM. *Scientific Basis of Transfusion Medicine: Implications for Clinical Practice*. Philadelphia: WB Saunders; 1994.

Auerbach P, ed. *Wilderness Medicine*. 3rd ed. St. Louis: Mosby-Yearbook; 1995.

Barson BJ, Scalea TM. Acute blood loss. *Emerg Med Clin North Am*. 1996; 14:1.

Beck WA. *Vascular Access: Emergency Medicine*. 4th ed. New York: McGraw-Hill; 1996:50.

Bickell WH, Wall MJ Jr, Pepe PE, et al. Immediate versus delayed fluid resuscitation for hypotensive patients with penetrating torso injuries. *N Eng J Med*. 1994; 331:17.

Bledsoe BE, Porter RS, Shade BR. *Brady Paramedic Emergency Care*. 2nd ed. Englewood Cliffs, N.J.: Prentice-Hall; 1994.

Callaham ML. *Current Practice of Emergency Medicine*. 2nd ed. Philadelphia: Decker; 1991; 61.

Capone AC, Safor P, Stezoski W, Tisherman S, Peitzman AB. Improved outcome with fluid restriction in treatment of uncontrolled hemorrhagic shock. *J Am Coll Surg*. 1995; 180:1.

Chang TMS. Recent and future developments in modified hemoglobin and microencapsulated hemoglobin as RBC substitute. *Art Cells Blood Subs Immob Biotech*. 1997; 25:1.

Coffland FI, Shelton DM. Blood component replacement therapy. *Crit Care Nurs*. 1993; 5:3.

Craig RL, Poole GV. Resuscitation in uncontrolled hemorrhage. *Ann Surg*. 1994:60:59.

DeChristopher PJ. Leukocyte reduction filtration: technologies, benefits, applications, and limitations. *Lab Med*. 1994; 25:2.

Dracker RA, Beadling W, Lauenstein K. The search for a clinically useful blood substitute. *Lab Med*. 1994; 25:11.

Falk JL, O'Brien JF, Kerr R. Fluid resuscitation in traumatic hemorrhagic shock. *Crit Care Clin*. 1992; 8:2.

Garratty G, ed. *Current Concepts in Transfusion Therapy*. Arlington, Va: American Association of Blood Banks; 1985.

Gursel E, Binns JH. Early management of burned patients. *Emerg Med Clin North Am*. 1983; 1:3.

Hamilton SM, Breakey P. Fluid resuscitation of the trauma patient: how much is enough? *Can J Surg*. 1996; 39:1.

Krausz MM, Landau EH, Klin B, Gross D. Hypertonic saline treatment of uncontrolled hemorrhagic shock. *Arch Surg*. 1992; 127:93.

Krone RL. Resuscitation of the multiple injured patient. *Med Clin North Am*. 1983; 1:3.

Lowe KC, et al. Perfluorochemicals and cell biotechnology. *Art Cells Blood Subs Immob Biotech*. 1997; 25:3.

Martin RR, Bickell WH, Pepe PE, Burch JM, Mattox KL. Prospective evaluation of preoperative fluid resuscitation in hypotensive patients with penetrating truncal injury: a preliminary report. *J Trauma*. 1992; 33:3.

Mayer K, ed. *Guidelines to Transfusion Practices*. Arlington, Va: American Association of Blood Banks; 1985.

Milzmorn DP, ed. Critical resuscitations. *Emerg Med Clin North Am*. 1996; 14:1.

Mollison PL. *Blood Transfusion in Clinical Medicine*. 9th ed. Oxford: Blackwell Scientific Publication; 1988.

Moore GP, Jordan R, eds. Hematologic/oncologic emergency. *Med Clin North Am*. 1993; 11:2.

Mosby's Paramedic Textbook: Shock. St Louis: Mosby-Year Book; 1994.

National Association of Emergency Medical Technicians, Prehospital Trauma Life Support Committee, American College of Surgeons, Committee on Trauma. *Prehospital Trauma Life Support: Shock and Fluid Resuscitation*. St Louis: Mosby-Year Book; 1994; 154.

Paquette ML. Blood substitutes: a risk free solution. *Adv Admin Lab*. 1995; 4:10.

Petz LD, ed. *Clinical Practices of Transfusion Medicine*. 2nd ed. New York: Churchill Livingston; 1989.

Piscotto PT, ed. *Blood Transfusion Therapy, a Physician's Handbook*. 4th ed. Bethesda, Md: American Association of Blood Banks; 1993; 65.

Popovsky MA. Strategies for limiting patient exposure to allogenic blood. *Lab Med*. 1994; 25:2.

Raichle LT, Paranto ME. Compatibility testing. In: Harmening DM, ed. *Modern Blood Banking and Transfusion Practices*. 3rd ed. Philadelphia: FA Davis; 1994; 257.

Rakel R, ed. *Conn's Current Therapy*. Philadelphia: WB Saunders; 1997.

Rea R, ed. *Trauma Nursing Core Curriculum*. 3rd ed. Chicago, Ill: Emergency Nurses Association, Award Printing Corporation; 1991.

Salit M. Artificial blood substitutes. Program at North Carolina Association of Blood Bankers. September 1996.

Spivey WH. Intraosseous infusions. In: Rosen P, Barkin R, eds. *Emergency Medicine: Concepts and Clinical Practices*. 3rd ed. St Louis: Mosby-Year Book; 1992; 364.

Stowell CP. When to pull the trigger, making the decision to transfuse red blood cells. *Lab Med*. 1995; 26:1.

Strauss R. Predicting the future of blood component therapy. Program at North Carolina Association of Blood Bankers annual meeting. September 1996.

Talbot-Stern JK. Gastrointestinal bleeding. *Emerg Med Clin North Am*. 1996; 14:1.

Thurer RL, Hauer JM. *Autotransfusions and Blood Conservation: Current Problems in Surgery*. Chicago, Ill: Year Book Medical Publishers; 1982; 97.

Verdile VP. Trends in IV therapy. *Emergency*. 1990.

Von Rueden KT, Dunham CM. Sequelae of massive fluid resuscitation in trauma patients. *Crit Care Nurs Clin North Am*. 1994; 6:3.

Walker RH, American Association of Blood Banks, eds. *Technical Manual*. 3rd ed. Bethesda, Md: JB Lippincott; 1993; 421.

Westphal RG. *American Red Cross Handbook of Transfusion Medicine*. 3rd ed. Washington, D.C.?: Robert's Press; 1990; 60.

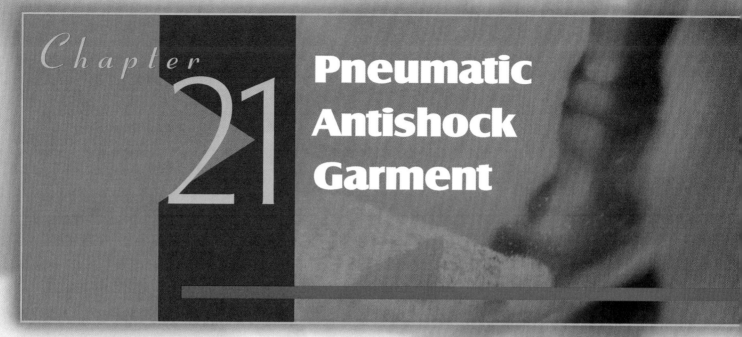

Chapter 21 Pneumatic Antishock Garment

OBJECTIVES

Upon completion of this chapter, the reader should be able to:

- Describe three key events in the development of the pneumatic antishock garment.
- Explain the physiological principles that account for the ability of the pneumatic antishock garment to raise blood pressure.
- Explain the physiological principles that account for the ability of the pneumatic antishock garment to control hemorrhage.
- List the indications and contraindications for use of the pneumatic antishock garment in trauma situations.
- Demonstrate three methods of application of the pneumatic antishock garment.
- Demonstrate the appropriate method of deflation and removal of the pneumatic antishock garment.

KEY TERMS

Bernoulli's law
Biophysics
Hemodynamics

Laminar
Laplace's law
Physiology

The pneumatic antishock garment (PASG) has been in use for nearly a century. For a medical device to generate controversy is not unusual. For it to have such a long history of use and still be controversial is most unusual.

INVENTION OF THE PASG

In 1903 George Crile, clinical professor of surgery at Western Reserve School of Medicine, informed his colleagues at a meeting in Boston of a device he had developed over the previous two years that restored and maintained blood pressure in surgical patients.[1]

The device was a double-walled rubber suit that, when laced, enclosed the patient's lower limbs and abdomen (Figure 21-1). Inflation of the suit developed a circumferential pressure in the covered body areas that Crile theorized increased peripheral vascular resistance, autotransfused blood from the lower body to the upper circulation, and resulted in a rise in blood pressure.

Born in Ohio in 1864, George Crile was a pioneer in understanding the nature and treatment of shock. He was one of the first to recognize the need to monitor blood pressure during surgery, to administer epinephrine for its vasoconstrictive properties, and to use blood transfusions to prevent surgical shock. However, it is his introduction of the PASG as a treatment for

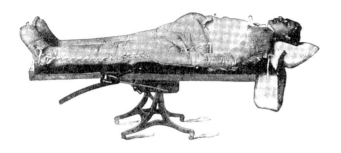

FIGURE 21-1 Original PASG developed by George Crile.
Source: Crile GW. *Blood Pressure in Surgery.* Philadelphia: JB Lippincott; 1903: 289. Dittrick Medical History Center of the Cleveland Health Sciences Library.

hypotension for which he is most often cited in prehospital literature. His early experiments initiated a patient care controversy that has yet to be resolved.

Crile's pneumatic suit was cumbersome and unreliable. He soon abandoned it in favor of other techniques he was developing for maintaining blood pressure, especially those for the transfusion of blood. The idea of the pressure suit would not resurface until 1941 when the plane on which Crile was a passenger was caught in a tornado and crashed when the crew lost consciousness. Crile theorized that their syncope was due to the loss of blood to the brain following the plane's rapid ascent in the funnel. He believed that his pneumatic suit could prevent this loss of consciousness by preventing the pooling of blood in the lower body experienced by pilots during rapid accelerations.[1] Thus was born the idea of the antigravity or G-suit.

DEVELOPMENT OF THE MODERN PASG

Not long after the development of the PASG by the military as the aviator's G-suit, the principle of external circumferential lower body pressure was once again being used in the care of patients and the device was undergoing modification. As early as 1952 W. James Gardner recognized the need for a PASG that could be easily and rapidly applied.[2] He developed a two-ply vinyl bag that was wrapped around the patient from the distal border of the ribs to the legs, laced up the front, and inflated. This bag could be placed under the patient at any time with the patient encased and the bag inflated when necessary, much as paramedics do today with the modern PASG. Gardner also recognized that an inflatable, double-walled bag made an effective splint.[3] Reports of the use of the antigravity suit to control hemorrhage began to appear in the literature. The G-suit was employed in surgically induced hemorrhage in animal studies and in the control of intra-abdominal bleeding in medical patients.[4] Although first suggested

by Crile early in the century, the use of a PASG in trauma situations was not employed to any extent until the Vietnam War. During this conflict military medical personnel adapted pilots' G-suits to patient use in order to maintain blood pressure and control hemorrhage, especially during long helicopter evacuations to surgical hospitals.

In 1973 Burton Kaplan and his colleagues reported on the development of the military antishock trouser (MAST) for use in the prehospital setting.[5] First employed by the City of Miami paramedics, this significant modification of the G-suit was manufactured by David Clark, Inc., and was similar to the PASG used on ambulances today. The MAST could be easily and rapidly applied, was recommended for patients experiencing medical or trauma-induced hypotension, and acted as an effective splint. It improved on the G-suit's ability to exert external lower body pressure allowing inflation to 104 mm Hg and applying this pressure to the body below the xiphoid process of the sternum. Kaplan's report also contained statements concerning autotransfusion volumes accomplished with MAST inflation, indications and contraindications for its use, patient care once MAST was inflated, and possible complications of MAST inflation, all of which served as the rationale for the estimated 2–3 million uses of MAST in the prehospital setting during the next decade and a half.[4]

Crile's version of the pneumatic suit enabled the user to inflate either or both legs and the abdomen singly or in combination. Early versions of the PASG for use in the prehospital setting were single-chambered devices with Velcro closures or heavy-duty zippers carried in metal cases. Current versions of the PASG are again the three-chambered device secured with Velcro and inflated with a foot pump to pressures monitored with a variety of gauges or relief valves and carried in plastic cases or soft-sided packs.

CONTROVERSIES

During the decades of the 1970s and 1980s numerous studies appeared in the literature concerning the responses of human volunteers and animals to the application of the PASG under varied conditions; yet, it was primarily the case studies and anecdotal reports of patient care successes with the PASG that maintained continued prehospital and in-hospital use of the garment. In the late 1980s, reports of the first large-scale prospective clinical study of prehospital PASG use were published.[6,7] The study involved approximately 1,000 hypotensive, urban trauma patients with penetrating injuries predominating. The findings heightened concern about the garment, as this study found no improvement in the prehospital condition of the patient nor in patient survival or length of hospital stay when the PASG was employed. Based upon this single study in an urban setting, the researchers recommended that the garment be abandoned as a prehospital treatment device. The protocol for this study had paramedics apply the PASG on alternate days to all patients with blunt or penetrating trauma in any body location when the patient presented with a systolic blood pressure of 90 mm Hg or less. On days when the PASG was not employed, standard protocols for trauma were employed. This research design included the use of the PASG with patients normally excluded by treatment protocols in most EMS systems by virtue of the systolic blood pressure or type and location of the wound. Some interpreted the results of this study to mean a more limited protocol for prehospital use of the PASG might be appropriate, one that excludes patients with thoracic trauma and those with short transport times. Recent studies lend support to the findings that the PASG does not appear to improve the condition of patients with transport times of under 30 minutes; and in the case of penetrating thoracic injuries, use of the PASG may actually be detrimental.[8,9] Injury above the level of the garment, such as a penetrating thorax wound, has always been, at the very least, a relative contraindication for PSAG use. It is possible that the time required to deflate the garment at the receiving facility may negate any benefit of PASG inflation when transport times are short.

Though a number of EMS systems have removed the device from their ambulances, this action is probably premature. There appear to be subsets of patients, such as those with ruptured abdominal aortic aneurysms or pelvic fractures, those with severe traumatic hypotension or refractory anaphylactic shock, and those with uncontrolled hemorrhage below the level of the garment, where the use of the PASG may be beneficial to the patient.[10] Almost a century after Crile surprised his colleagues with his success using a PASG, and even though current guidelines have been issued, the EMS community is still uncertain about the appropriate uses of this medical device.[11] The need for additional research seems evident.

BIOMECHANICS OF THE PASG

Hemodynamics is the study of the movement of blood and the forces and mechanisms that govern it. Blood flow, vascular resistance, and blood volume are regulated by biological control mechanisms and the physical laws of nature. When these physical laws are applied to biological problems, the study is referred to as **biophysics**. **Physiology** is the study of the func-

tion of living organisms and considers both the biological and physical processes involved. The principles of physiology and biophysics explain the effects seen with inflation of the PASG in trauma situations.[4]

CARDIAC OUTPUT AND BLOOD PRESSURE

Early researchers believed that the PASG exerted its influence on blood pressure by increasing the systemic vascular resistance (SVR) and autotransfusing as much as 1 liter of blood from the lower systemic circulation to the upper body circulation.[5] More recent studies reveal that autotransfusion is minimal and transient. The increase in SVR has a more pronounced and sustainable effect.[12] When the PASG is inflated, the pressure that develops is distributed through the underlying tissues to the blood vessels. This compression reduces the size of the vessels and the overall size of the vascular container that must be filled with blood. Blood flow through compressed vessels is significantly reduced.

Physiology and Biophysics

The explanation for the effect on blood flow was provided in the early part of the nineteenth century by Jean Louis Poiseuille (pronounced *PWAS ai ye*), a French physician who described the relationship of pressure and resistance to the flow of viscous fluids in tubes. When Poiseuille's findings are applied to the flow of blood in vessels, blood flow (F) is shown to be dependent on the difference in pressure between the ends of the vessel (ΔP), the length (L) and radius (r) of the vessel, and the viscosity (n) of the blood. The relationships of these factors along with the numerical constant $\pi/8$ are expressed in Poiseuille's equation:

$$F = \Delta P \times \frac{\pi}{8} \times \frac{1}{n} \times \frac{r^4}{L}$$

Assuming that at any given time blood viscosity and the pressure difference between the ends of the vessel are constant and the length of the vessel does not change, the factor that remains is the radius of the vessel. This equation demonstrates the remarkable relationship that exists between blood flow and vessel radius. Blood flow varies directly with the fourth power of the radius of the vessel (Figure 21-2). In practical terms this means that if the inflation of the PASG reduces the size of a vessel by one-half, the flow of blood through that vessel is reduced to one-sixteenth of the previous flow. Increased resistance in the smaller vessel is responsible. Poiseuille also described the factors influencing

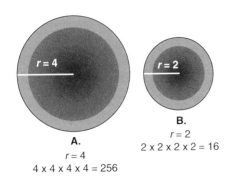

FIGURE 21-2 Radius of vessel B is one half that of vessel A. The blood flow (F) in vessel B (24) is 1/16th that of vessel A (44).

this resistance (*R*). Again it is the radius of the vessel that is the relevant factor as the other factors remain constant:

$$R = \frac{8}{\pi} \times \frac{n}{1} \times \frac{L}{r^4}$$

Here resistance is inversely proportional to the fourth power of the radius. Again in practical terms, when the PASG reduces a vessel by one-half, resistance to blood flow increases 16 times. This occurs because resistance to flow is greatest along the walls of a blood vessel and least in the center. In the larger vessel more of the blood will be further away from the vessel wall and less subject to resistance. In the smaller vessel most of the blood is in contact with the vessel wall or close to it, subjecting it to considerable resistance. This type of flow is described as **laminar**. The movement of the blood in laminar flow can be thought of as pulling open a telescope with the eyepiece. The eyepiece or innermost ring moves forward rapidly, leaving behind each concentric ring of the telescope tube in its turn. The closer a ring is to the outside of the tube when it is closed, the further behind it remains as it is opened. The closer blood cells are to the wall of the vessel, the slower they will flow in the vessel.

When the PASG is applied and inflated, the initial compression empties blood from the vessels in the lower body and returns it to the central circulation. This autotransfusion amounts to approximately 250–300 mL, or less than 5% of the total blood volume in an adult, far less than the 1,000 mL originally proposed.[10] A temporary increase in cardiac output is usually noted.[12] Applying Poiseuille's equation, continued compression of the vessels increases vascular resistance and restricts blood flow, decreasing the size of the vascular container. The effect is improvement of the usual measure of circulation, the blood pressure. The increased vascular resistance in the covered areas causes a rise in the SVR (the resistance provided by the systemic circulation to the output of the left ventricle).

Mean arterial pressure (MAP) varies proportionally with cardiac output (CO) and SVR:

$$MAP = CO \times SVR$$

When MAP increases, carotid artery pressure increases. Even though CO appears to fall over time when the garment is employed, the increased SVR from compression of the lower body should be sufficient to raise MAP and increase carotid artery blood flow in cases of hypotension. This would result in an increase in blood pressure with an accompanying increase in perfusion of the brain and heart. Empirical data of CO and SVR in the hypotensive trauma patient have not been obtained because of the difficulties involved in obtaining measurements requiring extensive invasive procedures in patients in need of immediate definitive medical care.

Concerns

Two issues have been raised concerning aspects of the hemodynamic responses to PASG inflation. The first is possible cardiac decompensation, which may follow if cardiac output falls during the time the patient is encased in the inflated PASG. The exact cause of the decreased CO following its initial rise has yet to be determined, but possible contributing factors are suggested from the hemodynamics involved.[12] The decrease in venous return from the lower body may contribute to an overall decrease in cardiac preload. Activation of baroreceptors and volume receptors in response to the increase in blood pressure is a possible mechanism. The PASG itself may affect filling pressure of the heart by increasing thoracic pressure through abdominal compression. Animal studies demonstrate that CO does decrease significantly over time when the PASG is inflated following hemorrhagic hypotension. Significant saline infusion restores CO to the prehemorrhage condition. If cardiac decompensation had occurred in these animals, the infusion would have caused further decreases in CO; instead the infusion increased CO to prehemorrhagic levels. In this experimental model the decrease in CO from PASG inflation did not result in cardiac decompensation in the healthy animal heart with sufficient cardiac reserve.[12] The caution raised by this study is the use of the PASG in patients with weakened hearts; the decrease in CO following PASG inflation may cause cardiac decompensation in these patients.

The second issue concerns the advisability of attempting to increase the blood pressure with the PASG or any other means in the hypotensive trauma patient. This practice has been central to the care of shock trauma patients for decades. Specific questions have recently been raised.[13] The most intriguing ask if hypotension might be a protective mechanism of the body in trauma and whether raising the blood pressure dislodges protective clots that are forming. The difficulty is that data are not available to answer these questions. The caution raised is that the inability to provide answers demonstrates a need for controlled studies. It should not necessarily mean the wholesale abandonment of a method of patient care. A second aspect of the same issue is the practice of relying on blood pressure to measure the success of the treatment of shock. Definitive treatment of symptomatic hypotension is elimination of the underlying cause whenever possible. For hypotension caused by hemorrhage this means closure of vessels by clot formation, surgical intervention, or other means. It has been demonstrated that the PASG can aid in hemorrhage control in certain patients. When definitive control of bleeding is not immediately possible, intervention strategies including PASG are used when the body's compensatory mechanisms are insufficient to keep blood pressure from reaching an irreversible state. The body uses blood pressure as a measure of the need to respond to hypoperfusion and does so through a series of negative-feedback mechanisms to maintain CO and arterial blood pressure. While blood pressure may not be the ultimate measure of success in the treatment of shock, it may be the indicator for intervention. Whether PASG is an appropriate prehospital intervention strategy and under what conditions this intervention should be undertaken remain to be definitively answered.

CONTROL OF HEMORRHAGE

Prehospital care providers are taught early on that direct pressure is a definitive measure for controlling bleeding from a wound. Inflation of the PASG and compression of the underlying tissues accomplish this in many instances of hemorrhage in tissues beneath the garment. Whether it is pressure applied directly to a wound or through inflation of the PASG, the explanation for the effects seen in the control of hemorrhage come from the physical laws of nature.

Two concepts are applicable, the laws of Bernoulli and Laplace. Eighteenth-century Swiss mathematician and physicist Daniel Bernoulli (pronounced *ber NOO lee*) demonstrated the relationship between pressure and the speed of moving liquids or gases. **Bernoulli's law** states that as the speed of a fluid increases, the pressure exerted by the fluid decreases. It explains a variety of phenomena, from the lift generated by air moving across the wing of a plane to the movement of fuel into an engine carburetor and the rate of leakage from a hole in a bucket:

$$Q = A(2T/P + V^2)^{1/2}$$

where Q is the rate of loss, P is the density of the fluid, T is the transmural pressure, and V is the velocity of fluid flow through the vessel. When applied to blood loss from a vessel laceration, the rate of hemorrhage is seen to be directly proportional to the transmural pressure, the pressure inside the vessel minus the external pressure. Increasing the external pressure by some form of vessel compression lowers the transmural pressure and slows the rate of hemorrhage from the wound. If, for example, the internal pressure of a vessel were 100 mm Hg and the external pressure were 20 mm Hg, then the transmural pressure would be 80 mm Hg. Increasing the external pressure to 50 mm Hg lowers the transmural pressure to 50 mm Hg, with a proportional reduction in blood loss (Q).

In 1821 Pierre Laplace (pronounced *lah PLAHS*), a French astronomer and mathematician, provided further explanation for the effects of increased external pressure on a bleeding vessel. **Laplace's law** states that for a cylinder like a blood vessel, the tension in the vessel wall (T) is equal to the transmural pressure (P) times the radius (R) of the vessel:

$$T = PR$$

If a laceration were made in a vessel wall, tension is the force that would cause the cut surfaces to separate or that would be necessary to bring them back together. According to the formula, anything that reduces the transmural pressure or the radius of the vessel will also reduce the vessel wall tension and decrease the flow of blood through the laceration. As has been shown, inflation of the PASG accomplishes a decrease in transmural pressure through increased external pressure. These laws of Bernoulli and Laplace are the physical principles that explain the action of the PASG in controlling hemorrhage beneath the area of the garment.

Concerns

The issue raised concerning the use of the PASG in hemorrhage focuses on those situations where hemorrhage is suspected above the level of the garment. This concern requires a further examination of these two laws. As has been demonstrated, the PASG increases SVR and raises blood pressure. The laws of both Bernoulli and Laplace demonstrate that the rate of hemorrhage is directly related to transmural pressure. While compression of a bleeding vessel directly under the PASG lowers transmural pressure and decreases blood flow from the wound, this same compression raises blood pressure in vessels not covered by the garment by raising the SVR. This increase in blood pressure raises the internal pressure in vessels outside the suit. Without a corresponding rise in external pressure, transmural pressure will increase and with it an accompanying increase in hemorrhage from any opening in a vessel wall will occur. In situations where the site of hemorrhage is above the level of the PASG and bleeding cannot be controlled by direct pressure, inflation of the garment may speed the loss of blood from lacerated vessels. For this reason, the PASG is not recommended in situations where bleeding is known or suspected above the level of the garment and such bleeding cannot be controlled by direct pressure.

INTERNET ACTIVITIES

Visit the National Library of Medicine Web site at http://www.ncbi.nlm.nih.gov/PubMed. Conduct a literature search on the use of the PASG in the setting of hemorrhagic shock. Review the abstracts of the search results. Ask your librarian to assist you in obtaining the journals with the five most relevant articles. Review these articles and summarize their findings.

IMMOBILIZATION OF FRACTURES

Immobilization of fractures through the use of splints is another basic concept of prehospital emergency care. The PASG is an effective splint for fractures of the pelvis and has been used for fractures of the femur associated with traumatic hypotension.

Physiology

Fractures of skeletal structures can be the cause of significant tissue disruption and hemorrhage. When the PASG is inflated, stabilization of the fracture site is accomplished and the control of hemorrhage in and around the fracture site can be significant. This is especially true in fractures of the pelvis following significant trauma. While significant blood loss can occur with a closed fracture of the femur, the space available for hemorrhage is limited by the density of the tissues of the thigh. Hemorrhage is less subject to these restrictions in pelvic fracture, especially when the fracture results in sufficient pelvic instability to increase the pelvic volume. In these cases the PASG can immobilize the pelvis and reduce the pelvic volume. Such treatment has been shown to control hemorrhage and reduce mortality from these severe pelvic injuries.[14]

Concerns

The issue raised with the prehospital use of PASG to immobilize fractures of the pelvis and femur concerns use of the garment in normotensive patients. For the patient with an isolated fracture of the femur where no significant bleeding is suspected and hypotension is not present or anticipated, another splinting device or method which effectively stabilizes the fracture site should be employed. Available methods for splinting an unstable pelvis in any patient are not as numerous. For the normotensive patient with a pelvic fracture, if necessary, the PASG can provide pelvic stabilization during transport.

USE OF THE PASG

In order for the patient to benefit from the PASG in the prehospital setting, patient assessment and application/inflation of the garment must occur as rapidly as possible. This is most urgent in incidents of significant trauma where on-scene time must be limited or when the signs and symptoms of shock are already present. The goal is for the PASG to be in place and the garment inflated in less than 2 minutes from the time the decision is made to employ the device.

INDICATIONS

The decision to employ the PASG requires the paramedic to recognize those situations where the garment may stabilize or improve the patient's condition. The National Association of EMS Physicians has issued guidelines on use of the PASG in trauma and medical situations (Table 21-1).[11] It follows from the discussion of the physiology and biophysics of the PASG that the use of the garment is acceptable in cases where hypotension is present and there is a need to:

● Control hemorrhage from vessels that can be compressed by the garment, including the abdominal aorta and femoral artery

● Stabilize pelvic fracture

● Raise blood pressure in severe traumatic hypotension and refractory anaphylactic shock

Though usually not a trauma situation, four case studies of the use of PASG in refractory anaphylactic shock have been reported.[10] While the data are limited, the successful outcome of these patients who failed to respond to the usual treatment protocol makes use of the PASG in refractory anaphylactic shock acceptable. An increase in SVR is the mechanism most likely responsible for these positive outcomes.[15]

Consideration must also be given to situations where use of the PASG may be helpful and is probably not harmful to the patient. These situations require judgment on the part of the paramedic. In many instances, data from controlled clinical trials are not available to support use of the PASG. Instead, reported patient case studies and an understanding of the physiological response mechanisms when the garment is employed make the PASG an acceptable, probably not harmful intervention in the following trauma patient presentations:

- Penetrating injury to the abdomen
- Urological and gynecological hemorrhage including ruptured ectopic pregnancy[16]
- Pelvic fracture without hypotension
- Spinal shock[17]

INTERNET ACTIVITIES

Visit the National Association of EMS Physicians Web site at http:\\naemsp.org/position papers.asp and review their position statement on the use of the PASG in the prehospital setting.

Table 21-1
Recommendations for Use of PASG in Trauma Situations

Usually indicated, useful, and effective:

- Hypotension due to ruptured abdominal aortic aneurysm

Acceptable, evidence favors usefulness:

- Hypotension from suspected pelvic fracture
- Severe traumatic hypotension
- Uncontrolled lower extremity hemorrhage
- Refractory anaphylactic shock

Acceptable, possibly helpful, probably not harmful:

- Penetrating abdominal injury
- Uncontrolled gynecological and urological hemorrhage
- Ruptured ectopic pregnancy
- Pelvic fracture without hypotension
- Spinal shock

Not indicated, may be harmful:

- Diaphragmatic rupture
- Penetrating thoracic injury
- Cardiac tamponade
- Abdominal evisceration
- Pulmonary edema
- Lower extremity splinting

Source: Adapted from O'Connor R, Domeier R. Use of the antishock garment (PASG) in various clinical settings. *Prehosp Emerg Care.* 1997; 1:36.

CONTRAINDICATIONS

It should now be clear that use of the PASG is not indicated and may be harmful to the patient with:

- Known or suspected bleeding or injury above the level of the garment, including diaphragmatic rupture, penetrating thoracic injury, and cardiac tamponade
- Pulmonary edema
- Lower extremity trauma without hypotension
- Abdominal evisceration

Rupture of the diaphragm is difficult to recognize in the prehospital setting. The PASG will likely worsen the condition of this patient as inflation of the abdominal compartment restricts the ability of the lungs to fully expand. In instances where the patient presents with severe respiratory distress following inflation, immediate deflation of the abdominal compartment is necessary. On-line medical direction should be advised of the patient's condition, and steps should be planned and taken to correct the patient's condition.

The contraindication of the PASG in evisceration is theoretical as no studies have been done that demonstrate it is harmful to the patient. However, the previous discussion of hemodynamics suggests that compression of the garment on exposed viscera may cause ischemia in these tissues, which are already at risk.[10]

GENERAL GUIDELINES

In deciding when use of the PASG is appropriate, consideration should be given to on-scene and prehospital transport time to definitive care. A recent study showed no delay in on-scene time when the PASG was employed in situations of major trauma.[18] This suggests that prophylactic application of the garment at the scene in situations where eventual need for the PASG is suspected should not delay patient transport and may benefit the patient should the patient's condition worsen and immediate inflation of the garment become warranted. Studies from one setting suggest that in urban areas with short transport times to major trauma centers, use of the PASG in penetrating abdominal trauma does not improve the long-term survival of the these patients.[6,7] However, note that no detrimental effects to the patient were demonstrated when the PASG was employed according to accepted indications and contraindications for use.

COMPLICATIONS OF USE

Paramedics who employ the PASG in the care of trauma patients must recognize and intervene if complications develop following inflation of the garment. Inflation of the abdominal compartment may limit diaphragmatic excursion with an accompanying reduction in vital capacity. Most patients appear to compensate through an increase in respiratory rate and chest expansion.[19] For those that do not, consultation with on-line medical direction regarding deflation of the abdominal compartment is advisable. Additionally, abdominal compartment inflation may cause nausea, vomiting, urination, and defecation from the compression of abdominal organs.

Although compartment syndrome (see Chapter 16) is a complication of PASG use, it occurs infrequently and almost always when the garment remains inflated longer than 2 hours. In almost every instance this is longer than the patient remains in the prehospital environment. It is imperative, however, that the paramedic inform the receiving facility of the time of inflation in order that this complication may be avoided.

Most serious of all the complications associated with inflation of the PASG is inadvertent deflation of the garment. Such an event can produce profound shock in the hemodynamically compromised patient. The patient is most at risk during movement from one location to another, and care must be exercised by the paramedic to avoid anything that might result in the inadvertent loss of pressure in one or more compartments of the garment. Paramedics are advised to clear the area under the garment of anything that might puncture or rip the garment, move the patient in such a way that nothing catches on the tube stems or stopcocks of the garment, and keep the garment away from sharp edges and objects. Should deflation occur in an intact garment, immediate reinflation is recommended. In the case of a damaged garment, another PASG should be employed. If this is not available, fluid resuscitation and other supportive measures must be initiated for the shock patient. Paramedics must also be able to advise individuals at the receiving facility who are not familiar with the deflation procedure of the proper sequence for deflation so that rapid deflation does not occur in this setting.

APPLICATION OF THE PASG

In serious traumatic injury, time works against patient survival. Application of the PASG, while relatively easy in the classroom setting with cooperative volunteer patients, can delay transport unless EMS partners have prepared in advance for the coordination required to apply the PASG effectively and efficiently. Although the fundamental components of application are unchanging, variations in the method of application have been developed by practitioners that many find improve efficiency under certain circumstances. Use of the garment is best accomplished by partners who practice the application sequence until only the changes demanded by the uniqueness of the trauma setting require verbal communication. New EMS partners should decide on a preferred application method prior to field use and practice the steps in the application sequence. Proper application and inflation should occur in less than 2 minutes.

If time and circumstances permit, removal of the patient's clothing beneath the garment is suggested. This is often necessary in order to complete an adequate patient assessment, to cover open wounds that will be covered with the garment, or to provide access for urinary catheterization postapplication. If clothing is not removed, a belt or any object in or on the clothing might puncture the garment or cause patient discomfort when the PASG is inflated.

Basic Application and Inflation Sequence

The basic sequence of events in the application and inflation of the PASG assumes that an appropriate trauma survey has occurred. This includes identification of life-threatening injuries with timely intervention, chest auscultation to rule out pulmonary edema, examination of the body area to be covered by the garment, and a check of pedal pulses. In the case of suspected spinal injury, spinal alignment must be maintained at all times during application. Once the patient has been cleared for application of the PASG, the following steps should be completed.

1. Prepare the garment for the patient.
2. Position the patient on the garment with the upper border of the abdominal compartment even with the posterior border of the ribs.
3. Enclose the patient in the garment with the Velcro fasteners until the garment is snug.
4. Connect the inflation tubing and foot pump to the garment and open the stopcock of each of the three compartments. If protocol requires inflation of the leg sections first, open only the leg stopcocks. Under no circumstances should the abdominal compartment be inflated before the leg compartments.
5. Inflate the chambers of the garment until an end point is reached. End points include crackling of the Velcro fasteners, release of air from the pressure relief valves, or return of the patient's systolic blood pressure to 100 mm Hg.
6. Close the stopcocks to maintain suit pressure.
7. Reassess the patient's blood pressure, lung sounds, and pedal pulses. Continue monitoring the patient's vital signs and the suit pressure.

Each of the following methods of PASG application involves a variation of the first two steps in the basic sequence, preparation of the garment and positioning of the patient. When these two are accomplished, each method concludes with the remaining five steps (3–7) in the basic sequence.

Log-Roll Method

1. Unfold the PASG patient side up on a long spine board. Secure the garment to the board by slipping the Velcro straps through the hand holds on each side and secure with tape.

   Using 2-inch tape, secure the top of the back portion of the abdominal compartment to the board.

2. With the presence of sufficient personnel to maintain spinal alignment, log roll the patient onto the backboard and garment simultaneously.

Trouser Method *(Figure 21-3)*

1. Assemble the PASG with all three chambers loosely secured by the fasteners. This may be done beforehand and the garment stored in this configuration.

2. After your partner passes a hand and arm through each lower leg opening, out the top of the garment, and grasps the patient's ankles, pull the garment into position on the patient as though pulling on a pair of trousers.

Diaper Method

1. Unfold the PASG patient side up at the patient's feet. Roll the three inner flaps of the leg and abdominal compartments toward the center of the garment. Other methods of folding the garment flaps so they will be easily accessible

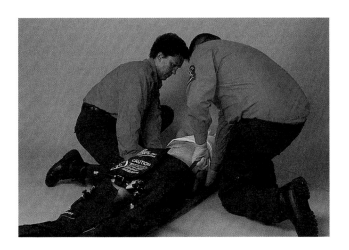

FIGURE 21-3 Trouser method of PASG application.

between the patient's legs when the garment is in position are acceptable.

2. Together lift the patient's legs and slide the garment up and under the legs. The lower leg borders of the garment should clear the patient's heels or the garment will catch on the next lift. Next lift the patient's hips and slide the garment into position under the patient. Then compartment enclosure flaps are pulled from between the patient's legs and secured. Care should be taken to ensure that spinal misalignment does not occur with this technique.

ENVIRONMENTAL EFFECTS

Temperature and pressure have an effect on the volume of gas in a closed chamber, such as an inflated PASG compartment. If a constant pressure is to be maintained in an inflated garment during patient transport, the paramedic must be aware of these effects. When the atmospheric pressure is constant, as it is at a relatively constant elevation above sea level, should the temperature of the environment increase, so will the volume of gas in the PASG compartments. When temperature decreases, the volume of gas will decrease. In cases where a patient is moved from a cold environment to the back of a warmed ambulance, the paramedic can expect an increase in pressure in the PASG as the air in the inflated compartments steadily warms and the volume of that air expands. The reverse occurs when the patient is moved from a warm environment into the back of a cooled ambulance. As air in the compartments steadily cools, its volume contracts and pressure in the PASG compartments falls.

Changes in atmospheric pressure also affect the volume of air in the PASG compartments. In cases where patients are transported by helicopter or nonpressurized fixed-wing aircraft, the paramedic can expect the volume of air in the PASG compartments to expand as altitude increases and to contract as the aircraft lands.

The paramedic must monitor the pressure in the PASG compartments to ensure a constant inflation pressure. Change in temperature or atmospheric pressure or leaks in the garment can all affect garment pressure. Some manufacturers equip the PASG with gauges for monitoring purposes. For suits without gauges and even for those that do have them, a simple hand squeeze of each chamber is a fast and effective method for monitoring the inflation pressure of the garment. When pressure in the compartments falls significantly, additional air should be added by means of the foot pump. Should pressure in the garment increase to a point where the security of the garment is at risk due to slipping of the fasteners, a small volume of air can be released from each chamber. Care must be exercised to ensure that total garment deflation does not occur.

DEFLATION AND REMOVAL OF THE PASG

Although removal of the PASG is usually accomplished at the facility that receives the patient, paramedics must be able to accomplish this task without compromising the patient. Paramedics must also be knowledgeable regarding deflation procedures should personnel at the receiving facility be unfamiliar with the PASG and its removal.

Given that the patient's condition is usually serious whenever the PASG is used, evaluation of the patient's vital signs and other indicators of patient stability should normally precede any attempt to deflate the garment. Preparation for deflation includes placement of at least one, and preferably two, large-bore intravenous catheters, delivery of an appropriate fluid volume, and the immediate availability of a surgical team should such intervention be warranted. X-rays need not be delayed, and these can be taken with the garment inflated. When it has been determined that deflation is appropriate, the following procedure should be used.

Method of Controlled Deflation

1. Release one-quarter to one-third of the air from the abdominal compartment by opening the stopcock for 1–2 seconds or until the pressure has dropped an equivalent amount on the abdominal pressure gauge.

2. Close the abdominal stopcock.

3. Reevaluate the patient's vital signs. If the heart rate increases by 5 beats per minute or the systolic blood pressure falls by 5 mm Hg, discontinue the deflation and take steps to stabilize the patient. A fluid challenge of 200–250 mL of normal saline or lactated Ringer's is appropriate. If the heart rate increases by more than 5 beats per minute or systolic blood pressure falls by more than 5 mm Hg, consider reinflating the compartment.

4. Repeat steps 1, 2, and 3 until the abdominal compartment is deflated.

5. Repeat steps 1, 2, and 3 for each leg separately. The total procedure may take 30–45 minutes.

SUMMARY

The PASG is the result of a desire on the part of George Crile to do something to maintain the blood pressure of trauma and surgical patients in shock. That same concern for the patient is evident in PASG research, especially that of the past 15 years. Though often controversial, this research dramatizes the need in prehospital emergency care for studies that confirm or refute the treatment protocols employed by paramedics in the care of patients. In the case of the PASG the evidence is not yet conclusive. Until that time an understanding of the hemodynamic mechanisms that affect cardiac output, blood pressure, hemorrhage, and fracture stabilization provides the paramedic with a rationale for employing the garment in the care of the trauma patient. The PASG requires that paramedics make judgments regarding use, employ appropriate assessment techniques, rapidly and accurately apply the garment, evaluate their actions and the reaction of the patient to inflation of the garment, recognize and react to developing complications, and advise others about the care of patients with the PASG inflated. The PASG is a medical device and, as such, demands that those who employ it understand all aspects of its use and role in patient care.

REVIEW QUESTIONS

1. The original development of a pneumatic garment to restore blood pressure in hypovolemic shock patients is credited to:
   a. David Clark
   b. George Crile
   c. W. James Gardner
   d. Burton Kaplan

2. According to the Poiseuille equation, reducing the size of a vessel by one-half should reduce the flow of blood through that vessel to:
   a. One-eighth of the previous flow
   b. One-fourth of the previous flow
   c. One-half of the previous flow
   d. One-sixteenth of the previous flow

3. Studies have demonstrated that the increase in blood pressure achieved by the PASG is primarily the result of:
   a. Autotransfusion from the lower extremities
   b. Rising thoracic and cardiac pressures
   c. Increased systemic vascular resistance
   d. Immobilization of the lower extremities

4. According to current guidelines, the use of the PASG is usually indicated, useful, and effective in only one situation, which is:
a. Ruptured abdominal aortic aneurysm
b. Penetrating abdominal injury
c. Refractory anaphylactic shock
d. Abdominal evisceration

5. According to current guidelines, the use of the PASG is not indicated and may be harmful when the patient presents with:
a. Ruptured ectopic pregnancy
b. Penetrating abdominal injury
c. Diaphragmatic rupture
d. Spinal shock

6. The PASG may be helpful and is probably not harmful to which of the following trauma patients?
1. Unstable pelvis with hypotension following a fall
2. Gunshot wound to the chest with hemorrhage
3. Severe hypotension and rigid abdomen from a mugging
4. Normotensive with fractures of both lower legs following a jump
  a. 1, 3
  b. 2, 3
  c. 1, 4
  d. 2, 4

7. Which of the following is an acceptable inflation sequence for the PASG?
1. All three chambers simultaneously
2. The abdominal compartment followed by both leg compartments
3. The leg compartments together followed by the abdominal compartment
4. Each leg compartment separately followed by the abdominal compartment
  a. 1 and 4
  b. 1 and 3
  c. 2 and 3
  d. 2 and 4

8. With one exception, all of the following are appropriate end points for inflation of the PASG. That exception is:
a. Crackling of the Velcro closures
b. Patient's blood pressure improves to 100 mm Hg systolic
c. Air releases from the pressure relief valves
d. Pedal pulses are no longer palpable

9. When the patient with PASG inflated is moved from a below-freezing environment to the back of a warm ambulance, the paramedic can expect the volume of air in the garment compartments to:
a. Increase
b. Decrease

10. Deflation of the PASG always begins with the _____ compartment.
a. Leg
b. Abdominal

CRITICAL THINKING

● Explain how compartment syndrome may result from the use of the PASG.

● Using your knowledge of the biophysics of the PASG, explain why the PASG is contraindicated in the setting of penetrating chest trauma.

● You are caring for a patient who has sustained blunt abdominal and chest trauma. You suspect intra-abdominal hemorrhage and have applied the PASG. Following inflation, your patient suddenly develops respiratory distress. What are the likely causes of the dyspnea? How will you manage this patient?

REFERENCES

1. Crile G., ed. *George Crile—An Autobiography.* Philadelphia: JB Lippincott; 1947.
2. Gardner WJ. The antigravity suit (G-suit) in surgery. *JAMA.* 1952; 162:274.
3. Gardner WJ. Circumferential pneumatic compression: effect of the "G-splint" on blood flow. *JAMA.* 1966; 196:117.
4. McSwain NE Jr. Pneumatic antishock garment: state of the art 1988. *Ann Emerg Med.* 1988; 17:506.
5. Kaplan BC, Civetta JM, Nagel EL, Nussenfeld SR, Hirschman JC. The military antishock trouser in civilian prehospital emergency care. *J Trauma.* 1973; 13:843.
6. Mattox K, Bickell WH, Pepe PE, Mangelsdorff AD. Prospective randomized evaluation of antishock MAST in post-traumatic hypotension. *J Trauma.* 1986; 26:779.
7. Mattox KL, Bickell WH, Pepe PE, Burch J, Feliciano D. Prospective MAST study in 911 patients. *J Trauma.* 1989; 29:1104.
8. Chang FC, Harrison PB, Beech RR, Helmer SD. PASG: does it help in the management of traumatic shock? *J Trauma.* 1995; 39:453.
9. Honigman B, Lowenstein SR, Moore EE, Roweder K, Pons P. The role of the pneumatic antishock garment in penetrating cardiac wounds. *JAMA.* 1991; 266:2398.
10. O'Connor RE, Domeier RM. An evaluation of the pneumatic antishock garment (PASG) in various clinical settings. *Prehosp Emerg Care.* 1997; 1:36.

11. Domeier RM, O'Connor RE, Delbridge TR, Hunt RC. Use of the anti-shock garment. *Prehosp Emerg Care.* 1997; 1:32.

12. Ali J, Duke K. Timing and interpretation of the hemodynamic effects of the pneumatic antishock garment. *Ann Emerg Med.* 1991; 20:1183.

13. Mattox KL. Editorial comment: "ideal" posttraumatic parameters. *J Trauma.* 1993; 34:734.

14. Flint L, Babikian G, Anders M, Rodriguez J, Steinberg S. Definitive control of mortality from severe pelvic fracture. *Ann Surg.* 1990; 211:703.

15. Perkin RM, Anas NG. Mechanisms and management of anaphylactic shock not responding to traditional therapy. *Ann Allergy.* 1985; 54:202.

16. Hall M, Marshall JR. The gravity suit: a major advance in management of gynecologic blood loss. *Obstet Gynecol.* 1979; 53:247.

17. Hopman MT, Kamerbeek IC, Pistonus M, Binkhorst RA. The effect of an anti-G suit on the maximal performance of individuals with paraplegia. *Int J Sports Med.* 1993; 14:357.

18. Karch SB, Lewis T, Young S, Ho CH. Surgical delays and outcomes in patients treated with pneumatic antishock garments. *Am J Emerg Med.* 1995; 13:401.

19. Riou B, Pansard JL, Lazard T, Grenier P, Viars P. Ventilatory effects of medical anti-shock trousers in healthy volunteers. *J Trauma.* 1991; 31:1495.

► **BIBLIOGRAPHY**

Allison EJ Jr. *Advanced Life Support Skills.* St Louis, Mo.: Mosby; 1994.

Burton AC. *Physiology and Biophysics of the Circulation* 2nd ed. Chicago, Ill.: Year Book Medical; 1972.

Cayten CG, Berendt BM, Byrne DW, Murphy JG, Moy FH. A study of pneumatic antishock garments in severely hypotensive trauma patients. *J Trauma.* 1993; 34:728.

Clark DE, Demers ML. Lower body positive pressure. *Surg Gynec Obstet.* 1989; 168:81.

Crile GW. *Blood Pressure in Surgery: An Experimental and Clinical Research.* Philadelphia: JB Lippincott; 1903.

Crile GW. The resuscitation of the apparently dead and a demonstration of the pneumatic rubber suit as a means of controlling blood pressure. *Trans South Surg Gynecol Assoc.* 1904; 16:362.

Cutler BS, Daggett WM. Application of the "G-suit" to the control of hemorrhage in massive trauma. *Ann Surg.* 1971; 173:511.

Ganong WF. *Review of Medical Physiology,* 12th ed. Los Altos, Calif.: Lange; 1983.

Guyton AC. *Human Physiology and Mechanisms of Disease,* 5th ed. Philadelphia: WB Saunders; 1992.

James ET, ed. *Dictionary of American Biography: Supplement Three, 1941–1945.* New York: Charles Scribner's Sons; 1973.

Rhoades RA, Tanner GA, eds. *Medical Physiology.* Boston: Little Brown; 1995.

Schneider PA, Mitchell JM, Allison EJ. The use of military antishock trousers in trauma—a reevaluation. *J Emer Med.* 1989; 7:497.

Townsend RN, Colella JJ, Diamond DL. Traumatic rupture of the aorta—critical decisions for trauma surgeons. *J Trauma.* 1990; 30:1169.

Chapter 22

Hazardous Material Incidents

OBJECTIVES

Upon completion of this chapter, the reader should be able to:

- Define the term "hazardous material."
- Discuss the importance of preplanning for a hazardous material incident.
- Identify eight methods of hazardous material identification.
- List four key scene size-up questions to be answered.
- Discuss the organization of a hazardous material scene.
- Identify three on-scene roles for properly trained EMS personnel.
- Outline six preliminary steps to be taken at the scene of a hazardous material incident.
- Discuss the four levels of personal protective equipment (PPE).
- Describe four problems associated with the use of PPE.
- Describe the purpose of patient decontamination.
- Discuss the three phases of patient decontamination.
- List the three zones of the hazardous materials scene and describe the activities that occur within each.
- Describe the medical care practices to be followed when caring for the victim of a hazardous material incident.

KEY TERMS

Bulk packaging
Definitive decontamination
Emergency technical decontamination
EMS/HM Level I
EMS/HM Level II
Gross decontamination

Hazard analysis
Hazardous material
Nonbulk packaging
Rule of thumb
Secondary decontamination

A tractor trailer overturns, spilling product on the roadway and injuring the driver. Vapors are rising from a derailed railroad tank car and heading toward a nearby apartment building. Hundreds of people run out of a subway station coughing and rubbing their eyes as an unusual odor begins filling the air. These are not Hollywood movie scenes. They are examples of an increasing type of incident emergency medical technicians (EMTs) and paramedics are being asked to assist with at the hazardous material (Hazmat) incident. A **hazardous material** is defined by the Department of Transportation (DOT) as "any substance or material in any form or quantity which poses an unreasonable risk to safety and health and to property when transported in commerce." However, since hazardous materials can be formed in homes, factories, and laboratories, Ludwig Benner's definition of a hazardous material as "any substance that jumps out of its container at you when something goes wrong and hurts or harms the things it touches" is more realistic. Currently, there are over 50,000 agents labeled as hazardous by government authorities. That number grows by 500 new products annually. Experts report that more than 10,000 incidents occur each year involving the release of dangerous solids, liquids, and gases. Injuries to nearby citizens may be secondary to inhalation, absorption, ingestion, and injection, producing a myriad of signs and symptoms depending upon the type of toxin involved.

To safely and effectively manage the medical problems posed by a hazardous material event and to avoid self-injury, prehospital providers must have a fundamental understanding of response planning, incident command, scene organization, toxicology, patient decontamination, and medical management of the contaminated victim.

PREPLANNING

Essential to an effective response is the performance of a **hazard analysis**, an inventory of the largest amounts of hazardous materials present in a community, their location, quantity, specific physical and clinical hazards, and risk of release. The ability of communities to create meaningful Hazmat response plans has been greatly aided by the 1986 Superfund Amendments and Reauthorization Act (SARA) Title III Act. SARA requires "right to know" information be made available to fire departments; it also calls for the creation of a Local Emergency Planning Committee (LEPC) in each community. Intended to include the participation of public safety agencies, industry, government, hospitals, and the public, this committee is charged with gathering and analyzing the hazard data, examining preventive measures, and planning for response and mitigation. EMS preplanning activities should effectively address medical management issues, transportation planning, and hospital preparedness for fires, industrial accidents, and transportation spills involving chemical, nuclear, and biological agents.

A general idea of the potential for a significant Hazmat-related incident can be gained by examining highway, waterway, pipeline, and air transport patterns to local and regional industrial, business, and government installations. Hazardous substances present at other sites, such as university research facilities, small businesses, households, and clandestine drug laboratories, also warrant specific preplanning in order to manage the danger and optimize the chance for a safe, effective, and integrated response by police, fire, EMS, and hospital personnel.

With this information a comprehensive community preplan can be developed by the local emergency services personnel that identifies problems and solutions, designates resources, and determines how to utilize and coordinate these resources in the event of an emergency. Each preplan must address the community's likely rescue, decontamination, and patient care problems, not simply fire hazards and property damage. Plans should be reviewed and updated annually to ensure accuracy and completeness. Plans need to be "user friendly" and quickly accessible in the event of an emergency. Frequent rehearsal by all personnel is essential to ensure familiarity with emergency plans and to build trusting relationships needed for successful emergency response.

TRAINING

As with preparing for any type of emergency, prehospital personnel must receive training on vital Hazmat areas, such as product identification, personal protective clothing, on-scene operations, patient decontamination, and treatment procedures. Current Occupational Safety and Health Administration (OSHA) 1910.120 regulations require police, fire, and EMS personnel to receive training based on the duties and functions performed by each responder of an emergency response organization. OSHA has outlined a tiered training scheme that requires that first-responder awareness training be given to each type of responder as a minimal level of training. More specialized training is required for personnel who assume a greater operational role (operations level, technician, and/or specialist level) or a command role (HazMat incident command). These requirements can be met by taking formal classroom training or by a responder demonstrating competency in pertinent skills in a HazMat incident. Each department or employer must "certify" that the standard has been satisfied by either a training program or by demonstration of competency. Emergency response personnel must also receive retraining annually to maintain their competencies.

The National Fire Protection Association (NFPA) has outlined training for EMS personnel in its document, *NFPA 473-Competencies for Medical Personnel at the Scene of a Hazardous Material Incident*. This document outlines two levels of EMS/HazMat responders.

EMS/HM Level I provides training requirements for EMS personnel who perform patient care in the cold zone of a hazardous material incident, provided the patient no longer poses a risk of secondary contamination. Competency requirements are outlined for both basic and advanced life support personnel. **EMS/HM Level II** targets personnel who perform patient care in the warm zone. Level II providers may render care to patients who still pose a significant risk of secondary contamination. Personnel at this level are expected to coordinate activities at a hazardous material incident and provide medical support for hazardous material incident response personnel.

ROLE OF EMERGENCY MEDICAL DISPATCH CENTER

Usually, the first indication for prehospital personnel that a hazardous material incident has occurred is a frantic phone call to the 911 operator from a victim, witness, or passerby. In this situation, the call taker has three responsibilities: (1) determine the exact incident location, the nature of the problem (including obtaining the names of the chemicals involved), the number of victims, and the types of injuries sustained; (2) reassure the caller, if necessary, and give explicit directions to ensure the caller's safety and that of anyone else nearby (first-aid instructions may also be given if indicated); and (3) relay all known details about the call to the police, fire, and EMS personnel responsible for managing the incident.

As additional information is obtained from other persons calling in to report the incident, or as first-arriving units provide initial "size-up" details, the updated information should be relayed by the dispatcher to all emergency response personnel as soon as possible. Whenever possible, the dispatcher should also provide information about safe routes of travel, wind direction, and speed. The preliminary information obtained from patients or witnesses of the incident and relayed by a properly trained emergency medical dispatcher is vital to protecting the emergency response personnel and beginning a safe and effective response.

METHODS OF HAZARDOUS MATERIAL IDENTIFICATION

Pulling up to the scene of an overturned, burning tractor trailer or a derailed railroad tank car with a vapor cloud forming above a broken valve, an EMT or paramedic should instantly recognize this situation as a "Hazmat call" and initiate an appropriate set of defensive actions. However, not every incident involving hazardous materials will be so obvious. The "man down" in a silo or the woman having seizures in the local hardware store may also prove to be the patient of a hazardous material exposure. Thus, the wise emergency care provider must realize that *any call can be a hazardous material call* and take proper precautions. Early identification of the risk is essential. Since saving lives and preserving property are the primary response objectives, the first task is to learn as much as possible about the situation from a safe distance. Binoculars or telescopes (10 × 35 power) and quick reference texts such as the *North American Emergency Response Guidebook* and *Hazardous Materials Injuries. A Handbook for Prehospital Care* are important tools to use in identifying what products may be involved. EMTs and paramedics should obtain expertise in effectively using these texts by practicing with them beforehand. There are eight basic methods for identifying a possible hazardous materials event (Table 22-1).

OCCUPANCY AND LOCATION

While hazardous materials can be found virtually everywhere, roughly three-quarters of all hazardous material incidents occur at sites where chemicals are manufactured, stored, or used. Frequently, the type of occupancy or design of a particular structure can indicate that hazardous materials may be found there. With the passage of "right to know" legislation and the implementation of SARA Title III in 1986, facilities are now required to notify the fire department of the hazardous materials they use and their location and quantity and provide material safety data sheets (MSDSs) for those chemicals either to a fire department's central database or in a secure lockbox at the periphery of the industrial site. The availability of this information is intended to assist the fire department/EMS agency in preplanning a response to that location. Compliance with this requirement is variable, especially for smaller businesses. Thus, response personnel may sometimes

Table 22-1
Basic Clues to a Hazardous Material Incident

1. Occupancy and location
2. Container shape
3. Markings and colors
4. Placards and labels
5. Shipping papers and documents
6. Material safety data sheets (MSDSs)
7. Monitoring and detection equipment
8. Senses and behavior

arrive at an incident involving a business using hazardous materials, only to find the owner or facility manager unable or unwilling to provide MSDS information.

Other locations of an incident should raise suspicions that hazardous materials are involved. Fuel terminals, railways, manufacturing plants, and research facilities are but a few of the common locations for hazardous material incidents to occur. In other situations, even without specific warnings, emergency response personnel can recognize a potential hazard by observing characteristic tools, equipment, or vehicles.

CONTAINER SHAPE

The size, shape, and construction features of a container can be useful in providing information about hazardous materials. Thus, emergency response personnel should familiarize themselves with characteristic containers commonly found in their area.

The packages and containers used for interstate transport of hazardous materials are regulated by the DOT. The containers are divided into two general groups. **Nonbulk packaging** has an internal volume of 119 gallons or less for liquids, 882 pounds (400 kg) or less for solids, or a water capacity of 1,000 pounds or less for gases. Many of these containers are 55-gallon drums, but they can also be cylinders and boxes of various sizes. **Bulk packaging** has an internal volume greater than the above dimensions. Unlike nonbulk packaging, which can be singly packaged or placed in other containers (overpacks) for transport, bulk packages may be an integral part of a transport vehicle, such as a tank car, or placed as a portable tank or container on a vehicle. In industrial sites, fixed bulk containers may include storage tanks or pools.

MARKINGS AND COLORS

Several types of hazardous material marking systems are in use today.

Fixed Facility

The square diamond NFPA 704 marking is increasingly used at fixed facilities such as bulk storage tanks and storage areas. It is not used on transport vehicles and does not specifically identify chemicals. Within the diamond shape are four sectors. The left, top, and right sectors numerically rate the substance's hazard in the categories of health risk, flammability, and reactivity, respectively. A scale of 1–4, least to most dangerous, is used. Pertinent "special information" may be provided in the bottom sector, which warns of the agent's reactivity to water, oxidation potential, radiation hazard, or required protective equipment.

Bulk liquid petroleum facilities that contain more than one product usually use an American Petroleum Institute (API) color code and symbol that denotes the different grades of gasoline and fuel oils. Color codes are also frequently found at liquefied petroleum gas facilities. Liquid product lines are color coded either dark blue or orange; vapor lines are light blue or yellow. The U.S. military uses its own marking system for identifying hazardous materials. This seven-symbol system identifies detonation, fire, and special hazards.

Bulk Transportation

The DOT requires that the names of approximately 42 hazardous materials be stenciled on both sides of "dedicated" railroad tank cars. Other railroad car markings, such as the DOT container specifications, specification number, tank registration, or serial numbers and the company name or logo, can identify the contents and their concentration and formulation.

Certain paint coloring schemes can also help identify the presence of specific hazardous materials. For example, hydrocyanic acid, a Class A poison, is commonly transported in a railroad tank car painted white with a red stripe running the length and around the ends of the car. Worth noting is that "Poison A" containers also lack pressure relief valves and are more likely to rupture if exposed to fire.

Cargo tank cars have company names, logos, identification numbers, and DOT tank specification plate information that can indicate a hazardous material is being transported. Their size and shape can sometimes identify the cargo they carry. In addition, the color scheme of the tank can be helpful. For example, corrosive tank trucks generally have a contrasting color band or rubber material in line with the dome covers and overturn protection.

Pipeline routes are identified by markers that identify the product, such as natural gas or propane, and a telephone number to contact in case of emergency.

Nonbulk Packages and Containers

Nonbulk packages and containers for pesticides and agricultural chemicals frequently display useful identification information. Markings fall into several categories:

- Toxicity signal words ("danger," "warning," "caution") indicate the relative degree of acute toxicity. The toxic categories are high toxicity, moderate toxicity, and low toxicity.

- A statement of practical treatment provides basic "first-aid" procedures for exposure.

- A physical or chemical hazard statement lists special flammability, explosion, or chemical hazards posed by the product.

- The product name is the brand or trade name. If followed by the term "technical," it generally indicates a highly concentrated percentage of active ingredients.

- An ingredient statement lists chemical ingredients by relative percentages or as pounds per gallon of concentrate.

- Environmental information includes how to properly store and dispose of the product and environmental considerations to keep in mind.

- The EPA registration number is a third way to positively identify a pesticide, in addition to the product name and chemical ingredient statements.

PLACARDS AND LABELS

The DOT Code of Federal Regulations Part 49 (49CFR) requires labels and placards be used when transporting certain types and quantities of hazardous materials. Approved labels are 4-by-4-inch markings with a distinctive black or white solid line border placed on certain packages of hazardous materials. The proper label (Figure 22-1) is determined by the hazard class of the product and is usually placed or printed near the content name on the manufacturing label. If the labels cannot be attached to the container, they are placed on tags or cards attached to the package. Because the law requires that each hazard be identified, some chemical containers may have multiple labels. Warning labels (e.g., "Dangerous When Wet," "Infectious Substances," "Radioactive Materials," "Poison," and "Inhalation Hazard") may also be required.

The $10^3/_4$-inch, diamond-shaped, weather-resistant identification marking applied to both ends and each side of freight containers, cargo tanks, and portable tank containers is known as a placard. The background color assigned to each placard indicates a general hazard. For example, the red background, for flammable or combustible and flammable gas, indicates that this material will burn; an orange background indicates an explosive; green, a nonflammable gas; yellow, a highly reactive substance; and blue, a water reactive substance. A combination of colors indicates multiple hazards. The size of individual packages and the quantity of the product will determine the placard used.

To assist the emergency response community to identify hazards more quickly and efficiently, the DOT modified the placarding requirements in 1981 to include the use of a four-digit identification number

referred to as the UN (United Nations) or NA (North American) identification code (Figure 22-2). This number is referenced in the *North American Emergency Response Guidebook* and other texts and in hazardous material computer databases (e.g., TOMES Plus) to access hazard information on that chemical or class of chemicals. The identification number is displayed either as 4-inch numbers on an orange 6-by-6-inch panel near the appropriate panel, a $3^1/_2$-inch number on the center of the hazardous material placard, or a $3^1/_2$-inch number in the center of a plain white placard with no hazard class symbols or notations (usually reserved for hazardous waste warnings). This numerical identification system is not used on placards for explosives, poisonous gas, or radioactive shipments.

While placarding and labeling regulations have made it easier for emergency response personnel to rapidly identify hazardous materials, serious limitations continue to exist that can put emergency personnel at risk. First, it is wrong to assume each transport vehicle is in full compliance with the law. Shippers and drivers may not be aware of the nature of their hazardous cargo; they may also choose to hide markings to evade route restrictions placed on hazardous materials transport. Second, under existing criteria, when a driver is carrying less than 1,000 pounds of aggregate gross weight of certain materials (e.g., nonflammable gas, such as chlorine or poison B), a placard is not required. Third, a "Dangerous" placard may be used in place of separate placards for two or more substances. When two or more placards are used, they are stacked according to a designated pecking order. Fourth, a vehicle may be placarded, but the placard may be incorrect or unreadable due to smoke, fire, or collision damage. Fifth, some materials like cryogenics are not considered hazardous under current regulations. In addition, each year the DOT grants hundreds of exemptions to its transportation rules. Finally, placards do not give information about how much product is on board or its physical properties or toxic risks, either alone or in combination with other substances present in the incident. They are simply a "warning" and a reminder to think carefully before undertaking rescue or clean-up.

SHIPPING PAPERS AND DOCUMENTS

Generally, any hazardous material being transported is required to be identified on a shipping paper. Each mode of transportation has a different title for their shipping paper [e.g., bill of lading (highway), dangerous cargo manifest (water), waybill/consist (rail), air bill (air)] and where it is kept also varies (cab, truck, with the conductor or engineer, the wheelhouse, or cockpit). Nonstandard locations are not infrequent. Conferring with the driver,

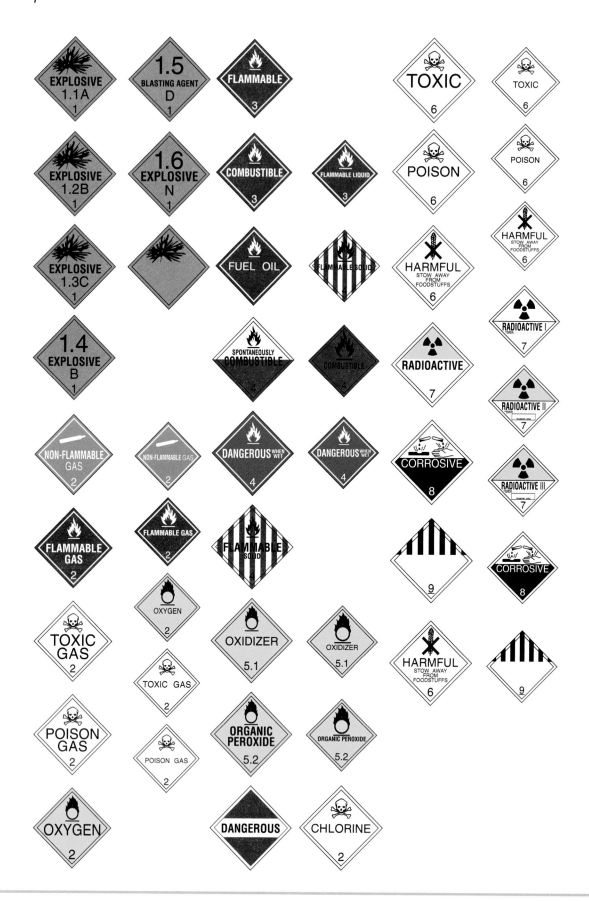

FIGURE 22-1 Hazardous materials warning placards—domestic placarding.

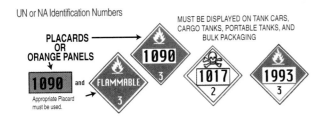

FIGURE 22-2 Hazardous materials warning placards—UN or NA identification numbers. (*Source:* Adapted from *Agency for Toxic Substances and Disease Registry: Managing Hazardous Materials Incidents,* Vol. I: *Emergency Medical Services: A Planning Guide for the Management of Contaminated Patients.* Washington, DC: US Government Printing Office; 1992:67.)

crew, shipper, distribution warehouse, or receiving company may provide valuable information.

Each shipping paper contains information on the proper shipping name (DOT), hazard classification (DOT), four-digit identification number(s), type of package, and total quantity by weight, volume, and/or packaging. Special wording may also be found in certain circumstances (e.g., "Waste," "Poison," "Oxidizer"), along with other authorized abbreviations. Hazardous materials being carried may be highlighted on the shipping papers by being listed first, through color highlighting, or by notation next to the substance entry in a column captioned "HM."

Never assume that "what you see is what you've got." Materials may have been delivered or picked up at intermediate points without change in the papers. Items may be mislabeled or not identified if they are present in small quantities. As costs of proper waste disposal increase, so do temptations to falsify records and to conduct illicit transport and disposal.

MATERIAL SAFETY DATA SHEETS

Material safety data sheets are used by manufacturers to meet legal requirements to address their employees' "right to know" what hazards are present in the workplace, to note the effects of overexposure, and to describe procedures for emergency care and spill containment. A basic understanding of chemical terminology and experience in reading similar data are useful, but physicians glean at least some useful points. The medical information provided is typically found in the Health Hazard Information section of each form and is usually limited to very basic first-aid measures. In addition, the quality and completeness of toxicologic data are highly variable and generally poor. Though the format may vary from business to business, these sheets

are required by law to be sent to each community's LEPC and fire department to assist with emergency response planning for that location. Through preplanning and cooperation, they can also be available to treating clinicians to provide at least a cursory understanding of the toxic agent and as a foundation for seeking further details about its health effects.

Problems with the MSDSs include the following: (1) there is no standardized format, (2) the producer or formulator does not consider the agent dangerous, (3) a chemical may not be listed, (4) the identity of an agent may be withheld if the manufacturer considers it a trade secret (though there are provisions to release information to physicians in an emergency), and (5) the accuracy and completeness of the data are variable at best. For instance, a hazardous substance may legally be omitted from the MSDS if it constitutes less than 1% of product weight (less than 0.1% if a carcinogen) but may still pose some risk. Receiving, updating, and storing MSDSs, along with providing rapid access to the information at the time of need, have proven to be significant challenges and legal issues for fire chiefs, emergency planners, and clinicians across the country.

MONITORING AND DETECTION EQUIPMENT

Monitoring and detection equipment can sometimes provide clues and data concerning the nature of the agents involved in a hazardous material accident. This "real-time" data can be used to assist in determining the location and size of an incident and to help with assessment of potential health effects and selection of proper personnel protective equipment (PPE). The concentration of hazardous materials can be identified by use of direct reading instruments and laboratory analysis of samples obtained through various collection methods. Industrial sites may also have records of routine industrial hygiene monitoring for hazards present at that site and a system of alarms to warn when ambient concentrations reach levels of concern.

Direct reading instruments generally provide information at the time they are used. They are employed to detect and monitor flammable or explosive atmospheres, oxygen deficiencies, certain gases and vapors, and ionizing radiation. Examples of direct reading instruments include combustible gas indicators (explosimeters), oxygen meters, calorimetric indicator tubes (e.g., Draeger tubes), pH meters or pH paper, and radiation survey instruments.

Even when available, calibrated, and used by trained personnel, such instruments have limitations: (1) they may detect or measure only specific classes of chemicals; (2) they are not usually designed to measure or detect airborne concentrations below 1 ppm; (3) false readings may result from interference from substances that the device is not designed to measure; (4) they are costly; and (5) employees or supervisors in workplaces may disable or fail to repair devices that they perceive as a nuisance, as alarms often generate paperwork and work interruptions.

SENSES AND BEHAVIOR

Sensory clues of sight, sound, and smell can help to determine that a dangerous substance is present and has, or is about to be, released into the environment. Determining the color of a smoke or vapor cloud can also prove helpful in identifying the products involved. Some chemicals are associated with characteristic smoke colors when they burn or form unique vapor clouds when accidently released. Unless properly protected, emergency personnel should avoid entering or being engulfed by smoke or a vapor cloud. Auditory clues may include the hissing of pressurized gas release, the sparking of downed power lines, or the groaning of metal containers under thermal or mechanical stress. Incidents involving more than one patient with common signs and symptoms should also be suspected of involving hazardous materials until proven otherwise.

Irritation of the eyes, nose, or respiratory tract is another sensory warning sign of a potentially dangerous environment, and the emergency responder should evacuate the area until the health threat is assessed and adequate protective equipment is employed. However, it must be remembered that the presence or absence of an odor, color, or irritation is not a reliable indicator of inhalation exposure. While certain chemicals have characteristic odors, not everyone can perceive these clues effectively. There is genetic variability in the ability to detect odors such as the "bitter almond" of cyanide. Nasal congestion due to colds or allergies also impair the responder's ability to perceive an odor until it is too late. For some substances like vinyl chloride, the odor or irritation threshold is higher than the toxic air concentration. Other chemicals (e.g., hydrogen sulfide) may "deaden" olfactory functioning in minutes and mislead the rescuer into thinking the risk has lessened when it has not. Finally, some very toxic compounds have no warning properties whatsoever, carbon monoxide being a classic example.

The behavior and symptoms of patients and rescuers can provide a vital clue to the presence of a hazardous substance. Beyond the symptoms described above, complaints such as cough and burning eyes, seizures, and unexplained unconsciousness should raise the question of a toxic substance, especially when more than one person is affected. Subtle changes, such as inappropriate euphoria, slurred speech, and altered gait, may be the first signs of the presence of a toxic substance or its penetration of protective gear. Parallel clues may occur in the behavior of animals or even in the sudden stalling or rough idling of engines on the scene. The World Trade Center bombings in New York City, the Sarin gas attack in Tokyo, and the Oklahoma City Federal Building bombing should remind all personnel that some incidents are not accidental.

SCENE OPERATIONS

While approaching the scene of the incident, EMS personnel should be alert to evidence of imminent danger, such as unusual clouds, spills, noises, or smells. Initial observation from a safe distance is vital, and binoculars are often useful. Sizing up an incident from a distance sufficient to cover the scene with one's outstretched thumb, the **rule of thumb** is sometimes suggested as a rough guide. Where the agents involved are known with certainty, the *North American Emergency Response Guidebook* offers more specific evacuation distances. Other field guides also provide easy, concise information on principal hazards, protective equipment, and basic therapy for many agents. Useful information can also be accessed through computer databases in response vehicles or by phone/fax links to resource centers like poison control centers and the Chemical Transportation Emergency Center (CHEMTREC) as well as local Hazmat teams.

EMS personnel should avoid driving through released product and be parked upwind, uphill, and in a safe position that allows for a quick exit. Wind shifts and back drafts pose additional threats and should be noted en route to the call and while on the scene.

THE INCIDENT COMMAND SYSTEM

Once on the scene, an incident command system (ICS) should be established immediately with one person, the incident commander, assuming ultimate responsibility and authority for managing all aspects of the operation. Using standard operating procedures, multiple tasks need to be quickly initiated and coordinated (Table 22-2).

The danger area and incident scene should be isolated with physical boundary markers, such as cones and tape, with the assistance of adequately protected personnel such as police. These personnel must be aware of changes in conditions, such as wind shifts or spread of fire to new containers. A command post (in the cold zone), hot (exclusion), warm (limited access, decontamination), and cold (support) zones, along with staging and treatment areas should be quickly established and be

Table 22-2
Essential Elements of Scene Operations

Isolation of the danger area and incident scene

Establishment of a command post and zones

Identification of the materials

Evaluation of material hazards and risks

Determination of initial response objectives

Selection of the proper protective clothing and equipment

Preparation of a decontamination area and staff

Organization of the medical surveillance and treatment areas

Preparation and coordination of transport vehicles

Search, extrication, and rescue

plainly visible, regardless of the time of day and weather conditions. The hot, warm, and cold zones should be of suitable size and configuration to allow for changes in conditions (such as wind direction) and to conduct activities in a safe and effective fashion.

Hazmat-trained and -qualified EMS personnel may be assigned to assume one of the several command positions, including EMS Hazmat Officer, Reference Officer, and Rehab Officer. All EMS agencies are mandated by OSHA to annually provide Hazmat awareness training to their personnel. In addition, EMS personnel should ideally be trained to either Level I or Level II of the *NFPA 473-Competencies for Medical Personnel at the Scene of a Hazardous Material Incident* standard. Concise, yet complete, "size-up" and periodic situation reports should be made by the incident commander or command post designee. Chemical names should be spelled out on the radio and not pronounced. There is a big difference between benzotrichloride and benzotrifluoride! Evaluation of the relative hazards and risks of the identified materials is performed through interpretation of available information and consultation with experts and reference materials and awareness of impending releases and nontoxic hazards. Changing weather conditions must be noted and considered when making decisions concerning sector size, work duration, decontamination location, and patient care activities.

Determination of initial response objectives should be based on analysis of the risk versus benefit. Is this a rescue or a body recovery situation? When no lives are threatened, by far the most prudent course may be to let a toxic fire burn itself out. Selection of the proper protec-

tive clothing and equipment can be done by using available reference material. Entry teams should not be sent in without having a backup team ready for support in case of trouble. Early interruption and control of continuing product release are of primary importance. Initial corrective strategies may include shutting off valves, setting aright overturned 55-gallon drums, and using tarps, patches, dikes, and absorbents to contain the escaping product. Preparation of a decontamination area includes setting it up in the warm zone, organizing equipment and supplies, and assigning personnel to the decontamination team. The decontamination area must be of sufficient size and a safe location to handle medical decontamination of exposed personnel and the cleaning of response personnel's protective clothing and equipment (technical decontamination). Organization of the medical surveillance and treatment areas in the cold zone is needed to handle pre- and postentry physical exams on response team members and treatment of injured personnel. Incident management and medical surveillance documentation are particularly important since acute exposures may pose immediate and delayed health implications. The absence of adequate documentation may hamper the responders' ability to justify a claim of work-related injury or illness. A decision must be made early in the incident's management as to whether the operation will be a rescue or recovery operation, and that decision must be shared with all on-scene personnel. Taking unnecessary and inappropriate risks compromises the success of the operation and the safety of response personnel.

Qualified sector officers wearing unique identification, such as command vests that identify their specific area of command responsibility, should coordinate the activities in each area. Using tactical work sheets, vital information about incident management should be organized and recorded. If casualties are suspected or found, alerting receiving hospitals should be done as soon as possible. A safety officer should be appointed and assume responsibility for identifying and correcting unsafe policies or practices. Continuous monitoring of the dynamics of an incident is needed so that new response plans can be quickly developed and efficiently implemented. In extraordinary circumstances, the off-site threat (e.g., an ammonia cloud rapidly approaching an elementary school with children outdoors) may take priority over on-scene rescue.

PERSONNEL AND SITE SAFETY

Safety is of paramount importance in all aspects of managing the hazardous material incident. Basic on-scene safety tenets are listed in Table 22-3. EMS personnel should not be operating in hot- and warm-zone activities unless properly trained and equipped. If an EMS unit arrives first on the scene and recognizes a life hazard exists, their initial actions should include (1) immediately requesting more expert assistance, such as a Hazmat team; (2) minimizing risk to themselves by remaining in a "safe" area; (3) organizing preliminary on-scene operations, such as establishing a command post and staging area; (4) trying to identify the material involved [e.g., obtaining the shipping papers or MSDS for the product(s) involved], present hazards, and number of injured persons; (5) determining whether immediate evacuation of nearby areas is indicated; and (6) directing injured personnel, by a public address system or bullhorn, to leave the danger area and relocate to a safe site, but still away from response personnel. *Unprotected personnel should not attempt to enter the hot zone to perform a rescue nor should they don personal protective clothing without appropriate training.*

PERSONAL PROTECTIVE EQUIPMENT

Hazardous material incidents typically require that at least some responders wear PPE, which is designed to protect body surfaces and the respiratory tract from contact and injury by toxic substances. The level of protection required depends on a number of factors, including (1) the material involved; (2) its physical properties under existing and foreseeable incident and weather conditions; (3) its form, concentration, and amount; and (4) the role of an individual in the response. Prior to donning PPE, all personnel should be given a preentry examination that evaluates blood pressure (BP), pulse, respiration, temperature (T), weight, and resting electrocardiogram (ECG). In addition, the responder should be asked about his or her current health and recent medication usage. Inclusion criteria (e.g., systolic BP less than 160, diastolic BP less than 90, pulse 50–110, respiration 12–20) should be followed. Personnel who do not meet the inclusion criteria should be precluded from suit work, which would put them at risk by wearing the PPE and working in danger areas. Initial physiological elevations are usually secondary to anxiousness that abates after a "rest period" in a quiet area. Postentry monitoring should be initiated after decontamination and significant variations from the earlier baseline values evaluated. Injured or ill responders should be promptly treated in accordance with the local protocol.

No single protective clothing material affords protection against all types of hazards, and use of such equipment imposes significant limitations on medical care. The selection of proper PPE is critical to the entry team, important to the field decontamination and scene control personnel, and must be individually considered for others. In general, prehospital medical

Table 22-3
Scene Safety Rules

1. Minimize the number of response personnel working in and near the contaminated area.

2. Avoid contact of personnel and equipment with contaminated surfaces.

3. Ensure that all tasks and responsibilities are identified before attempting entry into the hot zone. If necessary, practice unfamiliar operations prior to entry.

4. Monitor for atmospheres that are oxygen deficient or contain flammable or combustible vapors.

5. Use the buddy system for all entry operations and ensure properly equipped backup and decontamination crews are in place.

6. Maintain communication and visual contact between entry teams, backup crews, and the safety officers. Ensure all personnel are familiar with standard visual and audible communication practices.

7. Ensure that everyone knows the emergency evacuation signals and that the entrances and exits of the hot zone are clearly defined.

8. Observe for signs of breach of the suit, heat stress, and psychological distress.

9. Always have an escape route.

10. Work time and rest period schedules must be established and complied with by everyone. Keep a written log of personnel working in each area and the length of time that they are there.

11. Prohibit drinking, smoking, and any other practices that increase the possibility of hand-to-mouth contamination transfer in contaminated areas.

12. Appoint a safety officer to ensure that these safety practices are followed. In larger incidents, assign one safety officer to general-scene operations, with a second person assigned to just hot- and/or warm-zone operations.

Source: Adapted from Noll G, Hildebrand M, Yvorra J. *Hazardous Materials, Managing the Incident.* Fire Protection Publications. Stillwater, Okla: Oklahoma State University; 1996.

providers, unless they are part of the trained Hazmat entry or decontamination team, do not don PPE and do not enter the hot zone or decontamination corridor. Instead, they await patients at the cold-zone perimeter, with no special PPE except perhaps a basic communicable disease kit (gloves, disposable gown, mask, goggles). Disposable chemical-resistant jumpsuits, such as Saranex-coated Tyvek, can provide an extra measure of splash protection. It is essential that field personnel communicate effectively with the scene safety officer, poison control center, and/or medical control, and consult reference texts to assure proper protective clothing is worn by all on-scene personnel. The final decision concerning PPE is made when two or more resources agree on a common recommendation for that type of agent(s) and the incident situation.

PROTECTIVE EQUIPMENT CLASSIFICATIONS

There are three general types of personal protective clothing. Structural fire fighting clothing is designed to protect against temperature extremes, steam, hot water, hot particles, and ordinary hazards of fire fighting. Standard "turnout gear" falls in this category. High-temperature protective clothing protects against short-term exposure to high temperatures. Chemical protective clothing is designed to protect skin and eyes from direct chemical contact. A subclassification by the Environmental Protection Agency describes the four levels of chemical protective clothing, which are illustrated in Figure 22-3.

Level A

This optimum level of protection is used to enter areas that pose serious risks of inhalation, skin, mucous membrane, and eye exposure. The ensemble includes positive-pressure self-contained breathing apparatus (SCBA) or in-line air supply system, encapsulating chemical-resistant suit, multiple layers of chemical-resistant gloves, chemical-resistant boots, and airtight seals between the suit, gloves, and boots. Cooling vests are sometimes used to reduce heat stress and two-way radios using throat or ear microphones aid operations and medical surveillance for personnel dressed in either Level A or Level B gear.

Level B

Level B protection provides respiratory protection similar to Level A, but the suits lack full encapsulation and, thus, offer less protection to the skin, mucous membranes, and eyes. These suits are chemically resistant and prevent splash exposure. Level B protection includes positive-pressure SCBA, chemical-resistant, long-sleeved suit, multiple layers of chemical-resistant gloves, and chemical-resistant boots. Hard hats are often recommended at this and other levels because of the risk of head trauma in tight quarters or from falling debris.

Level C

This level of protective clothing is used when the type and air concentrations of hazardous materials fall within the capability of the chosen air purification filter and there is little likelihood of exposure to the skin, mucous membranes, or eyes. Safe use of all respirators requires fit testing, training, and equipment maintenance. Beyond these essentials, air purification respirators demand adequate ambient oxygen (O_2) and a known chemical substance with air exposure levels known to be below danger levels. This level of clothing protection includes a full-face, air purification respirator with appropriate canister, a chemical-resistant suit, chemical-resistant outer gloves, and chemical-resistant boots.

Level D

This level of clothing consists of common work clothes such as overalls or Nomex pants and shirt. It does not provide respiratory or skin protection. This clothing typically is worn underneath other types of protective clothing.

OSHA regulations and common sense dictate that personnel who use SCBA and air-purifying respirators must have specific training, be properly fitted for the equipment, and be physically fit. Fire departments and Hazmat teams have increasingly been using disposable suits at much less cost than the standard reusable suits. However, even with lower expense, there are major visibility, flexibility, and dexterity limitations when EMS personnel try to provide patient care while wearing Levels A, B, and C protective clothing. Suit wearers are also susceptible to heat illness and psychological stress while working.

The use of PPE is also associated with several other notable problems:

- Dexterity and vision: Auscultation and palpation skills are virtually eliminated and dexterity greatly reduced when a rescuer wears a suit and bulky gloves. Vision may quickly deteriorate in the smoke and mist of a hot zone or from fogging of the respirator face mask. Communication and physical coordination also suffer.

- Operational time: Air supply using SCBA is limited; a bottle rated at 1 hour may last only 20 minutes under extreme conditions. Bottle changes are not simple matters in the chaos of a major incident. In-line supplied air systems help to avoid these problems. "Time on air" limitations must take into account travel back and forth to the incident site and going through decontaminations, not just work-related considerations.

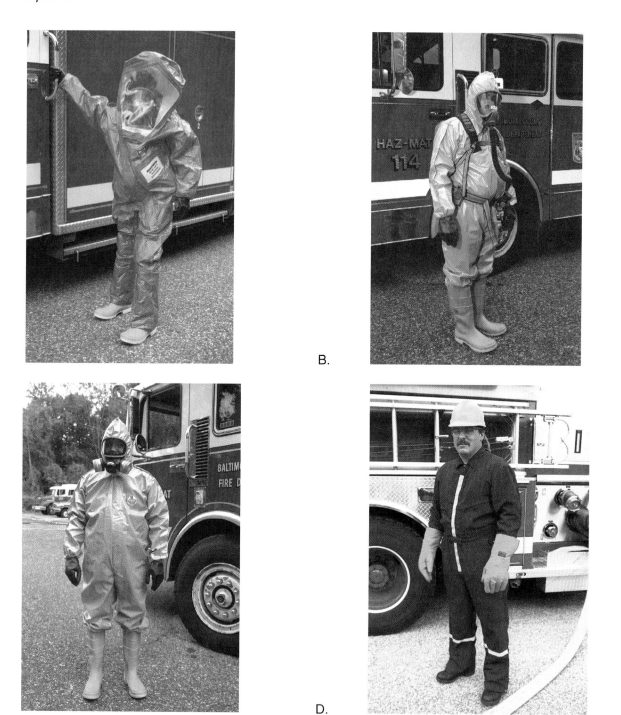

FIGURE 22-3 Levels of personal protective equipment: (A) Level A suit; (B) Level B suit; (C) Level C suit; (D) Level D suit.

- Respirator and cartridge function: Sophisticated support and maintenance are required for respiratory equipment, especially SCBA. Periodic fit testing is very important. Conventional eye glasses, gum chewing, dehydration, long hair, and even a few days of beard stubble may greatly compromise the seal of a mask on the face. Air-purifying cartridge respirators require adequate ambient oxygen. Appropriate cartridge utilization is not possible when substance identity and concentration are unknown, and cartridges may saturate with product and lose effectiveness.

- Rescuer injury: Fatigue, heat stress, and claustrophobic attacks are real risks. Hypothermia is also a risk when cryogenics are involved or environmental temperatures are cold. Not all temperaments lend themselves to functioning in PPE. In a setting of torn metal and uncertain footing, limited vision and altered balance from bulky gear can easily increase the risk of injury.

● Partial protection: Even if all of the above problems were surmounted, Level A suits provide only partial protection from radiologics, cryogenics, fire, and explosion. Inapparent tears can occur in suits, and a single product or one in synergy with other products can penetrate intact material. Chemical degradation occurs when the characteristics of the clothing material are altered through contact with chemical substances. Permeation is the process in which the chemical crosses through the protective barrier by passive diffusion, over a period of time known as "break-through time."

Despite these limitations, EMS personnel who are likely to be at risk for contamination should become familiar with working in Level B and C chemical protective clothing, particularly suits that are disposable. Thereafter, it is essential that comfort and competence be maintained by regular practice working in the attire and maintaining personal fitness year round.

Another important aspect of personnel protection is to prevent the spread of contamination from the toxin present at the primary exposure site to response personnel, their equipment, vehicles, and receiving hospitals. Failure to do so can create much anxiety on the part of staff and patients and, in extreme situations, may force the temporary closing of emergency departments. Important steps are listed in Table 22-4.

By necessity, these measures may delay the initiation of medical care. For example, a patient soaked with concentrated liquid Sarin, a highly toxic nerve agent used in the Tokyo subway terrorist act, must be decontaminated before endotracheal intubation, insertion of intravenous lines, or atropine and pralidoxime (2-PAM) administration. Otherwise, EMTs and paramedics face a serious risk of secondary contamination from accidental contact. Secondary contamination may also result from inhaling dusts or vapors given off by a volatile liquid on the patient's skin, hair, or clothing or contact with contaminated emesis. Risk for secondary contamination exists, particularly for agents that are highly toxic and likely to be carried on skin, in hair, or in clothing in sufficient quantities to create an exposure risk for downstream personnel and facilities. Serious hazards are also more likely for agents with systemic toxicity and modest warning properties, such as respiratory or skin irritation, since individuals will be less aware of ongoing exposure. It is important to remember that individuals posing a contamination risk to rescue and medical personnel remain at risk themselves because of continuing exposure. Similarly, failure at the scene to properly seal and dispose of contaminated clothing, shoes, watch bands, and tools can subsequently endanger emergency department personnel, coworkers, family, and the patients themselves. Table 22-5 lists some substances likely to pose a risk of secondary contamination.

On the other hand, many chemicals do not carry any significant risk of secondary contamination because they are not likely to remain on the patient in sufficient quantities to create a hazard to treatment personnel. In general, gases and vapors are considered to pose a very low risk for secondary contamination (unless they have condensed onto clothing or skin), since they are quickly dispersed into the surrounding atmosphere as soon as the patient is removed from the area of heavy exposure. For example, a person who has inhaled carbon monoxide or hydrogen cyanide gas may be extremely ill but does not normally carry enough toxic material to contaminate treatment personnel. Such a patient can be transferred immediately to EMTs or paramedics in

Table 22-4
Steps to Prevent the Spread of Contamination

1. Set up clearly marked and secured hot, warm, and cold zones.
2. Control public and media access to the incident.
3. Minimize the number of personnel working in the hot and warm zones.
4. Monitor entry, backup, and decontamination teams to ensure that their activities do not spread contamination.
5. Use disposable equipment when possible.
6. Prepare and line facility floors and vehicle interiors.
7. Follow prescribed decontamination processes for civilians, responders, equipment, facilities, and vehicles.
8. Have contingency decontamination plans for those contaminated and injured and for handling large numbers of contaminated persons.

Table 22-5
Examples of Substances with a Serious Risk of Causing Secondary Contamination

Organophosphate insecticides

Phenol and related compounds

Volatile solvents (xylene, trichloroethylene)

Radioactive dusts, oils, and liquids

the support zone, after gross decontamination. On the other hand, the presence of liquids, oils, dusts, or particles on the patient's clothing or body should be considered potentially contaminating. *The recognition of the potential for secondary contamination is essential for proper patient management.* A patient with serious potential for causing secondary contamination must be thoroughly decontaminated before invasive medical treatment is rendered.

The risk of secondary contamination can be reduced or eliminated by decontamination. Agents that are highly water soluble may be easy to remove or dilute with simple washing. On the other hand, oily or otherwise adherent materials may persist on the skin or in the hair and continue to pose a risk of secondary contamination, requiring repeated soap and shampoo washing. As previously noted, such materials represent a source of continued toxic absorption for the primary patient, which may make their removal a matter of some urgency. Internal contamination presents another set of considerations, including enhancing excretion, blocking internal absorption, and simple or isotopic dilution (the latter in the case of some radionuclides).

Regional poison control centers, toxicologists, and medical texts and databases can provide information about the potential for secondary contamination and degree of decontamination required. In general, the risks and benefits of decontamination must be balanced. Decontamination can lessen patient exposure and prevent the spread of contamination to emergency personnel and facilities. However, the time taken and the process itself may lead to the delay or neglect of more urgent medical needs, increase skin absorption through excessively scrubbed, abraded skin, and contribute to hypothermia, skin infection, and burn sepsis.

FIELD MANAGEMENT

Rescue and treatment is divided into the operational zones discussed earlier in this chapter and illustrated in Figure 22-4.

IN THE HOT ZONE OR EXCLUSION ZONE

A properly trained and equipped hazardous materials entry team, with appropriate backup, must quickly size up the situation (known as "recon") to determine the number of patients and the severity of their injuries. Because of the risk of imminent danger and the limitations on clinical examination imposed by their

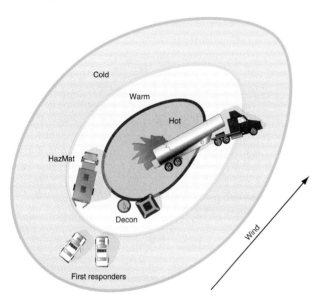

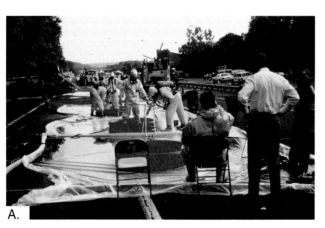

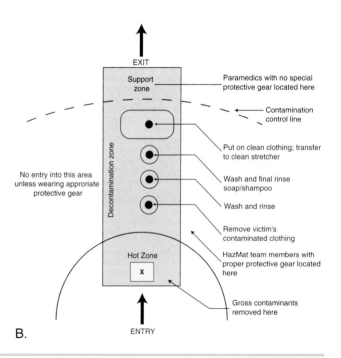

FIGURE 22-4 (A) Organization of a HazMat incident area. (B) Detail of decontamination zone.

protective clothing, rescuers should render only obvious, essential medical care while in the hot zone. This basic care includes (a) spinal stabilization if trauma is suspected, (b) corrective positioning of the head and neck to maintain an airway, (c) hemorrhage control, and (d) if extrication and a protracted rescue is required, administration of bottled air or supplemental oxygen. Isolation of the respiratory system from continuing toxic inhalation is of paramount importance in the hot and warm zones. "Escape packs" have simple hoods that slip over a breathing patient's head to provide clean air during extrication. Supplemental oxygen is rarely deleterious, the notable exception being severe cases of paraquat and diquat exposure where oxygen may exacerbate oxidative lung damage.

It is particularly important to establish rapid triage in a multicasualty incident. Ambulatory patients should be instructed where to move and to begin decontamination by removing their clothing and leaving it in the hot zone. Nonambulatory patients should be brought or dragged out of danger by the entry team. Ideally, this is done by means of strapping the patient to a backboard or portable stretcher with cervical spine support. Wire litter baskets (Stokes) are often useful and are relatively easy to decontaminate.

Contaminated clothing is to be removed by entry team personnel and obvious skin contamination brushed off, soaked up, and rinsed off prior to entering the decontamination area. This is known as **gross decontamination**. Rinsing off a contaminated patient before the removal of clothes is not generally a good idea since soaked clothing may hold contamination in direct contact with the skin. Patients who are obviously dead (i.e., not responsive, moving, or breathing) should not, as a rule, be moved until (a) all other living patients have been removed and cared for and (b) removal is approved by the police department or head of the incident investigation team. When the risk of secondary contamination exists, the dead should be decontaminated before being taken to the morgue.

IN THE DECONTAMINATION OR WARM ZONE

Initial decontamination has already begun in the hot zone as discussed above. The decontamination corridor is located in the warm zone and is usually staffed by trained hazardous materials team members wearing a lesser level of chemical protective gear than the entry team. Such gear usually consists of splash-resistant chemical clothing and either air-supplied respirators (SCBA) or air-purifying respirators that are Level B or Level C gear. Paramedics and other supporting medical personnel are generally not part of the decontamination team and will have to wait for the patient in the support (cold) zone. However, increasing numbers of hazardous materials teams are now including specially trained paramedics as part of the decontamination team so that initial clinical decision making and critical treatment, such as airway suctioning and assisted oxygen delivery, may be initiated while the patient is still undergoing decontamination.

As soon as possible, the decontamination team should determine the potential for secondary contamination and the necessity for further decontamination of patients. If the identity of the hazardous material is known with confidence, decontamination and other needed medical information can be obtained from department medical protocols and/or a regional poison control center or on-call medical toxicologist. In many cases, and as discussed earlier in this chapter, no further decontamination will be necessary if there is no secondary contamination risk. When the risk of secondary contamination does exist and the patient's clinical condition and other scene factors (e.g., number of patients and environmental conditions) allow, thorough, systematic washing with soft bristle brushes, soap (liquid hand or dishwashing), and water from head to toe is done at the scene to prevent further injury to the patient or to treatment personnel. This is known as **secondary decontamination**.

Ambulatory patients can perform much of the decontamination procedure themselves while nonambulatory/back-boarded patients must rely on decontamination team members to complete the process. Respiratory protection and multiple glove layers make it difficult to render medical care, particularly advanced life support (ALS) care. Generally, ECG monitors, pulse oximetry monitors, and other electronic equipment are not used in the decontamination area.

Some chemicals are labeled "water reactive" and rescuers may be hesitant to apply water during the decontamination process. However, the risk of water application producing an endothermic reaction, a toxic gas, or a caustic liquid has already been greatly reduced by transporting the patient out of the hot zone and removing clothing and gross contamination. Application of copious water at this point usually does not pose a threat to the patient or rescuers.

Preplans must address provision of an adequate supply of rinsing water, preferably heated to about 85°F. There are also a number of specialized decontamination solutions tailored for certain contaminating agents. Many of these solutions are designed for equipment decontamination and should not be applied to bare skin. Usually at least 90% of a contamination problem is reduced by removal of clothing and obvious dermal contamination. The availability of "the ideal solution" rarely determines ultimate clinical success.

Wastewater should be collected and disposed of after consultation with environmental officials or local water authority personnel.

Wherever possible, disposable medical equipment should be used in both the hot and warm zones. It is also important to remember that items initially used to treat patients in the warm zone generally should not come with patients once they are transferred into the cold zone. This "oneway flow" principle, that equipment remains in the most contaminated area until properly decontaminated, also applies to people. The individual briefly dropping off supplies in the warm zone and then attempting to leave without decontamination or shoe change may later cause contamination problems in his or her workplace or residence.

Definitive decontamination is the final washing and rinsing done to assure no product remains on the patient. Oftentimes, this determination is subjectively made. Radioactive agents and phosphorus are two exceptions because their presence can be determined using a Geiger counter and Wood's lamp, respectively. Definitive decontamination is most often done once the patient has reached the emergency department, rather than in the field.

"Emergency" technical decontamination will occasionally be required for a responder wearing protective equipment who suddenly collapses or runs out of air. The proper response to this emergency must be preplanned and rehearsed to assure the situation is properly managed. Once through decontamination, a quick assessment must be performed to determine whether the emergency is the result of a breach in the suit or other technical problem or whether it is a heat problem related to wearing the PPE.

Other supplies likely to be needed in the decontamination area include gowns, slippers, and blankets to wear after decontamination and tents or vans to shelter rescuers and patients in inclement or cold weather. Large barrels with plastic bags are useful for contaminated clothes and equipment. Clear freezer bags should be used for isolating and identifying personal items like rings and watches.

IN THE SUPPORT OR COLD ZONE

Rescuers in the support zone usually must wait for patients to be decontaminated in the warm zone before thorough evaluation and treatment can begin. Paramedical personnel in the cold zone must confirm that decontamination, if needed, has been properly carried out before they accept transfer of patients from the hot zone or decontamination area. If it has not been done before this point, the cervical spine should be stabilized with a cervical collar and lateral stabilization when there is a history of pain or trauma to the neck or head.

The airway should be rapidly evaluated and proper positioning, suctioning, airway adjuncts, and supplemental oxygen used, if indicated. Pulse oximetry may be helpful but must not be overly relied upon to indicate the severity of a patient's condition. Many toxins can cause serious injury to the respiratory tract (Table 22-6). Signs of such injury may include cough, tachypnea, labored breathing, stridor, or bronchospasm. It is important to remember that some inhaled agents, such as nitrogen oxides, can cause pulmonary edema after a relatively asymptomatic period of 4–12 hours. For symptomatic patients, high-flow supplemental oxygen via nonrebreathing face mask is usually indicated, though patients with existing obstructive disease should be observed for carbon dioxide retention and progressive somnolence. Bronchodilators have been shown to be beneficial. Early examination of the chest for external injury and auscultation of breath sounds helps to determine the severity of the patient's condition and serve as a baseline.

INTERNET ACTIVITIES

Visit the e-medicine Web site at http://www.emedicine.com. Click on the Emergency Medicine on-line book and select Toxicology.

- Click on Chlorine Gas. Review the chapter on the management of this exposure.
- Click on Ammonia. Review the chapter on the management of this exposure.
- Click on Carbon Monoxide. Review the chapter on the management of this exposure.
- Click on Cyanide. Review the chapter on the management of this exposure.
- Click on Organophosphates and Carbamates. Review the chapter on the management of these exposures.

If the patient is experiencing severe respiratory distress or is apneic, endotracheal intubation should be performed. Intubation is also often required in severe organophosphate pesticide exposures because of the profuse cholinergic secretions, mental status changes, and potential for life-threatening arrhythmias and seizures.

Pulse, obvious changes in perfusion, and signs of ongoing or extensive blood loss should be sought. Basic life support should be initiated, if required, and intravenous lines inserted to permit fluid resuscitation and medication administration. A cardiac monitor should be attached as soon as possible and the patient's ECG continuously monitored. Hypotension should be treated with boluses of saline (200–500 mL), especially if heat stress is suspected. Frequent premature ventricular contractions may be signs of hypoxia or ischemia from systemic toxins

Table 22-6
Selected Hazardous Material Agents

Agent	Synonyms, Trade Names	UN/NA Nos.	Physical Characteristics	Major Sources	Toxicity Effect	Signs and Symptoms	Treatment
Ammonia (NH_3)	Anhydrous ammonia; aqua ammonia; aqueous ammonia	2672, 2073, 1005	Odorless gas with pungent, suffocating odor	Fertilizers; explosives; petroleum producing; refrigerants	Local irritation	Conjunctivitis; respiratory tract irritation; pulmonary edema; chemical burns	Soap and water decontamination Oxygen Bronchodilators
Benzene (C_6H_6)	Benzol; phenyl hydride	1114	Colorless liquid; aromatic hydrocarbon odor; flammable	Industrial solvent; chemical manufacture of chemicals, dyes, nylon, varnishes, paint removers	Systemic toxic; local irritation; myocardial sensitization	Arrhythmia; seizures; respiratory depression; skin irritation; eye irritation; blood disorders; central nervous system (CNS) depression	Soap and water decontamination Respiratory support Cardiac support
Carbon monoxide (CO)	None	1016	Odorless, tasteless, very flammable gas	Exhaust gas; flue gas; foundry work; petroleum refining	Binds to hemoglobin, forming carboxyhemoglobin and causing cellular hypoxia	Dyspnea; headache; dizziness; nausea; seizures; altered mental status	Oxygen Hyperbaric O_2
Chlorine (Cl, Cl_2)	Molecular chlorine	1017	Greenish, yellowish, or orange gas or liquid; sharp odor; can be formed if acid cleaners are mixed with hypochlorite bleach cleaners	Bleaching of cloth and paper; plastic manufacturing; disinfection of sewage; swimming pools; water purification	Eye and respiratory irritation	Irritating to eyes, skin, and respiratory tract; sore throat; headache; cough; eye tearing; dizziness; skin burns	Soap and water decontamination Respiratory support
Cyanide salts (NaCN, KCN, CN)	Sodium cyanide; potassium cyanide; cyanide solution, NOS; cyanide inorganic, NOS; cyanide inorganic, solid NOS	1588, 1689, 1680, 1935	White granular or crystalline solids; colorless water solution; almond-like odor	Production of hydrocarbons; burning plastic byproduct; jewelry cleaning	Cellular asphyxiant	Cardiovascular and CNS dysfunction; nausea and vomiting (N/V); weakness; cardiac arrhythmias; hypotension; hypertension; altered mental status; seizures; skin burns	Soap and water decontamination Lilly antidote kit Amyl nitrite Sodium nitrite Sodium thiosulfate Oxygen Respiratory and cardiovascular support

(continues)

Table 22-6 (continues)
Selected Hazardous Material Agents

Agent	Synonyms, Trade Names	UN/NA Nos	Physical Characteristics	Major Sources	Toxicity Effect	Signs and Symptoms	Treatment
Dieldrin ($C_{12}H_8Cl_6O$)	HEOD; DDT	2761	White-brown crystal; odorless; when heated, decomposes to Cl fumes	Organochlorine insecticide	CNS stimulant	Headache; N/V; weakness; dizziness; seizures; altered mental status; pulmonary edema	Soap and water decontamination Airway support Respiratory support Cardiovascular support Antiseizure medication (i.e., Valium)
Hydrogen sulfide (H_2S)	Hydrosulfuric acid; sewer gas; sulfuretted hydrogen	1053	Colorless gas; strong rotten egg odor; flammable	Product of organic material decay and fossil fuel production	Cellular asphyxiant	Headache; cough; N/V; eye and respiratory irritation; dizziness; seizures	Soap and water decontamination Airway support Amyl nitrite Sodium nitrite Cardiovascular support Antiseizure medication (i.e., Valium)
Methyl bromide (CH_3Br)	Bromomethane; monobromomethane	1062	Colorless gas with chloroformlike odor; liquid below 38°; shipped as compressed gas	Fumigants; refrigerants; solvents	Local irritation; systemic toxicity	Pulmonary edema; headache; dizziness; N/V; seizures; tremors; dyspnea; skin, eye, and respiratory irritation; arrhythmias; renal and hepatic injury	Soap and water decontamination Respiratory support Cardiovascular support Antiseizure medication (i.e., Valium)
Parathion [($C_2H_5O)_2P(S)$ $OC_6H_4NO_2$, $C_{10}H_{14}NO_5PS$)]	Diethyl parathion; ethyl parathion; parathion-ethyl	2783, 1967	Yellow to dark brown liquid with garliclike odor; heating emits toxic fumes of sulfur, nitrogen, and phosphorus	Organophosphate insecticide	Cholinesterase inhibitor	Miosis; salivation, lacrimation, defication, gastric motility, emesis (SLUDGE); bronchoconstriction; muscle twitching; seizures	Soap and water decontamination Airway support Respiratory support Atropine Pralidoxime chloride (2-PAM) Antiseizure medication (i.e., Valium)

(continues)

Synonyms, Agent	UN/NA Trade Names	Physical Nos	Characteristics	Major Sources	Toxicity Effect	Signs and Symptoms	Treatment
Phosgene (CCl_2O, $COCl_2$)	Carbon oxychloride; carbonyl chloride; chloroformyl chloride	1076	Colorless gas or volatile liquid; odor of musty hay	Manufacture of insecticides, pharmaceuticals; metallurgy; chemical warfare	Local irritation	Throat and chest burning; dyspnea; pulmonary edema; N/V; skin burns; eye irritation	Soap and water decontamination Airway support Respiratory support Antiseizure medication (i.e., Valium)
Phosphorus (P_4)	Elemental white phosphorus; white phosphorus	1338, 1339, 1381, 2447	White to yellow, waxy or crystalline solid with acrid fumes; flammable; ignites suddenly on contact with air	Munitions; pesticides	Local irritation	N/V; irritant to eyes and respiratory tract; severe skin burns; hypoglycemia	Soap and water decontamination Dry decontamination Avoid skin contact with air Respiratory support Pain medication Cardiovascular support D_{50}
Sarin $[CH_3P(O)OCH(CH_3)_2]$	GB: isopropyl methyl phosphonofluoridate		Odorless gas or liquid	Nerve agent	Cholinesterase inhibition	SLUDGE; tremors; altered mental status; headache (H/A); respiratory depression; miosis	Soap and water or water with hypochlorite decontamination Airway support Respiratory support Atropine Pralidoxime chloride (2-PAM) Antiseizure medication (i.e., Valium)

such as carbon monoxide or cyanide or result from myocardial sensitization from solvents. Rescuers should be cautious about the use of epinephrine, dopamine, and related drugs in patients exposed to chlorinated or other halogenated hydrocarbons, since these drugs may aggravate myocardial irritability. While select toxins can be treated with antidotes, each drug has potential serious side effects and may not be suitable for field administration. Special Hazmat medical protocols should be developed to meet the unique medical problems identified from the hazard analysis and proper training given to assure prehospital provider familiarization with the expected standard of care.

The mental status of patients should be carefully noted and continuously monitored. Altered speech or gait, abnormal eye movements, and muscle twitching can provide crucial clues to the patient's toxin and should be documented. Hypoxia, heat stroke, head injury, and direct toxin effects may contribute to such changes. Patients should be carefully evaluated for possible trauma. A rapid but thorough secondary survey should be performed to rule out significant injury to the head, spine, thorax, abdomen, pelvis, or extremities.

When clinically indicated, unconscious patients should receive appropriate pharmacologic therapy (e.g., naloxone, dextrose 50%). Seizures are uncommon overall but may be related to respiratory or cellular hypoxia (cyanide, carbon monoxide, hydrogen sulfide) or cholinergic pesticides and should be treated with antiseizure medicines, such as diazepam.

Broken skin should be noted, both as a clue to underlying fracture or other injury and as a source of absorption and internal contamination. After decontamination, open wounds should have a dressing and bandage applied, and suspected fractures should be quickly immobilized using commercial splints, pillows, or padded board splints.

Patient cooperation may sometimes be an issue, particularly with ambulatory or combative patients. Brief, concisely worded directions spoken with authority by suited personnel via PA systems or bullhorns usually conveys the necessary message. Consideration of patient modesty and comfort with screens, sheets, and disposable gowns aids the process of appropriate decontamination. In cases where combativeness is believed to be secondary to the toxin, the use of paralytic agents followed by endotracheal intubation is indicated.

FIELD TRIAGE, COMMUNICATION, AND TRANSPORT

When an incident involves many potential patients, it may not be possible to perform a complete evaluation of each patient at the scene. Multicasualty protocols established for other mass casualty disasters may be difficult to use in hazardous materials incidents, because entrance by rescue personnel into the hot zone is restricted to a few individuals wearing bulky protective gear who can be quickly overwhelmed. Rescuers wearing Level A protective equipment also have limited visibility and cannot effectively auscultate or palpate a patient.

"Decon triage" should be instituted when multiple patients require decontamination, with the priority being given to decontaminating the least injured first to avoid deterioration and optimally utilize resources to do the greatest good for the greatest number. *No patient with the risk of secondary contamination should be transported without having undergone at least gross decontamination.* As soon as possible, communication should be established with the medical control hospital. Pertinent information should be relayed and consultation on medical management sought, when necessary.

Many hazardous materials protocols advise extensive measures to protect the ambulance from contamination by covering the floors and walls with plastic sheeting. However, if the hazardous materials incident is properly managed, all patients will have undergone at least gross decontamination before transport, thus reducing the risk of secondary contamination to downstream personnel or equipment. If the patient has not been decontaminated, plastic sheeting will not protect the ambulance crew (or the patient) from inhalation exposure to a volatile liquid that has soaked clothing, skin, or hair. Such considerations have also led a number of states to restrict the use of helicopter evacuation in hazardous materials incidents.

Transporting personnel must wear proper protective clothing (e.g., Tyvek or Saranex suit) and respiratory protection (e.g., cartridge respirators, if training permits). Maximum ventilation of the cab and patient compartment is essential. Only needed equipment and supplies should remain in the ambulance. Disposable equipment should be used as much as possible, and expensive items should be protected by plastic covering to the extent possible.

The alternative to stripping the vehicle is to place plastic sheeting throughout the patient compartment and seal compartments with tape. This will not protect personnel from inhalation risk. Rather, the primary purpose is to reduce contamination of the transport vehicle and keep it in service for subsequent runs. If secondary contamination is not a risk, this protection is unnecessary. In most cases, the time spent preparing a vehicle is better spent doing field decontamination, if it can be done safely. The slippery nature of wet plastic in a "cocooned vehicle" and restriction of access to supplies provide other incentives to avoid this process whenever possible.

The contaminated patient should be wrapped in a lined blanket or the equivalent, leaving only the face exposed. Body bags are sometimes used because they offer good control of contamination and rapid access should the patient deteriorate. However, these advantages should be balanced against enhanced skin absorption of some toxins, as bags trap the patient's body heat and placement in the body bag can be associated with emotional distress and claustrophobia. A more acceptable alternative may be wrapping the patient in a less expensive, nonporous, plasticized blanket.

En route, patients should be continuously monitored for respiratory distress, cardiovascular collapse, and neurological deterioration. Oxygen should be continued en route, if appropriate, and irrigation of eye burns should continue if initiated in the support zone. Finally, in cases involving ingestion of a poison, emesis during transport may create a hazard, especially if the ingested material is a volatile liquid (e.g., xylene, toluene) or has been converted into a toxic gas (e.g., hydrogen cyanide). When "toxic vomitus" is a possibility, carry several extra towels and plastic bags lining a large bucket so that, if the patient vomits, it can be quickly mopped up and isolated.

Periodic updates should be given to the hospital if transport from the scene is delayed. Hospitals may utilize alternative treatment locations or entrances when receiving contaminated patients. Thus, it is important to clarify where patients are to be taken once at the hospital. When multiple patients are involved, it is important to avoid overloading one facility or transporting to a hospital that is unprepared to handle patients. The use of triage tags is helpful in organizing transport priorities, documenting medical care, and keeping track of patient disposition. Make sure the hospital is informed before your arrival.

Local protocols or medical control should be consulted when trying to decide what antidotes or additional medical interventions are indicated. Medical control may also be helpful in assisting with patient disposition decisions and the coordination of multiple receiving hospitals. Med radio channels, cellular phones, computers with modems, and facsimile machines have proven useful as EMS communication tools in hazardous material incidents.

Once at the hospital, clearance for prehospital personnel to return to service should be given by the emergency department physician or the incident safety officer. In incidents involving secondary contamination and the use of police or private vehicles for patient transport, hospital security may need to be involved in keeping these vehicles isolated while awaiting decontamination.

In addition to completing a patient run report, each responder should submit to the appropriate supervisor a completed hazardous material exposure form. This form becomes part of the incident report and each individual's personnel record. This documentation can provide vital evidence if work-related illness later occurs.

Once the call is completed, a critique should be held and involve as many of the participants as possible. What went well and the problems that were encountered should be discussed. Needed revisions in the response plan and future training needs should also be identified. Because hazardous materials incidents are typically prolonged and stressful, consideration of the need for a critical incident stress debriefing (CISD) or defusing by a CISD team should be made by the incident commander or EMS officer.

INTERNET ACTIVITIES

Visit the e-medicine Web site at http://www.emedicine.com. Click on the Emergency Medicine on-line book and select Emergency Medical Systems. Then click on Hazardous Materials. Review the chapter on the management of hazardous materials incidents.

SUMMARY

The safe and effective response to a hazardous material incident requires the integration of planning personnel and equipment. On-scene operations must be organized and effectively supervised within hot-, warm-, and cold-zone sectors. Personnel must wear proper protective clothing while performing a rescue as well as patient decontamination. Tactical, as well as medical, decisions are based on accurate information obtained from textbooks, poison control centers, and medical control. The degree of patient decontamination performed is based on the risk of secondary decontamination, the patient's clinical condition, and other incident and environmental factors. All patients, regardless of their clinical condition, who pose a risk of secondary contamination must be, at a minimum, grossly decontaminated before transport to the hospital in appropriately prepared vehicles. Consideration must be given to the possibility that a contaminated patient may, in fact, also be a multiple-trauma patient. Receiving hospitals are to be prealerted and patient transport done by properly protected providers who continuously monitor the patient for signs of change and provide treatment according to local protocols or directions coming from medical control. Successful scene management and prehospital medical care of the Hazmat patient should happen by design and not by accident!

REVIEW QUESTIONS

1. A hazardous material is any substance that jumps out of its container when something goes wrong and hurts or harms anything that it touches.
   a. True
   b. False

2. Which of the following is a standard method for identifying a possible hazardous material incident?
   a. Occupancy and location
   b. Container shape
   c. Placards and labels
   d. Shipping papers
   e. All of the above

3. The toxic properties of carbon monoxide occur at the cellular level and require high concentrations of oxygen and possibly hyperbaric oxygen to reverse.
   a. True
   b. False

4. Discuss the three different zones commonly employed at the scene of a hazardous material incident and the activities that are conducted in each.

5. Discuss three possible roles to be played by properly trained EMS personnel on the scene of a hazardous material incident.

6. Outline the six preliminary steps to be taken upon arrival at the scene of a hazardous material accident.

7. Discuss the four different levels of personal protective equipment (PPE).

8. Outline four common problems associated with the use of PPE.

9. Discuss the difference between emergency technical decontamination and patient decontamination.

10. Outline the steps to be taken in decontaminating an ambulatory versus a nonambulatory patient.

11. When taking care of a chemically contaminated patient, the most important priority is the ABCs.
    a. True
    b. False

12. An antidote used for the treatment of organo-pesticide poisoning is:
    a. Atropine
    b. Narcan
    c. Penicillamine
    d. Eucamyst

13. Invasive advanced life support procedures are generally done in the:
    a. Hot zone
    b. Warm zone
    c. Cold zone
    d. None of the above

14. Which of the following is always true about an MSDS?
    a. Can be used to help identify a product
    b. Is found in the workplace and on transport vehicles
    c. Uniformly follows a format
    d. Always contains reliable information

15. Ambulatory patients can perform decontamination themselves if given instruction.
    a. True
    b. False

CRITICAL THINKING

- You are dispatched to the scene of a MVC. Upon approaching the scene, you are stopped by a military police officer who indicates that a military tanker has been involved in the collision and that the tanker contained Sarin. What is this agent? What signs and symptoms would you expect to see in exposed patients? What precautions must you take to protect yourself while working at this scene? What treatments are necessary for exposed patients?

- You are dispatched to the scene of a farming accident. Upon arrival, you are met by the farm owner, who states that one of his migrant workers became ill while working. You are led to the patient, whom you find seizing. Upon questioning his friends, you discover that he has no history of seizures, no significant past medical history, and no allergies and takes no medications. What possible toxic exposures are likely in this setting? What signs and symptoms would you expect to see? What are the treatments?

- Upon arrival at the scene of a "sick call," you are greeted by a distraught housewife. She is tearing, coughing, and retching. She indicates that she was cleaning the bathroom with an abrasive powder cleanser. When this did not clean to her satisfaction, she added bleach. It was at this point that she was "overcome by fumes." What gas was created by this chemical reaction? What is its toxicity? How should this patient be treated?

▶ BIBLIOGRAPHY

Agency for Toxic Substances and Disease Registry. *Managing Hazardous Materials Incidents*, Volume I: *Emergency Medical Services: A Planning Guide for the Management of Contaminated Patients*. Washington, DC: US Government Printing Office; 1992: 636–977.

Borak J, Callan M, Abbott W. *Hazardous Materials Exposure, Emergency Response and Patient Care*. St Louis, Mo.: CV Mosby; 1991.

Currance PL, Bronstein AC. *Emergency Care for Hazardous Materials Exposure*. St Louis, Mo.: CV Mosby; 1993.

Department of Transportation (DOT). *Emergency Response Guidebook*. DOT-P-5800.5. Washington, DC: U.S. Government Printing Office; 1996.

Ellenhorn MJ, Barceloux DG. *Medical Toxicology*. New York: Elsevier North-Holland; 1988.

Medical Research Institute of Chemical Defense. *Medical Management of Chemical Casualties Handbook*, 2nd ed. Frederick, Md.: Aberdeen Proving Ground; September 1995.

Noll G, Hildebrand MS, Yvorra JG. *Hazardous Materials, Managing the Incident*. Stillwater, Okla.: Fire Protection Publications, Oklahoma State University; 1996.

Ricks RC. *Hospital Emergency Department Management of Radiation Accidents*. Oak Ridge, Tenn.: Oak Ridge Associated Universities; 1984.

Sidell FR. *Management of Chemical Warfare Agent Casualties, A Handbook for Emergency Medical Services*. Bel Air, Md.: HB Publishing.

Stutz DR, Ulin S. *Hazardous Materials Injuries, A Handbook of Prehospital Care*. Greenbelt, Md.: Bradford Communications Corporation; 1993.

Sullivan JB Jr, Krieger GR. *Hazardous Materials Toxicology: Clinical Principles of Environmental Health*. Baltimore, Md.: Williams & Wilkins; 1992.

U.S. Army Medical Research Institute of Infections Diseases Handbook, 2nd ed. Frederick, Md.: Aberdeen Proving Ground; March 1996.

Chapter 23

Environmental Emergencies

OBJECTIVES

Upon completion of this chapter, the reader should be able to:

● Describe the continuum of care for selected land, sea, and air emergencies, including assessment, intervention, and rehabilitation or discharge as applicable.

● Describe the expected physiological response to heat and cold exposure, correlate it with adjustments in medications, and elaborate on its influence upon advanced life support interventions.

● Identify and list those factors that have the most influence on adverse outcomes as they relate to environmental emergencies.

● Describe possible educational efforts that could be used to decrease the incidence of injury due to environmental factors.

● List resources that can be accessed to support field treatment of diving emergencies, poisonings, or marine envenomations.

● Compare and contrast the treatment for ingestion of a caustic versus noncaustic toxic substance.

● Describe how carbon monoxide acts to interfere with the oxygen transportation system and list the interventions commonly used to treat a suspected victim.

● Discuss the pathophysiology, assessment findings, and management of insect bites and stings, animal bites, and snakebites.

● Describe the complications of animal bites, including rabies and tetanus.

● Discuss the pathophysiology, assessment findings, and management of ingestions and exposures to poisonous plants.

● Discuss the pathophysiology, assessment findings, and management of altitude illnesses including AMS, HAPE, and HACE.

● Discuss the pathophysiology, assessment findings, and management of heat-related illnesses including heat edema, cramps, tetany, exhaustion, and heatstroke.

● Discuss the pathophysiology, assessment findings, and management of cold-related illnesses including frostbite and hypothermia.

● Discuss the pathophysiology, assessment findings, and management of diving emergencies including decompression illness, air embolism, POPS, barotrauma, and nitrogen narcosis.

● Discuss the pathophysiology, assessment findings, and management of near drowning.

(continues)

(continued)

- Discuss the pathophysiology, assessment findings, and management of marine envenomations.
- Discuss the pathophysiology, assessment findings, and management of toxic marine ingestions.

KEY TERMS

Boyle's law	Gamow bag
Conduction	Heat tetany
Convection	Henry's law
Evaporation	Radiation

This chapter is designed to present an overview of selected environmental emergencies encountered across the varied practice venues of emergency services personnel. Environmental emergencies occur in a myriad of settings, under such a variety of climatic and topographical milieus, that covering each nuance is impossible within the parameters of this text. It is, therefore, the focus of this chapter to provide the individual with a solid basis for practice that is scientifically sound but allows for regional practice variations to accommodate those unique instances each practitioner will undoubtedly experience. To highlight the environmental backdrop that plays host to the specified emergency, this chapter has been divided into three sections: land, air, and sea. It is recommended that additional reading in current professional journals and research of local and regional standards be employed to maintain a current knowledge base.

LAND

HUMAN BITES

Human bites represent a challenge for emergency personnel. The human bite is often a complex pathophysiological occurrence involving laceration, avulsion, tear, puncture, or crush injury frequently made more complicated due to delay in reporting for treatment. Commonly, there is associated hematoma, ischemia, and microbial contamination from the oral cavity that can be linked with disease transmission, including such pathogens as hemolytic streptococcus, *Neisseria*, *Proteus*, actinomycosis, hepatitis B, *Clostridium tetani*, syphilis, tuberculosis, and human immunodeficiency virus (HIV). Theoretically, human-to-human rabies transmission via contact with infected saliva is also possible, although this has never been documented.

Statistics demonstrate that a human bite is most likely to involve a male between the ages of 15 and 30, peaking in incidence around age 25. Bites are more likely to occur on Saturdays and, not surprisingly, over 40% are associated with the use of alcohol.[1] Human bites are often the result of fights, sexual encounters, or contact sports. Bites may also be self-inflicted by individuals with psychiatric or behavioral disorders. Unintentional injury has been demonstrated to account for up to one-quarter of reported human bites.[1] Victims of human bites include health care workers who are bitten while restraining combative, mentally ill, confused, or frightened patients. Athletic competitions are another venue in which bites occur.[2] The most common site of a bite is the hand, specifically the third and fourth digits at the metacarpophalangeal joint following a closed fist punch.[1,2] The face, including the ears, nose, lips, and cheeks, is also a frequent site, although any part of the body may be involved. Not surprisingly, sexual assaults often involve bites to the breasts and genitalia, and frequently the victims are female.[1]

Treatment of human bites is often delayed because embarrassment or fear of legal consequences prevents the wounded individual from seeking care. For this reason, secondary infection is often a significant complication. When the bite involves a joint space, bone, or tendon, the resulting inoculation of oral flora, which can include up to 42 varieties of bacteria, often produces a soft tissue infection with significant potential for disability. The hand, inherently contaminated with a plethora of microbes and containing a plentiful blood supply, is significantly more prone to infection than the head or face. A facial scar may be somewhat disfiguring while a hand that has been infected can become contracted, limiting both motion and dexterity. While the most frequently seen complications are cellulitis, lymphangitis, and abscess formation, more severe infections may lead to tenosynovitis, osteomyelitis, septicemia, and amputation.

Initial assessment should include the 5 P's: pain, pallor, pulse, paralysis, and paresthesia.[3] Inspection of the wound should include scrutiny for foreign bodies, especially tooth fragments, which should be brought to the attention of both the emergency department (ED) physician and law enforcement officials. Retrieval of such fragments is best left to the physician, recalling that evidence (e.g., tooth fragments) must be handled using rigid chain-of-custody methods to preserve its validity in criminal proceedings. Bites involving the face may compromise or obstruct the airway and should be observed closely for signs of edema. Wound treatment on the scene should include flushing the involved area with sterile water, control of bleeding, retrieval and appropriate preservation of any amputated parts, application of a sterile dressing, splinting if appropriate, intravenous access, oxygen administration, maintenance of body heat, and emotional support.

Treatment for psychogenic and hypovolemic shock should be initiated per protocol for all trauma patients. Consideration must be given to emotional support of the victim, maintaining confidentiality, cooperation with law enforcement officials, and preservation of the crime scene. A health history includes tetanus immunization status, current medications, allergies, drug use, and underlying medical conditions. Any information available on the perpetrator, specifically health status, including current medical condition or illnesses and drug use, should be gathered if it does not compromise the care of the patient or delay transport. Lastly, objective, unbiased, and complete documentation by the paramedic is vital.

Rehabilitation specialist consultation may be required for bite victims. Contractures and scarring of hands and extremities must be minimized through rapid and aggressive surgical debridement, antibiotic use, and early physical and occupational therapy. Consultation and arrangement for cosmetic repair or plastic reconstruction should be an early consideration by the ED physician. Treatment and follow-up of emotional and psychological side effects are often shuffled aside or overlooked in the initial urgency to repair the physical damage caused by the bite. Mental health professionals, family violence and rape crisis centers, and other appropriate agencies should be involved early in the patient's treatment plan to enhance optimal recovery.

INTERNET ACTIVITIES

Visit the e-medicine Web site at http://www.emedicine.com. Click on the Emergency Medicine on-line book and select Environmental. Then click on Bites, Human. Review the chapter on the management of human bites.

ANIMAL BITES

The most prevalent animal bite is a dog bite. Dogs account for 90% of the bites seen in the ED.[2,3] The most frequent victim is a young child, often bitten on the face or hand due to the close physical proximity of that body part to the animal. Cats, gerbils, rabbits, ferrets, and other small animals kept as pets can generate

damaging bites that have significant potential for infection. Although the animal's bite may be smaller, it can present a very challenging scenario for emergency medical services (EMS) personnel who must treat both the hysterical child and frantic parents simultaneously.

Similar to human bites, the animal bite wound may be a puncture, jagged laceration, tear, crush, or avulsion and may be associated with scratches and abrasions as well as heavy contamination by dirt and oral flora. The likelihood of infection increases with extremes in the patient's age, often developing rapidly in those less than 4 years of age or over 50. Cat bites are especially prone to infection, signs of which can begin within a few hours of sustaining a bite. The isolation of *Pasteurella multocida* from an infected wound strongly suggests a cat bite and can be used to differentiate between the bite of a cat and a human if a question of child abuse is raised. An additional concern with animal bites is the possibility of rabies.

Clinical judgment and common sense are required when intervening in the treatment of a victim of an animal bite or attack. A patient mauled by a bear, mountain lion, bull, or large dog should be treated aggressively as a major trauma, with the possibility of blunt, internal trauma in addition to visible lacerations remaining an important consideration.

The initial treatment for animal bites is similar to that for a human bite. Observation and assessment of the airway, the 5P's, and control of bleeding take precedence. Wound inspection for bone and teeth fragments, irrigation, sterile dressings, and splinting should be accomplished rapidly. Oxygen administration, IV access, maintenance of body temperature, emotional support, and rapid transport should be performed in an orderly fashion. Proper preservation and transportation of any amputated or avulsed body part are critical and may mean the difference between a life of disfigurement or disability and the eventual return of unimpeded function. Complications involving tissue necrosis, nerve damage, and amputation must be considered a possibility in all animal bites.

Possible sequelae following animal bites include cellulitis, tenosynovitis, septicemia, osteomyelitis, rabies, and rarely, bubonic plague. Expected intervention by the ED physician includes copious irrigation, tetanus toxoid, repair of the laceration, wound culture, possible surgical debridement, antibiotic therapy, and rabies prophylaxis. The decision to close the wound is a clinical judgment best left to the ED physician. Small wounds are likely to be left open and allowed to heal by secondary intention. Larger wounds may be loosely sutured, dressed, elevated, and closely followed for signs of infection. Referral for evaluation of plastic or cosmetic surgical repair should be strongly considered for facial wounds or very large wounds.

Most states require the reporting of all animal bites and, while this is not the immediate concern of EMS personnel, the identification of the animal and its owner is important to both the receiving facility and law enforcement officials, often saving the patient anxiety and unnecessary administration of rabies vaccine. Without compromising patient care, gather what data are available at the scene, including a physical description of the animal, rabies vaccine status, the owner's name and address, and general health of the animal, if known. Try to obtain an idea of the animal's behavior immediately prior to the attack. It is important to know if the bite was provoked (e.g., stepped on the animal or hit it) or unprovoked. If it is a domestic animal, ask the owner to pen or tie up the animal and await instructions from the animal control officer. Strongly discourage killing the animal or disposing of it prior to the animal control officer's assessment. The animal may need to be transported to a facility for testing and observation.

INTERNET ACTIVITIES

Visit the e-medicine Web site at http://www.emedicine.com. Click on the Emergency Medicine on-line book and select Environmental. Then click on bites, animal. Review the chapter on the management of animal bites.

Snakebites

There are 120 species of snakes found in the United States, of which only 20 are poisonous.[4-6] The incidence of bites is highest in the southwestern and southeastern portions of the country. Pit vipers (family Crotalidae) account for 95% of bites while the coral snake (family Elapidae) account for 5%.[4,6,7] Statistical analysis demonstrates that two-thirds of all bites occur on the upper extremities, supporting the assertion that 57% of bites are due to handling of the snake.[6] An amazing 28% of cases involve a patient who is intoxicated.[6] This statistic is valuable due to the increased likelihood of complications found to occur in snakebite victims who are also intoxicated or given alcohol after the bite in a mistaken attempt to calm the patient. Alcohol causes vasodilation, which increases the circulation of venom and may contribute to hypotension. Alcohol also impedes the liver's effort at venom detoxification.

Physiological reaction to snakebite is variable, depending on factors such as age, weight, general physical health, location of bite, physical activity after being bitten, size of the snake, and the level of agitation of the snake. A provoked, angry reptile is more likely to inject venom. In general, bites to the hands and face are more

severe due to local tissue edema and necrosis accompanying the injection of venom into the patient.[6] It has been estimated that 25%–30% of bites are "dry bites," in which no venom is injected. Figure 23-1 shows the results of a dry bite: The fangs clearly penetrated the skin; however, no reaction ensued. This is true of both poisonous and nonpoisonous varieties. The greatest danger from snake venom is tissue damage caused by local necrosis, erythema, and edema. Figure 23-2 displays hemorrhagic blebs that formed 24 hours after envenomation occurred. Bites involving fingers and hands have the potential for extensive disability if untreated. Airway compromise secondary to systemic neurotoxin is the other major concern to EMS personnel. It is crucial to remember that psychological fright plays a significant role in the survival of the patient. It has been demonstrated that the fear of snakes is culturally almost universal among humans and that psychologically the potential to be "scared to death" exists subsequent to this premise.[4] Consequently, while initial airway, breathing, and circulation (ABCs) are of paramount importance, equally important is the need to provide as much emotional support and reassurance as possible.

Physical activity should be minimized, as should the manipulation of the bite site. If possible, the body area involved in the bite should be kept below the level of the heart. Cleansing with sterile water, light, loose sterile dressings, oxygen administration, IV access with infusion of isotonic crystalloid, cardiac monitoring, and rapid transport should not be delayed to retrieve the snake. A bite associated with a fracture should be splinted to prevent further muscle, nerve, and vessel damage. However, circulatory checks must be

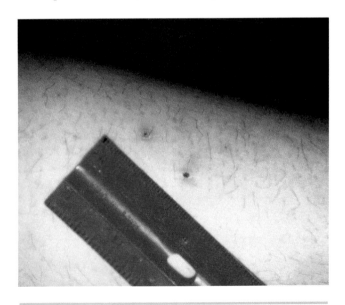

FIGURE 23-1 Fang marks on lower leg 3 days after a dry bite. Note lack of erythema or edema. (Courtesy of Mark Zeringue)

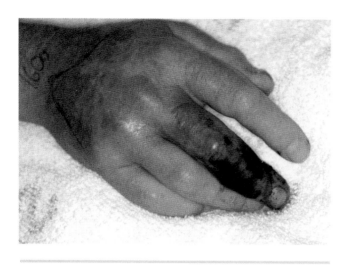

FIGURE 23-2 Hemorrhagic blebs 24 hours after envenomation by a rattlesnake. (Courtesy of Sean Bush, Loma Linda University Medical Center, Loma Linda, CA. Used with permission.)

performed every 5 minutes en route to ensure circulatory compromise secondary to edema does not ensue. Do not allow the patient to consume caffeine or alcohol; caffeine is a cardiac stimulant likely to increase the heart rate and circulation of venom within the body. Likewise, smoking should be avoided due to its vasoconstrictive effect, which decreases oxygen flow to body tissue already compromised by toxins producing necrosis. Removal of constrictive clothing and jewelry such as rings, bracelets, and necklaces should be carried out with a minimum of agitation to the affected site, but these must be removed as soon as possible to decrease the likelihood of circulatory compromise in the event of significant edema. The area of the bite demarcated by erythema should be marked with a felt tip pen and the circumference of the involved extremity measured for later comparison. The time of these measurements should be noted on the record.

A somewhat controversial intervention that is gaining popularity and acceptance is the application of a constricting band used to impede lymphatic flow but not compromise venous or arterial circulation.[2,4,6] The affected body part is wrapped with crepe or elastic bandage material at the same level of constriction used for sprains. Additionally, it must be stated that a tourniquet, popular in Western movies, is *never* to be used on the victim of snakebite for it only serves to increase the circulatory compromise already being experienced by the patient.

Commercial suction devices when used within the first 30 minutes of a bite may remove a small percentage of venom from the site. The systems consist of a syringe and suction cups of various sizes that are attached and positioned over the fang marks. An example of one such

device is shown in Figure 23-3. The plunger is drawn out, creating negative pressure that "pulls" the venom out of the punctures. Because no incision is made in the skin, this method does not increase the risk of infection or cause additional tissue trauma. The device must be left on for 20–30 minutes. While this method is not terribly effective, it is proven to do no harm.

Incision and suction are a rarely used interventions; their effectiveness is limited to use within the first 30 minutes or less of a bite. If used improperly, incision and suction can increase the spread of venom through the patient's system, cause increased edema and vascular compromise, and contaminate the wound. If the decision is made to use incision and suction, they should be performed by someone familiar with the technique to avoid excessive tissue damage. The following steps illustrate the order in which the procedure should be performed:

1. Wipe off any venom from the skin surface.

2. Make a small 0.25-inch linear incision across the fang bite, taking care not to penetrate too deeply into the dermis.

3. Apply a commercially prepared suction device and perform the suctioning per area protocol.

4. Consider using a light, constricting band to impede lymphatic flow (this should alternate on and off).

Under no circumstances are excision and suction, cryotherapy, or fasciotomy to be used in the field.[2,4–6] These methods are outdated and have been demonstrated to cause more tissue necrosis and damage by causing vasoconstriction and may decrease the flow of antivenin when administered. Additionally, never apply ice, which may cause frostbite injury and may result in a phenomenon known as rebound envenomation. This

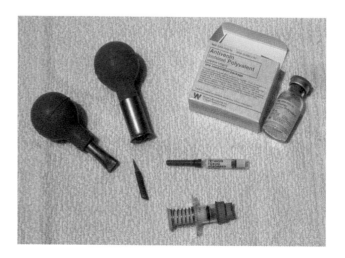

FIGURE 23-3 Suction device used following envenomation. (Courtesy of Johnsie Hubble)

condition occurs when the venom, restricted by vaso-constriction secondary to topical ice, is released into the vascular system as it opens back up during tissue rewarming, literally flooding the patient with venom and triggering shock.

Antibiotics designed to provide broad-spectrum gram-negative rod coverage are the most useful for moderate to severe envenomations. Cultures of snakebites have revealed that the most common organisms are *Proteus vulgaris* and *Escherichia coli.*

Systemic effects from venomous snakebite include diarrhea, vomiting, muscle cramps, fever, restlessness, coagulopathies, and circulatory collapse. Again, monitoring for the 5 P's is an important part of the assessment. Most venomous bites are very painful, with paresthesia and fasciculation common. Monitor the patient for disseminated intravascular coagulation (DIC), compartment syndrome, cardiac dysrhythmia, and cardiorespiratory compromise.

At the ED expect to be questioned about the snake. Identification of the species involved can prove very helpful to the medical team, but under no circumstances should you attempt to capture the snake. Even a recently decapitated snake is capable of injecting venom if the head is handled while muscular spasms are still occurring (up to 30 minutes after death). If the snake is still present in the immediate area, observe it from a safe distance, noting size, color, head shape, and scale patterns for later identification. Figure 23-4 compares venomous and nonvenomous snakes. Never delay transport of the patient to search for the reptile. If the patient is conscious, ask for a detailed description of the snake, eliciting as much detail as can be remembered. The copperhead, cottonmouth, rattlesnake, and coral snake each have a wide range throughout the United States and are the most likely snakes to be involved in a venomous bite (Figure 23-5). Regional variations in snake coloration are common. An excellent reference is the brochure published by the Department of Agriculture on the most common snakes found in each state, including habitat, range, pattern, and coloration.

Antivenin remains the mainstay of treatment for moderate to severe envenomations. Skin testing is always recommended prior to use, although it does not guarantee against anaphylaxis. The physician making the decision to administer antivenin should, therefore, be prepared for and skilled at treating anaphylaxis. While it is considered a rare complication, anaphylaxis is life threatening and requires immediate treatment with epinephrine, diphenhydramine, and hydrocortisone, as well as airway adjuncts and advanced cardiac life support (ACLS) measures.

Antivenin in the United States is polyvalent and made from horse serum. Best results from antivenin

Venomous snake

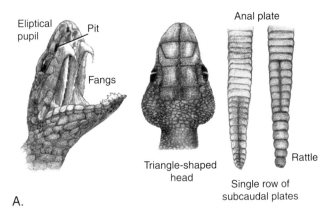

A.

Nonvenomous snake

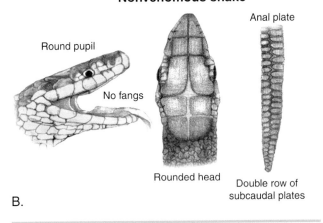

B.

FIGURE 23-4 Comparison of (A) venomous and (B) nonvenomous snakes.

are obtained if administered within 4 hours of the initial bite. After the skin test, 0.2 mL–0.5 mL of antivenin is injected intravenously over 5 minutes. The patient is observed closely, and if no reaction occurs, the remainder of the dose is given over a period of 30 minutes to 2 hours diluted in dextrose 5% and water (D_5W) or lactated Ringer's (LR).

Faced with a snakebite the ED physician will make the decision to treat with antivenin based on all the factors provided about the snake, the patient, and the circumstances surrounding the incident as well as the clinical progression of the patient. The amount of antivenin is based on the amount of venom injected and the potency of the snake. Pregnancy is not a contraindication for receiving antivenin; however, obtain expert obstetrical consultation early in the decision-making process. Snake venom can trigger uterine contractions resulting in spontaneous abortion. Table 23-1 provides guidelines to assist EMS personnel in determining levels of envenomation.

Determination of the severity of the bite is accomplished by observing the amount and progression of

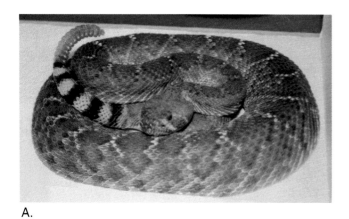

A.

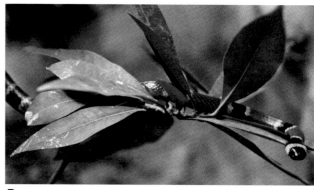

B.

FIGURE 23-5 (A) Western diamondback rattlesnake. (Courtesy of Sean Bush, Loma Linda University Medical Center, Loma Linda, CA.) (B) Coral snake. (Courtesy of PhotoDisc.)

Table 23-1
Grades of Envenomation

Grade I (mild)

Edema and erythema limited to immediate site

No systemic symptoms

No apparent spread of erythema or edema

Grade II (moderate)

Edema and erythema involving a portion of the extremity

Nausea, vomiting, oral paresthesia, tachypnea, tachycardia, blood pressure greater than 80 mm Hg

Slow spread of erythema and edema

Grade III (severe)

Edema and erythema involving the entire extremity

Rapid spread of the erythema and edema

Mental status changes, blood pressure less than 80 mm Hg, respiratory distress, coagulation abnormalities

edema and erythema. Physicians treating a snakebite should always consult with a specialist for the latest dosing and treatment regime. Exotic snakes, found in homes as pets and in zoos, have unique antivenin requirements. The Tucson, Arizona, Antivenin Index at (602) 626-6016 and the Boulder, Colorado, POISINDEX Central Office at (800) 332-3037 offer guidance on where to obtain a supply of local antivenin for common and exotic snake varieties. Regional zoos are another source of species-specific antivenin information.

Most antivenin is of equine origin and is highly immunogenic in nature. Recent research has been focused on deriving antivenin from sheep sources that demonstrate less reactivity in humans than the equine-based formulas currently in use. Another source of antivenin still unapproved by the Food and Drug Administration is a goat-derived serum being studied at Arizona State University. This is not for general use.

Few people die instantaneously as a result of a snakebite. Those who die usually do so 6–24 hours after the envenomation. For this reason, never delay transport of a snakebite victim for definitive care. ED treatment of snakebite, depending on the clinical severity, can range from observation and cardiac monitoring for several hours to transfusion with packed red blood cells (PRBCs), administration of fresh frozen plasma (FFP) or platelets, antivenin infusion, or surgical debridement requiring a hospital stay of several days.

Serum sickness generally occurs from 7 to 14 days after administration of antivenin and is dependent on the amount of antivenin given. It has been found that those receiving greater than 5 to 7 vials of antivenin have up to an 83% chance of experiencing serum sickness.[4,6,7] Symptoms include fever, rash, arthralgias, lymphadenopathy, cardiac arrhythmia, and coagulopathies. Rare complications are peripheral neuritis, pericarditis, and encephalitis. Treatment of serum sickness includes intervention for cardiac dysrhythmia, antihistamines, corticosteroids (such as a prednisone taper), and prophylactic antacids.

INTERNET ACTIVITIES

Visit the e-medicine Web site at http://www.emedicine.com. Click on the Emergency Medicine on-line book and select Environmental. Then click on various snake envenomations for snakes that are indigenous to your response area. Review the chapter on the management of these envenomations.

Spider Bites

Venomous spider bites are often painless and may go unrecognized for up to 12 hours. They are rarely fatal but can cause significant disability if not recognized and treated aggressively. Envenomations of the brown recluse and black widow spider are identified by characteristic lesions. Numerous spider species inhabit different geographic regions, and the recognition of the venomous species is particularly important for the EMS provider. Widow spiders often have the unique "hourglass" pattern on the body, as shown in Figure 23-6, but are not always black. The most poisonous of the "widow type" is the brown widow found in Florida. The brown recluse ranges from light tan to brown in color and has been described as having a "violin" shaped marking on its back.

Black Widow   The bite of the widow is felt as a pinprick or can be painless for up to 30 minutes, after which pain, localized redness, edema, piloerection, adenopathy, and urticaria alert the victim to the presence of a bite. The site has a surrounding border that is a red/blue color with a white center. Following the onset of pain at the site, abdominal cramping and pain in the chest and thighs develop. The abdomen may appear rigid but will be nontender and without rebound. Another finding is restlessness, a further clue that the abdomen is not a surgical one. The patient may demonstrate tremors and tonic muscle contractures, flushed, sweaty face, hypertension, and blepharoconjunctivitis, an inflammation of the eyelid and conjunctiva. It has been reported that the victim may experience significant feelings of fear and death. In the later stages of envenomation, bronchorrhea, vomiting, priapism, urinary retention, salivation, and diaphoresis occur. These symptoms may be quite pronounced for hours after envenomation.

Clinically, a thorough history is essential for correct diagnosis and appropriate treatment. Ask the patient and family about onset, observe the bite site, and determine what the patient was doing 30 minutes prior to the start of symptoms. Look for evidence of the spider, and if you can safely do so, bring the spider in for positive identification. Black widows inhabit dark, cluttered areas like garages, outhouses, barns, and other outbuildings.

Laboratory studies are generally not helpful in determining what type of bite is present. Chest radiographs should be obtained in moderate to severe envenomations to rule out pulmonary edema. A baseline electrocardiogram (ECG) is often helpful, particularly in the elderly, because myotonic contractions elevate creatinine phosphokinase (CPK) levels. Stimulation of the sympathetic nervous system frequently results in increased catecholamine circulation creating hypertension and dumping of glucose stores producing hyperglycemia. Administration of 10% calcium gluconate IV gives transient relief to the symptoms in a dramatic manner, although it only lasts for about 30 minutes. It can, however, support the definitive diagnosis. Field treatment consists of basic ABCs, oxygen administration, IV, cardiac monitoring, tetanus prophylaxis, immobilization of the affected area, emotional support, and rapid transport.

Antivenin is of equine origin, so skin testing prior to use is essential. One or two vials of antivenin is usually all that is required, with symptom resolution within 1 hour. Observe closely for anaphylaxis and use continuous cardiac monitoring. For severe reactions to venom, hospitalization is prudent. The following are suggested parameters for hospital observation: respiratory distress, cardiovascular signs and symptoms, hypertension, pregnancy, symptomatic individuals under 16 and over 65, preexisting hypertension or cardiovascular disease that is unstable, or prolonged distress after administration of muscle relaxants and calcium.[5,8]

Brown Recluse   The brown recluse, found in the southern United States, is nocturnal, nonaggressive, and smaller than the widows (Figure 23-7). The bite is rarely painful; however, it becomes severely necrosed and ulcerative over a period of hours to weeks. The venom is a phospholipid enzyme that works on cell membranes, the lipase triggering a cascade effect on the body systems. It begins as a red, edematous, or blanched lesion and progresses to a macular blue/gray halo encompassing the central puncture (Figure 23-8). This stage is followed by cyanotic-appearing pustules or vesicular bullous lesions with irregular surrounding purpuric discoloration. The formation of blebs and purpura herald the onset of necrosis. Eschar forms days later and it may be months before the wound is healed. Due to the poor blood flow in fatty body areas such as the thighs and abdomen, bites here often

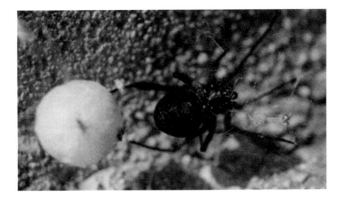

FIGURE 23-6 Black widow spider. (Courtesy of Sean Bush, Loma Linda University Medical Center, Loma Linda, CA.)

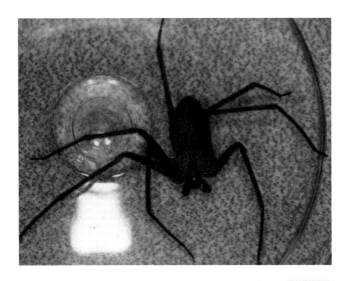

FIGURE 23-7 Brown recluse spider. (Courtesy of Sean Bush, Loma Linda University Medical Center, Loma Linda, CA.)

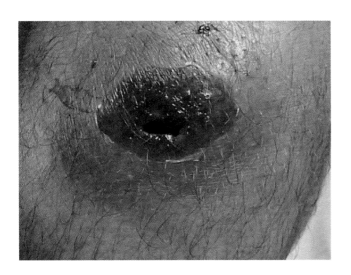

FIGURE 23-8 Typical cutaneous lesion following the bite of a brown recluse spider. (Courtesy of Deborah Funk, Albany Medical Center, Albany, NY.)

display extensive necrotic damage and require prolonged treatment and follow-up.

The brown recluse bite causes fever, malaise, nausea, vomiting, diarrhea, arthralgias, scarlatiniform rash, leukocytosis, hemoglobinuria, hypotension, DIC, and shock. There is no antivenin for the brown recluse bite; death, however, is rarely a result of this spider's bite. An important complication, however, is renal failure secondary to hemoglobinuria, which can contribute to secondary end-organ damage as the by-products of hemoglobin destruction crowd the small vessels. Prevention of acute renal failure is accomplished by fluid replacement and alkalization of the urine.

Initial scene treatment consists of basic ABCs, immobilization of the affected site, emotional support, IV crystalloid administration, nasal oxygen at 2–4 L/min, and cardiac monitoring. Cool compresses may be applied for comfort, but avoid ice, which can further compromise blood flow. Monitor blood pressure closely. An extraction tool may be used if the bite was witnessed and treatment begins within 3 minutes of the bite.[9] Beyond that time the venom is in the system and further manipulation will only spread the venom and damage surrounding tissues. Tetanus prophylaxis is recommended; however, antibiotics are not warranted unless there is evidence of skin infection. It is best to avoid injections around the site. Steroids have not been found to be helpful. Judicious surgical debridement is necessary after demarcation of necrosis is complete (which may take several weeks). Topical medications have little effect toward halting the extent of tissue damage. If available, hyperbaric oxygen, which forces oxygen into the body tissue under high pressure, may decrease tissue necrosis by alleviating ischemia.

INTERNET ACTIVITIES

Visit the e-medicine Web site at http://www.emedicine.com. Click on the Emergency Medicine on-line book and select Environmental. Then click on various spider envenomations for spiders that are indigenous to your response area. Review the chapter on the management of these envenomations.

Fire Ants, Wasps, and Bees

This section would not be complete without discussion of the plethora of flying and crawling insects that sting and bite, particularly in the spring and summer months. Wasps, hornets, yellow jackets, and other bees are familiar outdoor hazards that have been around for thousands of years. Those who are allergic to them are becoming better educated about avoidance and better equipped with medications to treat the all too frequent encounters. The use of commercial anaphylaxis kits (Anakits, Epipen) by both individuals and paramedics is a quick, efficient treatment for the anaphylactoid reactions that occur after a sting (Figure 23-9).

Within minutes of a sting bronchoconstriction and hypotension occur, placing the individual in a shock state. Frequently there is urticaria (hives), nausea, and chills. Emergency treatment is aimed at restoring airway patency and circulatory status. Establish an airway and provide high-flow oxygen, crystalloid IV fluids, subcutaneous epinephrine, and rapid transport to the nearest ED.

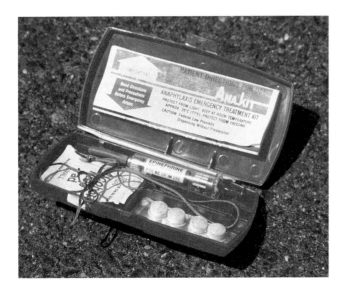

FIGURE 23-9 One type of commercially prepackaged anaphylaxis kit. (Courtesy of Johnsie Hubble)

Fire ants are a relatively new threat found in a large portion of the southern United States, having migrated from South America and entrenched themselves firmly in our warm soil. In 1994, 85,000 people were stung by fire ants, highlighting the potential for a significant number of injuries due to these aggressive and potentially fatal insects.[10] Fire ants are small, 2–5 mm in size, with a red-brown body (Figure 23-10). Their venom is an alkaloid-based protein injected into the victim through the mandibular teeth, which are used to grasp the body, allowing the fire ant to sting multiple times until it is physically dislodged. There is an immediate wheal, often 10 mm in size with pain, pruritus, fever, nausea, and malaise followed closely by the formation of vesicles that become pustules often

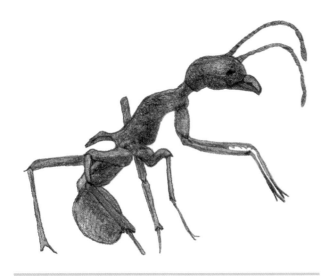

FIGURE 23-10 Fire ant.

lasting up to 10 days. An eschar forms over these eruptions with tissue damage and necrosis at the cellular level occurring within 30 minutes secondary to the alkaloid compounds and piperidines instilled by the ant. Underlying connective tissue may become necrosed within 72 hours if untreated. Anaphylaxis and life-threatening systemic symptoms usually begin within 30–45 minutes. There is flushing, hypotension, urticaria, angioedema, wheezing, dysphagia, chest tightness, abdominal cramps, nausea, vomiting, diarrhea, pruritus, and syncope. Sequelae include secondary skin infection, focal motor seizures, and, rarely, death secondary to anaphylaxis.

Interestingly, fatalities have been almost exclusively in adults and are twice as common in males. Five stings or less have been implicated in 32 deaths, suggesting that it is not the number of stings, but the individual's susceptibility and physiological response to the alkaloid compound introduced by the fire ant.[10] The paramedic's first action is to remove both the victim and himself from close proximity with the mounds. Fire ants have hives as large as 50 cm across. Clearly there should be no trouble seeing the mounds and thus avoiding the insects entirely. On-site treatment includes physical removal of the ants by brushing with a gloved hand or washing off, topical application of isopropyl alcohol, which may provide temporary pain relief, elevation of the affected part, and pain control. Daily wound care is necessary to prevent infection. While the use of topical or parenteral steroids, antibiotics, meat tenderizer, or antihistamines have met with only limited success, field treatment hinges on the use of these adjuncts. Airway maintenance, oxygen administration, subcutaneous epinephrine, IV crystalloid infusion, Benadryl, and dexamethasone are first-line interventions. The use of anaphylaxis kits may be helpful for those individuals with identified cross-sensitivity or anaphylaxis to yellow jackets and honey bees. Avoidance is the best protection against attack.

Tick Bites

The bite of the tick itself is often painless, becoming pruritic after removal. Benign as the site may appear, the tick as a vector is an efficient transmitter of disease-carrying organisms. Table 23-2 lists some of the more common tick illnesses and their reservoirs. Ticks are also responsible for transmission of relapsing fever and tularemia, both bacterial spirochetes; Colorado tick fever, a viral agent; Babesiosis, a protozoan; and tick paralysis, a neurotoxin. Various organisms are carried in different species of tick, and eliciting a complete history of tick exposure is often key to pinpointing a diagnosis. Each disease state manifests itself with a plethora of symptoms and diagnosis requires a

Table 23-2
Tick Illnesses and Reservoirs

Disease	Agent	Genus/Species	Reservoir
Rocky Mountain spotted fever	Rickettsia	*Rickettsia rickettsii*	Deer, dogs, rodents
Human ehrlichiosis	Rickettsia	*Ehrlichia chaffeensis*	Unknown
Lyme disease	Spirochete	*Borrelia burgdorferi*	Deer, mice

physician well schooled in the clinical presentations of the disease. EMS personnel need to be aware of likely settings in which ticks are endemic (wooded areas, recreational areas, and parks); be familiar with what a tick looks like and how to remove one; and know how to provide supportive care to the victim of advanced tickborne illness.

Suspect tickborne disease in anyone with a history of tick exposure. Most of the illnesses have 7–21 days incubation period. Ask about camping trips, hiking, or travel to other states where ticks are endemic. Inquire about the estimated time the tick was attached prior to removal. The likelihood of disease increases if it is attached and feeding for over 24 hours. Prime tick season is late spring, summer, and early fall. Ticks are generally dormant in the cold winter months and come in different sizes and patterns. Figure 23-11 shows a deer tick. A febrile illness in the summertime should always be suspect for tick illness. Removal of the tick is carried out by use of a tweezer to gently pull the tick straight out of the attachment site. Be cautious not to squeeze or crush the tick as this can cause regurgitation of the tick's stomach contents into the wound, increasing the likelihood of disease transmission.

Certain diseases do have characteristic signs, such as the erythema chronicum migrans, or "Bull's eye" rash seen around the wound of a tick carrying Lyme disease. Patients displaying this type of rash should be encouraged to seek treatment immediately. Ehrlichiosis may present with symptoms similar to those of toxic shock syndrome.[11] The most significant dangers with many of the more common tickborne diseases are the cardiac and neurological sequelae of unrecognized and untreated disease. Cases of Ehrlichiosis, Rocky Mountain spotted fever (RMSF), and Lyme disease can be fatal; death from hypotension, multisystem organ failure, respiratory failure, carditis, and encephalitis is not uncommon. In tick paralysis, a rare form of paralysis resulting from a tick bite, the simple removal of the tick will bring complete resolution of symptoms, including paralysis, within 48 hours. However, failure to discover the attached tick responsible for the paralysis can lead to death from res-

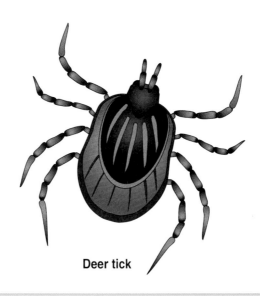

Deer tick

FIGURE 23-11 Deer tick.

piratory arrest. Rapidly intervene with basic and ACLS measures in the event of such a presentation. Rare will be the need for emergency tick removal. It is more likely EMS personnel will respond to a call involving a high fever, rash, altered mental status, or decreased level of consciousness in a person with advanced, hitherto unrecognized tick illness. Respiratory support, fluid resuscitation, and management of shock are the primary goals during transport. Once at the hospital, antibiotic therapy will be based on which tickborne illness is suspect. Fortunately, these illnesses generally respond well to aggressive antibiotic therapy if caught in time.

Public education for prevention and early detection of ticks is as follows: (1) frequent inspections for the purpose of discovering ticks on the clothing and body; (2) use of insect repellent if prolonged time out of doors is anticipated; (3) the wearing of light-colored, long-sleeved shirts and pants to discourage ticks and prevent attachment; (4) avoidance of tick habitats; (5) treatment of household pets known to harbor ticks (dogs, cats); and (6) showering or bathing immediately after prolonged exposure to likely tick habitats.

Scorpion Stings

Of the estimated 650 species of scorpions inhabiting temperate climates, only about 50 are harmful to humans. Envenomation, while painful and frightening, is rarely fatal. In the United States scorpions are found in Texas, Arizona, New Mexico, and the lower third of California. Scorpions are nocturnal, hanging upside down in lairs under rocky out croppings to rest during the day and becoming active at night in temperatures around 25°C (77°F). Scorpions vary greatly in size. *Centruroides sculpturatus*, the bark scorpion, named for its habitat, ranges from 13 to 75 mm in size and has a life span of about 5 years. This is the only scorpion in the United States known to be dangerous to humans.[2,5,8] For all its small size, *C. sculpturatus* can be deadly to humans. This species has a characteristically long, subtriangular sternum, slender pinchers, and a tubercle at the base of the stinger, as seen in Figure 23-12.

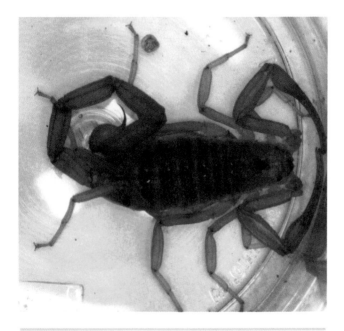

FIGURE 23-12 Bark scorpion. (Courtesy of Sean Bush, Loma Linda University Medical Center, Loma Linda, CA.)

Scorpion venom is a neurotoxin made of potent proteins and polypeptides. These compounds affect the sodium channels, prolonging action potential and triggering spontaneous nerve depolarization. Following the sting a localized area of erythema, or "flare," appears along with a wheal. There is generalized muscle pain, nausea, and vomiting. Both the sympathetic and parasympathetic systems are affected by proteins and polypeptides found in scorpion venom. Sympathetic nervous system stimulation may trigger hypertension, tachycardia, pulmonary edema, seizures, perspiration, hyperglycemia, and piloerection. Stimulation of the parasympathetic system can produce salivation, lacrimation, sphincter's relaxation, bradycardia, hypotension, and gastric distention. Symptoms result from releasing massive catecholamines into the bloodstream.

Treatment of a scorpion bite depends on determination of the species, if possible, and the amount of venom injected into the victim. A grading system, similar to that used for snakebite, aids in determining the need for antivenin (Table 23-3). The antivenin is derived from goats, is not approved for human use by the Federal Drug Administration (FDA), and is only available from Arizona State University.

Treatment of Grade I or II envenomations is local, cool compresses, analgesics, airway support, and IV fluids. Grade III or IV envenomations require antivenin although use is controversial (and *not* FDA approved).[8] Other drugs (antihistamines, corticosteroids, sympathomimetics) have been tried with little success. An extraction device can be utilized if applied within the first few minutes of a sting. As with snakebites, the lymphatic restricting band or wrap may be useful. No tourniquets are used. Intermittent ice

Table 23-3
Grading Scorpion Envenomations
Grade I: Local pain/paresthesia, a positive "tap" test (increased pain when you tap along the wound)
Grade II: All symptoms in Grade I, plus paresthesia expanding from around the site
Grade III: All symptoms found in Grades I and II, plus *either* (a) involuntary extremity jerking or skeletal muscle spasms (often mistaken for a seizure, but not seizure activity) *or* (b) cranial nerve dysfunction (blurred vision, hypersalivation, wandering-eye movements, dysphagia, tongue fasciculation, slurred speech, upper airway problems)
Grade IV: All symptoms in Grades I and II, plus both (a) *and* (b) symptomatology from Grade III

packs are mainly for pain control and must be monitored to prevent frostbite.

Primary prevention of scorpion stings is avoidance of their known habitats (woods, brush); wearing gloves and long-sleeved clothing when working or hiking in such areas; shaking out clothing and bedding prior to use if camping around habitats; and inspecting the area prior to sitting down. Interestingly, scorpions do fluoresce under ultraviolet light. A small Wood's light can locate them at night when they are active. Further information regarding up-to-date treatment of stings can be obtained from the Central Arizona Regional Poison Management at (602) 253-3334.

TETANUS

Clostridium tetani, the anaerobic bacillus responsible for the production of the exotoxin that causes tetanus, is ubiquitous in nature, being found in soil, manure, dust, skin surfaces, and the intestinal tract.[12–14] Although cases of tetanus in the United States have become rarer over the last decade due to aggressive immunization programs, persons from nonindustrialized, Third World countries where vaccinations are scarce remain at considerable risk. In the United States, adults over the age of 60 may lack primary tetanus prophylaxis and should be given tetanus immune globulin (TIG) followed by primary tetanus series unless contraindicated by a documented history of anaphylaxis. Any person with a contaminated wound should receive a tetanus booster unless there is proof of immunization within the last 5 years. Likewise, intravenous drug users and those who practice "skin popping," a method of administering drugs under the skin surface, are especially vulnerable to tetanus.

Administration of a tetanus toxoid booster is crucial to protecting a victim from the ravages of tetanus. Pregnancy, while not a contraindication to receiving tetanus vaccine, is a situation that should be considered on a case-by-case basis to determine if the theoretical risk, particularly in the first trimester, outweighs the expected benefit. There is no documented evidence that tetanus administration is harmful to the fetus, although studies are limited.[15] Certainly someone who has never been immunized against tetanus and presents with a high risk injury should always receive tetanus prophylaxis, for the alternative, tetanus disease, is almost always a death sentence. In general, any person age 7 years and older should receive the tetanus/diphtheria combined (Td), without the pertussis component of the vaccine, which is more likely to increase the risks of serious side effects. Soreness at the site of injection and self-limiting low-grade fever are the more common side effects and are never a reason to withhold tetanus prophylaxis. Severe reactions such as anaphylaxis or peripheral neuropathy from tetanus toxoid vaccine are rare.

The type of wounds most likely to harbor and nurture *C. tetani* are punctures with foreign bodies and contaminated lacerations that are irregular, stellate, or crushed in nature. In addition, wounds greater than 6–12 hours old and those that are ischemic or infected should be considered tetanus prone.[12–14] For this reason it is important to obtain an accurate history of tetanus prophylaxis on any patient with a wound, no matter how insignificant. Tetanus may enter the body through a break in the skin or other mucous membrane, including the eye or mouth. Other portals of entry that might be overlooked include skull fractures, otitis media, abortions, foreign bodies in the ear, nose, or eye, burns, and neonatal umbilical cord contamination.

The onset of tetanus is insidious, with gradual stiffness of the large muscles of the neck, back, abdomen, and legs. Characteristically, risus sardonicus, a bizarre, sneering grin due to facial muscle spasm, is seen in conjunction with dysphagia, trismus (lockjaw), and pain with chewing. As the disease progresses, there may be generalized malaise, headache, fever, chills, and hypertonicity of the muscles. This muscle rigidity progresses outward from the site of the wound. Opisthotonus, violent tonic contractions of the muscles causing the body to contort into a "C" shape, has been demonstrated to fracture vertebra and long bones and tear tendons from their insertion sites. Respiratory failure due to diaphragmatic spasms frequently results. Another common complication is laryngospasm that may be triggered during intubation attempts. Swelling, pain, and stiffness of the smaller joints are noticeably absent.

Once the muscle spasms become generalized, there is little that can be done other than supportive care. The disease carries an 80%–90% mortality rate.[12] Those rare survivors face a protracted rehabilitation and recovery period often lasting 4–6 weeks.

In rarer instances, tetanus may be localized to the area immediately surrounding the wound. This type of response carries a much better prognosis, although the spread of the disease is a distinct possibility and should be treated with the same attention as the generalized variety. The muscle rigidity caused by localized tetanus may last for months.

Cephalic tetanus is uncommon but may be the result of tetanus invading the body through a skull fracture or otitis media.[15] Neonatal tetanus, while rare in the United States, is still a significant factor in children born to unimmunized women delivering in poor, dirty conditions and in those living in underdeveloped countries for the reasons previously stated. For this reason, meticulous cord care and attention to hygienic practices during deliveries in the field is imperative. In 1993 estimates by the World Health Organization (WHO) gave a global mortality rate due to neonatal tetanus of 4.1 per 1,000 live births. Eighty percent of these deaths occurred in 12 countries.[16] Neonates developing signs of tetanus carry a poor prognosis for survival. The only hope for improvement in the survival rate is to aggressively immunize mother and baby while encouraging, teaching, and practicing sanitary deliveries.

Field treatment of a person suffering from suspected tetanus consists of airway maintenance, cardiac monitoring, minimal stimulation from light and noise, slow, gentle movement, and rapid transport to the nearest facility. A baseline neurological exam including the Glasgow Coma Scale (GCS) should be performed. Once the patient begins to display signs of cranial nerve involvement, prognosis is grave. Although tetanus interferes with the transmission of nerve impulses to the brain, it does not render its sufferer senseless. The patient hears, feels, and understands what is happening. For this reason, emotional support and attentiveness to the patient's psychological fear are paramount.

Opiates and other respiratory depressants should be avoided until an airway is established, either by endotracheal intubation or tracheostomy. Once a secure airway is in place, diazepam can be administered to control muscle spasms. Neuromuscular blocking agents are used in severe spasms only, and Nipride may be indicated for control of hypertension. Hospital treatment focuses on surgical debridement of any ischemic or infected tissue, drainage of abscess sites, and wound culture. The surrounding environment should be one of minimal light, noise, and movement, all of which can trigger violent muscle spasms. Due to autonomic dysfunction, the patient is at risk for cardiac dysrhythmia, including cardiac arrest, and labile blood pressure. For this reason, treatment and observation should be performed in an intensive care setting at a tertiary care facility.

RABIES

Rabies virus is epizootic in several areas of the United States, having spread out from foci in West Virginia and Virginia to include most of the eastern seaboard states.[17,18] In addition, three other foci involving the north central, south central, and mid-Atlantic states have been identified. While the dog is the global domestic reservoir, raccoons, bats, and skunks are the primary wild rabies sources found throughout the world. Domestic animals are generally thought to be infected by contact with wild animals, although there have been reported cases of domestic animals imported into the country with rabies.[18,19] Increasingly, cats are becoming a second source of domestic rabies. It is rare that rabbits, guinea pigs, or mice carry rabies.

Rabies is a rhabdovirus and is transmissible in three ways. The first, by direct inoculation through the bite or scratch of an infected animal, is the most common mode of transmission. Second, the disease can be conveyed from animal saliva coming in direct contact with an open wound or other area of nonintact skin or mucous membrane. Although rare, airborne transmission has been documented in laboratory workers and spelunkers.[19,20] Interestingly, in 1989 six cases of rabies transmission occurred in corneal graft transplant patients whose donors were unsuspected rabies victims.[19] Theoretically, transmission of rabies from an infected person's saliva is possible; however, there has never been a documented case of this occurring.[19,20] The advent of Standard Precautions and body substance isolation, if practiced meticulously, should preclude this method of transmission. It is important to note that contact with secretions other than saliva, such as urine, feces, or blood of infected animals, or having petted an infected animal is not considered an "exposure" and would not be grounds for rabies prophylaxis.

Once introduced into the body of its host, the rabies virus does not immediately begin to spread throughout the body; rather it replicates in the site for up to several days before migrating up the peripheral nervous system to the central nervous system (CNS), where it has been demonstrated to continue replication almost exclusively in the gray matter.[17,19] Viral behavior reinforces initial treatment by EMS personnel: copious irrigation with soap and water or saline and removal of any saliva from the patient's skin surface.

After establishing itself in the CNS, the virus disseminates to those sites that are highly innervated, such as the retina, cornea, and most especially, the salivary glands. The incubation period is prolonged, lasting 4–8 weeks on average, but may vary from a few days to 1 year. This tremendous variation in length often makes history-taking a challenge, particularly if the contact involves a young child or elderly person. A myriad of variables affect the incubation period: the age of the patient, body size, amount of inoculum, location of wound, type of tissue involved, the state of the patient's immune system, and, possibly, the distance the virus must travel to reach the CNS.

Classic rabies, the more common form of the disease, follows a clinical presentation similar to tetanus, since both attack the CNS. Initially, symptoms are vague: fever, myalgias, malaise, headache, sore throat, nausea, vomiting, and paresthesia, pain, fasciculation, or itching at the entry site, which may be present for several days. This is generally followed by the acute phase, in which the patient may alternate between hallucinations and aggressive, almost psychotic behavior with periods of rationality. Characteristically, the person is agitated, confused, and excitable and may display anorexia, dysphagia, and hydrophobia. Hydrophobia, a classic indicator of rabies, occurs when the patient attempts to swallow, invariably triggering violent diaphragmatic spasms, laryngospasm, facial grimacing, opisthotonus, and seizures. Occurring during a period of lucidness, this can be a terrifying experience for the patient. Other CNS symptoms that may be evident are diplopia, facial twitching, and coma. The respiratory muscles begin to fail due to brainstem dysfunction resulting in periods of apnea leading to respiratory arrest.

A second clinical picture may evolve, that of ascending, symmetric paralysis. Not as common as classic rabies, this form may mimic Guillain-Barré syndrome, poliomyelitis, and other forms of viral encephalitic diseases. Flaccid paralysis and decreased deep tendon reflexes are characteristic.[17] The paralysis evolves near the end of the acute neurological phase, confounding the clinical diagnosis, which is made more difficult by the lack of hydrophobia in this form of the disease. Persons suffering this form of rabies have been known to survive up to 1 month even without the benefit of intensive care, but survival from either form of the disease is extremely rare. Definitive diagnosis is made by brain biopsy, almost always postmortem, and several complex laboratory tests. To date, no rapid form of identification of the disease exists. Premortem diagnosis depends on early pinpointing of an exposure for any chance of recovery.

Treatment of rabies is optimally started within 72 hours following the exposure.[19] However, even after longer periods of delay, treatment should be administered aggressively for the patient to have any chance of survival. All bites of wild animals, especially raccoons, bats, skunks, and foxes, as well as those of feral (wild) dogs or cats, should be treated as an exposure to rabies. As mentioned earlier, immediate treatment consists of thorough washing of the wound with soapy water and copious irrigation. It is not necessary to use betadine or other antibiotic cleansers as a good soap scrub is adequate for cleansing. Aggressive cleansing should be continued in the ED, along with high-pressure irrigation, debridement, and foreign body removal.

If possible, obtain a description and identification of the animal. This helps animal control officers to track and trap the offending animal. Never expose yourself or others to the animal as the risk of being attacked and bitten is great if the animal is truly rabid. However, do your best to determine from onlookers if the attack was provoked or not. If any contact was made with the animal prior to it biting the patient, consider it a provoked attack. The bite of a chipmunk, squirrel, rabbit, mouse, hamster, or guinea pig is rarely suspect; however, the local health department should be consulted if the exposure is to one of these animals. If the animal is feral, it will be trapped, euthanized,

and sent for immediate rabies testing. A domestic animal may be isolated for 10 days and observed for the development of rabies signs and symptoms. As soon as it is determined that an animal does not have rabies, patient prophylaxis can be stopped. Initiation of prophylaxis should never be delayed awaiting laboratory results. If, however, the animal is a pet with a history of vaccination, it is reasonable to delay treatment pending the pet's 10-day quarantine.

Based on the site and size of the wound, the ED physician will make the determination to close the wound or allow it to heal by secondary intention. When at all possible, the wound should be left open to facilitate drainage. In lieu of sutures, steri-strips or surgical tape can be used to pull a large wound together to decrease the size of the scar. Passive immunization with human rabies immune globulin (HRIG) should be initiated in the ED simultaneously with active immunization using human diploid cell vaccine (HDCV) or rabies vaccine adsorbed (RVA). HRIG and the rabies vaccine must be given in separate sites. Dosing of HRIG is 20 IU/kg, half of which should be injected around the wound site if anatomically feasible, the other half given intramuscularly in the gluteus of adults or the anterolateral thigh of infants and small children.[20] This is a one-time dosing that is ineffective if given after the eighth day. HRIG should not be given in the deltoid. Individuals who have been previously immunized against rabies, such as animal control officers or zoo animal handlers, need only be given two doses of postexposure rabies vaccine. HRIG is not indicated in patients who have received the preexposure vaccination series unless there is a question of immune system compromise.

Rabies vaccine (HDCV or RVA) 1 cc intramuscularly in the deltoid is administered on days 0, 3, 7, 14, and 28.[19,20] The rabies vaccine series is never given in the gluteus because prophylaxis failure has been documented in cases in which this administration site was used.[19] New vaccines are being developed and tested that will require less vaccine and fewer injections with an increase in efficacy and a decrease in side effects. However, until they are approved for use in the United States, the mainstay of postexposure prophylaxis remains a combination of rabies immune globulin and rabies vaccine.

The advent of serious systemic or anaphylactic reactions to the vaccine must be weighed against the likelihood of rabies exposure. It may be necessary to premedicate the patient and continue the series despite reactions. Each case should be decided by the physician managing the patient, bearing in mind that the chance of survival following onset of rabies disease is slim. To date there is documentation of only three survivors of this disease responsible for 20,000 deaths per year worldwide.[18,19] Pregnancy is not a contraindication to receiving the vaccine when weighed against the possible outcome of untreated rabies disease, although there are only limited studies pertaining to the effects on the fetus.

INTERNET ACTIVITIES

Visit the e-medicine Web site at http://www.emedicine.com. Click on the Emergency Medicine on-line book and select Infectious Diseases. Then click on Rabies. Review the chapter on the management of rabies.

POISONOUS PLANTS

Unintentional ingestion of poisonous plants occurs primarily in children under the age of 6 years, while deliberate ingestion of toxic plants is most frequently seen in teenagers and young adults.[21–24] Many plants have been falsely labeled as being "deadly" when in fact the amount that must be ingested to cause death is quite large and unlikely to be consumed accidentally. The brightly colored berries, flowers, and leaves are frequently very bitter or sharp flavored and are usually spat out by the child who has been curious enough to take a bite. Vomiting or diarrhea, a part of the body's natural defense system, is also a common side effect of toxic plant ingestion. While unpleasant, it should be considered favorably by medical personnel.

As with any emergency, making the correct diagnosis in a timely fashion is of paramount importance. On the scene, EMS personnel should look for and obtain samples of the offending plant if it will not delay transport unduly. A copy of the plant's identifying properties (leaf, berry, stem) can be faxed or described over the telephone to the local poison control center to aid in identification. Treatment is dependent on the action of the poison. While some plants have specific antidotes, they should not be used without positive identification. Gastric lavage and use of activated charcoal is often the mainstay of treatment. Flushing the skin, eyes, and mucous membranes with water, particularly if there is a burning or itching sensation, is never harmful. Rehydration with crystalloid solution is often helpful in cases with copious fluid losses from excessive salivation, sweating, vomiting, or diarrhea. Oxygen administration should be initiated for anyone suffering dyspnea, dysphagia, wheezing, chest tightness, or edema of the oral mucosa.

Plants containing belladonna alkaloids, such as jimson weed or nightshade, cause anticholinergic symptoms and delirium. Expect dilated pupils; hot, dry, flushed skin; dry mouth; and urinary retention without nausea, vomiting, or diarrhea. Treatment is supportive.[21]

Castor beans are highly toxic but must be consumed in large quantities, although a small amount of the bean extract, being more concentrated and, therefore, more potent, has been used in underworld "hits." The castor bean contains ricin, which can cause headache, seizures, and shock. Treatment is supportive.[23]

Naturally occurring cardiac glycosides are found in foxglove and oleander. Used in the early 1900s by physicians for the beneficial effects on the heart, these plants were also used to murder individuals during those same times. Because of the narrow safety margin between toxicity and therapy, these plants were also responsible for inadvertent deaths caused by lack of sophisticated tests available to measure blood levels. Treatment includes ACLS protocols as necessary, pacemaker, atropine, and charcoal. Use of Digibind in the hospital setting is helpful.

Another group of plants frequently responsible for poisonings include tobacco, hemlock, peyote, morning glory, nutmeg, and mace and may cause CNS disturbances including seizures, hypotension, coma, respiratory distress, or hallucinations. The nicotine in tobacco is absorbed directly through the skin and has been responsible for illness and injury in farm laborers. In addition to being inhaled, pesticides and fungicides are also absorbed through contact with skin and are frequently implicated in poisonings. For this reason, any farmworker, produce worker, or orchard hand that presents with CNS symptoms and recent exposure to tobacco, pesticides, or other farm chemicals should be washed thoroughly (after life-threatening needs are met) to remove any residue from the skin surface.[22–24] Individuals handling these patients should wear gloves to protect themselves from the effects of the chemical toxins as well.

Fruit seeds, specifically the apricot, apple, almond, and cherry, as well as the hydrangea, contain enzymes that are converted by the body into cyanide. Silver polish and photography chemicals also contain cyanide. While the seeds need to be well chewed, often in significant amounts, to release the toxin, many of these plants or their compounds are found in herbal, folk, and other alternative medicines. The seeds are very bitter and not likely to be voluntarily eaten; however, amounts in sufficient quantity to do harm can be ingested in ground-up preparations. Burning of wool, silk, nylon, and polyurethane can release cyanide into the air.

Cyanide injures its victim by depriving the body of oxygen through blocking electron transport at the chemoreceptor cells. Cyanosis is not seen until very late in the progress of the illness, and oximetry will not demonstrate a drop in saturation because the hemoglobin molecule is not affected by cyanide. The first symptom is an increase in the respiratory rate followed by headache, dizziness, mental confusion, drowsiness, increasing dyspnea, ECG changes, hypotension, seizures, coma, and death. Characteristic of cyanide poisoning is a smell described as "bitter almonds," which may be apparent to the EMS provider, although 20%–40% of the population cannot detect this smell.[22,23] This is a medical emergency requiring immediate intervention to save the victim's life.

Respiratory support is important; oxygen should be administered at 100%. Commercially prepared cyanide antidote kits are available from Eli Lilly Company. Treatment consists of the rapid administration of nitrite via inhalation of amyl nitrite perles, which can be crushed and held under the nose of the victim or crushed and placed inside the mask being used to administer oxygen. As long as the blood pressure remains greater than 80 mm Hg, the perles can be administered at a rate of one every 2 minutes until an IV can be established, at which point administration of 3% sodium nitrite at a dose of 10 mL over 3–5 minutes should replace the amyl nitrite perles (pediatric dose: 0.15–0.33 mL/kg). This is followed by a 50-mL dose of 25% sodium thiosulfate at a rate of 10 mL/min (pediatric dose: 1.6 mL/kg). The sodium nitrite and sodium thiosulfate doses may have to be repeated and should be administered based on the methemoglobin level, which should not exceed 40%. Often, even with rapid treatment and 100% oxygen, the patient will suffer residual neurological damage.

Holiday plants have also been a source of concern for parents and emergency care providers with their brilliant colors, decorative and eye-catching bows, and lovely looking berries. The poinsettia is nontoxic; however, its leaves and berries can cause gastrointestinal distress if swallowed. Mistletoe, conversely, can be very toxic; as few as three berries may cause illness as it contains both alkaloids and cardiac toxins.[23] Symptoms include abdominal pain, vomiting, diarrhea, hypertension, seizures, and cardiac arrest. Treatment is supportive and patients should be rapidly transferred to the nearest ED.

Mushrooms are a dangerous and frequent toxic offender. Highly publicized accounts of illness and death, due to both deliberate and inadvertent poisonous mushroom ingestion, highlight the extent of this danger. While only a few species are responsible for deaths, many more are capable of causing serious gastrointestinal upset, seizures, or hallucinations. Identification of mushrooms is very tricky, and mistakes are made by "experts" who erroneously identify a toxic mushroom as edible. If a sample of the offending mushroom can be found, it should be brought with the patient when he or she is transported. Be sure to obtain the bulb, which grows beneath the soil surface, as it is necessary to correctly identify the mushroom.

A few species of mushrooms are responsible for the majority of deaths in the United States. *Amanita phalloides*, aptly named the "death cap," produces systemic symptoms within minutes to hours after eating even a small portion of the mushroom. The principal toxin is a cyclopeptide that inhibits ribonucleic acid (RNA) synthesis and produces cellular damage in the striated muscle cells and fatty degeneration. Multiple organs can be extensively damaged, including the kidneys, heart, liver, and brain. The patient exhibits symptoms of parasympathetic stimulation: pupil constriction; excessive salivation, lacrimation, and perspiration; nausea, vomiting, and diarrhea; hypotension and bradycardia; wheezing and dyspnea; and tremors, delirium, agitation, and mental confusion. *Amanita virosa* (destroying angel), *A. bisporigera*, and *A. muscaria* (fly agaric) and *Galerina venenata* cause symptoms similar to the death cap and are deadly. All three have a latent period of 6–20 hours, which is followed by cardiovascular collapse, convulsions, coma, hepatomegaly, jaundice, liver necrosis, dehydration, hypoglycemia, and renal failure. Approximately 50% of patients die within 5–8 days unless early, aggressive intervention is accomplished. Hemoperfusion (similar to hemodialysis) has been used with success in *Amanita* poisoning.[22,24,25]

Always encourage patients to be evaluated for toxic sequelae following any suspected poisonous plant ingestion. Obtain positive identification and samples of the plant to facilitate diagnosis and treatment. Attempt to establish how much of the plant matter was actually eaten and ascertain any underlying medical conditions the patient might have. Remember that supportive care is often all that is required as many of the symptoms are self-limiting. All EMS units should have an up-to-date text for identification of plants to assist them in the field.

HOUSEHOLD POISONS

The number and scope of poisonous chemicals commonly found in most households is astonishing. Cleaning supplies, medications, vitamins, distillates, paint, nail polish remover, analgesics, automotive supplies, and other toxic substances are literally lying about the house (Figure 23-13) and garage (Figure 23-14). The damage any one of these substances can do when ingested is frightening. Education regarding proper handling and storage of all chemicals must be stepped up to bring about awareness and behavioral changes among individuals. As much as 50% of all

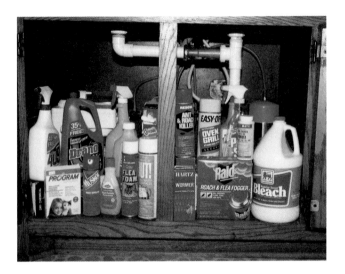

FIGURE 23-13 A look under the kitchen sink yields a number of poisonous items within reach of most children. (Courtesy of Mark Zeringue)

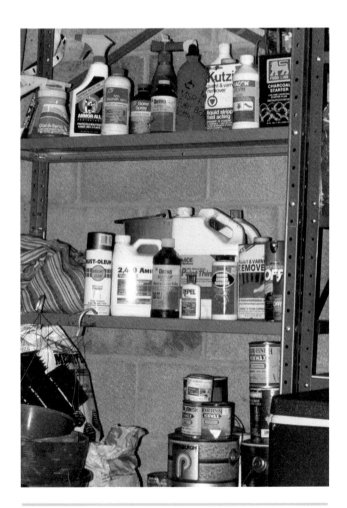

FIGURE 23-14 Most household garages or sheds contain a number of toxic poisons. (Courtesy of Elizabeth Zeringue)

poisonings occur in the home, with a common household substance responsible for the illness or injury afflicting the patient, a significant number of whom are children under 6 years of age.

Sources of unintentional poisoning that can be easily overlooked are the imported herbal and folk medicines found in health food stores and specialty markets. These products have gained increasing popularity as an alternative source of healing for conditions ranging from arthritis and headaches to cancer and AIDS. Many of these preparations contain ground parts from animals such as horns or hooves and desiccated gallbladders or livers. These preparations may contain high levels of heavy metals, particularly lead and arsenic, which produce toxic symptoms after prolonged use due to the cumulative effect of these chemicals. Because many of these products are imported illegally, the true contents may not be disclosed on the label as required by the FDA. This agency keeps extensive lists of such compounds and may be able to furnish the ED physician with a content analysis if the product label is available.

Alkaline poisons are such common items as lye, drain openers, enzymatic contact lens cleaner, and tablet-form reagents used to test diabetic urine. Contact with these substances produces a burn capable of destroying local tissue and causing severe pain of the lips, tongue, throat, and stomach. The damaged gastric mucosa sloughs off, producing bloody diarrhea or vomiting. Perforation and scarring of the esophagus and stomach are common; it may begin immediately or be delayed for hours or days. Treatment consists of administration of large amounts of water or milk without lavage. Never induce vomiting as regurgitation of the alkaline chemical will further damage tissue or could be aspirated. Be prepared to provide respiratory support as edema due to local tissue damage will be extensive and often compromises the airway. Flush the mouth and face with copious amounts of water; continue this en route to the ED. This is a "load and go" situation in which possible surgical intervention will likely be necessary depending on the extent of the damage. Esophagogastroduodenoscopy (EGD) should be performed by a physician within the first 24 hours to assess the injury. Treatment for shock and pain control is necessary. Rehabilitation following extensive esophageal destruction is a long, slow process often requiring multiple surgical procedures to mobilize and graft a piece of the colon to serve as an esophagus.

Acids are also extremely caustic substances that are as damaging as alkaline solutions. They are often ingested with suicidal intent; this is a very unpleasant and terribly painful way to die. Severe burns of the oral and gastric mucosal surfaces result in sloughing of tissue, scarring, perforation, peritonitis, and strictures. The mouth often shows black or brown charring. Some acids produce a yellow stain when ingested. Treatment is identical to alkaline substances with emphasis on the dilution of the acid by copious use of water or milk. Rehabilitation and reconstructive surgery will likely be similar, except the patient is more likely to die as a result of the extensive erosion and secondary infection following the acid burn.

Ingestion of acetaminophen either unintentionally or intentionally, is a common event with often deadly consequences. While touted as a "safe" alternative to aspirin, acetaminophen is extremely hepatotoxic when taken in a single dose of eight grams (8,000 mg) or more. Early symptoms are vague: nausea, vomiting, sweating, pallor, and fatigue. Hepatic dysfunction is often not apparent for 1 or 2 days. Symptoms of acute hepatic failure are decreased mental status, jaundice, hepatomegaly, coagulopathy, and coma causing a slow, unpleasant death. Treatment is gastric lavage and activated charcoal. Administration of N-acetylcysteine (Mucomyst) used to decrease liver toxicity is indicated if the acetaminophen ingestion is less than 24 hours old but should not be given with charcoal because absorption of the Mucomyst would be compromised.

Iron overdose is a serious condition that must be aggressively treated to avert death secondary to liver necrosis. Children are often the victims of this injury following the consumption of excessive amounts of multivitamins with iron.[24,26] These tablets are often attractive to children because they are brightly colored and fruit flavored and may depict favorite cartoon characters or heroes. Doses as small as 60 mg/kg have been reported as fatal, although larger amounts (300 mg/kg) are more likely to be responsible for deaths, particularly in children. Symptoms of iron toxicity are spread out over several stages shown in Table 23-4.

Early intervention using ipecac and gastric lavage assists in removal of iron from the system. To precipitate the iron, a solution of 5% sodium bicarbonate has been tried with varying success.[22,26] After obtaining an abdominal film, if any pill fragments are noted to have moved beyond the pyloric outlet, whole bowel irrigation should be employed. Use of a bowel preparation

such as Golytely (Braintree Laboratory) to cleanse the entire gastrointestinal tract is gaining acceptance. Although the preparation is usually ingested orally, it is not well tolerated in children. Therefore, it is acceptable to use the nasogastric tube previously employed for lavage to instill the laxative until the stool is clear. For those persons with serum iron levels greater than 350 µm/dL an iron chelating agent administered IV or intramuscularly (IM) will be necessary. The drug of choice is deferoxamine mesylate, given by slow IV infusion. It is important to monitor for hypotensive side effects, treating them acutely.

Rubbing alcohol is occasionally deliberately ingested by alcoholic individuals in addition to those unintentional incidents involving children. Isopropyl alcohol is metabolized into acetone. Rarely is this substance toxic; however, it is capable of inducing a coma that can last 12 hours or more. Supportive therapy is used along with induction of vomiting and gastric lavage. The primary effect is gastric irritation, nausea, and vomiting. Aspiration with subsequent pneumonia is a major concern in addition to intermittent gastritis, which is usually self-limiting. Acetone is also the primary component of fingernail polish remover, another common household chemical.

Ethylene glycol (antifreeze) is another common substance found in most households. This substance is responsible for the death of alcoholics, who may drink it. Fatal dosage is around 100 grams. Initial symptoms resemble alcohol intoxication. Metabolism of the glycol results in metabolic acidosis and hypocalcemia. Other commonly seen symptoms are tachypnea, bradycardia, vomiting, coma, and anisocoria. Large ingestion can result in pulmonary edema and acute tubular necrosis. Aggressive intervention to combat hypocalcemia, metabolic acidosis, and any hypothermia are necessary to decrease mortality. Additional treatment is supportive.

AIR

HIGH-ALTITUDE ILLNESSES

As more people explore the outdoors and challenge themselves physically and mentally with activities such as mountain climbing and high-altitude skiing, the chance of encountering illnesses related to high altitudes increases. Once a condition affecting only a small percentage of high-profile climbing teams, altitude illness is seen with increasing frequency in individuals who vigorously participate in these increasingly popular sports. As these activities continue to gain in popularity, accessibility, and affordability, EMS personnel will need to be familiar with the identification, treatment, and prevention of these unique illnesses.

Table 23-4 Symptoms of Iron Toxicity
Stage 1. Onset 30 minutes to 2 hours: nausea, vomiting, diarrhea, abdominal pain, restlessness, lethargy
Stage 2. Asymptomatic interlude
Stage 3. Onset 2–12 hours: fever, acidosis, shock
Stage 4. Onset 2–4 days: liver necrosis
Stage 5. Onset 2–4 weeks: bowel obstruction

At altitudes greater than 10,000–14,000 feet the oxygen-hemoglobin dissociation curve shifts to the right. If the body fails to make physiological adjustments or is so prevented by underlying medical conditions, the resulting "altitude sickness" may manifest itself in one or more of three conditions. The first, acute mountain sickness (AMS), may be experienced at altitudes greater than 8,000 feet and, while generally unpleasant, remains a benign, self-limiting, and reversible state when treated promptly. Ignored or unrecognized, AMS can progress rapidly over a period of hours to one or both conditions known as high-altitude pulmonary edema (HAPE) and high-altitude cerebral edema (HACE), which are life threatening and require rapid and aggressive treatment to prevent death.

Acute Mountain Sickness

Acute mountain sickness, generally seen at altitudes greater than 8,000 feet, is a collection of symptoms that often precedes HAPE and HACE and should be treated seriously. AMS is the body's response to hypoxia, which is triggered by a drop in oxygen saturation below 90%. This may start within 6 hours of ascent or after several days and is frequently described as feeling like a "bad hangover." It is difficult to predict who might be affected, but AMS appears to strike those between the ages of 1 and 20, with decreasing incidence at a later age.[27,28] It has been found that fit, healthy persons also seem to be more likely to be affected by AMS because they demonstrate the ability to ascend rapidly, without allowing the body to acclimate to the changes in oxygen concentration. Thus, AMS is frequently seen in skiers in the Rocky Mountain states and other mountain sports enthusiasts. AMS is divided into three stages: mild, moderate, and severe.

Initially, mild symptoms include a throbbing "hangover"-type headache—usually in the frontal area that is worse in the morning or with exercise—insomnia, anorexia, nausea, thirst, and dizziness. As the condition worsens, there may be vomiting, oliguria, dyspnea, chest pain, nightmares, lethargy, indigestion, edema, cough, retinal hemorrhage, and decreased coordination. This condition can be made worse by the intake of alcohol or sleeping medications, smoking, or increased exercise because they can decrease the already depleted oxygen concentration, thereby increasing the hypoxia. Descending 1,000 feet and resting for 24 hours usually resolves the symptoms. Slow ascent, frequent rest periods, and limited gains in altitude are necessary.

The second stage, moderately symptomatic AMS, includes all of the previous symptoms plus ataxia and mild confusion. A rapid descent of 2,000 feet is recommended followed by restricted physical exertion, fluids, and time to allow the body's natural adaptive mechanisms to effect the necessary changes. These changes include increased alveolar ventilation and red blood cell production, which will take place over a period of weeks. Continued ascent will change a transient, self-limiting condition into one that is an extreme medical emergency. The line of distinction between moderate and severe AMS is often unclear, progressing rapidly from one phase to the next. Untreated, severe AMS can rapidly lead to coma and death; it is characterized by cough productive of pink, frothy sputum, cyanosis, extreme dyspnea, orthopnea, increasing mental confusion, and coma.

The treatment of choice at this point is a rapid descent of at least 3,000 feet, supplemental oxygen at 4–6 L/min, warmth, and absolutely no exertion. While the symptoms of mild to moderate AMS usually peak in 24–36 hours and gradually resolve over 1–2 days, those suffering from severe AMS may require hospitalization. It is imperative that these symptoms not be ignored, and it is also important to rule out other possible causes, including exhaustion, hypothermia, dehydration, and carbon monoxide poisoning.

High-Altitude Cerebral Edema

HACE is a life-threatening condition seen at elevations greater than 9,000 feet with cardinal indicators being mental status changes and ataxia. Characterized by a cluster of neurological signs and symptoms, including severe headache, diplopia, paresthesia, vertigo, projectile vomiting, aphasia, seizures, disorientation, hallucinations, decreased judgment, focal neurological deficits, emotional lability, and frank psychosis, it is often preceded by AMS. Examination of the victim demonstrates retinal hemorrhage, papilledema, clonus, and cranial nerve deficits.

Physiologically, the body responds to hypoxia by increasing arterial blood flow to the brain in an effort to increase oxygen perfusion. This increased blood flow may increase the circulating volume by 25%–50% resulting in cellular edema. The ensuing cerebral edema is responsible for the decreased mental status and neurological findings.

Treatment is quick descent, oxygen at 2–6 L/min per nasal cannula, and bed rest for 2–3 days until the symptoms resolve. Ascent may be resumed gradually after resolution of symptoms. Dexamethasone, at a dose of 4–8 mg by mouth every 6 hours, can be used to decrease cerebral vasodilatation and blood flow, stabilize microvascular membranes, and increase diuresis. Be aware, however, that dehydration as a result of excessive diuresis can worsen all forms of altitude illness. Other side effects to be alert for include nausea, paresthesia, myopia, and polyuria.

High-Altitude Pulmonary Edema

Another possible sequelae of untreated, severe AMS is HAPE. It is recognized by distinct pulmonary presentation and should be suspected when the elevation is over 10,000 feet. Usually seen in young, healthy adults within 2–4 days of ascent, research suggests that susceptibility to HAPE increases after a person experiences one episode, with the recurrence rate estimated at 66%.[27,28] Unlike HACE, which affects only 1% of travelers, HAPE may affect 0.5%–15% of high-altitude visitors. Hallmark symptoms are rales, dyspnea, and pink, frothy sputum. A decrease in the partial pressure of oxygen leads to a decrease in the alveolar oxygen tension, which causes increased respiratory rate in an effort to compensate for the hypoxia. At sea level PaO_2 is 100 mm Hg but decreases to about 38 mm Hg at 15,000 feet. Failure of the body to compensate with greatly increased minute ventilation results in illness. The resulting alveolar leakage and overperfusion are related to fluid shifts from the vascular space to the intracellular space secondary to the failure of the adenosine triphosphate (ATP) dependent sodium pump.

Although there can be as much as a 20% decrease in blood volume, the interstitial space is severely fluid overloaded, producing the pulmonary edema. Those individuals with chemoreceptor sensitivity impairment due to smoking or an underlying pulmonary disease may not respond with an increase in the ventilatory rate and are, therefore, more prone to HAPE. Examination of the patient reveals a cough productive of pink, frothy sputum, flat neck veins, cyanosis, tachycardia, orthopnea, fever, hemoptysis, rales, decreased exercise tolerance, and severe fatigue with an inability to walk. Note that this is not adult respiratory distress syndrome (ARDS), as there is no inflammatory component. This is noncardiogenic pulmonary edema.

Radiographic examination demonstrates a normal cardiac silhouette and patchy, fluffy infiltrates. A high index of suspicion and early diagnosis supports swift intervention, for without rapid descent and supplemental oxygen the death rate from HAPE is 44%. Expeditious descent until the symptoms begin to improve and supplemental positive pressure oxygen may be all that are needed in mild cases. Other therapy includes maintenance of body temperature, emotional support, and judicious use of IV fluids.

Drugs, particularly diuretics, must be used carefully, because dehydration can worsen the overall condition of the victim. Dexamethasone is used to reduce cerebral vasodilation and cerebral blood flow and to promote diuresis. Acetozolamide is a carbonic anhydrase inhibitor that works by producing a mild metabolic acidosis by enhancing renal excretion of bicarbonate, stimulating the ventilation rate. A dose of 250 mg by mouth every 8–12 hours initiated 24 hours prior to ascent has been helpful in preventing the onset of HAPE. Diuretics, as already mentioned, are not recommended and must be used cautiously, if at all, due to the dehydration effect they can produce. Nifedipine, a calcium channel blocker, has been shown to improve the pulmonary hypertension frequently associated with HAPE by decreasing the work load of the right ventricle, decreasing vascular resistance, and reversing the pulmonary hypertension. Drugs are not a substitute for descent.

One method of avoiding the various forms of high-altitude sickness is to climb up during the day but return to a lower elevation at night to make camp and sleep.[27] It is best to avoid high-altitude sports if pregnant due to the risk of fetal hypoxia secondary to maternal hypoxia. Fetal oxygen supply is dependent on the maternal supply. A developing fetus is very sensitive to hypoxia, and intrauterine growth retardation can result from a lack of adequate oxygen. High altitudes can also increase the likelihood of maternal complications of hypertension, edema, and proteinuria. Those individuals who have sickle cell disease or sickle thalassemia are at grave risk for complications; the altitude causes sickling, which may result in death. Those with the sickle cell trait are at risk for splenic infarction and should avoid unpressurized high-altitude travel. Use of supplemental oxygen is recommended.

A word to rescue team members: If newly or temporarily assigned to a high-altitude duty station it would be wise to consult a physician prior to assignment regarding the need for prophylactic medication or the benefit of a 2–3 week acclimation period prior to assuming duties to prevent the occurrence of the aforementioned illnesses in EMS personnel.

CARBON MONOXIDE POISONING

It has been suggested that carbon monoxide (CO) is responsible for unrecognized morbidity and mortality frequently attributed to other causes due to its vague symptoms and insidious nature. It has been further implied that CO is the single leading cause of toxin-related death in the United States. [29–31] Carbon monoxide is an odorless, tasteless, invisible gas that results as a by-product of combustible fuels. It is also found in other sources such as wood stoves, kerosene heaters, gas water heaters or dryers, furnaces, and indoor charcoal grills. Fire fighters, the group with the single highest risk, are often victims of CO inhalation and not burns at fire scenes.[30]

With an affinity for hemoglobin 200 times that of oxygen, it is understandable that competition for binding sites is fierce. Cardiac myoglobin is especially affected by the oxygen transport impairment, leading to ischemia and dysrhythmia. Carbon monoxide kills by decreasing the oxygen-carrying capacity of hemoglobin and decreasing cellular respiration. Often the interval between injury and laboratory analysis of blood samples is quite long, allowing for normalization of CO levels through respiration. Oxygen administration on the scene can further obscure the true blood level. For this reason, it is suggested that a blood sample be obtained on the scene early in the treatment so that an accurate measurement of CO blood levels can be accomplished.

Environmental risk factors are given in Table 23-5.[29–31] Smokers are often compromised by the fumes coming from their own cigarettes; the smoke from cigarettes is very high in CO. Those factors most likely to affect the level of illness include concentration of CO, duration of exposure, activity level, and interval between insult and treatment.

Examination of the respiratory system, including appraisal of the nasal and eyebrow hair, should be rapidly accomplished when evaluating a victim for inhalation injury. With the multitude of chemicals used in textiles and commercial products, a myriad of toxic substances are released in fires and may rapidly poison those individuals who are exposed to them.

Initial treatment is to remove the patient from the source of the CO, followed by 100% oxygen via mask and limited activity until recovery is complete, usually within several hours. Systemic effects include cardiac dysrhythmia, respiratory distress, angina, ischemia with ECG changes, mental confusion, loss of consciousness, coma, seizures, and death. Bright red venous blood, demonstrated in the early stages of CO poisoning, fades and disappears in the later stages. Persons who smoke often tolerate higher levels of CO but will eventually succumb as CO reaches toxic levels. Normal blood carboxyhemoglobin (COHb) level is below 2%. Smokers demonstrate blood levels of between 5% and 9%. Symptoms of CO poisoning begin around 10%–20%. Profound symptoms (coma, seizures, death), often requiring hyperbaric oxygen therapy for resolution, manifest at COHb levels greater than 20%.[29–31]

Hyperbaric oxygen therapy to treat CO poisoning has been used by the U.S. military for many years. The treatment protocol used by the U.S. Air Force is summarized in Table 23-6. Due to lack of availability and accessibility, widespread use of hyperbaric chambers has not been seen outside of large urban centers.

Table 23-5
Activities with High Risk for CO Poisoning

Fighting fires

Warming of automobiles (winter months, garages)

Tractor pulls

Monster truck rallies

Indoor ice rinks that use propane- or gasoline-powered zambonis

Kerosene heaters

Tent camping

Auto mechanics working in closed bays

Table 23-6
Hyperbaric Treatment for Carbon Monoxide Poisoning

Depth	Time (min)	Oxygen Concentration (%)
Period 1		
3 ATA	23	100
3 ATA*	5	21
Period 2		
3 ATA	23	100
3 ATA*	5	21
Period 3		
2 ATA	25	100
2 ATA*	5	21
Period 4		
2 ATA	25	100
2 ATA*	5	21

Note: Continue 2 atmospheres of pressure (ATA) periods based on clinical picture. Final Phase is a 10-minute ascent to the surface.

* "Rest intervals" at room air have been demonstrated to decrease the risk of cerebral oxygen toxicity. Each period is separated by a rest interval. The periods at 2 ATA may continue for two to six cycles with 5-minute rest intervals.

Opponents criticize the use of hyperbaric chambers for CO poisoning because it may delay treatment of associated injury (burns).

Prevention of CO poisoning is aimed at increasing awareness and recognition of those activities prone to produce CO fumes. Carbon monoxide detectors are sold in most hardware stores and pharmacies. They are about the size of smoke detectors and are not difficult to install and maintain. Risk during outdoor activity is often overlooked. Farm workers who ride in a planting or harvesting seat (rear-facing seat at the level of the exhaust pipe) are far more likely to be victims of CO poisoning than the tractor driver. Allowing for adequate ventilation at events likely to generate fumes, like tractor pulls, auto racing events, or camp sites, can also prevent the senseless deaths that occur every year as a result of CO poisoning.

HEAT-RELATED ILLNESSES

Heat-related illnesses run the gamut in severity from mild, self-limiting conditions to those that are life threatening within minutes if untreated. The incredible complexity of the thermoregulatory process begins at the cellular level and progresses through the various body systems that must perform synchronously to produce the correct amount of heat energy for optimal body function. The uncompensated variation of just a few degrees too cool or too hot can be disastrous. Indeed, life depends on the meticulous balance of body temperature.

Heat Edema

Retention of sodium and water in response to aldosterone production is the underlying cause of heat edema, a very mild, self-limiting disease seen primarily in females. This condition results in the swelling of hands, feet, and ankles, which resolves spontaneously as the body acclimatizes to changes in ambient air temperature. Usually it takes around 2 weeks for the body to adjust to significant weather changes.

Heat Tetany

The condition known as **heat tetany** occurs in response to intense heat stress or heat exposure. It may be an early manifestation of heat exhaustion or heatstroke and should be monitored for resolution. Hyperventilation following a heat stress or high exposure causes respiratory alkalosis, paresthesia, carpopedal spasms, and tetany, causing the muscles in the hands to spasm, forming a characteristic clawlike appearance. Relief can be obtained by alleviating the heat stress and decreasing the hyperventilation. This, too, is a self-limiting condition.

Heat Cramps

Often suffered by those who exercise muscles strenuously and fail to replenish the body's supply of electrolytes and water, heat cramps are frequently seen in underconditioned sports enthusiasts who "overdo it" on the weekend; people who hike beyond their level of conditioning; and those who participate in competitive sports. Working muscles strenuously, often the calves, while sweating profusely and failing to drink enough results in hyponatremia, causing painful cramping of the muscles. Treatment of this condition is rest, fluids (preferably by mouth), salt replacement (a well-balanced sports drink), and a cool environment. If severe, heat cramps can require IV hydration with normal saline or 1% oral salt solution.

Heat Exhaustion

A more serious illness, heat exhaustion is due to loss of body water and electrolyte depletion resulting in headache, nausea, vomiting, lightheadedness, myalgias, and malaise. Dehydration is also commonly seen with this condition. It is vital to quickly distinguish heat exhaustion from the more deadly heatstroke. Some experts call heat exhaustion a "diagnosis of exclusion."[32] The excluding symptoms are changes in mental status and a core body temperature over 40°C (104°F). In other words, there is not enough evidence to support the diagnosis of heatstroke, the more deadly injury.

Treatment for heat exhaustion is rest in a cool environment and gradual rehydration over a period of hours. Treat with oral fluids if possible, but if symptoms are severe, an IV of normal saline or one-half normal saline should be used. The addition of 5% dextrose and water to the first liter (using 5% dextrose and normal saline) may also be used. The skin can be sprayed with tepid water and allowed to evaporate to gradually reduce the body temperature. Monitor the patient for about 12 hours and check a core temperature frequently. If the patient is very young or elderly or has a cardiac history, the use of IV fluids must be judiciously balanced against the cardiac status. It is vital to not miss the diagnosis of heatstroke, hence the caveat: *When in doubt, always treat for heatstroke.* It does not harm a person suffering from heat exhaustion to be treated for heat stroke, but it is fatal to treat heatstroke as heat exhaustion!

Heatstroke

Heatstroke is a medical emergency that carries a high morbidity and mortality rate if improperly treated or undertreated. A significant danger is overaggressive fluid therapy causing pulmonary edema and ARDS, due to a failure to realize the underlying pathology is distributive shock, not hypovolemia. " In heatstroke, patients suffer a redistribution of volume from the core to the periphery, not true hypovolemia.[32] A substantial shift from the periphery to the core occurs on cooling." *Begin cooling measures immediately.* Manifestations of heatstroke are mental status changes or CNS dysfunction, a core body temperature greater than 40°C (104°F), and a history of recent heat exposure or heat stress.

History reveals some activity immediately prior to symptoms that leads to suspicion for heat stroke. CNS disturbances are often present on the scene: irrational behavior, irritability, frank psychosis, seizures, syncope, or ataxia. Examination of the patient reveals tachycardia, tachypnea, or "panting dog" syndrome with a respiratory rate in the 60s, hypotension (due to distributive shock) with wide pulse pressures, a body temperature of 40.6°C or higher, and skin that is usually warm and dry but may be cool and clammy.[32] The patient should receive constant core temperature monitoring (urinary or esophageal), continuous cardiac monitoring and evaluation of cardiopulmonary status (rales and cyanosis are late signs), and a full neurological examination with frequent reevaluation of status. Look for posturing, seizure activity, obtundation, delirium, and coma. Although much of the organ system damage is reversible with cooling, there is always the risk of permanent damage. Frequent, devastating complications are ARDS, DIC, rhabdomyolysis, acute renal failure (ARF), liver failure, and brain damage.

Laboratory and ancillary data are important but should never be performed prior to initiation of cooling efforts. However, once these efforts are underway, arterial blood gas (ABG), chest radiograph, complete blood count (CBC), coagulation studies, electrolytes, blood urea nitrogen (BUN), creatinine, and urinalysis (UA) can be obtained. Always anticipate DIC in this situation. Renal failure is also a major concern due to the amount of hemolyzed red blood cells (RBCs) dumped into the system in response to tissue and organ damage.

Treatment is geared at rapidly and effectively lowering core body temperature to a nonlethal level. This can be accomplished in several ways, but generally a combination of methods is used. These patients are mortally ill, and research has shown that the same "golden hour" used in trauma applies to these patients. If effective cooling is not obtained, they die quickly. Effective cooling means a drop in body temperature exceeding the rate of 0.1°C–0.2°C per minute. Cooling continues until a core temperature of 39°C (102°F) is reached, with caution not to "overcool," resulting in rebound hypothermia.[32,33] For this reason constant temperature monitoring is essential. If the patient becomes hypothermic, the shivering mechanism may be triggered and result in a rebound rise in body temperature. The airway must be monitored and protected; oxygen should be administered. An IV of normal saline is reasonable, but fluid challenges, if used, must be for significant hypotension and should be small.

Cooling is optimally achieved by a light spray of tepid water over the naked body with constant air flow to promote evaporation. This convection/evaporation rather than conductive heat loss is significantly more effective. Ice packs can be placed in the axilla and groin (monitor for frostbite injury). Seizures during the cooling process are not unusual and should not interrupt the cooling process (up to 50% experience seizures). Use of diazepam and phenobarbital is usually sufficient to control the seizure activity. Seizure control is important because muscle activity during seizures increases body temperature. Never administer iced enemas to bring down core temperature. Stimulation of the vagus nerve may induce cardiac dysrhythmias. Iced peritoneal lavage is used only if body temperature is refractory to other methods. While iced gastric lavage has not been found to be harmful, it is not an efficient way to rapidly produce decreases in core temperature. The use of antipyretics is not beneficial as the causative mechanism in heatstroke is not the same as a febrile illness.

One important side note is the consideration of other causes of excessive body temperature shifts, particularly when the history is negative for heat stress exposure. If meningeal signs are present, differential diagnosis should include consideration for blackwater fever (falciparum malaria), late septicemia, and, rarely, cerebral vascular accident (CVA) affecting the hypothalamus. Certain poisons such as monoamine oxidase (MAO) inhibitors, lysergic acid diethylamid (LSD), salicylates, cocaine, amphetamines, cyclic antidepressants, and lithium can cause similar manifestations. Two rare syndromes, neuroleptic malignant syndrome and malignant hyperthermia, have demonstrable rigidity not seen in heatstroke; other disease processes such as thyroid storm, pheochromocytoma storm, or diabetic ketoacidosis (DKA) with septicemia can cause mental status changes with hyperthermia and should be considered in the differential diagnosis. It is important to recognize the value of a thorough history, which can make this diagnosis a very straightforward one.

INTERNET ACTIVITIES

Visit the e-medicine Web site at http:// www.emedicine.com. Click on the Emergency Medicine on-line book and select Environmental. Then click on Heat Exhaustion and Heatstroke. Review the chapter on the management of heat-related illnesses.

COLD-RELATED ILLNESS

The subtleties of early hypothermia, the aggressive interventions involved with rewarming, and the prevention of disability by careful handling of frostbite combine to make response to cold emergencies challenging and rewarding for the paramedic. As with other environmental emergencies, prevention and education are key in avoiding future morbidity and mortality. Although medical science has progressed rapidly in the treatment and care of cold-related injuries, many of the interventions, while not truly experimental, continue to be the subject of extensive study and research efforts. Early success with some procedures are balanced against dramatic failure or inconclusive results in others. Subsequently, it is recommended to be alert for new studies and to apply them cautiously in the practice of cold weather emergency care.

Regulation of body temperature and heat production is primarily the result of the action of the hypothalamus. The initial response to a drop in body temperature is shivering, which has been demonstrated to increase the basal metabolic rate (BMR) two to five times normal.[34] However, numerous factors can impair the ability to shiver, resulting in decompensation of the thermoregulatory system. As noted in the discussion of other environmental emergencies, the use of alcoholic beverages has been found to be a significant factor, increasing morbidity and mortality in hypothermic injuries. General circumstances that contribute to an increased risk of hypothermia are malnutrition, hypothyroidism, use of neuroleptic and other medications, dehydration, mental illness, homelessness, immobilization, and lack of adequate clothing. Physiological events such as trauma and burns, where large wounds or open abrasions allow heat loss that is uninterrupted by coverings, contribute to the development of hypothermia.

The body utilizes a combination of four external mechanisms for the transfer of heat:

1. **Conduction.** Heat energy is transferred by direct contact along a gradient from the warmer object to the cooler one. Responsible for as much as 15% of a body's heat loss, contact with cold water (e.g., immersion) or cold ground surfaces can swiftly carry body heat away.

2. **Evaporation.** Heat lost through perspiration and respiration is absorbed by the drier air. Responsible for 30% of the body's heat loss, insensible loss (5%) and sweating (25%) are the primary methods of cooling.

3. **Convection.** This method utilizes currents of air or water to transfer heat away from the body. In this situation, prolonged exposure to cool/cold water or air promotes rapid heat loss. It is an excellent method for those situations calling for immediate cooling but is less of a factor in hypothermia unless the temperatures are extreme.

4. **Radiation.** Infrared heat is transferred along the gradient from hot to cold objects. Radiation is the cause of up to 55% of heat loss.[35] Wearing a hat or covering the head and neck will conserve body heat.

Hypothermia

Hypothermia ranges along a continuum; measurement of core body temperature and mental status in conjunction with other clinical findings defines severity. By definition, a body temperature of 35°C (95°F) or below is defined as hypothermic with or without other clinical manifestations. Early systemic changes noted when the body temperature is 32°C (89.6°F) to 35°C (95°F) are tachypnea, tachycardia, and shunting of blood from the periphery to the core, often producing pale, cold extremities. Shivering, an unreliable sign, should not be used as a guide to treatment. As the body temperature continues to descend, moderately hypothermic persons, 30°C (86°F) to 32°C (89.6°F), experience a drop in heart and respiratory rate, loss of shivering, altered mental status, and decreased coordination. In severe hypothermia, a core body temperature less than 30°C (86°F), the victim will be very bradycardic and apneic, with a loss of reflexes, and exhibit acidemia, hypotension, and dysrhythmias. Often the victim is mistaken for dead.

Hypothermia has both negative chronotropic and inotropic effects on the heart, limiting cardiac output. Profound bradycardia increases the risk of thrombosis and embolism associated with hemoconcentration as a result of dehydration due to cold diuresis. A decrease in the spontaneous depolarization of pacemaker cells causes the bradycardia found in hypothermia to be refractory to atropine.[36] Both ventricular and atrial dysrhythmias are found in hypothermic patients due to the decrease in the fibrillation threshold. Researchers agree that atrial fibrillation is common, and like the more ominous ventricular fibrillation and asystole, usually converts spontaneously with rewarming.

Cold diuresis occurs in hypothermic individuals following an increase in blood flow to the core. Vasoconstriction increases resistance in the capillary beds, triggering diuresis in response to relative central hypervolemia. Cold diuresis hemoconcentrates the blood despite the overall decrease in glomerular filtration rate, increasing the risk of thromboembolism. Damage at the cellular level will occur if the body temperature drops below 35°C. Increased permeability of the capillary beds due to cold insult can produce crucial plasma loss into the interstitial space, worsening dehydration.

Initial tachypnea gives way to depressed respirations, retention of carbon dioxide, increased risk of aspiration due to bronchorrhea, and diminished cough and gag reflexes. Noncardiogenic pulmonary edema may develop.

Electrical activity in the brain slows and blood flow increases as hypothermia progresses. The central nervous system shuts down in an effort to conserve oxygen and energy, producing nonreactive, dilated pupils and coma on examination. It has been suggested that this response decreases oxygen need and may function as a protective mechanism to prevent further ischemic damage to the brain.[34] The usual treatment with Narcan, dextrose, and thiamine will not cause further harm to the patient. Never assume, however, that unresponsiveness is due to hypothermia.

Keep in mind the poor absorption rate of medications given intramuscularly secondary to vasoconstriction. The gastrointestinal tract also has impaired motility due to poor circulation, and medications will not be readily absorbed from this site. The liver in hypothermia is very slow to metabolize drugs; hence, toxic quantities can build up and be released during rewarming. Intravenous access is difficult in the severely hypothermic patient but is the preferred route for medications. However, most patients will respond to warming without the need to resort to drugs.

The degree of injury depends on the length of exposure time and the depth of the injury. Those people most prone to cold injury are the elderly, the very young, and hikers or those who have become hypothermic due to prolonged time out of doors in cool temperatures or wet conditions, particularly if they run short on food or become dehydrated. Hypothermia often has a gradual onset; however, it can be triggered abruptly by an event such as immersion in water.

Infants and young children, with their larger body surface area, lose heat more rapidly when exposed for even a short time to cool conditions. Of particular concern is the maintenance of infant body warmth during deliveries in the field or in a car or an unplanned home birth. Infants depend on heat production from a limited supply of brown fat, present only during the fetal and neonatal period. Usually not found in great supply in premature infants, brown fat contains mitochondria, an abundant energy source. Infants over 5 days of age have a limited supply of brown fat capable of doubling heat production; however, this form of nonshivering thermogenesis is accessed slowly by the infants' system. It is important to remember that infants do not shiver when they are cold; they simply become irritable, then lethargic.

Like neonates, the elderly frequently have little tolerance for prolonged cold due to failing thermoregulation and dwindling muscle mass, on which they rely for heat production. They are proportionally more vulnerable to heat loss due to impaired shivering mechanisms, decreased mobility, medication usage, and the inability to express the need for increased warmth. Elderly patients' perceptions of heat and cold may be dulled by chronic disease, peripheral neuropathy, or decreased vasomotor response. Cyclic antidepressants, neuroleptics, anti-Parkinson drugs, and barbiturates may impair the body's ability to shiver and thus the ability to produce heat.

For this reason, suspect and treat any patient exposed to cool, wet, or cold conditions as if they have hypothermia. Beware of transporting neonates and frail elderly in emergency vehicles that are overly cooled by air conditioning. While it frequently feels comfortable to the EMS provider, the passenger often requires additional covering to keep warm. Shivering, if present, increases oxygen consumption. For this reason, all hypothermic patients should receive warmed, humidified oxygen. Early recognition and aggressive intervention of the patient with mild hypothermia can ameliorate the progression of life-threatening hypothermia.

Recognition of hypothermia can be difficult. Initially, the patient may appear tired and express a vague feeling of malaise. Intervention at this point with rest, fluids, drying, and warmth can halt progression. The most common symptom of early hypothermia is an alteration in mental status. The patient may become confused and irritable, demonstrate irrational behavior and slurred speech, and eventually, lose consciousness. Ataxia or uncoordinated, stiff movements may be present along with loss of fine motor skills. Shivering may or may not be present and is an unreliable sign of hypothermia. Observe the skin for color changes and temperature. Is it red, pale, or cyanotic? Does it feel warm, cold, doughy, or wooden? A thermometer capable of registering low body temperature should be used for an accurate assessment of the core temperature. While rectal temperatures do not accurately reflect true "core" temperatures, few providers have the more sophisticated esophageal or urinary thermometers at their disposal. If you have them use them; otherwise use rectal temperatures, realizing that a probe inserted into frozen feces will not be accurate but may be your only option.

When severely hypothermic, the patient's heart is vulnerable to ventricular fibrillation, which can be triggered by rough handling or overstimulation. Respiration may be undetectable; therefore, the EMS provider is urged to check for pulse and respiration for 1–2 minutes. The medical caveat is "the patient is not dead until he is warm and dead."[34–36]

Treat the hypothermic patient by gently moving him or her to a sheltered, warm, dry area. Remove all wet clothing and surround the patient with dry covering. To conserve energy, cover the head and neck as these areas lose heat most rapidly. Do not rub the extremities; this only stimulates blood flow to the periphery, decreasing blood circulation to vital organs. Rubbing may also produce additional tissue damage if frostbite is present. In mild hypothermia, often all that is required is warm fluids and rest in a warm, dry environment. Avoid use of caffeine-containing beverages such as coffee or hot chocolate because of possible cardiac stimulation. Likewise, avoid alcohol, which can cause peripheral vasodilatation, shunting blood away from the core and further compromising vital organ function. The use of nicotine products, including patches, should also be avoided because they cause further vasoconstriction. Opt instead for warm soup unless the patient displays a decreased level of consciousness, which would require warm IV fluids and warmed, humidified oxygen.

It is important to establish the length of time the patient has been exposed, determine associated injuries, ascertain underlying medical conditions, and generally observe the setting in which the victim is found. Do not be deterred by the condition of the body; damage due to frostbite can cause deterioration of the skin, which may appear gruesome. If the victim is determined to be in respiratory arrest, warmed supplemental oxygen should be administered using a positive-pressure ventilation method. The field is not the optimal setting for intensive rewarming efforts so, unless the setting is a remote one with definitive care several hours or days away, rewarming is best limited to drying, insulating, oxygenating, and cardiac monitoring. Small-volume fluid challenges of 250–500 mL of warm 5% dextrose and normal saline should be judiciously administered.

Because the myocardium is so irritable, cardiac compressions should not be performed unless total absence of a pulse is determined. Remember that the hypothermic patient is in a state that requires very little oxygen; hence, circulation can be very minimal yet still sustain life. Defibrillation at 2 watt-seconds per kilogram may be performed once. If unsuccessful, cardiopulmonary resuscitation should be initiated and maintained throughout the trip to the ED. Successful defibrillation is rare until the body temperature is above 28°C (82.4°F) to 30°C (86°F). As the patient rewarms, oxygen consumption will increase proportionally. Be sure the airway is secure and the oxygen source adequate. Intubation is indicated to protect the airway and should not be withheld for fear of inducing dysrhythmias.

Once in the ED, continuous core temperature monitoring must be maintained, by esophageal, rectal, or urinary probe. Cardiac monitoring and cautious placement of central venous catheters and nasogastric tube with insertion of a Foley catheter and urometer should be performed. Anything touching or going into the patient should be warmed, including blankets, fluids, and oxygen. Laboratory data, including blood sugar, electrolytes, toxicology screen, ABGs, chemistry panel, coagulation profile, creatinine, and BUN, are all necessary to obtain a full clinical picture. If decreased level of consciousness continues after rewarming, thyroid studies, cardiac enzymes, and cortisol levels should be procured. Radiographic imaging of the chest and abdomen is necessary and, with suspected trauma, so are cervical spine films.

Dehydration is almost universal in moderate to severe hypothermia and rapid volume expansion is critical. Use warm, 40°C (104°F) to 42°C (107.6°F), boluses of 250–500 mL of 5% dextrose and normal saline, avoiding lactated Ringer's due to the hypothermic liver's inability to adequately metabolize lactate. Observe closely for fluid overload.

There are two primary methods for rewarming described in the literature. One or both may be used depending on factors such as availability of equipment, the patient's clinical status, and the degree of hypothermia involved in the injury. The first, passive external rewarming (PER), is always the treatment of choice for mildly hypothermic patients. Simply put, PER requires the patient to be covered with dry, warm, insulating material to minimize further heat loss and to transfer heat to the patient through radiation. It requires the ability to control ambient air temperature and prevent drafts. The patient must be able to shiver in order to raise the body temperature. A caution here: Glycogen stores are rapidly used up during shivering, and close monitoring of the blood glucose is essential. Temperature increases of 0.5°C–2.0°C per hour are usually adequate. This safe, easy method of rewarming can be performed almost anywhere.

The second form of rewarming is active rewarming, which is further distinguished as either active external rewarming (AER) or active internal rewarming (AIR). It becomes necessary to use one of the active methods when the patient demonstrates the following:

- Failure to rewarm passively or rewarming at an inadequate rate
- Cardiovascular instability
- Moderate to severe hypothermia (less than 32°C)
- Impaired thermoregulation due to CNS or endocrine malfunction
- Pharmacological impairment of thermoregulatory mechanism
- Acute spinal cord transection impairing thermoregulation

Active external rewarming remains somewhat controversial due to greater variation in survival rates, problems such as afterdrop (a rebound drop in core temperature as cold blood reenters circulation) and hypotension, and its more invasive nature. AER requires the use of exogenous heat sources such as hot water bottles, hot water immersion, plumbed garments, and heated water mattresses. Several large drawbacks are inherent, including special equipment, space constraints, and the difficulty of maintaining cardiopulmonary resuscitation (CPR) on a body floating in a hot water bath. As stated earlier, CPR may be a prolonged effort over several hours depending on the body temperature. The use of automated cardiac compression devices, such as the "Thumper," may be of help here. When the periphery begins to open up, the cold, pooled blood reenters active circulation. This can trigger afterdrop, a sudden drop in core body temperature, or embolic events due to clots formed by hemoconcentration that are freed into circulation. Afterdrop can be minimized by placing hot water bottles in the armpits and groin areas until cardiac output improves. AER is best used on moderately hypothermic individuals who have undergone sudden cold immersion injury and have no other known underlying health conditions, or

infants whose predictably rapid response to warming will minimize energy expenditure.

The last option, AIR, is by far the quickest method of rewarming but is invasive and carries significant risk. This method, however, is a necessity in severely hypothermic patients if they are to have any hope for survival. Table 23-7 displays several adjuncts that may be used in the process.

Predicting recovery in the event of cold injuries is difficult due to the vast physiological differences individuals display. In the field, EMS providers are likely to be called upon to perform passive rewarming and rapid transport of those persons suffering from hypothermia. Conditions or events that may impair CNS and hypothalamic responses include subdural hematoma, drug overdose, carbon monoxide poisoning, cerebrovascular accidents, and basilar skull fractures. Additionally, impaired metabolic response to cold can be seen in diabetes, epilepsy, hypothyroidism, and myxedema. Dementia due to alcoholism, Alzheimer's, or Parkinson's disease can alter appropriate responses to cold conditions, setting the stage for the development of hypothermia. Rapid recognition and intervention by EMS personnel can mean the difference between recovery and death.

Table 23-7
Methods of Active Internal Rewarming

1. Cardiopulmonary bypass (CBP): In a setting where CBP is available, it remains the treatment of choice for severely hypothermic patients. Requiring the use of a blood warmer and cannulation of the femoral veins, CBP produces a rapid, even increase in body temperature and blood volume eliminating afterdrop. Like peritoneal dialysis, it allows for correction of electrolyte imbalances. It is ideal in cases requiring prolonged cardiopulmonary resuscitation due to profound hypothermia. The disadvantage is that special equipment is necessary along with the personnel trained to perform the procedure. These are often not available outside of tertiary care facilities.

2. Peritoneal irrigation: The use of peritoneal irrigation is key in reversing hypothermia in the severely compromised patient. Its advantage lies in the ability to simultaneously correct electrolyte imbalances and rapidly rewarm the core organs, including the liver, which stimulates detoxification and release of glycogen stores. Two tubes must be introduced into the peritoneal cavity; warmed dialysate (40.5°C–42.5°C) is infused through one and removed through the other. This is essentially the same procedure as peritoneal dialysis. Risks are peritonitis and perforation. *Do not use* if abdominal trauma is suspected.

3. Airway rewarming: While not a significant source of heat, warm, humidified air facilitates clearance of secretions and mitigates the effects of afterdrop. *Do not use* if pulmonary edema is part of the clinical picture.

4. Pleural irrigation: This adjunct is used with open cardiac massage and may actually increase the heat loss due to the performance of open thoracotomy. This requires performance by highly trained professionals and is used to rewarm the heart directly.

5. Diathermy: This method of heat application employs the use of radio or microwave to the subcutaneous layers of the skin. It is cumbersome and expensive and requires special equipment and performance by trained personnel. *Do not use* if the patient is pregnant, has an implant of any kind, is known to have a malignancy, or has tuberculosis.

6. Gastrointestinal: Warmed irrigation of the colon or stomach is used cautiously. The danger of perforation, electrolyte imbalance, or ventricular fibrillation due to excessive stimulation is very real. *Do not use* if the patient has had recent gastric or colonic surgery.

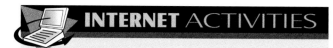

- Review the State of Alaska protocols for treating hypothermia at http://www.sarbc.org/hypo2.html.
- Visit the e-medicine Web site at http://www.emedicine.com. Click on the Emergency Medicine on-line book and select Environmental. Then click on Hypothermia. Review the chapter on the management of hypothermia.

Associated Cold Injuries

Because humans are physiologically constructed to lose heat, exposure to cold can result in injury. For homeostasis, living cells depend on blood circulation of nutrients and oxygen. When circulation is interrupted by vasoconstriction, cell injury and ischemia result, the extent of which depends on the type and length of exposure to the cold source. The protective mechanisms that result in shunting of blood from the periphery to the core, maintaining the heart, brain, and lungs, compromise the distribution of heat to vulnerable extremities. The associated cold-related injuries can range from mild, self-limiting frostnip to deep frostbite resulting in gangrene.

The same predisposing factors that make humans vulnerable to hypothermia are applicable to frostbite. Although homelessness has previously been considered a significant risk factor, the enthusiastic participation of young, otherwise healthy individuals in a plethora of cold weather sports has made frostbite and associated cold injuries commonplace in persons of varied socioeconomic backgrounds. When assessing the patient, recognize the need to prioritize interventions for hypothermia before that of caring for suspected frostnip or frostbite. Observe for constrictive or wet clothing and jewelry; remove it when possible. Immobility due to other underlying injury or entrapment further raises the likelihood of severe cold injury. Shock due to frostbite is rare and, if seen, alerts the provider to search for an underlying cause; treat shock before frostbite.

Immersion Foot More familiarly known as "trench foot," immersion foot is an injury that results not from freezing, but from prolonged exposure to wet conditions, which brings about decreased circulation, edema, and ischemia. The foot does not contain significant muscle or insulating fat and is, therefore, vulnerable to rapid cooling, even in warm water. While there is no freezing injury to the skin, muscle and nerve tissue are damaged by the exposure, and recovery may be hindered because of pain on weight bearing, ulceration, or superficial gangrene. Treatment consists of removal of the wet source, air drying, and elevation. Gentle handling of the waterlogged, swollen tissues is vital to prevent further injury. Constricting socks or foot coverings must be avoided.

Frostbite Frostbite, like hypothermia, evolves along a continuum dependent on type and length of exposure to cold elements. Lack of proper treatment can result in disability, pain, and loss of the affected body part. For this reason, rapid intervention and skilled handling by the EMS provider are essential. A most important caution is to *never thaw a frostbitten part unless one is certain that it will not be refrozen before arriving at a medical facility*. Refreezing of thawed tissue virtually guarantees death of that tissue.[34-36]

Frostbite occurs when tissue temperature reaches 0°C (32°F) and ice crystal formation begins. The formation of ice crystals within the tissue damages cellular structures and endothelium. Unstable cell membranes leak, resulting in intracellular dehydration and local edema secondary to electrolyte shifts. Stasis and thrombosis formation within the capillary beds decrease oxygen transportation and delivery resulting in tissue ischemia. Superficial frostbite affects the epidermis and subcutaneous layers of skin, while deep frostbite involves the deeper dermal structures, nerves, and muscles (Figure 23-15). The sites most frequently affected are the distal extremities; fingers and toes; face, nose, ears; and penis.

Frostbitten skin initially appears red and progresses to a white-gray color with a firm feel; pulses may still be palpable although capillary refill is delayed. As it progresses, there is complete loss of feeling in the affected part, pulses are absent, skin and underlying fat and muscle feel wooden to the touch, and movements are clumsy and uncoordinated. Blister formation is clinically indicative of a deep frostbite injury that has partially thawed, and while clear blebs carry a more favorable prognosis than hemorrhagic ones, determination of the full extent of tissue damage in frostbite is often delayed for 1–3 months.[37]

Experts universally agree that rewarming of frostbitten body parts is best performed under controlled circumstances frequently not possible in the field. Hence, if you are not in a position to rapidly rewarm the affected body part, provide pain control with narcotic analgesics and prevent any further cold exposure or likelihood of refreezing. *Do not attempt to thaw the injury*. The only exception to this is if the time to transport and rescue is likely to be prolonged and there is a reasonable expectation that thawing will begin prior to reaching a medical facility.

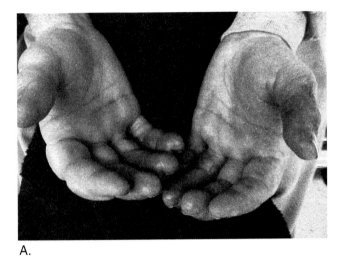

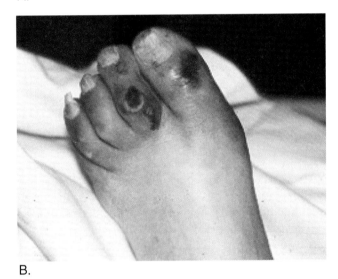

FIGURE 23-15 (A) Edema and blister formation 24 hours after frostbite injury. (Courtesy of Kevin Reilly, Albany Medical Center, Albany, NY.) (B) Deep frostbite results in permanent damage to tissue. (Courtesy of Deborah Funk, Albany Medical Center, Albany, NY.)

The paramedic, who may or may not be responsible for rewarming, shoulders a larger burden, that of assessing, packaging, protecting, and transporting the injured person. After ascertaining the type and extent of injuries present, gentle handling and protective packaging should be undertaken. Remove wet or constricting clothing and jewelry if it can be done without aggravating the injury. Treat for hypothermia and dehydration. Place dry gauze between affected digits and cover with a loose, sterile dressing. Erect a protective covering over the affected part to prevent secondary injury due to the weight of blankets. In the event of associated fractures, splint as necessary, but avoid constricting bandages, which can further compromise cir-

culation. Keep the extremity level with the heart; hands may rest on the chest. Never (1) break or attempt to aspirate blisters; (2) rub with snow or immerse the affected part in water; (3) attempt to warm the area by rubbing or chaffing the skin; (4) allow the patient to drink alcohol or use a nicotine product; or (5) warm the affected part with a dry heat source such as stove, hair dryer, or fire. The patient who has frostbitten extremities should be considered nonambulatory; however, if a life-threatening situation exists for either the patient or rescuer, walking on a frozen extremity usually will not harm it further. The greatest risk of damage is use after partial thawing has occurred.

Rewarming of the frozen body part should be accomplished rapidly, once initiated. Ideally, immersion of the affected part in a water bath constantly monitored for temperature (range of 39°C–42°C) for a period of 10–40 minutes will thaw the affected part. Slow, controlled patient movement rather than massage or manipulation hastens the thawing process. Thawing is exquisitely painful, though pain is generally a favorable indicator of reperfusion. Pain control during this early phase is necessary and is likely to be short term. Once rewarmed, avoid drying the affected part by hand; instead, allow it to air dry, thus avoiding further tissue damage. Separate fingers and toes with cotton or gauze to facilitate full drying of interdigital spaces.

Frostnip Frostnip occurs when only the topmost layers of the skin freeze and is generally reversible without significant damage. The skin surface appears pale and feels firm, but the underlying tissue remains soft to palpation. Treatment consists of gently warming the affected area by placing the body part, often the fingers, toes, earlobes, or cheeks, between two warm surfaces. A good method is to place the fingers under the arm pit or between the thighs, allowing body heat to gradually warm them. Untreated frostnip can progress to frostbite with continued cold exposure.

SEA

DIVING EMERGENCIES

Self-contained underwater breathing apparatus (scuba) diving, a recreational pastime enthusiastically embraced by people of all ages in a myriad of settings around the world, has led to an increase in the number of diving-related injuries faced by EMS personnel. Not only a sport, diving may be involved in construction, demolition, repair, underwater photography, search and rescue, as well as several scientific areas of study, including geology, oceanography, environmental research, archeology, geology, and biology. A wealth of argot, or jargon, litter the language of diving enthusiasts, creating a descriptive vocabulary unique to this sport. In this section, discussion centers on "the bends," "the chokes," "rapture of the deep," "the squeeze," "POPS," "gas in the gut," and "the staggers." Snorkeling is differentiated from diving because it does not involve submersion at depths of 1 atmosphere (33 feet) or below for a protracted period of time. In addition, understanding of two basic gas principles is crucial to comprehending the mechanism of injury involved in underwater emergencies:

- **Boyle's law:** The volume of a gas is inversely related to its pressure at a constant temperature. That is, the volume of gas will increase or decrease depending on the ambient pressure exerted by the environment. This same gas, however, expands the closer one gets to the surface.

- **Henry's law:** Gas will enter into a given volume of solvent in proportion to the partial pressure of the gas. In diving, nitrogen and oxygen will dissolve into the blood and tissue, being forced there by the increase in pressure. Reabsorption is slower, requiring ascent to be accomplished in stages to prevent embolism.

Compressed air is composed of 79% nitrogen and 21% oxygen, just like the air we breathe on the surface. The increase in pressure created by the density of water forces nitrogen and oxygen to dissolve from the lungs into blood and body tissue. Nitrogen, unlike oxygen, which is readily utilized by the body, accumulates in fatty tissue, particularly the myelin sheath and nervous system tissue. If adequate decompression is not obtained during ascent, nitrogen "bubbles out of the tissue," forming an air embolism that compromises circulation and may trigger multiple CNS and cardiovascular system disturbances. Mechanical injury of the vascular and lymphatic system is a result of obstruction, endothelial insult, transcapillary fluid losses, and increased blood viscosity leading to hypoperfusion and ischemia.

The use of diving tables allows a diver to calculate the amount of air and decompression time required to complete a dive within an allocated safety margin. A slow, methodical ascent allows sufficient time for the nitrogen to come out of the tissues and be transported to the lungs and exhaled. Decompression continues for several hours after reaching the surface with signs of decompression sickness occurring within 15 minutes to 12 hours after resurfacing. Several factors can influence development and severity of "the bends," including premature surfacing without use of decompression stops, obesity, advanced age, and alcohol consumption.

Cold water temperature can alter tissue perfusion and increase the likelihood of decompression sickness. Overall physical conditioning, exertion during the dive, and multiple dives occurring over several days can have a cumulative effect on the body.

Decompression Sickness

Decompression sickness (DCS) affecting the joints, known as "the bends," has the potential to become permanently disabling if unrecognized and untreated. Symptoms include severe joint pain, numbness, tingling, headache, fatigue, weakness, malaise, paralysis, and loss of bladder and bowel control. The large body joints, hip, shoulder, and knee are usually the first affected. A test for "the bends" utilizes a blood pressure cuff. When a cuff is placed over the affected joint and inflated to a pressure between 250 and 300 mm Hg, the joint pain will disappear, suggesting DCS. Maintain a high suspicion for decompression-related injury in anyone who reports diving within the last week.

Treatment is supportive with rapid transport to a decompression facility crucial. Oxygen should be administered at 100% and intravenous infusion of isotonic fluids titrated to a urine output of 1–2 mL/kg/hr. Immediate contact with a physician experienced in diving emergencies is imperative. If the victim must be air evacuated, the vehicle must have a pressurized cabin able to simulate sea level pressures. An element common to all diving emergencies is the need to treat the victim with 100% oxygen as expeditiously as possible. It is disheartening to note that as little as 33% of these victims actually receive oxygen in the field.[38] Significant disability could be avoided if this were improved. The **Gamow bag** is a portable hyperbaric chamber that can be used for temporary decompression while awaiting transport or space availability at a fixed site.

Other manifestations of DCS result when gas trapping causes a pressure differential that distorts the surrounding body structures, compromising blood supply, impinging on nerves, and effecting mucosal congestion. When "skin bends" occur, a marbling of the skin is seen, along with pruritis, burning, and rashes. Cutaneous manifestations can be precursors of further symptomatology of DCS. "The staggers" are used to describe the onset of CNS symptoms suggestive of cerebral impairment due to ischemia of the microcirculation in the brain. Seizures, scotomas (blind spots), diplopia, ataxia, vertigo, nystagmus, tinnitus (ringing in the ears), inappropriate behavior, and mental status changes are suggestive of this syndrome. Respiratory failure and shock can result from "the chokes," a variation of DCS affecting the pulmonary system. Cough, dyspnea, and chest pain are the most common presentations.

INTERNET ACTIVITIES

Visit the Virtual Naval Hospital Web site at
http://www.vnh.org/FSHandbook/11mgmt_dcs.html
and review the material on diving emergencies.

Arterial Gas Embolus

Arterial gas embolus (AGE), a life-threatening condition with a dramatic onset, occurs secondary to lung overpressurization and rupture when air is forced out of the alveoli and into the surrounding tissue or bloodstream because of the diver's failure to exhale on ascent. Underlying lung diseases such as asthma, emphysema, chronic obstructive pulmonary disease (COPD), or other air-trapping conditions play a significant role in the development of AGE. Symptoms are abrupt. Suspicion of AGE following the report of collapse immediately upon surfacing should be high. The air embolus may lodge in the brain, heart, or blood vessel, producing confusion, headache, tingling, numbness, weakness, convulsions, paralysis, unconsciousness, and death. A classic sign is asymmetrical multiplegia or paralysis. Sensory changes may include blindness, deafness, vertigo, and aphasia. Intracranial pressure rises rapidly. Any change in mental status or a decreasing level of consciousness should raise suspicion of embolus. The brain is the most common site of embolism because most divers ascend in a head-first position. Embolism to the left ventricle can cause cardiac arrest. Treat with ACLS protocols and rapid transport to a decompression facility.

Treatment hinges on immediate evacuation to a site where hyperbaric chamber decompression and intervention by a physician specializing in diving emergencies are located. Field administration of 100% oxygen by mask and maintenance of body temperature are supportive, with the oxygen used to create a gradient surrounding the bubbles, decreasing their size and forcing the nitrogen out. In the nonbreathing victim requiring intubation, hyperventilation may be used to decrease intracranial pressure. Circulation is further improved by decreasing tissue edema through vasoconstriction; this eases breathing by decreasing hypoxia. Those patients experiencing seizures should be treated with intravenous diazepam after securing the airway. The only way to halt the ischemic process caused by the embolus is to provide oxygen and recompress the victim. Always treat victims of suspected air embolus for DCS. Transportation of the victim is best accomplished supine, as extended transport in Trendelenburg or Durant's position (left lateral recumbent with head

down) increases cerebral edema and may compromise respiration.

Prevention of air trapping within the lungs is accomplished by forced exhalation throughout the surfacing procedure. In addition to air embolism, concomitant pneumothorax or subcutaneous emphysema may occur following overpressurization within the pulmonary cavity.

Pulmonary Overpressurization Syndrome

Pulmonary overpressurization syndrome (POPS), or "burst lung," may be seen with or without AGE. In this situation, an area in the alveoli weakens and ruptures secondary to the rapid expansion of gas within the lung. Associated physiological occurrences include pneumomediastinum, pneumopericardium, subcutaneous emphysema, pneumothorax, systemic air embolization, or pneumoperitoneum. Often called "the chokes," signs and symptoms include substernal chest pain, fullness in the throat, hoarseness, cough, dysphagia, dyspnea, and subcutaneous emphysema. In addition to the interventions for AGE, decompression of the chest with chest tube insertion must be accomplished rapidly. Rapid transport to a facility with decompression capabilities is essential.

Barotrauma of Descent

Barotrauma of descent comprises several syndromes collectively called "the squeeze syndromes." These syndromes, while not life-threatening emergencies, are painful, and if not treated promptly, have the potential to increase morbidity and disability. The ear squeezes are divided into three categories:

1. *Ear canal squeeze*: A result of trapped air in the ear canal, either natural (earwax) or man-made (earplugs). The tympanic membrane bulges *outward*, causing considerable pain. Ascent at the first sign of pain will "cure" this problem, while continuation of the dive will result in rupture of the eardrum. Examination often reveals rupture of the eardrum and petechia. Treatment consists of analgesics, keeping the ear canal dry, and no swimming or diving until healed. Antibiotics are only indicated if infection occurs.

2. *Middle-ear squeeze*: The most common of the syndromes, failure of the eustachian tubes to open during a Valsalva maneuver produced when yawning or swallowing can cause extreme vertigo, nausea, and disorientation. The principle is the same as used by individuals when flying: release the pressure, relieve the pain. Often due to

congestion, allergies, polyps, or trauma, diving with blocked eustachian tubes can be dangerous. It has been suggested that many near-drowning incidents can be linked to this syndrome. The tympanic membrane bulges *inward*, resulting in pain, usually severe enough to force the diver to the surface. Too rapid an ascent can result in cerebral air embolus as the tympanic membrane ruptures, releasing gas bubbles into the brain. Treatment includes decongestants, nasal spray, avoidance of water in the ear, and antihistamines if blockage is due to allergies. Antibiotics are only indicated if rupture occurred in polluted water.

3. Inner ear squeeze: Considered a medical emergency requiring immediate evaluation by an otolaryngologist, inner ear squeeze results in rupture of the oval or round window. This rupture forms a labyrinthine fistula with leakage of perilymph fluid. Permanent cochlear damage and hearing loss will result if untreated. The triad of hearing loss, vertigo, and tinnitus are classic symptoms of this condition. Other signs and symptoms include nausea, vomiting, disorientation, pain, ataxia, and a feeling of fullness. Nystagmus may or may not be present.

Other hollow spaces can be "squeezed" resulting in pain, disruption of membranes, and bleeding. The paranasal sinuses are subject to such occurrences, with treatment similar to that for middle-ear squeeze. Rarely barodontalgia, or "exploding tooth," can happen when an air pocket secondary to tooth decay or loose filling ruptures with descent or ascent. "Gas in the gut," or aerogastralgia, results when excessive amounts of air are swallowed during the dive, a person is chewing gum while diving, or a person has consumed carbonated beverages prior to diving. Symptoms include colicky pains, belching, and flatulence. This is seen more in inexperienced divers and is alleviated by freely passing flatus or belching during the dive.

INTERNET ACTIVITIES

Visit the e-medicine Web site at http://www.emedicine.com. Click on the Emergency Medicine on-line book and select Environmental. Then click on Barotrauma. Review the chapter on the management of barotrauma.

Nitrogen Narcosis

Nitrogen narcosis can occur when breathing compressed gas during a dive. The ensuing intoxication has effects similar to those of narcotics and has been nick-named "rapture of the deep" and is experienced by both novice and experienced divers. Symptoms include inappropriate behavior, euphoria, hallucinations, memory loss, delayed reflexes, and impairment of judgment and logic. Nitrogen narcosis is thought to play a significant role in near-drowning incidents. Treatment is ascending to safety.

It is vitally important that anyone who dives be properly educated and equipped. Never dive alone; always dive using the buddy system. Always use dive tables and allow adequate time for decompression stops. Duke University Medical Center is the home base for the Diver's Alert Network (DAN), an ongoing research and treatment center for all types of injuries related to diving mishaps. A physician specializing in diving-related injuries is available for consultation by phone for an emergency. The 24-hour hot line is (919) 684-8111. Multiple publications and an EMS video can be obtained by calling (919) 684-2948.

NEAR DROWNING

Drowning is asphyxiation following submersion in a liquid medium.[39–41] Near drownings are those incidents in which a patient survives greater than 24 hours after the episode of asphyxiation. Aspiration of water into the lungs with concomitant hypoxia is the end result of "wet" drowning. Laryngospasm, responsible for airway obstruction in "dry" drowning, is an infrequent occurrence, accounting for only 10%–15% of all deaths by drowning.[39–41] Even if ventilation is reestablished, cerebral hypoxic insult secondary to damage to the pulmonary system may be irreversible. Nevertheless, resuscitation of any drowning victim should be aggressive, providing the basis for the attempt to improve the outcome.

Several studies have demonstrated a bimodal age configuration of subjects most likely to be victims of near drowning. Children under 4 years of age account for 40% of all occurrences, with freshwater drowning in pools and lakes more common than saltwater.[2,39–41] The elderly, often drowning in the bathtub, are the other group at high risk. Alcohol consumption is a significant factor both in the circumstances surrounding the incident and in poor overall outcome following a submersion episode.[2,39–41] Any incident involving a bathtub drowning should engender suspicion of abuse or neglect rather than assume a chance event.

The effect of water aspiration on the alveolar surface is profound. Research has shown that although there are physiological differences in the mechanism of response in a freshwater aspiration versus saltwater aspiration, the terminal event is hypoxia due to compromised gas exchange. Table 23-8 compares the chain of events in these two types of drowning.

Emergency field treatment includes immediate assessment of the ABCs, with administration of 100% oxygen and CPR. Concurrent spine precautions are standard as a high incidence of neck injuries has been demonstrated to accompany near drowning. The Heimlich maneuver is only indicated for an obstructed airway and should not be used to facilitate drainage of water. In fact, attempts to remove water from the lungs is contraindicated because it can aggravate an existing spine injury, may delay or compromise administration of CPR, and has shown little efficacy in improving outcomes. Vomiting with concomitant aspiration is a larger concern. Suction should be set up and readily available. Dry the victim and provide for maintenance of body temperature. As discussed under cold injuries, hypothermia is a significant comorbidity in submersion injuries. Insertion of a Foley catheter to measure urinary output assists in assessment of fluid needs. Initiation of an IV line of warm isotonic fluid facilitates administration of drugs in the event of cardiac arrest. Those patients who are conscious require emotional support. If the near drowning involves a child, do not forget the emotional needs of the parents.

Maintain a high level of suspicion for postsubmersion syndrome if responding to a situation involving shortness of breath when there is a history of recent (72 hours) near drowning. Instances in which the victim initially showed no ill effects but deteriorated rapidly postinjury with complications of pulmonary edema and aspiration pneumonia are frequently seen. Attempt to elicit a history from bystanders or family about the length of time submerged, temperature of the water, underlying health problems, and alcohol or drug use.

Water-damaged lungs may initially demonstrate clear radiographs or can demonstrate aspiration pneumonia and pulmonary edema. Asymptomatic individuals without respiratory complaint should still have a full medical evaluation. Late respiratory complications following near drowning have been documented in a sufficient number of cases to warrant hospitalization and close observation for at least 24 hours following resuscitation.

As would be expected, the most frequent complications are aspiration pneumonia, pulmonary edema, and ARDS. Be alert for complaints of increasing shortness of breath, development of frothy sputum, cough, cyanosis, unconsciousness, and alteration in mental status. Take all cases of near drowning seriously. Cerebral hypoxia can result in permanent neurological impairment.

The most important fact about drowning is that most drownings are preventable. Encourage both children and parents to attend water safety and swimming classes designed specifically to prevent near drowning. Never leave young children unattended in the bathtub or pool for any reason. Obey warning signs at beaches and lakes; observe tidal activity notices. Do not participate in water sports without a life jacket. Observation of basic water safety rules can prevent disastrous outcomes and unnecessary tragedy.

MARINE ENVENOMATIONS

The vast oceans of the earth are home to thousands of species of marine animals, many of which are dangerous to humans. Increasingly over the last several decades, as advances in marine technology and interest in expanding our knowledge of the sea have grown, humanity's encroachment into the last great unknown wilderness has escalated the number of injuries following encounters with sea life. Research shows that the toxins and poisons found in sea life are among the most damaging and potentially injurious the world has ever known. Several factors influence the severity of the host response to marine envenomations: (1) amount and type of venom; (2) host response to the toxin; (3) age; (4) baseline health status; and (5) surface area involved.

It is not only poison that is a concern. Highly publicized accounts of shark attacks, while greatly exaggerated, do occur. Trauma in the form of bites, envenomations, lacerations, and punctures are common events to those EMS personnel who work in and near coastal areas, as well as those who perform duties in more nontraditional settings like cruise ships, university externships, or volunteer field work in other countries. A

Table 23-8 **Comparison of Freshwater versus Saltwater Drowning**	
Freshwater	**Saltwater**
Hypotonicity resulting in osmotic movement from within the lungs into the bloodstream	Hypertonicity creates osmotic gradient, drawing fluid into the lungs and causing hemoconcentration
Electrolyte dilution secondary to relative hypervolemia	Electrolyte concentration with relative hypovolemia
Surfactant function compromised by water influx resulting in atelectasis and alveolar collapse	Pulmonary edema
Impaired gas exchange	Impaired gas exchange
Hypoxia	Hypoxia

significant portion of the United States borders warm ocean waters, which harbor a variety of venomous sea life, although the colder waters off New England and the Pacific Northwest also host an array of marine creatures. While few marine animals are aggressive, human intrusion into their habitat engenders a fearful, often violent, response to that invasion. Most injuries to humans occur during handling of the creature or inadvertently stepping upon it.

Science has yet to uncover all the chemicals, proteins, polypeptides, and other substrates that combine to create marine toxins. Research has shown marine life toxins to be some of the most lethal known. Additionally, many marine animals cause injury by mechanical means, such as biting, lacerating, or crushing the victim. For the sake of simplicity and clarity, the mechanism of inflicting injury will be used to delineate treatment and guide field care. It is not vital to memorize an exhaustive list of marine creatures whose toxin or sting might be the source of painful or deleterious wounds, but rather it is important to be familiar with local marine life in one's area of practice and to recognize and respond to the detrimental effects of an encounter when it occurs. There are primarily three ways a marine animal can harm a human: bites, stings, and nematocysts.

Bites

Biting injuries are a mechanical means of producing trauma in a victim. The shark, barracuda, seal, sea lion, and eel are among the more common creatures that can administer traumatic wounds via multiple teeth and strong jaws. Shark bites appear rounded, in contrast to that of a barracuda, which is "V" shaped or in straight rows.[42] Bites of seals and sea lions, if unprovoked, should be considered for rabies prophylaxis as well. While the octopus does not have teeth, it does have a strong beak capable of delivering potent, occasionally fatal, venom stored in salivary glands. There is no antidote; treatment is supportive. Most of these injuries can be avoided by avoiding swimming and diving in areas known to be infested.

All sea snakes are poisonous, but fortunately in the United States, only in Hawaii and the southern Gulf of California are they endemic. Sea snakes can reach lengths of 3–4 feet or greater and have flat finlike tails. The bite of a sea snake should be assumed to be poisonous and is treated similarly to a bite experienced on land. Sea snake antivenin, however, is distinctly different from terrestrial antivenin (which is not effective for these envenomations). Initially there is no pain, but usually within 2 hours muscle stiffness, malaise, and euphoria or anxiety begin. Spastic or ascending paralysis can accompany other CNS and respiratory complications. Aggressive airway support and ACLS protocols may be necessary.

Establish an airway early, particularly if there are any signs of respiratory distress. Control of hemorrhage, wound irrigation and cleaning, splinting of fractures or dislocations, and treatment of shock are primary responsibilities. Initiate trauma lines of warm lactated Ringer's or normal saline for volume support. Tetanus prophylaxis, pain control, and rapid transport to the ED closely follow these measures. Contamination of the wound by organisms such as *Vibrio*, *E. coli*, *Staphylococcus*, and *Clostridia* is difficult to avoid, particularly with the level of water pollution found along many coastlines.

Stings

Stings are common in the water environment and basically involve piercing of the skin and injection with some form of venom. Most sea creatures use this as a form of defense as humans are far too large to be considered a meal. Stonefish, sea urchins, zebra fish, cone shells, starfish, catfish, scorpion fish, lionfish (Figure 23-16), and a host of others are capable of producing an excruciatingly painful wound. The spines often break off in the wound and must be removed carefully using forceps and always wearing gloves, as many of the spines are covered in a toxic, irritating slime. As expected, the site of injury is usually the foot and lower leg, although the hands and forearms can be damaged if the marine life was being handled, as is often the case.

Stingrays burrow in sand and are often stepped on. The animal becomes frightened and flings its barbed tail upward creating a tearing puncture loaded with venom. The Atlantic stingray, shown in Figure 23-17, is an example of the typical shape and configuration of rays.

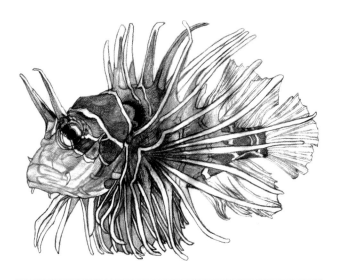

FIGURE 23-16 The lionfish.

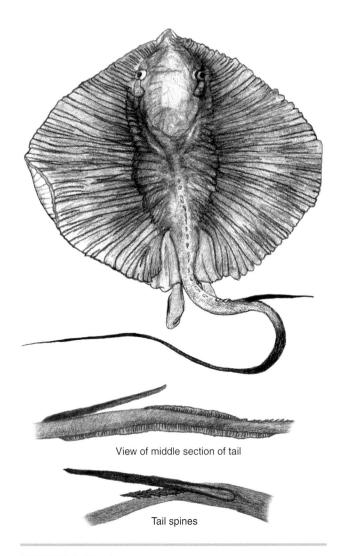

View of middle section of tail

Tail spines

FIGURE 23-17 Atlantic stingray.

Wounds to the abdomen or thorax by the larger species of rays amount to major trauma with retention of the spine and bits of organic matter. These injuries often require surgical intervention. Heat-labile toxin can be neutralized with hot water immersion. Avoidance is best, but unfortunately, rays and most other marine life enjoy the same shallow, warm water humans do.

Signs and symptoms of envenomation include pruritis, burning, and stinging, which usually occur immediately following contact. The development of blisters, edema, and petechial hemorrhage following stings are common with formation of skin ulcers and secondary skin infection in 1 or 2 weeks. Severe reactions can result in multisystem organ failure, CNS dysfunction, cardiac arrhythmia, delirium, coma, and death.

Treatment for this type of injury is supportive, as few antitoxins exist. Secure the ABCs, start oxygen, initiate IV therapy, control bleeding, place on a cardiac monitor, keep the victim warm and dry, and administer medication for pain control. A plethora of symptoms can follow the intense burning pain these envenomations engender, including nausea, vomiting, muscle fasciculation or paralysis, respiratory distress, seizures, cardiac arrhythmia, neurological disturbances, erythema, edema, and hypotension. Death, although rare, can occur in response to either the toxic envenomation or the hypersensitivity reaction/anaphylaxis resulting from the victim's physiological and immunological reaction. Any envenomation resulting in respiratory complications has the potential to be life threatening. Do not delay transport while attempting to remove retained spines; this may be more easily performed in the ED.

Ideally, removal of toxic slime and neutralization of the irritant should be performed at the scene for optimal outcome. Use of sea water rinse is advocated against that of fresh water due to certain chemical properties of the high molecular-weight toxins. Neutralization with 5% acetic acid (vinegar), isopropyl alcohol, or a baking soda paste, depending on the type of venom, has been somewhat effective in detoxifying the injury.

Following arrival in the ED the affected extremity will be further irrigated and the wound explored. Radiographs should be obtained as the spines, stingers, and barbs are radiolucent and are easier to identify on X-ray. Sea urchin spines will often stain the wound, creating the illusion of a retained foreign body. After X-ray and removal of foreign material the affected extremity should be plunged into a hot water bath (43°C–45°C) for 30–90 minutes. This will generally inactivate the heat-labile venom. Antihistamines, steroids, and analgesics should be dispensed following a period of observation. The decision to admit the patient should be based on symptomatology. Prophylactic antibiotics are not indicated unless wound infection occurs. It is important to schedule the patient for follow-up wound checks in 1 or 2 days to assess the need for antibiotics. If wound infection occurs, a culture should be obtained to identify the offending organism and guide antibiotic therapy. Tetanus status should be assessed on arrival to the ED and prophylaxis given if the patient is unable to document current status.

Nematocysts

Invertebrates such as the jelly fish, Portuguese man-of-war, corals, and sea anemones inject venom via specialized epithelial cells called nematocysts. The soft and "feathery" appearance of many of these creatures often tempts divers and snorkelers to touch them, resulting in intensely painful injuries. The nematocysts cover the tentacles of the creature and are discharged into the prey on contact. The mechanism is much like a harpoon. A barb covered with venom is attached to a long threadlike tube. When the tentacle brushes against the surface of the object, it fires the barb, injecting the venom. Most of the marine fauna with this type of defense mechanism have thousands or hundreds of thousands of these nematocysts. Consequently, the wounds and host responses to such envenomations can be overwhelming. The box jelly fish, found in the Indo-Pacific and Australian waters, can cause death in 30–60 seconds. There has been an antidote developed; however, administering it in a timely fashion is obviously difficult. Those species found in U.S. waters, while agonizing, are not fatal.

Signs and symptoms of envenomation include intense pain, pruritis, burning, and stinging, which usually occur immediately following contact. The development of blisters, edema, and petechial hemorrhage following stings are common with formation of skin ulcers and secondary skin infection in 1 or 2 weeks. Severe reactions can result in multisystem organ failure, CNS dysfunction, cardiac arrhythmia, delirium, coma, and death.

Treatment on the scene consists of irrigation with sea water (fresh water will cause further discharge from the nematocysts), removal of tentacles (always with gloves or forceps), and neutralization with vinegar; then, gently cover with either shaving cream or baby powder, and finally scrape off with a knife or razor blade. Immersion in hot water (discussed earlier) for 30–90 minutes affords further pain relief and detoxification. Importantly, tentacles that have washed up onto beaches have the same potential for discharging nematocysts, and small children and unwary beachcombers are injured by these remnants, too. Avoidance of known habitats and observation of all coastal warning signs can aid in evading an encounter.

Ingested Toxins

Tetrodotoxin poisoning, which results from eating contaminated fish, has been a relatively rare event in the United States. The advent of gourmet restaurants featuring Japanese, Taiwanese, and other ethnic dishes containing those species of fish or shellfish known to be toxic has created an environment in which such occurrences may become more commonplace. Fugu (puffer fish), a Japanese delicacy, requires skilled handling by a chef certified in its preparation. Even then, contamination during processing can lead to inadvertent poisoning with this potent neurotoxin. Sixty percent of persons consuming a product contaminated by tetrodotoxin will die.[43] Several species of fish and shellfish contain toxins that can produce violent and unpleasant gastrointestinal distress within minutes to hours following a meal containing even the smallest amount of these toxic substances. Surprisingly, several common foods can be implicated, including red snapper, grouper, mussels, clams, crabs, tuna, mahi mahi, anchovies, and mackerel.

Symptoms include the onset of paresthesia of the oral mucosa, vomiting, faintness, and weakness beginning within 10–45 minutes following ingestion. Initially, most victims will describe a tingling or numbness of the lips and tongue or tightness in the throat. Portions as small as one-quarter of an ounce have been demonstrated to cause significant illness.[43] Six to 24 hours after ingestion an ascending paralysis with secondary respiratory paralysis will occur. Other symptoms include hypotension, bradycardia, increased salivation, muscle fasciculations, dysphagia, diaphoresis, chest pain, convulsions, and fixed, dilated pupils.

Treatment is mainly supportive with no specific antidote. Rapid recognition following a history of recent seafood consumption and demonstrable symptoms facilitates diagnosis. Activated charcoal and aggressive gastric lavage should be administered as soon as possible. Intravenous hydration in those who have experienced significant vomiting and fluid loss is beneficial.

Eating raw fish or other seafood is never a good idea because the level of contamination in many of the world's oceans, rivers, and lakes is distressing. The protection afforded by cooking with heat applies only to those bacteria, viruses, and toxins that are heat labile. Educate the public to be sensitive to the need for strict food handling, storage, and preparation procedures. By raising awareness of this growing problem, EMS providers can impact the incidence of food contamination illnesses as the public becomes attuned to the danger.

The plethora of sea creatures capable of inflicting intensely painful or lethal injuries is enormous. It is important to remove the victim of any envenomation from the water. Drowning as a result of toxic envenomation is thought to be more common than previously realized. Few of these venomous species have an antidote, and the ones that do must often be obtained from distant sources, sometimes as far as Australia. Treatment that is supportive in nature is the mainstay of prehospital care. By recognizing and handling the type of injury appropriately from the start, especially neutralization of toxin and airway maintenance, the EMS provider is paving the way toward optimal patient outcomes.

▶ SUMMARY

The regional diversity of the United States supplies the paramedic with an assortment of environmental illnesses and injuries. A common thread is the vital need to be prepared and thoroughly familiar with regional variations and idiosyncratic occurrences particular to a practice area. Additionally, skills must be finely honed to successfully manage the variety of events likely to be part of the local scene. Obviously, no single paramedic, physician, or scientist is an expert in all areas of environmental emergencies. However, the astute paramedic possesses a fundamental knowledge of the local milieu and is adept at seeking and pinpointing expert resources before the need arises. The accumulation of up-to-date resources and a handy list of local experts can expedite emergency care when seconds count.

▶ REVIEW QUESTIONS

1. When examining any bite wound what are the five primary points of assessment?
   a. Pulselessness, paresthesia, pinkness, pain, paralysis
   b. Pain, pallor, paralysis, petechia, pulse
   c. Paresthesia, pallor, pulselessness, paralysis, paronychia
   d. Pain, pallor, pulse, paralysis, paresthesia

2. What is the most common location of a bite?
   a. Face
   b. Leg
   c. Hand
   d. Buttocks

3. The tourniquet is only a valid tool in the setting of:
   a. Snakebite
   b. Amputation
   c. An old Western movie
   d. An emergency room

4. Untreated acute mountain sickness can progress to which life-threatening illness(es)?
   a. HAPE only
   b. HACE only
   c. Both HAPE and HACE
   d. None of the above

5. Emesis is contraindicated in:
   a. Unconsciousness
   b. Age under 6 months
   c. Suspected caustic toxin ingestion
   d. All of the above

6. Discuss the treatment for heatstroke, including signs and symptoms.

7. List the interventions for hypothermia and briefly discuss the basis for each action.

8. All victims of drowning, near drowning, or diving accidents should receive what intervention first?

9. Describe the treatment for a patient who has encountered a large Portuguese man-of-war.

10. List and explain the four methods of heat transfer.

11. What should a person who has experienced a snakebite never be given?

12. What should a paramedic do when a plant is suspected of causing illness?

13. What is an excellent source of help and information when dealing with a poisoning victim?

14. Never induce vomiting in a victim who is _____.

15. What liquids can be given to a person who has ingested acid or alkaline substances?

16. High altitude pulmonary edema is a form of ARDS and should be treated the same.
    a. True
    b. False

17. A diver who collapses on board a boat and appears to be suffering from decompression sickness should be taken back down into the water with a new oxygen tank and decompressed.
    a. True
    b. False

18. A person suffering from carbon monoxide poisoning will appear cherry red and smell of almonds.
    a. True
    b. False

19. A child who is suspected of swallowing vitamins does not need evaluation unless he or she becomes symptomatic.
    a. True
    b. False

20. Few poisons have specific antidotes; therefore, symptomatic treatment is often the mainstay of treatment.
    a. True
    b. False

▶ CRITICAL THINKING

● You are dispatched to the scene of a person found lying beside the roadway. The ambient temperature is 22°F. Upon arrival you find a 22-year-old female. She is arousable only to pain. There is blood matted in her hair which is partially frozen. She is heavily clothed but appears to have been lying on the roadside overnight. Her skin is very cold to touch. Pupils are equal and reactive but slow to respond. Blood pressure is 108/palpation, heart rate is 54 with sinus bradycardia and frequent preventricular contractions, and respiration is 18. What treatments are indicated for this patient?

Environmental Emergencies **565**

Explain the underlying pathophysiology of this patient's presentation.

- Some experts suggest that CPR not be performed if a severely hypothermic patient should experience cardiac arrest. Explain the rationale of this recommendation.

- You are dispatched to the scene of a possible drowning at a local rock quarry. Upon arrival, you are met by several scuba divers who state that their friend was diving with them around some submerged excavating equipment at 300 feet. His air line became entangled in the equipment and was severed as he tried to free himself. After his air line was severed, the patient rapidly ascended to the surface. Upon reaching the surface, the patient began seizing and was pulled from the water by his diving buddies. You are led to the patient, where you find a 28-year-old male actively seizing. Explain the pathophysiology underlying this patient's presentation. What treatment will you provide?

► REFERENCES

1. Legge M, Murphy M. Human bite wounds. *J Emerg Nurs.* 1990; 16:145.
2. Jimmerson CL. Environmental emergencies. In: Sheehy S, ed. *Emergency Nursing Principles and Practice.* St Louis: Mosby; 1992.
3. King RC, Giles J. Dealing with animal bites. *RN* 1984; 47:31.
4. Gold BS, Barrish RA. Venomous snakebites. *Emerg Med Clin North Am.* 1992; 10:249.
5. Otten EJ. Venomous animal injuries. In: Rosen P, Barkin RM, Braen CR, et al., eds. *Emergency Medicine: Concepts and Clinical Practice.* St Louis: Mosby Yearbook; 1992.
6. Rydel JJ, Aks S, Lewis BB, Ferrano CG, Leikin JB. Management considerations in copperhead envenomation. *J Emerg Nurs.* 1993; 19:3.
7. Weaver D, Stroup DR, Slafka BA, Kuzniewski J, Hughes C. Timber rattlesnake bite to hand with secondary coagulopathy and serum sickness. *J Emerg Nurs.* 1991; 17:193.
8. Allen C. Arachnid envenomations. *Emerg Med Clin North Am.* 1992; 10:269.
9. McSwain NE. Brown recluse spider envenomation. *Emerg Med.* 1989; 21:39.
10. Hibel J, Clore ER. Prevention and primary care treatment of stings from imported fire ants. *Nurs Pract.* 1992; 17:6.
11. Fichtenbaum CJ, Peterson LR, Weil GJ. Ehrlichiosis presenting as a life-threatening illness with features of the toxic shock syndrome. *J Med.* 1993; 95:351.
12. Sebilia AJ. When was your last tetanus shot? *RN.* 1984; 47:18.
13. Angelucci D, Todaro A. Action stat! Tetanus. *Nursing.* 1990; 20:33.
14. Somerson SW. A 57 year old man with muscle spasms. *J Emerg Nurs.* 1991; 17:257.
15. Groleau G. Tetanus. *Emerg Med Clin North Am.* 1992; 10:351.
16. Centers for Disease Control. Progress toward the global elimination of neonatal tetanus, 1989–1993. *MMWR.* 1994; 43:48.
17. Doan-Wiggins L. Animal bites and rabies. In: Rosen P, Barkin RM, Braen CR, et al, eds. *Emergency Medicine: Concepts and Clinical Practice.* St Louis: Mosby Yearbook; 1992; 864.
18. Centers for Disease Control. Mass treatment of humans exposed to rabies—New Hampshire, 1994. *MMWR* 1995; 44:26.
19. Groleau G. Rabies. *Emerg Med Clin North Am.* 1992; 10:361.
20. Centers for Disease Control. Rabies prevention—United States, 1991, Recommendations of the immunization practices advisory committee. *MMWR.* 1991; 40:5.
21. Centers for Disease Control. Jimson weed poisoning—Texas, New York, and California, 1994. *MMWR.* 1995; 44:3.
22. Friedman PA. Poisoning and its management. In: Petersdor RA, et al, eds. *Harrison's Principles of Internal Medicine.* New York: McGraw-Hill; 1983.
23. Tomaszewski C. Toxicology of plants. Presented at the Fifteenth Annual East Coast Emergency Medicine Seminar; September 17, 1996; Morehead City, N.C.
24. Michener DC, Keller R, Kowalski RF. Poisonous plants. In: Tintinalli J, Ruiz E, eds. *Emergency Medicine—A Comprehensive Study Guide.* New York: McGraw-Hill; 1996.
25. Linden DH, Dowsett RP. Mushroom poisoning. In: Tintinalli J, Ruiz E, eds. *Emergency Medicine—A Comprehensive Study Guide.* New York: McGraw-Hill; 1996.
26. Deason JG. Acute iron ingestion in a 2-year-old child. *J Emerg Nurs.* 1995; 21:9.
27. Tso E. High altitude illness. *Emerg Med Clin North Am.* 1992; 10:231.
28. Yaron M, Honigman B. High-altitude illness. In: Rosen P, Barken RM, Braen CR, et al, eds. *Emergency Medicine Concepts and Clinical Practice.* St Louis: Mosby Yearbook; 1992.
29. Williams B. Carbon monoxide poisoning prevention. *Epi Notes.* 1995; 95:1.
30. Centers for Disease Control. Carbon monoxide poisoning at an indoor ice arena and bingo hall—Seattle, 1996. *MMWR.* 1996; 45:13.

31. Beckerman B, Gordon J, Brody, G. The challenge of managing carbon monoxide poisoning. *J Am Acad Phys Assistance*. 1993; 6:188.

32. Olshaker JS, Tek D. Heat illness. *Emerg Med Clin North Am*. 1992; 10:299.

33. Lee-Chiong TL, Stitt JT. Heatstroke and other heat-related illnesses. *Postgrad Med.* 1995; 98:26.

34. Krone R. Frostbite and other localized cold related injuries. In: Tintinalli J, Ruiz E, eds. *Emergency Medicine—A Comprehensive Study Guide*. New York: McGraw-Hill; 1996.

35. Jolly BT, Ghezzi KT. Accidental hypothermia. *Emerg Med Clin North Am*. 1992; 10:2.

36. Danzl DF. Accidental hypothermia. In: Rosen P, Barkin RM, Braen CR, et al. Eds. *Emergency Medicine: Concepts in Clinical Practice*. St. Louis: Mosby Yearbook; 1992.

37. Danzl DF. Frostbite. In: Rosen P, Barkin RM, Braen CR, et al, eds. *Emergency Medicine: Concepts in Clinical Practice*. St. Louis: Mosby Yearbook; 1992.

38. Shinnick MA. Recognition of scuba diving accident and the importance of oxygen first aid. *J Emerg Nurs*. 1994; 20:105.

39. Olshaker JS. Near drowning. *Emerg Med Clin North Am*. 1992; 10:339.

40. Knopp RK: Near-drowning. In: Rosen P, Barkin RM, Braen CR, et al, eds. *Emergency Medicine: Concepts in Clinical Practice*. St Louis: Mosby Yearbook; 1992.

41. Haynes BE. Near drowning. In: Tintinalli J, Ruiz E, eds. *Emergency Medicine—A Comprehensive Study Guide*. New York: McGraw-Hill; 1996.

42. Brown CK, Shepherd SM. Marine trauma, envenomations, and intoxications. *Emerg Med Clin North Am*. 1992; 10:385.

43. Centers for Disease Control. Tetrodotoxin poisoning associated with eating puffer fish transported from Japan—California, 1996. *MMWR*. 1996; 45:19.

◀▶ BIBLIOGRAPHY

Auerbach PS. Stings of the deep. *Emerg Med*. 1989; 21:12.

Brodeur V, Dennett S, Griffin L. Exertional hyperthermia, ice baths, and emergency care at the Falmoth road race. *J Emerg Nurs*. 1989; 15:5.

Brown CK, Shepherd SM, Marine trauma, envenomations, and intoxications. *Emerg Med Clin North Am*. 1992; 10:2.

Centers for Disease Control. Human granulocytic ehrlichiosis—New York, 1995. *MMWR* 1995a; 44:32.

Centers for Disease Control. Lyme disease—United States, 1994. *MMWR*. 1995b; 44:24.

Centers for Disease Control. Jimson weed poisoning—Texas, New York, and California, 1994. *MMWR*. 1995c; 44:3.

Centers for Disease Control. Lead poisoning among sand-blasting workers, Galveston, Texas, 1994. *MMWR*. 1995d; 44:3.

Centers for Disease Control. Necrotic arachnidism—Pacific Northwest, 1988–1996. *MMWR*. 1996a; 45:21.

Centers for Disease Control. Scopolamine poisoning among heroin users—New York City, Newark, Philadelphia, and Baltimore, 1995 and 1996. *MMWR*. 1996b; 45:22.

Dickey LS. Barotrauma. In: Rosen P, Barkin RM, Braen CR, et al, eds. *Emergency Medicine: Concepts in Clinical Practice*. St Louis: Mosby Yearbook; 1992.

Doyle CJ. Acute exposure to toxic agents. In: Tintinalli J, Ruiz E, eds. *Emergency Medicine—A Comprehensive Study Guide*. New York: McGraw-Hill; 1996.

Falco RC, Fish D. Potential for exposure to tick bites in recreational parks in a Lyme disease endemic area. *Am J Pub Health*. 1989; 79:1.

Ferrara T. More on tick bites. *J Emerg Nurs*. 1991; 21:277.

Guenin DG, Auerbach PS. Trauma and envenomations from marine fauna. In: Tintinalli J, Ruiz E, eds. *Emergency Medicine—A Comprehensive Study Guide*. New York: McGraw-Hill; 1996.

Hanson A. Management of pit viper bites. Lecture to Thursday Morning Intellectual Society of Chatham Hospital. August 17, 1995.

Huston CJ. Action stat! Caustic chemical ingestion. *Nursing*. 1990; 20:33.

Jerrard DA. Diving medicine. *Emerg Med Clin North Am*. 1992; 10:2.

Kizer KW. Diving into trouble. *Emerg Med*. 1989; 21:60.

Kizer KW. Dysbarism. In: Tintinalli J, Ruiz E, eds. *Emergency Medicine—A Comprehensive Study Guide*. New York: McGraw-Hill; 1996.

Kriegsman W, Peppers MP. Flumazenil for benzodiazepine overdose. *Emergency*. Jan 1994; 21.

Middleton DB. Not all tickborne illness is Lyme disease. *Emerg Med*. 1993; 25:20.

Norris MKG. Pediatric near drowning. *Nursing*. 1993; 23:5.

North Carolina Department of Environment, Health, and Natural Resources. Management of animal bites. Veterinary Public Health Program; 1994.

Reisdorff EJ, Wiegenstein JG. Carbon monoxide poisoning. In: Tintinalli J, Ruiz E, eds. *Emergency Medicine—A Comprehensive Study Guide*. New York: McGraw-Hill; 1996.

Russell M, Tomchic R. Seabather's eruptions, or "sea lice." *J Emerg Nurs*. 1993; 19:3.

Shannon BE. Poisoning and ingestions. In: Jenkins JL, Loscalzo J, eds. *Manual of Emergency Medicine.* Boston: Little, Brown and Company; 1990.

Steere AC. Lyme disease. *N Engl J Med.* 1989; 321:586.

Williams B. Carbon monoxide (CO) poisoning prevention. *Epi Notes.* 1995; 95:1.

Yarbrough B. Heat illness. In: Rosen P, Barkin RM, Braen CR, et al, eds. *Emergency Medicine: Concepts in Clinical Practice.* St Louis: Mosby Yearbook; 1992.

Chapter 24

Geriatric Trauma

OBJECTIVES

Upon completion of this chapter, the reader should be able to:

- Discuss the most common causes of geriatric trauma.
- Describe the physiological changes associated with aging.
- Discuss management of the geriatric trauma patient.
- List and describe the more common injuries of the elderly and describe their management.

It is estimated that approximately 12% of the population of the United States is over age 55.[1] As the "baby boom" generation matures, this age could increase to as much as 21%.[1] Trauma is the fourth leading cause of death in the over-55 age group and the fifth leading cause in those over 75.[1] While trauma may be ranked higher as a cause of death in other age groups, more than one-third of all resources allocated to trauma are spent on the geriatric age group.[1] As the aged population increases, so do the resources required to manage geriatric trauma.

The causes of trauma in the geriatric population differ from those of younger populations. Researchers note that 60% of emergency medical requests due to injuries in the geriatric population are for injuries resulting from falls.[2] Both physiological changes and environmental changes are major contributing factors to this large number of falls. Another major cause of injury is motor vehicle collisions (21%).[2] Because physiological changes can both contribute to the cause of injury and potentially increase mortality rates resulting from injuries, it is important for prehospital providers to have a general understanding of these changes.

PHYSIOLOGICAL CHANGES

A major contributing factor to the intolerance of trauma in the geriatric trauma patient is the physiological process of aging. The degree of physiological change varies greatly among age groups. While the most dramatic changes are usually seen in the older geriatric patient (80–90 years old), younger geriatric patients (60–70 years old) may have pronounced changes if their general health status is poor. The best way to understand the magnitude of these changes is to examine them by system.

RESPIRATORY SYSTEM

As the human body ages, the chest wall becomes less compliant, resulting in a decrease in vital lung capacity. This alteration in lung compliance and vital capacity decreases the patient's ability to compensate for the stress caused by trauma. Several microscopic changes also take place in the respiratory system. Respiratory ducts begin to enlarge, leading to a decrease in the size of alveolar subunits and in the surface area available for gas exchange. This may be apparent in arterial blood gas analysis, which can demonstrate a decreased partial pressure of oxygen and an increased partial pressure of carbon dioxide.

Another change that can decrease the geriatric patient's ability to compensate in trauma is a decrease in ciliary action. As ciliary action decreases, the ability to cough and swallow decreases, making it difficult for the patient to protect the airway. This helps to explain the high incidence of pneumonia in the critically injured and hospitalized geriatric trauma patient.

CARDIOVASCULAR SYSTEM

The cardiovascular system's ability to compensate during traumatic insults declines slowly with age. Both maximal heart rate (HR) and stroke volume (SV) decrease. Decreases in maximum heart rate are related to a slowing of electrophysiological conduction. In addition to this physiological decrease, the geriatric patient may be taking beta blockers, which prevent normal physiological increases in heart rate in response to increased cardiac demand. Decreases in SV are related to stiffening of the myocardium and decreases in myocardial cell mass and blood supply. It is estimated that both HR and SV decline approximately 1% per year after age 20.[3] Whereas cardiac output is a function of both HR and SV, cardiac output also declines by approximately 1% per year after age 20.

Reentry dysrhythmias are a common problem in the geriatric population; constant monitoring is required to detect and treat such dysrhythmias. This fact, in conjunction with atherosclerosis and decreased peripheral vascular resistance, makes the geriatric patient's cardiovascular system ill equipped to handle the increased demands imposed by traumatic injuries.

NEUROLOGICAL SYSTEM

Around age 30 neuronal mass begins to decrease in certain critical areas. This can result in up to a 10% reduction in total neuronal mass by age 70. Loss of neuronal mass combined with an increase in the adherence of the dura to the cranium leads to an increase in the subdural space. Increases in the subdural space and decreases in the epidural space result in an increased incidence of subdural hemorrhages and a decrease in epidural hemorrhages.

The velocity of neuronal impulses and vascular perfusion of the nervous system can also decrease with aging. As a result, mentation may be altered and responses may be blunted. Forgetfulness, disorientation, and memory loss, along with visual and hearing

loss, not only make assessment of these patients difficult but also increase the risk of unintentional injury. These factors also partially account for the large number of falls experienced in this age group.

Finally, the geriatric patient can experience neurological changes resulting in alteration of the body's thermoregulatory system. As a result, the geriatric trauma patient is more prone to hypothermia. Hypothermia can complicate resuscitation efforts by decreasing the ability of the blood to clot, making it extremely difficult to achieve hemostasis.

GASTROINTESTINAL SYSTEM

As the gastrointestinal system ages, the secretion of digestive enzymes decreases, as does the basal metabolic rate. This can result in a decrease in the supply of proper nutrients to bodily systems. In addition, intake is often altered as a result of atrophy of the olfactory glands, loss of taste buds, gum disease, and degeneration of the teeth. After initial stabilization in the hospital setting, proper attention must be given to the nutritional needs of these patients.

RENAL SYSTEM

Proper functioning of the renal system is essential to acid-base balance. After age 50, there is loss of kidney mass involving whole nephron units, and the glomerular filtration rate decreases. This results in a loss of the ability to concentrate urine, decreasing the total body water.

Two significant problems can arise from these age-related physiological changes in the kidney. First, as total body water decreases, water-soluble medication distribution may be altered, affecting therapeutic actions. In addition, the kidney's ability to regulate hydrogen ion concentration is altered, frequently resulting in acid-base disarrangements.

MUSCULOSKELETAL SYSTEM

Aging brings about numerous changes to the musculoskeletal system, including decreases in normal bone density and muscle mass. As a result, there is a general loss of strength and a decreased resistance to fracture. Osteoporosis is another common problem associated with aging. Osteoporosis has been linked to decreases in estrogen levels, physical activity, body mass, and alterations in the body's ability to utilize calcium.

As a result of this general decline in the integrity of the skeletal system, the geriatric patient may experience spontaneous vertebral compression fractures. When a fracture occurs in the thoracic or lumbar spine, it can produce a "hump," known as lower dorsal kyphosis. Kyphosis may be present, to some degree, in up to 68% of the geriatric population. These patients require special considerations in injuries requiring immobilization of the spine. Hip fractures are another common problem associated with declining skeletal strength. Up to 1% of males and 2% of females over the age of 85 sustain a hip fracture each year.[4] Hip fractures can result in significant morbidity and mortality among this group.

Finally, there is a decrease in the amount of lean muscle tissue and an increase in the amount of fatty tissue. As a result of the increase in fat tissue, medications that are fat soluble take longer to reach therapeutic levels and decrease the rate of elimination.

INTEGUMENTARY SYSTEM

The most significant physiological change associated with aging is loss of normal skin elasticity. Loss of elasticity makes the skin prone to tearing, resulting in a higher incidence of soft tissue injury. Special care must be taken in lifting and moving the geriatric patient in order to prevent unnecessary tearing of the skin. In addition, because the skin is a barrier to outside agents, the increased incidence of soft tissue injury raises the risk of foreign invasion. Special care should be taken when dealing with soft tissue injuries to maintain a clean environment.

IMMUNE SYSTEM

In the geriatric patient, both cell-mediated and humoral immune responses to foreign antigens are decreased, while the response to autologous antigens are increased. This, in conjunction with the increased incidence of soft tissue injury mentioned above, drastically increases the risk of sepsis.

MANAGEMENT OF THE GERIATRIC TRAUMA PATIENT

AIRWAY

While assessment and management priorities for the geriatric patient are the same as for younger patients, challenges exist in treatment interventions. Management of the airway with a bag-valve mask can be complicated by poor teeth, dentures, or atrophy of the muscular structure of the face, making it extremely difficult to obtain an adequate seal. Mask seal may be improved by decreasing the amount of air in the mask, which often increases the conformity of the mask.

Management of the airway may also be complicated by cervical arthritis or kyphosis. Both can make hyperextension of the neck and visualization of the vocal cords extremely difficult. Coupled with poor teeth or dentures, this action requires that special care be taken to avoid contact with teeth, which could easily be displaced, further complicating management.

While aggressive airway intervention should not be withheld from the unconscious, apneic, or distressed geriatric patient, elective endotracheal intubation is discouraged. Geriatric patients receiving endotracheal intubation are at increased risk of pneumonia and associated mortality.

BREATHING

Assessment of respirations can be complicated by both the physiological changes mentioned earlier and/or pathological processes. If the geriatric patient has emphysema, the chest may be barrel shaped; the patient may have air trapping, resulting in an increased effort to exhale. This can mimic respiratory distress from chest injuries, thereby complicating the assessment.

Due to decreases in the arterial partial pressure of oxygen (PaO_2) in the geriatric patient, oxygen saturations can quickly deteriorate. In order to compensate for this natural decrease, it is important that the geriatric trauma patient receive high concentrations of supplemental oxygen. If the patient has spontaneous respirations, this can be accomplished with a nonrebreather mask at 15 L/min flow. In the absence of spontaneous respirations, respirations should be assisted with 100% oxygen utilizing a bag-valve device or mechanical ventilator. The major advantage of the bag-valve device over mechanical ventilation is the ability to continually assess lung compliance.

CIRCULATION

When assessing circulation, remember that the patient may have a history of cardiovascular disease. Recall that maximal heart rate decreases with aging and many geriatric patients may be taking medications such as beta blockers or calcium channel blockers that can prevent increases in heart rate or vasoconstriction in response to blood loss. The inability of the heart to increase its rate, possible decreased myocardial strength, and decreased peripheral vascular resistance mean that the elderly trauma patient has limited ability to maintain adequate cardiac output, thereby worsening already inadequate tissue perfusion. For these reasons, it is imperative that the geriatric trauma patient receive aggressive management.

Hemostasis must be obtained as soon as possible. External bleeding can usually be controlled with external pressure, elevation of the injured part, pressure applied to a pressure point, and/or application of a pressure dressing. If all of these techniques fail, it may be necessary to apply a tourniquet. In the event that a tourniquet is applied, the time applied should be documented and the tourniquet should not be removed in the field.

Once attention has been given to hemostasis, intravenous access should be obtained and a crystalloid solution administered rapidly in an attempt to restore vascular volume. While these patients are in need of aggressive fluid resuscitation, it is important to avoid fluid overload. Since normal respiratory effort may already be compromised due to physiological changes, lung sounds should be monitored and fluids restricted if rales develop.

Finally, because the geriatric patient is more prone to cardiac dysrhythmias, a cardiac monitor should be applied. While prophylactic treatment for ventricular dysrhythmias is not recommended, if dysrhythmias develop in a hemodynamically unstable patient, they should be treated according to American Heart Association (AHA) Advanced Cardiac Life Support (ACLS) guidelines. When administering lidocaine to a geriatric patient, the dosage should be reduced. The AHA's ACLS standards recommend an initial loading dose of 1–1.5 mg/kg followed by a maintenance infusion that is 50% of the normal maintenance dosage.[5]

DISABILITY

Altered levels of consciousness can be difficult to assess in the geriatric trauma patient. Consciousness can be altered due to medications, neurological deterioration, or dementia. It is important to document baseline neurological status as early as possible. In the unconscious patient, either the AVPU or the Glasgow Coma Scale document neurological status. In addition, it is very important to obtain from relatives or friends the patient's normal level of mentation.

EXPOSURE

While it is important to expose the geriatric trauma patient to properly assess for injuries, remember that these patients have a decreased tolerance to heat loss. Assess for hypothermia and take steps to maintain normal body temperature. Actions include applying blankets immediately after assessment and administering warmed intravenous fluids. In addition, it may be emotionally uncomfortable for the geriatric patient to have their clothes removed by younger individuals. It is important that the reasons for removal of clothing be explained and that continued emotional support and encouragement be provided.

SHOCK

Management of the geriatric patient in shock is much the same as for younger patients. Patency of the airway is the first priority. If the patient is unconscious, the airway should be opened immediately with a jaw thrust, then secured with endotracheal intubation. Once patency of the airway is ensured, adequate oxygenation becomes the priority. In the spontaneously breathing patient, supplemental oxygen should be administered with a nonrebreathing mask at 15 L/min. In the apneic patient, 100% oxygen should be administered with a bag-valve device. While pulse oximetry can be a valuable adjunct to assessing oxygenation, remember that geriatric patients can have decreased peripheral circulation, which can affect the ability of the pulse oximeter to adequately monitor the amount of oxygen bound to hemoglobin.

Next, hemostasis should be achieved as soon as possible. External bleeding can be controlled as stated earlier. Adequacy of peripheral pulses should be serially assessed once a pressure dressing has been applied.

Expedient transport is the mainstay of care for the severely injured geriatric trauma patient. Once transport to a trauma center is underway, attention may be given to other treatment modalities. It is imperative to remember that definitive care of the geriatric trauma patient suffering from traumatic injuries is surgical intervention.

During transport, intravenous therapy may be initiated. As stated earlier, fluid resuscitation in the geriatric patient can be very challenging. While the patient needs rapid infusion of large quantities of crystalloid solutions, the geriatric patient, generally, has a decreased cardiac output and therefore can easily be overhydrated. For this reason, it is important to continually reassess hemodynamic status and lung sounds.

Aggressive fluid therapy consists of initiating two large-diameter, preferably 14- or 16-gauge, short peripheral catheters into large free-flowing vessels. The fluid of choice is lactated Ringer's (LR), with the second choice being normal saline (NS). Both fluids have theoretical concerns. The lactate in LR is converted by the liver to bicarbonate, which, theoretically, helps to buffer the metabolic acidosis that results from shock. In geriatric patients with liver damage, the lactate may not be converted to bicarbonate and can lead to increased lactate levels, leading one to believe that NS is a superior choice. However, NS, if given in large quantities, can result in hyperchloremia acidosis, adding to the already acidotic state of the system. So, while both have theoretical concerns, they are still the best fluids for initial prehospital fluid resuscitation.

If the patient has received 1–2 liters of crystalloid solution and continues to be hemodynamically unstable, blood products should be considered. In the prehospital environment, blood products are usually not available due to the difficulty in storage and short shelf-life in relation to their utilization. However, if available, they are very beneficial. Common problems associated with transfusion of blood to the geriatric patient include coagulopathies, hypothermia, and electrolyte imbalance.

As with any injured patient, it is important to continually reassess hemodynamic status. Other aspects of care consist of maintaining normal body temperature and keeping the patient calm and at rest in order to decrease metabolic demand.

HEAD INJURIES

Head injuries differ slightly in the geriatric patient from younger populations. Recall that due to physiological changes, the geriatric patient is less prone to epidural hematomas but has a threefold increase in the risk of subdural hemorrhage. Subdural hematomas are slow to progress, resulting in insidious changes or a lack of signs and symptoms. The only signs or symptoms present in the event of a subdural hematoma may be the history of a fall or head injury and a gradual decline in neurological status. One additional fact to consider is that 20–50% of these patients do not remember falling, so a high index of suspicion is essential.

Establishment of the patent airway should be accomplished as soon as possible in the geriatric head-injured patient. Oral tracheal intubation is the method of choice for managing the airway in the unconscious patient without a gag reflex. In the conscious patient, the patient with an intact gag reflex, or the patient with trismus (contraction of the muscles of the mouth), the use of neuromuscular blocking agents may be necessary to facilitate oral tracheal intubation. If rapid-sequence intubation is not available, then an alternative may be nasotracheal intubation.

In the event of rapid deterioration of neurological status, geriatric head-injured patients should be mildly hyperventilated to a $PaCO_2$ of 30 mm Hg. It is important to remember that hyperventilation is an increase in minute ventilation, which is a function of rate and tidal volume. Hyperventilation can be accomplished by increasing either side of the equation. Because most geriatric patients' tidal volume remains constant around 500 mL per breath, the increase in tidal volume associated with use of a 1,500–1,600 mL bag-valve device can increase the patient's minute ventilation, even if ventilations are given at their normal respiratory rate. One method of estimating the correct rate and depth of ventilations is to attempt to deliver approximately 15 mL/kg per breath at a rate of 16–18 breaths per minute (bpm).[6]

The second priority in management of the geriatric head-injured patient is to ensure adequate oxygenation. In the conscious and/or spontaneously breathing patient, administer supplemental oxygen by nonrebreather mask at 15 L/min flow. In the apneic and/or unconscious patient, bag-valve ventilation with 100% supplemental oxygen and use of a mechanical ventilator with 100% oxygen at the rates outlined above are the methods of choice.

Just as in other types of trauma, adequate tissue perfusion must be maintained in the geriatric head-injured patient. Inadequate perfusion can result in tissue hypoxia and increased intracranial pressure. While most head-injured patients do not experience shock as a result of head injuries, many have associated injuries to other body systems.

Several pharmacological agents, including mannitol, furosemide, lidocaine, and corticosteroids, have been utilized in the treatment of geriatric head injuries. The two that are utilized most often are the osmotic diuretic mannitol and the corticosteroid dexamethasone. These agents are discussed further in Chapter 11. The geriatric head-injured patient should be transported as soon as possible to a trauma center that has computerized tomography and neurosurgical capabilities.

MUSCULOSKELETAL INJURIES

Conditions such as osteoarthritis and osteoporosis can contribute to the complications of managing the cervical spine injury. Cervical arthritis and dorsal kyphosis can make it extremely difficult, if not impossible, for the patient's head to be lowered onto a spine board for immobilization. Spinal immobilization of this geriatric patient can be managed by placing padding underneath the head to maintain a neutral position. This position can vary with each patient so a variety of material such as sheets, pillows, and specially manufactured head padding should be available for use in such a situation.

Arthritis can also make it difficult to assess potential skeletal injuries. Many patients may have chronic arthritic pain or chronic deformity, making it extremely difficult to assess potential fractures. Splinting of joint and extremity injuries may also be difficult in these patients due to the deformity that frequently accompanies arthritis. Splinting material that can be configured to the patient works best for splinting fractures in these types of patients.

A Colles' fracture, fractures of the distal humerus that are commonly accompanied by a fracture of the ulnar styloid, results from falls onto an outstretched dorsiflexed hand.[7] Many refer to this as a "dinner fork" fracture.[3] In determining the severity of this type of fracture, it is important that the median nerve and motor function be assessed. Median nerve motor function can be assessed by placing an object, such as a pencil, upright in the palm of the patient's hand and then asking the patient to move the thumb from one side to the other side of the object. Median nerve motor function can also be assessed by testing the patient's ability to first touch the index finger and then the little finger.

BURNS

Burns are the third leading cause of traumatic death in the geriatric patient.[1] The mortality rate associated with burns ranges from 30% in patients with 6% burned body surface area (BSA) to 50% in patients with 40% burned BSA.[1] Even first-degree burns (superficial burns) and second-degree burns (partial thickness) can be life threatening to the geriatric patient and require aggressive care.

Alcohol and smoking in bed are the two most common causative factors related to geriatric burns. Other common etiologies of geriatric burns are falls against hot agents, unintentional ignition of loose clothing while cooking, and spillage of hot liquids due to muscle weakness. Another factor that can increase burn intensity is the decrease of nerve ending sensation (or decreased speed of feeling the burn), which can result in a longer exposure to the burning agent.

Aggressive management of the geriatric burn patient's airway is critical. Airways that are exposed to hot gas can rapidly become edematous and may lead to airway obstruction. Oral tracheal intubation should be performed immediately in any patient that has carbonaceous sputum or singed facial hairs, or been exposed to hot vapors in an enclosed area.

Loss of fluids through third spacing can be extremely severe in the geriatric burn patient. Large amounts of crystalloid solutions may be required to maintain adequate circulating blood volume. Following resuscitation, it is important to observe the geriatric patient for signs and symptoms of fluid volume overload since this lost fluid will be reabsorbed into the vascular space and can result in volume overload. For further discussion on burn care see Chapter 17.

INTERNET ACTIVITIES

Visit the National Library of Medicine Web site at http://www.ncbi.nlm.nih.gov/PubMed. Conduct a literature search on geriatric trauma. Review the abstracts of the search results. Ask your librarian to assist you in obtaining the journals with the five most relevant articles. Review these articles and summarize their findings.

ABUSE

An unfortunate cause of injury in the geriatric population is physical abuse. Since many of the etiologies mentioned above could result from physical abuse, it is important to maintain a high degree of suspicion to detect cases of abuse. In addition to physical abuse, financial and emotional abuse also exist; any suspected abuse should be reported to the appropriate authorities.

INTERNET ACTIVITIES

Visit the e-medicine Web site at http://www.emedicine.com. Click on the Emergency Medicine e-book, then the psychosocial chapter. Review the material on elder abuse.

HOSPITAL CARE AND REHABILITATION

Surgical care of the geriatric trauma patient is associated with several complications. First, transfusion of large quantities of blood can cause blood coagulopathy (see Chapter 20); in addition, many older patients may be taking oral anticoagulants (e.g., aspirin, Ticlid, Coumadin). A second complication that can be attributed to large volumes of blood transfusion is hypothermia. With an already diminished thermoregulatory ability from aging, this can result in severe cases of hypothermia. Finally, as a result of age-related cardiovascular system changes, patients can develop life-threatening dysrhythmias.

Intensive care following surgical intervention is also a critical time for the geriatric trauma patient. Patients who require endotracheal intubation and mechanical ventilation are very prone to pneumonia due to the age-related physiological changes of the respiratory system. In addition, they are at increased risk of deep vein thrombosis (DVT), pulmonary emboli, cerebral vascular accidents (CVA), disseminated intravascular coagulopathy (DIC), and sepsis. All of these potential problems not only add to the mortality and morbidity, but also add to the complexity of dealing with these patients during recovery in the intensive care unit.

▶ SUMMARY

As the number of geriatric patients continues to increase with aging of the baby boomers, the number of geriatric trauma patients will continue to rise. It is imperative that prehospital care providers be familiar with the physiological changes and the special procedures required to care for these patients. By understanding how the geriatric patient differs from the younger patient, prehospital providers can provide early aggressive care and allow the geriatric patient the best chance of survival and recovery.

▶ REVIEW QUESTIONS

1. Which of the following is NOT a common cause of traumatic injury to the geriatric patient?
   a. Falls
   b. MVC
   c. Stab wounds
   d. Burns

2. Which of the following physiological changes does NOT occur to the cardiovascular system with aging?
   a. Maximal heart rate decreases
   b. Stroke volume decreases
   c. Peripheral vascular resistance decreases
   d. Cardiac output increases

3. Due to atrophy of the brain, geriatric head-injured patients are prone to:
   a. Epidural hematomas
   b. Subdural hematomas
   c. Skull fractures
   d. Contusions

4. Fractures of the _____ are common in the geriatric patient and are associated with increased morbidity and mortality.
   a. Hip
   b. Ankle
   c. Wrist
   d. Forearm

5. Which of the following treatments can be complicated by the physiological changes that accompany aging?
   a. Airway management
   b. Fluid resuscitation
   c. Spinal immobilization
   d. All of the above

6. What are the common causes of traumatic injury to the geriatric patient?

7. What are the age-related physiological changes to the respiratory system?

8. Describe spinal immobilization of the geriatric patient with kyphosis.

9. Discuss the challenges in management of the geriatric patient's airway.

10. Discuss the importance of taking a past medical history, including current medications, in the geriatric trauma patient.

▶ CRITICAL THINKING

● You are treating a 74-year-old female involved in an MVC. She was the driver of a vehicle that was struck on the driver's side by a second vehicle. There is approximately 18 inches of crush to the driver's side door. The patient is conscious and alert, complaining of respiratory distress and chest pain. Upon physical examination, you discover instability to the left chest. Breath sounds reveal rales in the left lower lobe. Her skin is pale with circumoral cyanosis and cyanosis to the nailbeds. Blood pressure is 100/P, heart rate 70, respirations 36. The remainder of the physical examination is unremarkable. She has a past medical history of myocardial infarction, congestive heart failure, hypertension, arthritis, and atrial fibrillation. Her medications include Lopressor, Lanoxin, furosemide, and ibuprofen. How will her past medical history and medications affect her clinical presentation? How will it affect your treatment?

● You are called to the scene of a fall. Upon arrival, you find an 84-year-old female who has fallen down a flight of stairs. She complains of pain in the right hip. What changes associated with aging make her prone to such falls? What changes of aging make her more prone to injury? What injuries are possible in this patient? How will you manage her care?

● You are called to the scene of a fall. Upon arrival, you find a 70-year-old female who states that while she was walking "my leg gave out on me." You note that the left leg is shortened and externally rotated, and there is tenderness to palpation of the left thigh. Distal neurocirculatory function is intact. What injury do you suspect? What conditions predisposed this patient to this injury? How will you treat this patient?

▶ REFERENCES

1. Osler TM, Demarest, GB. Geriatric trauma. In: Mattox KL, et al, eds. *Trauma*. Stamford, Conn.: Appleton & Lange; 1988.
2. Spaite DW, Criss EA, Valenzuela TD, Meislin HW, Ross J. Geriatric injury: an analysis of prehospital demographics, mechanisms, and patterns. *Ann Emerg Med*. 1990; 19:12.
3. Fairman R, Rombeau JL. Physiological problems in the elderly surgical patient. In: Miller A, ed. *Physiologic Basis of Modern Surgical Care*. Washington, D.C.: Mosby; 1988.
4. Knowelden J, et al. Incidence of fractures in persons over 35 years of age. *Br J Prev Soc Med*. 1981; 18:130.
5. *Advanced Cardiac Life Support*. Dallas: American Heart Association; 1997.
6. Moore EE. *Early Care of the Injured Patient*. Toronto: BC Decker; 1990.
7. Bosker G, Schwartz GR, Jones JS, Sequeira M. *Geriatric Emergency Medicine*. St Louis, Mo.: Mosby; 1990.

▶ BIBLIOGRAPHY

Cardona VD, et al. *Trauma Nursing from Resuscitation through Rehabilitation*, 2nd ed. Philadelphia: WB Saunders; 1994.

Christ MA, Hohloch FJ. *Gerontological Nursing: A Study and Learning Tool*. Springhouse, Pa: Springhouse Publishing; 1988.

Feliciano DV, Moore ZE, Mattox KL. *Trauma*, 3rd ed. Stamford, Conn.: Appleton & Lange; 1996.

Hazzard WR. *Principles of Geriatric Medicine and Gerontology*. New York: McGraw-Hill; 1994.

Hoffer EP. *Emergency Problems in the Elderly*. Oradell, N.J.: Medical Economic Books; 1985.

Horst HM, Obeid FN, Sorensen VJ, Bivens BA. Factors influencing survival of elderly trauma patients. *Crit Care Med*. 1986; 14:8.

Osler TM, Hales K, Baack B, Bear K, Hsi K, Pathak D, et al. Trauma in the elderly. *Am J Surg*. 1988; 156(6):537.

PHTLS. *Basic and Advanced Pre-Hospital Trauma Life Support*, 3rd ed. St Louis, Mo.: Mosby; 1994.

Sanders MJ. *Mosby's Paramedic Textbook*. St Louis, Mo.: Mosby; 1994.

Shapiro MB, Dechert RE, Colwell C, Bartlett RH, Rodriguez JL. Geriatric trauma: aggressive intensive care unit management is justified. *Am Surg*. 1994; 60(9):695.

Zietlow SP, Capizzi PJ, Bannon MP, Farnell MB. Multisystem geriatric trauma. *J Trauma*. 1994; 37:6.

Chapter 25

Trauma in Pregnancy

OBJECTIVES

Upon completion of this chapter, the reader should be able to:

- Contrast the past epidemiology of pregnancy-related mortality and morbidity with the current and emerging etiologies of maternal deaths and differences in injury patterns and explain how these changes have implications for the paramedic, especially in an urban setting.

- Describe how the anatomy and physiology of the pregnant patient differ from those of the nonpregnant patient.

- Describe how the differences in the anatomy and physiology of the pregnant patient are relevant to the trauma assessment and explain the potential pitfalls of assessing the pregnant trauma patient.

- Discuss how the differences in the anatomy and physiology of the pregnant patient affect the out-of-hospital treatment of the pregnant trauma patient.

- Discuss how the differences in the out-of-hospital treatment of the pregnant trauma patient may affect basic trauma support (such as the differences in techniques of positioning), the method of notification of the receiving hospital, and how advanced life support may differ for the pregnant patient in traumatic arrest.

- Identify those factors that most threaten fetal survival.

- Describe the pathophysiology of the types of traumatic injury that are unique to the pregnant patient, including the pathophysiology of seemingly minor trauma.

- Discuss why the differences in the pathophysiology of minor trauma in the pregnant patient require in-hospital assessment and treatment to prevent adverse maternal and fetal outcomes.

- Discuss some of the differences in the out-of-hospital assessment of the pregnant patient, comparing these with in-hospital assessment of the pregnant trauma patient.

- Discuss some of the differences in the out-of-hospital treatment of the pregnant patient, comparing these with the nonpregnant trauma patient.

- Discuss some of the ways in which paramedic assessment and treatment of the pregnant trauma patient affects the in-hospital treatment.

KEY TERMS

Abruptio placentae
Fetomaternal hemorrhage

Paramedics frequently encounter trauma in female patients of child-bearing age. On occasion, in the approach to the trauma patient, in the intensity of the moment, it may be difficult to remember the possibility of pregnancy and pregnancy-related modifications of management. As is often true in medicine, the problem that is not exposed or considered is often the most severe. Just as with any injured patient, this "unexposed part" of the trauma patient may hide critical information needed for adequate stabilization.

Failure to recognize a gravid uterus may seem to be a gross oversight; but there are other, more subtle, pregnancy-related changes that may remain hidden unless considered. These potentially serious "hidden injuries" are the less obvious alterations of anatomy and physiology during pregnancy, the placenta, and the physiology of the fetus. The paramedic is expected to "expose" the critical, hidden information essential to the management of a variety of situations.

Certain situations raise practical questions regarding patient management. For example, which injuries are more common or more severe during pregnancy? In multisystem major trauma, how is fetal survival most affected? Are certain medications, which are usually safe in pregnancy, contraindicated in the pregnant trauma patient? Can the fetus be at risk if the mother is stable after her injury? Is it ever appropriate for the paramedic to estimate fetal age? In a motor vehicle crash (MVC), could a seat belt actually do more harm than good for the fetus? How are circulatory and respiratory failure treated in a way to minimize fetal injury? What is the paramedic's approach to traumatic arrest in the pregnant patient?

Fortunately, the approach to the pregnant trauma patient is fundamentally the same as for all trauma patients: treat hypoxia, treat shock. The mainstay of treatment for all trauma patients is the orderly and rigorous attention to the ABCs. Stabilization of the maternal ABCs is the most effective intervention a paramedic can make in the pregnant trauma patient—for the protection of both mother and fetus.[1,2] After initial stabilizing interventions, consideration is given to the hidden or subtle ways in which pregnancy modifies assessment and treatment of trauma.

EPIDEMIOLOGY AND ETIOLOGY OF INJURY

During the last half of the twentieth century, there has been a substantial decline in the maternal mortality rate in the United States. The obstetric-related death rate has decreased dramatically; unfortunately, the trauma-related maternal death rate has not. The leading causes of maternal deaths have shifted significantly in recent years in much the same way as in the pediatric population; unin-

tentional and intentional injuries have replaced other formerly common causes of death (Figure 25-1).

In years past, the leading causes of maternal death were infection, hemorrhage, and toxemia. In the United States, these three obstetric-related causes accounted for three-fourths of all maternal deaths. In 1942, a pregnant woman had a better chance of surviving the leading causes of maternal death if she resided in an urban locale (New York City).[1] But by 1992, in a similar urban setting (Chicago), a dramatic shift had occurred; trauma had become the leading cause of death during pregnancy. Today, a pregnant woman living in an urban setting is twice as likely to die from trauma than from all direct obstetric-related causes of death combined (Table 25-1). [1,3,4]

Fortunately, most trauma in pregnancy is minor trauma.[2] Major life-threatening trauma accounts for only a small percentage of all maternal injuries. The two most common causes of trauma (major and minor) during pregnancy are intimate partner violence and MVCs.[3,5,6] Major life-threatening blunt and penetrating trauma in pregnancy results from MVCs, assaults, falls, and burns. The prevalence of out-of-hospital maternal trauma has not been well described and needs further study. However, based on studies of pregnant patients in emergency department and primary care settings, it is predicted that the frequency and patterns of injuries in pregnancy encountered by an out-of-hospital paramedic will resemble those of the nonpregnant, age-matched population.[4,5,6]

Trauma is estimated to complicate from 7% to 23% of all pregnancies.[2,5] Prevalence studies vary widely regarding the frequency and patterns of trauma

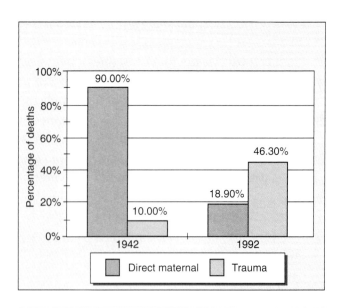

FIGURE 25-1 Changes in the leading causes of maternal death from 1942 to 1992.[1,3,4]

Table 25-1
Causes of Death During Pregnancy in the Urban United States: Changes in the Last Fifty Years

New York City (1942)[4]		Chicago, Cook County (1992)[3]	
Leading Causes of Direct Maternal Death	Percentage of Total	Leading Causes of Direct Maternal Death	Percentage of Total
Infection	22.80	Homicide	26.40
Hemorrhage	16.40	MVC	9.50
Toxemia	5.10	Burns	3.10
Abruptio placentae	3.80	Falls	2.10

during pregnancy. For example, some studies have shown MVCs to be, by far, the most common mechanism of injury during pregnancy, while other studies have found that fatal and minor maternal trauma is most often the result of intimate partner violence.[3,4,6] Some disparity is due to differences in research design, with some studies describing the total numbers of injuries and some reporting fatal injuries and mortality rates. There may also be inconsistencies in the method of reporting occurrences of trauma in pregnancy. These discrepancies may be due to a lack of consistency in defining, recognizing, and reporting all forms of maternal trauma.[4] Recent studies show a high rate of intimate partner violence occurring in female emergency department patients.[7] Some investigators have pointed out that domestic violence has become a public health problem of epidemic proportions.[8] Yet it has been well documented that emergency care providers often fail to report, or worse fail to even recognize, domestic violence.[5,9–11] It is reasonable to assume that the paramedic will encounter more maternal trauma due to intimate partner violence than has typically been predicted in the past.

Trauma during pregnancy may endanger both mother and fetus. Pregnant women who experience life-threatening injuries have the same survival rate as nonpregnant women.[2] Maternal survival depends upon those factors affecting severity of injury: critical force, presence of shock, and presence of head, chest, abdomen, or pelvic trauma. As with nonpregnant patients, pregnant trauma victims die primarily from hemorrhagic shock and head injury.[12,13] In this group of pregnant patients with major trauma, fetal survival correlates most precisely with the severity of maternal injury.[2,12] Adverse pregnancy outcome in severely injured pregnant patients approaches 100% in maternal death, 80% in maternal shock, and 50% in other maternal serious injuries.[14] An adverse pregnancy outcome may also occur in up to 25% of *minor* trauma.[15–17] Fetal demise or **abruptio placentae** (separation of the placenta from the uterine wall) may result from seemingly trivial maternal injury. In maternal trauma (major and minor), except for the death of the mother, the highest mortality for the fetus results from abruptio placentae.[6] Because nearly 90% of all trauma during pregnancy is minor, the greatest percentage of pregnancy losses are due to minor injuries.[14] This distinction between severity and frequency is illustrated in Table 25-2.

In addition to the common causes of trauma during pregnancy, MVCs and intimate partner violence, another very common cause of blunt maternal injury during pregnancy is a simple fall.[2] As with the minor trauma of MVCs and partner violence, a simple fall

Table 25-2
Maternal and Fetal Survival in Trauma During Pregnancy[12,18]

Type of Trauma	Relative Frequency	Maternal Mortality (%)	Fetal Mortality If Maternal Death Occurs (%)
Life threatening	Rare (<10%)	3.90	100.00
Shock	Rare (<10%)	2.20	≥75.00
Head trauma	Rare (<10%)	1.70	≤50.00
Minor trauma	Common (>90%)	≤4.00	≤02.50
"Trivial" trauma	Common (>90%)	0.00	≤05.00

may be complicated by abruptio placentae in 1% to 5% of patients.[2,12,13] Therefore, despite the fact that the majority of pregnant trauma patients have only minor injuries, it is critical that the paramedic be aware that even minor maternal trauma can have catastrophic results for the fetus.[13] An understanding of the epidemiology of injury as well as the normal anatomical and physiological changes during pregnancy, including fetal and placental responses to trauma, guide management and prevent the pitfalls of treatment of the pregnant trauma patient.

ANATOMIC AND PHYSIOLOGICAL CHANGES DURING PREGNANCY

During pregnancy almost every organ system of the body undergoes changes. The normal maternal and fetal physiological changes greatly impact the management and assessment of the pregnant trauma patient. For example, how accurately do vital signs reflect maternal and fetal well-being? How do maternal respiratory physiological changes, intra-abdominal anatomical, and uterine changes affect fetal and maternal oxygenation? It is important to have a basic understanding of the normal cardiovascular, respiratory, intra-abdominal, pelvic, and fetal changes during pregnancy and to know how these alterations are relevant to the management of maternal and fetal trauma.

CARDIOVASCULAR CHANGES

During pregnancy there is a tremendous increase in cardiac output (CO). Maternal blood volume expands by 50%, and the heart rate increases by 15–20 beats per minute (bpm). The resulting CO is 1,000–1,500 mL/min greater during pregnancy.[2] This extra reserve of CO makes detection of internal bleeding very difficult. As much as 35% of maternal blood volume may be lost before the usual signs of shock are exhibited.[19]

The large increase in maternal blood volume is not matched by a similar increase in total hemoglobin. Therefore, in order to maintain the same maternal and fetal oxygenation, this high output state must be maintained.

It is difficult to define the normal nonpreeclamptic pregnant blood pressure (BP); BPs have some normal variation prior to pregnancy. During the first 6 months of pregnancy, the BP will be lower than the prepregnant pressures. There is a drop in the systolic pressure of up to 4 mm Hg and a decrease in the diastolic pressure of up to 15 mm Hg—associated with a lowering of peripheral vascular resistance. During the last 3 months of pregnancy, the BP returns to prepregnant levels. A BP reading, by itself, is not a precise reflection of adequate perfusion and oxygenation, especially in the pregnant patient.

During the last half of pregnancy, the position of the enlarging uterus may greatly influence CO and BP. A gravid uterus' compression of the inferior vena cava reduces venous return and preload. After the eighth month, there may be total obstruction of caval venous return. This may reduce CO by as much as 28%, and systolic BP may fall 30% when the patient is supine.[20,21] Conversely, by removing the gravid uterus from the inferior vena cava (by displacing the uterus to the left or by placing the patient on her left side), CO may increase up to 25%.[22]

During early hypovolemia in the pregnant patient, there may be no significant increase in heart rate, drop in BP, or skin changes typical of shock. However, in maternal blood loss, uterine vasoconstriction occurs early, even before other signs and symptoms of blood loss are recognized.[19] The uterus has no ability to increase uterine blood flow by self-regulation. As a result, it is possible for life-threatening compromise of fetal oxygenation and perfusion to occur without evidence of maternal shock.[19] The fetal response to inadequate uterine blood flow may be bradycardia or tachycardia. The first indication of early maternal shock, therefore, may be an abnormal fetal heart rate.

RESPIRATORY CHANGES

During pregnancy there is a 20% reduction in maternal functional lung capacity and residual volume, resulting in a marked lowering of the oxygen reserve. The causes of this reduced reserve are the elevation of the diaphragm and a 15% increase in oxygen expenditure by the placenta, the fetus, and the maternal organs.[19] The reduction in oxygen reserve during pregnancy is partially compensated for by an increase in the respiratory rate and tidal volume. Therefore, the consequent normal respiratory state during pregnancy may also be thought of as "high output." One consequence of this increase in minute ventilation is a decrease in the $PaCO_2$. During the last half of pregnancy, the normal $PaCO_2$ is 30 mm Hg.[20] The normal increased minute ventilation and decreased $PaCO_2$ are compensated for by an increased excretion of bicarbonate by the kidneys. A $PaCO_2$ of 40 mm Hg, considered to be normal in the nonpregnant patient, reflects improper ventilation of the pregnant patient.[19] Inadequate ventilation may result in maternal acidosis, fetal acidosis, and fetal hypoxia.

GASTROINTESTINAL AND INTRA-ABDOMINAL CHANGES

During the course of pregnancy, the uterus grows from 7 cm (2.76 inches) to 36 cm (14.2 inches). In the first 3 months of pregnancy, the uterus is relatively protected by the pelvis and there is minimal displacement of the other intra-abdominal contents by the uterus. After the third month, the uterus extends out of the pelvis and displaces the intra-abdominal organs toward the diaphragm. The rate of growth of the uterus is roughly 1 cm per week of gestation, measured from the symphysis pubis. As this occurs, the uterus and bladder become abdominal organs and are more susceptible to injury. In blunt abdominal trauma, after the third month, the uterus may have a protective, "airbaglike" effect on the other intra-abdominal organs.[2,23]

The growing uterus causes a gradual expansion of the peritoneum and abdominal musculature. As a result, there may be significantly altered or even absent pain patterns, and the physical examination becomes unreliable. Major intra-abdominal organ injury may occur without the usual signs of peritoneal irritation: tenderness, guarding, and rigidity.[2,19]

During pregnancy the gastric muscle tone is decreased and there is delayed gastric emptying. This places the pregnant trauma patient at risk for aspiration, particularly the patient with an altered level of consciousness.

FETAL RESPIRATION AND CIRCULATION

Within 2 weeks after fertilization the embryo attaches to the uterine wall. Villi, or fingerlike projections, form an attachment between the uterine wall and the placenta. This uteroplacental connection is a "Velcro-like" vascular linkage. Through this vascular connection all gas exchange between fetus and mother occurs. Fetal survival depends upon maintaining both uterine blood flow and the anatomical integrity of the uteroplacental connection.

Two characteristics of this uteroplacental unit put the fetus at risk in trauma. First, there is no uteroplacental autoregulation of its circulation. That is, there is no fetal or placental method of increasing blood flow. Perfusion is dependent upon maternal systolic blood pressure. Second, the uteroplacental connection is at risk for separation because the placenta is relatively fixed and inelastic in relation to an elastic and compressible uterus.[2,19] Forces of direct trauma or deceleration cause differing placental and uterine rates and distances of movement. This results in a shearing disruption of the uteroplacental connection[19,24] (Table 25-3).

PATHOPHYSIOLOGY

Trauma is the leading cause of death in women of child-bearing age. The mechanisms of fatal injury are nearly the same for both the pregnant and the non-

pregnant populations. Maternal and fetal trauma may be blunt or penetrating, with hemorrhagic shock and head injury being the chief causes of maternal death.[2] Although certain injuries, such as uterine rupture, splenic rupture, and retroperitoneal hemorrhage occur more often during pregnancy, serious life-threatening trauma appears to have the same mortality rate in pregnant and nonpregnant women.[2]

Blunt and penetrating trauma may also result in premature rupture of membranes, uterine injury, premature labor, direct fetal injury, and fetomaternal hemorrhage. The two most common causes of fetal death as a result of life-threatening, major trauma are maternal death and abruptio placentae.[12,13] Abruptio placentae, which occurs in up to 50% of major trauma, is a more common cause of fetal death than direct fetal injury, maternal burns, penetrating abdominal injuries, and fetomaternal hemorrhage combined. Because of the frequency of minor trauma, fetal deaths due to minor trauma occur more often than those resulting from life-threatening trauma.[2,12] Minor trauma may result from falls, intimate partner violence, and seat belt injuries.

The first priority in managing the pathophysiology of maternal and fetal trauma is the stabilization of the pregnant patient. Regardless of how the different anatomic and physiological changes of pregnancy affect assessment and treatment, this patient needs aggressive ventilatory and circulatory interventions. Recognizing and treating the pathophysiology of maternal hypoventilation and shock, including vena caval occlusion, minimize fetal injury.

MAJOR TRAUMA

MATERNAL HEMORRHAGIC SHOCK

Major trauma resulting in life-threatening injury is rare in pregnancy. When maternal death does occur, the most frequent pathophysiology is hemorrhagic shock. In multisystem trauma, even with the presence of shock, maternal survival rate is very high (greater than 90%).[2,12,25] By contrast, fetal survival is low, with an adverse outcome in about 50% of major trauma.[2] If traumatic maternal hemorrhagic shock occurs, the fetal mortality rate is 80%.[2,25] In traumatic hypovolemia, the best chance of survival for the fetus is vigorous volume resuscitation of the mother, followed by definitive surgical intervention as indicated.

PLACENTAL ABRUPTION

Abruptio placentae is the separation of the placenta from its uterine attachment. Nontraumatic spontaneous abruptio placentae is extremely rare. In trauma,

Table 25-3

Anatomic and Physiological Changes During Pregnancy and Implications for Trauma Management

Anatomic or Physiological Parameter or Organ System	Nonpregnant Patient	Pregnant Patient	Pregnant Patient		
			Anatomic and Physiological Dynamics	Anatomic and Physiological Observations	Application in Management
Heart rate (HR)	80	95	High output	HR increases 5–10 beats	Increased HR cannot be used as an early reliable sign of hypovolemic shock
Blood pressure (BP)	110/70	100/50	Low peripheral vascular resistance	BP decreases 10%–15%	Evaluating hypovolemic shock is more difficult, particularly midtrimester
Respiratory rate (RR)	12–18	18–25	High O_2 demand, low O_2 reserve	RR increases 4–8 breaths/min, causing $PaCO_2$ to drop	"Normal" RR of 12 and $PaCO_2$ of 40 mm Hg may cause acidemia and hypoxia
Arterial blood gases (ABGs)	pH: 7.40; $PaCO_2$: 40	pH: 7.43; $PaCO_2$: 32	Low $PaCO_2$	Pregnant $PaCO_2$ should be 30–32 mm Hg	$PaCO_2$ of 40 mm Hg may mean acidemia
Circulation Vena cava	Normal venous return		Low venous return	Uterine compression of inferior vena cava decreases venous return	Placing patient in left lateral recumbent position or manual uterine displacement is necessary to prevent worsening shock
Blood volume	4.2 liters	6.0 liters	High output	Blood volume increases by 50%	Blood loss may be difficult to estimate
Red cell mass	37%	32%	High output	Plasma volume increases more than hemoglobin, causing "anemia of pregnancy"	"Decreased hemo-globin efficiency" is offset by a compensatory hyperventilation
Gastric	Normal gastric output		Low gastric output	Gastric motility decreases, causing delayed gastric emptying time	To minimize risk of aspiration, consider nasogastric tube and/or endotracheal airway
Abdomen: Fetal				Abdominal con-tents displaced from lower abdomen in later pregnancy	Penetrating trauma to the abdomen is likely to cause fetal and placental injury

unfortunately, the frequency of abruptio placentae is particularly worrisome. Complete abruptio placentae is universally fatal for the fetus unless an immediate cae-sarian section (C-section) is performed. Potentially lethal maternal risks associated with traumatic abruptio placentae are hemorrhage and disseminated intravas-cular coagulation (DIC).

Abruptio placentae is estimated to occur in up to 6% of minor trauma and in up to 50% of major mater-nal injury.[1,2,6,12] Fetal/neonatal death associated with maternal trauma is more commonly the result of abruptio placentae than any other injury in preg-nancy.[23] Only maternal death has as frequent an associ-ation with fetal death in trauma.[2]

In falls and blunt abdominal trauma, there may be deceleration or direct uterine deformation. This impacts both the uterus and the placenta. The uterus is made up of muscle fibers; the placenta has a consis-tency that is relatively stiff. When the movement of the elastic uterus becomes greater than that of the inflexi-ble placenta, it creates a shearing separation of the pla-centa from the uterus. This injury may occur with major or minor maternal trauma. Separation of the pla-centa results in fetal hypoperfusion leading to hypoxia, acidosis, and eventually death. Maternal complications include bleeding from the uteroplacental separation site and, rarely, release of placental or intrauterine material into maternal circulation. This injected mate-rial (tissue factor) may be thromboplastic and cause a rapid consumption of maternal clotting factors. This maternal bleeding disorder, known as DIC, has an associated mortality of 85%. Fortunately, this complica-tion is rare. If, however, a partial abruptio placentae goes unrecognized, then the incidence of this bleeding disorder is higher.[1]

Recognition of possible abruptio placentae begins with a clinical suspicion based on the patient presenta-tion. The single most important out-of-hospital finding is a mechanism of injury comparable with abruptio pla-centae; no other information is as valuable. The typical abruptio placentae signs and symptoms are vaginal bleeding, uterine tenderness, uterine rigidity, and fetal distress (tachycardia and bradycardia). These findings may be difficult to assess or even absent.

The typical signs and symptoms of abruptio pla-centae are also relatively inaccurate in the hospital set-ting. The most accurate assessment for abruptio placentae is in-hospital electronic monitoring for uter-ine contractions.[1,6,23,26] This monitoring is highly sensi-tive in detecting abruptio placenta.[1,6] Abruptio placentae usually occurs early after maternal trauma; therefore, electronic monitoring should begin as soon as the mother's condition is stabilized.[1] There are two guidelines for the paramedic. First, all pregnant patients (more than 20 weeks) with a mechanism of injury consistent with possible abruptio placentae should be transferred for electronic monitoring.[23] Second, in pregnant trauma patients, any medications that alter uterine contractions are contraindicated. Magnesium and terbutaline stop uterine contractions and therefore interfere with the ability of electronic monitoring to rule out abruptio placentae.[1,19]

INTERNET ACTIVITIES

Visit the e-medicine Web site at http://www.emedicine.com. Click on the Emergency Medicine on-line book and select Obstetrics and Gynecology. Then click on Abruptio Placentae. Review the chapter on the management of abrup-tio placentae.

BLUNT ABDOMINAL INJURIES

Blunt abdominal trauma in pregnancy may result in several serious intra-abdominal injuries: peritoneal bleeding resulting from laceration of the spleen or liver, retroperitoneal bleeding, abruptio placentae, uterine injury, and rarely, rupture of the diaphragm. Conversely, because of the hydraulic effect of the uterus, certain organs are less likely to be injured by blunt abdominal trauma.[1,2,23]

The likelihood of splenic injury and retroperi-toneal hemorrhage is greater in blunt abdominal trauma to the pregnant patient. Both of these injuries may lack the typical abdominal signs and symptoms of serious injury. However, the mortality rate for these life-threatening abdominal injuries appears to be the same in pregnant and nonpregnant women.[2] This may be the result of early recognition and aggressive treat-ment of the hemorrhagic shock associated with serious abdominal injuries.

Up to 40% of major maternal trauma with life-threatening abdominal injuries will have abruptio pla-centae.[14] Minor blunt abdominal trauma may occur in restrained/lap belt injury, unrestrained MVC injury, falls onto the abdomen, and intimate partner violence. As discussed earlier, up to 5% of minor trauma is com-plicated by placental abruption.[14] With respect to the placenta and the fetus, "minor" abdominal trauma is *never* minor.

PELVIC FRACTURE

In MVCs, pelvic fracture is especially dangerous in the pregnant patient. In pregnant women involved in fatal MVCs, pelvic fracture with hemorrhagic shock is the cause of death in nearly 20%.[25]

A marked increase in pelvic vascularity predisposes the pregnant trauma victim to both intra-abdominal and retroperitoneal life-threatening bleeding. There is an increased risk of hemorrhagic shock that is associated with blunt abdominal trauma and with pelvic fracture.[2] Retroperitoneal hemorrhage is commonly associated with pelvic fracture. The retroperitoneal space has the capacity for a volume of greater than 4 liters, accounting for the frequent correlation of hypovolemic shock with pelvic fracture.[14,23]

Pelvic fracture may cause uterine injury or direct fetal injury, and fracture of the maternal pelvis may be associated with many of the same injuries found in the nonpregnant female: laceration of the urethra, vagina, bladder, or ureter; fat embolism; and lumbar spine fracture.[2]

PENETRATING ABDOMINAL INJURY

Penetrating abdominal trauma during pregnancy has a surprisingly low incidence of nonuterine injury and a maternal mortality of less than 5%.[14] Nonuterine injuries occur in only 20% of penetrating maternal wounds (compared to an organ injury rate of 75% in the nonpregnant patient).[14,27] This may be explained by the fact that the uterus and fetus act as a defense for nonuterine maternal organs and/or by the fact that the trauma is frequently directed at the fetus. Not surprisingly the fetal injury rate is extremely high (93%) and the fetal mortality rate is 60%.[14,19] The most common wounds are knife and gunshot wounds, often associated with intimate partner violence, attempts to cause abortion, and aggravated assault.[1]

TRAUMATIC ARREST IN PREGNANCY

Traumatic arrest is always a difficult challenge for the paramedic. The clinical and ethical decisions and the pronouncement of death in the field are guided by accepted protocol. For the pregnant patient, the nature of the cardiopulmonary arrest and the decisions regarding cardiopulmonary resuscitation differ significantly from those of the nonpregnant patient. There are unique, out-of-hospital considerations for the second half of pregnancy.

Maternal traumatic arrest occurs when maternal vital signs have disappeared (and when an injury incompatible with life has occurred). Fetal vital signs may or may not be present immediately after maternal arrest. The best chance of survival for a fetus is aggressive resuscitation of the mother. If, however, the mother is in cardiopulmonary arrest, the paramedic should immediately determine if this patient is a candidate for emergency C-section upon hospital arrival.

Fetal viability is not the paramedic's sole concern; maternal resuscitation may be enhanced by emergency caesarian delivery.[1] Maternal survival has occurred after "postmortem" C-section.[28] A number of factors may favor maternal resuscitation, with removal of uterine vena cava compression probably being the most significant.[19] A perimortem C-section should be considered for any traumatic arrest during pregnancy. If after 1–4 minutes of advanced life support there is no return of maternal pulse and blood pressure, then emergency caesarian criteria should be considered. The two criteria favoring fetal (and perhaps maternal) survival are (1) time since the loss of maternal circulation and (2) fetal age. A shorter time from maternal arrest to delivery yields a greater chance for fetal survival and an improved chance of a neurologically intact newborn.[19] Fetal survival after 25 minutes of maternal arrest has not been reported.[29] The paramedic estimates fetal age by assessing the fundal height of the uterus (see Assessment). A fetal age of 25 weeks or greater is the gestational age considered viable.[1,19]

In the traumatic maternal arrest, as soon as possible, the paramedic should communicate with on-line medical direction and the receiving hospital. Immediate communication is essential. If maternal traumatic arrest is not specifically addressed in protocols and standing orders, in these instances the paramedic cannot legally or ethically terminate cardiopulmonary resuscitation (CPR) in the pregnant patient. In the event that an emergency caesarian delivery is to be performed, early notification of the receiving hospital facilitates preparations for determination of fetal viability, confirmation of fetal age, and surgery in the emergency department. The fetus has the highest chance of survival if an emergency C-section is performed within 5 minutes after loss of maternal vital signs.[2,23] But, if fetal vital signs are present in the emergency department, the procedure is indicated regardless of the duration of maternal arrest.[2,30]

MINOR MATERNAL TRAUMA

As discussed earlier, poor pregnancy outcomes occur in up to 5% of minor trauma.[2,14] The pregnant patient who sustains minor or even trivial injury often appears perfectly stable. Frequently, the patient is ambulatory at the scene and may even request to sign a refusal-of-transport release. In the pregnant patient, dismissing injuries as "minor" or "trivial" risks missing serious injury that may cause fetal death and, on rare occasion, maternal death. Failure to transport a pregnant patient is a decision weighted with serious medicolegal concerns.

Two common injuries often considered minor are falls and seat belt injuries. Because of the frequency of these injuries, they account for the greatest number of adverse pregnancy outcomes.[14]

FALLS

Falls during pregnancy are common; 80% of falls occur in the last 2 months of pregnancy, and falls occur more often during the last 2 months of pregnancy than during any other period in a woman's life.[2,12,19,23] The unsteadiness produced by a change in the center of gravity, a loosening of pelvic ligaments, respiratory alkalosis, and easy fatigability all contribute to the increased incidence of falls.[19,24] Approximately 2% of maternal deaths result from falls.[3] Fortunately, the majority of falls cause no significant maternal injury. However, as previously noted, abruptio placentae and fetal death may result from a simple fall on the buttocks.[2]

SEAT BELT INJURIES

Despite more than 25 years of scientific evidence, many of the nonparamedic public still have a total misunderstanding of the safety of seat belt use during pregnancy.[13] There is a misconception that the use of seat belt restraint systems may be of no help or may even be harmful to the fetus in MVCs during pregnancy. Nothing could be further from the truth. There have been repeated published reports specifically addressing the question of whether seat belt restraint systems are protective or harmful to the fetus in severely injured pregnant women.[12,13,23,31–33] Any (either two-point lap or three-point) use of seat belt restraints is a protection against maternal death, which is a leading cause of fetal death. The three-point restraint system further reduces the risk of both maternal and fetal injury during pregnancy.[33] Maternal and fetal injuries resulting from the seat belt itself do occur. Blunt abdominal maternal injuries have been previously discussed. Placental seat belt injuries may result in abruptio placentae and fetal death. However, the incidence of abruptio placentae is not increased by the use of seat belts.[13,23] In deceleration injuries, three-point restrained pregnant women are at a lower risk for abruptio placentae than those in a two-point or lap belt.[32] Proper use of the lap belt portion (across the pelvis, not the abdomen) of the three-point restraint during pregnancy may further reduce the risk of fetal injury.

OTHER TRAUMA

FETOMATERNAL HEMORRHAGE

Fetomaternal hemorrhage is the transplacental transfusion of fetal blood into the maternal circulation. The incidence and severity of fetomaternal transfusion are not necessarily correlated with the degree of maternal trauma.[2] Ninety percent of fetomaternal hemorrhage is uncomplicated; however, when complications occur, they may be lethal for the fetus. The principal complications are Rh sensitization of the Rh-negative mother and fetal hemorrhagic shock.[1] An early inhospital recognition of fetomaternal hemorrhage may prevent fetal exsanguination or an Rh incompatibility disorder in the mother. An Rh incompatibility disorder, which may be fatal for the fetus, can be easily prevented with administration of anti-Rh immunoglobulin.[19]

UTERINE INJURY

Isolated abdominal trauma or multisystem trauma during pregnancy may result in uterine injury that causes premature labor, premature rupture of the amniotic sac, uterine rupture, and the previously described abruptio placentae.

Uterine rupture is extremely rare, occurring in less than 1% of pregnant trauma patients.[1] This injury, which is unique to pregnancy, usually occurs only with major trauma. There are frequently other life-threatening injuries. Thus, patients with uterine rupture may present to the paramedic with signs of multisystem trauma, intra-abdominal bleeding, an asymmetrical abdomen, and an ill-defined uterine fundus.[23] If hypovolemia and concurrent injuries are well managed, maternal survival is likely. In uterine rupture, maternal mortality is less than 10%; however fetal mortality is nearly 100%, a much higher mortality than in the more commonly occurring abruptio placentae. Generally, uterine rupture occurs only after an enormous amount of direct uterine trauma.

SEXUAL ASSAULT

An estimated 2% of sexual assault victims are pregnant at the time of assault.[34] (The exact incidence of rape during pregnancy has not been well documented. It is estimated that more than 80% of all sexual assaults go unreported.[1]) The majority of assaults take place prior to the fifth month of pregnancy. Oddly, the traumatic injuries inflicted upon pregnant assault victims seem to be no more common than in nonpregnant rape victims.[34]

The paramedic caring for the pregnant rape victim should approach the patient in much the same way that nonpregnant rape victims are managed. The paramedic's responsibility is to care for both the physical and psychological needs of the patient. With the careful attention to the emotional well-being of the woman, the paramedic should determine if there is an indication for trauma assessment and treatment.

THERMAL INJURY

Rarely, a paramedic may care for a pregnant burn patient. Women who sustain burn injuries during pregnancy have the same (perhaps surprisingly) survival rate as nonpregnant women. If a pregnant patient's burn is greater than 50% total body surface area, then the maternal mortality is approximately 70%.[35]

Fetal survival usually parallels the percentage of burned surface area and survival of the mother; for the severely burned woman, fetal prognosis is very poor. Often the pregnant woman has spontaneous premature labor within several days and delivers a stillborn infant.[35] If the mother's prognosis is poor, the fetus has little chance of survival. However, in rare circumstances, a woman's deterioration may jeopardize a viable fetus. In these unusual cases, a C-section may be performed.[36] The potential maternal and fetal benefits of a perimortem cesarean delivery have been discussed earlier.[19,23] The chances for successful revival in any critically ill, hypovolemic pregnant patient may be improved by removal of caval compression by the fetus.[37] Emergency C-section may improve maternal venous return and cardiac output.[23,28] The implication is that the severely burned pregnant patient who appears to be terminal may respond to treatment. The out-of-hospital factors that contribute to poor maternal and fetal outcome are hypovolemia and pulmonary injury. Pregnant women tolerate smoke inhalation and chemical pneumonitis poorly.[1] In treating the pregnant burn patient, aggressive management of the airway, correction of hypoxia and hypercarbia, removal of caval compression, and vigorous fluid resuscitation may reduce maternal and fetal mortality.

ELECTRICAL AND LIGHTNING INJURIES

Maternal deaths as a result of electrical or lightning injury are rare.[1] However, fetal mortality and morbidity are high.[23] In minor maternal lightning injury, poor fetal outcome occurs in the overwhelming majority of cases, approximately 75%. The risk of spontaneous abortion and fetal demise is thought to result in part from the fact that the fluid and electrolyte content of amniotic fluid very effectively conducts current flow to the fetus.[23]

ASSESSMENT

Trauma during pregnancy presents the paramedic with two patients: the mother and the fetus. The trauma assessment of the pregnant patient with either major or minor trauma differs from assessment of the nonpregnant patient. It is appropriate to assess the fetus, and there are critical errors to be avoided. However, in the initial trauma assessment the paramedic's attention must focus on the evaluation and stabilization of the mother. The goal of evaluation and stabilization of maternal injuries is achieved by adhering to the familiar "ABCs" of assessment and treatment—the same as with the nonpregnant patient. Fetal survival depends upon stabilization of the mother's clinical condition. Of critical importance is the maternal circulatory status. Maternal shock, unrecognized and untreated, usually results in fetal demise.[2,25]

The overwhelming majority of pregnant trauma patients assessed by a paramedic are minor trauma.[2,14] The critical issue in these patients is the recognition of potential placental injury. The critical action is transfer to an appropriate facility. In these cases, initial assessment, vital signs, physical examination, and fetal assessment are usually uncomplicated and are accomplished in a matter of minutes.

By contrast, in the critically injured pregnant patient, the paramedic's only focus may be the initial assessment. The paramedic may use the entire out-of-hospital period completing the initial assessment and stabilization.

Assess the pregnant trauma patient just as any trauma patient: an initial assessment leading to a stabilization of vital signs. Next the maternal abdomen, uterine fundus, estimated fetal age, and fetal heart rate are considered, and then the physical examination is completed. The priorities of assessment and stabilization are first, initial assessment; second, fetal survey; and last, focused physical exam.

In the initial assessment, the order of priorities remains the same as always: C—cervical spine, A—airway, B—breathing, C—circulation, D—disability, and E—expose; then consideration may be given to F—fundus/fetal age estimate/fetal heart rate.

The paramedic should be aware of how anatomic and physiological changes of pregnancy may alter assessment and stabilization. Before an orderly integration of these differences into the initial and focused assessments, it may be helpful to review how those changes can contribute to difficulties in assessment. The cardiopulmonary changes of pregnancy can be summarized as high cardiac output, high oxygen demand, low blood pressure (plus or minus low peripheral vascular resistance), low or impeded venous return, and low oxygen reserve. The effects that these changes may have on maternal assessment are given in Table 25-4.

With these in mind, proceed with the familiar systemic progression of assessment and stabilization. In

Table 25-4
Anatomic and Physiological Changes of Pregnancy That Complicate Assessment

Change	Effect on Assessment	Difficulties in Assessment
High cardiac output	HR increases	Increased HR is NOT an early reliable sign of hypovolemic shock
High cardiac output	Increased blood volume	Significant blood loss may NOT be reflected by usual signs of shock
High O_2 demand, low O_2 reserve, low CO_2 normally	RR increases	RR ≤ 20 should NOT be considered adequate ventilation
Elevated abdominal contents	High diaphragm, decreased peritoneal responsiveness	Loss of landmarks for chest compressions; cannot rely on the usual signs of intra-abdominal bleeding

this chapter, the discussion of this process will emphasize how this assessment may be altered in pregnancy.

SCENE SIZE-UP

Before reaching the pregnant patient's side, the paramedic makes a preliminary 1–5-second assessment. While approaching the patient, observe for the presence or absence of labored or inadequate respirations, obvious hemorrhage or abnormal color, confusion or unresponsiveness, and an obviously gravid abdomen.

CERVICAL SPINE

The concern for possible spinal injury is no less important in the pregnant patient; the same indications for immobilization apply. In fact, hormones released during pregnancy to relax the ligaments of the pelvis also affect the ligaments of the cervical spine, predisposing the patient to cervical spine injury. Therefore, any pregnant patient with a severe mechanism of injury, neck pain, or altered level of consciousness should immediately receive in-line manual stabilization of the cervical spine. It is also important to tilt the long spine board to the left, once the patient is immobilized, to displace the uterus from the midline and off the inferior vena cava, reducing the risk for maternal supine hypotension syndrome. Alternatively, if tilting the spine board cannot be easily accomplished, manual displacement of the gravid uterus from the midline is acceptable.

AIRWAY

Aggressive airway management is particularly important in the pregnant trauma patient because of the risk of aspiration and the limited O_2 reserve. Appropriately

securing a protected airway may require rapid-sequence sedation or paralysis when indicated.

BREATHING

The paramedic assessing the adequacy of respiratory rate and depth should recall that the respiratory rate is normally hyperventilatory during pregnancy. A respiratory rate of less than 20 should always be considered potentially dangerous in the pregnant trauma patient. Chest auscultation may yield unequal breath sounds, suggesting pneumothorax, ruptured diaphragm, or unilateral pulmonary contusion. Pneumothoraces and hemothoraces during pregnancy become even more life threatening because of an elevation of the diaphragm and decreased O_2 reserve.

Tension pneumothorax may occur more precipitously in the pregnant patient as a result of hyperventilation combined with elevation of the diaphragm.[19] Timely management of a tension pneumothorax requires early recognition of unequal breath sounds, neck vein distension, and a declining blood pressure (tracheal deviation is a perimortem sign). Be aware that because of the 4-cm elevation of the diaphragm during latter pregnancy, a lateral needle thoracostomy risks causing an intra-abdominal injury.[38]

CIRCULATION

In a pregnant patient in the advanced stages of shock, the assessment may be straightforward: an absent radial pulse and altered level of consciousness. External hemorrhage assessment is performed in the usual fashion. However, *all* of the other usual estimates of circulatory status are subject to misinterpretation. Extensive hemorrhage may occur without the patient demonstrating the usual signs of shock. Heart rate, capillary refill, skin color and temperature, and blood pressure are poor predictors of the amount of blood loss. A pregnant trauma patient with a full pulse, normal skin, and slight confusion may have actually lost 30% of her blood volume.[1,23] In the latter half of pregnancy, circulatory assessment includes checking the position of the uterus. Failure to assess for inferior vena caval compression (and to relieve this compression) may result in a catastrophic drop in cardiac output.[2,14,23]

DISABILITY

The neurological assessment of the pregnant trauma patient is not significantly altered by the changes of pregnancy. Altered level of consciousness has the same significance as for the nonpregnant patient. The pupils are examined for asymmetry, indicating impending brain herniation and the need for hyperventilation. As with the nonpregnant patient, the usual alert, verbal, pain, unresponsive (AVPU) evaluation assesses the pregnant trauma patient for the same potentially reversible causes of altered level of consciousness: cerebral hypoxia, cerebral hypoperfusion, and hypoglycemia.

EXPOSURE

The gross error of failing to identify an obviously gravid uterus can be avoided by simply following the usual trauma life support practice of completely removing the patient's clothing. The patient is quickly inspected for any signs of penetrating or blunt injuries not already detected.

FETUS AND FUNDUS

One of the obvious ways in which the paramedic's evaluation of the pregnant trauma patient is different is the assessment of the uterus and fetus. As soon as the pregnant patient's condition is stabilized with adequate oxygenation, control of external hemorrhage, and adequate volume restoration, the paramedic begins the out-of-hospital obstetric assessment (before the continued assessment portion of the trauma assessment). This initial obstetric assessment consists of examination of the uterine fundus, a quick check for obvious vaginal blood or fluids, and a fetal evaluation.

The critical questions are (1) is there uteroplacental injury, (2) is the fetus of viable age, and (3) is there fetal distress? The critical actions are (1) palpate the uterine fundus, (2) estimate fetal age, and (3) attempt to auscultate fetal heart tones. All of these steps are, of course, inappropriate if maternal vital signs have not been adequately stabilized.

Before the paramedic proceeds with the uterine and fetal assessment, a brief (2–3-second) observation is made for any obvious vaginal blood or fluids. Then the uterus is palpated for tenderness and rigidity; the presence of these suggests serious uteroplacental injury, such as abruptio placentae.[6] Remember that vaginal bleeding and these uterine findings are not as sensitive or specific in confirming abruptio placentae as in-hospital fetal monitoring.[2,6]

In the latter half of pregnancy, the fundus of the uterus should be a well-defined dome on palpation. A nondefinable uterine fundus may indicate uterine rupture or significant intra-abdominal bleeding.

Next, the fundal height of the uterus should be estimated. The distance in centimeters from the pubic symphysis to the dome of the fundus approximates the age of the fetus in weeks (Figure 25-2). If the uterine fundus clearly extends above the umbilicus, the fetal age is estimated as greater than or equal to 26 weeks, and this is an indication of fetal viability.[2,19] The fetus is considered viable if the chance of newborn survival is greater than or equal to 50%. For most neonatal facilities, this occurs after 25 weeks, or at a weight of approximately 750 g.[19]

Prior to reaching the emergency department, the paramedic's methods of assessing fetal distress are limited. Briefly attempt to detect fetal heart tones (FHTs) and palpate the fundus for signs of fetal movement, which indicates potential viability. During the last month of pregnancy the fetal heartbeat can usually be detected using an ordinary stethoscope (the bell of the stethoscope is firmly placed in the periumbilical area). The availability of Doppler ultrasound may easily assess fetal heart rate after 20 weeks. The normal fetal heart rate is 120–160 bpm. An early sign of fetal distress may be tachycardia above 160 bpm. A sustained bradycardia below 110 bpm is an ominous sign that may signal abruptio placentae, fetal hypoxia, or fetal brain injury.[1,2,19]

In the emergency department, mandatory continuous fetal heart rate monitoring is begun in all pregnant trauma patients over 20 weeks gestation.[2,19,23] While continuous, or even frequent, fetal monitoring may not be feasible in the prehospital setting, a brief attempt by the paramedic to assess fetal distress is appropriate. In a number of pregnant trauma patients, fetal distress (not abdominal pain, tenderness, and vaginal bleeding) is the first indication of abruptio placentae.[1,2,19] Fetal distress may be the earliest sign of occult maternal hemorrhagic shock.[38] Since fetal distress is a more reliable sign of shock than other maternal vital signs, fetal heart rate is another "vital sign" useful for assessing maternal status.[1,38]

When the fetal assessment has been completed and maternal vital signs have been stabilized, the

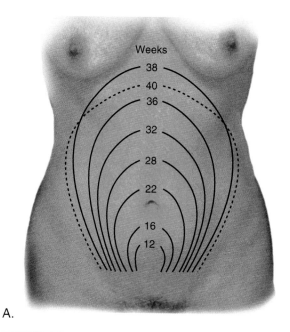

A.

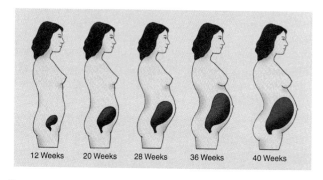

B.

FIGURE 25-2 (A) Estimation of uterine fundal height in centimeters and fetal age in weeks gestation. *Source:* Adapted from Estes, MEZ. *Health Assessment and Physical Examination.* Albany, N.Y.: Delmar Thomson Learning; 1998. (B) Gestational age and contour changes in the abdomen during pregnancy.

remainder of the assessment for fractures and internal injuries may proceed.

ONGOING ASSESSMENT

The ongoing assessment of the pregnant trauma patient is essentially the same as for the nonpregnant patient with a few differences: the abdomen and the pelvis.

Abdomen

Occasionally, the size of the near-term uterus obscures adequate assessment of the abdomen. Keep in mind that the nonpregnant signs of peritoneal irritation and intra-abdominal bleeding are frequently absent.[1,2,19]

Pelvis

The pelvic survey includes a check of the vaginal and perineal areas for blood and amniotic fluid. The bony survey of the pelvis is of critical importance, particularly in the MVC victim. Omission of an adequate bony pelvis examination may result in a failure to detect a pelvic fracture, which is a frequent cause of hypovolemic shock and death in MVC patients.[18,27]

During the course of and then again upon completion of the continued assessment, maternal vital signs should be reassessed, and, if possible, fetal heart rate is reassessed, keeping in mind that fetal assessment should never supersede maternal assessment and treatment. A concentration on the initial assessment directs the paramedic to the pathophysiology of the life-threatening maternal and fetal conditions.

MANAGEMENT

The essential management for all trauma in pregnancy is to ensure adequate maternal and fetal oxygenation and perfusion. Treatment of the pregnant trauma victim begins with the same order of priorities discussed in assessment: ABCDEF.

The pregnant trauma patient's care involves initial and definitive field care by the paramedic, emergency department care (including maternal and fetal diagnostic procedures), and finally, definitive surgical intervention when indicated. Throughout this process, the paramedic, emergency physician, obstetrician, and trauma surgeon must all adhere to the same disciplined clinical approach. The goal of therapy is to manage the traumatic injury in a way that optimizes maternal and fetal health. Critical therapeutic actions include competent assessment, intervention, communication with other members of the medical team, and emotional support of the patient and family. In a minor accident or in a life-threatening crisis, the paramedic needs a plan with rules and strategies. The first rule of trauma management is to treat the pregnant patient's ABCs. Vigorous attention to maternal oxygenation and circulation is the same priority for both the pregnant and nonpregnant patient.[1] The most common causes of fetal death are maternal hemorrhage, maternal death, and abruptio placentae. The most effective initial intervention is aggressive correction of hypovolemia and hypoventilation; maternal stabilization provides fetal stabilization.[2,14,19] Inadequate stabilization may result in the maternal circulation being maintained at the expense of the fetal circulation. Inadequate ventilatory stabilization results in maternal and fetal hypoxia. The critical actions in managing and stabilizing airway and breathing are to recognize and treat an absent gag reflex, a poor respiratory effort and/or rate, and a tension pneumothorax and to administer high-flow oxygen by the appropriate route[2] (Table 25-5).

In the pregnant trauma patient, airway and breathing interventions are indicated for a rate less than 18 and a tidal volume less than 800 mL. If the patient requires intubation, the controlled ventilatory rate of 25–30 produces the desired maternal $PaCO_2$ of 30 mm Hg.[19] The airway and cervical spine are managed simultaneously.

Upon recognition of a tension pneumothorax, a needle thoracentesis should be performed. A lateral

Table 25-5
Trauma Assessment and Treatment in Pregnancy: ABCDEF

Priority	Critical Decision	Altered in Pregnancy	Critical Action
1. C-spine	Does possibility of C-spine injury exist?	Yes, hormones relax C-spine ligaments	Immediately ensure in-line manual stabilization while securing the airway
2. Airway	How best to rapidly secure airway, endotracheal intubation and rapid induction	Yes; aspiration risk obstruction; check gag reflex	Check for foreign body airway reflex; vomitus present; intubate as indicated
3. Breathing	O_2 flow rate Assess breathing; Assess for tension pneumothorax	Yes (O_2 debt) Yes (RR >18/min) Yes (elevated diaphragm)	High O_2 flow rate Check rate and depth: assist if <18/min Check for neck vein distention; needle decompression at second intercostal space (ICS)/mid-clavicular line (MCL)
4. Circulation	Assess for shock	Yes (decreased pulse is a late sign)	Check pulses: carotid and radial
	Identify and treat blood loss	Yes	Apply direct pressure to external hemorrhaging sites
	IV therapy	Yes	Start two large-bore IVs of crystalloid; give 2 liters and reassess
	Vena caval release	Yes	Place patient in left lateral recumbent position
5. Disability	Is there an altered level of consciousness?	No	Check pupillary response and level of consciousness, patient response to pain stimuli
	Is there any risk of herniation?	Yes ($PaCO_2$ <25 mm Hg)	Place on hyperventilatory rate, no less than 20/min; choose rate of 25–30/min
6. Expose	Is the patient pregnant? Stabilize vital signs	Yes No	Completely remove patient's clothing Stabilize before proceeding
7. Fetus	Is there uteroplacental injury, fetal viability, fetal distress, or indication for 4-hr electronic monitoring?	Yes	Check blood and amniotic fluids; palpate uterine fundus; estimate fundal height and fetal age; attempt to detect fetal heart tones; transfer to appropriate facility

fourth or fifth intercostal site insertion may enter the abdominal cavity and is therefore discouraged.[19] An anterior second intercostal/midclavicular site avoids this complication.

While these interventions are proceeding, the other team members may be initiating circulatory stabilizing procedures: controlling major bleeding, starting two IVs, and positioning the patient on her left side. Keep in mind that failure to deflect the uterus away from the inferior vena cava markedly reduces cardiac output.[1,2] The patient should remain on her left side at all times unless this is absolutely impossible. A 6-inch rolled towel beneath the backboard will provide sufficient elevation to deflect the uterus from the vena cava.[14]

Circulation is stabilized in the usual manner: by placing two large-bore IVs with trauma tubing and rapidly infusing 2 liters of crystalloid solution while reassessing vital signs. While starting the IV lines, blood is drawn for rapid glucose testing and for other laboratory studies.

A potential pitfall in the management of circulation in the pregnant patient is the underestimation of internal bleeding (e.g., in a pelvic fracture). A life-threatening hemorrhage with 30%–35% blood volume loss (class III shock) may develop before obviously abnormal vital signs are detectable. In the second half of pregnancy, the volume of crystalloid used to resuscitate hypovolemia may need to be 50% greater. Aggressive volume resuscitation is not likely to result in volume overload (though this must be monitored).[2,14]

After or during the initiation of the IVs it is appropriate to consider using the pneumatic antishock garment (PASG) in the nonpregnant patient. In the pregnant patient, routine use of the PASG is not recommended. There are no studies demonstrating the effectiveness of the PASG for trauma in pregnancy.[2] Furthermore, the application of the abdominal compartment should be considered contraindicated after the 20th week of pregnancy when uterine compression of the inferior vena cava may decrease venous return and preload.[2,6,19,23]

The PASG may be used as a lower extremity air splint and may facilitate IV access. Inflating the PASG leg compartments increases peripheral vascular resistance (and afterload) in the pregnant trauma patient. Theoretically, this might benefit a pregnant patient with low peripheral vascular resistance, but this has not been studied in pregnant trauma patients.[19]

To complete the circulatory assessment, vital signs are obtained and recorded.

A quick neurological assessment of the pupils and AVPU directs the paramedic toward abnormal structural or metabolic conditions. If findings indicate any risk of uncal herniation, the patient should be hyperventilated. A hyperventilation rate over and above the usual tachypnea of pregnancy requires a ventilatory rate of 30 per minute, until arterial blood gases are available (goal: $PaCO_2$ between 25 and 30). If findings indicate hypoglycemia, 50 mL 50% dextrose in water $(D_{50}W)$ is given.

Next, adequately expose the patient and attach monitors (cardiac, BP, pulse oximetry). Reassess vital signs and the patient's response to initial therapy. If the patient has had no response to 2 liters of crystalloid, the patient requires the administration of O-negative blood upon arrival in the emergency department (ED).

After the airway, oxygenation, and fluid resuscitation are secured and completed, a brief obstetric evaluation may be performed, ideally prior to communication with the ED. The paramedic examines for "the four Fs": fluids, fundus, fetal age, and fetal distress, if possible, with the latter being more effectively accomplished in-hospital.

Communication with the ED should occur as soon as possible after the primary stabilization, the reassessment after therapy, and the brief obstetric observation. The paramedic's report to the ED should include (1) the patient's present condition, including interventions necessary; (2) the response to initial therapy; (3) the gestational age by history (if this is known) and/or the estimated fundal height (fetal age) by examination; and, of course, (4) the estimated time of arrival at the ED. This information facilitates ED preparation and mobilization of a multidisciplinary team, if indicated.

Once communication has occurred, reassess vital signs and complete the continued assessment portion of the trauma assessment. Paramedics providing critical care transport may perform gastric decompression with a nasogastric (NG) tube and urinary catheterization. Urinary catheterization provides valuable information regarding (1) renal output (reflective of adequate perfusion) and (2) the presence of blood in the urine. In the setting of traumatic maternal shock, gross hematuria suggests the diagnosis of pelvic fracture and/or a retroperitoneal hemorrhage.

All pregnant patients with *minor* trauma should (1) have high-flow O_2 administered; (2) be transported on their left side; and (3) have a large-bore IV of crystalloid started.

TRAUMATIC MATERNAL ARREST

By the time the paramedic completes the initial assessment and stabilization of the pregnant patient, it should be evident if maternal vital signs are not returning (or if maternal injuries are not compatible with life). After vigorous attempts to resuscitate the pregnant patient appear to have failed (or in a patient who would otherwise meet the criteria for field pronouncement of death), the paramedic should immediately assess the fetus. By this time in the assessment, the only pertinent question is: Is the fetal age 25 weeks or more? The paramedic may choose to document and communicate the fetal age qualitatively in terms of the fundal height, such as "below the umbilicus," "just above the umbilicus," or "well above the umbilicus." Unless specifically countermanded by protocol or by on-line medical direction, maternal resuscitation efforts should be continued until arrival at the ED. When chest compressions are indicated, performance of these may be facilitated by using the 6-inch backboard elevation method of maternal positioning. The hyperventilatory rate should be greater than 30 bpm to optimize PaO_2 and $PaCO_2$ levels.

Early communication with the ED is critical, allowing for mobilization of resources such as neonatology. Radio communication should be brief and blunt, such as: "We are transporting a pregnant traumatic arrest to your facility; fundal height is well above the umbilicus; CPR is in progress; ETA is 4 minutes."

Immediately upon arrival in the ED, a C-section should be performed if fundal height exceeds the umbilicus and clinical signs of fetal life are present (e.g., confirmation of fetal heartbeat). Maternal resuscitation efforts may continue after a perimortem delivery.

MINOR TRAUMA

Rarely is a paramedic confronted with major trauma in pregnancy and imponderables such as traumatic maternal arrest. However, paramedics are likely to encounter minor injuries. It is critical that the paramedic have a consistent and thorough approach to minor trauma in pregnancy. Potential pitfalls in caring for minor maternal trauma patients include (1) failure to do a paramedic obstetric examination; (2) failure to transport to a facility capable of conducting electronic obstetric monitoring; (3) failure to adequately give and document informed consent to a patient who refuses transport; (4) giving false reassurance that the pregnancy outcome will be good; and (5) administering inappropriate drugs to pregnant patients with minor trauma.

In the pregnant patient with minor injury, the maternal initial assessment and vital signs are easily and quickly obtained. Then, as indicated, the paramedic obstetric examination (fluids/fundus/fetal age/fetal heart rate) is performed. Every minor trauma pregnant patient with a fundal height above the umbilicus (25 weeks gestation or more) requires appropriate obstetric electronic monitoring (i.e., a minimum of 4 hours of uterine and fetal monitoring). This approach should include pregnant patients with no apparent signs of pelvic, low back, or abdominal injury. There may be significant fetal or uteroplacental injury without obvious injury.[6,19]

Informed consent for the patient who refuses transport is always problematic. By understanding the epidemiology of minor trauma in pregnancy, the paramedic is better equipped to inform the patient who wishes to refuse transport. The pregnant patient should be informed that even though her injury is minor, it may result in serious complications of pregnancy, such as fetal death, in 5%, or 1 in 20. Documentation should show that the risks and inadvisability of refusal were understood by the patient.

MEDICATIONS TO AVOID IN TRAUMA IN PREGNANCY

The paramedic will, on occasion, administer medications; these may include medications for pain, nausea, or asthma. The use of morphine for severe pain (e.g., ankle fracture) is acceptable. Ketorolac's (Toradol) safety in pregnancy has not been established and therefore should be avoided. Promethazine (Phenergan) has been used extensively in pregnancy; however, its safety, particularly in the first 3 months of pregnancy, has not been established. In the rare instance when a pregnant patient with minor trauma also has asthma, albuterol (Proventil) is probably safe. While albuterol has not been studied in trauma in pregnancy, its use in nontraumatic pregnancy has been. Fetal and placental blood flow alterations and fetal distress have not occurred with albuterol.[39] Two other medications sometimes used in asthma are terbutaline (Brethine) and epinephrine; both of these should be considered contraindicated for routine administration after blunt trauma in pregnancy.[19,23] Neither terbutaline nor epinephrine is the drug of choice for asthma; the former interferes with normal uterine contractions and monitoring, and the latter's vasoconstrictive effects may significantly decrease uterine blood flow and fetal oxygenation.[19,23]

Premature contractions are a common complication of trauma in pregnancy and may occur after minor trauma. Paramedic protocols that include the use of terbutaline or magnesium to arrest premature contractions should be amended to apply only to *nontraumatic* premature labor. The reason is that 90% of these premature contractions will spontaneously disappear and are usually benign.[6] Furthermore, those contractions that do not stop are often associated with uteroplacental injury such as abruptio placentae. In this setting, stopping the uterine contractions might limit the ability to diagnose serious complications.

EMOTIONAL CARE OF THE MATERNAL TRAUMA PATIENT

For the critically injured pregnant patient, the timely and appropriate initial stabilization does not allow for any more than basic emotional support. The paramedic employs the same focused, orderly, professional attention to critical life support decisions and actions.

For the pregnant patient with minor trauma the paramedic has the opportunity to provide more advanced emotional support. This attention to the patient's psychological needs is particularly important in cases of assault and domestic violence. But every pregnant patient has emotional needs. A potential problem for paramedics is the trauma patient who requests reassurance from them that "everything will be OK with my baby." While being emotionally supportive, the paramedic should avoid prognosticating. The paramedic may choose to respond with a comment such as: "The best thing you can do now for your pregnancy is to take care of yourself. While you are being evaluated and treated you'll be helping your baby," or "What the baby needs now is for us to help deliver more blood and oxygen. You can help by lying on your side." The anxious patient may easily interpret "most" as "always " and "not likely" as "never."

The pregnant patient's earliest response may involve denial, anger, guilt, and blaming. One of the healthiest coping responses of the pregnant patient is her involvement and participation in the care of her baby and of herself.

EMERGENCY DEPARTMENT CARE OF THE PREGNANT TRAUMA PATIENT

Once the paramedic presents the pregnant trauma patient to the ED, the process of stabilization and evaluation continues. Before a multidisciplinary team of neonatology, general surgery, and obstetrics can be utilized, the emergency physician proceeds in much the same way the paramedic does: initial, fetal, and continued assessment and treatment. One difference in the emergency physician's approach is that as the prioritized stabilization proceeds, definitive diagnostic evaluations and indicated emergent referrals are made. The

other principal difference from the prehospital approach is electronic monitoring of uterine contractions and fetal heart rate, which should be initiated as soon as the maternal condition is stabilized.

Once the primary stabilization and fetal evaluation have been accomplished, the definitive ED evaluation involve blood studies, x-rays, diagnostic peritoneal lavage, ultrasonography, and placement of NG tube and urinary bladder catheterization (if not already performed by the paramedic). Peritoneal lavage is no longer considered contraindicated in pregnancy.[19] Radiology studies (x-ray, computed tomography, magnetic resonance imaging) without fetal shielding (e.g., pelvis) are considered indicated if these are needed to rule out potentially life-threatening injuries.[19] Initial blood studies are complete blood cell count, including platelets, a DIC screen, type and cross match, routine chemistries and electrolytes, and possibly a Kleihauer Betke (KB) test. (This is a test for the presence of fetal blood in maternal circulation. This test determines the dosage of RhoGAM).

Electronic Obstetric Monitoring

All pregnant patients with direct or indirect abdominal trauma and with an estimated fetal age of greater than 20 weeks must have 4 hours of fetal and uterine electronic monitoring after the trauma event.[1,2,19,23] It is critical that monitoring be begun as soon as possible after maternal vital signs are stabilized in order to detect abruptio placentae, which occurs early after trauma.[1,23]

Monitoring for fetal heart rate abnormalities helps detect not only abruptio placentae but also maternal shock and fetal compromise. For ruling out adverse pregnancy outcomes, uterine monitoring appears to be even more important than fetal monitoring. Monitoring for uterine contractions (tocography) is extremely accurate in predicting abruptio placentae. If after 4 hours of uterine monitoring no abnormal uterine contraction activity is observed, the patient's chances of a normal pregnancy outcome are similar to that of an uninjured pregnant woman. Greater than four contractions in 1 hour is considered an abnormal contraction pattern.[14]

Fetomaternal Hemorrhage

As mentioned earlier in the chapter, a rare complication of trauma in pregnancy is the transfusion of fetal blood into the maternal circulation. The routine screening blood work done on pregnant trauma patients sometimes includes a KB test (for presence of fetal blood) and always should include type and Rh determination. In most cases, the KB test is useless because (1) it may fail to detect small but harmful amounts of fetal blood and (2) all Rh-negative mothers may safely receive an anti-Rh prophylactic injection. (This injection of anti-Rh immunoglobulin rids the maternal blood of Rh-positive fetal blood, thereby preventing maternal sensitization against and rejection of fetal blood.)[40] All Rh-negative pregnant women presenting after direct or indirect abdominal trauma should receive the standard anti-Rh injection.[19] It is not critical that this injection be given within 24 hours. However, to avoid mistakes in follow-up, it is most practical to administer the anti-Rh immunoglobulin injection prior to the patient's leaving the ED.

Emotional Support and Protective Services

The emergency physician continues the same attention to the pregnant patient begun by the field paramedic. In addition to anticipating the normal concerns and anxieties, the ED staff should be prepared to provide the initial emotional support for the patients with grief reactions or patients who have been victims of domestic violence or sexual assault. The ED is in a position to provide the patient with appropriate consultants and resources. This may involve consultation with mental health professionals, protective services, law enforcement, and crisis intervention counselors for victims of rape or domestic violence. The ED must comply with the state's requirements for reporting assault.

Admission Criteria

In some EDs that are staffed with ED paramedics, the paramedic will care for minor trauma patients. The appropriate role of the ED paramedic in managing minor trauma in pregnancy is to involve the ED physician early in the evaluation and in the disposition. For some EDs there is a policy to transfer all stable pregnant trauma patients to the labor and delivery department for further evaluation. If, however, the departmental policy is that some pregnant trauma patients are seen by the emergency physician and the ED paramedic, then there are admission criteria to be carefully observed. The pregnant trauma patient should *not* be discharged from the emergency department if any of these admission criteria are present. All pregnant trauma patients who are over 24 weeks pregnant should be admitted for 24 hours or more for the following: (1) vaginal bleeding; (2) rupture of membranes/amniotic fluid leak; (3) any evidence of maternal hypovolemia, even if the maternal vital signs are stable; (4) any serious maternal injury, even if the maternal vital signs are stable; (5) uterine or abdominal

pain and/or tenderness; (6) abnormalities (e.g., hematoma) found on uterine ultrasound; (7) abnormal uterine contraction pattern: over four contractions in an hour; and (8) abnormal fetal heart rate: (a) sustained tachycardia (greater than 160 bpm per minute), (b) sustained bradycardia (less than 120 bpm), (c) transient bradycardia occurring late after maternal contraction, and (d) loss of rate variability. The majority of these criteria can be detected by the field paramedic's 4F obstetric assessment.

The treatment of the pregnant trauma patient can be summarized with a priority setting: ABCDEF. A careful but rapid flow through the ABC process identifies critical actions needed to reverse unstable or lethal conditions. The chief differences from the treatment of nonpregnant patients are the fetal assessment and the circulatory critical actions: placing the patient in the left lateral decubitus position and more aggressive than usual fluid resuscitation (2 liters rapid infusion). In minor trauma, the treatment is to provide high-flow O_2, establish an IV, place in left lateral decubitus position, and transfer to an appropriate facility for 4-hour uterine and fetal monitoring.

In more serious trauma, the paramedic and ED protocols should thoroughly and efficiently advance the field and ED professionals through a system of mostly familiar priorities and critical actions (see Table 25-5).

INTERNET ACTIVITIES

Visit the British Trauma Society Web site at http://www.trauma.org/resus/pregnancytrauma.html and review the material on trauma in pregnancy.

SUMMARY

Trauma during pregnancy is common. A systematic approach for managing minor and major trauma in pregnancy is based upon familiar, core ABC management principals. The ABCDEF approach includes attention to clinically relevant pregnancy-related changes in anatomy and physiology; this system effectively addresses the maternal, fetal, and placental complications of trauma. The paramedic's role in trauma management of pregnant women is critical. The paramedic caring for the pregnant trauma patient may encounter anxiety-provoking and tragic circumstances. Early recognition of and intervention for life-threatening maternal, placental, and fetal conditions ensures the best chance for maternal and fetal well-being.

▶ REVIEW QUESTIONS

1. In the United States, the most common reported injuries in the pregnant trauma patient are:
   a. Physical assaults
   b. Motor vehicle crashes
   c. Industrial accidents
   d. Falls

2. In urban locales in the United States, such as Cook County, Illinois, the most common cause of death in pregnant patients is:
   a. Complications of pregnancy, labor, and delivery
   b. Motor vehicle crashes
   c. Gunshot wounds
   d. Stab wounds

3. Most trauma in pregnancy is a result of:
   1. Domestic violence
   2. Motor vehicle crashes
   3. Gunshot wounds
   4. Minor trauma
      a. 1, 2, 3
      b. 1, 3
      c. 2, 4
      d. 4 only
      e. All of the above

4. Adverse pregnancy outcomes in severely injured pregnant patients with maternal shock are:
   a. 100%
   b. 80%
   c. 50%
   d. 25%

5. In minor abdominal trauma, such as a simple fall:
   1. Abruptio placentae may occur.
   2. If there are no pelvic signs or symptoms, abruptio placentae may occur.
   3. Fetal demise may result.
   4. Direct fetal trauma is unlikely.
      a. 1, 2, 3
      b. 1, 3
      c. 2, 4
      d. 4 only
      e. All of the above

6. In the 1990s, a pregnant woman's highest mortality was associated with:
   a. Toxemia
   b. Postpartum hemorrhage
   c. Postpartum infection
   d. Trauma

7. Today, a pregnant woman's highest mortality is associated with:
   a. Obstetric-related diseases (such as toxemia) treated in an urban setting
   b. Urban trauma
   c. Obstetric-related diseases treated in a rural setting
   d. Rural trauma

8. Fetal mortality correlates most with:
   a. Presence of pelvic trauma
   b. Maternal mortality
   c. Presence of maternal shock
   d. Presence of head trauma

9. Anatomic differences between the nonpregnant and the obstetric patient include all the following except:
   a. Obstetric patient has a risk of decreased venous return causing a decrease in cardiac output.
   b. Obstetric patient has a cephalad displacement of her diaphragm.
   c. Obstetric patient has a decreased perfusion to the extrauterine pelvis.
   d. Obstetric patient has a greater size of pelvic vessels than the nonpregnant patient.

10. Physiological differences between the nonpregnant and the obstetric patient include all of the following except:
    a. In the pregnant patient, the resting heart rate is normally 10–15 bpm slower.
    b. In the pregnant patient, the resting respiratory rate is more rapid, thereby lowering the $PaCO_2$.
    c. In the pregnant patient, the blood pressure may be 10%–15% lower.
    d. In the pregnant patient, the gastric emptying rate is slower.

11. In penetrating midabdominal trauma during the latter months of pregnancy, visceral injuries to the mother:
    a. Occur in only 20% of pregnant patients as compared to over 70% of nonpregnant patients
    b. Occur in over 70% of pregnant patients as compared to only 20% of nonpregnant patients
    c. Occur in equal frequency in pregnant and nonpregnant patients
    d. Death is more likely due to nonobstetric injury and not uterine injury.

12. Unlike abruptio placentae, uterine rupture:
    a. Is more common
    b. May result from minor trauma
    c. May present without abdominal pain, tenderness, and hypovolemia signs
    d. Is more likely to be associated with maternal death due to the concurrent nonobstetric injuries

13. A multiple-trauma patient has an HR of 110, an RR of 26, anxiety and a confused mental status. The patient is 7 months pregnant. The class shock and estimated blood loss would be:

a. No shock; simple anxiety
b. Class I; 10% blood loss
c. Class II; 20% blood loss
d. Class III; 30% blood loss
e. Class IV; 40% blood loss

14. The most sensitive method of detecting possible abruptio placentae in the pregnant trauma patient is:
   a. Vaginal bleeding; if none, abruptio is unlikely
   b. Palpation of fundus by the paramedic; if nontender, abruptio is unlikely
   c. Fetal monitoring by the paramedic; if fetal heart tones (FHT) are greater than 120, abruptio is unlikely
   d. Electronic monitoring of uterine contractions

15. In trauma during pregnancy, fetomaternal hemorrhage, or fetal blood entering the maternal circulation:
   a. Is not of clinical significance after minor trauma
   b. Often results in maternal exsanguination
   c. Is more likely, depending upon the severity of injury
   d. Should always be treated with Rh immunoglobulin if the pregnant patient is Rh negative

16. In a 7-month pregnant multiple-trauma patient with an HR of 110, an RR of 26, anxiety and a confused mental status, the initial out-of-hospital treatment would be:
   a. D_5W, keep vein open (KVO) rate
   b. Crystalloid, KVO rate
   c. Crystalloid, 250 mL/hr
   d. Crystalloid, 1–2 liters infused rapidly
   e. None of the above

▶ CRITICAL THINKING

● Upon arrival at the scene of an MVC, you are led to a patient sitting on the curb. The patient is a 28-year-old female who was the driver of a vehicle that was struck head-on by a second vehicle. The impact was low speed and there is approximately 24 inches of crush to the front of the vehicle. The patient is obviously pregnant but has had no prenatal care and does not know her due date. She denies injury. Shoulder and lap restraints were worn. The car was not equipped with an airbag. Upon physical exam, the patient is conscious, alert, and oriented ×3. Skin is warm, dry, and normal in color. Capillary refill time is 2 seconds. Blood pressure is 136/P (palpation), HR 110, RR 36, and SpO_2 (oxygen saturation) 97%. Breath sounds are clear and equal bilaterally. The abdomen is soft and nontender, but there is a lap belt abrasion that extends across the abdomen at the level of the umbilicus. The fundus extends approximately 36 cm above the pubis. The patient refuses transport, stating she is uninjured. Based upon the physical examination, what is the gestational age of the fetus? Despite the lack of physical signs of injury, what injuries may exist? How reliable are the vital signs at predicting injury? Should this patient be encouraged to consent to transport? Explain the physiological changes of pregnancy that are relevant to this patient.

● You are dispatched to the scene of a gunshot wound. Your patient is a 32-year-old female who appears to be 36–38 weeks pregnant. She has sustained a gunshot wound to the left temple. The wound appears to be from a small-caliber handgun. There is minimal external hemorrhage. The patient is pulseless and apneic and cardiopulmonary resuscitation (CPR) is being performed by the first responders. The pupils are fixed and dilated. Witnesses to the shooting indicate that 10 minutes has elapsed since the shooting. Transport time to the hospital will be 12 minutes. Should CPR be discontinued on the scene? Why or why not? What treatment, if any, should be initiated on this patient?

● Recently the media reported the case of a perimortem C-section that was performed by two field paramedics on the order of their medical control. The mother was never resuscitated and expired at the scene and the infant survived only a few days. The paramedics then faced reprimands from their employer for performing a procedure outside their scope of practice. Evaluate the merits of performing a C-section in the field. If faced with the same situation, how would you respond?

▶ REFERENCES

1. Cunningham FG, MacDonald PC, Gant NF, eds. *Williams Obstetrics*, 19th ed. Norwalk, Conn: Appleton & Lange; 1993.
2. Pearlman MD, Tintinalli JE, Lorenz RP: Blunt trauma in pregnancy. *N Engl J Med.* 1990; 323:1609.
3. Fildes J, Reed L, Jones N, Martin M, Barnett J. Trauma: the leading cause of maternal death. *J Trauma.* 1992; 32:643.
4. Standler HJ. *Williams Obstetrics*, 9th ed. New York: Appleton-Century; 1945.
5. Helton AS, Aderson E, McFarlane J. Battered and pregnant: a prevalence study with intervention measures. *Am J Public Health.* 1987; 77:1337.
6. Pearlman MD, Tintinalli JE, Lorenz RP. A prospective controlled study of outcome after trauma

during pregnancy. *Am J Obstet Gynecol.* 1990; 162:1502.

7. Abbott J, Johnson R, Koziol-McCain J, Lowenstein SR. Domestic violence against women: incidence and prevalence in an emergency department population. *JAMA.* 1995; 273:1763.

8. The National Committee for Injury Prevention and Control. *Injury Prevention: Meeting the Challenge.* New York: Oxford University Press; 1989.

9. McLear SV. Education is not enough: a systems failure in protecting battered women. *Ann Emer Med.* 1989; 18:651.

10. Olson L, Anctil C, Fullerton L, Brillman J, Arbuckle J, Sklar D. Increasing emergency physician recognition of domestic violence. *Ann Emerg Med.* 1996; 27:741.

11. McLear SV, Anwar R. A study of battered women presenting in an emergency department. *Am J Public Health.* 1989; 79:65.

12. Rothenberger D, Quattlebaum FW, Perry JF, Zabel J, Fischer RP. Blunt maternal trauma: a review of 103 cases. *J Trauma.* 1978; 18:173.

13. Crosby WM, Costiloe JP. Safety of lap-belt restraint for pregnant victims of automobile collisions. *N Engl J Med.* 1971; 284:632.

14. Pearlman MD. Management of trauma during pregnancy. *Female Patient.* 1996;21:10.

15. Hoff WS, D'Amelio LF, Tinkoff GH, et al. Maternal predictors of fetal demise in trauma during pregnancy. *Surg Gynecol Obstet.* 1991; 172:175.

16. Agran PF, Dunkle DE, Winn DG, Kent D. Fetal death in motor vehicle accidents. *Ann Emerg Med.* 1987; 16:1355.

17. Stafford PA, Biddinger PW, Zumwall RE. Lethal intrauterine fetal trauma. *Am J Obstet Gynecol.* 1988; 159:458.

18. Crosby WM. Traumatic injuries during pregnancy. *Clin Obstet Gynecol.* 1983;26:902.

19. Neufield J. Trauma in pregnancy. *Emerg Med Clin North Am.* 1993; 2(1):207.

20. deSwiet M. The cardiovascular system. In: Hyten F, Chamberlain G, eds. *Clinical Physiology in Obstetrics.* Oxford: Blackwell Scientific Publications; 1980.

21. Waters W, MacGregor W, Hills M. Cardiac output at rest during pregnancy and the puerperium. *Clin Sci.* 1966; 30:1.

22. Ueland K, Hansen J. Maternal cardiovascular dynamics, posture, and uterine contractions. *Am J Obstet Gynecol.* 1969; 103:1.

23. Tintinelli J, Ruiz E, Krome RL. *Emergency Medicine: A Comprehensive Study Guide,* 4th ed. New York: McGraw Hill; 1996.

24. Crosby WM. Trauma during pregnancy: maternal and fetal injury. *Obstet Gynecol Surg.* 1974; 29:683.

25. Crosby WM, Snyder RG, Snow CC, Hanson PG. Impact injuries in pregnancy. *Am J Obstet Gynecol.* 1968; 10:100.

26. Kettel LM, Branch DW, Scott, JR. Occult placental abruption after maternal trauma. *Obstet Gynecol.* 1988; 71:449.

27. Buchsbaum HJ. *Trauma in Pregnancy.* Philadelphia: Saunders; 1979.

28. DePace NL, Betesh JS, Kotler MN. "Postmortem" caesarian delivery with recovery of both mother and offspring. *JAMA.* 1982; 248:971.

29. Weber CE. Postmortem caesarian section: review of the literature and case reports. *Am J Obstet Gynecol.* 1971; 110:158.

30. Katz VL, Dotters DJ, Droegemueller W. Perimortem caesarian delivery. *Obstet Gynecol.* 1986; 68:571.

31. American College of Obstetricians and Gynecologists. Automobile passenger restraints for children and pregnant women. *ACOG Tech Bull.* 1991; 151:1.

32. Crosby WM, King AI, Stout LC. Fetal survival following impact: improvement with shoulder restraint. *Am J Obstet Gynecol.* 1972; 112:1101.

33. Wolf ME, Alexander BH, Rivara FP, Hickok DE, Maier RV, Starzyk PM. A retrospective cohort study of seatbelt use and pregnancy outcome after a motor vehicle crash. *J Trauma.* 1992; 34:116.

34. Satin AJ, Hamsell DL, Stone IC, Theriot S, Wendel GD. Sexual assault in pregnancy. *Obstet Gynecol.* 1991; 77:710.

35. Amy BW, McManus WF, Goodwin CW, Mason A, Pruitt BA. Thermal injury in the pregnant patient. *Surg Gynecol Obstet.* 1985; 161:209.

36. Rode H, Millar AJ, Cywes S, et al. Thermal injury in pregnancy—the neglected tragedy. *J. S Afr Med.* 1990; 77:346.

37. Pimental L. Mother and child. *Emerg Med Clin North Am.* 1991; 9:549.

38. Scarletta TA, Schader JJ. *Emergent Management of Trauma.* New York: McGraw Hill; 1996.

39. Rayburn WF, Atkinson BD, Gilbert K, Tumbull GL. Short term effects of inhaled albuterol on maternal and fetal circulations. *Am J Obstet Gynecol.* 1994; 173:770.

40. Goodwin TM, Breen MT. Pregnancy outcome and fetomaternal hemorrhage after noncatastrophic trauma. *Am J Obstet Gynecol.* 1990; 162:665.

OBJECTIVES

Upon completion of this chapter, the reader should be able to:

- Describe the epidemiology and etiology of pediatric trauma.
- Describe the basic factors of growth and development from birth to adolescence.
- List the important factors of pediatric anatomy and physiology and describe the differences between children and adults.
- Outline the ABCDEF approach to pediatric trauma assessment.
- List the criteria for transfer of the pediatric trauma patient to a pediatric level I trauma center.
- Describe the airway management of the pediatric trauma patient.
- Discuss the fluid resuscitation management of the pediatric trauma patient.
- Describe the prehospital management of chest and abdominal injuries in the pediatric trauma patient.
- Describe the evaluation and treatment of pelvic and extremity injuries in the pediatric patient.
- Discuss the epidemiology of child abuse and neglect and the recognizable signs of abuse and neglect.
- Discuss the importance of integrating family members into the care of pediatric trauma patients.
- Discuss the importance of injury prevention for children.

KEY TERMS

Aerophagia	Kehr's sign
Commotio cordis	SCIWORA
Cullen's sign	Waddell's Triad

Caring for pediatric trauma patients is often a frightening experience for emergency providers, owing mostly to the infrequent contact with these patients. Although the assessment and management priorities do not differ greatly from those of adults, children do have unique anatomical and physiological characteristics that must be considered. This chapter highlights the distinct differences between the pediatric and adult trauma patient, enabling the EMS provider to address the specific needs of injured children. The reader is referred to the discussions of the general management of injured patients in earlier chapters for a complete understanding of pediatric trauma.

EPIDEMIOLOGY

Traumatic injuries kill more children between ages 1 and 18 than any other cause of death. Nearly half of all pediatric deaths in the United States are the result of trauma.[1,2] Each year, over 12,000 children between ages 1 and 19 die from unintentional injury, over 6 million are seen in emergency departments, 500,000 are hospitalized, and 50,000 are permanently disabled.[2-6] Fifty percent of child deaths from trauma occur within the first hour after injury. The most common mechanism of unintentional injury is motor vehicle–related trauma, accounting for about 40% of deaths, followed in descending order by drownings, pedestrian injuries, fires/burns, bicycle crashes, firearm wounds, and falls.[6-8] Blunt trauma is still the most prevalent mechanism (80%–90%); however, penetrating injury (gunshots and stabbings) accounts for 10%–20% of injuries and has become more common among children.[9] Blunt trauma often leaves minor external evidence of injury, so the paramedic must keep a high index of suspicion of underlying injuries, particularly if the mechanism of injury is known to result in internal injuries.

Intentional injuries kill over 5,500 more children between ages 0 and 19 each year. Homicide accounts for the largest portion of these deaths. Suicides are a significant cause of mortality for 10- to 19-year-olds, their third leading cause of all deaths. From 1980 to 1997, the rate of suicide among Americans aged 15–19 increased by 11% and among persons 10–14 years of age by 109%. Although suicide among young children is a rare event, the dramatic increase in the rate for 10- to 14-year-olds underscores the urgent need for prevention efforts for those in this age group. From 1980 to 1996, the suicide rate increased 105% for African-American males aged 15–19. Among 15- to 19-year-olds, firearm-related suicides accounted for over 60% of the increase from 1980 to 1997. The risk for suicide among young people is greatest among young white males; however, suicide rates are increasing most rapidly among young black males.[6]

Rates of homicide among youths 15–19 years of age reached record-high levels in the latter half of the 1980s, but in 1997, the rate of homicide among 15- to 19-year-old males declined 12.4% in 1 year. Despite this encouraging trend, current rates are distressingly high.[6]

Nonfatal injuries often occur during play activities both at home and in organized sports. Trampolines, for example, injure over 60,000 children each year, mostly leg and foot fractures and lower extremity sprains. Skates and skateboard crashes have caused at least 36 deaths since 1992, with wrist fractures and wrist sprains being the most prevalent nonfatal injury from this activity. Diving incidents can result in head and spinal cord injuries. Organized sports (baseball, basketball, football, soccer, hockey, skiing) send a quarter of a million children under age 15 to emergency departments every year, and lower extremity injuries predominate in all sports except basketball, where wrist and hand injuries are prevalent as well. Football, lacrosse, field hockey, and ice hockey may also cause significant head, spine, chest, and abdominal trauma. Proper protective sports gear can significantly reduce the severity of sport-related injuries. Because pediatric trauma deaths are a relatively rare occurrence while nonfatal injuries are common, the EMS professional can expect to care for many children with nonfatal injuries.

Each cause of traumatic death has a unique profile, depending upon the child's developmental level (e.g., toddler), a physical disability (such as hearing loss), the prevalence of a particular threat in a community (e.g., all-terrain vehicles, kerosene heaters), access to and use of preventive measures (e.g., seat belts, bicycle helmets), and level of supervision of the child (e.g., parent, another child). However, in general, males, those from low socioeconomic groups, and African-American and Native-American children are at highest risk for traumatic injury.[6] See Table 26-1 for common sources of trauma in children by age category.

MECHANISMS OF INJURY

Children often demonstrate amazing resilience in cases of trauma. Often, children do not appear "sick" immediately after suffering a significant injury. Treatment based on the mechanism of injury is more appropriate than care based solely on the child's presenting signs and symptoms or general appearance. Trauma in

Table 26-1
General Epidemiology of Pediatric Trauma by Age Groups

Age	Common Sources of Trauma
0–1	Child abuse, burns, falls, drowning
1–4	Motor vehicle crashes, drowning, burns, falls, pedestrian events
5–9	Motor vehicle crashes, pedestrian crashes, bicycle injuries, drowning, burns, falls, sports and recreational injuries
10–14	Motor vehicle crashes, bicycle crashes, drowning, sports and recreational injuries, gunshot wounds, suicide, burns
15–19	Motor vehicle crashes, pedestrian injuries, drowning, gunshot injuries, homicide, suicide, sports and recreational injuries

children differs from adult trauma for several reasons. A child's unique anatomical features often contribute to specific injury patterns. Also, a child's physiology responds to trauma slightly differently than an adult's, influencing the way traumatic injuries of children are managed. Children with internal injuries may present with normal baseline assessment findings and may rapidly decompensate after exhausting their natural compensatory mechanisms, chiefly tachycardia and increased systemic vascular resistance. High-risk mechanisms of injury include motor vehicle crashes, falls from moderate to high heights, diving injuries, pedestrian/motor vehicle collisions, unhelmeted bicycle crashes, and gunshot and stab injuries.

The pattern of injury associated with a high-speed motor vehicle crash typically includes serious head injuries, high cervical spine injuries, lacerations and abrasions (caused when unrestrained occupants are tossed around the passenger compartment), soft tissue injuries of the neck (caused by improperly worn shoulder belts), internal abdominal injury (caused when a lap belt is used without a shoulder belt or when a lap belt is improperly positioned above the iliac crest), and fractures of the lumbar spine (caused by hyperflexion at the waist when a lap belt is used without a shoulder belt). A history of being unrestrained significantly increases the risk of serious injury. A child's risk of life-threatening injury is usually minimal during lower speed vehicle crashes of 15 miles per hour or less—if the child is properly restrained. However, if the restraint is not properly positioned, then minor or moderate head and cervical spine injuries, lacerations and abrasions of the face and head, chest and abdominal injuries, and fractures of the lumbar spine can result.[10]

Passive supplemental restraint systems (SRSs) are designed to protect adult passengers. Due to their smaller stature, children are not optimally positioned in the seat and therefore may be seriously injured by a deploying air bag. Common SRS injuries include severe head injuries, high cervical spine injuries, and burns to the face and eyes.

High-risk pedestrian injury involves a vehicle moving at moderate or high speeds. Severe injuries occur when the child is thrown onto the hood or into the windshield of the car or if the child is projected any distance on impact. Typical injuries include severe head injuries, injuries of the torso, and fractures of the lower extremities. This series of injury is referred to as **Waddell's triad**. Waddell's triad includes three injuries: Injury to the femur and/or tibia/fibula occurs from striking the vehicle's bumper; a torso injury occurs from striking the grille and hood; and a closed head injury occurs when the child either rolls over the hood and strikes the head on the windshield or is projected away from the vehicle and strikes the head on the

ground. The head injury causes the highest mortality rate and must be addressed in the initial management period. The potential for an undiagnosed chest injury is very high. The flexible structures of the ribs provide little protection of the major organs and volume loss into to the abdomen and chest is likely. Finally, the lower extremity injury, while not life threatening, can cause long-term complications if not properly managed.

An infant or toddler who is "run over" by a car (e.g., while playing in a driveway) may sustain major injuries. Typical injuries include internal injuries of the chest, often without obvious external injury, resulting in respiratory distress or failure, abdominal injuries with hypotension, pelvic fractures, and fractures of the extremities.

In any fall, the seriousness of the injury depends on the height of the fall, the surface landed on, and the child's age. Injuries due to falls are particularly common in infants. An infant who falls 3 or 4 feet from a changing table onto a hard floor can sustain serious head injuries, injuries comparable to those seen in an older child falling 5 feet out of a bunk bed onto a similar surface. However, an infant falling 2 or 3 feet from a bed onto a carpeted floor is not as likely to suffer significant injury. Moderate falls of about 5–15 feet can result in injuries to the head, neck, and extremity fractures. Falls from greater than 15 feet (e.g., a fall from a second-story window) cause significant head, neck, chest, and abdominal injuries and often multiple fractures of the upper and lower extremities. A history of a fall greater than three times the child's height or when a child has been the victim of rapid-deceleration injury mandates immediate and aggressive therapy.

High-risk bicycle crashes occur when the child falls and lands on a hard surface. Typical injuries include head and neck trauma, lacerations and abrasions to the scalp and face, as well as fractures of the extremities. Failure to don a helmet increases the likelihood of serious head injury. A history of striking the handlebars during the crash increases the index of suspicion for internal injuries and hemorrhage. Bicycle crashes in which the child is wearing a helmet and traveling at low speeds typically result in small lacerations and abrasions and isolated fractures of the upper extremities.

The mechanism of injury is an important clue to the clinical picture of the pediatric patient. By understanding what to look for under certain circumstances, appropriate management can be initiated quickly and efficiently. The two greatest initial threats to the pediatric trauma patient's survival are respiratory failure and shock. Therefore, the key to pediatric trauma care is aggressive management of the airway and maintenance of circulation. Table 26-2 lists the major mechanisms of injury and their most commonly associated injuries.

Table 26-2
Common Injuries Based on Mechanisms of Injury

Mechanism	Injuries
Motor vehicle crashes	Blunt thoracoabdominal trauma, head injury
Pedestrian trauma	Head injury, chest injury, femur and tibia/fibula fractures
Near drowning	Hypoxia, coma, brain damage
Falls	Head injury, spinal and extremity fractures, internal chest and abdomen injury
House fires	Body burns, inhalation injury
Bicycle–motor vehicle collision or falling forward over the handlebars	Head and neck trauma, extremity fractures, abrasions and lacerations
Poisoning	Coma, kidney failure, hepatic failure
Gunshots and stabbings	Injury to organs and tissues in the direct path of the sharp or bullet; pneumothorax, hemothorax, tension pneumothorax, cardiac tamponade

CHILD ABUSE

Victimization of children has existed for centuries. The situation was so bad in Victorian England that attempts were made to improve the treatment of children using laws enacted to protect animals from cruelty. In the early 1960s Henry Kempe coined the term, "battered child syndrome."[11]

Homicide is the fourth leading cause of death in children under age 4 and ranks third among children from ages 10 to 14. Head injury is the leading cause of death among children who perish from child abuse. The need for a careful, timely review of child deaths remains a high priority of health care professionals.[12]

Child victimization remains a complex health and social problem that is not isolated to any socioeconomic group. Nearly 20% of all traumatic injuries seen in children under the age of 3 years are caused by maltreatment.[13] It is impossible to know the number of injuries that go unreported. Between 2,000 and 5,000 children are killed each year at the hands of a parent, guardian, or caregiver.[14] Most of these children are victims of repeated abuse. Physical abuse can manifest itself in

many ways: shaking, burns (see Chapter 17), beatings, binding, twisting extremities, gagging, poisoning, or starvation.

Sexual abuse is a form of exploitation of children and adolescents. This includes sexual activities that children do not fully understand, activities that are beyond their developmental level and to which they are unable to give informed consent, or activities that violate social taboos regarding roles and relationships within the family.

All suspected abuse must be reported to the appropriate agency. Suspicion is key to recognition; early recognition is the key to prevention. The indications that a child is being abused may be severe and obvious or deceptively mild. Clues such as a discrepancy between the history and the injury, a history of a repeated injury, or a contradictory history should raise suspicion. Look for multiple unexplained injuries or bizarre injuries such as bite marks, cigarette burns, or marks with a distinct pattern. Multiple bruises in various stages of healing can be a sign of abuse. A delay in seeking medical treatment, caregivers who are too eager to explain away an injury, or those who are resistant to providing information should increase the suspicion of abuse. Document the caregiver's story and any environmental clues so that child protective services can appropriately address the situation.

Since children have pliable bones, a great deal of force is required to cause a clean break. Long-bone fractures, particularly of the femur and humerus, are rare in infants and young children. The force necessary to fracture a long bone is usually beyond anything that happens unintentionally (e.g., a school-age child falling down the stairs or an infant rolling off a changing table).

An infant who is shaken violently can have severe head injuries, often without obvious external injury. In a typical scenario, EMS is called to the scene after a baby that has been shaken stops breathing or experiences a seizure secondary to the head injury. The coup-contrecoup injury to the brain damages the nerve tissue deep within the brain and tears the bridging veins between the brain and the dura, resulting in subdural or epidural bleeds. Repeated shaking, even if mild, significantly worsens this damage and leads to cerebral edema and subsequent neurological deficit. Consider this possibility in infants and children younger than 2 years who present in extremis without an obvious mechanism of injury.

Shaking can cause vertebrae to slide across each other and pinch, bruise, or transect the spinal cord without breaking any bones. This is due to the softness of the vertebrae and the flexibility of the connecting tissues. Symptoms such as numbness, tingling, and paralysis may develop over time.

Child abuse often leaves long-term sequelae even if the abuse is short term. Without appropriate entry into the health care system, these children are at risk for long-term complications.

GROWTH AND DEVELOPMENT

The assessment of children, while similar to adults, is very much an art form all its own. To ascertain the severity of a child's condition, the paramedic must swiftly determine several important parameters. Growth and development landmarks are important when deciphering the child's response to an emergency. The following brief descriptions of normal behavior refine the understanding of the injured child.

NEONATES (0–4 WEEKS)

Newborn babies are totally dependent upon others for survival. Without a caretaker to clothe, feed, change, warm, and nurture them, they quickly die. While neonates are a subgroup of infants, it is important to recognize the first 4 weeks of life as a very unique time in human growth and development. Infants born before 40 weeks gestation are less physically and neurologically developed. Pregnancy history of the mother and birth history of the infant are important. Because of underdeveloped thermoregulatory mechanisms and low amounts of subcutaneous fat, neonates must be kept warm.[15] Neonates and infants cry to express any type of pain or distress. Congenital anomalies and unintentional injuries are common causes of emergencies in this age group.

INFANTS (1 MONTH–1 YEAR)

An infant under 6 months of age will usually let you undress him, lay him on a warm, flat surface, and touch him with warm hands. Infants can recognize their caregiver's face and voice and are often fearful of separation from the caregiver. Older infants are particularly distressed by separation and almost always cry when separated from the parent. Infants over 6 months of age are more mobile, often understand some language, but possess a severely limited expressive vocabulary.[16] Stimulation around the highly sensory area of the head can create a sense of anxiety and fear in this age group. If possible, keep the infant with a parent and allow the infant time to become familiar with you before beginning physical examination or treatment. Reassure parents that everything possible is being done for their baby. If the parent remains calm, the infant experiences less anxiety.[17] Typical sources of trauma in infants are the improper use of equipment, such as cribs or car seats, burns, and foreign body aspiration. Child abuse is a leading cause of death under the age of 1 year.[15,17]

TODDLERS (1–3 YEARS)

Motor development and language development rapidly accelerate in this age group. Normally a toddler is constantly on the move; however, when hurt or in the presence of strangers, a toddler needs the comfort of a parent to feel safe. Toddlers fear strangers. Keep the child with a parent if possible. Toddlers do not like having clothing removed and resist being touched. Despite rapid development, they have limited language skills so use simple words and keep explanations brief. Separation from familiar environments can cause great distress. Let the toddler play with equipment, such as a stethoscope, until he or she becomes more comfortable with you and the strange environment.[17] Allow the child to hold security objects, such as a stuffed toy or blanket. Injuries in this age group are often associated with exploration and experimentation, such as falls, injuries from toys, foreign body aspiration, drowning, and burns.

PRESCHOOLER (4–5 YEARS)

Preschool children continue to develop language and fine motor skills. Children in this age group think concretely and literally interpret what is said. They have vivid imaginations and are often afraid of monsters and "the dark." While their vocabulary is more expanded, they may still confuse common words and often refuse to talk in the presence of strangers. Explain medical procedures slowly and in simple terms. Be honest but not detailed or graphic. Once again, allow the child to play with equipment and remain close to a caregiver. A preschooler is afraid of body mutilation and injury. Cover bleeding injuries as soon as possible and place bandaids or bandages on minor wounds. Explain how treatment procedures will make them look and feel better. Be sensitive to a child who is toilet trained and becomes overwhelmed by a bowel or bladder accident. Security objects are still important to preschool children. Typical sources of trauma in this age group are motor vehicle crashes, drowning or near drowning, injuries from toys, and falls.[15–17]

SCHOOL AGE (6–12 YEARS)

Usually children from this age group are cooperative and curious but still want parents close by in fearful situations. Legs are the fastest growing body part. Steady weight gain is the norm, with additional fat added before puberty.[18] At about age 7, the child develops reason and compromise and possesses complete language skills. Most school-age children have some idea of the function of EMS and are familiar with the 911 telephone number. They also have a simple understanding of anatomy and basic medical treatments, though their understanding of the human body may be incorrect or vague. They also have an incomplete understanding of death. School-age children are afraid of disfigurement, loss of body function, and death. Toward puberty, physical modesty emerges and they are more comfortable in clothes or covered. It is easy to engage their interest in procedures or equipment, but use nontechnical language in all explanations. Older children may ask for more detailed explanations than would be appropriate for a first-grade child. Keep in mind that injury may cause children to emotionally regress, but most children cope well if given the positive message that they can master the situation. Maturity levels are highly individualized at these ages. Honesty is very important with school-age children. Treat them with respect and try to make them partners in their care. Information is reassuring to them and may need to be repeated; it may be helpful to ask the child to explain what they understand. When possible, provide choices to the child to increase their sense of control. Typical sources of trauma are motor vehicle crashes, pedestrian injuries, bicycle crashes, sports injuries, drowning, and burns. Suicide and homicide increase in frequency as causes of death for those over age 10.[15–17]

ADOLESCENTS (13–18 YEARS)

Both the trunk and the legs lengthen during adolescence. Skeletal mass and organ systems double in size and adult sex characteristics begin to develop.[18] Peer relationships become of paramount importance. Issues of body image, disability, disfigurements, and modesty are all very important to this age group. Adolescents use concrete thinking and possess decision-making ability, so include them in decisions about their care. Although they have a realistic understanding of death, they feel immune to serious injury or death. Teens often exhibit emotional responses to pain that are out of proportion for the event. Most adolescents are reluc-

tant to disclose information about their sexual history, drug use, personal habits, and illegal activities, particularly in the presence of a parent. Record what an adolescent says and express no skepticism, even if it is obviously untrue. After an injury, adolescents often request the company of a friend or peer before asking for a parent. Acknowledge the patient's friends and let them help by notifying caregivers, holding equipment, or providing other support functions.

Adolescents are preoccupied with their bodies. An injury intensifies this preoccupation. Deliver information about their condition in a sensitive, yet honest manner. Typical sources of trauma among adolescents are motor vehicle crashes, drowning, bicycle crashes, sports injuries, and gunshot wounds. Homicide and suicide, particularly as a result of firearm wounds, increase significantly in the teen years.

INITIAL ASSESSMENT AND MANAGEMENT

The general management of children with traumatic injuries differs little from that of adult trauma patients; the highest priority is the identification of immediately life-threatening injuries. Assess children using an ABCDEF approach. Systematically look at airway and cervical spine, breathing, and circulation (ABC). Next consider disability or mental status (D). Expose, examine, evaluate, and consider the environment (E); then include the family (F) in the child's care as much as possible. The dramatic patient presentation coupled with the heightened anxiety level when dealing with children often results in missed findings on assessment. To avoid this pitfall, use a systematic approach to assessment. Frequent reevaluation is also crucial.

AIRWAY AND BREATHING

The initial priority in all pediatric trauma patients is to establish and maintain an open airway. Failure to manage the child's airway is a leading cause of preventable death. The National Pediatric Trauma Registry has reported that 30% of all pediatric trauma deaths are related to inappropriate airway management. To prevent spinal injury, trauma patients must have consideration given to maintaining alignment of the cervical spine at the same time that airway issues are treated.

The small mouth and narrow airway of young children is easily obstructed by blood, mucus, and loose teeth. Clear the mouth and upper airway with a rigid suction device, such as a Yankauer. Other foreign bodies, such as food and toys, predominantly obstruct the airways of infants and toddlers. Pediatric Magill forceps are sometimes used to remove these foreign bodies.

Most pediatric patients experience a period of compensated respiratory compromise prior to deteriorating or arresting. Physical signs of airway and respiratory compromise in the pediatric patient include tachypnea, tachycardia, bradycardia, cyanosis, mottled skin, drooling, nasal flaring, and intercostal, sternal, and supraclavicular retractions. Bradypnea, the abnormal decrease in respirations, is an ominous sign. Grunting, stridor, and wheezing indicate significant respiratory compromise. Changes in mental status, agitation, and somnolence may derive from airway and respiratory problems.[19,20] Normal vital signs for children vary significantly with age; a list of normal vital signs is given in Table 26-3. These normal vital signs are rarely recalled during an emergency, so referring to a chart ensures assessment accuracy.

A child's airway has significant anatomical differences from an adult's airway. These variations are most apparent in infants and become relatively unimportant by age 8. First, infants have larger heads relative to their bodies. To maintain an open airway or to prepare for intubation, the infant's head should be in the "sniffing position" and may require placing a folded towel under the shoulders. Excessive padding should be avoided because it results in misalignment of the spine and excessive flexion of the neck, promoting upper airway obstruction and hindering intubation. Second, an infant's tongue is relatively larger, such that upper airway obstruction occurs more easily and laryngoscopy becomes more difficult. Posterior airway obstruction

can be relieved with the jaw-thrust maneuver. Third, the larynx of an infant is located higher in the neck, at the level of C-3, compared to C-4 or C-5 for an adult. Fourth, the larynx is funnel shaped. The narrowest portion of the airway is in the subglottic area, not at the level of the vocal cords, as is found in an adult airway. Therefore, an endotracheal tube may pass easily through the vocal cords but meet with resistance distally. Fifth, the overall length of the trachea is shorter (4–5 cm in a newborn and 7–8 cm in an 18-month-old), setting the stage for right mainstem intubation. Lastly, the vocal cords of an infant are slanted anteriorly, not perpendicularly to the trachea, as in an adult. This characteristic can result in more difficult visualization of the vocal cords and a more challenging intubation.[7,19]

If the child is unconscious, an oral airway can be placed to assist with keeping an open respiratory passage. A nasopharyngeal airway can be used in the child who is conscious or has a gag reflex. Often, however, in small children and infants, their small nasal passages and hypertrophic adenoids make the placement of a nasal airway traumatic to the tissues.[21] Of course, all trauma patients should receive high-flow oxygen to prevent hypoxemia. A nonrebreathing mask is preferred but blow-by oxygen is acceptable for a child who does not tolerate a face mask. Monitor pulse oximetry constantly but remember that it is not a reflection of ventilatory status.[19,22]

Ventilatory assistance, if required, should be initiated early to prevent complications of hypoventilation

Table 26-3
Normal Vital Signs by Age

Age	Heart Rate (beats/min)	Respirations	Weight (kg)	Systolic Blood Pressure (mm Hg) by weight
Premature infants 1 kg 2 kg	140–160	<60	1–2 1 2	35–55 40–65
Newborns 1–6 weeks	100–160 100–160	<60 <60	3 4	50–70 60–80
Infants 6 months 1 year	90–120 90–120	24–40 20–30	8 10	80–105 80–105
Children 3 years 6 years 8 years 10 years 12 years 14 years	80–120 80–110 75–100 60–100 60–100 60–100	20–26 20–24 16–22 16–22 16–22 14–20	15 20 25 30 40 50	80–110 80–110 90–110 90–120 100–120 100–120

and hypoxemia. Ideally, a bag-valve mask is connected to a high flow rate of oxygen, 15 L/min, and the mask maintains a tight seal with the face. Child- and infant-sized self-inflating bags are available, but adult sizes may be used for the entire range of infants and children if special bags are not available.[19]

When the airway cannot be maintained by basic maneuvers or control of ventilation and oxygenation are required, endotracheal intubation is indicated. When possible, the most experienced paramedic should perform the intubation. There are a few special considerations in pediatric intubation. In children age 2 and under, a curved (MacIntosh) laryngoscope blade is not used for two reasons. First, the epiglottis is relatively large and flaccid and is not easily displaced by pulling on it from the vallecular space. Second, if a curved blade is used, it must be precisely sized to fit the curvature of the tongue. Intubating with the straight blade (Miller) is less dependent on blade size. The straight blade can be placed midline, with the tip underneath the epiglottis, lifting the epiglottis to visualize the trachea. Endotracheal tube sizes vary by age and patient size. Uncuffed tubes are used for children up to about age 8 because the narrowest part of the airway is in the subglottic area, and this area serves as the seal instead of a cuff. Choosing the proper size is important, and there are several formulas for determining correct tube size. The most accurate are based on body length and are determined by using resuscitation tapes such as the Broselow Pediatric Emergency Tape. The next most accurate is an age-based formula that can only be used in those 1 year old and above:

$$(\text{Age in years} \div 4) + 4$$

The diameter of the hand's fifth digit is the third method but has been found to be inaccurate. If the endotracheal tube fits loosely at the subglottic area, it can easily slip out of place. When the tube fits too tightly, the trachea can be injured, resulting in subglottic stenosis. However, in the prehospital setting an airway that is in place is preferable to no airway at all and the patient can be reintubated at the hospital after stabilization.[20]

Because of the short trachea, determining the depth of the tube can be difficult. First confirm the placement of the tube as for an adult. Be sure to listen to breath sounds at the axilla since the small child's chest easily transmits sounds. One technique of avoiding right mainstem intubation is to place the tube conservatively high by passing it until the second mark on the tube is just past the vocal cords. The disadvantage of this method is that the tube can easily become dislodged. Another technique is to deliberately place the tube into the right bronchus, then pull the tube back until it rests 1 cm above where breath sounds are heard

bilaterally. The disadvantage of this method is that the tube can move forward into the right bronchus, but there is less risk that the tube will be inadvertently dislodged.[19-21]

Once the endotracheal tube is in place, tape the tube on both sides of the face, but avoid wrapping the tape around the head. Tape can easily slip off the large occiput, causing the tube to become dislodged.[21]

Nasotracheal intubation is contraindicated in small children because of the difficulty in passing the tube through the vocal cords without direct visualization and because the larger adenoidal tissue is easily traumatized.[23]

Rapid-sequence intubation (RSI) is often the preferred method of intubation in critically ill children and may be a part of local protocols. This technique ensures airway access and minimizes complications. It involves preoxygenation and the administration of an intravenous anesthetic agent and a neuromuscular-blocking agent. Because children have relatively higher oxygen consumption rates, they experience more rapid desaturation with apnea than do adults. Thus, preoxygenation with 100% oxygen via a tight-fitting mask for 2 minutes or four vital capacity breaths is important, if time allows for it. Succinylcholine, a neuromuscular-blocking drug, can induce bradycardia in children. Because a child's cardiac output is significantly controlled by heart rate, premedication with atropine (0.20 mg/kg) is advised if succinylcholine is used in children under age 5 or if the heart rate is less than 120 beats per minute (bpm).[19]

If intubation fails, a laryngeal mask airway (LMA) can be used. Sizes for neonates to adults are available.[19] See Chapter 18 for further discussion of RSI and LMA.

The indications for a surgical airway do not differ from those of adults. In the rare event that such an airway is needed, the needle cricothyroidotomy is the preferred first choice in children. This is due to the small size of the airway structures and the high complication rates of other methods. The procedure does not differ from that of adults so the reader is referred to Chapter 18.

Just as in adults, during the breathing assessment look for signs of life-threatening conditions: apnea, hypoxia, tension pneumothorax, open pneumothorax, and hemothorax. Children are more rapidly compromised by a tension pneumothorax because of the increased flexibility of the mediastinum. The initial presentation of a tension pneumothorax is respiratory distress, tachypnea, and agitation related to hypoxia. Auscultate all lung fields to confirm any suspicions of unilaterally diminished or absent breath sounds. Tracheal deviation is a late finding and should not be relied upon for identifying a tension pneumothorax. Definitive management can be achieved by needle decompression of the chest with an 18-gauge or larger intravenous catheter. The preferred site of needle decompression in infants is along the midclavicular line at the second intercostal space.[23] Needle decompression only converts the tension pneumothorax to a simple pneumothorax, and the possibility of reoccurrence should not be overlooked. Constant evaluation of the airway is critical.

Gastric distention is very common in injured children, particularly those receiving bag-valve mask or invasive airway therapy. Because stomach distention severely limits diaphragmatic excursion, an orogastric or nasogastric tube should be placed as soon as possible by the paramedic. The gastric tube is often forgotten by prehospital personnel, yet it is an essential part of pediatric airway care. Airway and breathing assessment is summarized in Table 26-4.

CIRCULATION

The most frequently encountered problems a paramedic faces related to circulation are hypovolemia and hypovolemic shock. Assessing a child for shock or poor perfusion can be tricky. Children have exceptional vessel-constricting (catecholamine-release) properties that allow them to maintain a normal blood pressure until profound and often irreversible shock is reached; it is crucial to remember this fact. Because hypotension is such a late sign of shock in children, other signs must be used to evaluate a child. Better measures of circulation are capillary refill, mentation, skin color, pulses, skin temperature, heart rate, and respiratory status. These

Table 26-4
Assessment and Critical Interventions

Assessment	Critical Actions
Airway Summary	
Airway obstruction	Open airway, jaw thrust; needle cricothyroidotomy
Breathing Summary	
Apnea	Bag-valve mask, endotracheal intubation, gastric decompression with oro/nasogastric tube
Tension pneumothorax	Needle decompression
Massive hemothorax	Tube thoracostomy, blood transfusion
Open pneumothorax	Occlusive dressing, chest tube
Hypoxia	Oxygen therapy, endotracheal intubation

should be assessed and reassessed frequently.[7,20,21] A normal blood pressure in the context of an otherwise abnormal circulatory assessment is never reassuring.

Both bradycardia and tachycardia can be indicative of shock. Inadequate oxygenation is the most common cause of pediatric bradycardia. Bradycardia in a child is usually a foreboding sign, preceding cardiac arrest and representing impaired perfusion of the coronary arteries. In children, tachycardia represents an attempt to maintain cardiac output. Children in shock increase heart rates long before blood pressure falls. Tachycardia is a sign of shock; unfortunately it is a nonspecific sign. Heart rate is elevated as well with fever, pain, and anxiety.[20]

Palpate for the presence of a central pulse. For infants and younger children, the brachial pulse is usually the easiest central pulse to find. Alternatively, evaluate the femoral pulse in the groin. In older children, the carotid artery is the most appropriate for assessing a central pulse, whereas in infants the neck may be too chubby to feel the carotid pulse. If the central pulse is evident, evaluate its strength. Keeping one hand on the central pulse point, find the peripheral pulse with the other hand. Locate either the radial or the pedal pulse. Compare the peripheral pulse to the central pulse. A weak or absent peripheral pulse is indicative of poor peripheral perfusion and often accompanies uncompensated shock.

Capillary refill is extremely important to evaluate in children. It is abnormal if longer than 2 seconds. Capillary refill is not an accurate sign of shock if the patient is cold, however. Skin color is another important factor in pediatric assessment because poor skin perfusion is an early sign of shock. Pale or mottled skin suggests hypoperfusion. Cyanosis may or may not be present; with low levels of hemoglobin, which occurs with significant blood loss, cyanosis is not apparent.

Cool skin may indicate exposure to a cold environment or may be due to shock. The most important assessment of skin temperature is the line of demarcation between where the skin is warm and where it becomes cold. The line is easily felt and should be documented. This demarcation line roughly indicates the severity of the shunting process, which is the movement of blood from the extremities to the vital organs.

Level of consciousness can also be a clue to hypoperfusion because low cardiac output directly affects brain tissue. It is also a nonspecific sign because it can occur with head injury and hypoxia. In children, assess the ability to recognize parents. Failure to recognize parents is often an early sign of circulatory decompensation.[20]

Blood pressure should be measured only after the circulatory assessment has been completed. Do not delay treatment or transport to obtain a blood pressure reading. If treatment is delayed until the child's blood pressure drops, it may be too late to adequately restore the lost volume before the child slips irreversibly into a terminal condition. Blood pressure may remain constant until the child has lost 20%–25% of the body's circulating blood volume. The blood pressure may even be high during the compensatory stage of shock. Systolic blood pressure can be estimated for children over 1 year old with the following:

80 + 2 times the age in years

Because this formula results in a single number for the systolic blood pressure, it may be difficult to know whether the patient's blood pressure falls into an acceptable range. Nomograms or charts with ranges of blood pressures are much more useful tools. Remember that cuff size is important to determine accurate blood pressure in children, and bladder width should be two-thirds the length of the upper arm.[20]

Since children can temporarily compensate for volume loss better than an adult, consider treating any children that present with a significant mechanism of injury with intravenous fluids. Although children may look well initially, their condition can worsen suddenly and rapidly as compensatory mechanisms fail. The cornerstone of prehospital treatment of hypovolemic shock is crystalloid fluid boluses (Ringer's lactate or normal saline). Controversy exists regarding the ideal fluid for pediatric volume replacement; large volumes of normal saline can cause the child to become hypernatremic while the buffers in Ringer's lactate may be beneficial to the child's electrolyte balance. Follow local protocol. Rapid infusion of a fluid bolus of 20 mL/kg with a syringe attached to a three-way stopcock is delivered via a 20- or 30-cc syringe, followed by reassessment and additional boluses as indicated. Avoid depending on gravity or pressure bags to ensure fluid delivery. Children may require as much as 60 mL/kg in the first hour of treatment.[20]

Optimum therapy for hemorrhage in pediatric trauma patients is replacement of blood. Children have a circulating blood volume of 80–90 mL/kg (i.e., a newborn's total volume is equal to a 12-ounce can of soda), so compared to adults, less blood loss requires transfusion. Blood therapy is indicated for those who continue to show signs of hypovolemic shock after two 20-mL/kg boluses of crystalloid. Packed red blood cells are given in boluses of 10 mL/kg; reassessment is performed after each bolus. In young children for whom several transfusions are required, it is prudent to have the blood bank release small alliquots of blood from a single donor unit. This minimizes the chance of transfusion reactions, or reactions that would be possible if blood is given from different units of blood.[21–23] (For further discussion of blood transfusions see Chapter 20.)

The desire for aggressive fluid therapy must be balanced with the need to avoid fluid overload.

Frequent reassessment usually prevents the inadvertent development of overhydration.

In significant pediatric trauma, the placement of two large-bore intravenous lines ensures the rapid infusion of fluid. However, in children, obtaining one well-functioning intravenous line, though less than ideal, is often considered acceptable.[22] The antecubital fossa veins or the saphenous veins of the feet are appropriate sites for a trauma patient. Volume replacement should be initiated en route to the hospital to prevent delay in transport. Local providers should have protocols established to determine what sites, in what order, and in what time frame should be attempted for fluid access. In children under age 6, intraosseous lines, if not contraindicated, are used initially, or as a backup site if the first 90 seconds of intravenous attempts are unsuccessful. Complications of intraosseous lines include tibial fracture, infiltration, compartment syndrome, and osteomyelitis. Contraindications of intraosseous infusions are osteogenesis imperfecta (a rare bone disease in which bones easily fracture), placement through burned or infected tissue, and placement distal to a fracture site.[20,23] If peripheral access (IV or IO) is unattainable, femoral vein cannulation is recommended; the landmarks of this vein are easy to identify, its use is associated with a low complication rate, and it is located apart from most life-saving procedures.[23]

No matter which site is chosen, do not let the quest for vascular access divert attention from proper airway control. The time spent obtaining a fluid resuscitation line at the expense of an adequate airway is a critical error in pediatric trauma care.[21]

There have been limited studies regarding the value of the pneumatic antishock garment (PASG) in pediatric trauma. That fact notwithstanding, a PASG is never indicated for hemorrhagic shock in children, and this is true even in the face of long transport times and failure to obtain IV access. The abdominal compartment of the PASG has always been contraindicated in children because it interferes with breathing, especially in younger patients who rely on diaphragm muscles to breathe. Though once recommended for unstable pelvic fractures and control of bleeding of the lower extremities, experts no longer recommend the PASG for these injuries. The American College of Emergency Physicians lists the pediatric PASG as an "investigational" therapy. Table 26-5 summarizes the circulatory assessment.

INTERNET ACTIVITIES

Visit the British Trauma Society at http:// www.trauma.org/resus/paedmoulage/paed moulage.html and run the pediatric trauma resuscitation simulation.

Table 26-5
Assessment and Critical Interventions

Assessment	Critical Actions
Cardiac arrest	Assess for correctable cause, (e.g., tension pneumothorax) and treat; be aware that children have poor survival rates
Shock	Fluid boluses, blood transfusion
Pericardial tamponade	Pericardiocentesis, thoracotomy

DISABILITY AND MENTAL STATUS

Assessment of disability and mental status are summarized in Table 26-6. For a more complete discussion of this assessment, see the discussions of head trauma and spinal trauma in this chapter.

EXPOSURE AND ENVIRONMENT

Children possess a large surface area-to-body-mass ratio and lose heat more rapidly than adults, so hypothermia develops much more easily. Neonates are particularly vulnerable to heat loss, but hypothermia is a serious concern in all children. Signs of hypothermia are similar to those of shock states and include lethargy, coma, bradycardia, poor peripheral pulses, and bradypnea. As the body attempts to produce heat, shivering may be seen, except in newborns, whose thermoregulatory system is too underdeveloped. Shivering increases oxygen consumption and children already have higher

Table 26-6
Assessment and Critical Interventions

Assessment	Critical Actions
Serious head injury	Mild hyperventilation ($PaCO_2$ 30–34 mm Hg) Mannitol IV if ordered (0.5–1.0 g/kg)
Prolonged or repeated seizures	Lorazepam (0.1–0.2 mg/kg IV/IM) or diazepam (0.1–0.3 mg/kg IV/IM)
Spinal cord injury	Spinal immobilization Methylprednisolone (loading dose of 30 mg/kg IV)

metabolic rates, so oxygen therapy is important. Hypothermia can lead to hypoglycemia in neonates; therefore perform frequent fingerstick glucose measurements.[20] Rectal temperatures should be taken to determine body temperature.

It is extremely important to limit exposure during assessments and interventions and to cover the child as soon as possible. The patient compartment should be well heated, warmer than is comfortable for the provider. Do not leave doors open or the air conditioner running, even on moderately warm days. For example, the amount of heat loss the child experiences while lying on the roadway after being struck by a vehicle is significant. Even if the ambient air temperature is warm, the pavement quickly saps heat from the child. Remove wet clothing and use warm IV fluids when possible. Warm packs and warmed blankets are also helpful.[20,22]

Similar to the adult, respect the child's modesty, regardless of their mental status. Adolescents and children approaching puberty are particularly concerned with modesty and want to be covered.

During the exposure process any sites of exsanguinating hemorrhage are revealed and are treated identically to the care of these injuries in adults. A summary of this assessment can be found in Table 26-7.

INTERNET ACTIVITIES

Visit the University of Minnesota Department of Pediatrics Web site at http://www.peds.umn.edu/divisions/pccm/teaching/acp/trauma.html and review their guidelines for the initial assessment and resuscitation of the pediatric trauma patient.

FOCUSED ASSESSMENT AND UNIQUE CHARACTERISTICS OF CHILDREN

The focused assessment should be performed as it is in adults. With small children, a "toe-to-head" approach decreases anxiety. Remember, however, that valuable

Table 26-7
Assessment and Critical Interventions

Assessment	Critical Actions
Hypothermia	Warm blankets, remove wet clothing, warm IV fluids, warm packs
External hemorrhage	Direct pressure, air splints
Impaled objects	Stabilize, do not remove

scene time should not be wasted performing an exhaustive survey. Usually a quick examination that includes the head, chest, and abdomen is sufficient.

In each body system, infants and children have unique physiological and anatomical features, characteristics not found in adults, that present special challenges for the paramedic.

HEAD TRAUMA

Head injury is the leading cause of death among injured children and is responsible for between 30% and 50% of all trauma deaths.[7,20,21] Falls account for 37% of head injuries and are the predominant cause of these injuries in children age 4 and under.[22] This is followed by motor vehicle collisions (18%), pedestrian injuries (17%), and falls from bicycles (10%).[24] Motor vehicle crashes overtake falls in the teenage years.[22] After the head, the areas most often injured, listed in order of frequency, are the extremities, abdomen, and chest.

Small children have proportionately larger and heavier heads compared to adults. By the late teenage years the head is falling into proportion with the rest of the body. A heavier head, combined with underdeveloped neck muscles, leads to a relatively high incidence of head injury.[20] Since the brain is not fully myelinated, it is more susceptible to shearing forces during trauma.[22] When a child falls or is thrown, the head tends to strike the ground before the body. For this reason, head injury is the most common blunt injury in children. Serious head injuries are about five times more common than serious internal injuries in the pediatric population.

Primary head injury occurs at the moment of impact. Any loss of consciousness is indicative of damage to the central nervous system, whether from a direct blow or from secondary injuries. The large occiput automatically compromises a child's airway when in a supine position. Flexion, and conversely extension, of the neck can compromise the integrity of the airway by compressing the malleable tracheal rings and may result in a hypoxic insult. Secretions and other foreign bodies can quickly aggravate oxygen delivery to an already compromised patient by obstructing the airway. An infant's airway is the size of a straw (4–5 mm in diameter) and cannot compare with the "garden hose" size of the adult trachea (20 mm). A small amount of edema is proportionately more serious in a small child. Also recognize that the tongue is the most common obstruction in the unconscious child; a child's tongue is proportionately larger within the mouth than an adult's tongue. Simple maneuvers can relieve a tongue-obstructed airway.

Children develop cerebral edema more quickly in head injury than adults. In an adult, if blood is not adequately perfusing brain tissue, the body sends it more blood. In the pediatric patient increased cerebral blood flow exceeds metabolic demand, causing a diffuse cerebral edema. Nevertheless, children have better outcomes from head injury than do adults, succumbing to death from the injury half as often.[20] This is primarily thought to be due to a more cartilaginous skull and the presence of open sutures.[22]

Children do not usually become hypotensive from blood loss in a closed head injury. However, newborns and infants can develop hypotension from an isolated head injury, resulting from the loss of a significant portion of their blood volume into the subgaleal or epidural space. While hypotension from an isolated head injury is possible in infants, it is unusual. Any time an infant has a severe head injury and signs of shock, it is imperative that other possible sources of occult bleeding be investigated. In infants, the skull is thinner and softer than an adult's with open fontanelles anteriorly (closing between 12 and 18 months of age) and posteriorly (closing around 3 months of age). The sutures of the cranial vault are not completely locked until the child is around 2 years of age. This allows the skull to be more pliable and accommodates a small amount of edema or intracranial hemorrhage as a compensatory mechanism. Consequently, full fontanelles and split sutures are signs of increased intracranial pressure (ICP) in infants.[25]

The head is very vascular, feeding the rapidly maturing brain, and even seemingly small injuries can create large volume losses. In contrast to adults, intracranial hemorrhage may be of sufficient volume to induce shock in infants. Blood loss into the cranial vault, compared to an infant's small total blood volume (approximately 80 mL/kg), can result in shock. An infant's head is larger and much more vascular in proportion to the body, accounting for a greater percentage of total volume of blood. The soft cranial bones allow impact forces to be transmitted directly to the brain, resulting in acute edema and bleeding. The cranial sutures are not locked, and this allows edema and bleeding to occur within the skull without creating a terminal neurological event. This expansion of the skull serves as a protective mechanism that improves a child's potential outcome after a head injury, but also allows for more blood to collect in the third spaces of the head. If clinical signs of shock are present, it is particularly prudent to investigate sources of bleeding other than the head injury.[20]

Scalp lacerations can be life-threatening injuries due to the high vascularity of the pediatric scalp, particularly for infants.[20] Improperly managed or missed scalp lacerations have been documented to be the sole injury responsible for a child's hypovolemia.

Skull fractures in childhood indicate that a significant force has struck the head. Linear skull fractures are the most common skull fractures during childhood, and most heal well without intervention. However, epidural hematomas are often associated with linear skull fractures over the temporal or parietal areas of the head. In children under age 6, epidural bleeds often result from falls of less than 5 feet. It is noteworthy that epidural hematomas are rare in babies because the middle meningeal artery does not become imbedded into the temporal bone until about 2 years of age. Subdural hematomas are more common in children than epidural hematomas and are bilateral in 75% of the cases. Shearing forces, damaging the bridging venous vessels to the brain, commonly cause subdural bleeds. In newborns and infants, subdural hematomas most frequently present as focal seizures, bulging fontanelles, a weak cry, decreased level of consciousness, and vomiting. Children over ages 2 or 3 demonstrate symptoms similar to adults: pupillary changes, hemiparesis, altered level of consciousness, and restlessness. Pediatric subdural hematomas are associated with higher morbidity but less mortality than epidural hematomas.[20] Chronic subdural hematomas in children are most likely the result of "shaken baby syndrome." These children may present with a nonspecific symptom such as vomiting or failure to thrive. Seizures and level of consciousness changes are also common. Most victims are under 1 year old, and retinal hemorrhages are seen in 75% of the cases, so funduscopic examinations are a crucial component of the medical evaluation.[25]

In any child, the edema and possible hemorrhage resulting from a head injury can lead to a rapid buildup of pressure within the skull. This pressure compresses the vasculature within the skull, increasing ICP, and ultimately reduces blood flow to the brain. Reduced blood flow to the brain results in cerebral hypoxia and increasing edema, causing a cycle that leads to greater ICP. Children who are both poorly perfused and suffering from a head injury have a very high mortality rate. Aggressive management of the airway and maintenance of the circulatory status, combined with keeping the child warm, are the primary steps to resuscitation. Mild hyperventilation ($PaCO_2$ 30–34 mm Hg) with 100% oxygen may be helpful, just as it is in adults.[20] Aggressive hyperventilation is only used when signs of impending herniation are present, often signaled by pupillary changes.[22] Part of the child's neurological assessment includes using a Glasgow Coma Scale that has been modified for children (see Table 26-8) or use of the AVPU system (see Chapter 6 for AVPU). A GCS score of 8 or less is a sign of increased ICP, usually requiring intubation. A score that falls two points on reassessment is deteriorating significantly and requires urgent care and controlled intubation to maintain ventilation and oxygenation.[20,25] Older children can be assessed on the adult GCS (see Chapter 7 for the GCS). Although true for adults, decerebrate posturing and fixed pupils are rarely associated with isolated brainstem injury in children. These signs are more likely to be the result of diffuse cerebral swelling and hyperemia.[20] Other interventions include elevating the head of the bed 20°, while keeping the neck straight to promote venous drainage. Depending upon local

Table 26-8
Modified Glasgow Coma Score for Children

Activity	Score	>1 Year of Age	<1 Year of Age
Eye opening	4	Spontaneously	Spontaneously
	3	To verbal command	To shout
	2	To pain	To pain
	1	No response	No response
Motor response	6	Obeys commands	Spontaneously
	5	Localizes pain	Localizes pain
	4	Withdraws to pain	Withdraws to pain
	3	Flexion abnormal (decorticate rigidity)	Flexion abnormal (decorticate rigidity)
	2	Extension abnormal (decerebrate rigidity)	Extension abnormal (decerebrate rigidity)
	1	No response	No response
Verbal response	5	Appropriate words and phrases	Smiles, coos, babbles
	4	Disoriented, inappropriate words	Cries but is consolable
	3	Persistent cries and screams	Persistent cries, screams
	2	Grunts, meaningless sounds	Grunts, agitated, restless
	1	No response	No response
Total: 3–15			

medical control, IV mannitol, 0.5–1.0 g/kg, or furosemide, 1 mg/kg may be used to lower ICP.[22]

Between 10% and 25% of children develop seizures in the early posttraumatic period following head injury. These seizures, particularly if multiple or lasting more than a few minutes, demand aggressive treatment with lorazepam (0.1–0.2 mg/kg) or diazepam (0.1–0.3 mg/kg). Lorazepam is preferred because it has a longer duration of action and causes less venous irritation. If IV access is not available, both drugs can be given IO or IM. At the hospital a longer acting anticonvulsant agent, such as fosphenytoin (17 mg/kg IV/IM load), should be administered. Children also need an orogastric or nasogastric tube placed after head injury because spontaneous emesis in the first 30 minutes is common.[20,22]

INTERNET ACTIVITIES

Visit the University of Texas Health Science Center at San Antonio's Trauma Home Page at http://rmstewart.uthscsa.edu/fatal_brain/fatal brain.html. Review this case and follow the links to the sites evaluating the effectiveness of bicycle helmets.

SPINAL TRAUMA

Serious cervical spine (C-spine) injury is rare in children under age 15; less than 2% of all C-spine fractures occur in this age group. Over 60% of all pediatric C-spine fractures occur to children over age 12 and occur in the lower C-spine.[20,26,27] In the rare C-spine injury to those under age 12, two-thirds occur between the occiput and C-2.[22] Motor vehicle collisions are the most common cause of C-spine injury.[28] Diving injuries, falls, firearms, and sports injuries are the other major causes of spinal injuries in children.[1,20] Spinal cord trauma is also associated with a higher mortality rate in the pediatric population.[22]

Several anatomical features predispose children to spine injury. Rotation on the cervical axis is higher, usually at C-1 or C-2, compared to C-6 or C-7 in the adult.[25] This high rotation point combined with the immature and weaker musculoskeletal structures of the neck make overextension injuries and subluxation fractures common. Spinal injuries also tend to be higher than in adults, typically C-1, C-2, C-5, and C-6.[20] The spine of a child is more cartilaginous and elastic than an adult's. This allows a child to sustain severe cord damage without radiological signs of a fracture or dislocation. This type of injury is called **SCIWORA**, or spinal cord injury without radiographic abnormalities. However, if the child is alert and responsive and there are no neurological deficits or neck pain, SCIWORA is extremely unlikely.[20] Be aware, however, that 50% of children with SCIWORA have a delayed onset of paralysis, up to 4 days. But, at the time of injury, most of these children have some transient numbness or weakness.[22]

Mechanisms of injury that require cervical spinal immobilization are falls from heights, diving injury, ejection from a motor vehicle, or unrestrained passenger in a vehicle crash. Use in-line neutral positioning, not manual traction. Traction on the spine of a child can cause damage to the spongy, cartilaginous structures. Application of a rigid cervical collar is preferred but only if proper sizes are available. Estimate the distance between the angle of the jaw and the top of the shoulder to determine the width of the collar. A collar that is too short fails to provide adequate support. One that is too tall hyperextends the neck and compromises the airway. In an infant or child under 5 years old, rolled towels or blankets on either side of the head combined with 2-inch tape extending across the forehead to the backboard or car seat usually secures the C-spine.[20] Infants may also need padding behind the shoulders to prevent flexion from the larger head.[22] Methylprednisolone, a steroid, in a loading dose of 30 mg/kg IV, should be started for those with neurological deficits.[22,25]

CHEST TRAUMA

Serious chest injuries are rare, accounting for only about 6% of patients admitted to pediatric trauma centers; of these, fewer than 15% require intervention beyond chest tube placement.[1,29,30] Chest trauma is usually seen in combination with head or abdominal trauma or both, but rarely alone. Blunt trauma, most commonly from motor vehicle collisions, accounts for 83% of chest trauma, though penetrating trauma is increasingly frequent.[30] Despite their relative infrequency, chest injuries are the most underdiagnosed life-threatening injury in children and carry a mortality rate of up to 12%.[22]

The chest wall of a child is very compliant and can absorb a large amount of energy without fracturing bony structures. The ribs are more cartilaginous and flexible, and thus significant force is required to fracture them, making rib fractures a foreboding sign in children. The compliance of the structures of the thorax can transfer energy to the internal organs, resulting in significant internal injuries without obvious external indication. In addition, the pediatric chest has a much thinner layer of muscle and fat with which to protect underlying organs. Frequently children have no external marks yet have sustained serious thoracic injury.

The energy transmitted to the underlying structures of the torso can result in disruption of pulmonary system structures, the great vessels, and even the anatomically high liver and spleen, with little external evidence of injury. **Aerophagia**, or swallowing of air, is frequently seen in the injured child, causing stomach distention and compromise of the diaphragm's movement. This is important because the diaphragm is the primary respiratory muscle of small children. Intercostal muscle development does not begin until around 2 or 3 years of age and is not completed until age 8.[20]

The mediastinum is very flexible, allowing for a significant compression and shift of the heart to the unaffected side. Angulation of the great vessels and collapse of the pulmonary surface area can occur before obvious signs are evident. Tachypnea is the first, albeit vague, sign that oxygen requirements are not being met.

As noted, gross chest injuries are not always obvious because of the flexibility of the rib cage. Greenstick-type fractures of the ribs are the most common rib fracture and can cause significant injury to internal organs, without crepitus, flail segments, or disruption of the chest wall. Multiple rib fractures in children can be a significant source of blood loss if the intercostal arteries are lacerated, up to 125 mL of blood loss for each rib fracture.[31] Flail chest is uncommon in young children, once again because of the pliability of the ribs. It is more common that a young child will suffer a pulmonary contusion, especially if there is visible chest bruising. Pulmonary contusion is the most frequently seen thoracic injury in children. Often the child is without symptoms for the first few hours, then presents with hemoptysis, wheezes, crackles, and fever. Chest X-ray shows a fluffy infiltrate.[20,22,31]

Children are vulnerable to tracheal and bronchial tears, though tracheobronchial injuries are relatively rare in children. In blunt trauma about 80% of the injuries are to the mainstem bronchi, either at the junction with the trachea or within 2.5 cm of the carina.[31]

A tension pneumothorax is the most commonly missed life-threatening injury in the pediatric population. The signs and symptoms of this life-threatening injury are the same as for adults, with the addition of retractions. Be aware, however, that tracheal deviation, a very late sign, is difficult to evaluate in children.[20]

When a hemothorax occurs, it is most often the result of penetrating trauma but can occur after blunt trauma as well. For children a hemothorax can cause not only respiratory compromise but life-threatening blood loss as well. A child can lose as much as 40% of total blood volume in a single hemothorax. In addition to the placement of a chest tube, the child may need rapid replacement of blood with un-cross-matched O-negative blood.[20]

Cardiac tamponade is an infrequent injury in children but can occur after blunt trauma (though rare) as well as penetrating trauma (more common). Increases in pericardial fluid or blood are sometimes difficult to see on a chest X-ray. Children suffering from cardiac tamponade are hypotensive despite fluid resuscitation and have a narrowed pulse pressure, poor peripheral perfusion, tachycardia, and paradoxical pulse. Muffled heart sounds are a late sign. Just as with adults, life-saving treatment is needle aspiration of the pericardium.[20,31]

Commotio cordis is a problem of pediatric patients that follows the sudden impact of blunt force to the anterior chest wall (e.g., hit in the chest with a baseball). It causes sudden change in cardiac function and rhythm, often into ventricular fibrillation and, later, cardiogenic shock. In addition to usual therapy, these children may require extended antiarrhythmic therapy, a cardiac pacemaker, or inotropic agents.[25]

ABDOMINAL TRAUMA

Significant abdominal injuries occur in at least a quarter of all children with multisystem trauma.[32] Abdominal trauma is the third leading cause of traumatic death, following head and chest injuries.[25] Blunt trauma accounts for 85% of pediatric abdominal trauma.[25] Motor vehicle collisions, pedestrian injury, and falls account for the bulk of blunt abdominal injury.[7]

The child's anatomy predisposes the patient to certain types of injuries. Children have proportionately larger solid organs than adults, protuberant abdomens, and weaker abdominal muscles, all of which predispose them to solid organ injuries.[7,25] A child's abdomen is less protected than an adult's; there is less shielding by the ribs and less overlying muscle and fat tissue.[20] In addition, the child's relatively compact torso is less able to dissipate energy from blunt trauma.[7] Furthermore, diaphragmatic breathing by small children predisposes them to respiratory difficulties when the diaphragm is injured or irritated. Seemingly insignificant forces can injure the underlying abdomen.[20]

The liver and spleen are considered to be abdominal organs; however, in young children the compactness of the structures increase the suspicion of injury of those organs in both chest and abdominal trauma. The spleen is the most frequently injured abdominal organ in childhood, but children are often stable even after significant injury and usually can be managed without surgery. This is because a child's spleen has a thicker capsule and more elastin and smooth muscle than an adult's.[22,33] When possible, splenectomy is avoided due to its association with overwhelming sepsis in children.[20]

The second most commonly injured organ of the child's abdomen is the liver, and liver injuries can be difficult to diagnose. Unstable children need surgery while stable children are usually managed conservatively.

Traumatic injury to the pancreas occurs in less than 10% of children with abdominal trauma, is rarely the cause of death, but is frequently the cause of acute pancreatitis.[22] Motor vehicle crashes, child abuse, and bicycle handlebar injuries are the most common causes of traumatic pancreatic damage. The spleen and bowel are commonly injured along with the pancreas. A common blood test, amylase level, alerts the physician to possible pancreatic injury.[20] The hollow organs of the abdomen, the stomach and small and large intestines, are rarely injured in the pediatric population. When they are, it is usually the result of a motor vehicle lap belt injury, with the lap belt or the lap portion of the lap/shoulder belt incorrectly positioned over the abdomen.[20,22] Complications of hollow organ injury are peritonitis, obstruction, and intestinal strictures.

Abdominal tenderness, rigidity, distention, bruising, lacerations, gross hematuria, unexplained shock, and shoulder pain in the absence of shoulder injury all suggest intra-abdominal injury.[33] **Cullen's sign**, periumbilical ecchymosis, is indicative of a ruptured spleen. **Kehr's sign**, pain in the left shoulder from the irritation of the phrenic nerve, is caused by free blood in the abdomen. Bowel sounds should be assessed because their absence may stem from bleeding or perforation.[20,22]

If abdominal injury is suspected, placement of a nasogastric tube is strongly supported. As noted, children are prone to gastric distention, which can lead to vomiting, aspiration, and impaired lung expansion. In the emergency department, laboratory tests, an abdominal computerized tomography (CT) scan for the stable patient, or diagnostic peritoneal lavage (DPL) for the unstable child are often obtained because the physical assessment of the pediatric abdomen is often deceptive. DPL is very accurate in diagnosing serious abdominal trauma.[20,22]

PELVIC AND GENITOURINARY TRAUMA

The immature pelvis is very elastic. A tremendous amount of force is required to break the pelvic ring. Due to the compact nature of the child's abdominal anatomy, fractures of the pelvis often result in visceral, vascular, and neurological injuries. Pelvic anterior ring fractures are associated with urethral and bladder injury.[22] The presence of pelvic pain or tenderness on palpation cannot be overlooked during assessment. The propensity of concurrent injury as well as significant rehabilitative challenges make any pelvic fracture a

cause of great concern, and this is true despite the fact that children are less likely than adults to die from pelvic fracture hemorrhage.[34] Nevertheless, a pelvic fracture can result in the loss of 3,000 cc of blood in a child.[20] Prehospital treatment focuses on overall stabilization and fluid resuscitation.

Around 10%–15% of pediatric abdominal trauma includes injuries to the genital and urinary structures. The kidney is the third most frequently injured organ of the abdomen. When assessing for renal injury, ask about a history of renal abnormalities because about 25% of children with renal injury have a history of some preexisting abnormality.[20,22,34]

The kidneys in children are more vulnerable to injury than are an adult's for three reasons. First, their kidneys are less well anchored. Second, a child's kidney is not as heavily protected with perinephretic fat. Finally, the kidneys of a child are not shielded by the rib cage.[20] Tire marks on the flank, fractures of lower ribs, pelvic fractures, and severe skin abrasions should alert the paramedic to the possibility of renal trauma.[34] Dull back pain, flank ecchymosis, and hematuria are signs of renal injury.[25] Intravenous pyelogram (IVP) and CT scan are diagnostic tools used in the hospital setting. Almost all kidney trauma in children (85%) can be managed with IV fluids and conservative treatment rather than surgery.[20]

Ureteral injuries, though uncommon and difficult to diagnose, can occur in children. Due to the mobility and flexibility of a child's spine, extreme flexion of the trunk can cause the ureter to separate from the kidney. An IVP or retrograde pyelogram may be needed to diagnose this injury.[34]

Because the bladder is located more abdominally in children, it is more commonly injured than it is in adults. Abdominal pain and hematuria may be present.[20] Urethral injuries often accompany bladder injuries.

Urethral trauma is associated with straddle injuries, pelvic fractures, and insertion of foreign objects. Blood at the urinary meatus and perineal hematoma are signs of possible urethral injury. Cystourethrography is performed on these patients at the hospital before bladder catheterization. Straddle injuries are also linked with pubic fractures, testicular injuries, and labial or scrotal hematomas and lacerations.[7,22]

Emergency management of pediatric genitourinary trauma is the prevention and treatment of shock since these are rarely isolated injuries, instead occurring in the setting of multisystem trauma. Depending on the transport times, equipment, and medical direction, a urinary catheter may be placed en route but is more commonly done in the emergency department. Gross or microscopic hematuria is the hallmark finding in genitourinary trauma. However, the degree of hematuria does not necessarily correlate with the degree of injury, and some severely injured children show no hematuria.[7,20,22]

Genital trauma in children can occur in a variety of settings, from motor vehicle trauma to sports-related trauma to child abuse, and often presents challenging problems. Paraphimosis occurs when a tight penile foreskin is retracted into the coronal sulcus. Over time, swelling and pain develop. The application of ice and gentle traction usually reduces this condition. Testicular injuries are rare in children because of the relatively small size of the gonad and its mobility. However, zipper injuries to the penis are not unusual in young boys. Release of the tissue is best obtained by opening the zipper from the bottom upward. Without a clear-cut mechanism of injury, child abuse should be suspected in children with genital bruising, swelling, or laceration.[20,34]

MUSCULOSKELETAL TRAUMA

A child's extremities grow in length from the epiphyseal plates (growth plates) at each end of the bone. Bones are initially all cartilage and then ossify as minerals are deposited in the cartilage. Because of their cartilaginous structure, pediatric bones are much more pliable and porous than an adult's bones. Rather than completely fracturing, the bone often splinters or bends, producing buckle and greenstick fractures. The porous nature of the bone also makes fractures more common in children than in adults. The epiphyseal plate of a child's long bones is an area of relative weakness as well, and if not properly treated when fractured leads to disability and deformity. Children have a thick periosteum, and this thick bone covering often limits bony displacement of fractures. The periosteum also contains a generous supply of osteoblasts, cells that make new bone, so a child's fracture heals much faster than an adult's.[20,35]

All of a child's muscle fiber is present at birth; however the fibers lengthen and develop throughout childhood as the bones grow.[20]

Musculoskeletal trauma is treated much like it is in an adult, with immobilization occurring only after airway, breathing, and circulation issues are addressed. Hypovolemic shock can occur without systemic trauma with femur fractures (1,500 cc potential blood loss) and pelvic fractures (3,000 cc potential blood loss).[20]

PEDIATRIC TRAUMA CENTER CRITERIA

Once the primary assessment has been completed, decisions are made surrounding transportation and destination. The importance of regionalized pediatric trauma care cannot be overemphasized. The American College of Surgeons (ACS) has developed criteria for determining which pediatric trauma patients would benefit from a pediatric level I trauma center and these are listed in Table 26-9.[36]

FAMILY ISSUES

The pediatric lexicon includes the concept that "an injured child equals an injured family." This means that when a child is injured, the entire family is affected. When the incident involves multiple injuries and multiple parties, every effort should be made to locate the parents of the injured child. Keep family members together, transporting them to the same hospital if appropriate. If family members must go to different destinations, compile this information and disseminate it to relatives. Parents need to know what hospital is caring for their child, and the receiving hospital should be aware if injured parents have been taken elsewhere. If parents are not at the scene, find out how they can be contacted. If the parents are unavailable, a relative or close family friend should be contacted. Phone numbers and other essential information should be written down and given to the social worker or the receiving hospital nurse. When possible, give the name and phone number of the receiving hospital to a family member.

Throughout the care of the pediatric patient, it is important to provide adequate psychological support to the child and family. Provide frequent explanation of procedures. When possible, include parents in the assessment and management of the child; their presence is reassuring to the patient and comforting to the parents as well.

Regardless of the seriousness of the situation, families have real fears about what is happening to their child. Let parents know what steps are being taken to care for their child. Realistic answers delivered in a compassionate manner are the most effective. If the situation is critical, reassure them that everything possible is being done for their child. This approach does not create a false sense of security or make false promises regarding the outcome of the injury. During transport, allow a parent to accompany a child whenever possible. If this is not possible, be sure that parents are informed of the ambulance's destination.

▶ SUMMARY

Understanding the unique characteristics of children is paramount for the paramedic. The prehospital management of the injured child should be built upon a systematic and thorough assessment and rapidly initiated

Table 26-9
Criteria for Transport to a Level I Pediatric Trauma Center

Mechanism of Injury

- Unrestrained occupant of a vehicle traveling at speeds of 20 mph or greater
- Restrained occupant of a vehicle traveling at speeds of 40 mph or greater
- Struck by a vehicle traveling at speeds of 20 mph or greater or at an unknown speed
- Any child ejected from the vehicle
- Falls from a height of 10 feet or greater
- Prolonged extrication of 20 minutes or greater
- Any motor vehicle crash when another occupant is killed
- Pulled from or dragged underneath a vehicle or run over by a vehicle's wheels

Gross Location of Injury

- Any injury that produces shock or respiratory distress
- High suspicion of C-spine injury
- Uncontrolled hemorrhage
- Open fractures
- Severe maxillofacial injuries
- Unstable chest injuries and/or major pelvic injuries
- Penetrating or crush injury to the head, neck, chest, abdomen, or pelvis
- Neurological injuries producing prolonged loss of consciousness, altered mental status, posturing, seizures, or lateralizing signs of paralysis
- Amputations
- Tracheal or laryngeal injuries
- Burns greater than 20% total body surface area or any burn in which smoke inhalation is suspected

Physiological Distress

- Any child with a Pediatric Trauma Score (see Table 7-6) of 8 or less
- Any child with a Glasgow Coma Score (see Table 7-1) of 12 or less
- Any child with an Injury Severity Score (see Chapter 7) of 15 or greater
- Any child with a history of respiratory or cardiopulmonary arrest caused by the injury

interventions. The focus of treatment is on airway care, oxygen administration, and volume resuscitation. In pediatric trauma care, the paramedic must avoid these critical errors in judgment: (1) relying on blood pressure to measure circulatory status, since blood pressure stays normal until profound shock is reached; (2) failing to secure an adequate airway; (3) obtaining an intravenous line before securing an adequate airway; (4) withholding oxygen; (5) underestimating the detrimental effects of hypothermia; and (6) giving insufficient weight to the mechanism of injury.

▶ REVIEW QUESTIONS

1. Child abuse is a common source of traumatic injury in infants (age 0 to 1).
   a. True
   b. False

2. Waddell's triad can occur in pedestrian/vehicle collisions. What injuries does this triad include?
   a. Closed head injury, fractured humerus, injury to the femur
   b. Injury to the femur and tibia, closed head injury, foot fractures
   c. Injury to the torso, tibia or fibula fracture, foot and ankle fractures
   d. Closed head injury, injury to the torso, injury to the femur, tibia, and fibula

3. Indications of child abuse include:
   a. A history of repeated injury
   b. Multiple bruises in various stages of healing
   c. Unexplained or bizarre injuries such as bite marks or cigarette burns

d. A discrepancy between the mechanism of injury and the physical injuries

e. A caregiver who is very reluctant to give information related to the injury

   1. a, b, and c

   2. b, c, and d

   3. a, b, c, and d

   4. All of the above

4. An infant who suddenly stops breathing or experiences a seizure may be a victim of child abuse. This is typical of what mechanism of injury?

   a. Repeated violent shaking of the infant

   b. Sexual assault

   c. Verbal abuse

   d. Bouncing a baby on an adult's knee

5. The initial priority in all pediatric trauma patients is:

   a. To approach the child based on the child's developmental level

   b. To establish and maintain an open airway and effective respirations

   c. To make sure that a caregiver is with the child

   d. To watch for grunting, stridor, or retractions

6. Upper airway obstruction by the tongue occurs more easily in infants than in adults owing to the relatively larger size of the infant's tongue.

   a. True

   b. False

7. The narrowest portion of the infant's airway is the:

   a. Larynx

   b. Cricoid cartilage

   c. Posterior pharynx

   d. Subglottic space

8. Bag-valve masks of adult size can be adapted for use on children if special infant and child devices are not available.

   a. True

   b. False

9. The curved (MacIntosh) laryngoscope blade is the preferred blade used for intubations of children under the age of 2.

   a. True

   b. False

10. The most accurate way to determine endotracheal tube size for children is:

   a. An age-based formula

   b. A weight-based formula

   c. A length-based formula

   d. To look-at the diameter of the patient's fifth finger

11. The preferred site of needle decompression in infants is:

   a. Along the midclavicular line at the second intercostal space

   b. Along the midclavicular line at the first intercostal space

   c. Along the midclavicular line at the third intercostal space

   d. Along the midaxillary line at the fifth intercostal space

12. The best measures of pediatric circulation are:

   a. Blood pressure, heart rate, and skin color and temperature

   b. Heart rate, skin color and temperature, capillary refill, dry diaper

   c. Skin color and temperature, capillary refill, heart rate, mentation, and respiratory status

   d. Heart rate, blood pressure, capillary refill, mentation, and respiratory status

13. In assessing the heart rate, only tachycardia is indicative of shock in the pediatric patient.

   a. True

   b. False

14. The cornerstone of prehospital treatment of hypovolemic shock is crystalloid fluid boluses. The bolus should be given:

   a. Slowly in an amount of 20 mL/kg

   b. Rapidly in an amount of 20 mL/kg

   c. Slowly in an amount of 30 mL/kg

   d. Rapidly in an amount of 30 mL/kg via a syringe attached to a 3-way stopcock

   e. Rapidly in an amount of 20 mL/kg via a syringe attached to a 3-way stopcock

15. Cervical spine injuries in children tend to be at a higher level than in adults. The spine of a child is more cartilaginous and elastic than an adult's. This allows children to suffer from a spinal cord injury that does not show abnormalities on X-ray.

   a. True

   b. False

16. Aerophagia is frequently seen in injured small children. This is important because:

   a. Children have smaller stomachs than adults.

   b. Children use the diaphragm as the primary respiratory muscle and stomach distention prevents diaphragmatic excursion.

   c. Children use the diaphragm as the primary respiratory muscle and aerophagia causes over-inflation of the lungs.

   d. Children have smaller diaphragms than adults.

17. The most commonly missed life-threatening injury in the pediatric population is:

   a. Pulmonary contusion

   b. Tracheal tears

   c. Tension pneumothorax

   d. Hemothorax

18. A sudden impact of force to the anterior chest wall of a child, such as being hit with a baseball, can cause a sudden change in cardiac rhythm and function. This injury is termed:

a. Waddell's triad

b. Blunt trauma

c. Ventricular fibrillation

d. Commotio cordis

e. Baseball dysrhythmia syndrome

19. The paramedic should consider the prompt placement of an orogastric or nasogastric tube in the pediatric population in which of the following instances:

a. Closed head injury

b. Abdominal tenderness and significant distention

c. Gastric distention from aerophagia

d. All of the above

20. The kidneys of children are more vulnerable to injury than are adults' because:

a. A child's kidney is not as heavily protected with perinephretic fat.

b. A child's kidney is more rigidly anchored to surrounding structures.

c. The kidneys of a child are not shielded by the rib cage.

d. A child's kidney is smaller than an adult's.

e. A child's kidney is less well anchored to surrounding structures.

1. All of the above

2. a, b, c, and e

3. b, c, and e

4. a, c, and e

5. a, c, d, and e

▶ CRITICAL THINKING

1. You arrive at the home of a child care worker who is very upset. She directs you to the crib of a 3-month-old male infant she says she put down for a nap at 2 o'clock and "he was fine then." She states that she went back to the room to see if he was asleep and found him blue and not breathing. Your assessment reveals an apneic, pulseless infant and you begin CPR and resuscitation measures. The child care worker states that she knows of no medical problems, allergies, or recent illness or injuries, except that "he fell off his changing table about a month ago." Upon further assessment you note a purple bruise on the pad of both thumbs, but there are no other bruises. The fontanelles are soft and flat. The extremities are cool to the touch but the trunk is warm. The abdomen is flat and soft. There are no chest deformities. The extremities are normal in appear-

ance. Lung sounds are clear. What are the possible mechanisms of injury or causes of this arrest? What is the best way to determine endotracheal tube size and equipment sizes? What are normal vital signs for this 3-month-old? Is an orogastric tube a priority action, and if so why, and if not, what might change it to a priority intervention?

2. A 3-year-old child is hit by a car (traveling at about 30 miles per hour) while running into the road after a puppy. On your way to the scene you mentally prepare for the types of injuries you are likely to see. What are those types of injuries? What does Waddell's triad include? When you arrive at the scene you find a frightened child, weighing about 30 pounds, whose skin is pale, clammy, and damp. Capillary refill is 3 seconds. Respiratory rate is 42 and shallow, heart rate is 150, and systolic blood pressure is 100 mm Hg. There are diminished breath sounds on the right side. There is deformity of the left femur but the right leg is without deformity. Distal pulses are present in all extremities. What are your priorities in treating this child? What injuries do you suspect? What are the critical actions you need to take? Is this child showing signs of shock, and if so, what are they? How are you going to calm this child? You decide to initiate intravenous access to give crystalloid fluid. What kind of fluid would you give? What amount of fluid would you give initially and how would you give it? If you were unable to establish intravenous access what other options could you choose for fluid administration?

3. You are dispatched to the scene of a bicyclist/motor vehicle collision. Upon your arrival you observe a large pickup truck with a small deformity on the front bumper. Approximately 20 feet in front of the truck you note a badly mangled bicycle lying next to a 10-year-old child. The child appears unconscious. First responders greet you as you approach the scene. They inform you that your patient was struck at approximately 35 miles per hour and was pulseless and apneic upon their arrival to the scene. They have been performing CPR for approximately 10 minutes. You begin your physical examination and note the following: CPR in progress, no respiratory effort, and central pulses are absent. There is blood in the airway and efforts to suction are complicated by a dental appliance that has essentially wired the mouth closed and seems to be impossible to remove. Neck veins are flat and the trachea is midline. Bilateral breath sounds are diminished with crackles. Palpation of the anterior chest reveals multiple rib fractures and the abdomen is soft. The pelvis and long bones of the extremities are stable.

Pupils are 4 mm and nonreactive. ECG shows a wide complex pulseless electrical activity. What are the possible causes of cardiac arrest in this patient? Are any of these causes correctable? Based upon the physical examination what injuries do you suspect? What are the treatment priorities? How will you manage the airway? Assuming there is a parent at the scene what will you tell the parent regarding the child's condition?

▶ REFERENCES

1. Peclet M, Newman KD, Eichelberger MR, Gotschall CS, Guzetta PC, Anderson KD. Patterns of injury in children. *J Pediat Surg.* 1990; 25:85.

2. McCarthy DL, Surpure JS. Pediatric trauma: initial evaluation and stabilization. *Pediat Ann.* 1990; 19:584.

3. Haller J, Beaver B. Overview of pediatric trauma. In: Touloukian R, ed. *Pediatric Trauma.* St Louis, Mo.: Mosby; 1990.

4. Ramenofsky J. Emergency medical services for children and pediatric trauma system components. *J Pediat Surg.* 1989; 24:153.

5. Ribbeck BM, Runge JW, Thomason MH, Baker JW. Injury surveillance: a method for recording E-codes for injured emergency department patients. *Ann Emerg Med.* 1992; 21:37.

6. Centers for Disease Control and Prevention. National Center for Injury Prevention and Control. Internet: http://www.cdc.gov/ncipc; 2000.

7. Schafermeyer R. Pediatric trauma. *Emerg Med Clin North Am.* 1993; 11:187.

8. Sieben R, Leavitt J, French J. Falls as childhood accidents: an increasing urban risk. *Pediatrics.* 1971; 47:886.

9. National Pediatric Trauma Registry. Presented before the American Pediatric Surgical Association. Toronto; May 1986.

10. Angran P, Dankly D, Winn D. Injuries to a sample of seat-belted children evaluated and treated in a hospital emergency room. *J Trauma.* 1987; 27:58.

11. Clark JR. Child restraints: putting safety in the driver's seat. *JEMS.* 1991; 16(4):85.

12. American Academy of Pediatrics. Internet: www.aap.org; 2000.

13. Eichelburger MR, Randolph JG. Progress in pediatric trauma. *World J Surg.* 1985; 9:22.

14. Eichelburger MR. Trauma of the airway and thorax. *Pediat Ann.* 1897; 16(4):307.

15. Bledsoe BE, Porter RS, Shade BR. *Paramedic Emergency Care.* Englewood Cliffs, N.J.: Brady; 1994.

16. Paige CL, Wexler H. Prehospital management of pediatric trauma. *Emerg Care Q.* 1987; 3(7):15.

17. Sanders MJ. *Mosby's Paramedic Textbook.* St Louis, Mo.: Mosby Lifeline; 1994.

18. Seidel, HM, Ball JW, Dains JE, Benedict GW. *Mosby's Guide to Physical Examination.* St Louis, Mo.: Mosby Year Book; 1991.

19. Rubin M, Sadovnikoff N. Pediatric airway management. In: Tintinalli JE, Kelen GD, Stapczynski JS, eds. *Emergency Medicine: A Comprehensive Study Guide.* New York: McGraw-Hill; 2000.

20. Norwood SS, Zaritsky AL. *Guidelines for Pediatric Emergency Care.* Chapel Hill, N.C.: Emergency Medical Services for Children Project; 1992.

21. Hauda WE, II. Pediatric cardiopulmonary resuscitation. In: Tintinalli JE, Kelen GD, Stapczynski JS, eds. *Emergency Medicine: A Comprehensive Study Guide.* New York: McGraw-Hill; 2000.

22. Hauda WE, II. Pediatric trauma. In: Tintinalli JE, Kelen GD, Stapczynski JS, eds. *Emergency Medicine: A Comprehensive Study Guide.* New York: McGraw-Hill; 2000.

23. Chameides L, Hazinski MF, eds. *Textbook of Pediatric Advanced Life Support.* American Academy of Pediatrics. Dallas, Tex.: American Heart Association; 1994.

24. Lescholier I. Blunt trauma in children: consequences and outcomes of head vs. extracranial injuries. *Pediatrics.* 1993; 91:721.

25. Cantor R, Leaming J. Evaluation and management of pediatric major trauma. *Emerg Med Clin N Am.* 1998; 16:229.

26. Kisson N, Dreyer J, Walia M. Pediatric trauma: differences in pathophysiology, injury patterns and treatment compared with adult trauma. *Can Med Assoc J.* 1990; 142:27.

27. Pang D, Pollack I. Spinal cord injury without radiographic abnormality in children—the SCIWORA syndrome. *J Trauma.* 1989; 29:654.

28. Rachesky I, Boyce WT, Duncan B, Bjelland J, Sibley B. Clinical prediction of cervical spine injuries in children. *Am J Dis Child.* 1987; 141:199.

29. Bender T. Pediatric chest trauma. *J Thorac Imag.* 1987; 2:60.

30. Cooper A, Foltin G. Thoracic trauma. In: Barken R, ed. *Pediatric Emergency Medicine.* St Louis, Mo.: Mosby; 1992.

31. Brandt ML, et al. Thoracic trauma in children. *Emerg Care Q.* 1987; 3(7):45.

32. Inaba A, Seward PL. An approach to pediatric trauma. *Emerg Med Clin North Am.* 1991; 9:523.

33. Foltin G, Cooper A. Abdominal trauma. In: Barkin R, ed. *Pediatric Emergency Medicine.* St Louis, Mo.: Mosby; 1992.

34. Klauber GT. Genitourinary trauma in children. *Emerg Care Q.* 1987; 3(7):51.

35. Karlin L. Musculoskeletal trauma. *Emerg Care Q.* 1987; 3(7):57.

36. Moront ML, Williams JA, Eichelberger MR, Wilkinson JD. The injured child: an approach to care. *Pediat Clin N Am.* 1994; 41(6):1201.

▶ BIBLIOGRAPHY

Bourn MK. Intraosseous infusion: an innovation of the 1980s. *Emerg Nurs Rep.* 1988; 3(5):1.

Boyce MC, Melhorn KJ, Vargo G. Pediatric trauma documentation: adequacy for assessment of child abuse. *Arch Pediat Adolescent Med.* 1996; 150(7):730.

Bricker DL, Beall AC Jr. Trauma to the heart. In: Daughtry DC, ed. *Thoracic Trauma.* Boston: Little Brown & Co; 1980.

Clark JR. Where's my mommy. *The Gold Cross.* 1995; 66(2).

Clark JR, Valcourt GR. Family care. *Emergency.* 1992; 24(2):40.

Guerin, RT, Elling R. Prehospital pediatric care course: a continuing education course for paramedics. In: *Instructor Manual and Student Workbook.* Albany, N.Y.: New York State Department of Health EMS Program; 1990.

Henderson DP, Seidel JS. Approach to the pediatric patient. In: Seidel JS, Henderson DP, eds. *Prehospital Care of Pediatric Emergencies.* Sudbury, Mass.: Jones & Bartlett; 1997, 5B13.

Honigman B, Rohwederk K, Moore EE, Lowenstein SR, Pons PT. Prehospital advanced trauma life support for penetrating cardiac wounds. *Ann Emerg Med.* 1990; 19(2):145.

Kerns DL. Child abuse: emergency management of pediatric trauma. In: Mayer TA, ed. Philadelphia: WB Saunders Co; 1985.

Kram JA, Kizer KW. Submersion injury *Emerg Med Clin North Am.* 1984; 2(3):545.

Mack MG, Hudson S, Thompson D. A descriptive analysis of children's playground injuries in the United States 1990–1994. *Injury Prevention.* 1997; 3(2):100.

Martin TG. Near-drowning and cold water immersion. *Ann Emerg Med.* 1984; 13(4):263.

Morrisey MA, Ohsfeldt RL, Johnson V, Treat R. Trauma patients: an analysis of rural ambulance trip reports. *J Trauma.* 1996; 41(4):741.

Rivara FP, Grossman DC. Prevention of traumatic deaths to children in the United States: how far have we come and where do we need to go? *Pediatrics.* 1996; 97:791.

Chapter

27

Complications of Trauma

OBJECTIVES

Upon completion of this chapter, the reader should be able to:

- List the most important complications occurring in the trauma patient.
- Describe the pathophysiology of these complications.
- Recognize the clinical signs that are helpful in diagnosing these complications.
- List the diagnostic tests used to evaluate these complications.
- Identify those patients who are most susceptible to complicating factors.
- Explain the treatment modalities that may be used in caring for the victim of trauma complications.
- List the most common causes of traumatic cardiac arrest.
- Compare and contrast the underlying pathophysiological differences between traumatic versus nontraumatic cardiac arrest.
- Discuss the conclusions generated by current research related to expected outcomes following traumatic cardiac arrest.
- Based on an understanding of the current societal climate, expand upon the theme of ethical considerations in relation to use of resources, organ donation, and financial cost.

KEY TERMS

Adult respiratory distress syndrome (ARDS)
Air embolism
Disseminated intravascular coagulation (DIC)
Multiple-organ failure (MOF)

Sepsis syndrome
Spinal shock
Thromboembolism

A discussion of trauma would be incomplete without addressing those events that may occur following initial injuries. This chapter provides an overview of medical entities that are not initially present but when evolved can dramatically alter the trauma patient's prognosis. It is important for prehospital personnel to have some understanding of these late occurring complications so that measures can be taken toward prevention and,

should they already be present, understand their management in trauma care.

Complications of trauma encompass a very broad spectrum of medical problems. The complete coverage of this topic is certainly beyond the scope of this text. The focus here is on the most important complications, including respiratory conditions, blood-clotting disorders, shock, multiorgan failure, and cardiac arrest. The subject of shock itself consists of four categories: septic, neurogenic, hypovolemic, and cardiogenic. This chapter discusses septic and neurogenic shock. Hypovolemic and cardiogenic shock are covered in Chapter 9.

RESPIRATORY COMPLICATIONS

RESPIRATORY FAILURE

Respiratory insufficiency is a condition to be expected to some degree in most trauma patients. It is a product of the lungs' normal response to injury. Respiratory failure occurs when the lungs and muscles of inspiration are unable to provide efficient gas exchange to oxygenate and ventilate the tissues. What would otherwise be a trivial injury in the healthy person may cause respiratory failure in the susceptible patient who has previous lung pathology.

Many events can precipitate respiratory failure. Musculoskeletal injuries may cause structural damage disenabling the muscles of inspiration or otherwise limiting efficient air flow. Vertebral column injuries with spinal cord damage above cervical vertebrae 3, 4, and 5 may damage the phrenic nerves, which provide innervation to the diaphragm, thus preventing adequate ventilation. Aspiration of gastric contents may occur after trauma, leading to lung parenchymal damage, bronchospasm, and hypoxemia by destroying tracheal epithelial cells and alveolar pneumocytes. The damage incurred is dependent on the volume and pH of the aspirate. Because pain causes increased acidity of the gastric secretions and delays clearance by shunting blood away from the digestive tract, the pH is low. A pH of less than 2.5 or a volume greater than 1 mL/kg is likely to cause lung damage.[1] A trauma victim may also develop an aspiration pneumonia from bacteria contained in the aspirate.

Airway obstruction may be caused by trauma and cause respiratory failure. Structural damage to the patient's head, neck, or thoracic areas may produce mechanical obstruction. Solid objects may also be swallowed, with larger solids often lodging at the vocal cords, which is the narrowest part of the adult airway, while smaller objects may obstruct in the bronchi, producing lobar processes such as atelectasis and pneumonia distal to the obstruction.

The clinical signs of respiratory failure include visible nasal flaring, contraction of sternocleidomastoid and intercostal muscles on inspiration, and a rapid breathing rate. Stridor may be heard in airway obstruction. Skin pallor is associated with hypoxia due to inadequate ventilation, as are anxiety, inappropriate speech, and altered level of consciousness.

The treatments for these sources of respiratory failure include proper airway management with intubation and mechanical ventilation to ensure adequate air flow into the lungs. Aspiration may be treated and prevented by insertion of a nasogastric tube, upright body positioning, use of cricothyroid pressure, and a cuffed endotracheal tube.[1] Antibiotics are administered if aspiration pneumonia is a concern. The Heimlich maneuver is attempted if a foreign object is suspected. Bronchoscopic removal with a camera and instrumentation is required at the hospital if the object cannot be removed otherwise.

EMBOLIC DISEASES

Pulmonary Embolic Disease

Thromboembolism, or venous clot embolisms, are blood clots that form in the venous system, break loose, travel, and lodge elsewhere in the vascular system, often leading to fatal complications. Thromboemboli affecting the lungs are called pulmonary emboli. Saddle emboli are a form of pulmonary emboli that can cause instantaneous death by occluding the pulmonary arteries, thereby obstructing blood outflow from the right side of the heart. These emboli may occur early after injury or take days to weeks to develop in immobilized patients.

Pulmonary emboli are most often (greater than two-thirds of the cases) the result of deep venous thrombosis in the lower extremities, where venous stasis occurs due to a lack of muscular contractions, such as in immobilized trauma patients who require lengthy hospitalization. Other risk factors for developing deep venous thrombosis include cancer, elderly age group, lower torso or extremity trauma, surgery, oral contraceptive use, and as a postpartum condition. The pathology occurs when the clot formed in the deep vein breaks loose and travels downstream to the pulmonary arteries where it lodges occluding blood flow.

The clinical symptoms are tachypnea, chest pain, pulmonary infiltrates on chest radiograph, hypoxemia, and tachycardia. Diagnosis is made by ventilation/perfusion scanning, pulmonary arteriography, and Doppler studies of the femoral veins, which assess blood flow and diagnose obstructions. The chest radiograph is most often normal in these patients.

The treatment is 10,000 units of heparin, then a continuous drip of 25 units/kg/hr to reach a partial thromboplastin time (PTT) of about double the normal value, with supplemental oxygen given at 4–10 L/min.[2] Alternatively, enoxaparin (lovenox) 1 mg/kg may be administered subcutaneously every 12 hours. Thrombolytics and possibly angiographic removal are used in some cases. The use of pneumatic compression devices and heparin have been shown to be good prophylactic treatment to prevent deep vein thromboses.[3] Overall mortality of pulmonary embolism is low if diagnosed and treated appropriately, but if the diagnosis is initially missed, the survival rate drops to around 50%.

INTERNET ACTIVITIES

Visit the e-medicine Web site at http://www.emedicine.com. Click on the Emergency Medicine on-line book and select Cardiovascular. Then click on Pulmonary Embolism. Review the chapter on the management of pulmonary embolism.

Air Embolism

When an open vein is at or below atmospheric pressure, air may be sucked into the vessel to travel through the circulation and form an **air embolism**. This is an unusual event as empty veins usually collapse. However, veins that are stinted open (vertebral venous sinus, pulmonary vein) can entrain air. This air foams or forms tiny bubbles in the bloodstream and then collects in the right side of the heart, causing an obstruction of outflow and irritating the conduction system. Air embolization occurs with lacerations to the large veins of the neck, where pressure changes associated with respiration entrain air into the venous system. Air embolization may also occur with lung lacerations due to communications created between the bronchi and pulmonary veins. These lacerations allow air to pass through during positive-pressure ventilation. Because the air bypasses the pulmonary capillaries, systemic embolization may follow and lodge in the brain or heart, causing infarction. Symptoms are similar to those of a pulmonary embolism: tachycardia, tachypnea, and hypoxia.

Prevention of air embolism during external jugular vein cannulation is of paramount importance. If possible, the patient's head should be lowered to keep the jugular vein full and minimize the risk of embolization. The treatment for air embolization is the occlusion of the affected vascular structures in the lung,

INTERNET ACTIVITIES

Visit the e-medicine Web site at http://www.emedicine.com. Click on the Emergency Medicine on-line book and select Cardiovascular. Then click on Venous Air Embolism. Review the chapter on the management of venous air embolism.

endotracheal intubation, and the placement of the patient in the left lateral decubitus position in an attempt to prevent the air emboli from leaving the right side of the heart. In time, the air should be reabsorbed from the blood, barring other complications.

Fat Embolism

This is the second most common form of embolism causing vascular occlusion. The embolization of fat may take place after any major fracture and typically occurs with long-bone and pelvic fractures. They may also result from extensive trauma to fatty tissue.

The exact mechanism of fat embolization is not completely known. One theory is that the fractures may simply release globules of fat from the bone marrow or fatty tissue into venous channels at the location of injury. Other theories involve the aggregation of circulating chylomicrons (fat carried by protein) into fat droplets due to acute-phase reactants, and that damage from free fatty acids released by lipases (enzymes) results in the intravascular thrombi. The globules distribute throughout the circulation and cause obstruction in organs and thrombocytopenia secondary to adhesion of platelets to the fat emboli.

The classic presentation of fat embolism syndrome is thrombocytopenia, respiratory difficulty, skin and conjunctival petechiae, obtundation, and possibly coma and death. The pulmonary effects include hypoxia, pulmonary hypertension, and an increase in dead space, which is the area of the respiratory tract where gas exchange does not take place.

Modern management of bone injury has greatly reduced the incidence of fat embolisms. Early fixation of multiple fractures has decreased the incidence of fat emboli from 22% to 1.5%–4%. Treatment includes proper immobilization of fractures in the field and supportive care, such as oxygen administration and hemodynamic support.[1]

TENSION PNEUMOTHORAX

Tension pneumothorax is a common complication of blunt thoracic trauma and penetrating injury. The pneumothorax may occur acutely or may not develop until several days following the initial injury. Trauma may cause lung parenchymal or bronchial injury, which allows air to enter the intact pleural space through a one-way opening in the visceral pleura. As more air enters, a progressively increasing pleural pressure builds up, causing collapse of the lung, compromising venous return to the heart with subsequent circulatory collapse.

Clinical symptoms include unilaterally absent or decreased breath sounds and percussive hyperresonance on the affected side. Signs of respiratory distress and circulatory collapse such as poor peripheral perfusion, hypotension, and jugular venous distention may be seen. The diagnosis must be made quickly and is based primarily on the history and physical findings.

Suspected patients must have immediate large-bore (14–16-gauge) needle aspiration of the affected side. This is done through the second intercostal space at the midclavicular line. As the pleural space is entered, air rapidly escapes, yielding temporary relief of symptoms and confirmation of the diagnosis. It must be noted that a tension pneumothorax may be missed during an attempted needle thoracotomy, and therefore the lack of escaping air does not rule out a pneumothorax. Chest tube insertion should be performed following needle thoracotomy to prevent the re-formation of the pneumothorax. The patient needs supplemental 100% oxygen. See Chapter 13 for a more complete discussion of tension pneumothorax.

ADULT RESPIRATORY DISTRESS SYNDROME

Severe acute lung injury follows trauma in 20% of patients without primary pulmonary injuries. The mortality rate is approximately 50% and results from direct insult to lung parenchyma or from a systemic response to distant trauma.[4] **Adult respiratory distress syndrome (ARDS)** is an entity that occurs following trauma and involves the inability of the lungs to carry out proper gas exchange. It is a complication without a uniform definition; however, it consists of, at least, the following conditions:

1. The onset is acute, occurring within 24–48 hours after the precipitating incident.
2. Disturbances exist in oxygenation and ventilation.
3. Bilateral diffuse infiltrates are formed and visualized on radiograph.
4. Systemic manifestations are present, such as tachycardia, tachypnea, hyperthermia, and thrombocytopenia.
5. Left-sided heart failure is ruled out using a pulmonary artery catheter.[1]

The causes of ARDS are numerous and include trauma to the head or distant body sites, fractures, systemic inflammatory response secondary to tissue necrosis, aspiration, embolism, contusion, and pneumonia. ARDS is also highly associated with the development of sepsis.

The pathophysiology of ARDS can be divided into events taking place on a time scale. ARDS is a process of acute lung injury in which there is a loss of the integrity of the alveolar-capillary interface. The clinical course varies among patients. Some have transient deteriorations in oxygen saturation and an increase in minute ventilation. Others have precipitous oxygen deteriorations over a very short period of time progressing to pulmonary fibrosis and death.

Early Stage

The early phase occurs in the first 24 hours following injury, with interstitial and alveolar edema resulting from damage to endothelial cells. The pulmonary capillaries become clogged with fibrin and cellular debris. Pulmonary artery pressure rises, dead space increases, and a ventilation/perfusion mismatch results in hypoxemia. The patient becomes tachypneic with shallow breathing. Supplemental oxygen is usually all that is required at this time.

Moderate Stage

In the next 24 hours the transition to moderate ARDS occurs in which alveoli fill with blood, cell debris, and fibrin. Type I pneumocytes are injured while Type II pneumocytes, which secrete surfactant and are stem cells for production of the Type I's, proliferate in an attempt to repair and replace the injured cells. Lung compliance is poor and infiltrates may be seen on chest radiograph. The treatment at this stage may range from continuous positive airway pressure (CPAP) via mask to intubation with mechanical ventilation.

Severe Stage

The next stage is that of severe ARDS. If therapy is not begun, inflammatory cells (lymphocytes, macrophages, plasma cells) migrate into the lungs. This leads to further deterioration of gas exchange. The chest X-ray now shows diffuse white-out. Most of these patients require mechanical ventilation and positive end-expiratory pressure (PEEP).

End Stage

During the end stage of ARDS the body's immune response leads to fibroblast proliferation with collagen being formed around the air spaces. The severe fibrosis and emphysematous changes that follow lead to significant barotrauma and hemodynamic deterioration. This leads to severe pulmonary hypertension and right-sided heart failure. Figure 27-1 shows a microscopic view of normal lung tissue that includes alveoli filled with air. The alveolar walls are thin and contain blood vessels. Figure 27-2 is a microscopic section of lung with ARDS demonstrating the many changes that take place. Notice the alveolar spaces are congested, edematous, and full of red blood cells. The alveolar walls are thickened and

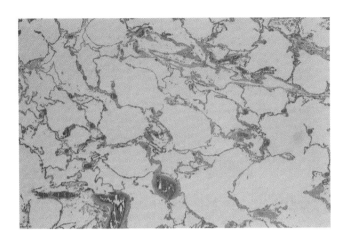

FIGURE 27-1 Microscopic view of a normal lung, including alveoli. (Courtesy of M. G. F. Gilliland, East Carolina University School of Medicine.)

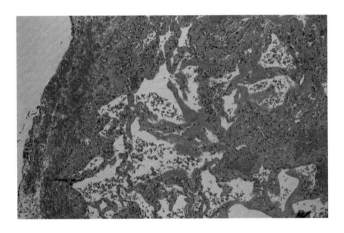

FIGURE 27-2 Microscopic view of an ARDS lung. Note the alveolar spaces are edematous and full of red blood cells. (Courtesy of M. G. F. Gilliland, East Carolina University School of Medicine.)

there is bleeding in the pleura near the edges of the tissue. These changes prevent the exchange of oxygen and carbon dioxide in the lungs and are associated with a high mortality rate (up to 70%).

Methods of treatment for ARDS are constantly being tested and evaluated. Recent studies using very low concentrations of nitric oxide appear to cause a decrease in pulmonary vascular pressure and a decrease in intrapulmonary shunting.[5] Superimposed high-frequency jet ventilation along with inhaled nitric oxide has also been tested with evidence of temporary improvement in the patient's condition.[6] The transbronchial application of exogenous surfactant, the body's substance that aids in keeping the alveoli open, has been tested in pilot studies and may have positive effects on gas exchange and pulmonary hemo-

dynamics.[7] These and further studies may produce a treatment formula to increase survival of the patient with ARDS.

It is helpful to keep in mind that respiratory injuries work together synergistically such that the combined effects are much worse than the injuries by themselves or simply added together. Because of this fact, even the young and physically fit may experience respiratory failure when there is a combination of injuries that would by themselves be well tolerated.

The long-term respiratory complications of trauma may be prevented by proactive airway management. Early intubation helps prevent exacerbations of increased intracranial pressure through avoiding hypercarbia and hypoxemia. Intubation also aids in the prevention of gastric content aspiration and its subsequent complications.

INTERNET ACTIVITIES

Visit the e-medicine Web site at http://www.emedicine.com. Click on the Emergency Medicine on-line book and select Pulmonary. Then click on Respiratory Distress Syndrome. Review the chapter on the management of ARDS.

DISSEMINATED INTRAVASCULAR COAGULATION

Disseminated intravascular coagulation (DIC) is a generalized activation of the body's clotting mechanism in which coagulation and fibrinolysis become unbalanced. This syndrome carries up to an 85% mortality rate, which is mostly due to the underlying cause, about half of those causes being obstetrical complications, one-third related to cancer, and about one-sixth trauma related. Traumatic causes include infection, tissue damage, and shock, with sepsis being the most common instigator. DIC is also caused by hemolysis from mismatched blood transfusions, snake venom, and Rocky Mountain spotted fever.

The common triggering event is the release of thromboplastic substances that initiate the coagulation cascade. Thrombin and plasmin are two very important enzymes involved in hemostasis. Thrombin converts fibrinogen to fibrin, digests factors V and VIII, and promotes platelet aggregation, all of which lead to blood coagulation. Plasmin acts to degrade fibrin to form fibrin split products, thus inhibiting normal coagulation of blood by delaying polymerization of fibrin, prolonging the thrombin time, and blocking platelet aggregation. Coagulation and fibrinolysis become unbalanced. Thrombosis may occur with thrombi formation in the microvasculature, consuming platelets, fibrin, and other coagulation factors. Bleeding may occur from the skin, mucous membranes, surgical and venipuncture sites, or intestinal or urinary systems due to depletion of elements needed for hemostasis.

The symptoms of DIC are bleeding, multiple petechiae, ecchymosis, microangiopathic anemia (due to red blood cell distortion by microthrombi), infarction of organs such as the kidney, which leads to oliguria (low urine output), mental status changes, gangrene, and ARDS.

DIC patients must be stabilized hemodynamically and given fluids, oxygen, and life support as needed. A primary concern is the treatment of the underlying cause. Blood and platelets are replaced as indicated by loss, and clotting factors are replenished with fresh frozen plasma. Antithrombin may be used to aid in thrombosis prevention. Experimental sepsis models associated with DIC have been developed and demonstrate that the hypercoagulable state, which is a necessary precursor to DIC, may be prevented by inactivating factor X or suppressing platelet activation.[8] The prognosis for DIC is variable and depends on the underlying cause. The severity of the syndrome depends on the vascular endothelium, the liver's ability to replace clotting factors, and platelet replacement by the bone marrow.

INTERNET ACTIVITIES

Visit the e-medicine Web site at http:// www.emedicine.com. Click on the Emergency Medicine on-line book and select Hematology. Then click on Disseminated Intravascular Coagulation. Review the chapter on the management of DIC.

SEPTIC SHOCK

Septic shock is a leading cause of death after trauma and carries a 50% mortality rate. There are nearly 500,000 cases of sepsis in the United States each year, half of which develop into septic shock. Of penetrating and blunt trauma deaths, 5% and 8%, respectively, are due to sepsis; most deaths occur in the first several days postinjury.[9]

Septic shock is a product of infection, which requires a susceptible host, immune system dysfunction, and bacterial colonization. Trauma incites a complex stress response with increases in adrenocorticotropic hormone, aldosterone, glucagon, antidiuretic hormone, catecholamines, and glucocorticoids, which predisposes the patient to infection. There are two sources of bacteria: introduction from the environment and the dissemination of native host bacteria. Bacteremia is defined as the invasion of bacteria into the blood. It occurs in 10%–20% of trauma victims.[10] The state of sepsis is the body's response to the bacteremia. The signs of sepsis are hypothermia (temperature less than 95°) or hyperthermia (temperature greater than 101°), tachycardia, and tachypnea. **Sepsis syndrome** (also termed systemic inflammatory response syndrome) is sepsis with signs of abnormal end-organ perfusion as evidenced by altered cerebral function, oliguria, hypoxemia, and elevated lactate levels secondary to tissue conversion to anaerobic metabolism in the absence of adequate oxygen. Septic shock describes the sepsis syndrome in the presence of hypotension.

Blunt injuries with soft tissue crushing and damage to vascular structures produce ischemia and a good culture medium for bacteria. Most posttraumatic infections are caused by the patient's own endogenous flora, which can become rapidly necrotizing.[11] Stab wounds usually produce minimal soft tissue damage and have only a 1%–2% incidence of sepsis. Gunshot wounds, especially shotgun, may cause massive tissue injury and carry debris into the wound, setting up a good nidus for infection. The highest infectious morbidity comes with abdominal injury involving the colon, where there are over 100 billion bacteria per gram of fecal mass. These bacterial cells are normally confined to the colon but may be released into the abdomen, pelvis, and bloodstream by trauma. The degree of fecal contamination determines the prognosis for developing sepsis. Overall, 12%–20% of septic cases are secondary to colon injury, with the chance of developing sepsis increasing as the amount of abdominal fecal content rises.[1] Other risk factors for incurring septic shock include diabetes, malignancy, immunosuppression, and extremes in age. Infants are more susceptible as their specific immune systems are incompletely developed, allowing bacteria to colonize and produce infection, while the elderly have blunted responses to infection.

The pathophysiology of septic shock is triggered by a cascade of events induced by the presence of bacteria, viruses, or fungi in the blood. These organisms stimulate the release of tissue necrosis factor (TNF), which starts the chain of events. Gram-negative bacterial endotoxin has been well studied because of its good laboratory reproducibility; it is the inciting organism in two-thirds of the cases of posttraumatic infections. Gram-negative bacteria produce an endotoxin (lipopolysaccharide) in their outer cell wall that stimulates the release of TNF from macrophages and other cells in the body. TNF is a pyrogen (produces fever) as well as a stimulator of other cytokines (polypeptides with hormonelike activity), platelet-activating factor, compliment, and the blood coagulation cascade. Nitric oxide is also released and causes vasodilatation and the hypotension associated with septic shock. The end result of the TNF-activated events is an alteration in organ systems, vascular endothelial cell damage, and sludging of blood in the capillaries.

The clinical presentation of sepsis is widespread. It most commonly produces a "warm" shock with an increased cardiac output and low systemic vascular resistance, decreased blood pressure, and warm, clammy skin. Tachycardia is usually present, but the heart's ejection fraction (the percentage of volume pumped out) may decrease due to the heart becoming dilated with poor muscular function. Tissue extraction of oxygen falls along with an increase in pulmonary vascular resistance. This inadequate oxygen delivery combined with a lower blood flow pushes the tissues into anaerobic metabolism and lactic acidosis. Renal insufficiency may occur most commonly as a result of acute tubular necrosis, with the cause not well understood, but it may be a result of the deposition of antigen-antibody complexes in the kidney. The most common feature of septic shock is fever, which is most likely the result of thermoregulatory center resetting mediated by prostaglandins released as part of the TNF cascade. Hyperventilation occurs secondary to hypoxia and the metabolic acidosis caused by lactic acid. Mental status changes may occur early, with initial mild anxiety and confusion progressing to lethargy and coma. The patient may develop ARDS as endothelial injury and capillary leakage continues. DIC may ensue with prolonged sepsis. The patient may also progress to multiple-organ failure.

Treatment of septic shock involves hemodynamic support, oxygen, antibiotics to kill bacteria, and surgery if indicated to remove sites of infection. Prevention of sepsis is maximized through aggressive resuscitation, debridement of devitalized tissue, removal of central lines and indwelling tubes as soon as possible, and specific management of injuries with sterile technique. Recent studies using hemofiltration and plasma filtration have been performed in children to treat severe sepsis. However, their effects on patient outcome have yet to be adequately determined.[12]

MULTIPLE-ORGAN FAILURE

Multiple-organ failure (MOF) is a complication that affects those patients who are severely injured, develop sepsis, or are "problem ridden" after surgery. The syndrome is the end result of a prolonged state of shock and accounts for 50% of late deaths in trauma patients.[1] Two broad categories of events precipitate MOF: those leading to regional blood flow abnormalities such as hypotension or fluid overload and those events that incite inflammatory responses such as sep-

sis and pancreatitis. No uniform definition of particular organ failure exists but rather many clinical and laboratory findings are used as evidence of organ dysfunction. Table 27-1 outlines data used to define failure in the organs or systems listed.

MOF is a nonspecific host response that is not aimed at any particular infection or injury but is a systemic response caused by a cascade of related events. Trauma or infection produces damage to macrophages, monocytes, T-cells, and endothelial cells. Each of these injured cell types releases various cytokines, which incite an inflammatory response. This response is a mechanism for host cellular defense. When the injury

Table 27-1
Signs of Organ/System Failure

Organ/System	Signs of Failure
Cardiovascular	Bradycardia of 54 beats per minute or less Mean arterial blood pressure less than 50 mm Hg Ventricular arrhythmia Extensive inotropic support
Respiratory	Ventilator support greater than 48 hours in duration Adult respiratory distress syndrome
Neurological	Glasgow Coma Scale under 15 uninfluenced by drugs
Gastrointestinal	Unable to tolerate oral feedings Gastrointestinal bleed of greater than 1 liter per 24 hours
Renal	Oliguria of less than 20 mL/hr over 8 hours BUN greater than 100 mg/dL Creatinine greater than 2 mg/dL
Metabolic	Hyperglycemia requiring administration of insulin at greater than 2 units/hr to keep glucose under 250 mg/dL Metabolic acidosis
Liver/biliary	Serum bilirubin greater than 2 mg/dL Either SGOT, SGPT, or GGT are double the normal value
Hematological	Thrombocytopenia with platelet count less than 60,000/mm³

Abbreviations: BUN, blood urea nitrogen; SGOT, serum glutamic oxaloacetic transaminase; SGPT, serum glutamic pyruvic transaminase; GGT, gamma-glutamyl transpeptidase.

Source: Adapted from Mattox KL, ed. *Complications of Trauma*. New York: Churchill Livingston Inc; 1994: 87.

or insult is severe enough, an uncontrolled release of the cytokines occurs that can cause injury to the host's organs. The coagulation, fibrinolytic, and kinin systems are also stimulated to initiate their cascade of events. Neutrophils aggregate in small vessels impeding blood flow. Microcirculatory arrest is a critical event in the evolution of MOF in the septic patient. Reactive oxygen metabolites such as superoxide are produced and released secondary to the ischemia that results from the blockage of blood flow. These oxygen-free radicals have been associated with provoking cellular injury. Focal necrosis (death) occurs with the summation of the necrosis becoming greater as the process progresses until there is compromise in function of the organ system. Figure 27-3 shows a microscopic section of normal kidney with small, round glomeruli and pale, oval lumens of cross sections of tubules. In Figure 27-4

we see a higher power microscopic slide of a kidney that has undergone acute tubular necrosis, a complication of shock and MOF in which injury occurs to the glomeruli, tubules, and renal vessels by the means listed above. This figure shows that the tubules have become dilated, with necrosis of some lining cells. The round structure comprising about one-third of the photo is the glomeruli, seen here containing pathological fibrin thrombi. Figure 27-5 is a photograph of a dissected slice of a normal liver. The color is a uniform light brown. Figure 27-6 is a specimen of a "shock" liver that has the characteristic appearance called nutmeg liver. A back-up of venous blood caused by the effects of shock on the cardiovascular system has led to congestion and pooled blood around the liver's central veins. This leakage of blood into the tissue has given it a dark color as compared to the normal liver. The

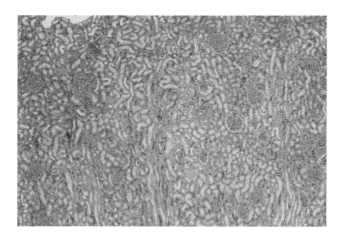

FIGURE 27-3 Microscopic view of a normal kidney. (Courtesy of M. G. F. Gilliland, East Carolina University School of Medicine.)

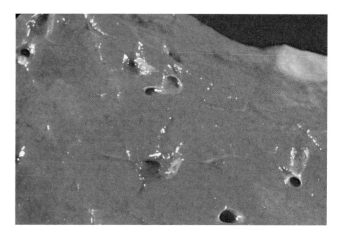

FIGURE 27-5 Dissected slice of a normal liver. (Courtesy of M. G. F. Gilliland, East Carolina University School of Medicine.)

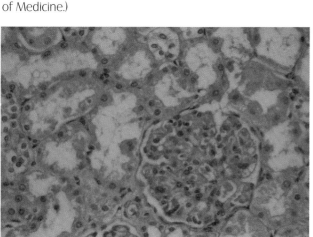

FIGURE 27-4 Microscopic slide of an MOF kidney. (Courtesy of M. G. F. Gilliland, East Carolina University School of Medicine.)

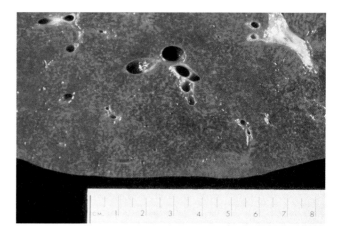

FIGURE 27-6 A specimen of "shock" liver often called "nutmeg" liver due to its appearance. (Courtesy of M. G. F. Gilliland, East Carolina University School of Medicine.)

congestion and decreased circulation lead to death of cells around the central vein.

Metabolic changes also take place in MOF with the transition of amino acids from constituents of protein synthesis to substrates for oxidation to meet cellular needs. The effects include hypermetabolism, increased gluconeogenesis in the liver, increased loss of nitrogen in the urine, and insulin resistance. This net catabolic response is not reversed with the administration of exogenous glucose or amino acids.

Age greater than 55 years, more than six units of packed red blood cells administered within 12 hours, high lactate levels, sepsis, severe trauma, preexisting chronic illness, and decreased pH are all predictors of MOF.[13,14]

Measures to prevent and treat MOF include ensuring adequate prehospital ventilation and oxygenation, fluid administration, and maintenance of hemodynamics. In the intensive care unit the goal is to prevent MOF by maximizing oxygen consumption at the tissue level through providing proper ventilation and fluid balance. Specific organ system support must also be provided, with emphasis on acute renal failure, which occurs late in MOF. Patients with MOF-induced acute renal failure have a poor prognosis even when adequately dialyzed. Plasma exchange with colloidal replacement fluid has been used to reverse the effects of MOF and has inspired clinicians to recommend plasma exchange to reverse late-stage MOF.[15]

NEUROGENIC SHOCK

Traumatic injury to the spinal cord may produce **spinal shock**, which consists of a loss of vascular tone and a loss of sympathetic nerve input to the heart. This is caused by traumatic impairment of the descending sympathetic nerves along the spinal cord. These sympathetic nerves innervate the blood vessels and produce the constriction (or tone) inherent in the vessels. When this innervation is lost, the vessels dilate, which causes a decreased return of blood to the heart, pooling of blood in the lower extremities, and hypotension. The sympathetic nerves are also responsible for stimulating the heart to beat at a faster pace. This stimulus is offset by the parasympathetic input, which acts to slow the heart beat. Thus, the loss of the sympathetic stimulus produces a bradycardia induced by the parasympathetic input from the vagus nerve.

The usual clinical presentation is a decreased heart rate with a wide pulse pressure. The skin is warm and dry and may be flushed. Cardiac output is reduced secondary to the decreased venous return of blood to the heart. As neurogenic shock progresses, blood flow to the organs is reduced, producing symptoms similar to those seen in hypovolemic shock.

Initial treatment of the patient with a possible spinal cord injury involves the assessment of the airway, breathing, circulation, and immobilization of the spine. Every patient with acute spinal cord injury should be given an intravenous bolus of methylprednisolone at 30 mg/kg body weight within the first 8 hours after the injury. During the next 23 hours the patient should receive 5.4 mg/kg methylprednisolone.[16] The purpose of the steroid administration is to decrease swelling around the injured cord, thus reducing further injury. In treating neurogenic shock, it is important to remember that the hypotension is from the loss of vascular tone, not fluid loss. The preferred initial treatment is volume expansion with 1 liter of crystalloid fluid if there are no signs of blood loss. However, attempting fluid resuscitation may cause a fluid overload. Therefore, treatment requires careful monitoring and the judicious use of vasopressors, such as Neo-Synephrine and phenylephrine, to restore tone in the vessels. Atropine is a parasympatholytic drug that may be used to block the parasympathetic input to the heart, increase the electrical conduction through the heart's atrioventricular (AV) node, and push the pulse rate toward normal. The recommended dosage is 0.5–1.0 mg intravenously given every 1–2 hours as needed.[17,18] The symptoms of neurogenic shock are often reversible with treatment and time, depending on the extent of injury.

TRAUMATIC CARDIAC ARREST

The advent of rapid transit, the growth in popularity of athletic competition, and the risk of violent crimes against individuals have contributed to an ever-increasing number of traumatic injuries. Many researchers and physicians agree that cardiac arrest secondary to blunt or penetrating trauma is likely to be a terminal event.[19–24] The encroachment of managed care, discussion of resource allocation, cost containment concerns, and burgeoning health care costs have resulted in many health care providers reexamining outcomes following traumatic injuries. Weighing the cost of providing extensive, sophisticated care for a few against the need to provide a broad range of comprehensive, preventative services for many has led to increased media attention and much ethical debate on this topic.

While 15% of all trauma victims experience a cardiac injury, not all patients require costly, heroic measures.[19] This is part of the current conflict under discussion in emergency departments (EDs) and ambulance stations and at professional organizational meetings across the country. Do we continue to use precious, limited resources (i.e., blood, organs) at great expense to save a small fraction of the population or do we draw an arbitrary, albeit well-researched line at prolonging life for hours or days just because we can? Can we justify the high cost and personal risk involved in medical evacuation missions when the outcomes are more often than not dismal? Many argue that the high mortality, significant health care worker (HCW) exposure, and low donor yields do not justify often extraordinary attempts to reverse the inevitable.

OUTCOME PREDICTORS

Successful resuscitation following prolonged cardiopulmonary resuscitation (CPR; greater than 30 minutes) whether the arrest occurs at the scene, en route to the facility, in the ED, or in the operating suite is doubtful. In one survey, no patient who arrested more than once survived.[22] Studies have looked at age, mechanism of injury, ambulance crew configuration (all three showing no difference), and cardiac rhythm [only correctable caused pulseless electrical activity (PEA) has a more favorable outcome]. Rapid correction of the underlying cause of arrest has the greatest impact on survival rates.[19,22]

Researchers participating in a 10-year, retrospective review of 12,518 missions in which 320 patients received air medical transport requiring CPR following blunt or penetrating trauma found dismal outcomes for these patients that are consistent with other reports.[23] Prolonged scene or transport times delayed definitive treatment and worsened neurological outcomes. They concurred that there is no "golden hour" for these patients. To make a critical difference intervention must occur within the first 10 minutes.[23]

PATHOPHYSIOLOGY

Cardiac arrest in the setting of trauma is one of the most challenging situations the EMS provider will encounter. It is one of the most difficult situations to process and accept on both a professional and personal level. Generally working under hazardous and stressful conditions, the EMS provider devotes a significant amount of time, energy, and skill attempting to resuscitate an individual with a prognosis experts agree is dismal at best.[19–24]

Cardiac arrest resulting from ischemic heart disease or ventricular fibrillation due to an irritable myocardium is treated in a straightforward manner using advanced cardiac life support (ACLS) protocols. However, these same protocols are inappropriate, and may even be harmful, in the setting of traumatic arrest until the underlying cause of the arrest is corrected.[21,23–25] That said, it is important to obtain a history to determine whether cardiac symptoms were present prior to the traumatic event. Because of the distinctly different treatment approaches between medical and traumatic arrest, always ascertain the underlying mechanism causing the arrest. The scene often offers clues to an underlying medical arrest in a trauma situation, such as a single-vehicle MVC into a tree without roadway skid marks present. A comparison of underlying factors contributing to medical and traumatic arrest is provided in Table 27-2.

MECHANISMS OF ARREST IN TRAUMA

When caring for victims of traumatic arrest, there is no golden hour. The paramedic's patient care in the first 10 minutes determines the outcome. Keep on-scene times short and have the patient at the trauma facility for definitive surgical intervention in under 60 minutes.[23,25] Remember that CPR is of little value in traumatic arrest until the underlying cause of the arrest is identified and treated.[24] Many of the underlying causes can be treated, often preventing the development of cardiopulmonary arrest. This is the goal.

Circulatory

Decreased cardiac output following penetrating or blunt trauma may be the result of exsanguination, tension pneumothorax, or pericardial tamponade. Other less common causes are rupture of the chambers of the heart and bronchial or esophageal disruption.

Table 27-2
Causes of Medical Cardiac Arrest Versus Traumatic Cardiac Arrest

Medical*	Traumatic
Ischemia	Exsanguination
Thrombus	Hypovolemia
Plaque	Hemorrhagic shock
Vasospasm	Pericardial tamponade
Myocardial failure	Cardiac contusion
Acute pulmonary edema	Tension pneumothorax
Arrhythmia	Aortic dissection
Congestive heart failure	Sheering injury to great vessels
Septic shock	

*Risk factors often associated with cardiac disease: obesity, male gender, smoking, diabetes, hypertension, emotional stress, elevated cholesterol.

Deceleration injuries are more likely to result in shearing of the great vessels, such as the aorta, and require immediate surgical treatment.

Exsanguination is a correctable cause of cardiac arrest. The resulting hypovolemia and hemorrhagic shock have left the "pump" empty. The first thought in cardiac arrest is to begin external cardiac massage; however, CPR is useless until volume is replaced. In fact, in chest trauma patients external cardiac massage is probably harmful.[24] These patients' hypovolemic state translates into ineffective cardiac compressions and possible injury to the heart, lungs, liver, and great vessels. In one study, 12% of chest trauma arrest victims treated by paramedics with forced ventilation and external cardiac compressions died of air embolisms in the coronary arteries.[24]

The cardiac monitor may display a rhythm, but further assessment often reveals PEA. Begin treatment with control of hemorrhage, establish and maintain a patent airway, and start volume replacement via two large-bore IV lines with warm crystalloid and colloid fluids. Large amounts, up to 3 liters, may need to be rapidly infused before a pulse is palpable.

The volume replacement of choice, however, is blood.[21] Ground EMS units rarely carry blood for emergency transfusion; therefore, rapid transportation of the victim to an ED is vital. Additionally, the administration of un-cross-matched blood carries serious risks and should never be administered without thoughtful and deliberate consideration by the emergency physician. Once arrived at the ED, emergency release of O-negative blood is generally obtained pending type and screen specific units (see Chapter 20).

Pericardial tamponade, discussed in Chapter 13, is a treatable cause of traumatic arrest readily identified by Beck's triad: hypotension, muffled heart sounds, and distended neck veins. Prior to cardiac arrest, pulsus paradoxus is often found in these patients. Tamponade is the most common result of penetrating trauma.[26,27] Treatment of this surgical emergency is pericardiocentesis performed by a specially trained provider or physician. Those services without this capability serve the best interest of the patient through rapid transportation to the closest ED.

Tension pneumothorax (see Chapter 13) occurs when the lung collapses and compresses the heart within the chest to the extent that it can no longer fill with blood to circulate to the vital organs, resulting in tissue hypoxia and ischemia leading to cardiac arrest. Symptoms include dyspnea, facial flushing, and distended neck veins. Tracheal deviation is a late sign. Decompression of the chest is accomplished by needle insertion into the second or third intercostal space at the midclavicular line. Release of this pressure usually restores circulation.

Left untreated, a large pneumothorax or hemothorax can lead to cardiac arrest via impaired ventilation and venous return or exsanguination. A chest tube is the definitive treatment.[24]

It is no longer standard practice to perform a resuscitative ED thoracotomy (surgical incision of the chest wall to control bleeding, cross-clamping the aorta, and performing internal cardiac massage) on all trauma arrest patients. This procedure is most likely to be helpful in patients who arrive at the ED within 5 minutes of arrest and who sustain penetrating trauma to the chest, neck, or extremities.[24] It is rarely useful in patients who suffer blunt trauma, penetrating abdominal trauma, or head injuries.[24] Neither is resuscitative thoracotomy of benefit to patients with penetrating trauma who arrest at the scene, unless the injuries are isolated penetrating chest or extremity wounds.[24,28]

Myocardial contusion occurs when the heart is compressed between the spine and the sternum, as frequently occurs in MVCs and falls when the patient hits a steering wheel or other immovable object. The most common injury following nonpenetrating trauma, myocardial contusion is often undetected among the plethora of traumatic injuries, yet is the most frequent cause of death.[29] Unlike ischemic chest pain, the chest pain from cardiac contusion is unrelieved by nitrates. A history assists the EMS provider in determining if the chest pain began before or after the injury. Patients suspected of having a myocardial contusion must be monitored by electrocardiogram (ECG). Serial ECGs are necessary to demonstrate cardiac injury, although changes are often very subtle, occurring 24–72 hours after injury. These ECG changes are due to decreases in cardiac output as a result of abnormal wall movement that impairs proper pumping action. Early recognition of ECG changes and intervention with medication can prevent the development of cardiac arrest. Necrosis following injury of the myocardium can produce ischemia and can lead to arrhythmias. Nonexsanguinating tachyarrhythmias should be treated with cardioversion as patients experiencing this readily correctable complication are salvageable.[19]

Blunt cardiac trauma has been found to be more common in children than previously thought.[30] A study conducted in Ontario, Canada, suggests that cardiac rupture is as common as aortic transection in the pediatric population. Because the heart and great vessels move freely in the mediastinum, they are more susceptible to sheering forces. Additionally, children's rib cages are more flexible, allowing compression of the heart by sternum and spine more easily than adults. Researchers suggest that as much as 90% of traumatic cardiac injuries in children are due to deceleration forces.[30] Cardiac injury is common, occurring in 15% of all trauma patients.[19] Index of suspicion must be high, cardiac monitoring initiated early, and correction of underlying injuries swiftly identified and treated.

Respiratory

Airway compromise leading to hypoxia is another readily treatable cause of cardiac arrest in the trauma patient. Obstructed airway and impaired gas exchange are corrected using the ACLS algorithm with special attention to maintaining cervical spine alignment. Rapid restoration of breathing and supplemental oxygen administration ensure improved tissue perfusion. Time is critical; brain injury after 4 or 5 minutes is often irreversible. Failure to ventilate is rapidly fatal in these patients. Intubation should not be delayed if basic interventions do not produce adequate ventilation. Surgical airway may be required if intubation fails or is not possible. Be aware that trauma patients are likely to vomit, especially children and those with a head injury. Cardiac arrest can be prevented in these patients with early recognition and intervention.

Neurological

Unfortunately, neurological impairment is frequently present in trauma patients. The literature is very clear on the prognosis for those individuals who fail to demonstrate intact neurological function at the scene. Researchers agree that patients conforming to specific criteria are not likely to benefit from extensive resuscitative efforts (see Table 27-3).[20–25] There is strong support for the assertion that sustained neurological function is the most critical predictor of survival.[20–22]

Table 27-3
Suggested Criteria Useful in Determining the Relative Benefit of Cardiopulmonary Resuscitation Following Trauma

Beneficial	Not Beneficial
No brain injury or head trauma	Penetrating cranial trauma with primary brain injury
Lack of vital signs but intact neurological function	Lack of neurological response
Glasgow Coma Scale score greater than 9	Prolonged (>30 minutes) cardiac arrest
Cardiac arrest due to treatable cause (exsanguination, tamponade, airway obstruction, tension pneumothorax)	Multiple episodes of cardiac arrest
Hypothermia	Obviously dead at the scene (decapitated)

Head injury and neurological trauma represent up to 80% of traumatic injuries in children.[31] High cervical fracture, a fracture at or above C-5, results in respiratory failure, which leads to cardiac arrest. Resuscitation in these cases entails intubation and support of both the respiratory and cardiac function in addition to treatment of concurrent injuries.

Table 27-4 provides a guideline for the paramedic facing a traumatic arrest situation. The reader is also encouraged to review the section on Maternal Cardiac Arrest in Chapter 25.

INTERNET ACTIVITIES

Visit the University of Texas Health Science Center at San Antonio's Trauma Home Page at http://rmstewart.uthscsa.edu/default.html. Click on the Patient Case Presentations link, then select the case entitled Stab Wound to the Left Chest with Prehospital Cardiac Arrest. Review the case. How does this case correlate with the material in Chapter 13 on penetrating cardiac trauma? Did the cardiac tamponade serve a protective role in this patient?

ETHICAL CONSIDERATIONS

It is difficult to abandon a patient in cardiopulmonary arrest particularly when time and effort have been invested. Often however, it is the most appropriate management.[23] Most trauma victims are healthy, young people in the prime of life. The societal climate is rife with debate over the need to perform heroic, life-prolonging measures on one of the most dismal of cases, traumatic arrest. Scientific research on traumatic arrest needs further investigation to help all members of the emergency team make decisions about when, and when not to, resuscitate.

To complicate matters, the hotly contested controversies over the allocation of precious resources rage onward in a milieu controlled and influenced by managed care organizations. Economic uncertainty, hospital downsizing, and lagging availability of technology in rural areas "muddy the waters." One of the most precious, yet finite, resources is blood. Thousands of units of type O blood are used in traumatic resuscitation each year. This severely curtails the availability of this blood type for patients having simpler, routine procedures. If decisions were based on the best chance for survival, then trauma cases, by and large, would go wanting.

Another hazard of trauma is the possibility of the worker contracting fatal diseases such as HIV or hepatitis B. Hundreds of needle-stick injuries happen every

Table 27-4
Guidelines for Paramedic Traumatic Resuscitation

1. Systematically identify the most lethal injuries. ABCs. Load and go. If the patient is in cardiac arrest at the scene, consider terminating care. If not done before your arrival, engage first responder to begin cutting off all clothing.

2. *Airway–C-spine:*

   a. Assess for airway patency: chin lift, maintain cervical spine alignment.

   b. Airway obstruction: manually clear the airway, suction, and maintain the airway via endotracheal intubation or surgical airway.

3. *Breathing:*

   a. Ventilate and administer 100% oxygen; monitor oxygen saturation.

   b. Examine chest and neck for chest movement, breath sounds, crepitus, open wounds, treacheal deviation, and fractured sternum and ribs.

   c. Tension pneumothorax: needle decompression.

   d. Sucking chest wound: occlusive dressing.

   e. Pneumothorax: chest tube.

   f. Hemothorax: chest tube with evaluation of blood loss.

   g. Incorrect tube placement: withdrawal from right mainstem bronchus or esophagus, reintubate, recheck breath sounds.

4. *Circulation:*

   a. Assess carotid pulse, heart tones, jugular venous filling, blood pressure, cardiac rhythm, pulsus paradoxus, and Beck's triad; apply pressure to sites of exsanguination; if pregnant, place roll under right hip; Pneumatic Antishock Garment (PASG) as indicated or per protocol.

   b. Hypovolemia: establish 2 large-bore IVs; rapidly infuse 2 liters crystalloid; in children give two 20-mL/kg boluses; use warm IV fluid if available; if arm sites not possible, per protocol perform saphenous vein cutdown, central line, or intraosseous line.

   c. Pericardial tamponade: pericardiocentesis (thoracotomy in ED).

   d. PEA EKG rhythm: treat hypovolemia and diligently search for correctable cause.

4. Notify the trauma center or ED:

   a. Mechanism of injury and traumatic arrest or near-arrest situation. If arrest: time elapsed from injury to arrest and arrest to present time and location of arrest—at the scene, en route.

   b. Sex and age of patient.

   c. Patient injuries: blunt trauma, penetrating injury, location of injuries.

   d. Airway patency and your actions to maintain the airway: intubation, surgical airway.

   e. Breathing and circulation: pulse, respiration, blood pressure, and heart tones now and if ever present; ventilation with 100% O_2, IV lines established and amount of fluid infused, EKG rhythm, O_2 saturation, breath sounds, PASG.

   f. Underlying causes of the arrest or near arrest and actions taken to remedy these causes.

   g. Estimated blood loss.

   h. Estimated time of arrival to hospital.

Note: Assessment and quick actions can prevent an impending arrest or rapidly restore breathing and circulation.

year with an increased number occurring during traumas and cardiac arrests.[20]

Does the percentage of organ donations received from trauma victims justify the cost to society, the health risks to medical personnel, and the use of finite resources? Studies differ slightly in percentages, but between 8% and 13% of trauma victims donate organs.[20,22] In one study of 138 trauma cases in which 70% (96) sustained blunt trauma and 30% (42) sustained penetrating trauma, only 8% (11 people) were organ donors (donating corneas only). The aggregate cost of care was $871,186.00.[20] This is a miniscule number of individuals donating organs when comparing the numbers of those waiting, sometimes futilely, for the liver or heart that never arrives (see Chapter 30).

SUMMARY

A multitude of complications can occur following the primary injuries in the trauma patient. The onset of these entities is more the rule than the exception. Therefore, treatment not only involves the initial resuscitation and care of specific injuries but also includes taking immediate steps toward the prevention, identification, and treatment of complicating factors as they occur. Keep in mind that the seriously injured trauma patient may have more than one of these complicating processes at the same time and that these factors act together in a cumulative fashion to make the patient's condition more severe than if only one of the processes existed alone.

Prevention is the most important point to be stressed. If the factors causing the complications of trauma discussed here can be stopped before they progress to a full-blown state, the patient's outcome will be dramatically improved. The paramedic can assist in the prevention of later complications by aggressively tending to the ABCs of trauma care. It is obviously not always possible to prevent all complications from occurring, but through recognition of the etiology and pathogenesis of the complications the healthcare provider is better prepared to diagnose them early and provide adequate treatment.

Traumatic cardiac arrest differs from medical cardiac arrest in that the paramedic treats the underlying causes rapidly and aggressively, rather than focusing on cardiac rhythms and drug interventions. Conditions the paramedic may recognize and treat successfully include hemorrhage, tension pneumothorax, pericardial tamponade, myocardial contusion, pneumothorax, hemothorax, and airway obstruction and compromise.

Many of the individuals suffering from trauma are young, adding to the emotional cost of an untimely death and raising concerns about our own mortality.

Research is needed to clarify and illuminate decision criteria on when to treat traumatic cardiac arrest and to justify such decisions in a sound scientific base.

REVIEW QUESTIONS

1. The initial treatment of pulmonary embolism is:
   a. Sublingual nitroglycerin (0.4 mg)
   b. Propanolol (beta blocker) 80 mg orally
   c. Heparin 10,000-unit bolus
   d. Activase (thrombolytic) 10 mg IV bolus

2. Risk factors for pulmonary embolism include all except:
   a. Immobilization
   b. Excessive physical activity
   c. Extremity trauma
   d. Elderly age

3. The most immediate complication of steam and hot vapor inhalation is:
   a. Adult respiratory distress syndrome
   b. Tension pneumothorax
   c. Obstruction due to upper airway edema
   d. Pulmonary embolism

4. All of the following are effects of carbon monoxide poisoning except:
   a. Shortness of breath
   b. Cyanosis
   c. Mental confusion
   d. Decreased respiratory rate

5. A passenger involved in a motor vehicle collision is found to have no breath sounds and hyperresonance in one lung field. The passenger is also in respiratory distress. The most likely diagnosis for these symptoms is:
   a. Adult respiratory distress syndrome
   b. Pulmonary embolism
   c. Tracheal obstruction
   d. Tension pneumothorax

6. Needle aspiration for the relief of a tension pneumothorax is normally performed through which intercostal space?
   a. Second ICS, midclavicular line
   b. Third ICS, midaxillary line
   c. Fourth ICS, midclavicular line
   d. First ICS, midaxillary line

7. Lungs with poor compliance, interstitial and alveolar edema, severe fibrosis, and emphysematous changes are consistent with which condition?
   a. Disseminated intravascular coagulation
   b. Adult respiratory distress syndrome
   c. Septic shock
   d. Neurogenic shock

8. Plasmin is an important enzyme in disseminated intravascular coagulation due to its ability to:
   a. Convert thrombin to antithrombin.
   b. Convert fibrin to fibrinogen.
   c. Convert fibrinogen to fibrin.
   d. Convert fibrin to split products.

9. Septic shock is differentiated from sepsis syndrome by the presence of:
   a. Tachycardia
   b. Elevated lactate levels
   c. Hypothermia
   d. Hypotension

10. The highest rate of infectious morbidity occurs with injury to the:
    a. Head
    b. Colon
    c. Extremities
    d. Lungs

11. Metabolic acidosis may occur when:
    a. Cellular metabolism is aerobic in nature
    b. Cellular metabolism is anaerobic in nature
    c. Excessive vomiting occurs
    d. The patient is hyperventilating

12. Trauma to the spinal cord produces neurogenic shock with which set of clinical symptoms?
    a. Warm, dry skin with a decreased pulse rate
    b. Warm, dry skin with an increased pulse rate
    c. Cool, sweaty skin with a decreased pulse rate
    d. Cool, sweaty skin with an increased pulse rate

13. All of the following are predictors of multiple-organ failure except:
    a. Increased blood pH
    b. Age greater than 55 years old
    c. Receiving more than 6 units of packed red blood cells
    d. Increased blood lactate levels

14. Chest pain in trauma patients that does not respond to administration of nitrates is likely due to:
    a. Cardiac ischemia
    b. Pericardial tamponade
    c. Cardiac contusion
    d. Sheering forces

15. All of the following are causes that can be treated to prevent the development of traumatic cardiac arrest except:
    a. Exsanguinating hemorrhage
    b. Pericardial tamponade
    c. Blocked airway
    d. Blunt abdominal trauma

16. The leading cause of death in persons age one to 39 is:
    a. Drowning
    b. Cardiac arrest
    c. Congenital birth defects
    d. Trauma

17. Beck's triad, used to identify cardiac tamponade, consists of:
    a. Hypertension, distended neck veins, and red face
    b. Hypotension, flat neck veins, and bounding pulse
    c. Hypotension, distended neck veins, and muffled heart sounds
    d. Muffled heart sounds, pulsus paradoxus, and distended neck veins

18. The patient finding most likely to indicate a poor prognosis for recovery is:
    a. No respiration
    b. No pulse
    c. No spontaneous neurological function
    d. Multiple fractures

19. The most common nonpenetrating traumatic injury that causes cardiac arrest is:
    a. Cardiac contusion
    b. Tension pneumothorax
    c. Acute pulmonary embolus
    d. Hypothermia

▶ CRITICAL THINKING

● You are preparing to transport a patient from your local hospital to a tertiary care center. The patient is a 22-year-old male who sustained multisystem trauma two weeks ago in an MVC. He later developed DIC and ARDS. He weighs 190 pounds. He is medicated with Diprovan and is being ventilated with the following settings:

Mode: control

Rate: 18

Tidal volume: 90

PEEP: 0

F_1O_2: 0.5

En route, his SpO_2 declines and his heart rate increases. Breath sounds reveal scattered rales bilaterally and equal breath sounds. You obtain an arterial sample and run an arterial blood gas (ABG). The values from this ABG are:

PaO_2:   68

PCO_2:   37

pH: 7.2

Explain the pathophysiology of ARDS and DIC. What changes should be made to ventilator settings?

● You are dispatched to a private residence regarding a patient with respiratory distress. You arrive to find a 32-year-old male who states he experienced an acute onset of dyspnea approximately 2 hours ago. He is conscious and alert but restless. His skin is pale with circumoral cyanosis. Bilateral breath sounds are clear and equal. Blood pressure is 110/60, heart rate 140, and respirations 46. Upon further questioning, you discover that this patient suffered a tibia/fibula fracture 2 days earlier and was sent home with a long-leg cast. His ABGs at the scene are pH 7.20, PCO_2 68, PO_2 62, and HCO_3 26. What is your impression of this patient? Explain the underlying pathophysiology. What treatments will you administer? What other complications is this patient at risk for?

● Upon arrival at the scene of an MVC, you find a 23-year-old male who was ejected from a vehicle that struck a second vehicle head on. There is massive deformation to the front of both vehicles. The patient is lying supine on the roadway with first responders performing CPR. A quick assessment of the carotid pulse confirms the patient is pulseless. There are no signs of external trauma other than abrasions to the back, where the patient landed on the roadway. Once intubated, the breath sounds are confirmed revealing clear and equal air exchange. The abdomen is soft and the rib cage is intact. The cardiac monitor reveals a wide complex PEA at a rate of 40. What injuries may be the cause of the cardiac arrest? How will you manage this patient? What is the likelihood of survival for this patient? Which pathologies leading to cardiac arrest have the best chances for treatment and a positive outcome?

REFERENCES

1. Mattox KL, ed. *Complications of Trauma.* New York: Churchill Livingston Inc; 1994.
2. Isselbacher KJ, Harrison TR. *Harrison's Principles of Internal Medicine*, 13th ed. New York: McGraw-Hill, Inc; 1995.
3. Kakkar VV, Adams PC. Preventive and therapeutic approach to venous thromboembolic disease and pulmonary embolism—can death from pulmonary embolism be prevented? *J Am Cardiol.* 1986; 8(6 Suppl B):146B.
4. Zapol WM, Lemaire F, eds. *ARDS.* New York: Marcel Dekker; 1991.
5. Barie PS. Organ specific support in multiple organ failure: pulmonary support. *World J Surg.* 1995; 19(4):581.
6. Schragl E, Donner A, Kashanipour A, Ullrich R, Aloy A. Superimposed high-frequency jet ventilation in the administration of NO: technical basis and early clinical results with ARDS. *Anaesthetist.* 1995; 44(12):843.
7. Temmesfeld-Wollbruck B, Walmrath D, Grimminger F, Seeger W. Prevention and therapy of adult respiratory distress syndrome. *Lung.* 1995; 173(3):139.
8. Sakon M, Kabayashi J. Treatment of multi organ failure. *Nippon Rinsho.* 1993; 51(1):107.
9. Carmona R, Catalona R, Trunkey DO. Septic shock. In: Shires GT, ed. *Shock and Related Problems.* New York: Churchill Livingston, 1984.
10. Stillwell M, Caplan ES. The septic multiple-trauma patient. *Crit Care Clin.* 1988; 4:345.
11. Moore FA, Moore EE. Postinjury shock and early bacteremia: a lethal combination. *Arch Surg.* 1992; 127(8):893.
12. Reeves JH, Butt WW. Blood filtration in children with severe sepsis: safe adjunct therapy. *Intens Care Med.* 1995; 21(6):500.
13. Sauai A, Moore FA, Moore EE, Haenel JB, Read RA, Lezotte DC. Early predictors of postinjury multiple organ failure. *Arch Surg.* 1994; 129(1):39.
14. Toninelli A, Agapiti C, Terenghi P, Latronico N, Candiani A. Gastric intramucosal pH in trauma patients: an index for organ failure risk? *Minerva Anestesiologica.* 1995; 61(1–2):9.
15. Stegmayr BG, Jacobson S, Rydvall A, Bjorsell-Ostling E. Plasma exchange in patients with acute renal failure in the course of multiorgan failure. *Int J Artif Organs.* 1995; 18(1):45.
16. Fehlings MG, Louw D. Initial stabilization and medical management of acute spinal cord injury. *Am Fam Phys.* 1996; 54(1):155.
17. Data Pharmaceutica Inc. *Physicians' genRx.* Smithtown, NY: Data Pharmaceutica Inc; 1996.
18. American Medical Association. Division of Drugs and Toxicology. *Drug Evaluations Annual.* Milwaukee, WI: American Medical Association; 1995.
19. Cotter G, Moshkovitz Y, Barash P, Baum A, Faibel H, Segal E. Ventricular fibrillation in the patient with blunt trauma: not always exsanguination. *J Trauma.* 1996; 41(2):345.
20. Rosemurgy AS, Norris PA, Olson SM, Hurst JM, Albrink MH. Prehospital traumatic cardiac arrest: the cost of futility. *J Trauma.* 1993; 35(3):468.
21. Jones TK, Barnhart GR, Greenfield LJ. Cardiopulmonary arrest following penetrating trauma: guidelines for emergency hospital management of presumed exsanguination. *J Trauma.* 1987; 27(1):24.

22. Fulton RL, Voigt WJ, Hilakos AS. Confusion surrounding the treatment of traumatic cardiac arrest. *J Am Coll Surg*. 1995; 181(3):209.

23. Falcone RE, Herron H, Johnson R, Childress S, Lacy P, Scheiderer G. Air medical transport for the trauma patient requiring cardiopulmonary resuscitation: a 10 year experience. *Air Med J*. 1995; 14(4):197.

24. Wilson RF, Steiger Z. Thoracic trauma. In: JE Tintanalli, RL Krone, E Ruiz, eds. *Emergency Medicine: A Comprehensive Study Guide*. New York: McGraw-Hill Book Co; 1988.

25. American Heart Association. Special resuscitation situations. *JAMA*. 1992; 267:2242.

26. Brader AH. Chest trauma. In: TC Kravis, CG Warner, LM Jacobs, eds. *Emergency Medicine*. New York: Raven Press; 1993.

27. Hammond SG. Chest injuries in the trauma patient. In: BM Beavers, DM Cooper, eds. *The Nursing Clinics of North America*. Philadelphia: WB Saunders Co; 1990.

28. Jorden RC. Multiple trauma. In: P Rosen, et al, eds. *Emergency Medicine: Concepts and Clinical Practice*, 3rd ed. St Louis: Mosby Year-Book; 1992.

29. Alexander JB, Delrossi AJ, Cilley JH. Vascular emergencies. In: TC Kravis, CG Warner, LM Jacobs, eds. *Emergency Medicine*. New York: Raven Press; 1993.

30. Scorpio RJ, Wesson DE, Smith CR, Hu X, Spence LJ. Blunt cardiac injuries in children: a postmortem study. *J Trauma*. 1996; 41(2):306.

31. Keen TP. Nursing care of the pediatric multi trauma patient. In: BM Beavers, DM Cooper, eds. *The Nursing Clinics of North America*. Philadelphia: WB Saunders Co; 1990.

Chapter 28

Medical Management During Extrication and Rescue

OBJECTIVES

Upon completion of this chapter, the reader should be able to:

● List desirable qualities of rescue personnel.

● Describe operational constraints of the rescue environment.

● Describe the requirements of a litter used for patient evacuation.

● List several considerations for the selection of a transport device.

● Discuss the advantages and disadvantages of various litters available for patient evacuation.

● Describe methods and considerations of proper patient packaging for a specific litter and environment.

● Explain methods of airway control and oxygen administration in the uncontrolled environment.

● Describe the signs, symptoms, and emergency management of hypothermia in the uncontrolled environment.

● Delineate the signs, symptoms, and emergency management of heat stress in the uncontrolled environment.

● Describe the assessment of pain in the uncontrolled environment.

● Describe techniques of pain control in the uncontrolled environment.

● Describe specific techniques of care for the rescue patient.

● Explain the adaptation of common medical items to alternative uses in the uncontrolled environment.

Rescue is defined as the removal from danger or peril. Victims may or may not require medical care, yet special rescue techniques and equipment must be employed to effect the safe return of those in jeopardy. This is the interface of medical care and technical rescue.

The qualities of a good rescuer are difficult to define. A good paramedic may not necessarily have or need good rescue skills. But a good rescuer must possess adequate patient care skills, for he or she may be the only help the patient has for an extended period. Rescuers must serve as patient advocates and be able to safeguard themselves in uncontrolled conditions,

since any mishap during the course of a rescue can have insurmountable consequences.

THE RESCUE ENVIRONMENT

The environment of field care in EMS is uncontrolled and sometimes hostile and uncooperative. A seemingly trivial occurrence can result in tragedy. Inexperience, lack of training and proper equipment, faulty equipment, and failure to recognize and act upon a serious life threat can quickly lead to disaster. Once an injury has occurred, a time fuse is triggered that immediately initiates a physical and mental deterioration of the victim. With the "golden hour" perilously at risk, speed and efficiency are essential in rescue efforts. With the multitude of mechanisms to injure patients, this environment brings with it medical, ethical, and legal challenges that rescuers must resolve in a matter of seconds.

Most protocols are written for the usual time frames and constraints placed on EMS. Extended care has been defined as greater than 1 hour, certainly easily exceeded in some rural areas even when the patient is accessible![1] In extended rescue situations paramedics may find it physically and ethically impossible to adhere to accepted protocols. Do paramedics perform cardiopulmonary resuscitation (CPR) on a hunter suffering a gunshot 2 miles from the ambulance? If this patient is viable on our arrival, what are our procedures, and to what extent should resuscitative efforts be pursued? What about impaled objects that may further delay transport or result in infection if left in place for extended periods? What are our options if paramedics are unable to directly contact medical control? If your agency operates under these conditions, then a set of protocols addressing these issues are needed to guide decision making in the field.

Unfortunately, the very act of treating an injured patient sometimes negatively impacts patient comfort. Paramedics remove an injured patient from a wrecked vehicle, place him or her on an unyielding spine board, apply a collar around the neck, place head blocks on each side of the head, and position straps across the body. Now, add a few therapeutic modalities involving needles, and the treatment may be perceived as being worse than the injury! Emergency medical devices are normally designed for brief intervals of use and tolerance. When these devices must stay in place for extended periods of time, alterations to standard techniques may be necessary to avoid patient injury and discomfort. Proper packaging is vital to the efficient care of the rescue patient. Given a basic means, virtually anyone could physically carry someone from one point to another, but it is proper patient packaging that makes patient treatment possible, more efficient, and comfortable.

PATIENT TRANSPORT

The perfect stretcher does not exist. Just as in any other therapeutic modality, advantages and disadvantages of available devices must be weighed, and the appropriate equipment selected for the task at hand. Situational constraints may force the use of a less than ideal device, for it may be the only equipment that will adapt to the confines of a particular environment. In other cases, isolation may limit equipment selection. Unfortunately, most of the time paramedics must make the patient match the stretcher as opposed to the stretcher matching the patient.

LITTER REQUIREMENTS

A patient litter should fulfill three requirements. First, it must protect the patient from further injury. This may very well dictate the type of device paramedics use and may alter the manner in which the patient is packaged. This theory emphasizes the "do-no-harm" basis of good medical care. Second, it must provide for a degree of patient comfort. Realize that the patient is already injured and possibly quite uncomfortable. Additionally, the patient may be placed in a device that was not designed for comfort and must stay in the device for an extended period of time while being hand carried from the wilderness and exposed to the elements. Often, proper packaging techniques permit greater patient comfort and ease of treatment. Third, the device should complement the evacuation effort. If the patient is to be hand carried, then the device should have adequate handholds. If the patient is to be air evacuated, a low-profile stretcher that fits into the confines of the helicopter must be chosen. Once again, select equipment suited to the task at hand.

CONSIDERATIONS FOR TRANSPORT DEVICES

Several considerations should come to mind as a patient transport device is chosen. Over what type of terrain must the patient be moved? Does it involve a hand carry or must it float in the water? The nature of the patient's injuries may alter our choice; maybe the patient must be supine due to leg fractures or modified Trendelenburg position for the treatment of shock. What is the evacuation time? Longer evacuations force us to consider the personal needs of the patient. Paramedics must provide for nutrition as well as elimination. Preplanning is necessary if secondary transport is to be utilized. Further injury may result if the patient must be moved to a different stretcher in order to fit into the helicopter or ambulance. The environment may dictate stretcher selection. The open wire mesh of the Stokes basket is notorious for getting hung on roots and rocks, but it may be ideal in a hot environment to allow circulation of air around the patient. Regardless of what is best for the situation, you may be forced to use what is available, so knowledge of several different devices is essential.

TYPES OF LITTERS

Spine boards are the mainstay in patient movement devices. Normally intended to limit spinal movement, the long spine board is often used to move a patient from one point to another. Spine boards are intended to restrict movement of the entire body, keeping the spine in alignment. They may serve to limit the movement of other injuries, such as leg and pelvic injuries. However, they are generally difficult to maneuver and are certainly uncomfortable, even for short periods of time.

There are a variety of techniques and devices for securing patients to spine boards. Although there appears to be no "standard" strapping technique, a recent study explored several techniques.[2] Figure 28-1 illustrates the method that produced the largest reduction in motion.

There are several styles of commercial short spine board devices. Most are made of an outer fabric material with a series of internal wooden slats. The flexibility of the fabric between the slats allows the device to conform to the patient's upper torso, and the handhold straps effectively put "handles" on the patient. Some models have rated attachment points specifically designed for lifting with a high angle rope system, making them ideal for confined-space or limited-access rescue. These units can also be inverted, with the torso area secured around the pelvis and the neck area extending toward the leg, for use as a pelvic/leg splint.

The scoop stretcher is an aluminum device that separates into left and right halves. It is adjustable to different patient heights, making it more manageable in tight quarters. There are, however, some limitations of this device. The metal adopts the temperature of the surrounding environment, a problem in cold climates. Although there are models that have a solid metal head plate, many models have a Velcro attached head pad that does not give the patient's head a firm base on which to rest. In addition to the flexibility of the fabric, the Velcro is unpredictable in holding power, especially after field use. This may cause an unexpected failure, hyperextending the patient's head. Also, the device does not support the spine where the two halves meet in the middle. For these reasons, the scoop stretcher is not recommended for spinal immobilization. It is best suited for use in intermediate patient movement, such as "scooping" the patient from the roof of an overturned vehicle, then

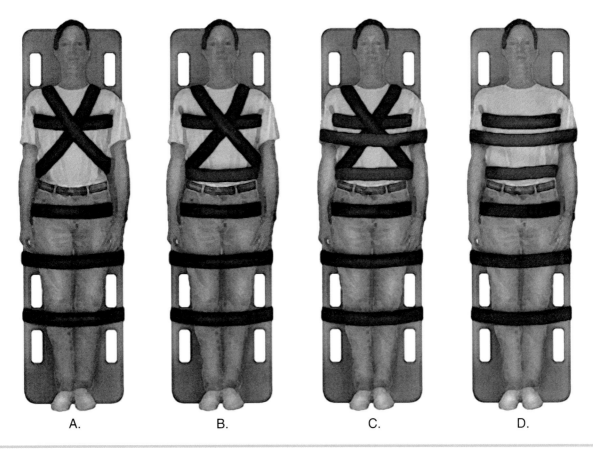

A. B. C. D.

FIGURE 28-1 A comparison of four strapping techniques. Technique C provided the largest reduction in motion. *Source:* Manix T. The tying game: how effective are body-to-board strapping techniques? *J Emerg Med Services.* 1995; 20:45.

depositing the patient onto a long spine board. When using this unit, make absolutely certain that the latches are properly secured prior to moving a patient.

Although not well designed for any particular type of rescue, the basket stretcher has become a staple in the rescue field. Since the rescue field is saturated with these devices, anyone directly involved in rescue would be well advised to become competent in its use. The basket stretcher was originally designed by Charles Stokes in 1895.[3] Currently there are several different styles and designs. Most are tapered near the bottom, taking on a coffin-style shape. Conventional rectangular spine boards do not fit inside, so these stretchers need a spine board specifically designed to conform to the basket. This allows easy movement of the immobilized patient into the basket. Most metal baskets have an open wire mesh design that is prone to catching on objects. The sharp wire ends can also prove annoying to rescuers, who receive small cuts as they work with the basket. This open mesh design makes proper patient packaging vital, as there is minimal physical and thermal protection. Figure 28-2 illustrates the proper blanketing technique.

Several styles of rescue baskets warrant caution. One authority recommends caution in using a metal Stokes design manufactured for the military by Medisco-Federal.[3] These are prone to breakage and are not acceptable for patient transport, especially high-angle evolutions. Some end users have modified these devices by strengthening their weak points.

The second basket style has a plastic tub and aluminum rail. It is tapered into the shape of a coffin and has the aluminum rail secured to the ABS basket by side-set rivets. The ABS plastic is brittle and prone to breakage, and the side-set rivets may come into contact with abrasive surfaces as the basket is moved. This wear eventually files the rivet head off, effectively detaching that section of the handle from the basket.

The newer plastic baskets are constructed of high-density polyethylene, and the aluminum rail is secured with top-set rivets that are less prone to abrasion. These style baskets incorporate a larger diameter hand rail as opposed to the all-metal baskets. This requires a wide gate carabiner that will fit over the rails to allow attachment of ropes and harnesses.

PACKAGING THE PATIENT

There are several items necessary to properly package a patient. First, any patient care items should be prepared. This may involve changing the configuration of the item,

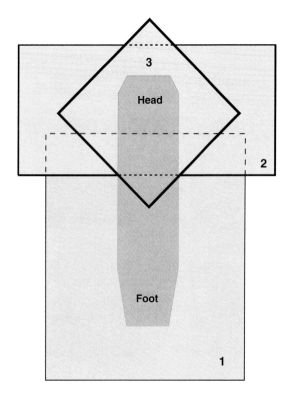

A.

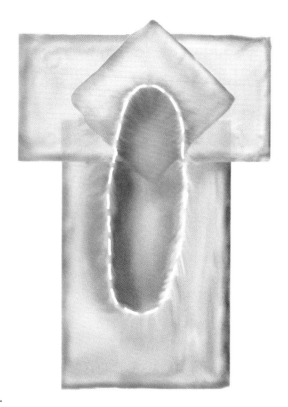

B.

FIGURE 28-2 Proper blanketing technique. Blanket #3 is folded around the patient's head, followed by blanket #2. Upon folding blanket #1, a complete hypothermia wrap is created.

such as using a bag-valve mask for inflating the pneumatic antishock garment and leaving the pump and gauges behind. Also, preapplying certain medical devices to the patient, such as those required for monitoring vital signs, proves to be very helpful. Think ahead for items you may need in the future, including a longer than anticipated evacuation time. The fall of darkness can change the operational environment entirely. Some type of vapor barrier is needed, both to prevent moisture entry as well as a barrier to wind. A sleeping bag works well as an insulator, or if the climate is more temperate, a thin blanket will suffice.

Protection of the patient's skin is often neglected. Carefully consider the environment and choose appropriate protection. An exposed patient is as likely to be sunburned as a rescuer. Simple packaging with a sheet to cover the patient blocks the sun, and sun block may be warranted for exposed areas around the face and lip balm will help to protect the lips.

Eye protection provides protection from the sun and dirt. Eye protection from debris can be supplied by a pair of goggles. A vented pair, with antifog solution, will protect patients' eyes and allow them to see their surroundings. Likewise, patients carried in a stretcher have their eyes exposed to the sun. The glacier-style sunglasses with side covers work well in this situation.

Head protection must be provided. If the patient's cervical spine is immobilized secondary to potential injury, then head protection must be designed into the package. Helmets that would provide any protection at all have a suspension system in place. This requires the head to remain in a neutral position with the helmet in place and may require firm padding behind the occiput. Some rescuers advocate the removal of the suspension system to avoid this situation. In order to provide protection, helmets must have a suspension system, so any modification must be carefully considered. Helmets can also be fitted with face shields to protect the face, and there are commercially available plastic shields that attach to basket stretchers to provide protection.

Arrangements for urinary elimination allow longer, uninterrupted transport times and afford the patient a greater degree of comfort. Since there are several risks associated with catheters inserted through the urethra, an excellent option for male patients in an uncontrolled environment is the condom catheter. The condom catheter is suitable for patients who still have complete and spontaneous bladder emptying. The soft, pliable sheath slips over the penis, with the end forming into a tube that empties into a collection bag. Specially designed elastic tape secures the condom in place. This tape is designed to expand with changes in penis size, so use of other tapes should be avoided. The collection bag can be attached to the stretcher but is more secure if attached to the patient's leg. Special attention should be given to properly securing the tip of the condom tube just beyond the distal end of the penis. Twisting motions of the tubing can cause skin irritation and may obstruct urine flow. Condom catheters should be changed daily, with the penis and urethral meatus cleansed at the same time.

Alternatives for women are limited. The indwelling catheter is the most effective but requires training for insertion. Other options are disposable undergarments or absorbent pads. These leave the skin surface wet and may result in skin irritation, infections, or unpleasant odors.

An appropriate lashing line is needed to secure the patient safely and comfortably in the stretcher. It may be of rope or web construction and must be of lifeline quality. Environmental needs should also be considered, such as flashlights, radios, hot packs, food, and water.

While considering the proper packaging and protection of the patient, understand that there may be technical reasons for using a particular evacuation technique. Consider a horizontal versus a vertical lift. The patient's body area exposed to falling rocks in a horizontal lower is approximately 70 by 20 inches, equaling 1,400 square inches. In a vertical lower, about 5 inches of the patient's head protrudes above the basket handle and the shoulders usually protrude 2 or 3 inches, equaling less than 10 square inches of patient exposure to falling debris.

SPECIFIC CONCERNS OF THE RESCUE PATIENT

This section highlights several environmental concerns specific to the rescue patient and how patient care is rendered.

AIRWAY CONTROL

The very act of caring for a patient's medical needs in an uncontrolled environment presents the need to improvise and adapt. Of paramount importance, the patient's airway must be maintained and controlled. Airway control techniques may need to be modified to accommodate patients who are in awkward positions (see Chapter 18).

Intubation of the seated patient is possible through several approaches. The most conventional would be the approach from the patient's back, employing techniques common to the patient lying supine. While another rescuer may have to stabilize the head, landmarks remain oriented as we are used to seeing them. The same technique can be used by standing at the patient's side. Generally, being positioned toward the patient's right makes intubation easier, as the laryngoscope is held in the left hand. Suctioning of foreign material must be emphasized, due to the fact that gravity now works to move debris freely into the trachea.

If the patient's back is inaccessible, perhaps a frontal approach would be in order. Depending on the available surface, a standing or lying approach can be used. This technique calls for a reversal in the hands from conventional intubation techniques. Holding the laryngoscope in the right hand allows the tongue to be swept to the left of the patient's mouth and, depending on the blade used, leaves the open area of the blade to the right. This allows for visualization and passage of the tube with the right hand.

There are several commercially available adjunctive devices that may aid in airway control. One is transillumination of the trachea through the use of a lighted stylet. This technique uses a light source at the end of a conventionally designed stylet, permitting the endotracheal tube to be maneuvered according to the appearance of the light through the soft tissues of the neck. Transillumination works well in trauma patients, as very little manipulation of the neck is needed and it can be performed in close quarters while positioned at awkward angles around the patient.

Sometimes it is preferable to alter the position and configuration of an endotracheal tube after actually visualizing the airway structures. This can easily be accomplished by the use of a directional stylet, which allows the operator to change the curvature of the distal end of the tube by varying pressure on the stylet. Endotracheal tubes are available that have a small wire embedded in the wall of the tube permitting such manipulation of the tube.

Retrograde intubation is useful in cases where trauma or anatomical difficulties prevent airway control by conventional means. Access to the airway is made using the Seldinger technique and a 110-cm wire as a guide for the endotracheal tube (see Chapter 18).

Suction Units

Hand-powered suction units are now available that provide excellent suction capability, are lightweight, and are completely portable. They also have disposable reservoirs to satisfy infection control concerns yet can be carried in an emergency field pack. These units are small enough for an attendant to keep conveniently nearby on a basket stretcher during lowers.

In high-angle evacuations performed with an attendant, a "barf line" is commonly attached. This line is attached to the side of the stretcher and is rigged so that the attendant can apply body weight and tilt the stretcher. This tilting aids clearing of the airway if the patient vomits.

OXYGEN ADMINISTRATION

As in all aspects of patient care, airway is of paramount importance. Protection of the cervical spine complicates this task, and the rescue situation introduces positional or environmental constraints.

Portable oxygen cylinders are most commonly utilized for oxygen administration in the field. D and E cylinder sizes are used most often and aluminum cylinders are more lightweight than traditional steel tanks. Also, C tanks are available that are slightly smaller than the common D size. Yet another variation is the Jumbo D, a larger capacity D tank. The oxygen from tanks can be very uncomfortable to the patient due to drying of the mucosa. Several gauze dressings can be dampened with water and placed inside the mask for humidification. However, use caution in covering the patient's airway from your view, especially in the unconscious patient.

Many nonrebreathing oxygen masks are supplied with only one valve. This allows the patient to partially breathe outside air, diluting the oxygen concentration. To maximize the oxygen concentration, the open valve can be covered with a piece of tape. However, it is important that the oxygen supply be carefully monitored. The oxygen supply tube will be the only passage for air supply, and the patient could be asphyxiated if a crimp in the tubing goes unnoticed.

Due to time and weight constraints, several rendezvous points may need to be established along the evacuation route for integration of fresh personnel and replenishment of supplies.

HYPOTHERMIA

Systemic hypothermia is the term used to describe a generalized cooling of the body. Although paramedics tend to associate hypothermia with cold temperatures, the condition can develop when temperatures are well above freezing. Persons who have had little nourishment and are injured or fatigued are especially susceptible to hypothermia. Likewise, people who are exposed to a cold environment for extended periods of time are likely victims.

Signs and Symptoms

Hypothermia leads to physiological changes in all body systems. There is progressive deterioration with apathy, poor judgment, ataxia, dysarthria, drowsiness, and eventually coma. Shivering, the body's attempt to increase metabolism and thereby heat, may be suppressed temperatures below 90°F. In severe cases, peripheral pulses may be undetectable. Cardiac irregularities may develop secondary to hypoxemia and acidosis.

Emergency Management

Monitor the patient's temperature with a hypothermic thermometer. Standard glass thermometers generally only read down to 96°F, whereas hypothermia units have an extended range of 75°F–105°F. Several models of electronic units are available. Rectal monitoring would be ideal but is not practical for field evacuations. Move the patient out of the wind. Remove wet clothing, replacing with dry if possible. Provide external heat by any means available. This may be from a fire, a portable stove, or even another person's body heat. Immersion in water at a temperature of 105°F–110°F is also effective. If possible, monitor the patient's cardiac rhythm. Myocardial irritability can be cold induced and may lead to ventricular fibrillation. Ventilatory support with heated humidified oxygen is an excellent means for rewarming.[4] Data indicate that dry air has little effect on the rewarming process, so the ability to humidify the air is vital.[5] This is possible with a commercially available device that operates from 12 volts DC or 115 volts AC. A rechargeable nicad battery pack is available, giving the unit about 1 hour operating duration. The unit is packaged in a backpack, weighing about 4 pounds. Heated IV fluids may also be administered in the field. One warming device holds two 1-liter bags of fluid, heating them to body temperature. The fluids can be administered directly from the heated bag, and insulated sleeves are available to reduce heat loss as fluid travels through the tubing. This device is powered by a 12-volt DC vehicle connection or 115 volts AC. Internal warming by oral hot liquids also provides warmth as well as a measure of nutrition.

HEAT STRESS

Heat stress is defined as the strain placed on the human body as it attempts to cope with excess internal heat. Generally, the emergency service occupation requires that protective gear be worn for a variety of situations. The human body generally rids itself of heat by radiation and convection to the cooler surroundings. Paramedics cover the body with an insulating layer, effectively blocking much of this mechanism. If the surrounding air temperature becomes the same or higher than body temperature, then body heat must be lost by vaporization. This is further complicated as the humidity of the air rises, since this effectively slows down vaporization.

Signs and Symptoms

The physical effects of heat stress can range from minor to fatal. All signs of heat stress warrant monitoring, regardless of their apparent severity. Each person varies in their ability to tolerate heat. Age, weight, physical condition, metabolism, and present state of health are all factors in heat tolerance. Some people can become acclimatized, but everyone is susceptible to heat's ill effects. Mentally, heat raises the potential for mishaps by decreasing concentration and diminishing motor skills. Weak and thready pulse, rapid and shallow breathing, general malaise, pale and clammy skin, profuse perspiration, dizziness, extreme thirst, nausea, vomiting, and unconsciousness are among the signs and symptoms.

Emergency Management

Self-monitoring should be the first line of defense, especially by emergency personnel. The institution of work practices to reduce heat stress include proper training, fluid replacement programs, rehabilitation, and on-scene health monitoring. Protective equipment should be specific for the environment, being the lightest and coolest while affording proper protection.

If signs and symptoms of heat stress are noted, immediately reduce the patient's physical activity. Move the patient to a cool area and remove as much clothing as possible. Apply wet compresses or towel-wrapped cold packs to high-heat-transfer areas of the body. These are the head, neck, armpits, and groin. Water gently applied in a stream works well. Have the patient drink plenty of water. If there is not a noticeable improvement in the patient's condition within 30 minutes, then transportation to a medical facility is warranted. The intake of water proves to be among the most effective means of combating heat exhaustion.

PAIN MANAGEMENT

Often, pain management is neglected in the prehospital setting. In the extended incident, failing to manage pain may negatively affect the patient's hemodynamic status. Reluctance to treat a patient's pain may be based on the fear of masking certain symptoms or the inability to handle any untoward effects of the medication.

Assessment

Several parameters are helpful in assessing a patient's pain. The characteristics of pain include location, duration, rhythmicity, and quality. Generally, there are two types of pain: chronic and acute. Chronic pain is defined as pain lasting 6 months or longer, and acute pain is of recent onset and associated with a specific injury or departure from normal health. Although both definitions are fairly arbitrary, it is important for the field clinician to know whether a specific pain complaint is associated with an acute problem or part of a chronic health problem.

The response to pain may include physiological as well as psychological manifestations. The patient's response to pain may be altered by the physical environment, certainly of particular concern in the uncontrolled environment. Various observations can be used to identify the patient's behavioral response to pain. Intensity relates to the degree of pain. It is useful to ask the patient to rate his or her pain using a scale of 0–10. Rating a change in the level of pain, such as from a 7 to a 3, provides the clinician with a trend and a means to evaluate interventions.

Tolerance is the maximum intensity of pain the patient is willing to endure. The patient's perception of pain is influenced by a range of factors. These factors may very well be situational and are handled best by proper psychological support. Being acutely traumatized and exposed to an uncontrolled environment in itself can cause great distress. The human body manufactures its own supply of morphinelike substances called endorphins and enkephalins. These substances have several implications for the rescue patient. Certain psychological stimuli promote the excretion of endorphins, such as mental imagery. This also explains why different people have different levels of pain tolerance; there are individual differences in endorphin levels.

Pain Control

Pain may be reduced to a tolerable level by simple emergency care procedures. The splinting of injured limbs, proper packaging and immobilization techniques, as well as appropriate transport all enhance patient comfort. Certainly psychological support should not be overlooked, as many pain responses occur at the subconscious level. Properly conducting these activities may allow you to forego pain medication or, if needed, to administer a smaller dosage.

If drug administration is warranted to control pain, any of the conventional routes may be used. Obviously, IV administration ensures the most rapid and controlled effect. Certainly the paramedic selects the most convenient and effective route available. However, the field environment may prove to be very challenging for the majority of administration techniques.

Nitrous oxide (Nitronox) mixtures are self-administered and very effective for musculoskeletal trauma. Mixed at a 50:50 ratio of oxygen and nitrous oxide, the drug is equivalent to 10–20 mg of morphine and has a very rapid onset. The greatest advantage is that the effects are short-lived once administration is stopped. Studies have shown that 80–90% of patients achieved relief of moderate to severe pain when using nitrous oxide. Due to self-administration, the concern of over-

medication is minimized and there are no direct effects on the respiratory system. Most importantly, there are no effects on the cough and gag reflexes. Because of the tendency of the gas to settle in dead air spaces, caution is urged in the setting of chest or abdominal trauma. Due to potential effects on personnel, the gas should be administered in a well-ventilated area.

The majority of EMS systems carry morphine sulfate; however, its primary use is in the setting of congestive heart failure. Whereas opiates can be used to control pain, caution is certainly urged in the setting of respiratory or hemodynamic compromise. Morphine is probably more suited to use in the isolated injury where secondary effects are not a concern.

Fentanyl is a synthetic opioid that has several advantages for prehospital use. The duration is 30–60 minutes, and it is 75–200 times more potent than morphine due to its solubility in lipids. It has minimal cardiac depressant effects, making hypotension rare. Of particular interest for extended control of pain, fentanyl is available in a transdermal (Duragesic) system. This consists of a skin patch that is applied to a nonirritated area on the upper torso. The dosage is varied by the size of the patch and is designed to be worn for 72 hours.

Nalbuphine (Nubain) and butorphanol (Stadol) have limited effects on the respiratory and circulatory systems, making these agents ideal for field use. Nalbuphine is comparable to morphine in strength, yet is not classified as a controlled substance. This relaxed degree of medical control required to administer nalbuphine makes it favorable for extended events where direct orders under medical control may not be possible. The usual IV dosage is 5–10 mg.

Butorphanol is available as a nasal spray, with 2 sprays being equivalent to 75 mg of demerol. Certainly this option is worth considering when faced with the difficulty of vascular access. The usual IV dosage is 0.5–4 mg every 3 hours.

Nonsteroidal anti-inflammatory agents can be used independently or to potentiate the effects of other opiate agents. Toradol (ketorolac tromethamine) is an example of one such agent, available in oral and parenteral forms. With Toradol, the patient does not experience the sedation that accompanies narcotic analgesia. Pain management studies have shown the overall effect of 30 mg of Toradol was equivalent to 6–12 mg of morphine. These drugs must be avoided in patients with blood-clotting abnormalities.

CARE OF THE RESCUE PATIENT

As mentioned earlier, the environment paramedics are forced to operate in is uncontrolled and therefore can be hostile at times. The environment may negate proper communications. Working around a waterfall or in a plant with running machinery may make hearing difficult, and poor lighting may make seeing hand signals impossible. Paramedics have to adapt to the environment. A system of hand or light signals may suffice, a portable public address unit may work, or the simple tug system on a lifeline may be adequate. A whistle may relay a message just fine. Most major radio manufacturers provide a system of attaching remote speaker-microphones or portable earphones to the radio set. If this is not adequate, there are aftermarket manufacturers that will engineer a headset system to work with your radio. There are even confined space and underwater supplied air line systems with a communications cable hardwired into the system for constant two-way communications. If communications in your operations is a link to safety or efficient patient care, devise a means to maintain communications in your particular environment.

Operating at the scene of a vehicle collision in inclement weather can prove very challenging, particularly if you are determined to provide some degree of patient comfort. A salvage cover hooked to the vehicle with straps serves as an excellent windbreak. The free end can be extended over one end of the vehicle and supported with pike poles and rope to provide a type of "lean-to" protection. Covering the patient to prevent heat loss can be accomplished with ordinary blankets, protective clothing, an aluminized survival blanket, or even a rain cover to prevent water and wind penetration.

Commercial-style ventilation fans are also available, some with warming units. These are available through most industrial suppliers. This is the type of fan typically used by utility contractors to provide ventilation in a confined space; with the heating option, it can provide a temperate climate inside a chilly confined area, such as an underground pipe (Figure 28-3). They are manufactured in gas and electric styles and come with a variety of accessories such as ducting to provide selective direction of the air flow.

A hair dryer serves as an excellent patient warmer. Although an electrical supply is needed, generally in the neighborhood of 1,000 to 1,500 watts, its purpose is well defined at vehicle accidents where patients are trapped. Consider the plight of the trapped patient with his or her shirt cut off, the roof of the vehicle removed, all in a 35°F rain. Why compound the patient's condition with hypothermia? Careful use of a hair dryer under the protective blanket goes a long way toward proper patient care, not to mention comfort. If used cautiously to prevent burns and fire hazards, floodlights can also provide warmth inside the vehicle. Special caution should be given to flammable hazards, and any AC electrical device used on an emergency scene should be operated with a ground-fault interrupter to protect personnel.

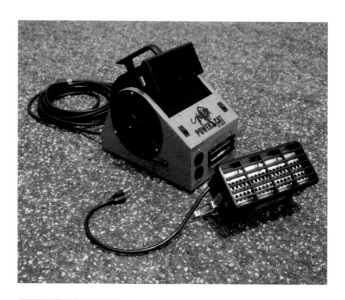

FIGURE 28-3 Ventilation fans can provide heat as well as ventilation.

A chemically activated style of pocket warmer is available, some even with the ability to be reused. Although they are not designed for mass rewarming, they are portable and economical and have the ability to warm the hands and feet. Several placed in the pockets and high-heat-transfer areas of the body help make patients comfortable.

If you must care for a patient placed on the ground, take measures to prevent the loss of body heat to the ground. A tarp, blanket, additional clothing, brush from nearby vegetation, or even rope flaked back and forth can provide some degree of insulation from the cold ground.

A golf-style umbrella serves well to keep rain off a working area as well as provides shade. A simple plastic sheet can be stored under the stretcher mattress to serve as an impenetrable barrier. It is quickly available, weighs very little, and is economical.

A body bag provides excellent protection for a patient exposed to the environment. As well as the insulating properties, the heavy vinyl provides a degree of protection. For further insulation, a sleeping bag placed in the body bag further insulates the patient. Commercial body pouches are also available. These are designed with patient care specifically in mind, with features such as full-length zippers, arm access, and provisions for urinary catheters. Coverage of a patient's head is vital to the prevention of hypothermia. At 40°F a patient's exposed head radiates up to 50% of the body's total heat production. At 5°F, the heat loss increases to 75%.[6]

A commercially designed aluminized blanket provides excellent protection from debris as well as a degree of protection from fire. Many agencies rely on fabric sheets and blankets for patient protection. Besides having very little fire resistance and thermal protection, glass and metal shards can find their way into their fibers. It is doubtful that these particles are easily washed out. Even using a dedicated blanket has drawbacks; what was the "glass" side during the last use may very well be the "patient" side next time. The smooth surface of the aluminized blanket can be washed without penetration of debris into the fibers and its heavy design will last for years.

Proper documentation during extended care is essential. A flow sheet should be established that provides for documentation of the patient's vital signs, interventions performed, and any changes in condition. This allows for sequential following, so that trends may be noted. This makes it much easier if patient attendants must be changed during the course of the rescue, and it gives the emergency facility a complete picture of the patient's treatment. Due to situational constraints of the particular rescue, continuous, direct medical control may not be possible. Medical control may have to be contacted periodically at control points established along or during the rescue, and patient flow sheets will prove valuable. The flow sheets also set the stage for obtaining qualifying advance orders from a physician in anticipation of patient conditions, enhancing overall patient care.

ADAPTATION OF ITEMS FOR MEDICAL CARE

An important part of providing care to patients in an uncontrolled environment is the ability not only to adapt one's attitude to the situation but also to adapt and use equipment in a variety of situations. Inventing multiple uses from one piece of equipment is an example. Many medical care items can be adapted and improvised to serve multiple duties. This allows the load to be lightened for manual transport packs and perhaps to render more efficient patient care by realizing the duplicate equipment capabilities.

Proper equipment preparation is vital to a successful operation. This serves several purposes. First, if paramedics have prepared their equipment, they are familiar with the equipment and any deficiencies that may exist. Second, preparing equipment before an incident saves valuable time when needed. Plan what actions could shorten the delivery time of this procedure to a patient. The packaging and storage methods paramedics use on the ambulance may not prove adequate for the rigors of use in the wilderness, a cave, or the passageways of a confined space. Paramedics must learn to streamline their equipment, making every item as useful as possible.

Compare this ideology to the fire service. The fire department has several variations of hose packages stored on the apparatus, each with a specific job in mind, but all *preconnected.* This means that the hose is connected and ready—just pull it off, pump the water, and go. For this reason, paramedics should design a system so that their equipment is at its point of use. You may do this systematic organizing now and not realize it. Most units tend to have cervical collars, head immobilizers, and spine boards stored together; likewise, the IV fluids, IV catheters, and IV sets are packaged together. Just take this a step further and anticipate what is needed for the type of rescue environment in which you will function.

The pneumatic antishock garment (PASG) is in a state of controversy. However, it can serve to splint the lower extremities, can hold direct pressure, and is relatively light and takes up little space. For small patients, the garment can be inverted and placed between the patient and the immobilization straps. Inflation of the leg sections fills the void space and firmly secures the patient. For the models with soft bags, there is usually additional room for some basic trauma supplies, an IV setup, and a bag of IV fluid. The same holds true for models stored in the rigid plastic boxes; the room in the lid can be used to great advantage, and the entire box can be used as an emergency cooler for amputated parts. Consider the convenience of grabbing the PASG and having basic supplies and an IV setup available. Otherwise, the garment can be removed and included as part of another pack. Unless it is absolutely necessary for the garment operation, consider leaving the inflation pump and gauges behind to lighten the load. Experimentation with various adapters allows you to utilize a bag-valve mask for inflation. An endotracheal tube adapter works well (Figure 28-4).

Many of the short spine-board-style devices have been on the market for several years. These devices modify the concept of the rigid board and are designed to mold around the patient's thorax while immobilizing

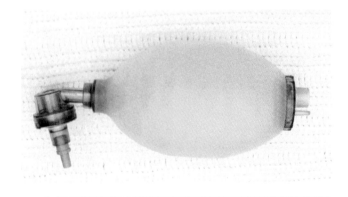

FIGURE 28-4 The PASG may be inflated with the bag-valve device with an attached endotracheal tube adapter.

the upper body as one unit. These devices provide a moderate profile when applied to a patient, and some are even designed with rated lift points for the attachment of lifting slings. Some of these devices can easily be used in an inverted fashion around the pelvis, effectively serving as a splint.

Ladder splints are very useful in rescue situations. They are economical and lightweight, can be formed into a variety of shapes to match the situation, and can be folded around the inside perimeter of soft-packs, providing a degree of structure for the pack, and easily removed when needed. You can carry this one step further by padding the splints with dressing and bandaging material. "Stockinette"-style fabric tubing can be used to cover the splint, and sterile bandage dressings can be stored inside. The bandage and dressing material could then be removed as needed, getting double duty out of one item as well as minimizing the storage area.

Intravenous bags serve as excellent head immobilizers, once again giving us multiple uses for a single item. A patient's shoes serve well in the same manner. Although contraindicated with a suspected spinal injury, it is also worthwhile to mention that placing an IV bag behind the adult patient's occiput often provides the correct "sniffing" position for intubation.

Intravenous therapy in the uncontrolled environment can pose several problems. First, explore whether the line is needed; heparin or saline locks can provide almost instantaneous access to venous circulation if periodic access is indicated. If the line is needed for a steady infusion, then a means to keep the IV bag elevated should be devised. A ladder splint folded over and taped to the litter structure will free hands. If the environment is not favorable to elevating the bag, the IV system can be purged of all air and placed under the patient's body weight or an infuser or blood pressure cuff can provide the necessary pressure. The purging of air from the system can be accomplished by "spiking" the bag, then inverting and forcing the residual air out, with the tubing and drip chamber fully filled with fluid. This allows the set to flow in any position as long as pressure is sufficient for flow. Of course, exact fluid flow rates cannot be determined, but if fluid infusion is needed, it does provide a means to do so without the risk of air embolism.

If the patient is properly packaged, access for monitoring of vital signs may prove difficult. Design a blood pressure cuff system where the cuff stays in place on the arm and the inflation bulb and gauge can be disconnected. One particular blood pressure cuff design has the gauge and inflation bulb combined into one unit. Design extensions to the tubing so it reaches out of the patient packaging system, and label or color code to avoid confusion. Tape a stethoscope head in place over the brachial artery, being mindful of excessive circum-

ferential pressure, and extend that tube out also. Several modified stethoscope heads allow you to place several on the chest, particular to the patient's condition, and with the use of a single earpiece, be able to monitor breath sounds and blood pressure (Figure 28-5).

If you can obtain a section of tubing from a ventilator circuit, it will fit between the bag unit and the nonrebreathing valve of the bag-valve mask (BVM). This allows you to provide ventilation assistance away from the immediate area of the patient. Of course, if a mask is used, someone must position and seal the unit; however, if the patient is intubated, this may free up valuable room around the patient. Some oxygen tubing used in the hospital on humidified oxygen mask units suffice for this purpose also. Experiment and be inventive; put together a system that works for you (Figure 28-6).

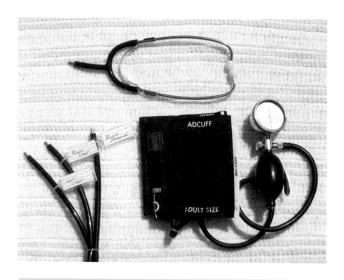

FIGURE 28-5 Example of a modified stethoscope for monitoring breath sounds and blood pressure.

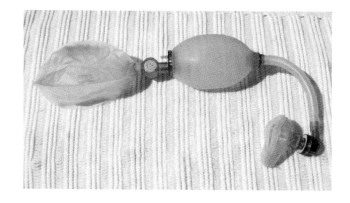

FIGURE 28-6 Ventilator tubing can be used to extend the interface between the bag-valve device and the endotracheal tube.

The ski patrol has modified the modern style of the Stokes basket by fitting the underside with extra long skis. This effectively supplies them with a large container to carry emergency equipment to the patient's side as well as providing an easy way to move an injured patient. As an additional suggestion, an exposure-type bag could be used to cover the whole package, allowing the equipment to arrive by the patient's side in dry condition.

INTERNET ACTIVITIES

- Visit the National Library of Medicine Web site at http://www.ncbi.nlm.nih.gov/PubMed. Conduct a literature search on wilderness search and rescue. Review the abstracts of the search results. Ask your librarian to assist you in obtaining the journals with the five most relevant articles. Review these articles and summarize their findings.
- Search the World Wide Web for sites related to wilderness search and rescue (SAR). Locate organizations dedicated to SAR and visit their home pages. Look for on-line educational material related to the medical management of patients during prolonged extrication and rescue.
- Visit the National Association for Search and Rescue (NASAR) Web site at www.nasar.org and read about current search and rescue missions by clicking on the News Archive site under General Information.

SUMMARY

Special rescue training, techniques, and equipment must be incorporated to safely rescue those in jeopardy. Patient care and technical rescue must mesh, minimizing the effects of a sometimes hostile and uncooperative environment. Once an accident occurs in an isolated area, the golden hour extends into overtime, initiating a physical and mental deterioration of the victim. Speed and efficiency are essential in rescue efforts, mitigating the medical, ethical, and legal pitfalls present.

REVIEW QUESTIONS

1. Discuss the various environmental factors that may hinder or alter the ability to care for a patient in the uncontrolled environment.

2. Discuss methods of adapting equipment and patient care techniques to the demands of the uncontrolled environment.

3. Discuss the requirements and considerations for the selection of a patient transport device.

4. Describe several methods of airway control in the rescue patient.

5. Discuss the methods of proper patient packaging compatible with the environment and patient care requirements.

6. What stretcher is best suited for intermediate movement of a patient who does not require spinal immobilization?
   a. Stokes basket
   b. Spine board
   c. Commercial short spine device
   d. Scoop

7. Which of the following is not a consideration for a horizontal versus a vertical patient lower?
   a. Ambient temperature
   b. Danger of falling debris
   c. Patient injuries
   d. Patient comfort

8. What part of the body has the greatest heat loss potential?
   a. Groin
   b. Head
   c. Armpits
   d. Abdomen

9. Which of the following drugs may be favorable when parenteral routes are not available?
   a. Nalbuphine
   b. Butorphanol
   c. Fentanyl
   d. Morphine sulfate

10. Which of the following is untrue regarding nitrous oxide?
    a. Suppression of the cough reflex may result in airway compromise.
    b. The gas tends to settle in dead air spaces.
    c. The oxygen-to-nitrous ratio is 50:50.
    d. The effects are short lived once administration is stopped.

CRITICAL THINKING

- You are part of a high-angle rescue team that has been summoned to a popular rock face for an injured climber. You are led to the scene where a 22-year-old male who was free climbing a rock face without a belay and slipped and fell approximately 30 feet onto a ledge. He is accessible only by rapelling roughly 150 feet from above. Upon reaching the patient, you find that he has suffered a major head injury and requires intubation and positive-pressure ventilation. Extrication from the rock face requires a horizontal lift using a Stokes basket. During this procedure, how will you continue ventilation? What other treatments will you provide? How will you manage this patient during the ascent to the top of the rock face?

- Upon arrival at the scene of a motor vehicle collision, you find a 37-year-old male pinned in the front seat of a large truck he was driving. The patient is accessible only from the nipple line up, the remainder of his body being pinned by the dashboard. The patient is unconscious and shows signs of a head injury. His respirations are agonal at a rate of 4 per minute. Bilateral breath sounds are clear and equal. The neck veins are flat and the trachea is palpable in the midline. Blood pressure is 220 by palpation, heart rate 43, and SpO_2 77%. Extrication is expected to take at least 30 minutes. How will you manage this patient while rescue personnel attempt to extricate him from the vehicle?

- As part of a confined-space rescue team, you are led to the scene of an injured spelunker. Your trip into the cave took approximately 4 hours. You anticipate extricating the patient will require 18–24 hours. The patient, a 29-year-old male, fell approximately 15 feet while doing a vertical descent into a large cavern. He landed on his left side, fracturing his femur and humerus. How will you manage this patient's injuries during the prolonged extrication?

REFERENCES

1. Vines T. Rescue medicine. *Rescue.* 1995; 8:6.
2. Manix T. The tying game: how effective are body-to-board strapping techniques? *J Emerg Med Services.* 1995; 20(6):44.
3. Hudson S, ed. *Manual of U.S. Cave Rescue Techniques,* 2nd ed. Huntsville, Ala.: National Speleological Society; 1988.
4. Ignatavicius DD, Workman ML, Mishler MA. *Medical-Surgical Nursing,* 2nd ed. Philadelphia: WB Saunders; 1995.
5. Grandy J. Hypothermia. *Emergency.* 1995; 27:1.
6. Rescue Training Associates. *Action Guide for Emergency Service Personnel.* Bowie, Md.: Brady Communications Co.; 1985.

BIBLIOGRAPHY

Byers E. Saved but not safe. *Emergency.* 1994; 26(3):40.

Dickinson E. Small spaces, big challenges: treating the entrapped victim. *J Emerg Med Services.* 1991; 16(11):56.

LaValla R, Stoffel S. Bring unique rescue problems. *Rescue Squad Q Mag.* 1988; 2(2):21.

Leduc T, Desphante J. Retrograde intubation for difficult airways. *J Emerg Med Services.* 1996; 21(9):57.

Leduc T, Paris P. Relieving the pain. *J Emerg Med Services.* 1996; 21(12):74.

Perry A, Potter P. *Clinical Nursing Skills and Techniques,* 3rd ed. Baltimore, Md.: Mosby Lifeline; 1994.

Pons P, Cason D. *Paramedic Field Care. American College of Emergency Physicians.* St. Louis, Mo.: Mosby Lifeline; 1997.

Valcourt G. Basket stretchers. *Rescue.* 1993; 6(5):36.

Vines T. Industrial rescue. *Emergency.* 1994; 26(10):64.

Wilkerson J, ed. *Medicine for Mountaineering,* 2nd ed. Seattle: The Mountaineers; 1975.

Chapter 29

Air Medical Transport of the Traumatized Patient

OBJECTIVES

Upon completion of this chapter, the reader should be able to:

- Discuss the development of air medical services in the United States.
- Discuss the advantages and disadvantages of air medical transport of the traumatized patient.
- Describe the preparation of the trauma patient for air medical transport.
- Describe the effects imposed on the body by changes in altitude.
- Describe the potential effects of altitude on various pieces of medical equipment.
- Describe the preparation and safety aspects associated with landing a helicopter at the scene of a traumatic incident.
- List the criteria for transporting patients by medical helicopter.

KEY TERMS

Barotitis media
Boyle's law
Dalton's law

Henry's law
Third spacing

As early as the Napoleonic Wars (1803–1814), the need for rapid transport of sick and injured soldiers from the front line to medical attention was recognized. Dominique Jean Larrey, considered the greatest military surgeon of his time, is credited with developing the first ambulance.[1] It was a two-wheeled vehicle in which the patient was wheeled to a safe area to receive medical attention. Because of its ability to move patients rapidly, Larrey called his invention the "flying ambulance."[1] Air medical transport followed years later during the Franco-Prussian War. The first air medical transport occurred on November 16, 1915, in a hydrogen-filled balloon. The balloon transported 160 sick and injured soldiers out of Paris.[2]

With the flight of the first airplane by the Wright brothers in 1903, a new era of air medical transport was on the horizon. During World War I the first military air ambulance was developed but saw little use.[3] The primary function of this plane was to transport sick and wounded soldiers over long distances. The mortality rate was so high that few patients benefited from this service. During World War II, the use of air ambulances continued to develop. However, there was no standardization or organization to the use of these services.

In the 1950s the Korean War spawned further development of air medical transport. During the Korean conflict, Sikorsky YH-5 helicopters were utilized to evacuate injured soldiers from the front line.[3]

In addition, in May 1954, the first C-131 airplane designed especially to evacuate wounded soldiers was assigned to routine air medical evacuation.[4]

In the mid-1960s, the Vietnam conflict produced a rapid expansion of air medical evacuation. For the first time, plans were developed for the air evacuation of sick and wounded soldiers. During the course of the conflict, more than 349,000 patients were evacuated.[3] It was also during this time that the C-131 was replaced by the larger C-141.[3] Development of air medical transport for civilians in the United States soon followed.

In 1969, R Adams Cowley persuaded the Maryland legislature to fund a statewide air medical transport program. Cowley argued that if patients could be rapidly transported from the scene of traumatic accidents to the Maryland Shock Trauma Center, mortality could be significantly reduced. The legislature agreed to fund a program serving both the air medical transport and law enforcement needs of the state. This became the first statewide coordinated air medical system. It is still a model system today.[4]

Other states were slower to adopt air medical transport. One option available for air medical transport began in 1970 and was called the Military Assistance to Safety and Traffic Program.[3] Under this program, military aircraft could be used to transport civilians in need of air medical transport. However, this service suffered from slow response due to a lack of coordination through local agencies. While this met some of the needs of interfacility transport, it failed to meet the needs of acutely injured patients who needed rapid transport from the scene.

Many hospitals recognized the need for local air medical transport systems and began to develop hospital-based helicopter programs. The first hospital-based air medical program was established at St. Anthony's Hospital in Denver, Colorado, in the early 1970s.[5] By 1996, hospital-based air medical transport programs had exploded to more than 200 across the nation.[6]

ADVANTAGES AND DISADVANTAGES OF AIR MEDICAL TRANSPORT

Air medical transport offers some distinct advantages over ground transport of trauma patients, the most obvious of which is speed. Air ambulances also have the ability to travel in a straight line between two points, decreasing the distance that must be traveled.

Another advantage of air medical services is the ability to bring advanced procedures to the scene of an injury. Examples of these advanced procedures include advanced airway procedures, such as rapid-sequence intubation utilizing neuromuscular blockades and surgical cricothyroidotomies (which are not performed in all out-of-hospital systems). Air medical programs also have the ability to establish central venous catheters and administer medications not normally carried on ground ambulances. Finally, one of the most beneficial aspects of air medical services is the ability to carry and administer blood products.

While all of these advantages make air medical transport sound like the perfect mode of transport, there are some drawbacks. There are four major disadvantages of air medical transport. First, air medical transport may not be possible due to adverse weather conditions such as rain, fog, or ice storms. Second, air medical resources are limited. Air services are not available to respond when they are on another transport. For this reason, alternate courses of action must be planned in the event that air medical transport is not available. Another disadvantage is that aircraft are very maintenance intensive; not only do these aircraft require daily inspection, they also require replacement of parts after a specified number of flight hours. Finally, air medical services are very expensive, costing five to ten times that of ground transport. In health care today, more emphasis is being placed on patient outcomes and cost. For this reason, it is increasingly important that air medical transport be utilized solely for patients needing this type of transport or for those transported over long distances.

GUIDELINES FOR AIR MEDICAL TRANSPORT

Access of air medical services differs throughout the United States. In some areas, helicopters are dispatched by local 911 communications centers while in others they are dispatched by hospital communications centers. Different types of communications centers require different types of predispatch information. All centers require the type of request, number of patients, and type of injuries. Table 29-1 outlines an example of the information required by an air medical service.

While the criteria for interhospital transport varies from area to area according to local resources, criteria for scene response are better defined. The National Association of EMS Physicians has developed criteria for scene response as outlined in Table 29-2.

PREPARING THE PATIENT FOR AIR MEDICAL TRANSPORT

Several aspects of care should be instituted while awaiting the arrival of an air ambulance and are summarized in Table 29-3. Transport of the trauma patient should not be delayed for anything other than establishing a

Table 29-1
Information Required by Air Medical Service

a. Name of requesting agency

b. Location of incident and landing site (nearby highways, intersection, major landmarks, and road numbers or names)

c. Name and radio contact frequency with continuous tone squelching system (CTSS) tone of the landing zone coordinator

d. Nature of the incident and if possible the number of patients and their extent of injury

e. Potential hazards at the scene and landing site

f. Special situations that may require special resources, such as mass casualty incidents

Source: Carolina Air Care. University of North Carolina. Chapel Hill, NC.: 1996.

Table 29-2
Criteria for Scene Response

Trauma score < 12

Glasgow Coma Scale < 10

Adults with the following vital signs:

    Systolic blood pressure < 90

    Respiratory rate < 10 or > 35

    Heart rate < 60 or > 120

    Unresponsive to verbal stimuli

Penetrating injury to chest, abdomen, pelvis, neck, or head

Spinal cord or vertebral column injury or trauma that produces paralysis of a limb or any localizing neurological signs

Amputation of any limb, whether partial or total (except finger and toes)

Fractures of two or more long bones

Crush injury to chest, abdomen, or head

Burns greater than 10% total body surface area (TBSA) or burns to face/hands/feet/perineum or burns with inhalation injury, or major electrical/chemical burns

Children less than 12 and adults over 55 years old

Mechanism of injury:

    Vehicle roll overs with unbelted passenger

    Vehicle striking pedestrian at > 10 mph

    Falls from greater than 15 feet

    Motorcycle victim ejected at > 20 mph

    Multiple patients

Difficult-access situations

    Wilderness rescue

    Ambulance egress or access impeded at the scene by road conditions, weather, or traffic

Time/distance factors

    Transportation time to the trauma center greater than 15 minutes by ground ambulance

    Transport time to local hospital by ground greater than transport time to trauma center by helicopter

    Patient extrication time > 20 minutes

    Utilization of local ground ambulance leaves local community without ground ambulance coverage

Source: National Association of EMS Physicians. *Air Medical Dispatch: Guidelines for Trauma Scene Response.* Lanexa, Kansas: 1992.

Table 29-3
Care While Awaiting Arrival of Aircraft

Airway management

Adequate circulation

  a. Two large-bore (14–16-gauge) peripheral IVs of lactated ringers or normal saline

  b. Placement of PASG (per local protocol)

Spinal immobilization

Cover wounds and control hemorrhage

Apply splints as necessary

Use restraints as indicated

Keep patient warm

Source: Carolina Air Care, University of North Carolina Hospital. Chapel Hill, NC.: 1996.

patent airway. Once the airway is maintained, attention can be focused on controlling hemorrhage, establishing two large-bore peripheral catheters, and spinal immobilization. In some situations, the special skills of the air medical team may be required to accomplish these tasks. Completing as many of these tasks as possible prior to the arrival of the air medical team shortens the amount of time the air medical crew stays on the ground. The goal for many air medical teams is to keep the time on the ground to less than 10 minutes. It is important to remember that definitive care for the deteriorating trauma patient is surgery.

HELICOPTER SAFETY

It is imperative that personnel involved in air medical scene operations be aware of the requirements for safe operations. Most air medical services require a landing area of at least 100 by 100 feet. This area should be as flat and firm as possible. In the event that a rotor wing aircraft must land on an uneven surface, it is important to remember that personnel must approach from the downhill side; this prevents walking into a low turning rotor.

Not only does the landing area need to be flat and firm, but it is essential that ground operations assist the air medical pilot in making sure that the landing area is clear of utility lines, debris, and bystanders. During certain hours of the day and during night operations it is extremely difficult to see obstacles from the air.

When landing an aircraft at night, ground units need to light the landing area. One commonly used method is to cross the headlights of two emergency units across the landing area. While many air medical services prefer ground units to leave their rotating lights on to assist in locating the area, all strobe lights

must be shut off. Strobe lights are too bright and can blind the pilot, making it impossible to land.

As the aircraft nears the ground, the rotorwash can create winds in excess of 100 mph. This is enough wind to blow off hats or sheets, topple safety cones, scatter debris, or overturn stretchers. It can create problems for both the pilot who is trying to land and ground personnel who are trying to care for patients. It is important to ensure that all loose objects are secured until the aircraft is on the ground and has decreased its engine speed.

Once the aircraft has landed, no ground personnel should approach the aircraft from the rear or approach while the aircraft is running, unless accompanied by a member of the air medical crew (Figure 29-1). As soon as possible after landing, a member of the air medical team leaves the aircraft to meet the ground crews.

Some air medical services advocate the use of a three-point guard system. When using this system, three individuals are assigned to the security of the aircraft. One individual assumes the role of landing zone commander and conducts all communications with the aircraft, including advising the crew of potential obstacles. Once the aircraft lands, the medical team meets the landing zone commander for a condition update on the patient. The other two point guards secure the landing area from bystanders, ensuring that no one gets near the turning aircraft rotors. To ensure that air medical operations are carried out in a safe, timely, and efficient manner, all personnel involved should abide by these safety measures.

INTERNET ACTIVITIES

Review the air evacuation protocols of the North Central Texas Trauma Advisory Council at http://www.dfwhc.org/ncttrac/protocols.htm.

FLIGHT PHYSIOLOGY

In order to properly manage the trauma patient in the air medical environment, it is essential to have an understanding of the natural laws governing gases. Not only can alterations in gases lead to physiological changes, they can also alter medical equipment. The gas laws that exert the greatest effect on trauma patients during air medical transport are Boyle's law, Dalton's law, and Henry's law. **Boyle's law** states that the volume of a gas is inversely related to the pressure of a gas. As an aircraft ascends in altitude and atmospheric pressure decreases, the volume of gas increases. This can lead to significant problems in the trauma patient. If the patient has a pneumothorax, the volume

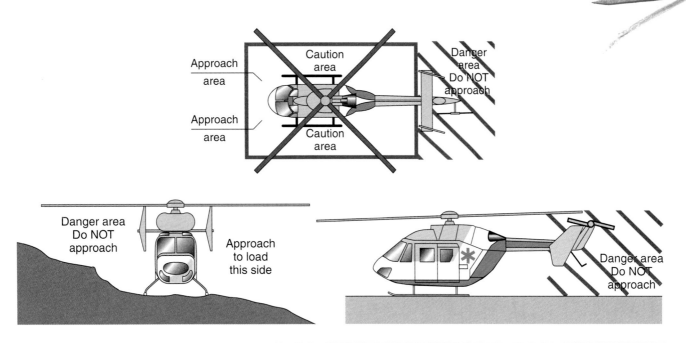

FIGURE 29-1 Safe zones for approaching a helicopter.

of air that has accumulated in the pleural space can expand during ascent, causing the pneumothorax to progress into a tension pneumothorax.

The second gas law of significance is **Dalton's law**. Dalton's law states that the partial pressure of a gas decreases as altitude increases. Everyone has experienced this law if they have traveled to a mountainous location that is at a higher altitude and then experience air hunger while involved in physical activity. This same principle holds true for the air-transported trauma patient. As the aircraft increases in altitude, the partial pressure of oxygen decreases, resulting in increased work of breathing and possibly hypoxemia in the trauma patient.

The final law that can affect the trauma patient in the air medical setting is **Henry's law**, which states that the amount of gas dissolved in a liquid is proportional to the partial pressure of the gas. More simply stated, as that partial pressure decreases, the amount of gas dissolved in the liquid decreases. As altitude increases, the partial pressure of oxygen decreases, resulting in a decrease in the amount of oxygen that is dissolved in the blood volume, further decreasing tissue oxygenation.

STRESSES OF FLIGHT

Air medical transport can create both physical and psychological stress on both trauma patients and medical crew. Browne and colleagues outlined nine such stressors of flight that have been widely accepted by air medical services throughout the United States.[7] These stressors include barometric pressure, hypoxia, noise, vibration, gravitational forces, thermal considerations, dehydration, third spacing, and fatigue.

Barometric pressure, caused by changes in altitude, are directly related to both Dalton's law and Boyle's law. These changes in pressure can affect both the physiological status of the trauma patient and medical equipment and may result in injury to various bodily organs.

The first such condition that can develop is **barotitis media**. Barotitis media results from an increase in the pressure in the middle ear. The problem is compounded when the eustachian tubes, which connect the middle ear and the external atmosphere, become blocked due to inflammation. This tube usually functions as a one-way valve, allowing gas to exit easily to the external environment but preventing gases from returning to the middle ear. This etiology is explained by the effects of Boyle's law. As an aircraft ascends, the volume within the middle ear increases and excess gases and pressure are allowed to escape from the eustachian tubes. Then, as the aircraft descends, a negative pressure is created within the middle ear, and as a result, the volume of air decreases. This negative pressure results in an inward pressure on the tympanic membrane. The tympanic membrane becomes inflamed and, in rare cases, can perforate. Common signs of barotitis media are a feeling of fullness in the ear, severe pain, tenderness, vertigo, nausea, tinnitus, perforation of the eardrum, and bleeding.[8]

When the eustachian tubes are blocked, it may be difficult to equalize pressure in the middle ear. There are several techniques that can assist in equalizing this pressure. One technique is to shift the mandible from side to side or open the mouth in a yawn. These techniques open the eustachian tubes as much as possible and usually allow pressure to equalize. A second method is simply to pinch the nostrils and blow gently. It is important not to blow too hard as this can increase the pressure in the middle ear, enough to damage the eardrum. A common manner of equalizing pressure is to chew gum during flight. Chewing can, however, result in the swallowing of air. The air that is swallowed during ascent can expand and create nausea or gastric distention.

Flying should be prohibited in conditions that could lead to blocking of the eustachian tubes, such as allergies and upper respiratory tract infections. In the event that flight is necessary, patients and air crew members should use a topical vasoconstrictive nasal spray 15 minutes prior to liftoff and landing. Topical agents are safer than oral agents. Oral agents can become ineffective during flight and ear damage could result during landing. If oral agents are used, topical agents should also be available. If at any time a patient or air crew member feels any discomfort, the pilot should be advised so that he or she can descend slowly to allow more time for the equalization of pressure. The most commonly used oral agent is pseudoephedrine (Sudafed).

Treatment for mild irritation of the tympanic membrane consists of anti-inflammatory agents, decongestants, and analgesics. In the event that the tympanic membrane is injured, flying should be restricted until it is healed.

Barometric changes can also affect medical equipment, which includes all tube bulbs filled with air. The bulb of an endotracheal tube is inflated with air. During ascent, the volume of air in the bulb can increase due to decreased barometric pressure. If the pressure of the bulb is not corrected, it can impair the vascular supply to the walls of the trachea, leading to necrosis. Luckily, rotor wing aircraft usually fly at lower altitudes for relatively short distances, so patients are only exposed to mild increases of pressure for a short period of time. However, fixed-wing aircraft usually fly at high altitudes for longer periods of time, exposing the trachea to increased pressure for longer periods. One solution for managing endotracheal tubes during fixed-wing flights is to fill the bulb of the endotracheal tube with water; because it is a liquid instead of a gas, barometric pressure does not create a noticeable change in the volume of the water, thus preventing increased pressure on the inner surface of the trachea.

Another piece of medical equipment affected by barometric pressure changes is the pneumatic anti-shock garment (PASG). During ascent the pressure

within the PASG increases and is able to escape through pop-off valves or through loosening of Velcro straps. The problem arises during descent when the volume of air within the PASG decreases, resulting in decreased circumferential pressure and hemodynamic decompensation of the patient. For this reason the PASG pump should be readily available and additional air added as needed to maintain the integrity of the PASG.

Hypoxia is a condition of inadequate supply of oxygen to the tissues of the body. Hypoxia can occur in the trauma patient during air medical transport as a result of traumatic injuries such as pneumothorax or hemothorax. Dalton's law, which states that the partial pressure of a gas decreases as altitude increases, also contributes to hypoxia. As the partial pressure of oxygen decreases, the amount of oxygen diffusing from the alveoli into the bloodstream decreases, and ultimately there is a decrease in the supply of oxygen to bodily tissues. Hypoxia in the trauma patient leads to an altered level of consciousness, agitation, or restlessness. In an attempt to compensate for hypoxia, the depth and rate of respirations, as well as the heart rate, may increase.

Patients with hemothoraces can also be affected by a decrease in the partial pressure of oxygen. While the hemothorax does not expand as a result of decreased barometric pressure, the decrease in partial pressure of oxygen can cause the patient to deteriorate as a result of decreased diffusion from the alveoli to the bloodstream and from the bloodstream to the tissues. Some air medical services are capable of inserting chest tubes to evacuate the blood that is accumulating in the pleural space. It is important that blood only be removed when blood is available for replacement; otherwise hemostasis can be delayed and blood loss may be increased.

Treatment of hypoxia in the air medical environment revolves around correcting the underlying cause and addressing the effects of a decrease in the partial pressure of oxygen. In the event that a patient has a simple pneumothorax, the air medical crew must be ready to perform a needle thoracentesis if a tension pneumothorax develops. The treatment for hypoxia, resulting from a decrease in partial pressure of oxygen and from traumatic injuries, is simply to administer high concentrations of oxygen, making more oxygen available for diffusion into the tissues. All unconscious or apneic patients should have their airways secured with an endotracheal tube and ventilations should be assisted with 100% oxygen. In the conscious and/or spontaneously breathing patient oxygen should be administered at 15 L/minute via a nonrebreather mask.

Noise during air medical transport can be a stressor to both patients and air medical crew members. The noise associated with an aircraft can intensify a patient's anxiety. One way to decrease the noise level for patients is to place disposable ear plugs in their ears.

Noise can also add to the difficulty of properly assessing a trauma patient. The level of noise created by an aircraft makes it virtually impossible to auscultate lung sounds. For this reason, it is best to secure a patent airway by inserting an endotracheal tube, prior to flight, in patients that are experiencing respiratory difficulty. In the event that endotracheal intubation has to be performed in flight, it is imperative that tube placement be ensured by observing symmetrical chest expansion, condensation in the endotracheal tube, and positive color change or reading with a carbon dioxide detector.

Short-term exposure to aircraft noise can cause symptoms such as headaches, nausea, and fatigue or temporary hearing loss. Long-term exposure to aircraft noise can result in permanent hearing loss. For this reason, it is essential that air medical crew members always wear adequate hearing protection and keep noise exposure to a minimum.

The level of *vibration* associated with air medical transport can be enormous. Vibration can affect both patients and air medical crew members. Vibration can increase basal metabolic rate in the trauma patient, resulting in an increase in both respiratory rate and cardiac rate. These changes can lead to rapid decompensation in the already physiologically stressed trauma patient.

Another complication arising from aircraft vibration is alterations in the body's thermoregulatory system, seen in both hypothermic and hyperthermic patients. In the hypothermic patient, vibration can lead to lowering of body temperature. In the hyperthermic patient, vibration results in vasoconstriction, leading to further increases in body temperature.

As atmospheric pressure decreases, so does *temperature*. Temperature changes can result in physiological alterations to both the patient and air medical crew members. Both increases and decreases in body temperature can result in increases in metabolic demand and oxygen demand. In the critically injured trauma patient this increase in oxygen demand further compromises the body's already taxed physiological systems. To prevent this deterioration, it is imperative that normal body temperature be maintained. It is important to remember that the body loses and gains heat in four distinct ways: convection, conduction, evaporation, and radiation. In the hypothermic patient, maintaining normothermia can be accomplished by properly applying blankets, administering warmed IV fluids, and using onboard aircraft heaters.

Trauma patients suffering from head injuries can be adversely affected by both rotor and fixed-wing transport. The most dramatic effects are experienced during liftoffs and landings. During these times *gravita-*

tional forces can increase intracranial pressure, especially if the patient is improperly placed in the aircraft. Head-injured patients should be placed with their head toward the front of the aircraft. By placing the head toward the front, the amount of gravitational force is decreased during critical times. Another method for decreasing intracranial pressure is to elevate the head of the aircraft stretcher 30°. This may be difficult because the mechanisms that cause head injuries can also result in injuries to the cervical spine, requiring spinal immobilization. In these situations the patient can be placed in a reverse Trendelenburg position by simply raising the head of the spinal immobilization device.

Air medical transport exposes the trauma patient to decreasing humidity levels, pushing the patient toward *dehydration*. Humidity changes result from the decrease in temperature as altitude increases; as gases cool, they lose moisture. This, in conjunction with administration of supplemental medical oxygen, can lead to thirst, dry mouth, dry mucus membranes, sore throat, hoarseness, and dry or scratchy eyes.[8] In an attempt to compensate for this decrease in humidity, the body increases its production of mucosecretions by increasing the metabolic rate, which may be detrimental in the critically traumatized patient.

In order to prevent the complications that can result from dehydration associated with flight, the trauma patient should receive humidified oxygen (if possible) and be closely monitored for hydration level throughout transport. This is accomplished by continually monitoring heart rate for increases and blood pressure for decreasing pulse pressure or decreases in systolic pressure. In addition, air medical crew members should consume adequate amounts of fluids. By following these simple guidelines, dehydration can be prevented.

Third spacing results when fluid is lost from the intravascular space into the extravascular space. During air medical transport, the decrease in ambient pressure allows fluid to leak from the intravascular space into the extravascular space. In addition, late-stage shock can result in alterations in normal cellular permeability and loss of intravascular fluids. Whereas third spacing can result in fluid and electrolyte disturbances, it is important to monitor for early signs and symptoms of third spacing. These signs and symptoms consist of generalized edema, increased heart rate, decreased blood pressure, and dehydration.[8] Treatment for third spacing of the acute trauma patient consists of administration of crystalloid solutions.

All of the stressors of flight outlined above can result in *fatigue* of air medical crew members. For this reason, it is imperative that air medical crew members maintain a high level of health. It is also important that air medical crew members prepare for flight by maintaining good physical condition, eating healthy foods, and avoiding tobacco products and alcoholic beverages.

SUMMARY

Air medical transport of the trauma patient can decrease the time to definitive care. However, air medical transport can create physiological stresses on both patients and air medical crew members. It is essential that prehospital care providers have an understanding of flight physiology and the stresses that can result from air medical transport. Finally, to ensure the safety of everyone involved with air medical operations, out-of-hospital providers must be educated in air medical safety procedures.

REVIEW QUESTIONS

1. The first trauma patient transported by air was transported by:
   a. Lear jet
   b. BK117 helicopter
   c. Hot-air balloon
   d. None of the above

2. Which of the following is a disadvantage of air medical transport?
   a. Speed of transport
   b. Cost
   c. Advanced procedures
   d. Expertise of the medical crew

3. Which of the following pieces of information is important to supply when requesting the services of an air medical service?
   a. Number of patients
   b. Types of injuries
   c. Type of incident
   d. All of the above

4. Changes in barometric pressure can affect:
   a. PASG
   b. Endotracheal tubes
   c. Urinary catheters
   d. All of the above

5. During descent from altitude the air contained within a body cavity will:
   a. Increase in volume
   b. Decrease in volume
   c. Stay the same
   d. None of the above

6. Boyle's law can account for:
   a. Gastric distention
   b. Expansion of a pneumothorax to a tension pneumothorax
   c. Pressure in the ears
   d. All of the above

7. Air medical transport of hemodynamically unstable patients should be delayed to:
   a. Place urinary catheters
   b. Splint simple fractures
   c. Establish a patent airway
   d. All of the above

8. As a result of the partial pressure of oxygen _____ at altitude air medical patients should be placed on oxygen.
   a. Increasing
   b. Decreasing

9. What is needed to prepare a trauma patient who requires air medical transport?

10. Describe the three-point landing system for securing a landing zone.

11. Discuss the complications that can arise from transporting a patient by air with a pneumothorax.

12. Why is it essential that all objects in close proximity to the landing zone be secured prior to an aircraft landing?

13. What actions should be taken in the event that pain develops in the ear during a descent?

CRITICAL THINKING

● As part of an air medical crew, you are called to the scene of a MVC. You are presented with a patient whose injuries include a pneumothorax, head injury, abdominal hemorrhage, and radius/ulna fracture. The paramedics have placed an endotracheal tube, started two large-bore IVs of normal saline, applied and inflated the pneumatic anti-shock garment, and applied an air splint to the fractured arm. The IVs are being pressure infused with a pressure infuser inflated to 300 mm Hg. What precautions must you take during air medical transport of this patient? Using your knowledge of the physics of altitude changes, describe how these changes will affect your equipment and your treatment of this patient.

- Describe the circumstances under which air medical transport is superior to ground transport. Discuss the safety risks and financial costs of using air medical transport of patients who could be effectively transported by ground.

- What specialized equipment and procedures are provided by the air medical services in your area? Are they capable of search and rescue as well as patient transport? How many patients can be transported in their aircraft? What is the protocol for summoning the flight team to the scene?

▶ REFERENCES

1. Odom JW, Jarl RW, Boyd CR, Swan KG. The first flying ambulance: the beginning of rapid transport of the trauma patient. *J Air Med Trans*. 1990; 12(11):11.

2. Macnab AJ. Air medical transport: "hot air" and a French lesson. *J Air Med Trans*. 1992; 14(8):15.

3. Merwin CA. U.S. Air Force patient airlift: from balloon to high-speed jets. *J Air Med Trans*. 1990; 12:18.

4. Hoffman J. Coverage by air. *911 Magazine*, March/April 1991:11.

5. Jacobs LM, Bennett BR. Helicopter EMS. *Emerg Care Q*. 1986; 2:3.

6. Mayfield TY. 1996 annual transport statistics and transport fees survey. *Air Med*. 1996; 2(4):14.

7. Browne L, Bodenstedt R, Campbell P, Nehrenz G. The nine stresses of flight. *J Emerg Nurs*. 1987; 13(4):232.

8. Blumen IJ, Rinnert KJ. Altitude physiology and stresses of flight. *Air Med J*. 1995; 14(2):90.

Chapter 30

Tissue and Organ Donation

OBJECTIVES

Upon completion of this chapter, the reader should be able to:

- Discuss the historical progression of organ donation.
- Explain the role of immunology and histocompatibility in organ and tissue transplantation.
- Describe the federal legislative impact on both organ donation and transplantation.
- Explain the role of the United Network for Organ Sharing in the organ donation and transplantation process.
- Define brain death.
- Discuss donor evaluation and management.
- Describe the role of out-of-hospital professionals in the donation process.
- Explain the inequities between supply and demand.
- Describe some emerging technologies in tissue and organ donation.

KEY TERMS

Cellular immune response
Cellular rejection
Heterotopic
Histocompatibility
Humoral immune response

Hyperacute rejection
Immunology
Orthotopic
Xenografts

The concept of organ and tissue transplantation dates back to ancient times. Some of the earliest documented cases ranged from attempting to transplant a leg from a dead soldier to a patient suffering a traumatic amputation to the Chinese attempting a heart transplant for the purpose of curing emotional ailments.[1–3] Progress was either nonexistent or not well documented until the twentieth century. In the early 1900s renal and heart transplantation experiments began on animal subjects.[1,3] With the early attempts came the recognition of the transplant rejection process and future attempts at utilizing kidneys from other species, known as **xenografts**.[1] In the 1940s, the first successful cadaver transplant occurred in the United States, with the donor kidney functioning for a full 9 months.[2,3] It was not until 1954 that the first living-related kidney transplant of identical twins was performed.[1,3,4] Success at **orthotopic** heart transplantation in animals came in the early 1950s by transplanting an organ into the location it would normally be found in the body.[3] By the mid-1950s there were attempts at **heterotopic** liver transplant, which is a procedure where the donor liver is placed next to (not in place of) the diseased liver.[1,3] As more transplants were attempted, rejection rapidly became a major complication, and by the end of the decade, total-body radiation was implemented in an attempt to decrease rejection by disabling the immune system.[1,3] Significant contributions continued into the 1960s with increased use of steroids and the advent of *donor/recipient matching.* The decade ended with the first implantation of an artificial heart in 1969.[1,3] The 1970s brought transplantation of long bones for trauma and osteosarcoma patients. The single most important immunosuppression finding came in 1978 with cyclosporine, which is a fungal metabolite first thought to be an antibiotic.[1,3]

The 1980s were progressive years, starting with the first successful heart-lung transplant, followed by the first long-term use of an artificial heart, the Jarvic 7, in patient Barney Clark in 1984.[1,3,5] Ventricular assist devices (VAD) were developed as a bridge to transplantation.[1,5] The VAD using pig heart valves prolonged life for up to a year while the recipient awaited a transplant organ. Split-liver transplantation was successfully performed with one lobe to a child and the remainder of the liver to a small adult.[1] The 1990s showed significant growth in heart transplantation with approximately 2,000 transplants done in the United States annually.[1,6] The survival rate for heart transplants in 1990 was 90%, up from 65% in 1980 and 20% in 1970.

Continued work and research in all areas of transplantation, including immunosuppression therapy and organ management and preservation techniques, make what will be possible during the next century not even imaginable now.

THE ROLE OF EMS PROFESSIONALS

Early identification and detailed documentation are essential first steps of the organ and tissue donation process. The management of a patient thought to be a candidate for organ donation is the same as for any patient before brain death has been declared and confirmed. These same life-saving measures serve to prevent dysfunction of any organs appropriate for donation. This is accomplished through adequate oxygenation and tissue perfusion as well as overall hemodynamic stability. A patient pulseless in the field should be treated without regard to donation potential. If cardiac death occurs, the patient may then be evaluated for tissue donation potential. A patient suffering brain death may be considered for organ and/or tissue dona-

tion, while a patient suffering cardiac death is currently only considered for tissue donation. The time from death to tissue recovery is significantly longer with tissue donation than with organ donation. Aside from the current medical situation, it is of great importance to obtain a detailed past medical history and social history. Both the past medical history and social or behavioral histories are essential in determining a patient's suitability for organ and tissue donation.

The evaluation of patients as potential organ or tissue donors is an extensive and ever-changing process. Because the process is extremely involved and the number of donors any one area receives on a regular basis is minimal, organ recovery personnel should be contacted early to screen for donation potential and to manage care when appropriate.

As the average life span increases in the United States, so does the age range for organs to be considered for donation. Because criteria for organ and tissue donors change with increased knowledge and medical advances, organ recovery agencies find that it is very difficult for EMS and hospital professionals to remain current with the changing parameters. Thus they rely more on organ and tissue recovery agencies for screening potential donors.

EMS and hospital professionals play a vital role in the donation process. Without early recognition and referral of a potential donor to an organ recovery agency, the process never begins. When tragedy strikes and a patient is critically injured, medical professionals exhaust all resources in an attempt to create a positive outcome. When those resources have been depleted within the context of this emotional situation, the option of donation may not be remembered. When families and friends are devastated, organ and tissue recovery personnel can offer an opportunity that can turn a tragic situation into something positive—organ donation. One individual's tragic death can enhance or save the lives of many others.

IMMUNOLOGY AND ADVANCEMENTS IN HISTOCOMPATIBILITY

Immunology and histocompatibility play a vital role in the success of organ and tissue transplantation. **Immunology** deals with the body's response to a foreign substance while **histocompatibility** deals with tissue typing and matching. The body reacts to transplanted organs and tissues as foreign substances, thus activating the immune system. The objective is to decrease the immune response, first by utilizing donor organs and tissues that match the recipient's tissue type as closely as possible and then by using immunosuppressive therapy.[5]

IMMUNOLOGY

After transplantation, the immune system is activated when human leukocyte antigens (HLA) from the donor organ or tissue are recognized by the recipient's lymphocytes as a foreign substance. The transplanted organ or tissue can then be rejected through two different mechanisms. The first mechanism is the **humoral immune response**, which pertains to the production of antibodies.[7] This response can completely destroy the transplanted graft through **hyperacute rejection**. Hyperacute rejection takes place as T-helper cells influence B cells to produce an antibody in response to the foreign substance or antigen recognized. The **cellular immune response** is the second mechanism and pertains to the production of cytotoxic T cells.[1] The T cells seek out and destroy any cells containing the foreign antigen identified by the T-helper cells. This type of response, called **cellular rejection**, can be acute or chronic in nature.[7] With either form of rejection there are cells remaining in the circulation known as *memory cells*. These memory cells can be activated at any time the same foreign antigen is recognized. In an immune response, typically both the humoral and cellular immune responses are involved (Figure 30-1). In transplantation it is imperative that these responses be muted or suppressed in order for the donor organ or tissue to be accepted by the recipient. This is accomplished through an aggressive immunosuppressive regimen. Immunosuppressive medications can be broken down into four classifications: (1) antibodies against lymphocytes, which adhere to the surface of lymphocytes rendering them inactive; (2) lymphocyte-specific drugs, which inhibit the function of lymphocytes; (3) antimetabolites, which block production of DNA, preventing cells from rapidly dividing in response to foreign tissue; and (4) corticosteroids, of which the mechanism of action is not clearly understood.[1]

Administration of immunosuppressives must be accurately balanced with histocompatibility considerations. Inadequate dosages may lead to rejection while excessive dosages may leave the recipient vulnerable to infecting organisms: Opportunistic infections are the most common cause of death among immunocompromised patients.[8]

HISTOCOMPATIBILITY

The closer an organ donor's tissue matches the recipient's, the less chance there is of rejection, and thus the need for immunosuppression is decreased. With the advent of histocompatibility testing, the donor antigens are evaluated against the recipient antibodies. The two major genetic systems impacting organ and tissue transplantation are the ABO red cell system and the HLA system.[3,5] The ABO system is present on red blood cells and vascular endothelial cells, making ABO compatibility between the donor and the recipient necessary for transplantation of most organs and tissue. The far more intricate HLA system is composed of two classes of antigens: class I are located on white cells, while class II are found primarily on vascular endothelial cells. Transplanted organs have been found to function longer when the recipient and donor are closely matched for HLA.[5]

LEGISLATIVE IMPACT

Dating as far back as 1968 federal legislation and regulations have played a vital role in both organ recovery and transplantation.

UNIFORM ANATOMICAL GIFT ACT

Before organs or tissue can be recovered for transplantation, consent must be obtained. Prior consent may come from the donor or may be obtained from legal next of kin at or near the time of death. The Uniform Anatomical Gift Act has, in part, resolved

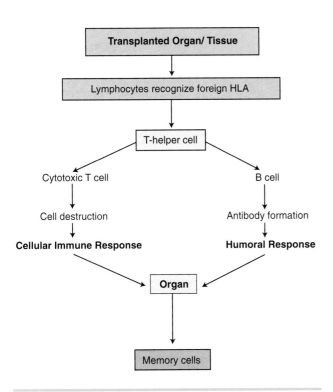

FIGURE 30-1 Immunological response to an antigen.

some of the issues involving consent. In 1968, this act, being adopted by all states, authorized the gift of all or part of a human body at death for the purpose of transplantation, research, education, or other therapies.[3] This act includes information on who may donate, how to execute the process, and who is eligible to receive the donation. A revision to the act in 1987 eliminates the requirement of a witnessed donor signature and prohibits the next of kin from revoking the donor's authorization.[3] The revision also requires hospitals, on admission, to document on the patient's chart wishes about donation and, if necessary, to search for documentation of the patient's wishes regarding donation.

UNIFORM DETERMINATION OF DEATH ACT

In 1959 the clinical aspects of brain death were described for the first time by physicians in France.[3] Defining brain death was the first step toward addressing a growing problem involving an imbalance between supply and demand. In the 1960s there was an explosion in the utilization of cardiopulmonary resuscitation and ventilators.[3] These well-intentioned measures were used much too often in cases with poor prognosis in a time of limited resources. With moral and ethical dilemmas surrounding brain death, legislation was sought to make the definition of brain death less ambiguous. This was accomplished in 1980 through the Uniform Determination of Death Act, which recognizes death as either irreversible cessation of circulatory and respiratory functions or irreversible cessation of all functions of the entire brain, including the brain stem.[9]

NATIONAL ORGAN TRANSPLANT ACT

The National Organ Transplant Act evolved as the need for transplantable organs and tissue grew while the supply of available donors remained fairly constant. This trend continues today with a widening gap between those donating organs and those awaiting organs. In 1984, the act provided for a task force on organ transplantation and grants for planning, establishing, and expanding organ recovery organizations.[9] It also required a contracted agency to develop and operate the organ recovery and transplantation network, with services to include a scientific registry of organ transplant recipients. To address public concern, the National Organ Transplant Act also specifically prohibits the buying and selling of organs.[9]

OMNIBUS BUDGET RECONCILIATION ACT OF 1986

Due to the widening gap between the need for transplantable organs and the donor organs available for transplantation, the Omnibus Budget Reconciliation Act evolved. This act mandates hospitals receiving financial reimbursement from Medicare and Medicaid to develop policies that ensure potential donor families are approached and organ recovery organizations are notified. Under this act, transplant hospitals must become members of the Organ Procurement and Transplantation Network and follow the rules set forth by the network.[9]

UNITED NETWORK FOR ORGAN SHARING

The subjects of organ donation and transplantation have raised many ethical, social, and economical questions over the years. The National Organ Transplant Act appointed an agency to develop and maintain the organ recovery and transplantation network.[9] The United Network for Organ Sharing (UNOS) was awarded the contract and has maintained it as of this writing. In obtaining the contract, UNOS was charged with maximizing the recovery of potential organs and ensuring that the distribution be equitable.[9] UNOS implemented a concise and organized system of listing recipients nationally. This system ensures that donated organs and tissues are allocated according to genetic matching, medical urgency, waiting time, and geographical location.[6]

According to the national patient waiting list developed by UNOS, as of June 1996, there were greater than 40,000 registrants awaiting organ transplants[6] (Figure 30-2).

In 1995 there were 19,024 transplant operations performed nationwide to include 10,793 kidney transplants (3,114 from living donors), 3,915 liver transplants, 2,358 heart transplants, 916 kidney-pancreas transplants, 863 lung transplants, 110 pancreas transplants, and 69 heart-lung transplants.[6] One-third of those on the waiting list die before they receive a lifesaving organ, and every 20 minutes a new name is added to the list.[10]

BRAIN DEATH

Before making the transition between treating a patient and managing a donor, brain death must be confirmed clinically and diagnostically and be documented by two attending level physicians.[3] Until fairly recently brain

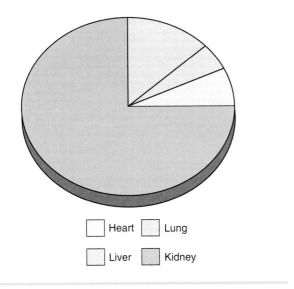

FIGURE 30-2 Recipients waiting. Distributive comparison by organ.

Heart ☐ Lung ☐

Liver ☐ Kidney ■

death was not clearly defined, and even now the chosen methods to confirm brain death vary by institution. According to the President's Commission report on brain death, the accepted definition is an irreversible loss of cerebral hemisphere and brain stem functions.[3] An extensive clinical examination for spontaneous movement, response to painful stimuli, brain stem reflexes, and spontaneous respirations must be done in conjunction with diagnostic testing.[1] The diagnostic confirmation may include any of the following or a combination of electroencephlograms, cerebral blood flow studies, and apnea testing.

The pathophysiology as well as the physiological manifestations of brain death must be clearly understood in order to anticipate changes in condition and to be able to manage donor care. The process starts with an insult to the brain that causes the destruction of tissue and the loss of cell membrane integrity (Figure 30-3). With the loss of cell membrane integrity, fluid moves from the intracellular and/or intravascular fluid compartments into interstitial spaces. These fluid shifts cause an increase in intracranial pressure with compression of the microvasculature and a decrease in cerebral blood flow. A decrease in cerebral blood flow leads to tissue ischemia and an accumulation of carbon dioxide. As capillary pressure increases, there is arteriolar dilatation causing further edema and a continued increase in intracranial pressure. When the intracranial pressure reaches a point that there is no further room for expansion, brain stem herniation occurs. With herniation, there is brain death and a loss of all regulatory mechanisms.[1]

The body's response to this cascade of events starts before herniation and brain death. Increasing

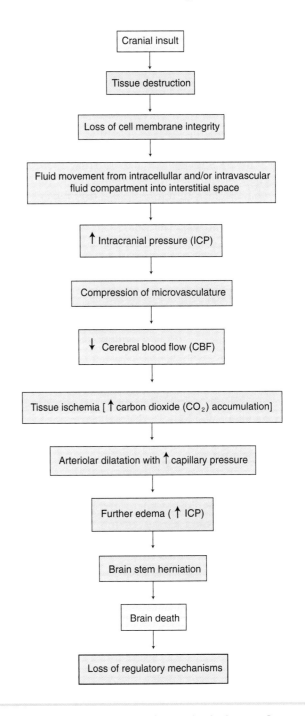

FIGURE 30-3 Pathogenesis of brain death. *Source: Organ Donor Management: Pathophysiologic Principles.* East Hanover, N.J.: Sandoz Pharmaceuticals.

intracranial pressure resulting from brain ischemia causes a systemic hypertension and tachycardia. The normal catecholamine release that occurs with injury may result in ventricular dysfunction or complete failure and neurogenic pulmonary edema. Prior to brain death hypothalamic function is irregular and hyperthermia is typically seen, with an initial spike that may continue due to meningeal irritation but subside with complete herniation.[1]

After herniation there is a loss of circulatory regulation and spontaneous respiration, followed by hypothermia. The sympathetic nervous system stops functioning, leading to a decrease in systemic vascular resistance and complete vasodilation. There is then a decrease in preload and cardiac output, leading to a distributive hypovolemia and resultant hypotension (Figure 30-4). After brain death the pituitary becomes nonfunctional and the lack of antidiuretic hormone results in polyuria, dehydration, serum hyperosmorality, hypokalemia, and hypernatremia, all indicative of diabetes insipidus, which occurs in 50%–70% of brain dead patients.[11] The hypothalamus stops functioning after brain death, and the control of temperature is lost, causing hypothermia that can lead to a decrease in oxygen delivery to the tissue and ventricular fibrillation (Figure 30-5). As the brain becomes necrotic, tissue fibrinolytic agents are released, causing coagulopathies. Almost 90% of patients with a fatal head injury develop disseminated intravascular coagulation.[3] Because no two patients progress to brain death in the same amount of time or with the same clinical manifestations, an organized plan of management should be developed early.

DONOR EVALUATION

The success of organ and tissue donation depends on early recognition by medical personnel and speedy referral to the organ recovery agency. Failure to refer a potential organ and tissue donor denies a family the right to make an informed decision about donation and denies a recipient the chance to receive life-saving organs or life-enhancing tissues.[5] Due to the fact that criteria for organ and tissue donation are constantly changing, a routine referral system is critical. Routine referral is a quick-and-easy system that involves organ recovery agencies in the screening process for identifying potential organ and tissue donors (Figure 30-6).

Often the first evaluation for the recovery agency is to differentiate between a potential organ donor and a potential tissue donor. With a potential organ donor, brain death has occurred or is imminent and the patient is being maintained through mechanical ventilation. This is a patient who has suffered a catastrophic brain injury or other cerebral event.[5] With a potential tissue donor, cardiac death has already occurred. Cardiac death is straightforward—the heart has stopped beating. Although brain death criteria and the numerous mechanisms for its verification vary by institution, irreversible cessation of functions of the brain, including the brain stem, must take place.[3]

The donor evaluation process occurs in three distinct stages. First the recovery personnel obtain a detailed history and perform a physical assessment. Next diagnostic studies are conducted in consultation with specialists. The final evaluation is conducted during surgery by the recovery surgeons, who visually inspect and physically examine the organs for abnormalities. Failure to identify any abnormalities in these three stages may lead to mistakes in management of the potential donor as well as possible damage to the organs.

After an extensive medical history has been obtained (to include the current hospital course), brain death has been declared, and consent for organ donation has been obtained from the legal next of kin, a detailed social/behavioral history must be documented. Even if there are no medical contraindications to donation at this point, a social history can rule out a potential donor. The questions in the social history are based on the Centers for Disease Control guidelines and include questions on cigarette smoking, alcohol intake, sexual orientation and practices, legal and/or illegal drug use, criminal imprisonment, and travel outside the United States.[1,3,5]

DONOR MANAGEMENT

Management of a donor is focused on therapeutic modalities that maximize organ function and viability. Prior to brain death, hypertension, tachycardia, and hyperthermia should be managed conservatively because these responses are usually short term and subside after herniation.[1] Not only do these responses subside, but usually the reverse response occurs after herniation, compounding the effect if treated too aggressively. The hyperthermia is often treated with cooling blankets because antipyretics have little effect on central nervous system (CNS) mediated temperatures. If hyperthermia persists, consider the presence of an infectious process. If the hypertension and tachycardia require treatment, short-acting calcium blockers and beta blockers are normally effective.[1]

Subsequent to brain death, the focus shifts to hypotension, hypothermia, and electrolyte disturbances. Hypotension is usually significant with systolic pressures in the 40s necessitating volume replacement with 5 cc/kg crystalloid boluses to obtain a central venous pressure (CVP) and/or pulmonary capillary wedge pressure (PCWP) of greater than 8 mm Hg (or cm H_2O) but not to exceed 2 L/hr.[1,3,10,12] Maintenance fluids should infuse at 2 mL/kg/hr and each mL of urine output should be replaced with a mL of crystalloid fluid. If there is not the benefit of central venous pressure (CVP) or pulmonary capillary wedge pressure (PCWP) measurements, intake and output can be calculated to maintain a positive balance. If the CVP is less than 2 mm Hg (or cm H_2O) and the systolic blood pressure is less than 90 mm Hg, consider albumin to rapidly

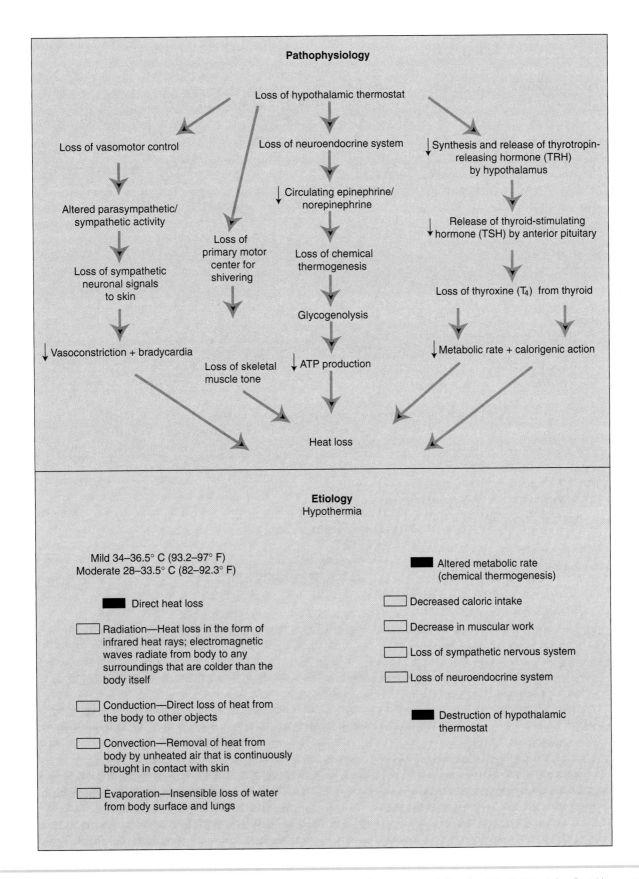

FIGURE 30-4 Pathophysiology of hypothermia. *Source: Organ Donor Management: Pathophysiologic Principles.* East Hanover, N.J.: Sandoz Pharmaceuticals.

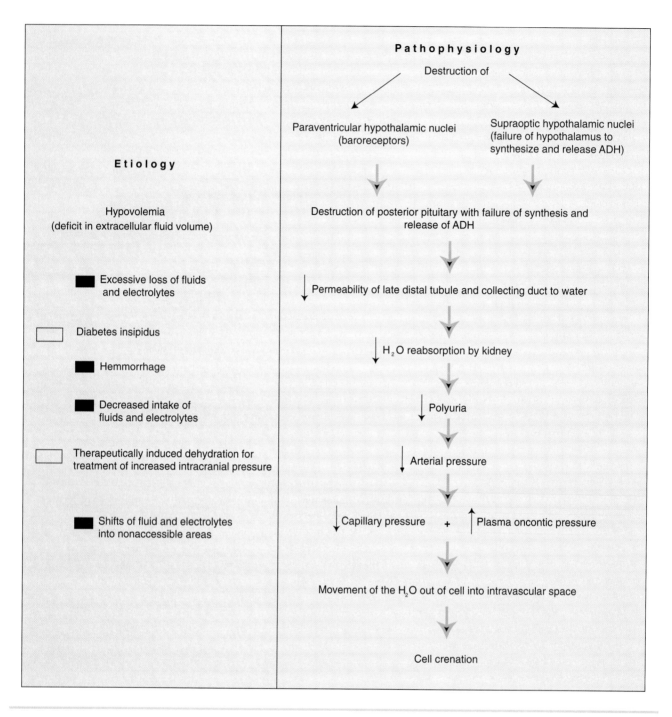

FIGURE 30-5 Pathophysiology of hypovolemia. *Source: Organ Donor Management: Pathophysiologic Principles.* East Hanover, N.J.: Sandoz Pharmaceuticals.

expand the intravascular volume. Hespan may also be used, but possible developing coagulopathies are a concern.[1] If dilutional effects develop with a hematocrit of less than 30%, administer packed red blood cells (one unit increases the hematocrit by 3%–5% and the hemoglobin by 1 g/dL). When the CVP remains above 10 mm Hg (or cm H_2O) with a systolic blood pressure of less than 100 mm Hg, dopamine should be started at 5 µg/kg/min in an attempt to obtain and maintain the

systolic blood pressure above 100 mm Hg. If dopamine does not maintain the blood pressure, utilize hormone replacement of thyroxine.[1,3] Central nervous system ischemia with brain death depletes hormone stores and metabolism converts to anaerobic, further depressing myocardial function. The anaerobic metabolism and subsequent production of lactic acid negatively affect all organs and tissues. Thyroxine replaces a hormone no longer produced after brain death, enhancing cellular

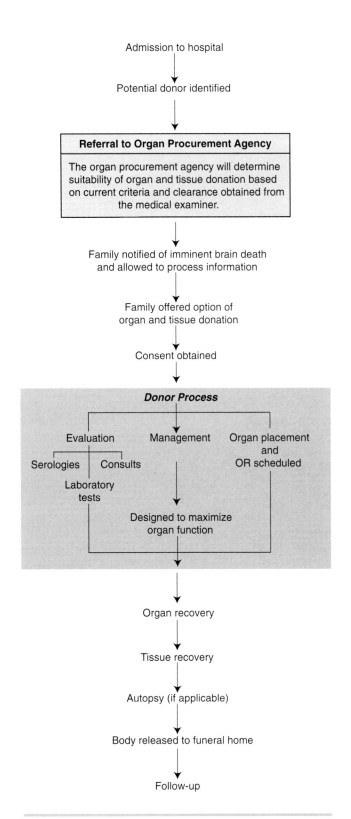

Admission to hospital

↓

Potential donor identified

↓

Referral to Organ Procurement Agency

The organ procurement agency will determine suitability of organ and tissue donation based on current criteria and clearance obtained from the medical examiner.

↓

Family notified of imminent brain death and allowed to process information

↓

Family offered option of organ and tissue donation

↓

Consent obtained

↓

Donor Process

Evaluation   Management   Organ placement and OR scheduled

Serologies   Consults

Laboratory tests

↓

Designed to maximize organ function

↓

Organ recovery

↓

Tissue recovery

↓

Autopsy (if applicable)

↓

Body released to funeral home

↓

Follow-up

FIGURE 30-6 Organ and tissue donation process. (Courtesy of Carolina Organ Procurement Agency, Greenville, N.C.)

metabolism by converting back to aerobic metabolism. If difficulty in maintaining an adequate systolic blood pressure continues, consider a combination of dopamine and dobutamine, not to exceed a combined total of 20 µg/kg/min.[3,10] If all regimens at this point prove to be ineffective, consider other vasopressors, such as epinephrine, norepinephrine, or Aramine, while being cognizant of potentially compromised hepatic and renal perfusion. A fine line exists between preventing prolonged hypotension, which causes organ damage from hypoperfusion states, and utilizing minimal drug therapy, which can also lead to organ damage through vasoconstrictive effects.

Hypothermia should be anticipated and preventative measures instituted early. If the temperature drops significantly, rewarming should occur no faster than 2°F per hour due to the risk of cardiac dysrhythmias.[1,3] During rewarming, insulin production returns and potassium shifts intracellularly, leading to hypokalemia that may produce the cardiac dysrhythmias. Warming methods include hyperthermia blankets, warmed air through the ventilator, and fluid warmers.

Anticipated electrolyte disturbances include hypernatremia, hypokalemia, and hypomagnesemia typically due to volume replacement, dehydration from keeping the patient "dry" before herniation to decrease intracranial pressure, and altered renal function consistent with diabetes insipidus. The goal is to normalize electrolytes.

Hypernatremia is corrected by utilizing a hypotonic solution in treating a volume deficit. Early correction is important because hypernatremic hepatocytes rupture in the presence of isotonic serum and the degree of sodium elevation is a direct correlation with primary liver dysfunction. Hypokalemia and hypomagnesemia are both treated through replacement of these electrolytes and, when normalized together, lessen the chance of cardiac dysrhythmias. Since increased intracranial pressure is no longer a concern after brain death, dehydration is corrected with fluid replacement. An altered renal function is treated with an antidiuretic hormone inhibitor such as desmopressin or pitressin.[1] Consideration must be given to some antidiuretic hormone inhibitors' vasoconstrictive effects that may cause damage to the liver. If urinary output exceeds 4 mL/kg/hr, consider the use of desmopressin. Maintenance fluids should be administered on the basis of a milliliter replacement of the hourly urinary output.[3,10]

Since sepsis is a major concern both in the management of the donor and in rendering the organs and tissue unsuitable for donation, donors are treated prophylactically with antibiotics. In addition to the administration of antibiotics, blood for cultures and serological testing is obtained. Other aspects of donor management focus on early recognition and treatment. Be alert to signs of hypoxemia, hypoxia, acid-base disturbances, diabetes insipidus, sepsis, and coagulopathies.

SUPPLY AND DEMAND

Public awareness and support of donation have increased significantly over the last several years. This increase has not followed through with an increase in actual donors. Over the last several years the annual number of donors has stagnated while the number of those awaiting life-enhancing and life-saving organs continues to grow each year.[10] Current figures indicate that well in excess of 40,000 people are awaiting organ transplants in the United States.[6] Even more alarming is that every 20 minutes someone new is added to the waiting list.[13] With these figures in mind, consider to what extent the donor-recipient gap has widened with fewer than 5,000 donors a year providing transplantable organs for less than 20,000 people on the waiting list.[6] A single organ donor can provide up to seven organs for transplant.

Fairly conservative estimates from the Center for Disease Control and Prevention (CDC) in Atlanta indicate that approximately 20,000 people annually meet the criteria to be organ donors.[14] Nearly 12,000 people die annually from brain death alone, with only one out of every three becoming an organ donor.[10] The small number of potential donors is believed to be the result of families declining the option to donate, failure of medical personnel to involve organ recovery personnel in the screening process, delays in declaring the patient brain dead, and the patient becoming too unstable.

Organ recovery agencies spend endless hours in public education programs in an attempt to narrow the gap between those donating organs and those awaiting organs. Education can help to remove the mystery that surrounds donation as well as to correct misconceptions. With a better understanding of brain death, the public will be assured that everything medically is done to save the critically injured or ill before the option of donation is explored. In addition, the fear that donation causes pain or suffering to the donor or that it prevents a normal funeral or open casket ceremony can be dispelled. Many people have religious concerns regarding donation, yet all major religious faiths support organ donation (Figure 30-7).[15] Education efforts about the benefits of donation focus not only on the recipient but also on the donor family who gains solace from a positive aspect of an otherwise tragic, unexpected loss.

Another side of transplantation, not often realized, is the financial savings that can occur. Two examples are that a kidney transplant costs less than sustaining the same patient 2 years on dialysis and a lung transplant costs less than the care of an advanced cystic fibrosis patient for even 1 year.[10] In both cases, the quality of life has been significantly improved.

INTERNET ACTIVITIES

- Visit the Internet site www.organdonor.gov and find the most frequently asked questions about organ donation. Read about the myths surrounding organ donation.
- Find the latest changes in federal legislation concerning organ donation. Check the Web site at www.transweb.org and the UNOS (United Network for Organ Sharing) Web site www.unos.org/frame_Default.asp.
- Using the Web site for UNOS, discuss the role of UNOS and its role in organ donation.

▶ SUMMARY

Work continues to refine virtually every aspect of the donation and transplantation field as well as to develop new methods of expanding the donor pool. Preservation solutions are being explored to prolong the time to transplantation, allowing organs to be utilized more globally. Work continues with xenografts, recovering and utilizing tissue from other species for transplantation into humans. Further work is being done with non-heart-beating donors to develop ways to utilize organs after cardiac death has occurred.

Tissue and organ donation as well as transplantation are very new specialties within the field of medicine and much more research needs to be done. Organ donation science changes quickly. The miracles of yesterday are today's technology, while the dreams of today will become commonplace in the years ahead.

▶ REVIEW QUESTIONS

1. Define:
   a. Xenograft
   b. Orthotopic
   c. Heterotopic
2. What was the single most important immunosuppression finding and in what year did it occur?
3. How is the immune system activated after transplantation?
4. Describe the two mechanisms by which a transplanted organ or tissue may be rejected.

How Religions View Organ Donation and Transplantation

People considering organ and tissue donation and transplantation often wonder if such acts are compatible with their religious beliefs. Research conducted by the American Council on Transplantation has found that while answers vary from faith to faith, a majority of religions support donation and transplantation. Here are the thoughts of some representatives of the major religions.

AMISH: The Amish will consent to transplantation, but would be reluctant to donate their organs if the transplant outcome was known to be questionable. John Hostatler, an authority on Amish religion, says in his book, *Amish Society*, that "...the Amish believe that since God created the human body, it is God who heals; however, nothing in the Amish understanding of the Bible forbids them from using modern medical services including surgery, anesthesia, hospitalization, dental work, blood transfusions or immunization."

BUDDHISM: The Buddhists believe organ donation is a matter of individual conscience. According to the faith's leaders, there is no written resolution in this issue. Leaders have said they honor people who donate bodies and organs to the advancement of medical science and to saving lives.

CATHOLICISM: Catholics view organ donation as an act of charity, fraternal love and self-sacrifice. Transplants are ethically and morally acceptable to the Vatican. Pope John Paul II has expressed concern about donors' "psychological and physical integrity," but has taken no position against organ transplantation. According to Father Leroy Wiechowski, director of the office of health affairs of the Archdioceses of Chicago, "We encourage donation as an act of charity. It is something good that can result from a tragedy and a way for families to find comfort by helping others. We do caution, however, that the organs are removed only after death and that people's wishes are respected."

CHRISTIAN SCIENTISTS: The Church takes no specific position on transplants or organ donation as distinct from other medical or surgical procedures. Church members usually rely on spiritual rather than medical means of healing. They are free, however, to choose the form of medical treatment they desire, including organ transplantation. The decision of organ donation is left to the individual.

HINDUISM: Hindus are not prohibited by religious law from donating their organs, according to the Hindu temple Society of North America. The act is an individual decision.

ISLAM: The Moslem Religious council initially rejected organ donation by followers of Islam in 1983. It has reversed its position, however, provided the donor's consent is written in advance. The organs of Moslem donors must be transplanted immediately and not stored in organ banks. Moslem officials say they have no policy against organ donation as long as it is done with respect for the deceased and for the recipient.

JEHOVAH'S WITNESSES: Jehovah's Witnesses do not encourage organ donation, but believe it is a matter of individual conscience, according to the Watch Tower Society, the legal corporation for the religion. Although the group is often assumed to ban transplantation because of its taboo against blood transfusion, it does not oppose donation or receiving organs. All organs and tissues, however, must be completely drained of blood before transplantation.

JUDAISM: Judaism teaches that saving a human life takes precedence over maintaining the sanctity of the human body. A direct transplant is preferred, however. Jewish officials have stated that if a member is in the position to donate an organ to save another's life, it is obligatory to do so, even if the donor never knows who the beneficiary will be. The basic principle of Jewish ethics—

the infinite worth of the human being—also includes donation of corneas, since eyesight restoration is considered a life-saving operation. They have also noted donors must be brain dead in accordance with standards set by the Harvard University criteria and the President's Commission on brain death.

MENNONITE: There is no prohibition against organ donation and transplantation in the Mennonite faith. Church officials state such decisions are individual ones.

PROTESTANTISM: Protestantism encourages and endorses organ donation. The Protestant faith respects individual conscience and a person's right to make decisions regarding his/her body. Officials for the various denominations which compose Protestantism say organ donation enables more abundant life, alleviates pain and suffering, and is an expression of life in times of tragedy.

SEVENTH-DAY ADVENTISTS: Seventh-Day Adventist officials have stated organ donation and transplantation to be acceptable practices for members. The decision is an individual one.

QUAKERS: Officials for the Quaker faith do not oppose donation and transplantation. The decision, they say, is an individual one.

LATTER-DAY SAINTS (Mormons): Latter-Day Saints are not prohibited by religious law from donating their organs or receiving transplants, according to the church leaders. The decision is a personal one. Burial of the body is customary, but the final decision remains with the next of kin.

From: "Organ and Tissue Donation: Reference Guide for Clergy," United Network for Organ Sharing, 1990. Richmond, Va.

FIGURE 30-7 How religions view organ donation and transplantation. *Source: Organ and Tissue Donation: Reference Guide for Clergy.* United Network for Organ Sharing; 1990. Reprinted with permission.

5. Name the two major genetic systems impacting organ and tissue transplantation.

6. What information does the Uniform Anatomical Gift Act address?

7. What does UNOS stand for and what is its role?

8. Define brain death.

9. List some of the diagnostic tests performed to confirm and document the presence of brain death.

10. Name some of the clinical manifestations that occur after herniation and brain death.

11. List the three stages of the donor evaluation process.

12. What information should be elicited from a social/behavioral history?

13. Explain why hypertension, tachycardia, and hyperthermia should be managed conservatively prior to brain death.

14. What donation potential exists with a patient suffering:
    a. Brain death?
    b. Cardiac death?

15. Currently, what is the general feeling of all major religious faiths toward organ donation?

CRITICAL THINKING

● Discuss the implications of chronic cyclosporin and steroid therapy in transplant patients.

● Describe the role of the paramedic in managing a potential organ and/or tissue donor.

● Are you an organ or tissue donor? What ethical, moral, philosophical, and religious beliefs led you to this decision?

REFERENCES

1. NATCO. Unpublished material. The Organ and Tissue Donation Process: An Introductory Course for Transplant Coordinators. University College, University of Minnesota; 1995.

2. Carolina Organ Procurement Agency. What's changed in 10 years. In: *Horizons.* Durham, N.C.: Carolina Organ Procurement Agency; 1995.

3. Phillips M. *Organ Procurement, Preservation and Distribution in Transplantation.* Richmond, Va.: William Byrd Press, Inc.; 1991.

4. Carolina Organ Procurement Agency. A little history. In: *Horizons.* Durham, N.C.: Carolina Organ Procurement Agency; 1995.

5. Nolan M, Augustine S. *Transplantation Nursing. Acute and Long-Term Management.* Norwalk, Conn.: Appleton and Lange; 1995.

6. Carolina Organ Procurement Agency. *Facts about Transplantation in the US and North Carolina.* Greenville, N.C.: Carolina Organ Procurement Agency; 1996.

7. Flye M. *Principles of Organ Transplantation.* Philadelphia: WB Saunders Co.; 1989.

8. Smith S. Immunologic aspects of transplantation. In: Smith S, ed. *Tissue and Organ Transplantation: Implications for Professional Nursing Practice.* St. Louis: Mosby; 1990.

9. Carolina Organ Procurement Agency. *Federal Legislation and Regulations Relevant to Organ Procurement and Transplantation.* Greenville, N.C.: Carolina Organ Procurement Agency; 1995.

10. Detterbeck F, Williams W, Egan T. *From the Despair of Brain Death to New Hope through Multiple Organ Donation.* Chapel Hill, N.C.: Division of Cardiothoracic Surgery, University of North Carolina School of Medicine; 1993.

11. Bodenham A, Park G. Care of the multiple organ donor. *Intensive Care Med.* 1989; 15:340.

12. Flye M. *Atlas of Organ Transplantation.* Philadelphia: WB Saunders Co.; 1995.

13. Delaware Valley Transplant Program. *Organ & Tissue Donation: Some Facts to Know.* Philadelphia: Delaware Valley Transplant Program; 1995.

14. Peters T. Organ donation and emergency medicine: the golden hour. *Top Emerg Med.* 1990; 12:64.

15. Carolina Organ Procurement Agency. *How Religions View Organ Donation and Transplantation.* Greenville, N.C.: Carolina Organ Procurement Agency; 1990.

Chapter

31

Forensics in Trauma

OBJECTIVES

Upon completion of this chapter, the reader should be able to:

- Discuss the types of body tissue injuries and their forensic significance.
- List the major types of weapons used to inflict injury and the forensic importance of each.
- Define "physical evidence."
- Explain the basic principles of evidence preservation and how the paramedic can participate in evidence collection.
- Define "chain of custody" and outline the steps the paramedic must take to preserve it.
- List the basic tenets of documentation and photography in forensic cases.

KEY TERMS

Clinical forensic medicine
Forensic pathology
Forensic toxicology

Intradermal bruising
Physical evidence

Violence has always been present in American society. However, in recent decades escalating violence has increased the number of patients, both victims and criminals, treated by EMS personnel. This is particularly true regarding gun violence. While society struggles to deal with violence and trauma, it is more and more aware of how laws, while designed to protect the innocent, seemingly provide loopholes for the guilty. It is increasingly important, then, to narrow the gap between medicine and law and to work cooperatively to provide the best care possible while preserving and protecting legal evidence. There exists an unavoidable overlap in the duty to care for a patient and the duty to protect, handle, secure, and document legal evidence. A cooperative effort from both law enforcement and health care personnel serves to enhance patient care and ensure justice.

In order to cooperate, EMS personnel must incorporate into their practice an understanding of forensic medicine. Health care professionals are called upon not only to preserve and collect evidence but also to provide testimony in a court of law. In the past, forensic education of health care professionals has been sporadic and, in general, neglected. This chapter introduces EMS personnel to the basic forensic issues they may face while performing their duties.

The word *forensic* has its roots in the roman word *forum*, which was the Roman marketplace where lawyers conducted business.[1] The term **forensic pathology** refers to the part of forensic science that deals with the deceased. **Clinical forensic medicine**, *clinical forensics*, and *living forensics* are terms associated with living patients. In trauma, the degree of injury separating fatal from nonfatal wounds is often minimal, causing the science of forensic pathology to overlap with clinical forensics. **Forensic toxicology**, the study of the effect of poisons and other chemicals on the body, is also a specialty and helps to unravel many mysteries surrounding illness and death.

It is not always easy to know when a particular case will have medicolegal significance. However, most countries have in place a system to investigate events that are criminal, suspicious, suicidal, sudden, unexpected, or unexplained. Persons most often involved in these situations include coroners, police surgeons, law enforcement officers, criminalists, and forensic medical specialists. EMS personnel should have a policy that lists all the types of situations that require the notification of law enforcement personnel. They should also have in place protocols for securing, handling, and documenting evidence. Unfortunately, these protocols are often missing from EMS organizations.[2]

INJURIES

In the study of trauma and its forensic application, injuries are often categorized based upon the type of injury or type of weapon inflicting an injury. No matter how they are classified, they all involve damage to body tissue. This chapter discusses injuries based on both aspects. It is important to remember that every injury, no matter how small or seemingly insignificant at the time, should be noted and documented. Often, as in blunt trauma, small external injuries may be the only indicator of more severe internal injuries. It is important to document the wound exactly as it appears on first inspection, as treatment often alters the appearance.

ABRASIONS

Abrasions are superficial injuries involving the epidermis and sometimes a small amount of the dermis. Although the least life-threatening of all wounds, forensically they are often the most informative. They note the precise impact of blunt or sliding forces. Each of us has easily observed this on our knees, elbows, or knuckles. Abrasions may appear along with bruises or lacerations, and they may exhibit patterns, such as tire or radiator marks. It is precisely the fact that abrasions may show patterns that make them so important.[3] Abrasion patterns can often be explained by the object(s) contacting the patient, such as a rope or piece of clothing. For example, on one female victim five circular abrasions were found on her back. These abrasions were formed by hooks on the brassiere she wore when she was pressed against the floor at the time of her death.[1] The direction of force against the skin can be determined by examining the skin. The epidermis is

pulled toward the distal end of the wound and will appear rough and shredded. Abrasions are often particularly important in assaults, homicides, and "hit-and-run" motor vehicle crashes.[3]

BRUISES AND CONTUSIONS

Bruises are the result of a blunt trauma that causes the underlying arterioles and venules to leak blood into the tissues along fascial planes. Therefore, bruises usually do not produce the pattern of the offending object, nor do they necessarily lie at the point of impact as abrasions do. One exception is called **intradermal bruising**, where there is bleeding between the dermis and epidermis. This bruise may show a pattern and is most often seen when the skin is compressed between two objects, such as the tread of a vehicle's tire.[3] Of course, bruises change color with time. They also may change position as they progress, as blood moves within tissue planes. For instance, a bruise on the forehead may become a "black eye" with the passage of time. Forensic pathologists often view bruises at different time intervals to check color and position progression and for the appearance of new bruises. New bruises that were deep at the time of initial injury or death can later become visible on the surface of the skin.[3]

Bruise location can be very significant. Bruising around the neck can often indicate choking, throttling, or strangulation (Figure 31-1). Along the shoulder blades, bruises are often the result of pressure against a hard surface, such as holding a rape victim against a concrete floor. Sexual assault victims may also have bruises on the inner thighs or genitalia. Bruises on the arms are common in physical assaults, such as domestic violence, where grabbing frequently occurs.

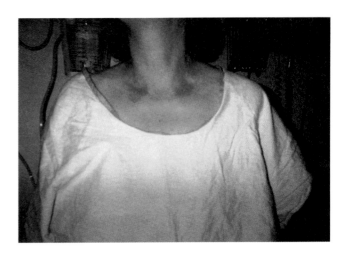

FIGURE 31-1 Bruising of the neck of a victim of strangulation.

Bruises change color with time, but do not do so on a set schedule. In general, bruises progress from red to blue, purple, or black, then to green and yellow. Color change is the result of the breakdown of hemoglobin and the tracking of blood outward toward the skin during hemolysis. The rate at which a bruise changes color varies with each individual, so much so that dating bruises accurately by color is not possible.[3] The young generally recover more quickly from a bruise, whereas the elderly patient may retain a bruise for weeks or months. However, it is possible to compare bruises on one individual at a given time and make some judgment on which bruises are recent and which are older by color, providing that they are of similar severity.[3] In most people, a bruise of red, black, or blue color is recent, usually not more than 1–5 days old. Once again, this can also depend on the depth of the bruise.[1] Also, a bruise that has progressed to a green color cannot be less than 24 hours old.[3]

LACERATIONS AND INCISED WOUNDS

Technically speaking, lacerations are a jagged tearing or splitting of the skin caused by a blunt force, whereas incised wounds are clean-edged wounds caused by sharp objects, such as scalpels, knives, glass, or razors. Lacerations are most common over bony areas where the force of the blunt object sandwiches the skin between the object and the bone, such as the skull, knees, elbows, or extremities. The trauma causes bruising of the edges of the wound and underlying tissues.[3] Lacerations commonly result from falls against concrete, pavement, stairs, furniture, or other hard objects, from motor vehicle injury, or from intentional injury with pistol butts, hammers, fists, stones, shovels, and the like. Lacerations inflicted before death bleed and bruise, whereas those inflicted after death do not bruise and bleed very little.[1]

Incised wounds or sharps injuries can be of the slash or stab type. Slash wounds are longer and less deep than stab wounds, but stab wounds are generally more life threatening. Stab wounds to the chest, where essential life support structures are easily damaged, are the most frequently fatal, followed by those to the neck and abdomen (Figure 31-2).[3]

Stab wounds directed upward are usually homicidal wounds, whereas those directed downward can be either suicidal or homicidal. It is much easier to stab oneself with downward thrusts. Some wounds, such as stab wounds to the back, are inaccessible to the victim and are usually not self-inflicted. Stabbing to the heart area can be either, but homicidal wounds are more often inflicted at a higher point on the chest.[1] Forensic specialists can determine a wealth of information about the type and

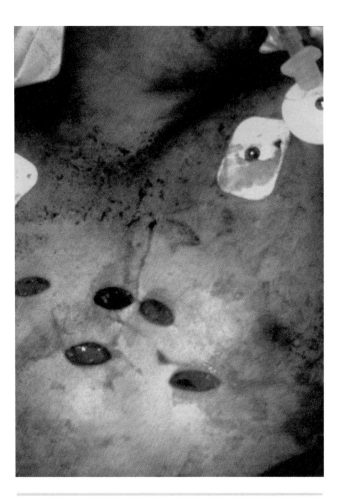

FIGURE 31-2 Appearance of a stab wound. (Courtesy of Deborah Funk, Albany Medical Center, Albany, NY.)

size of a weapon by the characteristics of the stab wound.[4] If the stabbing instrument, such as a knife, is inflicted with force, it is possible for the wound to be deeper than the length of the knife. If the knife is twisted or rocked, the underlying wound may be of greater size or have an irregular shape on the skin. Scissor wounds are most commonly inflicted by women and have a characteristic Z-shape or star diamond shape.[3]

Attempt to leave all stab wounds intact. Do not incorporate them into incisions, drains, or other procedures unless necessary.[5] It is best to describe the wound in detail rather than surmise that you note a "stab wound." Some experts contend that a stab wound is an alleged stab wound, even when a knife is in place.[2]

PUNCHING

Punching another person with clenched fists is common during fights and can result in severe injury. Injuries from punching are most often seen on the upper part of the body. Black eyes, bruises, abrasions, lip and tongue lacerations, loose teeth or tooth avulsions, and fractures of the jaw and nose are frequently seen with fist-inflicted injury. In cases of child abuse, the injuries can be located anywhere, and punches to the abdomen can result in serious injury to the liver, spleen, or intestine.[3]

KICKING

The trauma inflicted with kicking during assault or homicide is often more severe than that seen with punching. This is due to the greater strength of the legs over the arms and the presence of shoes. The victim is often lying on the ground or floor at the time of assault, thereby allowing the assailant to stomp or grind into the victim with full body weight. Frequent sites for kicking assaults are the head, neck, chest, abdomen, and groin. Soft tissue wounds, fractures of the skull, ribs, and sternum, lacerations with heavy bleeding, and abdominal organ injury can result from kicking during assaults.[3]

DEFENSE INJURIES

Persons who find themselves being assaulted by punching, kicking, or knifing usually try to shield or defend themselves. Victims reflexively attempt to protect vital areas of the body: the head, face, neck, chest, abdomen, and perineal area. Victims shield with less vital and more mobile structures: the hands, arms, and legs. The shielding process often produces specific injuries called *defense injuries*. The hands and forearm can be abraded, bruised, or lacerated, and fingers or hands may be fractured in an attempt to protect vital regions. Bruises on the thigh are seen when the victim tries to shield the perineal area by crossing the legs or by turning the back toward the assailant. Knife attacks often result in wounds to the flexor surface of the fingers at the joints and cuts in the web space between the forefinger and thumb.[3]

BITING

The teeth are able to survive the body's total decomposition because they are the hardest, toughest structure in the human body. The teeth can survive even fire and high heat and thus are often used to identify the deceased. High-impact crashes, such as airline disasters, frequently leave few remains of the crew and passengers, leaving forensic odontologists to identify the dead based on teeth and dental records. The teeth, along with dental records, serve as a fingerprint of sorts because every individual has a unique set of teeth and subsequent dental intervention. The teeth can also be

used to help identify the age, sex, and race of an individual and are sometimes used in living persons to identify age for immigration and adoption.[3]

Because of the strength of the teeth and power of the jaw, teeth can become a weapon. Teeth marks and saliva left from a biting injury can be used in criminal investigation to identify an offender. Defensive bite marks of the victim can also be identified on an assailant. Bite mark evidence has been used for over a century. Nowhere in the United States has bite mark evidence been inadmissible in court.[6]

Bite mark patterns may be left in food, skin, or other soft objects, on the victim or the assailant. The most commonly bitten areas are the nose, nipples, ears, neck, breasts, and thighs, although bite marks may be found anywhere on the body. Thigh, breast, and head bite marks are often the result of sexual assault. Unlike using teeth for identification, which can often be done with a high degree of certainty, bite marks can only be used to give a *reasonable probability* of the identity of the person inflicting the bite mark.[3,7]

Research has shown that social workers who receive bite mark detection training significantly increase the number of reports of this type of injury (associated with abuse), yet most paramedics and emergency health care workers have never received such training.[8] It is easy to mistake other pattern injuries to the skin with bite marks, and if they are suspected, an expert in forensic odontology or criminology should be notified. It is recommended that not even a forensic pathologist handle bite mark analysis, but that it be done by a bite mark expert. Animal bites are easily distinguished from human bites due to the differences in tooth and jaw structure.[7] Pattern injuries that resemble bite marks are listed in Table 31-1.

In addition to bite mark patterns, evidence can be obtained from saliva that is left during the biting process. Eighty-five percent of the human population secrete a saliva substance (these persons are called

| **Table 31-1** |
| **Causes of Injuries Resembling Bite Marks** |
| ECG and defibrillator pads |
| Pebbles, gravel, seashells |
| Postmortem insect activity |
| Resuscitation trauma |
| Watchbands, rings, bracelets, and other jewelry |
| Clothing |
| Belt buckles |
| Shoe heels |

secretors) that contains the concentrated blood group proteins A, B, and O.[7] Saliva samples should be collected before wounds are cleansed and as soon as possible because saliva breaks down rapidly. Avoid areas that are contaminated with the victim's blood, and be sure to take samples from the victim's skin for a control. Salivary swabs must be air dried.[6,7]

Photographs are also used to preserve evidence of bite marks and are best done by those with forensic training. However, there is no reason why paramedics cannot photograph them too, especially if time only permits pictures to be taken by EMS personnel before wounds are treated or cleansed. First photograph without a scale, then shoot another photograph with a ruler or scale; be careful not to cover evidence. Photographs are best done by a four-by-five-inch camera (although 35-mm or Polaroid cameras are sometimes used) and can be taken in both black and white and color. Black-and-white photographs show more detail, but color photographs taken over several days show progression of the bite mark. The American Board of Forensic Odontology (ABFO) has established scales to be used in photographing bite mark evidence. The ABFO scales photograph well; some scales do not. Retain any scale used so that its accuracy can be verified in court.[6] Paramedics should have written protocols to handle bite mark evidence in order to ensure that the evidence is handled and preserved in the best possible way. If you frequently care for victims of abuse or violence, encourage your employer to provide forensic training or assistance.

GUNSHOT WOUNDS

Firearm fatalities increased by about 25% from 1985 to 1995 in the United States.[9] These grim statistics make it likely that the paramedic will care for many victims of gunshot injuries. The large amount of kinetic energy transferred to body tissues causes firearm injuries.[3] *Ballistics* is the term for the science of the firing characteristics of firearms.[5]

There are two types of firearms: (1) smooth-bore weapons, or shotguns and sporting guns, and (2) rifled weapons, which include revolvers, automatic pistols, rifles, and many kinds of military weapons. Shotguns are designed for use from 30 to 50 meters and are not likely to kill at distant ranges.[3] They fire a large number of small lead pellets that spread in a cone shape upon leaving the barrel.[5] Shotguns are sometimes illegally shortened and called "sawn-off" or "sawed-off" shotguns. Shotgun cartridges consist of a metal base beneath a plastic tube, the tube being filled with propellant charge and topped with a plastic cap called the wad. Shotgun wounds are affected by the hot gas, flame, smoke, propellant, wad, and shot, and their appearance is a result of the distance between these items and the victim. The farther the victim is from the firearm blast, the larger the wound pattern will be.[3]

At contact, a shotgun entrance wound causes blackening inside the tissues and possible pink coloring around the site from carbon monoxide gas discharge. The wound will be round unless over bone, which produces a ragged appearance. Close to medium ranges (near skin to 1 meter) cause burning of the skin, and the wads will be located in the wound. Powder tattooing from burning flakes of propellant may be seen on the skin. At longer ranges (2–3 meters) the wound will be surrounded by smaller pellet holes, and at farther distances there is solely uniform peppering of shot (rarely fatal).[3]

Rifled weapons fire one projectile through a spiral grooved barrel, which creates a gyroscopic spin on the bullet, helping to maintain an accurate trajectory. Most rifled weapons have mechanisms to automatically reload another bullet into the firing chamber. There are numerous types of bullet designs, including air tips, which distort the bullet on impact, and explosive tips, which explode on impact.

Contact entrance wounds from rifled weapons are round but, like shotgun wounds, may be irregular if impacted over bony areas. There may be a muzzle mark, burning, redness, or bruising around the wound (Figure 31-3). At close range (20 cm) there will be a circular or oval hole with 1–2 mm of abrasion around the edge, perhaps some smoke and powder burns, and bruising. However, the extent of these characteristics is dependent on the type of weapon and ammunition. At long ranges there will not be burning, smoke soiling, or powder tattooing, and the bullet may even strike sideways, leaving a linear entrance wound.[3]

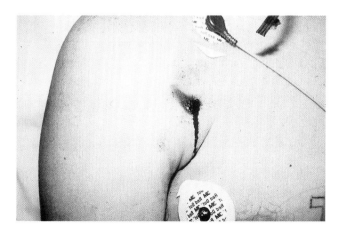

FIGURE 31-3 An entrance wound typically is identified by its round or oval shape and the narrow (1–2 mm) area of abrasion and burns from the weapon. (Courtesy of Deborah Funk, Albany Medical Center, Albany, NY.)

Bullet exit wounds are usually everted and often have a ragged slitlike appearance (Figure 31-4). They are frequently larger than entrance wounds, but not always. Tight clothing, belts, brassieres, or the victim being pressed against a wall or firm surface may leave an exit wound that is not everted and is as small as the entrance wound.[5] Table 31-2 lists some causes of variations in bullet exit wounds. It is also possible to have more than one exit wound per entrance wound. This can result from fragmentation of the bullet in the body, the splintering of bone causing bone to be shot out through the body, or two bullets entering at the same point but leaving at different points.[4] Frequently there is no exit wound at all because the bullet's energy is completely dissipated while still in the body. When bullets hit solid organs, such as the liver, heart, kidneys, or bone, the organs themselves may splinter and form new projectiles.[5]

Distinguishing between entrance and exit wounds is critical to future legal proceedings. However, unless you are an expert in examining these injuries, it is best

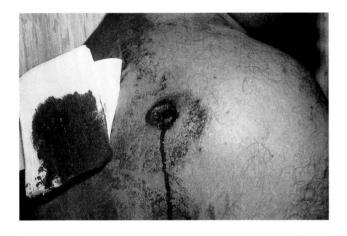

FIGURE 31-4 Exit wounds are typically slitlike, stellate, or irregular in shape. (Courtesy of Deborah Funk, Albany Medical Center, Albany, NY.)

Table 31-2
Causes of Variations in Bullet Exit Wounds

Velocity of the bullet on exit

Surface area of the bullet on exit

Deformation of the missile

Yawing and tumbling of the bullet

Fragmentation of the bullet

Bone fragments

Objects pressing against the skin (e.g., car seat, wall, chair)

not to speculate or call any particular wound an "entrance" or "exit" wound. Research has shown that emergency physicians and trauma surgeons misinterpret and confuse entrance and exit wounds a high percentage of the time.[10] This is particularly true in multiple gunshot victims. It is better to describe the wounds rather than identify them as "entrance" or "exit" wounds. Documentation should include the dimensions of the wound, its location, and the presence of powder, soot, bruises, redness, or other characteristics.[10] Drawings and photography supplement documentation. If the wounds must be cleaned before photographs can be made, then document/draw the wound's appearance before the cleansing process.[5]

If a bullet is recovered, surgically or otherwise, place it in a paper envelope. Never place it in plastic or formalin or clean the bullet. This can destroy evidence. Avoid contact of the bullet with metal objects when recovering them. The contact can mar the bullet's longitudinal markings for ballistics examination, which links the bullet to a specific gun.[4,5,11]

The clothing of firearm victims can also contain valuable evidence. Fibers may be carried into the wound. Chemical markings in the clothing can give information about the range of the gunfire. Smoke, fire, and powder residues may be embedded in clothing.[4] When removing garments, avoid cutting through bullet holes and their surrounding area to prevent destruction of evidence. Always keep articles of the victim's clothing for law enforcement personnel.

Never assume that any two bullet holes are matched, for example, two shoulder and two hip wounds. It is possible that a bullet could have entered the hip and exited the shoulder and the other entered the shoulder and exited the hip, rather than entering and exiting at the two closest points. The paramedic should assume the worst trajectory, then assess and prepare accordingly.[10]

Do not assume that any firearm injury is a suicide or homicide. Although there are some general guidelines the paramedic may be familiar with (such as a weapon in arm's reach is a *suicide*; the presence of multiple wounds is a *homicide*),[3] there are exceptions to every rule. Therefore, leave these determinations to the forensic specialist.

EXPLOSIVE DEVICES

The magnitude of what was once reserved for military warfare has now spread to the civilian population, and therefore the paramedic may one day be faced with responding to this type of incident. The release of high levels of energy from explosives can cause injury and destruction over a wide area. (See Chapter 5 for the injuries produced by explosives.) Evidence is often scattered over a wide area, making investigation for law enforcement difficult.[3] Often the paramedic will be searching for small remains of bodies for identification, particularly teeth and parts of bone containing teeth.

ASPHYXIA

Asphyxia is a general term to describe a variety of conditions in which oxygen and carbon dioxide fail to undergo adequate exchange. This can be accomplished four ways: (1) compression of the neck, such as hanging or "throttling," which means to choke or strangle; (2) obstruction of the airway, as in smothering, in aspiration, or following a blow to the neck; (3) compression of the chest preventing air exchange; and (4) exclusion of oxygen, such as carbon dioxide poisoning, carbon monoxide poisoning, or cyanide poisoning.[7]

In any of these cases death may be slow, causing cyanosis, congestion, and petechiae, or be rapidly fatal, leaving a pale-colored facial skin. Manual strangulation is a common means of homicide in male sexual attacks against women and children but is rare in male-versus-male attacks due to the disparity in physical strength and size required. There may be bruises, abrasions, and fingernail marks around the neck of the victim.[3]

MOTOR VEHICLES AND PEDESTRIANS

Paramedics treat pedestrian victims of hit-and-run crashes. Motor vehicle crashes can also involve suicide or homicide. Care should be taken to preserve any evidence left at the scene. Save all clothing. The victim should be undressed on a clean sheet when possible, leaving the clothing in the folded sheet for evidence. Clothing can contain tire impressions and vehicular debris. That same clothing may leave fibers on the vehicle when it is torn or ripped, so carefully note the locations of damaged clothing.[5]

EVIDENCE PRESERVATION

Physical evidence includes any object, no matter how small, that places or connects the perpetrator to the crime scene.[12] The classic dilemma facing prehospital care providers is treating the patient while simultaneously collecting and preserving key evidence. Neither law enforcement nor health care personnel have found an acceptable way to preserve evidence from crimes discovered well after the patient has been treated. In other cases, advanced planning and protocols can make a significant difference.[13] As the first person on the scene of a medicolegal situation, your actions can "make or break" a law enforcement investigation. With a bit of foresight the paramedic can save

critical pieces of evidence without compromising patient care.[14] Remember that how the evidence is collected is just as important as what is collected.[4]

No one expects the paramedic to be a criminologist or forensic pathologist. However, it is the paramedic's responsibility as a health care professional to be familiar with basic tenets of collecting and preserving evidence. Each case is unique, and the individual circumstances will influence the actions you take. Follow these basic guidelines:

1. Law enforcement subscribes to the *transfer theory*, that is, everyone who enters the scene leaves something at the scene, and everyone at the scene takes something with them when they leave.[12] The paramedic should enter and leave the scene as directed by law enforcement officials and in as narrow a path as possible. Keep personnel to a minimum. Confine the crime scene as much as possible, and limit what is touched. Do not use the phone at the scene or house; the last call made is often traceable. Do not use the water, sinks, or drains because they often contain trace evidence.[12]

2. Observe and document the patient's appearance and behavior.[4] Note body position. The position of the victim furnishes important clues about what happened.[12]

3. Try to remove the victim's clothing without cutting it off. If you must cut the clothes, then follow it seams if possible. Do not cut into or through bullet or knife wounds or through rips and tears that already exist. The characteristics of tears and holes give police information about the size and type of weapon. Remember, too, that clothing can alter the appearance of wounds.[4]

4. Avoid touching and washing in a "sea of wound cleansing liquid" soot, gunshot residue, blood splatters, or other debris.[14] Gunshot residue examinations are done on hands and weapons. The residue test is very sensitive, and evidence is easily destroyed. If a weapon is in a victim's hand, avoid using that hand or washing it until law enforcement can collect evidence. If a weapon must be moved, carefully do so, noting where it is located and in what position relative to the victim and other objects. Weapon location is very important in distinguishing a homicide from a suicide.[12] Allow law enforcement personnel to photograph the victim before cleansing if possible, and if not, then document the patient's appearance before treatment begins. Remember that the police may need the patient's consent before photographing or searching, depending on the circumstances.[14]

5. Be especially careful with knife and gunshot wounds. These wounds are often the only evidence of the weapon used, bullet or blade trajectory, and any evidence lying between the bullet or knife and the assailant or victim. Once again, *if possible,* allow the police to photograph before injuries are treated. However, do not delay life-saving treatment for photographs.

6. Save all clothing, medicine, and other objects no matter how trivial they seem initially.[12]

7. Depending on the circumstances, photographs may be taken of a wound with a ruler or scale beneath it before treatment begins. This can document valuable evidence.

8. Carefully document all procedures, especially invasive sites, such as intravenous attempts, even if unsuccessful. This helps the medical examiner or other expert to determine which wounds resulted from the crime and which from medical intervention. Mark any surgical incisions you must make into a wound site, such as a chest tube into a knife wound, with ink or sutures and document carefully. If the patient dies, leave all tubing and lines intact.[4]

9. Place paper bags on hands, feet, or head as appropriate to preserve trace evidence.[4] Gunshot powder or residue and skin or hair fibers are often found under the nails, so avoid cleansing them if possible. Secure the paper bags with tape or rubber bands. Do not use plastic bags because the trapped moisture causes bacterial and fungal growth, which causes evidence to dissolve.[5]

10. Clothing should be placed in separate paper bags. It may be necessary to enclose it in an unclosed plastic bag to comply with universal precautions (or body substance isolation), but do so only for the brief period needed to turn the clothing over to law enforcement officials. Eventually, all bloody clothing should be air dried out of direct sunlight and over a paper liner. Air drying of body fluids is important because it prevents decomposition, allowing blood typing and DNA testing. The liner is also saved to collect trace evidence dropped from the clothing. Evidence from clothing is often as important as the evidence acquired from wounds themselves.[4,5]

11. Place any bullets, fibers, or other objects in separate paper envelopes. The same applies to broken fingernails, glass fragments, and paint chips. Fingernails can be used to determine race, sex, and ABO blood group. The striations are unique to each individual, making them a valuable piece of evidence. Glass fragments can often be matched to headlights, windows, or mirrors. Paint chips are also traceable to specific vehicles. Do not handle bullets with metal objects such as forceps because they may mar the identifying surface. Use a gloved hand. Sharps should be enclosed in cardboard containers or placed in paper envelopes and then into cardboard.[4,5]

12. Do not leave friends or family members alone with the patient or body. This ensures that none of the evidence is altered while the patient is in your care.

13. Do not manipulate the patient's body any more than necessary. Handle all evidence with clean gloves, especially blood and tissue. This prevents the transfer of ABO factors to the evidence by those of us who are ABO secretors.[4]

14. When collecting a saliva sample, allow it to air dry, then seal it in a paper envelope.

15. If hanging is the mechanism of injury, do not cut through any part of the knot or close to it. The type of ligature provides important clues to law enforcement.[12]

16. Collaborate with local law enforcement agencies to establish on-scene evidence collection and preservation protocols.

CHAIN OF CUSTODY

The best efforts at collecting evidence can be for naught if the chain of custody is broken. The chain of custody is the pathway the evidence travels from the time it is collected until it is "booked" by law enforcement officials. Establishing a chain of custody is also called authenticating the evidence or laying a proper foundation for admission into court.[11]

Of course, common sense tells us the fewer transfers of evidence the better and that once collected, evidence should remain in the possession of the collector. Each transfer must be well documented. All items and specimens should be put in separate containers and sealed. Each piece of evidence must be labeled with the patient's name, the identification number assigned to each patient (or prehospital care report number), the item enclosed, the date and time of enclosure and transfer, the signature of the person releasing, and the signature of the person receiving. Establishing a written log which contains this information can also be helpful.[4,5] Organizational protocols, particularly when prepared in cooperation with local law enforcement departments, are extremely valuable in facilitating an unbroken chain of evidence.

DOCUMENTATION

Although not as exciting as collecting and preserving forensic evidence, EMS documentation is definitely as important. The EMS report is critical and is often brought into court as evidence. The paramedic is often called as a witness or as part of the chain of evidence. Paramedics frequently render the first treatment and stabilization to the patient; therefore their documentation is critical. At least one study found that prehospital providers often fail to provide a general statement of the victim's appearance and condition upon arrival to the scene.[2] They also frequently fail to document the mechanism of injury or do so incompletely. Other studies have shown the existence of a widespread lack of adequate forensic documentation.[5,10] The following is a list of suggestions to improve the quality of the documentation:

1. Include a descriptive note on the initial general appearance of the victim(s), including body position. Body diagrams may be helpful. Be sure to include the patient's behavior.

2. Use objective, descriptive terminology. Avoid such labels as "entrance" "or exit" wound, "drunk," or "problem patient." Instead document such things as "puncture wound with tattooing" or "breath smelling of alcohol." You may have to defend yourself in court over which is an entrance wound and which an exit wound. Do not label wounds unless you are prepared for legal scrutiny.[2]

3. Write legibly. If you have to interpret your notes in court, you will need to be able to read them.

4. Include the mechanism of injury if possible, and completely document the chain of custody.

5. Note any care that is rendered before your arrival, such as first-responder care.

6. Record the use, or lack thereof, of helmets or restraint devices.

7. Keep a record of the disposition of the patient and who received the patient from you. Be sure to note the condition of the patient at final disposition.[5]

8. Carefully describe wounds, noting precise location and characteristics such as soot, powder, or bruising.[10] Document all bruises, no matter how small or seemingly insignificant.[14]

9. If the patient is wearing clothing that is on "inside out," make a note of this fact.[4]

10. Carefully and completely document the care you give. Include all interventions such as failed intravenous punctures or finger-stick blood glucose sites.

11. Note your point of entry to the crime scene, your path through the scene, your contact with the scene, and your place of exit. Tire and foot impressions are often crucial pieces of evidence and must not be confused with or covered by medical or legal personnel as they enter and leave the crime scene.[12]

12. Make sure the EMS call report includes the date and time of the dispatched call; scene arrival time; location of the ambulance at the scene as well as its entrance and exit paths; and destination of the ambulance or where the patient was taken for further medical treatment.[12]

13. Note any clothes or valuable items that are given to family or medical team members.[12]

PHOTOGRAPHY

A picture is worth a thousand words. True to the old saying, photographs can add powerful detail and force to your documentation. As a supplement to written words, they can also serve as valuable evidence during legal proceedings, effectively saving evidence that may otherwise be destroyed or changed. Failure to photograph evidence can sometimes ruin a victim's chances in court.[15]

Establish a written policy to ensure that the pictures are admissible for court proceedings and that all patient consent issues are treated properly. Consult with law enforcement personnel to establish how photographs will become an official part of the patient's legal record and therefore admissible in court. Permission is usually needed to photograph a patient's injuries. Written consent as well as the date, patient's name, photographer's name, your organization's name, patient's signature, and the signature of a witness are the basic items required. Any limitations to the photograph, such as not showing the face, should also be included.[15]

The minimum equipment needed is an instant camera with close-up attachments.[15] Thirty-five millimeter cameras can also be used.[6] Scales are often placed in a photograph to document size. When using a scale, photograph the evidence without the scale first, then with the scale; lawyers have argued successfully in court that the ruler contaminated or destroyed evidence.[12] Often it is best to call police photographers to take expert photographs. If you must take the photographs, take the best pictures you can. There have been many legal cases won based on the worst photographs. Photographs provide a large amount of information instantly, whereas it takes a lot of documentation to describe the injuries of a multiple stab victim.[15]

INTERNET ACTIVITIES

Find the Web site for the International Association of Forensic Nurses at www.forensicnurse.org and discover links to other forensic Web sites.

SUMMARY

If you are interested in learning more, the International Association of Forensic Nurses (IAFN) has established the Council of EMT/Paramedic Forensic Specialists. The council is concerned with educating EMS providers in the recognition, preservation, and collection of evidence and with assisting EMS organizations to develop forensic protocols. The council is also interested in working with the U.S. Department of Transportation to include forensic medicine in the EMT curriculum.[16] Anyone interested in further information can contact the IAFN at East Holly Avenue, Box 56, Pitman, NJ 08071-0056 (phone: 856-256-2425) or the Clinical Forensic Consultants at P.O. Box 892723, Oklahoma City, OK 73189-2723.

REVIEW QUESTIONS

1. Which type of injury often provides the most clinical forensic information?
   a. Bruises
   b. Abrasions
   c. Lacerations

2. Intradermal bruising is:
   a. Bruising in the dermis
   b. Bleeding between the dermis and the epidermis
   c. A bruise pattern

3. Bruises change color with time and it can be accurately determined by color exactly how old a bruise is.
   a. True
   b. False

4. If saliva is obtained from a bite wound and forensically tested, the saliva will always show the blood type of the perpetrator.
   a. True
   b. False

5. Name five actions the paramedic can take to preserve evidence.

6. Name five ways to improve documentation in forensic cases.

CRITICAL THINKING

● You are dispatched to the scene of an assault. Upon arrival, you discover your patient sitting in the back of the police cruiser. She has a large hematoma to the left temple and abrasions on her wrists. She states that she was sexually assaulted about an hour ago. How will you manage the physical and emotional needs of this patient? How will you examine this patient? What steps will you take to preserve evidence?

● Develop a plan for taking photographs at trauma scenes such as motor vehicle collisions and gunshot wounds. How can this be accomplished without interfering with patient care?

REFERENCES

1. Polson CJ, Gee DJ. *The Essentials of Forensic Medicine*, 3rd ed. Oxford: Pergamon Press; 1973.
2. Carmona R, Prince K. Trauma and forensic medicine. *J Trauma*. 1989; 29:1222.
3. Knight B. *Simpson's Forensic Medicine*, 10th ed. London: Edward Arnold; 1991.
4. Meserve KL. Preserving medicolegal evidence: a guide for emergency care providers. *J Emerg Nurs*. 1992; 18:120.
5. Schramm CA. Forensic medicine: what the perioperative nurse needs to know. *AORN J*. 1991; 53:669.
6. Johnson LT, Cadle D. Bite mark evidence: recognition, preservation, analysis, and courtroom presentation. *NY State Dent J*. 1989; 3:38.
7. Spitz WU. *Spitz and Fisher's Medicolegal Investigation of Death*, 3rd ed. Springfield, Ill: Charles C. Thomas; 1993.
8. Malestic SL. Fight violence with forensic evidence. *RN*. 1995; 1:30.
9. www.cdc.gov/nchs/fastats/firearms.htm. Hyattsville, Md.: National Center for Health Statistics (NCHS); 1994.
10. Randall T. Clinicians' forensic interpretations of fatal gunshot wounds often miss the mark. *JAMA*. 1993; 269:2058.
11. Mittleman RE, Goldberg HS, Waksman DM. Preserving evidence in the emergency department. *Am J Nurs*. 1983; 83:1652.
12. Tulley P. Lecture at the Emergency Medicine Today '97 Conference; September 30, 1997; Greensboro, N.C.
13. Lynch VA. Forensic nursing in the emergency department: a new role for the 1990s. *Crit Care Nurs Q*. 1991; 14:69.
14. Descheneaux K. Death investigations: how you can help. *Nursing*. 1991; 9:52.
15. Pasqualone GA. The importance of forensic photography in the emergency department. *J Emerg Nurs*. 1995; 2:566.
16. Rooms R. New council formed: council of EMT/paramedic specialists. *On the Edge, IAFN Newsletter*. 1995; 1(2):4.

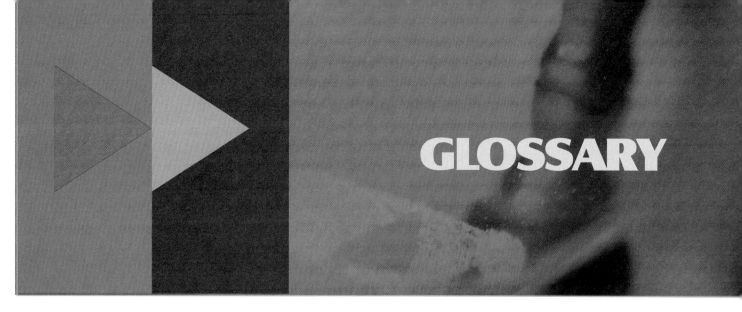

Abbreviated Injury Scale (AIS) An assessment tool that rates injuries numerically by body region affected.

Abruptio placentae Separation of the placenta from the uterine wall.

Accident An unexpected event that occurs by chance.

Active intervention Method of protecting an individual when the individual plays a part in protecting him- or herself.

Acute stress disorder The response of the body to a traumatic experience similar to PTSD but not as severe; symptoms usually occur within a month after the event and last less than a month.

Acute stress reaction The body's response immediately following an incident; usually occurs within 24 hours.

Adult respiratory distress syndrome Condition following trauma that prevents the lungs from carrying out proper gas exchange.

Aerophagia Swallowing of air.

Afterload The amount of resistance that the heart must overcome to eject fluid from the ventricle.

Air embolism An air bubble traveling through the circulatory system.

Albumin A biological protein derived from human blood.

Anisocoria Unequal pupils.

Anterior branch A branch of the spinal nerves that innervates the front and sides of the trunk and limbs.

Anterior cord syndrome Pressure on the anterior portion of the spinal cord or damage to the anterior artery resulting from hyperextension injury.

Aortic disruption An injury resulting in shearing of the aorta from the supporting vessels.

Arterial blood pressure (BP) The pressure of fluid found within the arterial side of the circulation.

Ascending tract The communication pathway in the spinal cord that conducts sensory information to the brain.

Assist control ventilation (ACV) Ventilation that provides a patient with a set respiratory rate and ensures that tidal volume is delivered with each spontaneous breath.

Atlas The cervical vertebra that supports and balances the head.

Autotransfusion Reuse of one's own blood as replacement for blood loss.

Axial loading Spinal compression as the result of forces transmitted directly through the spinal column.

Axis The cervical vertebra that allows the head to pivot.

Barotitis media An increase in pressure in the middle ear.

Basilar skull fracture An injury to the brain that is usually open, with damage extending into the cranial vault.

Beck's triad The classic presentation of cardiac tamponade: increased venous pressure, decreased arterial pressure, and muffled heart tones.

Bernoulli's law As the speed of a fluid increases, the pressure exerted by the fluid decreases.

Biophysics The study of physical laws applied to biological problems.

Blast wave An impulse of extreme pressure that radiates from the epicenter of the blast.

Blunt trauma A nonpenetrating injury that occurs as the result of forces being applied to the body.

Body The portion of the stomach that is long and curving; most food contents lie here during digestion.

Boyle's law The volume of gas is inversely related to its pressure at a constant temperature.

Brain An organ within the central nervous system that is divided into three sections: the cerebrum, cerebellum, and brain stem.

Brain stem The part of the brain consisting of the midbrain, pons, and medulla that is responsible for lower brain functions.

Brown-Sequard's syndrome A rarely occurring partial cord lesion that involves half of the spinal cord.

Bulk packaging A container of 119 gallons or more of liquids, 882 pounds or more of solids, 1,000 pounds or more of water capacity for gases.

Burn shock A type of hypovolemic shock in which smaller components of blood are lost from the vascular space.

Capnography A waveform measurement of the partial pressure of carbon dioxide in a gas sample.

Cardia The portion of the stomach surrounding the gatroesophageal junction.

Cardiac output (CO) The volume of blood pumped by the heart in 1 minute.

Cardiac tamponade A penetrating injury to the heart resulting in excessive fluid in the pericardial sac, causing compression of the heart and decreased cardiac output.

Category-specific rate A rate presented for a specific group.

Cauda equina The descending spinal nerves; called the horse's tail.

Cecum A small sac from which the appendix forms that functions to maintain fluid and electrolyte balance.

Cellular immune response Activation of the immune system in response to the production of cytotoxic T cells.

Cellular rejection The destruction of transplanted organs as a result of cellular immune response.

Cellular respiration The transfer of gases between the red blood cells and body tissues.

Central cord syndrome Pressure or damage to the central portion of the spinal cord resulting from hyperextension and flexion injuries.

Central herniation syndrome An injury to the brain that occurs when a lesion in one of the spaces displaces both cerebral hemispheres, pushing them downward toward the tentorial notch.

Cerebellum The part of the brain responsible for subconscious fine tuning of skeletal musculature.

Cerebral laceration Injury to the brain's surface caused by rotational injury.

Cerebral perfusion pressure The level of the blood that is transported through the brain; can be calculated by subtracting the mean arterial pressure from the mean intracranial pressure.

Cerebrum A portion of the brain that is divided into two hemispheres and serves to process information entering and leaving the brain.

Cervical vertebrae Bones of the spinal column that consist of the atlas, which supports and balances the head, and the axis, which allows the head to pivot around a point.

Ciliary body A structure within the iris made up of ligaments and muscles that attach the lens to the eye.

Circumferential burn A burn that completely surrounds a body part.

Clinical forensic medicine Examination and discovery of evidence in a crime when the victim is living.

Coccyx The bones found in the lowest part of the vertebral column.

Colles' fracture A break involving the distal radius.

Colloid solutions Large-molecule compounds that act primarily in the intravascular space by drawing fluid from both the intracellular and interstitial spaces into the bloodstream.

Colon The organ that makes up the majority of the large intestine and that functions to maintain fluid and electrolyte balance.

Coma A failure of arousal.

Combitube An airway adjunct with a double lumen, double balloon system, similar to the PTLA.

Commotio cordis An injury following sudden blunt force to the anterior chest wall that causes a sudden change in cardiac function and rhythm such as ventricular fibrillation and cardiogenic shock.

Compartment syndrome An injury characterized by increasing tissue pressure that compromises circulation and neuromuscular function.

Complete lesions An injury to the spine usually resulting from a fracture or dislocation in which the spinal cord is fully transected.

Compression A change in dimension related to forces being applied to tissue in a manner in which the tissue's density is increased or the tissue's volume is decreased.

Concussion The mildest form of diffuse brain trauma resulting in temporary disruption of normal neurological function without structural damage to the brain.

Conduction Heat loss as a result of energy transfer by direct contact from a warmer object to a colder one.

Contractility The heart's ability to forcibly contract, or shorten its muscle fibers, to eject blood.

Controlled mandatory ventilation (CMV) Ventilation that delivers a preset tidal volume at a time-triggered respiratory rate.

Contusion The mildest form of focal brain injury, indistinguishable from a concussion.

Convection Heat loss as a result of currents of air or water transferring heat away from the body.

Corium The second layer of skin composed of collagen and fibrous tissue; also known as the dermis.

Cornea The thin transparent surface covering the sclera.

Coup/contrecoup The ability of the brain to recoil and strike the skull at a point opposite the initial impact point; this is due to the mobility of the brain within the skull.

Coxae The hipbone.

CRAMS score An assessment tool that combines scores from physiological, historical, and anatomical variables to pinpoint severity of injury based upon circulation, respiration, and abdominal, motor, and speech function.

Cricothyrotomy An opening established in the trachea at the level of the cricothyroid membrane to allow for ventilation.

Crisis The situation that occurs when stressors push an individual beyond the normal range of his or her coping mechanisms.

Critical incident Any significant emotional event that has the power to cause distress in healthy, normal people.

Critical incident stress debriefing (CISD) A structured group process utilizing both crisis intervention and educational techniques to lessen the effects of a traumatic event.

Critical incident stress management (CISM) An intervention to help people deal with the stress of a critical incident.

Crude rate A rate presented for an entire population.

Crush injury A type of extremity trauma resulting from continuous and prolonged pressures on the limb.

Crush syndrome Multiple systemic complications of soft tissue injury and the disruption of muscle integrity.

Crystalloid solutions A balanced salt product used for volume resuscitation.

Cullen's sign Periumbilical ecchymosis.

Cumulative stress The body's response to stressors that occur over time due to numerous exposures.

CUPS classification system A method used to assign priority to patients: critical, unstable, potentially unstable, stable.

Cushing's triad Increased blood pressure, decreased pulse, and irregular respirations exhibited when intracranial pressure increases.

Dalton's law The partial pressure of a gas decreases as altitude increases.

Decerebrate Rigid extension of the arms and legs; the back and neck may also be arched.

Decorticate Rigid flexion of the arms and extension of the legs.

Deep cervical fascia The muscle layers that support the structures of the neck.

Definitive decontamination The final washing and rinsing to assure no contaminants remain on the body.

Defusing A short, less formal, less structured critical incident stress debriefing.

Demobilization An intervention that serves to allow a period of transition between the traumatic event and return to routine duty or home.

Depressed skull fracture An injury to the brain with underlying intracranial hematoma.

Dermatomes Areas of the skin in which sensory nerve fibers of a particular spinal nerve innervate.

Dermis The second layer of skin composed of collagen and fibrous tissue; also known as the corium.

Descending tract The communication pathway of the spinal cord that conducts motor impulses to motor neurons that extend to muscles and glands.

Dextran A synthetic glucose polymer used to expand intravascular blood volume by shifting fluid from the interstitial and intracellular spaces into the vascular space.

Diagnostic peritoneal lavage (DPL) A minimally invasive surgical procedure used to detect abdominal trauma in the emergency room.

Diplopia Double vision.

Disseminated intravascular coagulation (DIC) A generalized activation of the body's clotting mechanism in which coagulation and fibrinolysis become unbalanced.

Dorsal root A branch of the spinal nerves that is responsible for sensory function.

Down-and-under pathway The mechanism of injury in a frontal collision whereby the occupant may move forward while sliding under the steering wheel and impacting the floor and the dashboard with the feet and knees.

Duodenum A C-shaped portion of the small intestine that manufactures enzymes and receives bile from the gall bladder.

Dural sinuses Collecting areas for venous blood from the brain that are found in the folds of the dura mater.

Early death Victims who die as a result of their injuries within a few hours of injury.

Electron transport Cellular metabolism in which molecules produced in glycosis and the Krebs cycle react with oxygen molecules to produce energy.

Emergency technical decontamination Decontamination of a responder who has collapsed while on scene.

EMS/HM Level I An EMT trained in providing patient care in the cold zone of a hazardous materials incident.

EMS/HM Level II An EMT trained to provide patient care in the warm zone of a hazardous materials incident.

Enophthalmos Recession of the globe into the orbit of the eye.

Epidemiology The study of the distribution and causal factors of injury (and disease) in human populations.

Epidermis The outer layer of skin composed of five cellular layers: stratum corneum, stratum lucidum, stratum granulosum, stratum sponsor, and stratum germinativum.

Epidural hematoma A collection of blood between the skull and the dura mater.

Epidural space The space between the dura mater and the skull that contains the middle meningeal arteries.

Epistaxis Nosebleed.

Equity The fairness or justness of an intervention.

Esophageal gastric tube airway (EGTA) An airway adjunct that resembles an elongated cuffed endotrachial tube with a tube that passes into the stomach to aid in gastric decompression.

Esophageal obturator airway (EOA) An airway adjunct that resembles an elongated cuffed endotrachial tube with perforations in the proximal one-third of the tube.

Evaporation Heat loss as a result of perspiration and respiration absorbed by drier air.

Event phase The period in the injury process when forms of energy (kinetic, chemical, electrical, thermal, or radiation) are transferred to body tissues.

Expiratory center Respiratory control center in the nervous system that synchronizes with the inspiratory center to produce forceful inhalation and exhalation in times of respiratory distress.

Facial nerve The cranial nerve responsible for control of facial musculature, lacrimination, and salivation.

Falx cerebri A double-layered vertical projection of dura mater from the superior portion of the skull that separates the two cerebral hemispheres of the brain.

Fascia A tough, inelastic membranous connective tissue.

Fetomaternal hemorrhage The transplacental transfusion of fetal blood into the maternal circulation.

Fick principle The amount of a substance taken up by an organ is the product of the blood flow to the organ and the difference in concentrations of the substance in the precapillary and postcapillary beds.

Fight or flight The body's response to a threat by either standing ground or running from harm.

First-degree burn A burn injury in which only the epidermis has been damaged; also known as a partial-thickness burn.

Flail chest An injury to the chest wall characterized by a segment of ribs becoming detached from the remainder of the chest wall and moving freely and paradoxically.

Forensic pathology Examination and discovery of evidence in a crime when the victim is deceased.

Forensic toxicology Examination and discovery of evidence in a crime related to poisons and chemicals on the body.

Fracture A break in bone or cartilage

Full-thickness burn A burn injury that involves the subcutaneous tissue and may involve muscle and bone; also known as a third-degree burn.

Fundus The portion of the stomach superior to the cardia.

Galea aponeurotica A tough fibrous sheet spanning the cranium and connecting the frontalis muscles over the forehead with the occipital muscles at the back of the skull.

Galeazzi's fracture A radioulnar joint dislocation.

Gallbladder A pear-shaped organ that functions as a repository for bile until the bile is needed in the duodenum to process fatty materials.

Gamow bag A portable hyperbaric chamber used for temporary decompression.

Glasgow Coma Scale (GCS) An assessment tool that provides a quantitative analysis of consciousness through eye opening, verbal response, and motor response.

Glossoptosis Downward displacement of the tongue.

Glycosis Cellular metabolism in which monosaccharides are converted into energy molecules.

Golden hour Accepted as the national standard in trauma care; asserts that a patient has 60 minutes from initial injury to care in a trauma center for optimal outcome.

Gray matter Brain tissue composed of nerve cell bodies.

Grey-Turner's sign Ecchymosis over the flank near the eleventh and twelfth ribs indicating retroperitoneal bleeding and possible kidney damage.

Gross decontamination Removal of contaminated clothing and removal of contaminants from skin.

Hamman's sign A crunching sound heard during systole upon auscultation of the heart that usually indicates air within the mediastinum.

Hazard analysis An inventory of the largest amounts of hazardous materials present in a specified area.

Hazardous material Any substance or material in any form or quantity that poses an unreasonable risk to safety and health and to property when transported in commerce.

Heat tetany A condition that results from extreme heat stress or exposure.

Hemodynamics The study of the movement of the blood and the forces and mechanisms that govern it.

Henry's law Gas will enter into a given volume of solvent in proportion to the partial pressure of the gas.

Hering-Breuer reflex Regulation of normal respiratory rhythm and depth.

Heterotopic Transplantation of an organ next to the diseased organ.

Histocompatibility Tissue typing and matching.

Horizontal equity All groups are provided interventions in the same way.

Human tolerance The amount of energy human tissue can withstand without resulting in injury.

Humoral immune response Activation of the immune system in response to the production of antibodies.

Hydrostatic force The physical pressure of fluid.

Hydrostatic pressure The pressure of the blood, which drives fluid out of the capillary bed and into the interstitial space.

Hydroxyethyl starch A synthetic macromolecule used to expand plasma volume; also known as hetastarch.

Hyperacute rejection The complete destruction of transplanted graft as a result of humoral immune response.

Hypercapnia Elevated $PaCO_2$.

Ileum A portion of the small intestine that is about 12–13 feet in length and that serves to absorb nutrients and maintain electrolyte balance.

Immediate death Death as a result of injury within the first hour that the injury occurs; usually 50% of all trauma fatalities.

Immobilization Prevention of movement of the body to protect the spine.

Immunohematology The study of antigens and antibodies and their relationship to blood.

Immunology The study of the body's response to a foreign substance.

Incidence A measure of the number of new cases of an injury (or disease) in a population of people at risk during a specific time period.

Incident command system (ICS) The coordinated and controlled management of responding resources, so that limited expenditure of those resources can produce the greatest positive effect.

Incomplete lesions An injury to the spine in which a portion of the spinal cord remains intact.

Injury biomechanics Investigation of the physical responses to impact injury.

Injury prevention All actions taken to achieve reduction of or elimination of injury or trauma.

Injury severity score (ISS) An assessment tool that sums the squares of the highest of the seven AIS scores.

Inspiratory center Respiratory control center in the nervous system that causes contraction of the diaphragm and intercostal muscles.

Intentional injury An injury resulting from an intent to cause death or harm.

Intermittent mandatory ventilation (IVM) Ventilation that delivers breaths at a set rate and volume.

Intervertebral disks Tough cartilaginous disk-shaped material that separates the vertebrae.

Intracerebral hematoma An injury to the deep tissues of the brain that may not exhibit signs until days after the injuring event; usually surgically correctable.

Intradermal bruising Bleeding between the dermis and the epidermis.

Iridodialysis Tearing of the iris from the ciliary body.

Iris A thin sheet of pigmented tissue; eye color.

Jejunum A portion of the small intestine that is about 8 feet long and that serves to absorb nutrients and maintain electrolyte balance.

Joule's law The amount of heat produced is directly related to current, resistance, and time (duration of contact).

Kehr's sign Pain in the left shoulder from the irritation of the phrenic nerve caused by free blood in the abdomen.

Kidneys Paired organs, reddish brown in color and bean-shaped, that function to eliminate wastes and balance electrolyte levels.

Kinematics Determining injury as a result of the forces of motion.

Kinetic energy The energy of motion.

Kussmaul's sign Increased jugular venous distension with spontaneous inspirations.

Lacrimal glands Found in the orbits of the eyes and responsible for lubrication of the eyes.

Laminar The closer the blood cells are to the wall of the vessel, the slower they will flow.

Laplace's law The tension in a vessel wall is equal to the transmural pressure times the radius of the vessel.

Large intestine The organ that surrounds the periphery of the small intestine and that serves to continue the absorbtion of nutrients and begin the process of eliminating wastes.

Laryngeal mask airway (LMA) An alternative to endotracheal intubation; a short endotrachial tube with an oval-shaped mask on the end.

Laryngospasm Forceful contraction of the laryngeal muscles to expel foreign bodies that may enter the larynx.

Late death Death as a result of injury several days after the injury occurs.

Le Fort I fracture Category of fractures exhibiting a separation of the hard palate and lower maxilla from the remainder of the skull.

Le Fort II fracture Category of fractures exhibiting a separation of the nasal skull and lower maxilla from the facial skull and the remaining cranial bones.

Le Fort III fracture Category of fractures exhibiting a separation of the entire midface from the cranium.

Level I trauma center A medical care facility that offers the entire spectrum of care for trauma patients from prevention to research.

Level II trauma center A medical care facility capable of managing most trauma cases and often offering prevention programs.

Level III trauma center A medical care facility located in a community-based hospital that offers initial resuscitation and stabilization.

Level IV trauma center A medical care facility established in a remote rural area that offers advanced life support.

Level V trauma center A medical care facility established in a desolate area offering only initial resuscitation while waiting for transport to another facility.

Life years lost A measure of the number of years a person would have lived if no fatality had occurred; it is found by subtracting the age at premature death from the current life expectancy for someone of the deceased's age.

Linear fracture An injury to the brain with a small amount of underlying brain tissue damage; there are usually no specific signs.

Liver The largest organ in the abdomen, which functions as the processing center for nutrients absorbed by the digestive system.

Load and go Rapid packaging and transport of high-priority patients to appropriate medical facilities.

Local crush injury An injury that occurs when weight is allowed to push on tissue for hours, resulting in the crushing of musculoskeletal structure.

Lumbar vertebrae The largest bones of the spinal column that support weight.

Lund and Browder Chart Age-related anatomical scale or diagram used to estimate the percentage of burn.

Mandatory intervention Method of protecting an individual as a requirement of law.

Mangled Extremity Severity Score (MESS) A guideline for assessing the viability of severely injured limbs.

Massive hemothorax An injury to the chest that allows a collection of about 1,500 cc of blood in the pleural space.

Mediastinum The central region of the thorax.

Meningeal branch Branches of spinal nerves that reenter the vertebral canal to supply the meninges and blood vessels of the cord.

Meninges The connective tissue that covers the external surface of the brain; consists of three layers: dura mater, pia mater, and arachnoid.

Menisci Two semilunar cartilages in the capsule of the knee joint that act as shock absorbers by lubricating the joint and distributing the weight more evenly.

Minute ventilation (MV) A calculated or measured volume of air exchanged by the lung in 1 minute; the product of tidal volume and respiratory rate.

Moderate-deep partial-thickness burn A burn injury that involves epidermal and varying degrees of the dermal layer of the skin; also known as a second-degree burn.

Monro-Kellie principle An increase in volume of one element must be compensated by a decrease in the volume of the other elements within a closed container.

Morbidity rate An incidence rate, measuring the number of new cases of a nonfatal injury or disease (numerator) divided by the total population at risk (denominator) during a specific time period.

Mortality rate A measure of the incidence of death (all deaths or deaths from a specific cause) in a specific population during a given period of time.

Multiple-organ failure (MOF) A complication affecting patients who are severely injured, develop sepsis, and have problems after surgery, usually resulting in death.

Multisystem trauma Injury that involves more than one body system resulting in life threats to the patient.

Myocardial concussion An injury resulting from a blow to the midanterior chest resulting in brief dysrhythmia, hypotension, or loss of consciousness.

Myocardial contusion An injury from a blow to the chest resulting in necrotic myocardial fibers, edema, and hemorrhage.

Myocardial rupture An acute traumatic perforation of the ventricles, atria, and intraventricular septum, intra-atrial septum, chordae, papillary muscles, or valves.

Nasopharyngeal airway (NPA) An airway adjunct inserted through the nasal passages; is well tolerated in conscious patients and trauma patients.

Needle thoracentesis A procedure that will result in relieving pressure in the intrathoracic space.

Neurogenic shock An interruption of nervous system control between the brain and the rest of the body; also known as spinal shock.

Nonbulk packaging A container of 119 gallons or less of liquids, 882 pounds or less of solids, 1,000 pounds or less of water capacity for gases.

Ohm's law Electrical current is directly proportional to voltage and inversely proportional to resistance.

Olecranon process The prominent body projection of the ulna.

Oncotic force The chemical pressure to attract fluid.

Oncotic pressure The force exerted by the large protein molecules in the blood that regulates the movement of water across a selectively permeable membrane.

On-scene support Intervention provided at the time that a critical incident is occurring.

Open fracture A break in bone in cartilage with a break in skin integrity as well.

Open pneumothorax An injury to the chest wall that allows air to enter the thoracic space.

Open skull fracture An injury to the brain that exposes the brain and meninges to the external environment, making these structures prone to infection.

Oropharyngeal airway (OPA) An airway adjunct designed to overcome soft tissue obstruction; it also serves as a bite block.

Orthotopic Transplantation of an organ in the place where the diseased organ was housed.

Osteofascial compartments Areas of the body formed when fascia connects with bone; typically these areas contain skeletal muscle, nervous system tissue, and vascular structures.

Outcome evaluation Assessing the effectiveness of a program based upon the results or the "big picture."

Pancreas An elongated organ that functions to manufacture and deliver enzymes to the gastrointestinal system and create insulin to regulate glucose.

Parietal pleura The thin tough membrane that lines the chest wall.

Parkland formula A method of calculating fluid replacement for the burn victim based upon the patient's weight and percentage of total body surface area injured.

Parotid gland A paired serous gland anterior to the auditory canal and inferior to the zygomatic arch that is responsible for salivation.

Partial-thickness burn A burn injury in which only the epidermis has been damaged; also known as a first-degree burn.

Passive intervention Method of protecting an individual without the individual's participation.

Pediatric trauma score (PTS) An assessment tool designed for the special circumstances of pediatric patients through evaluation of six parameters in determining severity of injury: size, airway, blood pressure, level of consciousness, skeletal assessment, and cutaneous.

Pedicles The structures that form the sides of the vertebral foramen.

Peer counseling An intervention that promotes discussions among co-workers to combat stress and deal with traumatic events.

Pelvic sacral foramina Structure found on the ventral surface of the sacrum that provides a pathway for nerves and blood vessels.

Pendelluft Movement of air between the injured and uninjured lung with each breath.

Penetrating abdominal trauma index (PATI) An assessment tool that uses a numeric risk factor correlated to each abdominal organ to assess severity of penetrating trauma.

Penetrating trauma Injuries that create either a temporary or permanent communication with the atmosphere.

Perfluorocarbons A man-made product designed to transport oxygen and remove carbon dioxide from cells.

Pericardiocentesis Needle penetration of the pericardial sac to remove accumulated blood or fluid.

Pericardium The tough fibrous sac that contains the heart.

Permanent cavitation The formation of a cavity that occurs as a result of the tissues being recoiled after the passing of a bullet; the tissues do not retain their original shape.

Pharyngeotracheal lumen airway (PTLA) An airway adjunct with a double-lumen tube and a twin-balloon system.

Physical evidence Any object, no matter how small, that places or connects the perpetrator at or to the crime scene.

Physiological dead space The volume of air in structures that cannot exchange oxygen and carbon dioxide, such as the trachea.

Physiology The study of the function of living organisms.

Platinum ten minutes The period of time it should take to get the multisystem trauma patient packaged and to definitive care to ensure a positive outcome for the patient.

Platysma muscle A thin, superficial muscle that originates in the deep fascia of the upper chest.

Plexus Complex networks of spinal nerves.

Pneumotaxic center The area of the brain that is thought to control respiratory rhythm during times of labored breathing.

Pneumothorax An injury in which air enters the pleural space.

Poikilothermy Condition in which the body temperature assumes the temperature of the environment.

Postevent phase The period in the injury process in which actions are taken to treat, minimize, or rehabilitate an injury.

Posterior branch A branch of the spinal nerves that innervates the muscles and skin of the back; also called posterior ramus.

Posttraumatic stress disorder (PTSD) The response of the body to a severe traumatic event exhibited by intrusive thoughts, nightmares, reliving the event, and avoidance; symptoms can occur more than 6 months after the event.

Preevent phase The period in the injury process before energy is exchanged.

Prehospital index (PHI) An assessment tool that assigns numeric values to the findings of blood pressure, pulse, respiratory status, and level of consciousness to determine injury severity and patient priority.

Preload The filling pressure and volume of the ventricles at the end of diastole.

Prevalence A measure of the number of cases of injury or disease in a population at a given point in time, and a function of both incidence and the duration of an injury or disease.

Priaprism Sustained erection of the penis.

Primary brain injury An injury that occurs at the moment of impact as a result of transfer of kinetic energy.

Process evaluation Assessing the effectiveness of a program based upon the details of how the program was implemented.

Proprioception Sense of position.

Pseudocoarctation syndrome An injury characterized by acute upper extremity hypertension with absent or diminished femoral pulses.

Pulmonary contusion An injury to the chest resulting in bruising or edema in the lungs.

Pulmonary respiration The transfer of gases between the alveoli and the red blood cells in the lungs.

Pulsus paradoxus A decrease in systolic blood pressure by greater than 10 mm Hg with inspiration.

Pylorus The portion of the stomach that allows food to pass into the duodenum.

Radiation Heat loss as a result of energy transfer form hot to cold objects.

Rectum The last portion of the large intestine that is a conduit for the elimination of wastes from the body.

Reflex A response to a stimulus.

Reticular activating system (RAS) The primary structural element located in the brain stem that regulates arousal and consciousness.

Retina The innermost layer of the eye that is photoreceptive.

Retrograde tracheal intubation (RTI) Creation of an airway by passing a catheter through a tracheostomy into the pharynx and the subsequent use of the catheter as a guide for passing the endotracheal tube.

Revised trauma score (RTS) An assessment tool that assigns a numeric value to represent the extent of injury based upon respiratory rate and chest expansion, capillary refill, and blood pressure ranges; also known as the trauma score (TS).

Rhabdomyolysis The destruction of skeletal muscle cell membranes.

Rule of nines A universal guide to determining the extent of a burn injury.

Rule of thumb Distance from which an outstretched thumb can cover the scene.

Sacrum A triangular-shaped structure at the base of the vertebral column.

Scalp The skin of the head consisting of five vascular superficial layers.

SCIWORA Spinal cord injury without radiographic abnormalities.

Sclera The outer fibrous coat of the eye made up of an opaque white material.

Secondary brain injury An injury that occurs minutes, hours, or days after the initial transfer of energy.

Secondary decontamination Systematic washing with soft bristle brushes from head to toe.

Second-degree burn A burn injury that involves epidermal and varying degrees of the dermal layer of the skin; also known as a moderate-deep partial-thickness burn.

Seldinger technique A venous access technique that uses a guide wire to thread the catheter into the vein allowing the user to insert a standard IV catheter into a peripheral vein and convert the site to a much larger bore catheter.

Sepsis syndrome Infection with signs of abnormal end-organ perfusion as evidenced by altered cerebral function, oliguria, hypoxemia, and elevated lactate levels.

Shear strain A change in dimension related to application of forces to tissue from opposing directions.

Shock A condition resulting from serious injury in which insufficient amounts of oxygen are carried to tissues; characterized by weak, rapid, pulse; pale, cool skin; and listlessness.

Simple triage and rapid treatment (START) An evaluation system used to make quick assessments of patients involved in mass casualty incidents.

Singular system trauma Injury that involves only one body system and that does not compromise the patient.

Skull The bones covering the brain.

Small intestine An organ that is 21–23 feet in length, made up of three sections—the duodenum, jejunum, and ileum—that functions to absorb nutrients from digestion.

Smith fracture A break resulting from a direct blow to the hand while it is in a flexed position.

Spalling The mechanism of injury related to blast injuries resulting from a wave passing through a tissue of high density adjacent to a tissue of lower density, resulting in the surface tissue of higher density being disrupted.

Spinal column The structure that houses the spinal cord; it is separated into five regions: cervical, thoracic, lumbar, sacral, and coccygeal.

Spinal cord The structure found within the spinal column that extends from the foramen magnum to the lower border of the first lumbar vertebra.

Spinal nerves Communications pathways for the spinal column and brain.

Spinal shock Condition exhibited by a loss of vascular tone and a loss of sympathetic nerve input to the heart.

Spleen A purplish, highly vascular organ that functions as a filter for the circulatory system.

Splenorrhaphy Surgical repair of the spleen.

Stabilization The process of making firm or steady; securing an arm in a splint, for example.

Starling equation Determines the direction and rate of fluid flow through the capillaries based upon the permeability of the capillary wall, hydrostatic forces, and oncotic forces.

Starling's law of the heart Over a physiological range increased filling of the heart ventricle results in better emptying.

Stick-em-up position The position a patient suffering from spinal injury assumes: arms are flexed and extended above the head.

Stomach A highly mobile organ that functions to initiate the digestion of food.

Stratum corneum A cell layer in the epidermis that acts as a vapor barrier to the body to protect it from microorganisms.

Stress The nonspecific response of the body to any demand placed upon it.

Stressor Any event that invokes the fight-or-flight response.

Stroke volume (SV) The amount of blood ejected from the left ventricle with each contraction.

Stroma-free hemoglobin A product designed to carry large amounts of oxygen to the cells of patients who have lost significant amounts of blood.

Subarachnoid hemorrhage An injury to the brain that occurs secondary to the small arterial vessels in the outermost surface of the brain; occurs as the brain moves across the uneven surface of the cranial vault.

Subarachnoid space The area that separates the arachnoid layer and the pia mater that is filled with cerebral spinal fluid.

Subcutaneous tissue The skin layer that lies below the dermis composed of areolar, adipose, and loose connective tissue; also known as the superficial fascia.

Subdural hematoma A collection of blood in the space between the dura mater and the arachnoid membrane.

Subdural space The area that separates the arachnoid layer and the dura mater that is crossed by small venous vessels that empty into the dural sinuses.

Sublingual gland A paired gland at the base of the tongue, responsible for salivation.

Submandibular gland A paired gland medial to the mandibular, ramus and inferior to the angle of the mandible, responsible for salivation.

Superficial cervical fascia The thin layer of connective tissue that lies immediately beneath the skin.

Surveillance The systematic collection of population-based information on the occurrence and cost of injury and disease.

Synchronized intermittent mandatory ventilation (SIMV) Ventilation that delivers mechanical breaths at or near the beginning of a spontaneous breath.

Systemic crush syndrome An injury that occurs when muscle tissue disintegrates and myoglobin, potassium, and phosphorus leak into the circulation.

TCA (Krebs) cycle Cellular metabolism in which molecules are catalyzed by certain enzymes to produce carbon dioxide and ATP molecules.

Temporary cavitation The formation of a cavity that occurs as the result of tissue being stretched by the shock wave produced by a bullet.

Tensile strain A change in dimension related to the length of an object.

Tension pneumothorax An injury to the chest resulting in a one-way valve allowing air to enter the pleural space but not exit, resulting in collapse of the affected lung and compression of the mediastinum.

Tentorium cerebelli A horizontal projection of the dura mater arising from the posterior cranial fossa and the cerebellum.

Third spacing A condition that results when fluid is lost from the intravascular space into the extravascular space.

Third-degree burn A burn injury that involves the subcutaneous tissue and may involve muscle and bone; also known as a full-thickness burn.

Thoracic vertebrae The larger bones of the spinal column that serve to support the weight.

Thromboembolism Blood clots that form in the venous system, break loose, travel, and lodge elsewhere in the vascular system.

Tidal volume (TV) The volume of air inhaled and exhaled.

Torsion A change in dimension related to one end of tissue being twisted while the other end remains motionless.

Transillumination intubation Orotracheal intubation using a lighted malleable stylet.

Transtracheal jet insufflation (TJI) An airway technique that involves insertion of a cannula through the cricothyroid membrane with it connected to an intermittent high-pressure oxygen source.

Transverse process The portion of the spinal column that originates between the pedicle and the laminae and extends laterally and posteriorly.

Trauma score (TS) An assessment tool that assigns a numeric value to represent the extent of injury based upon respiratory rate and chest expansion, capillary refill, and blood pressure ranges; also known as the revised trauma score (RTS).

Trauma systems An interconnected source of services and providers with the resources and expertise to manage life-threatening, traumatic injuries.

Traumatic iridosyclitis Inflammation of the iris or iris ciliary body, usually a result of blunt trauma; also called traumatic iritis.

Traumatic iritis Inflammation of the iris or iris ciliary body, usually a result of blunt trauma; also called traumatic iridosyclitis.

Traumatic miosis Constriction of the ciliary body.

Traumatic mydriasis Dilation of the ciliary body.

Triage The allocation of resources based on the number and severity of patient injuries in relation to the health care system's ability to manage a given incident.

Trigeminal nerve The cranial nerve responsible for control of chewing and the sensory function of the face.

TRISS method An evaluation method used for patients sustaining multisystem trauma; compares the outcomes of a trauma center's patients to the outcomes of other trauma centers' patients with similar injuries.

Tube thoracostomy A procedure by which a large-bore plastic drainage tube is inserted into the pleural cavity.

Two-point discrimination Sensory test of patient's ability to distinguish between two sharp objects placed against the skin. The objects are moved closer together until the patient can no longer tell if there are one or two objects.

Uncal herniation An injury to the brain that occurs when a lesion in one of the spaces displaces one of the cerebral hemispheres.

Unintentional injury An injury resulting from events that are inadvertent or accidental.

Up-and-over pathway The mechanism of injury in a frontal collision whereby the occupant continues to move forward, traveling over the steering wheel.

Ventilation The mechanical process of moving atmospheric gases into and out of the lungs.

Ventilation-perfusion (V/Q) matching Pulmonary blood that is directed to areas of the lung that are well ventilated.

Ventral root A branch of the spinal nerves that is responsible for motor function.

Vertebrae The bones that make up the spinal column.

Vertebral column Bones making up the spine that extend from the base of the skull to the pelvis.

Vertical equity Unequal groups are provided unequal interventions in an attempt to make the groups more equal.

Vestibulocochlear nerve The cranial nerve that is responsible for the senses of hearing and equilibrium.

Victim blaming The view that the cause and responsibility of the injury lies solely with the host or victim.

Visceral branch A branch of the spinal nerves that innervates the thoracic and lumbar region and is part of the autonomic nervous system.

Visceral pleura The membrane that lines the outer surface of each lung.

Voluntary intervention Method of protecting an individual in which the individual takes the responsibility on him- or herself.

Waddell's triad Injury to the femur and/or tibia/fibula, a torso injury, and a closed head injury as a result of a pedestrian versus motor vehicle collision.

White matter Brain tissue composed of myelinated nerve axons that act as insulated nerve pathways.

W-statistic The sample population treated at a facility compared to other facility patient populations; $W = (A - E)/(n/100)$.

Xenograft Transplantation of kidneys from other species.

Years of productive life lost (YPLL) A measure of a person's productivity lost, found by subtracting the age at premature death from retirement age.

Zone of coagulation The innermost layer of a burn wound.

Zone of hyperemia The superficial outer layer of a burn wound.

Zone of stasis The middle layer of a burn wound.

Z-statistic A comparison of the actual number of survivors (A) in a facility with the number of expected survivors (E) based on current industry data. Statistical variation is measured by s; $Z = (A - E)/s$.

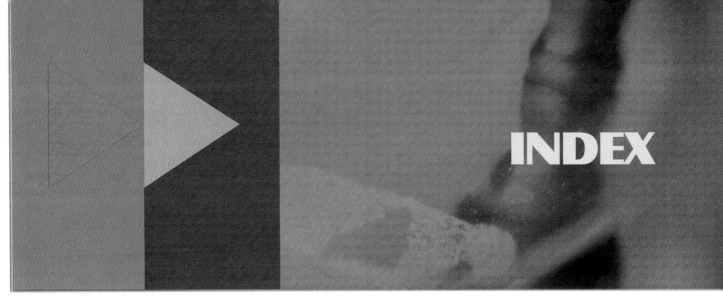

INDEX

B

F

N

O

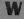

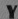